Roach's Introductory Clinical Pharmacology

Susan M. Ford, MN, RN
Nursing Faculty
Tacoma Community College
Tacoma, Washington

Sally S. Roach, MSN, RN, AHN-BC
Associate Professor
University of Texas at Brownsville and Texas Southmost College
Brownsville, Texas

EDITION 9

Wolters Kluwer | Lippincott Williams & Wilkins
Health
Philadelphia · Baltimore · New York · London
Buenos Aires · Hong Kong · Sydney · Tokyo

Acquisitions Editor: Elizabeth Nieginski
Project Managers: Betsy Gentzler and Michelle L. Clarke
Director of Nursing Production: Helen Ewan
Art Director: Brett MacNaughton
Design Coordinator: Joan Wendt
Manufacturing Coordinator: Karin Duffield
Senior Manufacturing Manager: William Alberti
Production Service: Spearhead Global
Printer: RRD Shenzhen

8 7 6 5 4 3 2

9th Edition

Library of Congress Cataloging-in-Publication Data

Ford, Susan M.
Roach's introductory clinical pharmacology / Susan M. Ford, Sally S. Roach. — 9th ed.
    p. ; cm.
  Rev. ed. of: Introductory clinical pharmacology / Sally S. Roach, Susan M. Ford. 8th ed. c2008.
  Includes index.
  ISBN-13: 978-1-60547-633-9
  ISBN-10: 1-60547-633-1
  1. Clinical pharmacology. 2. Nursing. I. Roach, Sally S. II. Roach, Sally S. Introductory clinical pharmacology.
III. Title. IV. Title: Introductory clinical pharmacology.
  [DNLM: 1. Pharmacology, Clinical—Nurses' Instruction. 2. Drug Therapy—Nurses' Instruction. 3. Pharmaceutical Preparations—administration & dosage—Nurses' Instruction. QV 38 F711r 2010]
  RM301.28.S34 2010
  615.5′8—dc22

2009023146

LWW.com

RRS1002

This book is dedicated to two very special women in my life,
Sylvia Jones and Viola Oberholtzer.
Sylvia is the first nurse I ever met, because she is my mother—
and encouraged me to become a nurse, too.
Aunt Vi (Viola O.) is the person who told me to look at alternative
routes to the Registered Nurse pathway, encouraging me to start
at the community college and advance from there.
Without the support of these two women in my life,
I would not be authoring this book now!
Susan M. Ford, RN, MN

Reviewers

Mary Ann Ambrose, BSN, MSN, FNP-C
Program Director and Instructor, Licensed Vocational
    Nursing
Cuesta College
Paso Robes, California

Marjorie Bessette, MSN, RN
Assistant Professor, Practical Nurse Certificate Program
Holyoke Community College
Holyoke, Massachusetts

Kathy Bredberg, MSN, RN
Director, Vocational Nursing Program
Grayson County Junior College
Van Alstyne, Texas

Carol Buttz, BS, RN, CEN
Nursing Instructor
Dakota County Technical College
Rosemount, Minnesota

Ingrid Chen, RN
Instructor
McFatter Vocational Center
Davie, Florida

Virginia Christensen, ADRN, MSN (c)
Faculty Instructor, Pediatrics, Pharmacology,
    and IV Therapy
Tennessee Technology Center at Livingston
Livingston, Tennessee

Maryann Cosgarea, BSN, BA, RN
Practical Nursing Coordinator
Portage Lakes Career Center—W. Howard Nicol School of
    Practical Nursing
Green, Ohio

Cassandra Dansby, BSN, BA, RN
Practical Nursing Instructor
Atlanta Tech
Atlanta, Georgia

Heather Deane-Clark, BN, MAEd, RN, GNC(c)
Instructor, Practical Nursing Programs
Camosun College
Victoria, British Columbia, Canada

Elizabeth DeMarsh-Smith, BA, RN
Course Coordinator/Curriculum Chairperson
Robert T. White School of Practical Nursing
Alliance, Ohio

Kathleen Doline, MSN, RN
Associate Professor of Nursing
Northampton Community College
Bethlehem, Pennsylvania

Linda Douglas, BSN, RN
Nursing Instructor
Crowder College—Nevada Campus
Nevada, Missouri

Marion Doyle, MSN, MS, RN
Associate Professor of Nursing
Northampton Community College
Bethlehem, Pennsylvania

Sherlyn Farrish-Barner, MSN, RN
Nursing Educator for the Practical Nursing Program
Germanna Community College
Locust Grove, Virginia

Penny Fauber, PhD, MS, BSN
Director
The LPN School of Nursing
Carilion Stonewall Jackson Hospital and Rockbridge
    County Schools
Lexington, Virginia

Denise Fowler, MSA, MSN
Practical Nursing Instructor
Augusta Technical Institute—Thomson
Thomson, Georgia

Kathy Fukuyama, ESN, MEd, RN
Department Head, BSN Program
Vancouver Community College
Vancouver, British Columbia, Canada

Shari Gould, RN, MSN (c)
Instructor, Vocational Nursing Program
Victoria College
Gonzales, Texas

Janis Grimland, BSN, RN
Site Coordinator
Hill Junior College
Clifton, Texas

Kathleen Gudgel, MSN, RN
Assistant Professor, Nursing
Pennsylvania College of Technology
Williamsport, Pennsylvania

Donna Hage, BS, MSN (c)
Nursing Faculty/Clinical Coordinator
Minnesota West Community and Technical College
Worthington, Minnesota

Rosemary Hathaway, BSN, MSN, BS
PN Program Coordinator
Hillyard Technical School
St. Joseph, Missouri

Tina Hawley, MS, BSN, RN
Coordinator
Wood County School of Practical Nursing
Parkersburg, West Virginia

Robbin Hutton Argentine, BA, BS
Master Instructor
Board of Cooperative Educational Services/
Consortium of Continuing Education—
    Madison and Oneida Counties
Verona, New York

Mary Ellen Gallagher, MSN, RN
Instructor
St. Margaret School of Practical Nursing
Blawnox, Pennsylvania

Helena Jermalovic, MSN, RN
Assistant Professor
University of Alaska, Anchorage
Anchorage, Alaska

Linda Johnson, MSN, FNP, CRNP
Faculty, Practical Nursing Program
Mercyhurst College
Northeast, Pennsylvania

Melissa Jones, BSN, RN
Practical Nursing Coordinator
Waynesville Technical Academy School of Practical Nursing
Waynesville, Missouri

Denise Kampfhenkel, BSN, RN
Vocational Nursing Instructor
Schreiner University
Kerrville, Texas

Raina Lively, RN
Vocational Nursing Instructor/Site Coordinator
Hill Junior College
Cleburne, Texas

Dianne Lucy, MSN
Former Director, Practical Nursing Program
Rappahannock Community College
Glenns, Virginia

Christine Miller, BSN, RN, AASN
Assistant Professor/Vocational Nursing Instructor
Victoria College
Victoria, Texas

Laura Moskaluk, BSN, RN
Nursing Faculty
Somerset County Technology Institute
Bridgewater, New Jersey

Robbie Murphy, BSN, ANCC Certification in Gerontology, GNC
Faculty
San Jacinto College North Campus
Houston, Texas

Diana Mustacchio, BSN, RN
Second Level Course Coordinator and Clinical Coordinator
The Robert T. White School of Practical Nursing
Alliance, Ohio

Amy Nieporent, BSN, RN
Instructor
Holy Name Hospital School of Practical Nursing
Teaneck, New Jersey

Lisa Nolan, BSN
LPN Instructor
Mercer County Technical School
Trenton, New Jersey

Laurie Pierce, BSN, MSN, RN
Instructional Faculty
Medical Careers College
Richmond, Virginia

Virginia Radom, BSN, MSN, RN, MSHA
Professor
Johnson County Community College
Merriam, Kansas

Sandra Reider, BA, BSN, MSN, RN
Associate Professor
Reading Area Community College
Reading, Pennsylvania

Susan Roth, BS, RN
Lead Instructor
HFM Boces School of Practical Nursing
Johnstown, New York

Carolyn Santiago, MSN, RN, NP-C
Director of Nursing Programs
Santa Barbara Business College
Bakersfield, California

Patricia Schrull, MSN, MBA, MEd, RN, CNE
Associate Professor/Program Director
Lorain County Community College
Elyria, Ohio

Joanne Scorci, MS, RN, ANP/BC, CD
Associate Professor and Clinical Instructor
Trocaire College
Buffalo, New York

Cathrine Shafer, BSN, RN
Director, Vocational Nursing Program
San Diego City College
San Diego, California

Greg Sherrill, RN
Senior Practical Nursing Instructor
AAS Roane State Community College
Tennessee Technology Center at Crossville
Crossville, Tennessee

Carol Snyder, ADS, ADN, BSN
Associate Professor, Nursing, Health, and Human Services
Central Florida Community College
Ocala, Florida

Ann Thurman, BSN, RN
Coordinator Practical Nursing
Tennessee Technology Center at Hartsville
Hartsville, Tennessee

Sheila Upshaw, ADN
Practical Nursing Program Chair
University of Arkansas – Monticello
Crossett, Arkansas

Ercelle Vann, BSN, MSN, RN
Program Director
Southampton Memorial Hospital School of Practical
   Nursing
Franklin, Virginia

Rose Veith, MSN, FNP-BC, CNE
Practical Nursing Coordinator
Assabet Valley Regional Technical School
Marlborough, Massachusetts

Brenda Washington, BSN, MSN, RN
Nurse Educator
Robert Morgan Educational Center
Miami, Florida

Christina Wilson, BAN, PHN, RN
Faculty, Practical Nursing Program
Anoka Hennepin Technical College
Anoka, Minnesota

Margaret Yoder, MS, MHA, RN
Associate Professor Nurse Education/Practical Nursing
   Program Coordinator
Quinsigamond Community College
Worcester, Massachusetts

Joan Zarra, BSN, MSN, RN
Professor
Dover Business College School of Practical Nursing
Clifton, New Jersey

Preface

The ninth edition of *Roach's Introductory Clinical Pharmacology* reflects the ever-changing science of pharmacology and the nurse's responsibilities in administering pharmacologic agents. All information has been updated and revised according to the latest available information to prepare nurses to safely administer medications. The text prepares the nurse to meet the challenges of the 21st century by promoting critical thinking and problem solving when administering medications.

Purpose

This text is designed to provide students with a clear, concise introduction to pharmacology. The basic explanations presented in this text are *not* intended to suggest that pharmacology is an easy subject. Drug therapy is one of the most important and complicated treatment modalities in modern health care. Because of the frequent additions and changes in the field of pharmacology, it is imperative that health care professionals constantly review and update their knowledge.

Current Drug Information

Information regarding drugs in this book was gathered primarily using the latest update of *Facts and Comparisons*. The student and practitioner should remember that information about drugs, such as dosages and new forms, is constantly changing. Likewise, there may be new drugs on the market that were not approved by the U.S. Food and Drug Administration (FDA) at the time of publication of this text. The reader may find that certain drugs or drug dosages available when this textbook was published may no longer be available. For the most current drug information and dosages, the practitioner is advised to consult references such as the most current *Physician's Desk Reference,* yearly-updated drug handbooks, or the package inserts that accompany most drugs. Internet resources should always be verified for their reliability when used. The clinical pharmacist or physician should be contacted for information concerning a specific drug, including dosage, adverse reactions, contraindications, precautions, interactions, or administration.

Special Features

A number of features have proven useful for students in their study of basic pharmacology. The following features appear in the ninth edition:

- **Key Terms** listed at the beginning of each chapter highlight the important words defined in each chapter.

- **The Nursing Process** is used as a framework in most chapters for presenting care of the patient as it relates to the drug and the drug regimen.
- **Nursing Alerts** identify urgent nursing considerations in the management of the patient receiving a specific drug or drug category.
- **Lifespan Alerts** alert the nurse to problems for which particular populations are at increased risk. Alerts are specific to these populations, such as pediatric or gerontologic patients. While the text does not specifically address administration of medication to children, it is important to recognize some of the common precautions or considerations when administering medications to children. The nurse is alerted to situations that may arise during drug therapy for patients with chronic illnesses, such as diabetes, hypertension, or epilepsy.
- **Contraindications, Precautions, and Interactions** of the most commonly used drugs in the category under discussion are included in each chapter. While limited space prevents listing every contraindication, precaution, and interaction, the more common ones are included. Interactions of the most commonly used drugs are presented in a table format so that the student can see at a glance how interactions with other drugs or even foods may affect a patient's progress.
- **Patient Teaching for Improved Patient Outcomes** highlight specific issues that the patient or family may encounter while undergoing drug therapy. These features provide must-know information that empowers the family to participate knowledgeably and accurately in the patient's drug regimen. As more and more patients are cared for outside the hospital, it becomes increasingly important for the nurse to know what information the patient or family needs to obtain an optimal response to the drug regimen.
- **Summary Drug Tables** contain commonly used drugs representative of the class of drugs discussed in the chapter. Important drug information is provided, including the generic name, pronunciation guide for generic names, trade names, adverse reactions, and dosage ranges. In these tables, generic names are followed by trade names; when a drug is available under several trade names, several of the available trade names are given. When a drug is available only by its generic name, of course, no trade name is given. The most common or serious adverse reactions associated with the drug are listed in the table's adverse reaction section. It should be noted that any patient may exhibit adverse reactions not listed in this text. Because of this possibility, the nurse, when administering any drug, should consider any sign or symptom as a *possible* adverse reaction until the cause of the problem is determined by the primary health care provider.

The adverse reactions are followed by the dosage ranges for the drug. In most cases, the adult dosage *ranges* are given in these tables because space does not permit the inclusion of all possible dosages for various types of disorders. Likewise, space limitations do not permit an inclusion of pediatric dose ranges, due to the complexity of determining the pediatric dose of many drugs. Many drugs given to children are determined on the basis of body weight or body surface area and have a variety of dosage schedules. When drugs are given to the pediatric patient, the practitioner is encouraged to consult references that give complete and extensive pediatric dosages.

- **Medication Dosage Problems** provide the student an opportunity for immediate application in medication administration. Because calculation of medication dosage is an important aspect of medication administration, Chapter 3 reviews the mathematics involved in dosage calculation and formulas used to calculate medication dosages. To ensure the student's understanding and application of this type of problem, two or more medication dosage problems are included at the end of most chapters and deal with specific medications discussed in the chapter. Answers to these questions are provided in Appendix E.
- A **Glossary** at the end of the book lists and defines key terms and other drug-related terms.
- **Herbal** or **Health Supplement Alerts** provide important information on common herbs and supplements not regulated under the auspices of the FDA. **Appendix C** lists select herbs and natural products with examples of their common and scientific name(s). While not all of the common or scientific names are given, the most commonly used names (both common and scientific) are included. With more and more individuals using herbs as a part of their health care regimens, it is critical that the nurse be aware of the more common herbs currently in use. The nurse must consult appropriate sources when patients indicate they are using herbs as part of their health care regimen.
- **Key to Abbreviations** provides a list of abbreviations used in this text, particularly in the Summary Drug Tables.

New Features

- **Chapter 3** focuses on the reduction of medication errors due to mathematical issues rather than the traditional arithmetic exercises. The nurse learns how and why math accountability is critical in administering medications.
- **Pharmacology in Practice** case studies are introduced in each unit. These patient scenarios are introduced in chapter 5 and are placed in each subsequent unit introduction throughout the book. Patients present to the providers with typical questions or issues seen by nurses when caring for different populations of patients.
- **Think Critically: Pharmacology in Practice** are exercises that provide realistic patient care situations to help students apply the material contained in the chapter by exploring options and making clinical judgments related to the administration of drugs. These critical thinking exercises are related to the Pharmacology in Practice case studies and are based upon the select group of clients introduce in Chapter 5. Care for these individuals is presented like a group of puzzle pieces so that students appreciate the complex issues in providing care to both individuals and families.
- **Review Questions** at the end of each chapter were written to help students determine whether they understand both the content of the chapter and the NCLEX-PN question format. This provides the student an opportunity to answer questions specifically about the drugs covered in the chapter as well as to practice testing in the NCLEX-PN format. These questions enable the student to practice answering questions concerning medication therapy and administration of drugs. Questions in each chapter are keyed to specific components of the current NCLEX-PN test blueprint. Answers to these questions are provided in Appendix E.

Organization

The text contains 55 chapters, which are divided into 13 units covering general areas. Units 4 through 12 are organized in a 'head-to-toe' fashion. This gives the student an easier way to find information as well as to organize his or her understanding of how drugs impact the human body. Organization of the text in this manner allows the student to move about the text when these general areas are covered in the curriculum. Although pharmacologic agents are presented in specific units, a disease may be treated with more than one type of drug, requiring consultation of one or more units. Each unit begins with an overview of the unit content and a intriguing patient case study.

Unit I presents a foundation for the study of pharmacology in five chapters that cover general principles of pharmacology, the administration of drugs, calculation of drug dosages, a discussion of the nursing process as applicable to pharmacology, and a review of the teaching–learning process where the nurse is introduced to a group of clients in the clinic setting. This establishes the priority of educating the patient and family maintained in subsequent chapters.

Unit II contains eight chapters presenting the anti-infective drugs, grouped according to classification. The antibacterial chapters are grouped to help the student better understand drugs that work in similar ways. Other chapters focus on drugs to treat viral, tubercular, and fungal/parasitic infections. Shorter chapters allow more-inclusive coverage of the different types of anti-infectives and of the appropriate nursing considerations for each classification.

Unit III includes five chapters covering the various types of drugs used to manage pain: the nonopioid analgesics (salicylates, nonsalicylates, and nonsteroidal anti-inflammatory drugs), the opioid analgesics, and the opioid antagonists. The reduction of pain during surgical procedures is a major component of anesthesia, so anesthetic drugs are included in this unit.

Drugs affecting the central and peripheral nervous systems have been divided between two separate units (IV and V).

Unit IV includes five chapters beginning with the central nervous system stimulants and progressing through antianxiety drugs, sedatives and hypnotics, antidepressants, and the antipsychotic drugs—drug categories with a primary focus in the central nervous system.

Unit V drug categories affect the peripheral nervous system, where brain and body messages connect. These four chapters cover the adrenergic drugs, adrenergic blocking drugs, the cholinergic drugs, and the cholinergic blocking drugs.

Unit VI is a new unit covering the drug categories with mind and body connections. The four chapters in this unit discuss cholinesterase inhibitors, antiparkinsonism drugs, anticonvulsants, and drugs used to treat disorders of the musculoskeletal system.

Unit VII contains three chapters concerning drugs that affect the respiratory system. The first chapter in this unit discusses antitussives, mucolytics, and expectorants; the second chapter covers antihistamines and decongestants; and the last chapter deals with bronchodilators and antiasthma drugs.

Unit VIII has been expanded to include all drugs that affect the cardiovascular system. This unit is divided into five chapters, progressing from drugs used to minimize heart disease—antihyperlipidemics and antihypertensives—to those used in the treatment of coronary heart disease—anticoagulants and thrombolytic drugs, antianginals, cardiotonics and miscellaneous inotropic drugs, and antiarrhythmic drugs.

Drugs used to treat the gastrointestinal tract and the urinary systems have been divided between two separate units to better illustrate the head-to-toe concept of the book.

Unit IX's two chapters cover drugs that affect the upper and lower gastrointestinal tracts.

Unit X discusses drugs that affect the endocrine system and consists of five chapters: antidiabetic drugs, pituitary and adrenocortical hormones, thyroid and antithyroid drugs, male and female hormones, and drugs acting on the uterus.

Unit XI's two chapters cover diuretics and urinary tract anti-infectives, antispasmodics, and other urinary drugs.

Unit XII discusses drugs that affect the immune system. The unit consists of three chapters: immunologic agents, antineoplastic drugs, and a new chapter on immunostimulants (drugs that affect the hematological system and agents used in the treatment of anemia).

Unit XIII consists of three chapters that discuss types of drugs not previously discussed or not belonging to a particular class or group. Chapters in this unit include topical drugs used in the treatment of skin disorders, otic and ophthalmic preparations, and fluids, electrolytes, and parenteral therapy. In this last chapter, concepts dealing with the parenteral administration of fluids and medications are concentrated for quick and easy reference.

Chapter Content

Each chapter opens with learning objectives and a listing of key terms used and defined in the chapter. Less commonly used medical terms are also defined within the chapter and may be found in the Glossary. Chapters 1 through 5 provide introductory information concerning general principles of pharmacology, medication administration, a review of arithmetic and calculation of drug dosages, the nursing process, and patient and family teaching. Each chapter ends with critical thinking questions and several chapter review questions.

The remaining chapters discuss specific drug classifications and follow a common format. In addition to the learning objectives and key terms, the remaining chapters each contain at least one table indicating the drug classifications

and drugs discussed in the chapter. The body of each chapter contains the actions, uses, adverse reactions, contraindications, precautions, and interactions of the class or type of drug being discussed, followed by a section devoted to the nursing process. These chapters end with critical thinking questions, several chapter review questions, and two or more medication dosage problems. To promote easy retrieval of information, each area is identified by a large-type heading.

- **Actions**—a basic explanation of how the drug accomplishes its intended activity.
- **Uses**—the common uses of the drug class or type. No unlabeled or experimental uses of drugs are given in the text (unless specifically identified as an unlabeled use) because these uses are not approved by the FDA. Students should be reminded that, under certain circumstances, some physicians may prescribe drugs for a condition not approved by the FDA or may prescribe an experimental drug.

  In discussing the use of antibiotics, this text does not list specific microorganisms. Microorganisms can become resistant to antibiotic drugs very rapidly. Because of this, the author feels that listing specific microorganisms or types of infections for an antibiotic may be misleading to the user of the text. Instead, when antibiotics are needed, the author recommends consulting culture and sensitivity studies to indicate which antibiotic has the most potential for controlling the infection.
- **Adverse Reactions**—the most common adverse drug reactions are listed under this heading.
- **Contraindications**—contraindications for administration of the drug or drugs discussed in the chapter.
- **Precautions**—precautions to take before, during, or after administration.
- **Interactions**—more common interactions between the drug(s) discussed in the chapter and other drugs.
- **Nursing Process**—with a few exceptions, the nursing process is used in every chapter of the book and is geared specifically to the administration of the drugs discussed in the chapter. The assessment phase is divided into two distinct parts to include a preadministration and ongoing assessment. This division assists the reader in determining what assessments to perform before administration of specific drugs in various drug categories and what important assessments to perform during the entire time the drug is administered. Nursing diagnoses related to the administration of the drug are highlighted in a nursing diagnoses checklist. Under "Implementation," three sections are included when applicable: "Promoting an Optimal Response to Therapy," "Monitoring and Managing Patient Needs," and "Educating the Patient and Family." These sections provide invaluable information to ensure that the drug is properly administered and that effective nursing interventions are used when certain adverse reactions occur.

Comprehensive Teaching/ Learning Package

- **Student Study Guide**—*Study Guide to Accompany Introductory Clinical Pharmacology*, 9th Edition, correlates with the textbook chapter by chapter. For every chapter in the textbook, the study guide contains a corresponding chapter, each with the following three sections: Learning Objectives, Assessing Your Understanding, Applying Your Knowledge, and Practicing for NCLEX. In Assessing Your Understanding, students are provided with matching and fill-in-the-blank questions, short-answer questions, and dosage calculations while in Applying Your Knowledge, students are asked to complete case studies. Practicing for NCLEX gives students the opportunity to engage in that very activity: our NCLEX-style multiple-choice questions are presented in the same format as that used in the NCLEX examinations and provide students with at least 10 questions per chapter, complete with full rationales.

- **Student CD-ROM**—Free and bound in the book, this learning tool supplies an NCLEX alternative-format tutorial, **WATCH&LEARN** videos on preventing medication errors, **CONCEPTS** in action **ANIMATION** 3-D animated depictions of pharmacology concepts, a Spanish-English audio glossary, and monographs of the 100 most commonly prescribed drugs.
- **Instructor's Resource CD-ROM**—This CD-ROM contains additional information and activities that will help you engage your students from the semester's beginning to its end. To begin, the CD-ROM gives you and your students even more NCLEX-style questions, this time presented within a test generator that allows you to create and edit your own exams. Additionally, the Instructor's Resource CD-ROM supplies an image bank, PowerPoint presentations to accompany each chapter, and the Answers to the Review Questions and Medication Dosage Calculations from the textbook.
- **thePoint** http://thepoint.lww.com—This web-based course and content management system provides every resource instructors and students need in one easy-to-use site. Advanced technology and superior content combine at thePoint to allow instructors to design and deliver on-line and off-line courses, maintain grades and class rosters, and communicate with students. ThePoint offers a sample syllabus and an extensive collection of materials for each chapter, which consists of the following five components: Pre-Lecture Quizzes and Answers, which are quick, knowledge-based assessments that allow you to check students' reading; PowerPoint presentations; Guided Lecture Notes, which walk you through the chapters, objective by objective, and provide you with corresponding PowerPoint slide numbers; Discussion Topics (and suggested answers), which can be used as conversation starters and are organized by objective; Assignments (and suggested answers), which are broken up into four categories—written, group, clinical, and web—and also map back to the chapters' learning objectives; and Case Studies, with multiple questions and answers for each chapter. Students can visit thePoint to practice for the NCLEX with five additional NCLEX-style review questions per chapter, access supplemental multimedia resources to enhance their learning experience, check the course syllabus, download content, upload assignments, and join an on-line discussion. ThePoint … where teaching, learning, and technology click!

Acknowledgments

I wish to thank everyone involved in the creation of this ninth edition of *Roach's Introductory Clinical Pharmacology*. A special thanks to Sally S. Roach for trusting and believing in my efforts to continue the legacy of her book; to Elizabeth Nieginski, Acquisitions Editor, and Betsy Gentzler, Associate Managing Editor, for teaching and mentoring my efforts to become an author over the development of the last two editions; and to Susan Rockwell, Red Act Group, for her support and editorial assistance with manuscript preparation and development. My gratitude also goes to all those associated with Lippincott Williams & Wilkins who worked in any way on the design, production, and preparation of this book.

Contents

Foundations of Clinical Pharmacology

This unit provides a foundation for our study of pharmacology by discussing the general principles of pharmacology, reviewing the administration of medication and the mathematics involved in dosage calculation, illustrating the nursing process, and discussing patient and family teaching.

Basic principles are covered in Chapter 1, starting with how drugs are derived from natural sources, such as plants, or made synthetically. Drug categories are based upon the body system they influence or the way they are made chemically. Some drugs require a prescription (those given under the supervision of a licensed health care provider) or may be purchased as nonprescription (those obtained over the counter and designated as safe when taken as directed). When taken by a patient, drugs undergo a series of steps to be processed, utilized, and eliminated by the body—this is the basis for the study of pharmacology by health care providers.

Administration of a drug is primarily the responsibility of the nurse and is discussed in Chapter 2. Nurses have the duty to safely provide patient care by correctly administering the medication prescribed by the primary health care provider. This is achieved by learning and following the principles of drug administration, proper technique, and using medication systems correctly.

The nurse's ability to correctly calculate mathematical problems is one of the most important steps in providing safe care to patients. Multiple steps in drug administration and delivery help to ensure accuracy in those math calculations. Chapter 3 provides both the opportunity to practice calculation and an overview of the tasks that nurses undertake to be sure doses of drugs are correct before administration.

Most patients experience problems of anxiety or deficient knowledge regarding new medication routines. The nursing process is used to help members of the health care team provide effective patient care. This process is used to develop an individualized care and teaching plan for the patient. These concepts are covered in Chapter 4.

It is crucial that the patient understand the important information about the medication prescribed, including the dosage, how to take the medication, the expected effect, and adverse reactions. In Chapter 5, a group of individuals receiving nursing care in an ambulatory setting are introduced. Their stories are designed to help nurses understand how all this information is used in the nursing care of patients receiving drug therapy. Nurses will learn how concepts are put into practice using case studies throughout the textbook.

By understanding the basic principles of pharmacology, nurses can build a sound knowledge base of the drugs used to help patients maintain their highest levels of wellness.

General Principles of Pharmacology

additive drug reaction
adverse reaction
agonist
allergic reaction
anaphylactic shock
angioedema
antagonist
antibodies
antigen
biotransformation
controlled substances
cumulative drug effect
drug idiosyncrasy
drug tolerance
first-pass effect
half-life
herbal medicine

hypersensitivity
metabolite
nonprescription drugs
pharmaceutic
pharmacodynamics
pharmacogenetics
pharmacokinetics
pharmacology
physical dependency
polypharmacy
prescription drugs
psychological dependency
receptor
synergism
teratogen
toxic

LEARNING OBJECTIVES

On completion of this chapter, the student will:

1. Define pharmacology.
2. Identify the different names assigned to drugs.
3. Distinguish between prescription drugs, nonprescription drugs, and controlled substances.
4. Discuss drug development in the United States.
5. Discuss the various types of drug activity and reactions produced in the body.
6. Identify factors that influence drug action.
7. Define drug tolerance, cumulative drug effect, and drug idiosyncrasy.
8. Discuss the types of drug interactions that may be seen with drug administration.
9. Discuss the nursing implications associated with drug actions, interactions, and effects.
10. Discuss the use of herbal medicines.

Pharmacology is the study of drugs and their action on living organisms. A sound knowledge of basic pharmacologic principles is essential if the nurse is to administer medications safely and monitor patients who receive these medications. This chapter gives a basic overview of pharma-cologic principles that the nurse must understand when administering medications. The chapter also discusses drug development, federal legislation affecting the dispensing and use of drugs, and the use of **herbal medicine**s as they relate to pharmacology.

Drugs have changed the way in which health professionals treat patients over the last century. In the early 1900s, individuals died of infections, both medically and surgically caused, due in part to lack of sanitary conditions and the fact that medicines to combat infection did not exist. The discovery of drug substances has changed infections into deviations in health rather than death sentences. Additionally, patients lacking certain substances in their bodies, such as insulin, or diagnosed with cancerous tumors can now live long and productive lives due to drug therapy.

Medications are both derived from natural sources, such as plants and minerals, and synthetically produced in a laboratory. Examples of natural sources include digitalis, which is an extract from the foxglove plant that acts as a potent heart medication. On the other hand, mipomersen is a chemically engineered drug being studied to target specific cell components in people with high cholesterol.

Drug Names

Throughout the process of development, drugs may have several names assigned to them: a chemical name, a generic (nonproprietary) name, the official name, and a trade or brand name. This can be confusing, and the nurse must have a clear understanding of the different names used. The chemical name is the scientific term that describes the molecular structure of a drug; it typically is the chemical components of the drug. The generic name is the general name given to a drug that can be made or marketed by any company; it is non-proprietary. This name is typically written in lower case letters. Often the generic name is also the official name that is given a drug by the U.S. Food and Drug Administration (FDA). It also is the name found in the *National Formulary* or the *U.S. Pharmacopeia* for an accepted drug. When a drug name is capitalized, this signifies that it is the trade or brand name. The trade name is selected by a specific company for marketing purposes. In fact, a drug can have several trade names. To avoid confusion, it is best to use the generic name. Table 1.1 identifies the various names and provides an explanation of each.

Table 1.1 Drug Names

Drug Name	Example	Explanation
Chemical name (scientific name)	Example: ethyl 4-(8-chloro-5, 6-dihydro-11*H*-benzo[5,6] cyclohepta[1,2-*b*]-pyridin-11-ylidene)-1- piperidinecarboxylate	Gives the exact chemical makeup of the drug and placing of the atoms or molecular structure; the chemical name is not capitalized.
Generic name (nonproprietary)	Example: loratadine	Name given to a drug before it becomes official; may be used in all countries, by all manufacturers; the generic name is not capitalized.
Official name	Example: loratadine	Name listed in *The United States Pharmacopeia–National Formulary*; may be the same as the generic name.
Trade name (brand name)	Example: Claritin®	Name that is registered by the manufacturer and is followed by the trademark symbol; the name can be used only by the manufacturer; a drug may have several trade names, depending on the number of manufacturers; the first letter of the trade name is capitalized.

Drug Classes and Categories

A drug may be classified by the chemical type of the active ingredient or by the way it is used to treat a particular condition. Each drug can be classified into one or more drug classes. In Unit II, drugs that retard or destroy pathogens are classified as anti-infectives. In each chapter, these drugs are further categorized by the way they work (such as antivirals) or their chemical structure (e.g., penicillins). Once a drug is approved for use, the FDA assigns it to one of the following categories: prescription, nonprescription, or controlled substance.

Prescription Drugs

Prescription drugs are designated by the federal government as potentially harmful unless their use is supervised by a licensed health care provider, such as a nurse practitioner, physician, or dentist. Although these drugs have been tested for safety and therapeutic effect, prescription drugs may cause different reactions in some individuals.

In institutional settings, the nurse administers the drug and monitors the patient for therapeutic effect and **adverse reactions**. Some drugs have the potential to be **toxic** (harmful). The nurse plays a critical role in evaluating the patient for toxic effects. When these drugs are prescribed to be taken at home, the nurse provides patient and family education about the drug.

Prescription drugs, also called *legend drugs,* are the largest category of drugs. Prescription drugs are prescribed by a licensed health care provider. The prescription (Fig. 1.1) contains the name of the drug, the dosage, the method and times of administration, and the signature of the licensed health care provider prescribing the drug.

DEA# _____

CHARLES FULLER, M.D.
SUSAN LUNGLEY, FNP-BC
1629 TREASURE HILLS
HOUSTON, TEXAS 79635

_____

NAME _____

ADDRESS _____ DATE _____
R$_x$

Lasix 20 mg
orally every morning

☐ Another brand of drug, indentical in form and content, may be dispensed unless checked.

Refill _____ times PRN

Susan Lungley, FNP-BC M.D.

Figure 1.1 Example of a prescription form.

Nonprescription Drugs

Nonprescription drugs are designated by the FDA as safe (when taken as directed) and can be obtained without a prescription. These drugs are also referred to as over-the-counter (OTC) drugs and may be purchased in a variety of settings, such as a pharmacy, drugstore, or the local supermarket. Over-the-counter drugs include those given for symptoms of the common cold, minor aches and pains, constipation, diarrhea, and heartburn.

These drugs are not without risk and may produce adverse reactions. For example, acetylsalicylic acid, commonly known as aspirin, is potentially harmful and can cause gastrointestinal (GI) bleeding and salicylism (see Chapter 14). Labeling requirements give the consumer important information regarding the drug, dosage, contraindications, precautions, and adverse reactions. Consumers are urged to read the directions carefully before taking OTC drugs.

Controlled Substances *Marajuana-Medicinal*

Controlled substances are the most carefully monitored of all drugs. These drugs have a high potential for abuse and may cause physical or psychological dependency. **Physical dependency** is the habitual use of a drug, in which negative physical withdrawal symptoms result from abrupt discontinuation; it is the body's dependence on repeated administration of a drug. **Psychological dependency** is a compulsion or craving to use a substance to obtain a pleasurable experience; it is the mind's desire for the repeated administration of a drug. One type of dependency may lead to the other.

The Controlled Substances Act of 1970 established a schedule, or classification system, for drugs with abuse potential. The act regulates the manufacture, distribution, and dispensing of these drugs. The Controlled Substances Act divides drugs into five schedules, based on their potential for abuse and physical and psychological dependence. Appendix A describes the five schedules.

Prescription practices of the primary health care provider for controlled substances are monitored by the Drug Enforcement Agency (DEA). Under federal law, limited quantities of certain schedule V drugs may be purchased without a prescription, with the purchase recorded by the dispensing pharmacist. In some cases, state laws are more restrictive than federal laws and impose additional requirements for the sale and distribution of controlled substances. In hospitals or other agencies that dispense controlled substances, the scheduled drugs are counted every 8 to 12 hours to account for each injectable, tablet, or other form of the drug. Any discrepancy in the number of drugs must be investigated and explained immediately.

Drug Development

Drug development is a long and arduous process that can take from 7 to 12 years, and sometimes longer. The FDA has the responsibility for approving new drugs and monitoring drugs currently in use for adverse or toxic reactions. The development of a new drug is divided into the pre-FDA phase and the FDA phase. During the pre-FDA phase, a manufacturer discovers a drug that looks promising. In vitro testing (testing in an artificial environment, such as a test tube) using animal and human cells is done. This testing is followed by studies in live animals. The manufacturer then makes application to the FDA for Investigational New Drug (IND) status.

With IND status, clinical (i.e., human) testing of the new drug begins. Clinical testing involves three phases, with each phase involving a larger number of people (Fig. 1.2). All effects, both pharmacologic and biologic, are noted. Phase 1 involves 20 to 100 individuals who are healthy volunteers. If Phase 1 studies are successful, the testing moves to Phase 2, in which tests are performed on people who have the disease or condition for which the drug is thought to be effective. If those results are positive, the testing progresses to Phase 3, in which the drug is given to large numbers of patients in medical research centers to provide information about adverse reactions. Phase 3 studies offer additional information on dosing and safety.

A New Drug Application (NDA) is submitted after the investigation of the drug in Phases 1, 2, and 3 is complete and the drug is found to be safe and effective. With the NDA, the manufacturer submits all data collected concerning the drug during the clinical trials. A panel of experts, including pharmacologists, chemists, physicians, and other professionals, reviews the application and makes a recommendation to the FDA. The FDA then either approves or disapproves the drug for use. After FDA approval, continued surveillance is done to ensure safety.

Postmarketing surveillance (Phase 4) occurs after the manufacturer places the drug on the market. During this surveillance, an ongoing review of the drug occurs with particular attention given to adverse reactions. Health care professionals are encouraged to help with this surveillance by reporting adverse effects of drugs to the FDA by using MedWatch (Display 1.1) or the Institute for Safe Medication Practices (ISMP) Medication Errors Reporting Program (MERP).

Special FDA Programs

Although it takes considerable time for most drugs to get FDA approval, the FDA has special programs to meet different needs. Examples of these special programs include the orphan drug program and accelerated programs for urgent needs.

Orphan Drug Program

The Orphan Drug Act of 1983 was passed to encourage the development and marketing of products used to treat rare diseases. The act defines a "rare disease" as a condition affecting fewer than 200,000 individuals in the United States or a condition affecting more than 200,000 persons in the United States but for which the cost of producing and marketing a drug to treat the condition would not be recovered by sales of the drug. The National Organization of Rare Disorders reports that there are more than 6000 rare disorders that affect approximately 25 million individuals. Examples of rare disorders include multiple myeloma, cystic fibrosis, and phenylketonuria.

The act provides for incentives, such as research grants, protocol assistance by the FDA, and special tax credits, to

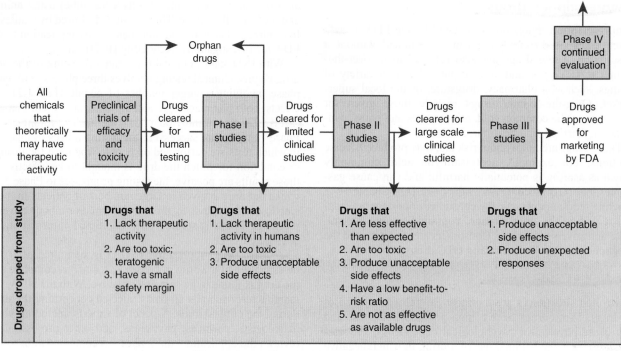

Figure 1.2 Phases of drug development.

encourage manufacturers to develop orphan drugs. If the drug is approved, the manufacturer has 7 years of exclusive marketing rights. More than 100 new drugs have received FDA approval since the law was passed. Examples of orphan drugs include Valortim for anthrax infection, FK778 for acute organ transplant rejection, and Atiprimod for the treatment of multiple myeloma.

DISPLAY 1.1 MedWatch and Reporting Adverse Events

The FDA established a safety information and adverse event reporting program called MedWatch, by which nurses or other health care professionals can learn about or report observations of serious adverse drug effects. Anyone can access the website (http://www.fda.gov/medwatch/index.html) to obtain safety alerts on drugs, devices, or dietary supplements.

A drug must be used and studied for many years before all of the adverse reactions are identified. Nurses play an important role in monitoring for adverse reactions. The website provides a standardized form for reporting which can be submitted electronically or downloaded, filled out, and mailed/faxed in to the program. It is important to submit reports, even if there is uncertainty about the cause–effect relationship. The FDA protects the identity of those who voluntarily report adverse reactions.

The FDA considers serious adverse reactions those that may result in death, life-threatening illness, hospitalization, or disability or those that may require medical or surgical intervention. This form also is used to report an undesirable experience associated with the use of medical products (e.g., latex gloves, pacemakers, infusion pumps, anaphylaxis, blood, blood components).

Accelerated Programs

Accelerated approval of drugs is offered by the FDA as a means to make promising products for life-threatening diseases available on the market, based on preliminary evidence and before formal demonstration of patient benefit. The approval that is granted is considered a "provisional approval," with a written commitment from the pharmaceutical company to complete clinical studies that formally demonstrate patient benefit. This program seeks to make life-saving investigational drugs available before granting final approval to treat diseases that pose a significant health threat to the public. One example of a disease that qualifies as posing a significant health threat is AIDS. Because AIDS is so devastating to the individuals affected and because of the danger the disease poses to public health, the FDA and pharmaceutical companies worked together to shorten the IND approval process for some drugs that show promise in treating AIDS. This accelerated process allows primary care providers to administer medications that indicate positive results in early Phase 1 and 2 clinical trials, rather than wait until final approval is granted. If the drug continues to prove beneficial, the process of approval is accelerated.

Drug Activity Within the Body

Drugs act in various ways in the body. Oral drugs go through three phases: the *pharmaceutic* phase, *pharmacokinetic* phase, and *pharmacodynamic* phase (Fig. 1.3). Liquid and parenteral drugs (drugs given by injection) go through the latter two phases only.

A is safest

competitive agonists bind reversibly with receptor sites, administering larger doses of an agonist can overcome the antagonist effects. The noncompetitive antagonist binds with receptor sites and always blocks the effects of the agonists. Administering larger doses of the agonists will not reverse the action of the noncompetitive antagonist.

Receptor-Mediated Drug Effects

The number of available receptor sites influences the effects of a drug. When only a few receptor sites are occupied, although many sites are available, the response will be small. When the drug dose is increased, more receptor sites are used, and the response increases. When only a few receptor sites are available, the response does not increase when more of the drug is administered. However, not all receptors on a cell need to be occupied for a drug to be effective. Some extremely potent drugs are effective even when the drug occupies few receptor sites.

Alteration in Cellular Environment

alters cellular movement

Some drugs act on the body by changing the cellular environment, either physically or chemically. Physical changes in the cellular environment include changes in osmotic pressure, lubrication, absorption, or the conditions on the surface of the cell membrane. An example of a drug that changes osmotic pressure is *mannitol*, which produces a change in the osmotic pressure in brain cells, causing a reduction in cerebral edema. An example of a drug that acts by altering the cellular environment by lubrication is sunscreen. An example of a drug that acts by altering absorption is activated charcoal, which is administered orally to absorb a toxic chemical ingested into the GI tract. The stool softener *docusate* is an example of a drug that acts by altering the surface of the cellular membrane. Docusate has emulsifying and lubricating activity that lowers the surface tension in the cells of the bowel, permitting water and fats to enter the stool. This softens the fecal mass, allowing easier passage of the stool.

Chemical changes in the cellular environment include inactivation of cellular functions or alteration of the chemical components of body fluid, such as a change in the pH. For example, antacids neutralize gastric acidity in patients with peptic ulcers.

Other drugs, such as some anticancer drugs and some antibiotics, have as their main site of action the cell membrane and various cellular processes. They incorporate themselves into the normal metabolic processes of the cell and cause the formation of a defective final product, such as a weakened cell wall, which results in cell death, or produce a lack of a needed energy substrate that leads to cell starvation and death.

Pharmacogenomics

The Human Genome Project was a study to determine the different components of the human genetic code. One discovery from this project was that the genetic make-up of a person can affect the pharmacodynamics of a drug. Pharmacogenomics is the study of how people's responses to medications are variable due to individual genetic variation. The study of pharmacogenetics is the creation of individualized drug therapy that allows for the best choice and dose of drugs.

Drug Use, Pregnancy, and Lactation

The use of any medication—prescription or nonprescription—carries a risk of causing birth defects in the developing fetus. Drugs administered to pregnant women, particularly during the first trimester (3 months), may have teratogenic effects. A **teratogen** is any substance that causes abnormal development of the fetus, often leading to severe deformation. Some drugs are teratogens.

To prevent teratogenic effects, the FDA has established five categories suggesting the potential of a drug for causing birth defects (Appendix A). Information regarding the pregnancy category of a specific drug is found in reliable drug literature, such as the inserts accompanying drugs and approved drug references. In general, most drugs are contraindicated during pregnancy and lactation unless the potential benefits of taking the drug outweigh the risks to the fetus or the infant.

During pregnancy, no woman should consider taking any drug, legal or illegal, prescription or nonprescription, unless the drug is prescribed or recommended by the primary health care provider. Smoking or drinking any type of alcoholic beverage also carries risks, such as low birth weight, premature birth, and fetal alcohol syndrome. Children born of mothers using addictive drugs, such as cocaine or heroin, often are born with an addiction to the drug abused by the mother. Women who are pregnant should also be very careful about the use of herbal supplements because these products can act like drugs. Women should not take an herbal supplement without discussing it first with her primary health care provider.

heroin increases surfactant

When a mother breastfeeds, her child risks exposure to harmful medications. A number of drugs can be excreted in breast milk. Therefore, if a mother is lactating (breastfeeding), some of the drug she is taking may be ingested and absorbed by the infant or breastfeeding child. It is important for both mothers and nurses to know the potential of exposure to a breastfeeding child when the mother is taking a drug.

The National Library of Medicine provides a free online database with information on drugs and lactation called LactMed (http://toxnet.nlm.nih.gov/cgi-bin/sis/htmlgen?LACT). This website is geared to the health care practitioner and nursing mother and contains over 450 drug records. It includes information such as maternal levels in breast milk, infant levels in blood, and potential effects in breastfeeding infants. A pharmacist, Dr. Thomas Hale, from Texas Tech University has developed a system of lactation risk categories similar to that of the FDA pregnancy risk categories for drugs. Drugs are assigned an L1 to L5 risk according to the drug's transmission in breast milk and the effect it may have on the child. Hale's listing of certain drugs may differ from those published by organizations such as the American Academy of Pediatrics, yet it is a good starting point for discussion with mothers who are breastfeeding.

Drug Reactions

Drugs produce many reactions in the body. The following sections discuss adverse drug reactions, allergic drug reactions, **drug idiosyncrasy**, **drug tolerance**, **cumulative drug effect**, and toxic reactions.

Adverse Drug Reactions

Patients may experience one or more adverse reactions or side effects when they are given a drug. Adverse reactions are undesirable drug effects. Adverse reactions may be common or may occur infrequently. They may be mild, severe, or life-threatening. They may occur after the first dose, after several doses, or after many doses. Often, an adverse reaction is unpredictable, although some drugs are known to cause certain adverse reactions in many patients. For example, drugs used in treating cancer are very toxic and are known to produce adverse reactions in many patients receiving them. Other drugs produce adverse reactions in fewer patients. Some adverse reactions are predictable, but many adverse drug reactions occur without warning.

Some texts use both the terms *side effects* and *adverse reactions*, using *side effects* to explain mild, common, and nontoxic reactions and *adverse reactions* to describe more severe and life-threatening reactions. For the purposes of this text, only the term *adverse reaction* is used, with the understanding that these reactions may be mild, severe, or life-threatening.

Allergic Drug Reactions

An **allergic reaction** is an immediate **hypersensitivity** reaction. Allergy to a drug usually begins to occur after more than one dose of the drug is given. On occasion, the nurse may observe an allergic reaction the first time a drug is given, because the patient has received or taken the drug in the past.

A drug allergy occurs because the individual's immune system responds to the drug as a foreign substance called an **antigen**. When the body responds to the drug as an antigen, a series of events occurs in an attempt to render the invader harmless. Lymphocytes respond by forming **antibodies** (protein substances that protect against antigens). Common allergic reactions occur when the individual's immune system responds aggressively to the antigen. Chemical mediators released during the allergic reaction produce symptoms ranging from mild to life-threatening.

Even a mild allergic reaction produces serious effects if it goes unnoticed and the drug is given again. Any indication of an allergic reaction is reported to the primary health care provider before the next dose of the drug is given. Serious allergic reactions require contacting the primary health care provider immediately, because emergency treatment may be necessary.

Some allergic reactions occur within minutes (even seconds) after the drug is given; others may be delayed for hours or days. Allergic reactions that occur immediately often are the most serious.

Allergic reactions are manifested by a variety of signs and symptoms observed by the nurse or reported by the patient. Examples of some allergic symptoms include itching, various types of skin rashes, and hives (urticaria). Other symptoms include difficulty breathing, wheezing, cyanosis, a sudden loss of consciousness, and swelling of the eyes, lips, or tongue.

Anaphylactic shock is an extremely serious allergic drug reaction that usually occurs shortly after the administration of

Body System	Symptoms
Respiratory	Bronchospasm Dyspnea (difficult breathing) Feeling of fullness in the throat Cough Wheezing
Cardiovascular	Extremely low blood pressure Tachycardia (heart rate >100 bpm) Palpitations Syncope (fainting) Cardiac arrest
Integumentary	Urticaria (hives) Angioedema Pruritus (itching) Sweating
Gastrointestinal	Nausea Vomiting Abdominal pain

Table 1.2 **Symptoms of Anaphylactic Shock**

a drug to which the individual is sensitive. This type of allergic reaction requires immediate medical attention. Symptoms of anaphylactic shock are listed in Table 1.2.

All or only some of these symptoms may be present. Anaphylactic shock can be fatal if the symptoms are not identified and treated immediately. Treatment is to raise the blood pressure, improve breathing, restore cardiac function, and treat other symptoms as they occur. Epinephrine (adrenalin) may be given by subcutaneous injection in the upper extremity or thigh and may be followed by a continuous intravenous infusion. Hypotension and shock may be treated with fluids and vasopressors. Bronchodilators are given to relax the smooth muscles of the bronchial tubes. Antihistamines and corticosteroids may also be given to treat urticaria and angioedema (swelling).

Angioedema (angioneurotic edema) is another type of allergic drug reaction. It is manifested by the collection of fluid in subcutaneous tissues. Areas that are most commonly affected are the eyelids, lips, mouth, and throat, although other areas also may be affected. Angioedema can be dangerous when the mouth is affected, because the swelling may block the airway and asphyxia may occur. Difficulty in breathing and swelling in any area of the body are reported immediately to the primary health care provider.

Drug Idiosyncrasy

Drug idiosyncrasy is a term used to describe any unusual or abnormal reaction to a drug. It is any reaction that is different from the one normally expected from a specific drug and dose. For example, a patient may be given a drug to help him or her sleep (e.g., a hypnotic). Instead of falling asleep, the patient remains wide awake and shows signs of nervousness or excitement. This response is idiosyncratic because it is different from what the nurse expects from this type of drug. Another patient may receive the same drug and dose, fall asleep, and ~~after 8 hours~~ be difficult to awaken. This, too, is abnormal and describes an over-response to the drug.

The cause of drug idiosyncrasy is not clear. It is believed to be due to a genetic deficiency that makes the patient unable to tolerate certain chemicals, including drugs. **Pharmacogenetics** is the study of ways that specific genes can enhance sensitivity or resistance to certain drugs. A pharmacogenetic disorder is a genetically determined abnormal response to normal doses of a drug. This abnormal response occurs because of inherited traits that cause abnormal metabolism of drugs. For example, individuals with glucose-6-phosphate dehydrogenase (G6PD) deficiency have abnormal reactions to a number of drugs. These patients exhibit varying degrees of hemolysis (destruction of red blood cells) when these drugs are administered. More than 100 million people are affected by this disorder. Examples of drugs that cause hemolysis in patients with a G6PD deficiency include aspirin, chloramphenicol, and the sulfonamides.

Drug Tolerance

~~Drug tolerance~~ is a term used to describe a decreased response to a drug, requiring an increase in dosage to achieve the desired effect. Drug tolerance may develop when a patient takes certain drugs, such as opioids and tranquilizers, for a long time. The individual who takes these drugs at home ~~increases the dose~~ when the expected drug effect does not occur. The development of drug tolerance is a sign of physical drug dependence. Drug tolerance may also occur in the hospitalized patient. When the patient begins to ask for the drug at more frequent intervals, the nurse needs to assess whether the dose is not adequate based upon the disease process or whether the patient is building a tolerance to the drug's effects.

Cumulative Drug Effect

A ~~cumulative drug effect~~ may be seen in those people with liver or kidney disease because these organs are the major sites for the breakdown and excretion of most drugs. This drug effect occurs when the body is ~~unable to metabolize~~ and excrete one (normal) dose of a drug before the next dose is given. Thus, if a second dose of the drug is given, some drug from the first dose remains in the body. A cumulative drug effect can be serious because too much of the drug can accumulate in the body and lead to toxicity.

Patients with liver or kidney disease are usually given drugs with caution because a cumulative effect may occur. When the patient is unable to excrete the drug at a normal rate, the drug accumulates in the body, causing a toxic reaction. Sometimes, the primary health care provider lowers the dose of the drug to prevent a toxic drug reaction.

~~Toxic Reactions~~

Most drugs can produce toxic or harmful reactions if administered in large dosages or when blood concentration levels exceed the therapeutic level. Toxic levels build up when a drug is administered in dosages that exceed the normal level or if the patient's kidneys are not functioning properly and cannot excrete the drug. Some toxic effects are immediately visible;

others may not be seen for weeks or months. Some drugs, such as lithium or digoxin, have a narrow margin of safety, even when given in recommended dosages. It is important to monitor these drugs closely to detect and avoid toxicity.

Drug toxicity can be reversible or irreversible, depending on the organs involved. Damage to the liver may be reversible, because liver cells can regenerate. However, hearing loss from damage to the eighth cranial nerve caused by toxic reaction to the anti-infective drug streptomycin may be permanent. Sometimes drug toxicity can be reversed by administering another drug that acts as an antidote. For example, in serious instances of digitalis toxicity, the drug Digibind may be given to counteract the effect.

Nurses must carefully monitor the patient's blood level of drug to ensure that the level remains within the therapeutic range. Any deviation should be reported to the primary health care provider. Because some drugs can cause toxic reactions even in recommended doses, the nurse should be aware of the signs and symptoms of toxicity of commonly prescribed drugs.

Minimizing Drug Reactions Through Pharmacogenomics

Drug developers are also researching ways to target cell structures and selected cells to minimize reactions in other body tissue, thereby reducing or eliminating adverse reactions. Pharmacogenomics is the search for genetic variations associated with drug efficiency. The goal of pharmacogenomics is the creation of drugs that can be tailor-made for individuals, target specific cells in the body, and adapt to each person's own individual genetic makeup.

Drug Interactions

It is important for the nurse administering medications to be aware of the various drug interactions that can occur, especially *drug–drug interactions* and *drug–food interactions*. This section gives a brief overview of drug interactions. Specific drug–drug and drug–food interactions are discussed in subsequent chapters.

Drug–Drug ~~Interactions~~

A drug–drug interaction occurs when one drug interacts with or interferes with the action of another drug. For example, taking an antacid with oral tetracycline causes a decrease in the effectiveness of the tetracycline. The antacid chemically interacts with the tetracycline and impairs its absorption into the bloodstream, thus reducing the effectiveness of the tetracycline. Drugs known to cause interactions include oral anticoagulants, oral hypoglycemics, anti-infectives, antiarrhythmics, cardiac glycosides, and alcohol. Drug–drug interactions can produce effects that are additive, synergistic, or antagonistic.

Additive Drug Reaction
An **additive drug reaction** occurs when the combined effect of two drugs is equal to the sum of each drug given alone. For example, taking the drug heparin with alcohol will increase bleeding. The equation $1 + 1 = 2$ is sometimes used to illustrate the additive effect of drugs.

Synergistic Drug Reaction

Drug **synergism** occurs when drugs interact with each other and produce an effect that is greater than the sum of their separate actions. The equation $1 + 1 = 3$ may be used to illustrate synergism. Drug synergism is exemplified when a person takes both a hypnotic and alcohol. When alcohol is taken simultaneously or shortly before or after the hypnotic is taken, the action of the hypnotic increases considerably. The individual experiences a drug effect that is greater than if each drug was taken alone. On occasion, the occurrence of a synergistic drug effect is serious and even fatal.

Antagonistic Drug Reaction

An antagonistic drug reaction occurs when one drug interferes with the action of another, causing neutralization or a decrease in the effect of one drug. For example, protamine is a heparin antagonist. This means that the administration of protamine completely neutralizes the effects of heparin in the body.

Drug–Food Interactions

When a drug is given orally, food may impair or enhance its absorption. A drug taken on an empty stomach is absorbed into the bloodstream more quickly than when the drug is taken with food in the stomach. Some drugs (e.g., captopril) must be taken on an empty stomach to achieve an optimal effect. Drugs that should be taken on an empty stomach are administered 1 hour before or 2 hours after meals. Other drugs—especially drugs that irritate the stomach, result in nausea or vomiting, or cause epigastric distress—are best given with food or meals. This minimizes gastric irritation. The nonsteroidal anti-inflammatory drugs and salicylates are examples of drugs that are given with food to decrease epigastric distress. Still other drugs combine with a food, forming an insoluble food–drug mixture. For example, when tetracycline is administered with dairy products, a drug–food mixture is formed that is unabsorbable by the body. When a drug is unabsorbable by the body, no pharmacologic effect occurs.

Factors Influencing Drug Response

Certain factors may influence drug response and are considered when the primary health care provider prescribes and the nurse administers a drug. These factors include age, weight, sex, disease, and route of administration.

Age

The age of the patient may influence the effects of a drug. Infants and children usually require smaller doses of a drug than adults. Immature organ function, particularly of the liver and kidneys, can affect the ability of infants and young children to metabolize drugs. An infant's immature kidneys impair the elimination of drugs in the urine. Liver function is poorly developed in infants and young children. Drugs metabolized by the liver may produce more intense effects for longer periods. Parents must be taught the potential problems associated with administering drugs to their children. For example, a safe dose of a nonprescription drug for a 4-year-old child may be dangerous for a 6-month-old infant.

Elderly patients may also require smaller doses, although this may depend on the type of drug administered. For example, the elderly patient may be given the same dose of an antibiotic as a younger adult. However, the same older adult may require a smaller dose of a drug that depresses the central nervous system, such as an opioid. Changes that occur with aging affect the pharmacokinetics (absorption, distribution, metabolism, and excretion) of a drug. Any of these processes may be altered because of the physiologic changes that occur with aging. Table 1.3 summarizes the changes that occur with aging and their possible pharmacokinetic effects.

Polypharmacy is the taking of numerous drugs that can potentially react with one another. This is seen particularly in elderly patients who may have multiple chronic diseases; polypharmacy leads to an increase in the number of potential adverse reactions. Although multiple drug therapy is necessary to treat certain disease states, it always increases the possibility of adverse reactions. The nurse needs good assess-

Grapefruit

Table *1.3* Factors Altering Drug Response in Children and Elders		
Body System Changes	**Children/Infants**	**Elderly**
Gastric acidity	Higher pH—slower gastric emptying resulting in delayed absorption	Higher pH—slower gastric emptying resulting in delayed absorption
Skin changes	Less cutaneous fat and greater surface area—faster absorption of topical drugs	Decreased fat content—decreased absorption of transdermal drugs
Body water content	Increased body water content—greater dilution of drug in tissues	Decreased body water content—greater concentration of drug in tissues
Serum protein	Less protein—less protein binding creating more circulating drug	Less protein—less protein binding creating more circulating drug
Liver function	Immature function—increased half life of drugs and less first-pass effect	Decreased blood flow to liver—delayed and decreased metabolism of drug
Kidney function	Immature kidney function—decreased elimination, potential for toxicity at lower drug levels	Decreased renal mass and glomerular filtration rate—increased serum levels of drugs

one of eight agencies in the Public Health Service in the U.S. Department of Health and Human Services (DHHS). NCCAM explores complementary and alternative healing practices through scientific research. It also trains complementary/alternative medicine (CAM) scientists and disseminates the information gleaned from the research it conducts. Among the various purposes of the NCCAM, one is to evaluate the safety and efficacy of widely used natural products, such as herbal remedies and dietary and food supplements. The Center is dedicated to developing programs and encouraging scientists to investigate CAM treatments that show promise. The NCCAM budget has steadily grown, reflecting the public's interest and need for CAM information that is based on rigorous scientific research.

The NCCAM defines CAM as a "group of diverse medical and health care systems, practices, and products that are not presently considered to be part of conventional medicine." Examples of complementary therapies are therapies such as relaxation techniques, massage, aromatherapy, and healing touch. Complementary therapies are often used with traditional health care to "complement" conventional medicine. Alternative therapies, on the other hand, are therapies used in place of or instead of conventional or Western medicine. The term *complementary/alternative therapy* often is used as an umbrella term for many therapies from all over the world.

THINK CRITICALLY: PHARMACOLOGY IN PRACTICE

1. Mrs. Moore, aged 85 years, is receiving a low dose of meperidine (Demerol), an opioid analgesic, for postoperative pain. Her family questions the use of such a low dose. Determine what information you would give her family when they voice concerns that the dosage will not adequately relieve their mother's pain. Analyze what patient assessment, if any, you would need to make before talking with the family.

● Test Your Knowledge

1. Mr. Carter has a rash and pruritus. You suspect an allergic reaction and immediately assess him for other more serious symptoms. What question would be most important to ask Mr. Carter?

A. Are you having any difficulty breathing?
B. Have you noticed any blood in your stool?
C. Do you have a headache?
D. Are you having difficulty with your vision?

2. Mr. Jones, a newly admitted patient, has a history of liver disease. In planning Mr. Jones' care, the nurse must consider that liver disease may result in a(n) _____.

A. increase in the excretion rate of a drug
B. impaired ability to metabolize or detoxify a drug
C. need to increase the dosage of a drug
D. decrease in the rate of drug absorption

3. A patient asks the nurse to define a hypersensitivity reaction. The nurse begins by telling the patient that a hypersensitivity reaction is also called a(n) ____ ____.

A. synergistic reaction
B. antagonistic reaction
C. drug idiosyncrasy
D. allergic reaction

4. In monitoring drug therapy, the nurse is aware that a synergistic drug effect may be defined as _____.

A. an effect greater than the sum of the separate actions of two or more drugs
B. an increase in the action of one of the two drugs being given
C. a neutralizing drug effect
D. a comprehensive drug effect

● Prepare for the NCLEX

1. Under the Controlled Substances Act, schedule II to V drugs are typically accounted for in the health care setting. Which of the following drugs would the nurse least expect to be counted during change of shift duties?

A. Opioids
B. Antidiarrheals with codeine
C. Anabolic steroids
D. Heroin

To check your answers, see Appendix E.

the**Point** *For more NCLEX questions, log on to http://thepoint.lww.com to access more than 1000 questions.*

Administration of Drugs

drug errors
inhalation
intradermal
intramuscular
intravenous
parenteral

Standard Precautions
subcutaneous
transdermal
Unit dose
Z-track technique

On completion of this chapter, the student will:

1. Discuss the five + 1 rights of drug administration.
2. Discuss general principles of drug administration.
3. Identify the different types of medication orders.
4. Describe general guidelines the nurse should follow when preparing a drug for administration.
5. Discuss how the Joint Commission's National Patient Safety Goals and Institute for Safe Medication Practices website help nurses reduce medication-related errors.
6. Describe the various types of medication-dispensing systems.
7. Discuss the administration of oral and parenteral drugs.
8. Discuss the administration of drugs through the skin and mucous membranes.
9. Discuss nursing responsibilities before, during, and after a drug is administered.

The administration of a drug is a fundamental responsibility of the nurse. An understanding of the basic concepts of administering drugs is critical if the nurse is to perform this task safely and accurately. In addition to administering the drug, the nurse monitors the therapeutic response (desired response) and reports adverse reactions. In the ambulatory setting, the nurse is responsible for teaching the patient and family members the information needed to administer drugs safely in an outpatient setting.

The (Five + 1) Rights of Drug Administration

The nurse preparing and administering a drug to a patient assumes responsibility for this procedure. Responsibility entails preparing and administering the prescribed drug. There are five "rights" in the administration of drugs:

1. Right patient
2. Right drug
3. Right dose
4. Right route
5. Right time

In recent years, the concern for increasing medication errors has produced a sixth right for nurses to heed:

6. Right documentation

Right Patient

When administering a drug, the nurse must be certain that the patient receiving the drug is the patient for whom the drug has been ordered. It is important to use two methods to identify the patient before administering the medication. Identifiers can include visual as well as verbal methods. A visual identifier may include checking the patient's name on his or her wristband (Fig. 2.1). If there is no written identification verifying the patient's name, the nurse obtains a wristband or other form of identification before administering the drug.

Figure 2.1 In following the "six rights" of medication administration, the nurse always verifies that the "right patient" is receiving the medication by using two identifiers, one of which is checking the patient's identification bracelet.

The nurse may also ask the patient to identify himself and request another unique identifier such as his date of birth. However, the nurse should not ask, "Are you Mr. Jones?" Some patients, particularly those who are confused or have difficulty hearing, may respond by answering "yes" even though that is not their name. Some long-term care or rehabilitation care facilities have pictures of the patient available, which allows the nurse to verify the correct patient. If pictures are used to identify patients, it is critical that they are recent and bear a good likeness of the individual.

Right Drug

Drug names are often confused, especially when the names sound similar or the spellings are similar. Nurses who hurriedly prepare a drug for administration or who fail to look up questionable drugs are at increased risk for administering the wrong drug. Appendix B identifies examples of drugs that can easily be confused. The nurse compares medication, container label, and medication record as the item is removed from the cart, compared to the Medication Administration Record (MAR) and before the actual administration of the drug (Fig. 2.2).

Right Dose, Route, and Time

The nurse should obtain a primary health care provider's written order for the administration of all drugs. The primary health care provider's order must include the patient's name, the drug name, the dosage form and route, the dosage to be administered, and the frequency of administration. The primary health care provider's signature must follow the drug order. In an emergency, the nurse may administer a drug with a verbal order from the primary health care provider. However, the primary health care provider must write and sign the order as soon as the emergency is over.

If a verbal order is given over the telephone, the nurse writes down the order, repeats back the information exactly as written, and then asks for a verbal confirmation that it is correct. Any order that is unclear should be questioned, par-

Figure 2.3 The nurse always documents the medication immediately after the drug is administered.

ticularly unclear directions for the administration of the drug, illegible handwriting on the primary health care provider's order sheet, or a drug dose that is higher or lower than the dosages given in approved references.

Right Documentation

After the administration of any drug, the nurse records the process immediately (Fig. 2.3). Immediate documentation is particularly important when drugs are given on an as-needed (PRN) basis. For example, most analgesics require 20 to 30 minutes before the drug begins to relieve pain. A patient may forget that he or she received a drug for pain, may not have been told that the administered drug was for pain, or may not know that pain relief is not immediate, and may ask another nurse for the drug again. If the administration of the analgesic was not recorded, the patient might receive a second dose of the analgesic shortly after the first dose. This kind of situation can be extremely serious, especially when opioids or other central nervous system depressants are administered. Immediate documentation prevents accidental administration of a drug by another individual. Proper documentation is essential to the process of administering drugs correctly.

Considerations in Drug Administration

General Principles of Drug Administration

The nurse must have factual knowledge of each drug given, the reasons for use of the drug, the drug's general action, the more common adverse reactions associated with the drug, special precautions in administration (if any), and the normal dose ranges.

Some drugs may be given frequently; in this case, the nurse becomes familiar with pharmacologic information about a specific drug. Other drugs may be given less frequently, or a new drug may be introduced, requiring the nurse to obtain information from reliable sources, such as the drug package insert, internet sources, or the hospital department of pharmacy. It is of utmost importance to check current and approved references for all drug information.

Figure 2.2 Before administering the medication, the nurse compares the medication, the container label, and the medication record to ensure that the patient received the "right drug" and the "right dose."

The nurse also needs to take patient considerations, such as allergy history, previous adverse reactions, patient comments, and change in patient condition, into account before administering the drug. Before giving any drug for the first time, the nurse should ask the patient about any known allergies and any family history of allergies. This includes allergies not only to drugs but to food, pollen, animals, and so on. Patients with a personal or family history of allergies are more likely to experience additional allergies and must be monitored closely.

If the patient makes any statement about the drug or if there is any change in the patient, these situations are carefully considered before the drug is given. Examples of situations that require consideration before a drug is given include:

- Problems that may be associated with the drug, such as nausea, dizziness, ringing in the ears, and difficulty walking. Any comments made by the patient may indicate the occurrence of an adverse reaction. The nurse should withhold the drug until references are consulted and the primary caregiver contacted. The decision to withhold the drug must have a sound rationale and must be based on knowledge of pharmacology.
- Comments stating that the drug looks different from the one previously received, that the drug was just given by another nurse, or that the patient thought the primary health care provider discontinued the drug therapy.
- A change in the patient's condition, a change in one or more vital signs, or the appearance of new symptoms. Depending on the drug being administered and the patient's diagnosis, these changes may indicate that the drug should be withheld and the primary health care provider contacted.

The Medication Order

Before a medication can be administered in a hospital or other agency, the nurse must have a physician's order. Medications are ordered by the primary health care provider, such as a physician, dentist, or, in some cases, an advanced nurse practitioner. Common orders include the standing order, the single order, the PRN order, and the STAT order. See Display 2.1 for an explanation of each.

DISPLAY 2.1 Types of Medication Orders

Standing Order: This type of order is pre-established and approved for use by nurses and other professionals under specific conditions in the absence of a health care provider. They may be drug orders for pre-surgical/procedure or post-surgical/procedure nursing care. *Example:* Cefotetan 1 gm IV 30 minutes preoperatively

Single order: An order to administer the drug one time only. *Example:* Valium 10 mg IM at 10:00 am.

PRN order: An order to administer the drug as needed. *Example:* Percocet 1-2 tablets orally q 4 hr PRN for pain.

STAT order: A one-time order given as soon as possible. *Example:* Morphine 10 mg IV STAT for cardiac pain.

Preparing a Drug for Administration

When preparing a drug for administration, the nurse should observe the following guidelines:

- Always check the health care provider's written orders and verify any questions with the primary health care provider.
- Be alert for drugs with similar names. Some drugs have names that sound alike but are very different (see Appendix B). To give one drug when another is ordered could have serious consequences.
- Wash hands immediately before preparing a drug for administration. Do not let hands touch medication, especially topical preparations that the nurse may absorb through the tissue of the hands.
- Always check and compare the label of the drug with the MAR three times: (1) when the drug is taken from its storage area, (2) immediately before removing the drug from the container, and (3) before administering the drug to the patient.
- Never remove a drug from an unlabeled container or from a package whose label is illegible. Do not remove the wrappings of the unit dose until the drug reaches the bedside of the patient who is to receive it. After administering the drug, the nurse charts immediately on the MAR drug record.
- Never crush tablets or open capsules without first checking with the clinical pharmacist. Some tablets can be crushed or capsules can be opened and the contents added to water or a tube feeding when the patient cannot swallow a whole tablet or capsule. Some tablets have a special coating that delays the absorption of the drug. Crushing the tablet may destroy this drug property and result in problems such as improper absorption of the drug or gastric irritation. Capsules are gelatin and dissolve on contact with a liquid. The contents of some capsules do not mix well with water and therefore are best left in the capsule. If the patient cannot take an oral tablet or capsule, consult the primary health care provider because the drug may be available in liquid form.
- Never give a drug that someone else has prepared. The individual preparing the drug must administer the drug.
- Place drugs requiring special storage to the storage area immediately after they are prepared for administration. This rule applies mainly to drugs that need refrigeration, but may also apply to drugs that must be protected from exposure to light or heat.

Preventing Drug Errors

Drug errors include any event or activity that can cause a patient to receive the wrong dose, the wrong drug, an incorrect dosage of the drug, a drug by the wrong route, or a drug given at the incorrect time. Errors may occur in transcribing drug orders, when the drug is dispensed, or in administration of the drug. Nurses, as the drug administrators, serve as the last defense against drug errors. When a drug error occurs, it must be reported immediately so that any necessary steps to counteract the action of the drug or any observation can be made as soon as possible. In most institutions, the nurse must complete an unusual occurrence report and notify the primary care provider. It is important to report errors even when the patient suffers no harm.

Drug errors occur when one or more of the five + 1 rights have not been followed. Each time a drug is prepared and administered, the five + 1 rights must be a part of the procedure. In addition to consistently practicing the five + 1 rights, the nurse should adhere to the following precautions to help prevent drug errors:

- Confirm any questionable orders.
- When calculations are necessary, verify them with another nurse.
- Listen to the patient when he or she questions a drug, the dosage, or the drug regimen.
- Never administer the drug until the patient's questions have been adequately researched.
- Avoid distractions and concentrate on only one task at a time.

A significant number of errors can be made during administration of a drug. Errors most commonly occur because of a failure to administer a drug that has been ordered, administration of the wrong dose or strength of a drug, or administration of the wrong drug. Two drugs often associated with errors are insulin and heparin. A number of agencies have instituted policies and practices to help in the reduction of errors.

National Patient Safety Goals

To evaluate the safety and the quality of care provided at various accredited health care organizations, the Joint Commission establishes National Patient Safety Goals (NPSG) on a yearly basis. These goals are established to help accredited organizations address specific areas of concern with regard to patient safety. Several of these goals directly affect medication administration. For example, the 2009 NPSG required improvement in the accuracy of patient identification. At least two methods must be used to identify the patient (other than the patient's room number) when administering medication or blood products. Another important standard that institutions desiring accreditation must follow is to compile a list of abbreviations, symbols, and acronyms *not* to be used throughout the institution. The Joint Commission has developed its own list of abbreviations that may no longer be used in any written medical documents (e.g., care plans, medical orders, nurses' notes). This list is referred to as the "minimum list." See Table 2.1 for the official "Do Not Use" list. Table 2.1 also

Table 2.1 Joint Commission Official "Do Not Use" List

Abbreviation	Potential Problem	Use Instead
Official "Do Not Use" List* U (unit)	Mistaken as 0 (zero), 4 (four), or "cc"	Write "unit"
IU (international unit)	Mistaken as IV (intravenous) or 10 (ten)	Write "international unit"
Q.D., QD, q.d., qd (daily)	Mistaken for each other	Write "daily" and "every other day"
Q.O.D., QOD, q.o.d, qod (every other day)	The period after the "Q" can be mistaken for an "I" and the "O" can be mistaken for "I"	
Trailing zero (X.0 mg)†	Decimal point is missed	Write X mg
Lack of leading zero (.X mg)		Write 0.X mg
MS	Can mean morphine sulfate or magnesium sulfate	Write "morphine sulfate" or "magnesium sulfate"
MSO_4 and $MgSO_4$	Confused for one another	
Additional Abbreviations, Acronyms, and Symbols (For Possible Future Inclusion in the Official "Do Not Use" List)		
> (greater than) < (less than)	Misinterpreted as the number "7" or the letter "L"; confused with one another	Write "greater than" or "less than"
Abbreviations for drug names	Misinterpreted because of similar abbreviations for multiple drugs	Write drug names in full
Apothecary units	Unfamiliar to many practitioners; confused with metric units	Use metric units
@	Mistaken for the number "2" (two)	Write "at"
cc (cubic centimeter)	Mistaken for U (units) when poorly written	Write "mL" for milliliters
μg (microgram)	Mistaken for mg (milligrams), resulting in one thousand–fold overdose	Write "mcg" or "micrograms"

*Applies to all orders and medication–related documentation that is handwritten (including free-test computer entry) or on preprinted forms.
†Exception: A "trailing zero" may be used only where required to demonstrate the level of precision of the value being reported, such as for laboratory results, imaging studies that report size of lesions, or catheter/tube sizes. It may not be used in medication orders or other medication-related documentation.
From Joint Commission Resources. *Official "Do Not Use" List*. Retrieved July 31, 2008, from the Joint Commission website: http://www.jointcommission.org/Patient Safety/DoNotUseList/. Reprinted with permission.

lists additional abbreviations, acronyms, and symbols for possible addition to the official "Do Not Use" list in the future. Facilities accredited by the Joint Commission are required to be in compliance with the National Patient Safety Standards. Current information on these standards can be found at the Joint Commission website (http://www.jointcommission.org/PatientSafety/).

The Institute for Safe Medication Practices

The Institute for Safe Medication Practices (ISMP) is a nonprofit organization devoted to the study of medication errors and their prevention. In addition to offering safety and educational information, it contains a section called the Medication Errors Reporting Program. This program is designed to identify the number and type of drug errors occurring around the country. It is a program similar to the MedWatch program of the U.S. Food and Drug Administration (FDA). The goal of this voluntary reporting system is to collect data and disseminate information that will prevent such errors in the future. A link to the report form may be found online at http://www.ismp.org/. Nurses are urged to participate in this important program as a means of protecting the public by identifying ways to make drug administration safer.

Drug Distribution Systems

Primary or specialty providers order drugs for administration. Pharmacists dispense the medications and nurses carry out the actual administration. Several drug distribution systems are available to be used by the nurse to facilitate the administration of medication after it has been ordered for the patient. A brief description of three methods follows.

Unit Dose System

The **unit dose** system is a method in which drug orders are filled and medications dispensed to fill each patient's medication orders for a 24-hour period. The pharmacist dispenses each dose (unit) in a package that is typically labeled by the manufacturer and contains one tablet or capsule, a premeasured amount of a liquid drug, a prefilled syringe, or one suppository. Enough packaged drug for one day is placed in drawers in a special portable medication cart with a drawer for each patient. If the drug does not come individually packaged, a clinical pharmacist also may prepare unit doses. The pharmacy restocks the cart each day with the drugs needed for the next 24-hour period. If the cart is portable, the nurse takes the drug cart to each patient's room. Once every 24 hours, it goes back to the pharmacy to be refilled and for new drug orders to be placed.

In facilities where patients may stay for a long time, such as long-term care, the drug may be packaged using a multi-unit dose method. With this system, individual doses are 'bubble' packed onto a card that may hold up to 60 individual doses (Fig. 2.4). Cards are labeled for individual patients and may hold 1 to 2 months' supply of a drug. These cards are then stored in slots for individual patients in a locked medication cart. When administering a drug, the nurse obtains the patient's card and pops the individual dose out of the card, returning the card with its remaining doses to the medication cart.

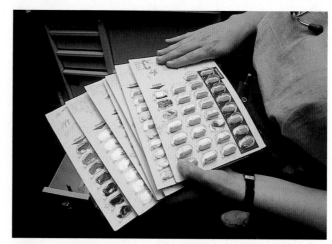

Figure 2.4 Multi-unit dose packs, frequently used for medication administration in long term care settings.

Automated Medication Management System

Automated or computerized management systems (Fig. 2.5) are used in most hospitals or agencies distributing drugs. Drug orders are managed in the pharmacy from physician orders that are sent from the individual floors or units. Each floor or unit has a medication station in which medications are placed in specific drawers. Once the order is entered into the system, nurses enter the patient's name and the drug to be administered at the unit's automated medication station. The drawer with the specific drug opens for the nurse to remove the drug, and then using a computer touch screen, the dose is automatically recorded into the computerized system. This information is then printed out for individual patients as their MAR.

Figure 2.5 An automated medication system.

Figure 2.6 Bar-coded, point-of-care patient wrist bands used for medication administration.

Bar-Coded Point-of-Care Medication System

Some hospitals use a bar-code scanner in the administration of drugs. To use this system, a bar code is placed on the patient's hospital identification band when the patient is admitted to the hospital (Fig. 2.6). The bar codes, along with bar codes on the drug unit dose packages, are used to identify the patient and to record and charge routine and PRN drugs. Additionally, provider identification badges are scanned during the procedure, thus identifying the nurse giving the medication. The scanner also keeps an ongoing inventory of controlled substances, which eliminates the need for controlled substance counts at the end of each shift.

Due to the serious consequences of administering the wrong drug, newer and more sophisticated automated systems to administer drugs are being constantly researched to provide the best safety to patients.

Administration of Drugs by the Oral Route

The oral route is the most frequent route of drug administration and rarely causes physical discomfort in patients. Oral drug forms include tablets, capsules, and liquids. Some capsules and tablets contain sustained-release drugs, which dissolve over an extended period. Administration of oral drugs is relatively easy for patients who are alert and can swallow.

Nursing Responsibilities

The nurse should observe the following points when giving an oral drug:

- Verify that the patient is able to swallow and is not nauseated or vomiting. Place the patient in an upright position. It is difficult, as well as dangerous, to swallow a solid or liquid when lying down.
- Assess the patient's need for assistance in holding the tablet or capsule or holding a glass of water. Some patients with physical disabilities cannot handle or hold these objects and may require assistance.
- Make sure that a full glass of water is readily available. Advise the patient to take a few sips of water before placing a tablet or capsule in the mouth.

- Instruct the patient to place the pill or capsule on the back of the tongue and tilt the head back to swallow a tablet or slightly forward to swallow a capsule. Encourage the patient first to take a few sips of water to move the drug down the esophagus and into the stomach, and then to finish the whole glass.
- Give the patient any special instructions, such as drinking extra fluids or remaining in bed, that are pertinent to the drug being administered.
- Never leave a drug at the patient's bedside to be taken later unless there is a specific order by the primary care provider to do so. Some units, such as postpartum, may offer self-administered medications. A few drugs (e.g., antacids or stool softeners) may be ordered to be left at the bedside.
- Patients with a nasogastric feeding tube or gastrostomy tube may be given their oral drugs through the tube. Before administration, check the tube for placement. Dilute and flush liquid drugs through the tube. However, crush tablets and dissolve them in water before administering them through the tube. Flush the tube with water after the drugs are placed in the tube to clear the tubing completely.
- Instruct the patient to place buccal drugs against the mucous membranes of the cheek in either the upper or lower jaw. They are absorbed slowly from the mucous membranes of the mouth. Examples of drugs given buccally are lozenges and troches.
- Certain drugs are also given by the sublingual (placed under the tongue) route. These drugs must not be swallowed or chewed and must be dissolved completely before the patient eats or drinks. Nitroglycerin is commonly given sublingually.

Infrequent Dosing of Drugs

Soon, many drugs will be available for once-a-week, or even once-a-month, administration. The doses are designed to replace daily doses of drugs. One of the first was alendronate (Fosamax), a drug used to treat osteoporosis (see Chapter 31). In 2001, the FDA approved two strengths for this drug to be given once a week. In clinical trials, once-a-week dosing showed no greater adverse reactions than the once-daily regimen. Since that time other drugs have been developed for dosing infrequently. A similar product, ibandronate (Boniva), is administered once a month for the treatment of osteoporosis. Infrequent dosing may prove beneficial for those experiencing mild adverse reactions in that the reactions would be experienced less frequently than every day.

Administration of Drugs by the Parenteral Route

Parenteral drug administration entails giving a drug by the **subcutaneous** (subcut), **intramuscular** (IM), **intravenous** (IV), or **intradermal** route (Fig. 2.7). Other routes of parenteral administration that may be used by the primary health care provider are intradural (into the dural space of the spine), intra-arterial (into an artery), intracardiac (into the heart), and intra-articular (into a joint). In some instances, intra-arterial drugs are administered by a nurse. However, administration is

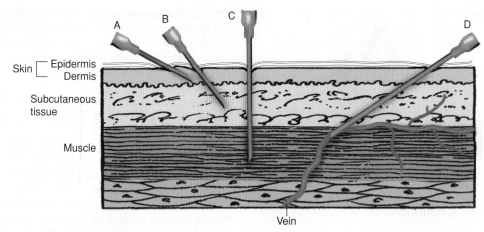

Figure 2.7 Needle insertion for parenteral drug. (**A**) Intradermal injection: a 26-gauge, 3/8-inch long needle is inserted at a 10-degree angle. (**B**) Subcutaneous injection: a 25-gauge, 1/2-inch long needle is inserted at an angle (45 to 90 degrees) that depends on the size of the patient. (**C**) Intramuscular injection: a 20- to 23-gauge, 1- to 3-inch long needle is inserted into the relaxed muscle at a 90-degree angle with a quick (dart-throwing) type of hand movement. (**D**) Intravenous injection: the diameter (18 to 26 gauge) of the needle used depends on the substance to be injected and on the site of injection.

not by direct arterial injection but by means of a catheter that has been placed in an artery.

Nursing Responsibilities

The nurse should observe the following points when giving a drug by the parenteral route:

- Wear gloves for protection from the potential of a blood spill when giving parenteral drugs. The risk of exposure to infected blood is increasing for all health care workers. The Centers for Disease Control and Prevention (CDC) recommends that gloves be worn when touching blood or body fluids, mucous membranes, or any broken skin area. This recommendation is referred to as **Standard Precautions**, which combine the Universal Precautions for Blood and Body Fluids with Body Substance Isolation guidelines.
- After selecting the site for injection, cleanse the skin. Most hospitals have a policy regarding the type of skin antiseptic used for cleansing the skin before parenteral drug administration. Cleanse the skin with a circular motion, starting at an inner point and moving outward.
- After inserting the needle for IM administration, pull back the syringe barrel to aspirate the drug. Aspirate for 5 to 10 seconds. If blood is in a small vessel, it takes time for the blood to appear. If blood appears in the syringe, remove the needle so the drug is not injected. Discard the drug, needle, and syringe and prepare another injection. If no blood appears in the syringe, inject the drug. Aspiration is not necessary when giving an intradermal and most subcutaneous injections.
- After removing the needle from an IM, subcut, or IV injection site, place pressure on the area. Patients with bleeding tendencies often require prolonged pressure on the area.

- Most hospitals use needles designed to prevent sticks. This needle has a plastic guard that slips over the needle and locks in place as it is withdrawn from the injection site.
- Do not recap syringes, and dispose of them according to agency policy. Discard needles and syringes into clearly marked, appropriate containers to prevent needle-stick injuries. Most agencies have a "sharps" container located in each room for immediate disposal of needles and syringes after use. Proper disposal protects the nurse and others from injury and contamination.

Administration of Drugs by the Intradermal Route

Drugs given by the intradermal route are usually those for sensitivity tests (e.g., the tuberculin test or allergy skin testing; see Fig. 2.7A). Absorption is slow and allows for good results when testing for allergies.

Nursing Responsibilities
The nurse observes the following points when administering drugs by the intradermal route:

- The inner part of the forearm and the upper back may be used for intradermal injections. The area should be hairless; areas near moles or scars or pigmented skin areas should be avoided. The nurse should cleanse the area in the same manner as for subcutaneous and IM injections.
- A 1-mL syringe with a 25- to 27-gauge needle that is 1/4 to 5/8 inch long is best suited for intradermal injections. Small volumes (usually smaller than 0.1 mL) are used for intradermal injections and administered with the bevel up.
- The nurse should insert the needle at a 15-degree angle between the upper layers of the skin. The nurse should not aspirate the syringe or massage the area. Injection produces

a small wheal (raised area) on the outer surface of the skin. If a wheal does not appear on the outer surface of the skin, there is a good possibility that the drug entered the subcutaneous tissue, and any test results would be inaccurate.

Administration of Drugs by the Subcutaneous Route

A subcutaneous injection places the drug into the tissues between the skin and the muscle (see Fig. 2.7B). Drugs administered in this manner are absorbed more slowly than IM injections. Drugs for blood thinning and diabetes are commonly given by the subcut route.

Nursing Responsibilities

The nurse should observe the following points when giving a drug by the subcut route:

- A volume of 0.5 to 1 mL is used for subcut injection. Larger volumes (e.g., more than 1 mL) are best given as IM injections. If a volume larger than 1 mL is ordered through the subcut route, the injection is given in two sites, with separate needles and syringes.
- The sites for subcut injection are the upper arms, the upper abdomen, and the upper thighs. The back is less frequently used (Fig. 2.8). Rotate injection sites to ensure proper absorption and minimize tissue damage.
- When giving a drug by the subcut route, insert the needle at a 45-degree angle. However, to place the drug in the subcutaneous tissue, select the needle length and angle of insertion based on the patient's body weight. Obese patients have excess subcutaneous tissue, and it may be necessary to give the injection at a 90-degree angle. If the patient is thin or cachectic, there usually is less subcutaneous tissue. For such patients, the upper abdomen is the best site for injection. Generally, a syringe with a 23- to 25-gauge needle that is 3/8 to 5/8 inch in length is most suitable for a subcut injection.
- When administering a subcut medication, often aspiration is not required. If the nurse does use the aspiration technique, it involves pulling back on the plunger of the syringe. If blood appears in the syringe, withdraw the needle, discard the syringe, and prepare a new injection. If blood does not

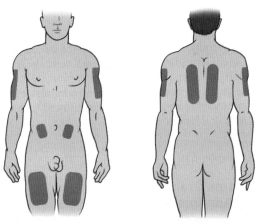

Figure 2.8 Sites on the body at which subcutaneous injections can be given.

appear, continue to inject the medication by depressing the plunger with a slow, even pressure.

Administration of Drugs by the Intramuscular Route

An IM injection is the administration of a drug into a muscle (see Fig. 2.7C). Drugs that are irritating to subcutaneous tissue can be given by IM injection. Drugs given by this route are absorbed more rapidly than drugs given by the subcut route because of the rich blood supply in the muscle. In addition, a larger volume (1 to 3 mL) can be given at one site.

Nursing Responsibilities

The nurse should observe the following points when giving a drug by the IM route:

- If an injection is more than 3 mL, divide the drug and give it as two separate injections. Volumes larger than 3 mL will not be absorbed properly.
- A 22-gauge needle that is 1½ inches in length is most often used for IM injections.
- The sites for IM administration are the deltoid muscle (upper arm), the ventrogluteal or dorsogluteal sites (hip), and the vastus lateralis (thigh; Fig. 2.9). The vastus lateralis site is frequently used for infants and small children because it is more developed than the gluteal or deltoid sites. In children who have been ambulating for more than 2 years, the ventrogluteal site may be used.
- When giving a drug by the IM route, insert the needle at a 90-degree angle. When injecting a drug into the ventrogluteal or dorsogluteal muscles, it is a good idea to place the patient in a comfortable position, preferably in a prone position with the toes pointing inward. When injecting the drug into the deltoid, a sitting or lying-down position may be used. Place the patient in a recumbent position for injection of a drug into the vastus lateralis.

Z-Track Technique

The **Z-track** technique of IM injection is used when a drug is highly irritating to tissues or has the ability permanently to stain the skin. The nurse should adhere to the following procedure when using the Z-track technique (Fig. 2.10):

- Draw the drug up into the syringe.
- Discard the needle and place a new needle on the syringe. This prevents any solution that may remain in the needle (that was used to draw the drug into the syringe) from contacting tissues as the needle is put into the muscle.
- Pull the plunger down to draw approximately 0.1 to 0.2 mL of air into the syringe. The air bubble in the syringe follows the drug into the tissues and seals off the area where the drug was injected, thereby preventing oozing of the drug up through the extremely small pathway created by the needle.
- Place the patient in the correct position for administration of an IM injection.
- Cleanse the skin.
- Pull the skin, subcutaneous tissues, and fat (that lie over the injection site) laterally, displacing the tissue to the side (approximately 1 inch).

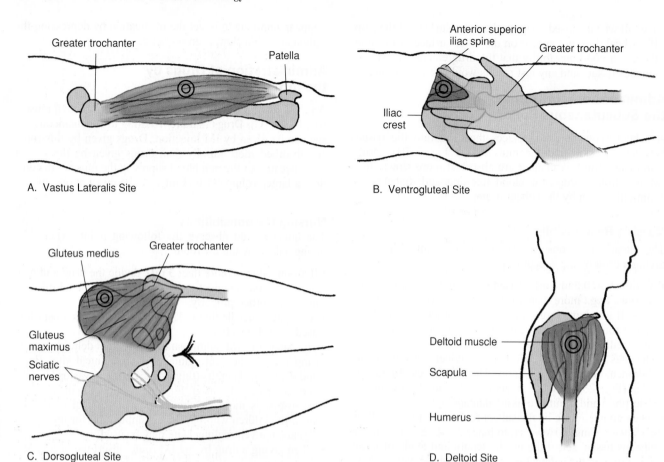

Figure 2.9 Sites for intramuscular administration. (**A**) Vastus lateralis site: the patient is supine or sitting. (**B**) Ventrogluteal site: the nurse's palm is placed on the greater trochanter and the index finger is placed on the anterior superior iliac spine; the injection is made into the middle of the triangle formed by the nurse's fingers and the iliac crest. (**C**) Dorsogluteal site: to avoid the sciatic nerve and accompanying blood vessels, an injection site is chosen above and lateral to a line drawn from the greater trochanter to the posterior superior iliac spine. (**D**) Deltoid site: the mid-deltoid area is located by forming a rectangle, the top of which is at the level of the lower edge of the acromion, and the bottom of which is at the level of the axilla; the sides are one third and two thirds of the way around the outer aspect of the patient's arm.

• While holding the tissues in the lateral position, insert the needle at a 90-degree angle and inject the drug.
• After the drug is injected, wait 10 seconds to permit the medication to disperse into the muscle tissue, then release the tissue while withdrawing the needle. This technique prevents the backflow of drug into the subcutaneous tissue.

Administration of Drugs by the Intravenous Route

A drug administered by the IV route is injected directly into the blood by a needle inserted into a vein. Drug action occurs almost immediately. Drugs administered by the IV route may be given:

• Slowly, over 1 or more minutes
• Rapidly (IV push)
• By piggyback/syringe pump infusions (drugs are mixed with 50 to 100 mL of compatible IV fluid and administered during a period of 30 to 60 minutes piggybacked onto the primary IV line)
• Into an existing IV line (the IV port)
• Into an intermittent venous access device called a *heparin lock* (a small IV catheter in the patient's vein; the catheter is connected to a small fluid reservoir with a rubber cap through which the needle is inserted to administer the drug)
• By being added to an IV solution and allowed to infuse into the vein over a longer period

For explanation of the procedure and nursing responsibilities see Chapter 55.

Other Parenteral Routes of Drug Administration

The primary care provider may administer a drug by the intracardial, intra-arterial, or intra-articular routes. The nurse may be responsible for preparing the drug for administration.

Figure 2.10 Z-track injection. (**A**) The tissue is tensed laterally at the injection site before the needle is inserted. This pulls the skin, subcutaneous tissue, and fat planes into a "Z" formation. (**B**) After the tissue has been displaced, the needle is thrust straight into the muscular tissue. (**C**) After injection, tissues are released while the needle is withdrawn. As each tissue plane slides by the other, the track is sealed.

A   B   C

The nurse should ask the primary health care provider what special materials will be required for administration.

Venous access ports are totally implanted ports with a self-sealing septum that is attached to a catheter leading to a large vessel, usually the vena cava. These devices are most commonly used for chemotherapy or other long-term therapy and require surgical insertion and removal. Drugs are administered through injections made into the portal through the skin. These drugs are administered by the primary health care provider or a registered nurse.

Administration of Drugs Through the Skin and Mucous Membranes

Drugs may be applied to the skin and mucous membranes using several routes: topically (on the outer layers of skin), transdermally through a patch on which the drug has been implanted, or inhaled through the membranes of the upper respiratory tract.

Administration of Drugs by the Topical Route

Most topical drugs act on the skin but are not absorbed through the skin. These drugs are used to soften, disinfect, or lubricate the skin. A few topical drugs are enzymes that have the ability to remove superficial debris, such as the dead skin and purulent matter present in skin ulcerations. Other topical drugs are used to treat minor, superficial skin infections. The various forms of topical applications and locations of use are described in Display 2.2.

Nursing Responsibilities

The nurse considers the following points when administering drugs by the topical route:

• The primary care provider may write special instructions for the application of a topical drug—for example, to apply the drug in a thin, even layer or to cover the area after application of the drug to the skin.

• Other drugs may have special instructions provided by the manufacturer, such as to apply the drug to a clean, hairless area or to let the drug dissolve slowly in the mouth. All of these instructions are important because drug action may depend on correct administration of the drug.

• Ointments are sometimes used and come with a special paper marked in inches. Measure the correct length (onto the paper), place the paper with the drug ointment side down on the skin, and secure it with tape. Before the next dose, remove the paper and tape and cleanse the skin.

Administration of Drugs by the Transdermal Route

Drugs administered by the **transdermal** route are readily absorbed from the skin and provide systemic effects. This type of administration is called a *transdermal drug delivery*

DISPLAY 2.2 Topical Applications and Locations of Use

• Creams, lotions, or ointments applied to the skin with a tongue blade, gloved fingers, or gauze
• Sprays applied to the skin or into the nose or oral cavity
• Liquids inserted into body cavities, such as fistulas
• Liquids inserted into the bladder or urethra
• Solids (e.g., suppositories) or jellies inserted into the urethra
• Liquids dropped into the eyes, ears, or nose
• Ophthalmic ointments applied to the eyelids or dropped into the lower conjunctival sac
• Solids (e.g., suppositories, tablets), foams, liquids, and creams inserted into the vagina
• Continuous or intermittent wet dressings applied to skin surfaces
• Solids (e.g., tablets, lozenges) dissolved in the mouth
• Sprays or mists inhaled into the lungs
• Liquids, creams, or ointments applied to the scalp
• Solids (e.g., suppositories), liquids, or foams inserted into the rectum

Figure 2.11 Transdermal drug delivery system. (**A**) Find and remove a previously placed patch. (**B**) Cleanse application site. (**C**) Record date, time, and initials on the new patch. (**D**) Remove protective covering. (**E**) Apply new patch to hairless area of skin.

system (Fig. 2.11). The drug dosages are implanted in a small, patch-type bandage and the drug is gradually absorbed into the systemic circulation. This type of drug system maintains a relatively constant blood concentration and reduces the possibility of toxicity. In addition, the administration of drugs transdermally causes fewer adverse reactions, and administration is less frequent than when the drugs are given by another route. Duragesic (used to treat severe pain) and Ortho Evra (used as birth control) are two drugs given frequently by the transdermal route.

Nursing Responsibilities

The nurse observes the following points when administering drugs by the transdermal route:

- Assess the skin for patches currently in use; remove all old patches to prevent added dosing of the drug (see Fig. 2.11A).
- Choose a dry, hairless area of intact skin large enough for the patch to fit smoothly and cleanse (see Fig. 2.11B).
- Document the time and date and your initials on the back side of the patch (see Fig. 2.11C).

- Remove the backing and apply the patch to the skin (see Figs. 2.11D, 2.11E).
- Rotate sites for transdermal patches to prevent skin irritation. The chest, abdomen, buttocks and upper arm are the most commonly used sites. Do not shave the area to apply the patch; shaving may cause skin irritation.

Administration of Drugs Through Inhalation

Drug droplets, vapor, and gas are administered through the mucous membranes of the respiratory tract using a face mask, nebulizer, or positive-pressure breathing machine. Examples of drugs administered through inhalation include bronchodilators, mucolytics, and some anti-inflammatory drugs. These drugs primarily produce a local effect in the lungs.

Nursing Responsibilities

The primary nursing responsibility with drugs administered by inhalation is to provide the patient with proper instructions for administering the drug. For example, many patients with asthma use a metered-dose inhaler to dilate the bronchi and make breathing easier. Without proper instruction on how to use the inhaler, much of the drug can be deposited on the tongue, rather than in the respiratory tract. This decreases the therapeutic effect of the drug. Instructions may vary with each inhaler. To be certain that the inhaler is used correctly, the patient is referred to the instructions accompanying each device. Figure 2.12 illustrates the proper use of one type of inhaler.

Nursing Responsibilities After Drug Administration

After the administration of any type of drug, the nurse is responsible for the following:

Figure 2.12 A respiratory inhalant is used to deliver a drug directly into the lungs. To deliver a dose of the drug, the patient takes a slow, deep breath while depressing the top of the inhaler's canister.

- Recording the administration of the drug. The nurse should complete this task as soon as possible. This is particularly important when PRN drugs (especially opioids) are given.
- Recording (when necessary) any information concerning the administration of the drug. This includes information such as the IV flow rate, the site used for parenteral administration, problems with administration (if any), and vital signs taken immediately before administration.
- Evaluating and recording the patient's response to the drug (when applicable). Evaluation may include such facts as relief of pain, decrease in body temperature, relief of itching, and decrease in the number of stools passed.
- Observing the adverse reactions. The frequency of these observations depends on the drug administered. The nurse must record all suspected adverse reactions and report them to the primary care provider. The nurse must immediately report serious adverse reactions to the primary care provider.

Patient Teaching for Improved Patient Outcomes

Assessing the Home for Safe Drug Use

For most patients, drugs will be prescribed after discharge to be taken at home. Because the home is not as controlled an environment as a health care facility, the nurse should assess the patient's home environment carefully to ensure complete safety. It is important to keep in mind the following when making a home safety assessment:

✓ Does the home have a space that is relatively free of clutter and easily accessible to the patient or a caregiver?
✓ Do any small children live in or visit the home? If so, is there a place where drugs can be stored safely out of their reach?
✓ Does the drug require refrigeration? If so, does the refrigerator work?
✓ If the patient needs several drugs, can the patient or caregiver identify which drugs are used and when? Do they know how to use them and why?
✓ Does the patient need special equipment, such as needles and syringes? If so, where and how can the equipment be stored for safety and convenience? Does the patient have an appropriate disposal container? Will the refuse be safe from children and pets?
  - Suggest using plastic storage containers with snap-on lids made especially for home syringe disposal.
  - Advise the patient to use an impervious container with a properly fitting lid, such as a plastic milk jug, for safe disposal of needles.
  - Advise the patient of Sharps Disposal Programs in the area. These may be at local pharmacies, police and fire stations, or local healthcare centers.

Administration of Drugs

Administration of Drugs in the Home

Often, drugs are not administered by the nurse in the home setting, but rather by the patient or family members serving as caregivers. When this is the case, it is important that the patient or caregivers understand the treatment regimen and are given an opportunity to ask questions concerning the drug therapy, such as why the drug was prescribed, how to administer the drug, and adverse reactions of the drug (see Chapter 5 for information concerning patient and family education). When a patient is taking a drug at home, special equipment or items may be needed in the home to administer the drug. Patient Teaching for Improved Patient Outcomes: Assessing the Home for Safe Drug Use gives some guidelines to follow when drugs are administered in the home by the patient or caregiver, rather than by the nurse.

THINK CRITICALLY: PHARMACOLOGY IN PRACTICE

1. After administering a drug to a patient, you find that the incorrect dosage was given. The dose that you administered was two times the correct dosage. Analyze what action, if any, you would take.

2. Discuss why the sixth right, right documentation, is important in drug administration.

● Test Your Knowledge

1. The nurse correctly documents administration of a drug _____.

 A. at the beginning of the shift
 B. when preparing to give the drug
 C. immediately after giving the drug
 D. at the end of the shift

2. The nurse correctly administers an IM injection by _____.

 A. displacing the skin to the side before making the injection
 B. using a 1-inch needle
 C. inserting the needle at a 90-degree angle
 D. using a 25-gauge needle

3. When preparing a drug for subcut administration, the nurse is aware that the usual volume of a drug injected by the subcut route is _____.

 A. less than 0.5 mL
 B. 0.5 to 1 mL
 C. 2 to 5 mL
 D. 3 to 4 mL

4. The nurse explains to the patient receiving an IV injection that the action of the drug occurs _____.

 A. in 5 to 10 minutes
 B. in 15 to 20 minutes
 C. within 30 minutes
 D. almost immediately

● Prepare for the NCLEX

1. When administering a drug, the nurse _____.

 A. checks the drug label two times before administration
 B. asks the patient to identify themselves
 C. may administer a drug prepared by another nurse
 D. may crush any tablet that the patient is unable to swallow

To check your answers, see Appendix E.

thePoint *For more NCLEX questions, log on to http://thepoint.lww.com to access more than 1000 questions.*

Calculation of Drug Dosages and Mathematical Review

Accurate dosage calculations are critical to the health of a patient who is receiving medications. When drugs are administered, it is important that the numbers used and the answers obtained are correct. Unlike an error on a math test in school, there is no partial credit for simple arithmetic errors or incomplete answers in dosage conversions and calculations. Harm, and even death, can result from an error in a drug dosage calculation.

Systematically Checking Accuracy

It has been estimated that 1 in 10,000 hospital deaths occur each year in the US due to mistakes made *specifically when calculating the drug dose*. Often these miscalculations are due to human error. Factors in the work environment often contribute to errors made by people. These factors include poor lighting, noise, interruptions, and a taxing workload. We should be aware of all of these elements of our environment when calculating drug doses.

Technological changes such as computerized order entry and bar coding systems can detect errors made by health care providers. However, the best method of error detection is the

manual redundancy system. This is a system in which each person in the process of medication prescription and delivery checks the drug dosage for accuracy. Nurses perform the "5 rights and 3 checks" to catch a potential error in drug preparation. Although nurses may not be responsible for the initial mixing, packaging, or delivery of a medication, 95% of potential dose calculation errors are found during manual redundancy checks. When a nurse checks the dose calculation of a drug, during preparation or at bedside, a serious error can be detected before it reaches the patient.

Calculating Drug Doses Safely

To calculate drug doses safely, the nurse needs to systematically look at the process of drug delivery. First, the nurse must recognize how drugs are packaged and how to look for the information on the labels needed to calculate drug doses. Then, the nurse looks at the orders and how these are presented on the medication administration record (MAR). The mathematical ability of the nurse is important as one looks at the MARs and labels. The nurse asks, Am I able to check the dose calculation using my head, my hand, or with a calculator?

Nurses will find that mathematical calculations are performed using various methods when preparing drugs for administration. Sometimes the math is relatively simple, and a calculation can be done quickly in the nurse's head. When distractions are present or if conversions are involved, the nurse may use a pen and paper to handwrite out the mathematical equations needed to determine the correct dose. A nurse may use a number of steps in the calculation of a medication and find that a calculator is helpful to hasten the process. When using any of these methods, it is important for the nurse to understand the basic concepts of the dose calculation to ensure the right answer is obtained.

Information about the process of dose calculation is examined in this chapter. Many textbooks are designed to teach the methodology of dosage calculations; this chapter is meant as a review and supplement to that instruction. Examples of drug dose calculations are provided throughout the chapters to test your ability to properly complete the math. Answers can be found in Appendix E.

Reading Drug Labels

Drug labels give important information the nurse must use to obtain the correct dosage. Although labels contain a great amount of information about the drug being given, three specific items are needed to administer a drug: the name, form, and dosage strength.

Drug labels may contain two names: the trade (brand) name and the generic or official name (see Chapter 1). The trade name is usually capitalized, written first on the label, and identified by the registration symbol. The generic name is written in smaller print, often in parentheses, and usually located under the trade name. Drugs may be prescribed by either the trade name or the generic name. Often the generic drug is less expensive than the brand name drug. If the primary health care provider does not specify that a substitution _cannot_ be made, it is likely that a generic version of the drug will be dispensed to reduce the cost to the patient. Problems can arise if a patient recognizes the brand name of a drug but does not know the generic name and refuses the medication (since companies that make generic-only drugs do not include a trade name on the label). Therefore, it is important for the nurse to know the generic name of drugs and always check for brand name versions if the patient questions the prescription.

QUESTION #1

Looking at the label in Figure 3.1, what are the brand and generic names of this drug? _(See Appendix E for answer.)_

The unit dose is the most common type of labeling seen in hospitals. The unit dose is a method of dispensing drugs in which each capsule or tablet is packaged separately. On the label, the type of preparation will be specified; in other words, it will list the drug as a capsule, tablet, or other form of the drug.

At times the drug will come to the nursing unit in a container with a number of capsules or tablets or as a solution. The nurse must then determine the number of capsules/tablets or the amount of solution to administer. Therefore, the nurse must know the amount of drug in each tablet or capsule (**dosage strength**). The dosage strength is also given on the

container. The dosage strength is used to calculate the number of tablets or the amount of solution to administer.

QUESTION #2

Looking at the label in Figure 3.1, find the form of the drug and the dosage strength. _(see Appendix E for answer)_

Basic Formula Method of Dosage Calculation

Once the nurse has identified the basic information about the drug, the calculation can be performed to prepare the drug.

CALCULATION #1

Looking at the label in Figure 3.1, use this information to solve the following dose problem:

The primary health care provider orders: 400 mg of cimetidine after each meal. How many tablets will the nurse administer following breakfast? _(see Appendix E for answer)_

Although most hospital pharmacies dispense drugs as single doses or in a unit dose system, on occasion the nurse must compute a drug dosage because it differs from the dose of the drug that is available. This is particularly true of long-term care facilities, outpatient clinics, and in the home where the dose may be changed periodically or in situations in which having multiple dosage strengths of a particular drug for the patient would be costly.

CALCULATION #2

Looking at the label in Figure 3.1, use this information to solve the following dose problem:

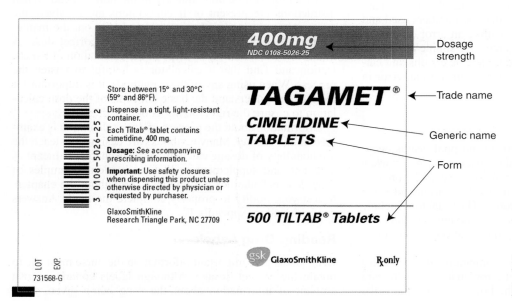

Figure 3.1 Drug label for Tagamet. (Courtesy of GlaxoSmithKline.)

The primary health care provider changes the order after late morning rounds: 800 mg of cimetidine after each meal. How many tablets will the nurse administer after meals? (*see Appendix E for answer*)

Some nurses can do this type of calculation in their heads; others find it helpful to do the problem by hand on paper. This is especially helpful when the dosage ordered by the primary health care provider may not be available.

Basic Formula Method by Hand

To find the correct dosage of a solid oral preparation, the following formula may be used:

$$\frac{\text{dose desired}}{\text{dose on hand}} = \text{dose administered (the unknown or X)}$$

This formula may be abbreviated as:

$$\frac{D}{H} = X$$

When the dose ordered by the primary health care provider (dose desired) is written in the same *measurement* as the dose on the drug container (dose on hand), they are both milligrams, then these two figures may be inserted into the formula without changes.

EXAMPLE

The primary health care provider orders cimetidine 800 mg (milligrams). The drug is available as cimetidine 400 mg (milligrams).

$$\frac{D}{H} = X$$

$$\frac{800 \, \text{mg (dose desired)}}{400 \, \text{mg (dose on hand)}} = 2 \text{ tablets of 400 mg cimetidine}$$

QUESTION #3

Use the label in Figure 3.2 to solve the following problem.

Looking at the label, find the drug name, form, and dosage strength (*see Appendix E for answer*)

Figure 3.2   Drug label for Zyprexa. (Courtesy of Lilly Company.)

CALCULATION #3

Looking at the label in Figure 3.2, use this information to solve the following dose problem:

The primary health care provider orders: 10 mg Zyprexa daily. How many tablets will the nurse administer? (*see Appendix E for answer*)

Understanding the Metric System of Measurement

If the primary health care provider orders ascorbic acid (Vitamin C) 0.5 g, and the drug container label reads ascorbic acid 250 mg, a *conversion of grams to milligrams* (because the drug container is labeled in milligrams) would be necessary before the basic formula can be used. Therefore it is important for the nurse to understand the **metric system** of measurement.

There are three systems of measurement associated with drug dosing: the metric system, the apothecary system, and household measurements.

The metric system is the most commonly used system of measurement in medicine. The metric system uses decimals (or the decimal system). In the metric system, the **gram** is the unit of weight, the **liter** the unit of volume, and the **meter** the unit of length. Display 3.1 lists the measurements used in the metric system. The abbreviations for the measurements are given in parentheses.

The apothecary system at one time was used for weight measurement. In 1994, recommendations were made by the Institute for Safe Medication Practices (ISMP) to eliminate this system due to the high rate of medication errors it produced (information about this system can be found in Appendix D). The household system is rarely used in a hospital setting but may be used to measure drug dosages in the home.

Ratio and Proportion Method of Dosage Calculation

Converting Units for Calculation

When using the Basic Formula, the **numerator** and the **denominator** must be of like terms—for example, milligrams over milligrams or grams over grams. To set up a problem, a fraction must be stated in *like terms;* therefore, proportion may be used to convert grams to milligrams.

> **! NURSING ALERT**
>
> Errors made by nurses in using this and other drug formulas will be reduced if the entire dose is labeled rather than just writing the numbers.
>
> $$\frac{0.5 \, \text{g}}{250 \, \text{mg}} \text{ rather than } \frac{0.5}{250}$$
>
> This will eliminate the possibility of using unlike terms in the fraction.

In the aforementioned example, where the order read ascorbic acid 0.5 g and the drug container was labeled ascorbic

DISPLAY 3.1 Metric Measurements

Weight
The unit of weight is the gram.
1 kilogram (kg) = 1000 grams (g)
1 gram (g) = 1000 milligrams (mg)
1 milligram (mg) = 1000 micrograms (mcg)

Volume
The unit of volume is the liter.
1 deciliter (dL) = 10 liters (L)
1 liter (L) = 1000 milliliters (mL)
1 milliliter (mL) = 0.001 liter (L)

Length
The unit of length is the meter.
1 meter (m) = 100 centimeters (cm)
1 centimeter (cm) = 0.01 meter (m)
1 millimeter (mm) = 0.001 meter (m)

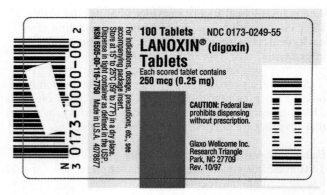

Figure 3.3 Drug label for Lanoxin. (Courtesy of Glaxo-SmithKline.)

acid 250 mg, a conversion of grams to milligrams is necessary to perform the dose calculation. A nurse may be able to perform this calculation in his or her head. If it is done by hand, the proportion and a known equivalent are set up in a ratio and used for this type of conversion.

Ratio and Proportion Method by Hand

EXAMPLE

Convert 0.5 gram (g) to milligrams (mg); using proportion and the known equivalent 1000 mg = 1 g, set up the ratio:

$$1000 \text{ mg:1 g::X mg:0.5 g}$$
$$X = 1000 \times 0.5$$
$$X = 500 \text{ mg}$$

or

$$\frac{1000\,mg}{1\,g} = \frac{X\,mg}{0.5\,g}$$
$$X = 1000 \times 0.5$$
$$X = 500 \text{ mg}$$

Therefore, 0.5 gram (g) equals 500 milligrams (mg). After changing 0.5 g to 500 mg, use the basic method formula:

$$\frac{D}{H} = X$$

$$\frac{500\,mg}{250\,mg} = 2 \text{ tablets of 250 mg ascorbic acid}$$

Safeguard in Preventing Errors

To prevent dose calculation errors, many manufacturers include both levels of measurement (grams and milligrams) on the label if the drug is frequently ordered in doses different from the size dispensed (Fig. 3.3). This is very important when doses are in small amounts such as micrograms (mcg). Again, manufacturers typically include the dose

strength in both units of measurement (milligrams and micrograms). Even when both are included, the nurse should perform the calculation to double check that the dose is correct.

Errors are a frequent problem when zeros (0) are involved. When there is no number to the left of the decimal, a zero is written, for example, 0.25. Although in general mathematics the zero may not be required, it should be used in the writing of all drug doses. _Use of the zero lessens the chance of drug errors,_ especially when the dose of a drug is hurriedly written, and the decimal point is indistinct.

For example, if a drug order is written as digoxin (Lanoxin) **.25 mg** instead of digoxin **0.25 mg**, the order might be interpreted as **25 mg**, which is 100 times the prescribed dose.

QUESTION #4

Use the label in Figure 3.3 to understand the following example.

Looking at the label, find the drug name, form, and dosage strength in both units of measurement (_see Appendix E for answer_)

CALCULATION #4

Looking at the label in Figure 3.3, use this information to solve the following dose problem:

The primary health care provider orders: 0.50 mg of digoxin daily. How many tablets will the nurse administer? (_see Appendix E for answer_)

Drugs in Liquid Form

Drugs may be ordered in liquid form for many reasons. The patient is a child, the drug is to be put in a feeding tube, injected directly into the tissues or intravenous (IV) line, or the patient is too ill to swallow a solid form of the drug like a tablet. In these situations, the drug is made in a solution form.

Figure 3.4 Drug preparations in solution form: (top row) vials and ampules; (middle-bottom rows) prefilled cartridges and holders.

Solutions

A solute is a substance dissolved in a **solvent.** Usually, water is used as the solvent for preparing a solution unless another liquid is specified. Today, most solutions are prepared by a clinical pharmacist or the manufacturer and not by the nurse. It is important for the nurse to understand how the solutions will be prepared and labeled.

Examples of how solutions may be labeled include:

- 10 mg/mL—10 mg of the drug in each milliliter
- 1:1000—a solution denoting strength of 1 part of the drug per 1000 parts of solvent
- 5 mg/teaspoon—5 mg of the drug in each teaspoon of solution (home use)

Parenteral Drug Dosage Forms

Drugs for parenteral use must be in liquid form before they are administered. Parenteral drugs may be available in the following forms (see Fig. 3.4 for examples):

1. As liquids in disposable cartridges or disposable syringes that contain a specific amount of a drug in a specific vol-

ume; for example, meperidine 50 mg/mL. After administration, the cartridge or syringe is discarded.
2. In ampules or vials that contain a specific amount of the liquid form of the drug in a specific volume. The vials may be single-dose vials or multidose vials. A multidose vial contains more than one dose of the drug.
3. In ampules or vials that contain powder or crystals, to which a liquid (called a diluent) must be added before the drug can be removed from the vial and administered. Vials may be single-dose or multidose vials.

Dose Calculations with Liquids

In liquid drugs, there is a specific amount of drug in a given volume of solution. Look at Figure 3.5. In this example, the dosage strength of Augmentin is 125 mg/5 mL solution. Instead of labeling the drug in one unit of measure (tablet or capsule), the drug is written as a specific amount in a specific *quantity* of solution. For example, if the label states that there is 125 mg/5 mL, 5 mL is the *quantity* (or volume) in which there is 125 mg of this drug.

NURSING ALERT
Use "mL" instead of "ml" when writing the abbreviation for milliliters. This prevents the error of ml being misread as m 1 or meter 1.

The basic formula for computing the dosage of liquids is:

$$\frac{\text{dose desired}}{\text{dose on hand}} \times \text{quantity} = \text{volume administered}$$

This may be abbreviated as

$$\frac{D}{H} \times Q = X$$

The quantity (or Q) in this formula is the amount of liquid in which the available drug is contained.

QUESTION #5

Use the label in Figure 3.5 to understand the following example. **Looking at the label, find the drug name, form, and dosage strength** (*see Appendix E for answer*)

Figure 3.5 Drug label for Augmentin. (Courtesy of GlaxoSmithKline.)

CALCULATION #5

Looking at the label in Figure 3.5, use this information to solve the following dose problem:

The primary health care provider orders: Augmentin 125 mg – 4 times daily. How many mL (milliliters) will the nurse administer in each dose? (*see Appendix E for answer*)

As with tablets and capsules, the prescribed dose of the drug may not be the same as what is on hand (or available). For example, the primary health care provider may order 500 mg Augmentin and the drug is labeled as 125 mg/5 mL. The 5 mL is the amount (quantity or Q) that contains 125 mg of the drug.

$$\frac{D}{H} \times Q = X \text{ (the liquid amount to be given)}$$

$$\frac{500\,mg}{125\,mg} \times 5 = X$$

$$\frac{4}{1} \times 5 = 20\,mL$$

Therefore, 20 mL contains the desired dose of 500 mg of Augmentin.

Parenteral Drugs in Disposable Syringes or Cartridges

In some instances a specific dosage strength is not available and it will be necessary to administer less than the amount contained in the syringe.

EXAMPLE

The physician orders diazepam 5 mg IM. The drug is available as a 2-mL disposable syringe labeled 5 mg/mL.

$$\frac{D}{H} \times Q = X$$

$$\frac{5\,mg}{10\,mg} \times 2\,mL = X$$

$$X = \frac{1}{2} \times 2 = 1\,mL$$

Note that because the syringe contains 2 mL of the drug and that *each* mL contains 5 mg of the drug, there is a total of 10 mg of the drug in the syringe. Because there is 10 mg of the drug in the syringe, half of the liquid in the syringe (1 mL) is discarded, and the remaining half (1 mL) is administered to give the prescribed dose of 5 mg.

Parenteral Drugs in Ampules and Vials

If the drug is in liquid form in the ampule or vial, the desired amount is withdrawn from the ampule or vial. In some instances, the entire amount is used; in others, only part of the total amount is withdrawn from the ampule or vial and administered.

Whenever the dose to be administered is different from that listed on the label, the volume to be administered must be calculated. To determine the volume to be administered, the formula for liquid preparations is used. The calculations are the same as those given in the preceding section for parenteral drugs in disposable syringes or cartridges.

EXAMPLES

The physician orders chlorpromazine 12.5 mg IM.

The drug is available as chlorpromazine 25 mg/1 mL in a 1-mL ampule.

$$\frac{D}{H} \times Q = X$$

$$\frac{12.5\,mg}{25\,mg} \times 1\,mL = X$$

$$\frac{1}{2} \times 1\,mL = \frac{1}{2}\,mL\,(or\,0.5\,mL)\,volume\,to\,be\,administred.$$

The physician orders hydroxyzine 12.5 mg. The drug is available as hydroxyzine 25 mg/mL in 10-mL vials.

$$\frac{D}{H} \times Q = X$$

$$\frac{12.5\,mg}{25\,mg} \times 1\,mL = \frac{1}{2}\,mL\,(or\,0.5\,mL)$$

Therefore, 0.5 mL is withdrawn from the 10-mL multidose vial and administered. In this example, the amount in this or any multidose vial is *not* entered into the equation. What is entered into the equation as quantity (Q) is the amount of the available drug that is contained in a specific volume.

Parenteral Drugs in Dry Form

Some parenteral drugs are available as a crystal or a powder. Because these drugs have a short life in liquid form, they are available in ampules or vials in dry form and must be made a liquid (reconstituted) before they are removed and administered. Often the drug is in a container with both the powder and liquid separated by a barrier that is broken right before mixing and administering. If the drug is not dispensed in this form, the product directions for reconstitution on the label or on the enclosed package insert should be included with the drug. The manufacturer may give the following information for reconstitution: (1) the name of the diluent(s) that must be used with the drug, or (2) the amount of diluent that must be added to the drug.

In some instances, the manufacturer supplies a diluent with the drug. If a diluent is supplied, no other stock diluent should be used. Before a drug is reconstituted, the label is carefully checked for instructions.

EXAMPLES

Methicillin: To reconstitute 1-g vial, add 1.5 mL of sterile water for injection or sodium chloride injection. Each reconstituted milliliter contains approximately 500 mg of methicillin. If there is any doubt about the reconstitution of the dry form of a drug, and there are no manufacturer's directions, the clinical pharmacist should be consulted.

Once a diluent is added, the volume to be administered is determined. In some cases, the entire amount is given; in others, a part (or fraction) of the total amount contained in the vial or ampule is given.

After reconstitution of any multidose vial, the following information *must* be added to the label:

• Amount of diluent added
• Dose of drug in mL (500 mg/mL, 10 mg/2 mL, etc.)
• Date of reconstitution
• Expiration date (the date after which any unused solution is discarded)

Dosage Calculation Using Dimensional Analysis

Dimensional analysis (DA) is a method to perform calculations where the focus is on the units of measure, thereby eliminating the need to memorize equations. Because the units are set up in a specific order, it eliminates the need to be concerned about setting up proportions correctly. When using DA to calculate dosage problems, dosages are written as common fractions. For example:

$$\frac{1\,mL}{4\,mg} \quad \frac{5\,mL}{10\,mg} \quad \frac{1\,tablet}{100\,mg}$$

When written as common fractions, the numerator is the top number. In the example above, 1 mL, 5 mL, and 1 tablet are the numerators.

The numbers on the bottom are called denominators. In the example above, 4 mg, 10 mg, and 100 mg are denominators.

EXAMPLE

The primary health care provider orders 10 mg of diazepam. The drug comes in dosage strength of 5 mg/mL. How many milliliters would the nurse administer?

Step 1. To work this problem using DA, always begin by identifying the unit of measure to be calculated. The unit to be calculated will be milliliters if the drug is to be administered parenterally. Another drug form is the solid, and the unit of measure would be a tablet or capsule. In this problem, the unit of measure to be calculated is milliliters.

Step 2. Write the identified unit of measure to be calculated, followed by an equal sign. In this problem, milliliters is the unit to be calculated, so the nurse writes:

$$mL =$$

Step 3. Next, the dosage strength is written with the numerator *always expressed in the same unit that was identified before the equal sign.* For example:

Step 4. Continue by writing the next fraction with the numerator having the same unit of measure as the denominator in the previous fraction.

For example, our problem continues:

$$mL = \frac{1\,mL}{5\,mg} \times \frac{10\,mg}{X\,mL}$$

Step 5. The problem is solved by multiplication of the two fractions.

$$mL = \frac{1\,mL}{5\,mg} \times \frac{10\,mg}{X\,mL} = \frac{10\,mg}{5X\,mL} = 2\,mL$$

NOTE: Each alternate denominator and numerator cancel, with only the final unit remaining.

EXAMPLE

Ordered: 200,000 U

On hand: Drug labeled 400,000 U/mL

$$mL = \frac{1\,mL}{400,000\,U} \times \frac{200,000\,U}{X\,mL} = \frac{1}{2}\,mL\,or\,0.5\,mL$$

Metric Conversions Using Dimensional Analysis

Occasionally, the primary health care provider may order a drug in one unit of measure, whereas the drug is available in another unit of measure.

EXAMPLE

The physician orders 0.4 mg of atropine. The drug label reads 400 mcg per 1 mL. This dosage problem is solved by expanding the DA equation, by adding one step to the equation.

Step 1. As above, begin by writing the unit of measure to be calculated, followed by an equal sign.

Step 2. Next, express the dosage strength as a fraction with the numerator having the same unit of measure as the number before the equal sign.

Step 3. Continue by writing the next fraction with the numerator having the same unit of measure as the denominator in the previous fraction.

$$mL = \frac{1\,mL}{400\,mcg} \times \frac{mcg}{mg}$$

Step 4. Expand the equation by filling in the missing numbers using the appropriate equivalent. In this problem, the equivalent would be 100 mcg = 1 mg. This will convert micrograms to milligrams.

$$mL = \frac{1\,mL}{400\,mcg} \times \frac{mcg}{mg}$$

Repeat Steps 3 and 4. Continue with the equation by placing the next fraction, beginning with the unit of measure of the denominator of the previous fraction.

$$mL = \frac{1\,mL}{400\,mcg} \times \frac{1000\,mcg}{1\,mg} \times \frac{0.4\,mg}{X\,mL}$$

When possible, cancel out the units, leaving only mL.

Step 5. Solve the problem by multiplication. Cancel out the numbers when possible.

$$mL = \frac{1\,mL}{400\,mcg} \times \frac{1000\,mcg}{1\,mg} \times \frac{0.4\,mg}{X\,mL} = \frac{400}{400X} = 1\,mL$$

Solve the following problems using DA. Refer to the equivalents table if necessary (see Display 3.1).

EXAMPLE

Ordered: 250 mg

On hand: Drug labeled 1 g per 1 mL

$$mL = \frac{1\,mL}{1\,g} \times \frac{1\,g}{1000\,mg} \times \frac{250\,mg}{X\,mL} = \frac{1\,mL}{4} = \text{or } 0.25\ mL$$

Selected Methods Used in Calculation of Drug Dosages

Pediatric Dosages

The dosages of drugs given to children are usually less than those given to adults. The dosage may be based on age, weight, or body surface area (BSA). Today, most pediatric dosages are clearly given by the manufacturer, thus eliminating the need for formulas, except for determining the dosage of some drugs based on the child's weight or BSA.

Drug Dosages Based on Weight

The dosage of an oral or parenteral drug may be based on the patient's weight. In many instances, references give the dosage based on the weight in kilograms (kg) rather than pounds (lb). There are 2.2 lb in 1 kg.

When the dosage of a drug is based on weight, the primary health care provider or clinical pharmacist, in most instances, computes and orders the dosage to be given. However, errors can occur for any number of reasons. The nurse should be able to calculate a drug dosage based on weight to detect any type of error that may have been made in the prescribing or dispensing of a drug whose dosage is based on weight.

EXAMPLES

To convert a known weight in kilograms to pounds, multiply the known weight by 2.2.

Patient's weight in kilograms is 54:

$$54 \times 2.2 = 118.8 \text{ (or 119) lb}$$

To convert a known weight in pounds to kilograms, divide the known weight by 2.2.

Patient's weight in kilograms is 61.5:

$$61.5 \times 2.2 = 135.3 \text{ (or 135) lb}$$

CALCULATION #6

Determine the patient's weight in kilograms when the patient weighs 142 pounds (*see Appendix E for answer*)

Determine the child's weight in kilograms when the child weighs 43 pounds (*see Appendix E for answer*)

Once the weight is converted to pounds or kilograms, this information is used to determine drug dosage.

EXAMPLES

A drug dosage is 5 mg/kg/day. The patient weighs 135 lb, which is converted to 61.2 kg.

$$61.2\text{ kg} \times 5\text{ mg} = 306.8\text{ mg}$$

Proportions also can be used:

$$5\text{ mg:}1\text{ kg::X mg:}61.2\text{ kg}$$

$$X = 306.8\text{ mg}$$

A drug dosage is 60 mg/kg/day in three equally divided doses.

The patient weighs 143 lb, which is converted to 65 kg.

$$65\text{ kg} \times 60\text{ mg} = 3900\text{ mg/day}$$

$$3900\text{ mg} \div 3\text{ (doses per day)} = 1300\text{ mg each dose}$$

If the drug dosage is based on body surface area (m^2), the same method of calculation may be used.

Body Surface Area (BSA)

Charts (called nomograms, see Appendix D) are used to determine the BSA in square meters according to the child's height and weight. Once the BSA is determined, the following formula is used:

$$\frac{\text{surface area of the child in square meters}}{\text{surface area of an adult in square meters}} \times \text{usual adult dose} = \text{pediatric dose}$$

EXAMPLE

A drug dosage is 60 to 75 mg/m^2 as a single IV injection.

The body surface area (BSA) of a patient is determined by means of a nomogram for estimating BSA and is found to be 1.8 m^2. The physician orders 60 mg/m^2.

$$60\text{ mg} \times 1.8\ m^2 = 108\text{ mg}$$

Proportion can also be used:

$$60\text{ mg: }1\ m^2\text{::X mg:}1.8\ m^2$$

$$X = 108\text{ mg}$$

Temperatures

Two scales used in the measuring of temperatures are Fahrenheit (F) and Celsius (C) (also known as centigrade). On the Fahrenheit scale, the freezing point of water is 32°F, and the boiling point of water is 212°F. On the Celsius scale, 0°C is the freezing point of water and 100° C is the boiling point of water.

To convert from Celsius to Fahrenheit, the following formula may be used: F = 9/5 C + 32 (9/5 times the temperature in Celsius, then add 32).

EXAMPLE

Convert 38C to Fahrenheit:

$$F = \frac{9}{5} \times 38° + 32$$
$$F = 68.4° + 32$$
$$F = 100.4°$$

To convert from Fahrenheit to Celsius, the following formula may be used: C = 5/9 (F − 32) (5/9 times the temperature in Fahrenheit minus 32).

EXAMPLE

Convert 100°F to Celsius:

$$C = \frac{5}{9} \times (100 - 32)$$
$$C = \frac{5}{9} \times 68$$
$$C = 37.77 \: or \: 37.8°$$

Household Measurements

When used, household measurements are for volume only. In the hospital, household measurements are rarely used because they are inaccurate when used to measure drug dosages. On occasion, the nurse may use the pint, quart, or gallon when ordering, irrigating, or sterilizing solutions or stock solutions. For the ease of a patient taking a drug at home, the physician may order a drug dosage in household measurements. Display 3.2 lists the more common household measurements.

Mathematical Review

The remainder of the chapter contains various mathematical concepts. This portion is included should the drug dosage calculations in the earlier sections cause confusion or if they are hard to understand. Practice of calculations is important to help the nurse practice safe medication administration (Fig. 3.6).

DISPLAY 3.2 Household Measurements

3 teaspoons = 1 tablespoon
2 tablespoons = 1 ounce
2 pints = 1 quart
4 quarts = 1 gallon

Figure 3.6 Nurses are involved in the administration component of drug therapy, yet they hold great responsibility in helping the entire team provide safe patient care and correct calculation of drug doses.

Fractions

The two parts of a fraction are the numerator and the denominator.

$$\frac{2}{3} \begin{matrix} \leftarrow \text{numerator} \\ \leftarrow \text{denominator} \end{matrix}$$

A proper fraction may be defined as a part of a whole or any number less than a whole number. An improper fraction is a fraction having a numerator the same as or larger than the denominator. For example,

proper fraction $\frac{1}{2}$

improper fraction $\frac{7}{3}$

The numerator and the denominator must be of *like entities or terms,* that is:

Correct (like terms)	Incorrect (unlike terms)
$\dfrac{2\,acres}{3\,acres}$	$\dfrac{2\,acres}{3\,miles}$
$\dfrac{2\,grams}{3\,grams}$	$\dfrac{2\,grams}{5\,milliliters}$

Mixed Numbers and Improper Fractions

A mixed number is a whole number and a proper fraction. A whole number is a number that stands alone; 3, 25, and 117 are examples of whole numbers. A proper fraction is a fraction whose numerator is *smaller than* the denominator; 1/8, 2/5, and 3/7 are examples of proper fractions.

These are mixed numbers:

22/3   2 is the whole number and 2/3 is the proper fraction
31/4   3 is the whole number and 1/4 is the proper fraction

When doing certain calculations, it is sometimes necessary to change a mixed number to an improper fraction or change an improper fraction to a mixed number. An improper fraction is a fraction whose numerator is *larger than* the denominator; 5/2, 16/3, and 12 3/2 are examples of improper fractions.

To change a *mixed number to an improper fraction,* multiply the denominator of the fraction by the whole number, add the numerator, and place the sum over the denominator.

EXAMPLE Mixed number 3 3/5

1. Multiply the denominator of the fraction (5) by the whole number (3) or 5 ×3 = 15:

$$3 \times \frac{3}{5}$$

2. Add the result of multiplying the denominator of the fraction (15) to the numerator (3) or 15 + 3 = 18:

$$3 \times \frac{3}{5}$$

3. Then place the sum (18) over the denominator of the fraction:

$$\frac{18}{5}$$

To change an *improper fraction to a mixed number,* divide the denominator into the numerator. The quotient (the result of the division of these two numbers) is the whole number. Then place the remainder over the denominator of the improper fraction.

EXAMPLE Improper fraction 15/4

$$\frac{15}{4} \begin{matrix} \leftarrow \text{numerator} \\ \leftarrow \text{denominator} \end{matrix}$$

1. Divide the denominator (4) into the numerator (15) or 15 divided by 4 (15 ÷ 4):

$$\begin{array}{r} 3 \leftarrow \text{quotient} \\ 4\overline{)15} \\ \underline{12} \\ 3 \leftarrow \text{remainder} \end{array}$$

2. The quotient (3) becomes the whole number:

$$3\frac{3}{4}$$

3. The remainder (3) now becomes the numerator of the fraction of the mixed number:

$$3\frac{3}{}$$

4. And the denominator of the improper fraction (4) now becomes the denominator of the fraction of the mixed number:

$$3\frac{3}{4}$$

Adding Fractions With Like Denominators

When the denominators are the *same,* fractions can be added by adding the numerators and placing the sum of the numerators over the denominator.

EXAMPLES

2/7 + 3/7 = 5/7
1/10 + 3/10 = 4/10
2/9 + 1/9 + 4/9 = 7/9
1/12 + 5/12 + 3/12 = 9/12
2/13 + 1/13 + 3/13 + 5/13 = 11/13

When giving a final answer, fractions are *always* reduced to the lowest possible terms. In the examples above, the answers of 5/7, 7/9, and 11/13 cannot be reduced. The answers of 4/10 and 9/12 can be reduced to 2/5 and 3/4.

To reduce a fraction to the lowest possible terms, determine if any number, which always must be the same, can be divided into both the numerator and the denominator.

4/10: the numerator *and* the denominator can be divided by 2

9/12: the numerator *and* the denominator can be divided by 3

For example: $\dfrac{4 \div 2}{10 \div 2} = \dfrac{2}{5}$

If when adding fractions the answer is an improper fraction, it may then be changed to a mixed number.

2/5 + 4/5 = 6/5 (improper fraction)

6/5 changed to a mixed number is 1 1/5

Adding Fractions With Unlike Denominators

Fractions with *unlike denominators* cannot be added until the denominators are changed to like numbers or numbers that are the same. The first step is to find the *lowest common denominator,* which is the lowest number divisible by (or that can be divided by) all the denominators.

EXAMPLE Add 2/3 and 1/4

$$\frac{2}{3}$$
$$\frac{1}{4}$$

The lowest number that can be divided by these two denominators is 12; therefore, 12 is the lowest common denominator.

1. Divide the lowest common denominator (which in this example is 12) by each of the denominators in the fractions (in this example 3 and 4):

$$\frac{2}{3} = \frac{}{12} \qquad (12 \div 3 = 4)$$

$$\frac{1}{4} = \frac{}{12} \qquad (12 \div 4 = 3)$$

2. Multiply the results of the divisions by the numerator of the fractions ($12 \div 3 = 4 \times$ the numerator $2 = 8$ and $12 \div 4 = 3 \times$ the numerator $1 = 3$) and place the results in the numerator:

$$\frac{2}{3} = \frac{}{12} \qquad \frac{8}{12}$$

$$\frac{1}{4} = \frac{}{12} \qquad \frac{3}{12}$$

3. Add the numerators $(8 + 3)$ and place the result over the denominator (12):

$$\frac{8}{12}$$

$$\frac{3}{12}$$

$$\frac{11}{12}$$

Adding Mixed Numbers or Fractions with Mixed Numbers

When adding two or more mixed numbers or adding fractions and mixed numbers, the mixed number is first changed to an improper fraction.

EXAMPLE Add 3 3/4 and 3 3/4

$3\frac{3}{4}$ changed to an improper fraction $\rightarrow \frac{15}{4}$

$3\frac{3}{4}$ changed to an improper fraction $\rightarrow \frac{15}{4}$

The numerators are added $\rightarrow \dfrac{30}{4} = 7\,2/4 = 7\,1/2$

The improper fraction (30/4) is changed to a mixed number (7 2/4) and the fraction of the mixed number (2/4) changed to the lowest possible terms (1/2).

EXAMPLE Add 2 1/2 and 3 1/4

$2\frac{1}{2}$ changed to an improper fraction $\frac{5}{2}$

$3\frac{1}{4}$ changed to an improper fraction $\frac{13}{4}$

In the example above, 5/2 and 13/4 cannot be added because the denominators are not the same. It will be necessary to find the lowest common denominator first.

$\dfrac{5}{2}$ the lowest common denominator is 4 $\quad\dfrac{10}{4}$

$$\frac{13}{4} \qquad\qquad \frac{13}{4}$$

$\dfrac{23}{4}$ changed to a mixed number $= 5\dfrac{3}{4}$

Comparing Fractions

When fractions with *like* denominators are compared, the fraction with the *largest numerator* is the *largest* fraction.

EXAMPLES

Compare: 5/8 and 3/8 Answer: 5/8 is larger than 3/8.

Compare: 1/4 and 3/4 Answer: 3/4 is larger than 1/4

When the denominators are *not* the same, for example, comparing 2/3 and 1/10, the lowest common denominator must first be determined. The same procedure is followed when adding fractions with unlike denominators (see above).

EXAMPLES Compare 2/3 and 1/10 (fractions with unlike denominators)

$$\frac{2}{3} = \frac{20}{30}$$

$$\frac{1}{10} = \frac{3}{30} \quad \text{lowest common denominator}$$

The largest numerator in these two fractions is 20; therefore, 2/3 is larger than 1/10.

Multiplying Fractions

When fractions are multiplied, the numerators are multiplied *and* the denominators are multiplied.

EXAMPLES

$$\frac{1}{8} \times \frac{1}{4} = \frac{1}{32} \qquad \frac{1}{2} \times \frac{2}{3} = \frac{2}{6} = \frac{1}{3}$$

In the above examples, it was necessary to reduce one of the answers to its lowest possible terms.

Multiplying Whole Numbers and Fractions

When whole numbers are multiplied with fractions, the numerator is multiplied by the whole number and the product is placed over the denominator. When necessary, the fraction is reduced to its lowest possible terms. If the answer is an improper fraction, it may be changed to a mixed number.

EXAMPLES

$$2 \times \frac{1}{2} = \frac{2}{2} = 1 \text{ (answer reduced to lowest possible terms)}$$

$$2 \times \frac{3}{8} = \frac{6}{8} = \frac{3}{4} \text{ (answer reduced to lowest possible terms)}$$

$$4 \times \frac{2}{3} = \frac{8}{3} = 2\frac{2}{3} \text{ (improper fraction changed to a mixed number)}$$

Multiplying Mixed Numbers

To multiply mixed numbers, the mixed numbers are changed to *improper fractions* and then multiplied.

EXAMPLES

$$2\frac{1}{2} \times 3\frac{1}{4} = \frac{5}{2} \times \frac{13}{4} = \frac{65}{8} = 8\frac{1}{8}$$

$$3\frac{1}{3} \times 4\frac{1}{2} = \frac{10}{3} \times \frac{9}{2} = \frac{90}{6} = 15$$

Multiplying a Whole Number and a Mixed Number

To multiply a whole number and a mixed number, *both* numbers must be changed to improper fractions.

EXAMPLES

$$3 \times 2\frac{1}{2} = \frac{3}{1} \times \frac{5}{2} = \frac{15}{2} = 7\frac{1}{2}$$

$$2 \times 4\frac{1}{2} = \frac{2}{1} \times \frac{9}{2} = \frac{18}{2} = 9$$

A whole number is converted to an improper fraction by placing the whole number over 1. In the above examples, 3 becomes 3/1 and 2 becomes 2/1.

Dividing Fractions

When fractions are divided, the *second* fraction (the divisor) is inverted (turned upside down) and then the fractions are multiplied.

EXAMPLES

$$\frac{1}{3} \div \boxed{\frac{3}{7}} = \frac{1}{3} \times \frac{7}{3} = \frac{7}{9}$$

$$\frac{1}{8} \div \frac{1}{4} = \frac{1}{8} \times \frac{4}{1} = \frac{4}{8} = \frac{1}{2}$$

$$\frac{3}{4} \div \frac{1}{2} = \frac{3}{4} \times \frac{2}{1} = \frac{6}{4} = 1\frac{1}{2}$$

In the above examples, the second answer was reduced to its lowest possible terms and the third answer, which was an improper fraction, was changed to a mixed number.

Dividing Fractions and Mixed Numbers

Some problems of division may be expressed as (1) fractions and mixed numbers, (2) two mixed numbers, (3) whole numbers and fractions, or (4) whole numbers and mixed numbers.

Mixed Numbers and Fractions

When a mixed number is divided by a fraction, the whole number is first changed to a fraction.

EXAMPLES

$$\boxed{2\frac{1}{3}} \div \frac{1}{4} = \frac{7}{3} \div \frac{1}{4} = \frac{7}{3} \times \frac{4}{1} = \frac{28}{3} = 9\frac{1}{3}$$

$$2\frac{1}{2} \div \frac{1}{2} = \frac{5}{2} \div \frac{1}{2} = \frac{5}{2} \times \frac{2}{1} = \frac{10}{2} = 5$$

Mixed Numbers

When two mixed numbers are divided, they are both changed to improper fractions.

EXAMPLE

$$\boxed{3\frac{3}{4}} \div \boxed{1\frac{1}{2}} = \frac{15}{4} \div \frac{3}{2} = \frac{15}{4} \times \frac{2}{3} = \frac{30}{12}$$

$$= 2\frac{6}{12} = 2\frac{1}{2}$$

Whole Numbers and Fractions

When a whole number is divided by a fraction, the whole number is changed to an improper fraction by placing the whole number over 1.

EXAMPLE

$$\boxed{2} \div \frac{2}{3} = \frac{2}{1} \div \frac{2}{3} = \frac{2}{1} \times \frac{3}{2} = \frac{6}{2} = 3$$

Whole Numbers and Mixed Numbers

When whole numbers and mixed numbers are divided, the whole number is changed to an improper fraction and the mixed number is changed to an improper fraction.

EXAMPLE

$$4 \div 2\frac{2}{3} = \frac{4}{1} \div \frac{8}{3} = \frac{4}{1} \times \frac{3}{8} = \frac{12}{8} = 1\frac{4}{8} = 1\frac{1}{2}$$

Ratios

A ratio is a way of expressing *a part of a whole* or *the relation of one number to another.* For example, a ratio written as 1:10 means 1 in 10 parts, or 1 to 10. A ratio may also be written as a fraction; thus 1:10 can also be expressed as 1/10.

EXAMPLES

1:1000 is 1 part in 1000 parts, or 1 to 1000,
     or 1/1000

1:250 is 1 part in 250 parts, or 1 to 250, or 1/250

Some drug solutions are expressed in ratios; for example, 1:100 or 1:500. These ratios mean that there is 1 part of a drug in 100 parts of solution or 1 part of the drug in 500 parts of solution.

Percentages

The term *percentage* or *percent* (%) means *parts per hundred.*

EXAMPLES

25% is 25 parts per hundred

50% is 50 parts per hundred

A percentage may also be expressed as a fraction.

EXAMPLES

25% is 25 parts per hundred or 25/100

50% is 50 parts per hundred or 50/100

30% is 30 parts per hundred or 30/100

The above fractions may also be reduced to their lowest possible terms:

25/100 = 1/4, 50/100 = 1/2, 30/100 = 3/10.

Changing a Fraction to a Percentage

To change a fraction to a percentage, divide the denominator by the numerator and multiply the results (quotient) by 100 and then add a percent sign (%).

EXAMPLES

Change 4/5 to a percentage

$$4 \div 5 = 0.8$$
$$0.8 \times 100 = 80\%$$

Change 2/3 to a percentage

$$2 \div 3 = 0.666$$
$$0.666 \times 100 = 66.6\%$$ or ? 66.7%

Changing a Ratio to a Percentage

To change a ratio to a percentage, the ratio is first expressed as a fraction with the first number or term of the ratio becoming the numerator and the second number or term becoming the denominator. For example, the ratio 1:500 when changed to a fraction becomes 1/500. This fraction is then changed to a percentage by the same method shown in the preceding section.

EXAMPLES

Change 1:125 to a percentage

1:125 written as a fraction is 1/125
$$1 \div 125 = 0.008$$
$$0.008 \times 100 = 0.8\%$$
adding the percent sign = 0.8%

Changing a Percentage to a Ratio

To change a percentage to a ratio, the percentage becomes the numerator and is placed over a denominator of 100.

EXAMPLES

Changing 5% and 10% to ratios

$$5\% \text{ is } \frac{5}{100} = \frac{1}{20} \text{ or } 1 : 20$$

$$10\% \text{ is } \frac{10}{100} = \frac{1}{10} \text{ or } 1 : 10$$

Proportions

A proportion is a method of expressing equality between two ratios. An example of two ratios expressed as a proportion is: 3 is to 4 as 9 is to 12. This may also be written as:

3:4 as 9:12
or
3:4::9:12
or
$$\frac{3}{4} = \frac{9}{12}$$

Proportions may be used to find an unknown quantity. The unknown quantity is assigned a letter, usually X. An example of a proportion with an unknown quantity is 5:10::15:X.

The first and last terms of the proportion are called the *extremes.* In the above expression 5 and X are the extremes. The second and third terms of the proportion are called the *means.* In the above proportion, 10 and 15 are the means.

means

5:10::15:X

extremes

$$\text{extreme } \frac{5}{\text{mean } 10} = \frac{15 \text{ mean}}{X \text{ extreme}}$$

To solve for X:

1. Multiply the extremes and place the product (result) to the *left* of the equal sign.

$$5:10::15:X$$
$$5X=$$

2. Multiply the means and place the product to the *right* of the equal sign.

$$5:10::15X$$
$$5X = 150$$

3. Solve for X by dividing the number to the right of the equal sign by the number to the left of the equal sign ($150 \div 5$).

$$5X = 150$$
$$X = 30$$

4. To prove the answer is correct, substitute the answer (30) for X in the equation.

$$5:10::15:X$$
$$5:10::15:30$$

Then multiply the means and place the product to the left of the equal sign. Then multiply the extremes and place the product to the right of the equal sign.

$$5:10::15:30$$
$$150 = 150$$

If the numbers are the same on both sides of the equal sign, the equation has been solved correctly.

If the proportion has been set up as a fraction, cross-multiply and solve for X.

$$\frac{5}{10} = \frac{15}{X}$$

$$5 \text{ times } X = 5X \text{ and } 10 \text{ times } 15 = 150$$
$$5X = 150$$
$$X = 30$$

To set up a proportion, remember that a sequence *must* be followed. If a sequence is not followed, the proportion will be stated incorrectly.

EXAMPLES

If a man can walk 6 *miles* in 2 *hours,* how many *miles* can he walk in 3 *hours?*

miles is to *hours* and *miles* is to *hours*

or

miles:hours::miles:hours

or

$$\frac{miles}{hours} = \frac{miles}{hours}$$

The unknown fact is the number of miles walked in 3 hours:

6 miles:2 hours::X miles:3 hours

$$2X = 18$$
$$X = 9 \text{ miles (he can walk 9 miles in 3 hours)}$$

If there are 15 *grains* in 1 *gram,* 30 *grains* equals how many *grams?*

15 grains:1 gram::30 grains:X grams

$$15X = 30$$
$$X = 2 \text{ grams (30 grains equals 2 grams)}$$

Decimals

Decimals are used in the metric system. A decimal is a fraction in which the denominator is 10 or some power of 10. For example, 2/10 (read as two tenths) is a fraction with a denominator of 10; 1/100 (read as one one hundredth) is an example of a fraction with a denominator that is a power of 10 (i.e., 100).

A power (or multiple) of 10 is the *number 1 followed by one or more zeros.* Therefore, 100, 1000, 10,000 and so on are powers of 10 because the number 1 is followed by two, three, and four zeros, respectively. Fractions whose denominators are 10 or a power of 10 are often expressed in decimal form.

Parts of a Decimal

There are three parts to a decimal:

	1.25	
number(s)	**d**	number(s)
to the	**e**	to the
left of	**c**	right of
the	**i**	the
decimal	**m**	decimal
	a	
	l	

Types of Decimals

A decimal may consist only of numbers to the right of the decimal point. This is called a decimal fraction. Examples of decimal fractions are 0.05, 0.6, and 0.002.

A decimal may also have numbers to the left *and* right of the decimal point. This is called a mixed decimal fraction. Examples of mixed decimal fractions are 1.25, 2.5, and 7.5.

Reading Decimals

To read a decimal, the position of the number to the left or right of the decimal point indicates how the decimal is to be expressed.

0 hundred thousands
0 ten thousands
0 thousands
0 hundreds
0 tens
0 units

DECIMAL POINT
0 tenths
0 hundredths
0 thousandths
0 ten thousandths
0 hundred thousandths

Adding Decimals

When adding decimals, place the numbers in a column so that the whole numbers are aligned to the left of the decimal and the decimal fractions are aligned to the right of the decimal.

EXAMPLE

20.45 + 2.56   2 + 0.25

is written as: is written as:

$$\begin{array}{r} 20.45 \\ +\ 2.56 \\ \hline 23.01 \end{array} \qquad \begin{array}{r} 2.00 \\ +\ 0.25 \\ \hline 2.25 \end{array}$$

Subtracting Decimals

When subtracting decimals, the numbers are aligned to the left and right of the decimal in the same manner as for the addition of decimals.

EXAMPLE

20.45 − 2.56   9.74 − 0.45

is written as: is written as:

$$\begin{array}{r} 20.45 \\ -\ 2.56 \\ \hline 17.89 \end{array} \qquad \begin{array}{r} 9.74 \\ -\ 0.45 \\ \hline 9.29 \end{array}$$

Multiplying a Whole Number by a Decimal

To multiply a whole number by a decimal, move the decimal point of the product (answer) as many places to the left as there are places to the right of the decimal point.

EXAMPLE

$$\begin{array}{r} 500 \\ \times.05 \\ \hline 2500. \end{array}$$ ← there are two places to the right of the decimal — the decimal point is moved two places to the left

After moving the decimal point, the answer reads 25.

$$\begin{array}{r} 250 \\ \times.3 \\ \hline 750. \end{array}$$ ← there is one place to the right of the decimal — the decimal point is moved one place to the left

After moving the decimal point, the answer reads 75.

Multiplying a Decimal by a Decimal

To multiply a decimal by a decimal, move the decimal point of the product (answer) as many places to the left as there are places to the right in *both* decimals.

EXAMPLE

there are two places to the right

$$\begin{array}{r} 2.75 \\ \times.05 \\ \hline 1375. \end{array}$$ ← of the decimal ← plus two places to the right of the decimal, move the decimal point four places to the left

After moving the decimal point, the answer reads 0.1375.

Dividing Decimals

The divisor is a number that is divided into the dividend.

EXAMPLE

$$0.69 \div 0.3 \qquad\qquad 0.3\overline{)0.69}$$

↑   ↑   ↑   ↑

dividend   divisor   divisor   dividend

This may be written or spoken as 0.69 divided by 0.3. To divide decimals:

1. The *divisor* is changed to a whole number. In this example, the decimal point is moved one place to the right so that 0.3 now becomes 3, which is a whole number.

$$0.3\overline{)0.69}$$

2. The decimal point in the *dividend* is now moved the *same number of places* to the right. In this example, the decimal point is moved one place to the right, the same number of places the decimal point in the divisor was moved.

$$0.3\overline{)0.69}$$

3. The numbers are now divided.

$$3\overline{)6.9} = 2.3$$

When only the dividend is a decimal, the decimal point is carried to the quotient (answer) in the same position.

EXAMPLES

$$2\overline{)0.750} = .375 \qquad 2\overline{)3.472} = 1.736$$

To divide when only the divisor is a decimal, for example,

$$.3\overline{)66}$$

1. The divisor is changed to a whole number. In this example, the decimal point is moved one place to the right.

$$.3\overline{)66}$$

2. The decimal point in the dividend must also be moved one place to the right.

$$.3\overline{)66.0}$$

3. The numbers are now divided.

$$3\overline{)660} = 220$$

Whenever the decimal point is moved in the dividend it must *also* be moved in the divisor, and whenever the decimal point in the divisor is moved it must *also* be moved in the dividend.

Changing a Fraction to a Decimal

To change a fraction to a decimal, divide the numerator by the denominator.

EXAMPLE

$$\frac{1}{5} = 5\overline{)1.0}^{\,.2} \qquad \frac{3}{4} = 4\overline{)3.00}^{\,.75} \qquad \frac{1}{6} = 6\overline{)1.000}^{\,.166}$$

Changing a Decimal to a Fraction

To change a decimal to a fraction:

1. Remove the decimal point and make the resulting whole number the numerator: 0.2 = 2.
2. The denominator is stated as 10 or a power of 10. In this example, 0.2 is read as two tenths, and therefore the denominator is 10.

$$0.2 = \frac{2}{10} \text{ reduced to the lowest possible number is } \frac{1}{5}$$

ADDITIONAL EXAMPLES

$$0.75 = \frac{75}{100} = \frac{3}{4} \qquad 0.025 = \frac{25}{1000} = \frac{1}{40}$$

THINK CRITICALLY: PHARMACOLOGY IN PRACTICE

1. On your unit, one of the nurses states the following: "because we use the new computer system, we don't need to do the 5 rights and 3 checks anymore." Describe how you would respond to this nurse.

● Test Your Knowledge

1. Manual redundancy activities help the nurse provide:

   A. Control over dangerous drugs
   – B. Safety by recognizing error

   C. Reassurance to the patient
   D. Feedback to other providers

2. What percentage of potential drug errors is found when nurses check medication calculations for accuracy?

   A. 25%
   B. 49%
   C. 67%
   – D. 95%

3. Knowing both trade and generic drug names is important because:

   A. Cost is reduced using generic drugs.
   B. Only one name is provided on the drug label.
   C. Primary health care providers do not know the differences.
   – D. Patients may think the drug is incorrect.

4. The ISMP discourages use of which measurement system?

   A. Household
   B. Metric
   – C. Apothecary
   D. Body Surface Area

● Prepare for the NCLEX

1. Which of the following drug doses is written correctly?

   A. Lanoxin .25 mg orally
   B. Lanoxin .250 mg orally
   – C. Lanoxin 0.25 mg orally
   D. Lanoxin 0.250 mg orally

To check your answers, see Appendix E.

the**Point** *For more NCLEX questions, log on to http://thepoint.lww.com to access more than 1000 questions.*

The Nursing Process

analysis
assessment
evaluation
expected outcome
implementation
independent nursing actions
initial assessment

nursing diagnosis
nursing process
objective data
ongoing assessment
planning
subjective data

LEARNING OBJECTIVES

On completion of this chapter, the student will:

1. List the five phases of the nursing process.
2. Discuss assessment, analysis, nursing diagnosis, planning, implementation, and evaluation as they apply to the administration of drugs.
3. Differentiate between objective and subjective data.
4. Discuss how the nursing process may be used in daily life, as well as when administering drugs.
5. Identify common nursing diagnoses used in the administration of drugs and nursing interventions related to each diagnosis.

The **nursing process** is a framework for nursing action consisting of problem-solving steps that help members of the health care team provide effective patient care. It is a specific and orderly plan used to gather data, identify patient problems from the data, develop and implement a plan of action, and then evaluate the results of nursing activities, including the administration of drugs.

The five phases of the process are used not only in nursing, but in daily life. For example, when buying a computer one may first think about whether it is really needed, shop in several different stores to find out more about computers (**assessment**), and then determine what each store has to offer (**analysis**). At this point, one decides exactly what computer to buy and how to pay for the computer (**planning**); then the computer is purchased (**implementation**). After purchase and use, the computer is evaluated (**evaluation**).

Using the nursing process requires practice, experience, and a constant updating of knowledge. The nursing process is used in this text only as it applies to drug administration. It is not within the scope of this textbook to list all of the assessments, nursing diagnoses, plans, implementations, and evaluations for the medical diagnosis that requires the administration of a specific drug.

The Five Phases of the Nursing Process

Although the nursing process can be described in various ways, it generally consists of five phases: assessment, analysis (or formation of the **nursing diagnosis**), planning, implementation, and evaluation. Each part is applicable, with modification, to the administration of medications. Figure 4.1 relates the nursing process to administration of medications.

Assessment

Assessment involves collecting objective and subjective data. **Objective data** are facts obtained by means of a physical assessment or physical examination. **Subjective data** are facts supplied by the patient or the patient's family.

Assessments are both initial and ongoing. An **initial assessment** is made based on objective and subjective data collected when the patient is first seen in a hospital, ambulatory setting (clinic or health care provider's office), or long-term care facility. The initial assessment usually is more thorough and provides a database (sometimes called a *baseline*) against which later data can be compared and decisions made. The initial assessment provides information that is analyzed to identify problems that can be resolved or alleviated by nursing actions.

Objective data are obtained during an initial assessment through activities such as examining the skin, obtaining vital signs, palpating a lesion, and auscultating the lungs. A review of the results of any recent laboratory tests and diagnostic studies also is part of the initial physical assessment. Subjective data are acquired during an initial assessment by obtaining information from the patient, such as a family history of disease, allergy history, occupational history, a description (in the patient's own words) of the current illness or chief complaint, a medical history, and a drug history. In addition to the prescription drugs that the patient may be taking, it is important to know the over-the-counter drugs, vitamins, or herbal therapies that the patient uses. For women of childbearing age, the nurse needs to ask about the woman's pregnancy status and whether or not she is breastfeeding.

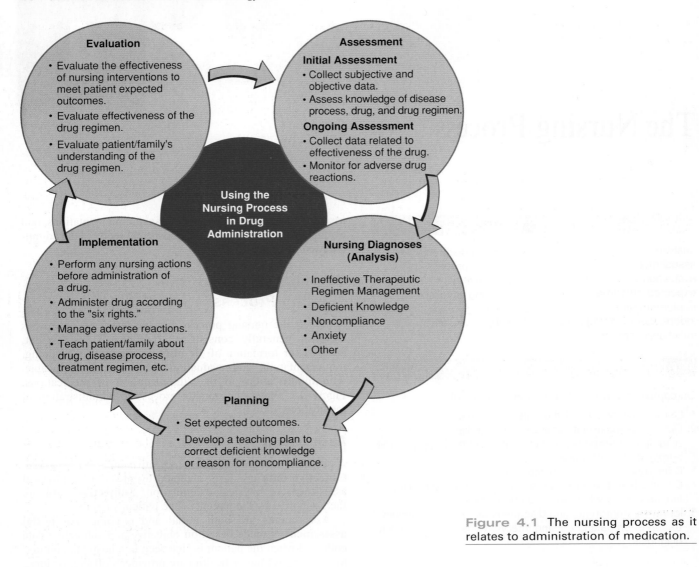

Evaluation
- Evaluate the effectiveness of nursing interventions to meet patient expected outcomes.
- Evaluate effectiveness of the drug regimen.
- Evaluate patient/family's understanding of the drug regimen.

Assessment

Initial Assessment
- Collect subjective and objective data.
- Assess knowledge of disease process, drug, and drug regimen.

Ongoing Assessment
- Collect data related to effectiveness of the drug.
- Monitor for adverse drug reactions.

Using the Nursing Process in Drug Administration

Implementation
- Perform any nursing actions before administration of a drug.
- Administer drug according to the "six rights."
- Manage adverse reactions.
- Teach patient/family about drug, disease process, treatment regimen, etc.

Nursing Diagnoses (Analysis)
- Ineffective Therapeutic Regimen Management
- Deficient Knowledge
- Noncompliance
- Anxiety
- Other

Planning
- Set expected outcomes.
- Develop a teaching plan to correct deficient knowledge or reason for noncompliance.

Figure 4.1 The nursing process as it relates to administration of medication.

An **ongoing assessment** is one that is made at the time of each patient contact and may include the collection of objective data, subjective data, or both. The scope of an ongoing assessment depends on many factors, such as the patient's diagnosis, the severity of illness, the response to treatment, and the prescribed medical or surgical treatment.

The assessment phase (including the initial and ongoing assessment) of the nursing process can be applied to the administration of drugs, with objective and subjective data collected before and after to obtain a thorough baseline or initial assessment. This allows subsequent assessments to be compared with the baseline information. This comparison helps to evaluate the effectiveness of the drug and the presence of any adverse reactions. Ongoing assessments of objective and subjective data are equally important when administering drugs. Important objective data include blood pressure, pulse, respiratory rate, temperature, weight, appearance of the skin, appearance of an intravenous infusion site, and pulmonary status as assessed by auscultation of the lungs. Important subjective data include any statements made

by the patient about relief or nonrelief of pain or other symptoms after administration of a drug.

The extent of the assessment and collection of objective and subjective data before and after a drug is administered depends on the type of drug and the reason for its use.

Nursing ~~Diagnosis~~ (Analysis)

Analysis is the way nurses cluster data into similar groupings to determine patient need or a nursing diagnosis. The data collected during assessment are examined for common threads; the nurse identifies the patient's needs (problems) and formulates one or more nursing diagnoses. A nursing diagnosis is not a medical diagnosis; rather, ~~it is a description of the patient's problems~~ and their probable or actual related causes based on the subjective and objective data in the database. A nursing diagnosis identifies problems that can be solved or prevented by **independent nursing actions**—actions that do not require a physician's order and may be legally performed by a nurse. Nursing diagnoses provide the framework for selections of nursing interventions to achieve expected outcomes.

The North American Nursing Diagnosis Association (NANDA) was formed to standardize the terminology used for nursing diagnoses. NANDA continues to define, explain, classify, and research summary statements about health problems related to nursing. NANDA has approved a list of diagnostic categories to be used in formulating a nursing diagnosis. This list of diagnostic categories is periodically revised and updated.

In some instances, nursing diagnoses may apply to a specific group or type of drug or a particular patient. One example is Deficient Fluid Volume related to active fluid volume loss (diuresis) secondary to administration of a diuretic. Specific drug-related nursing diagnoses are highlighted in each chapter. However, it is beyond the scope of this book to discuss all possible nursing diagnoses related to a drug or a drug class.

Some of the nursing diagnoses developed by NANDA may be used to identify patient problems associated with drug therapy and are more commonly used when administering drugs. The most frequently used nursing diagnoses related to the administration of drugs include:

- Effective Therapeutic Regimen Management
- Ineffective Therapeutic Regimen Management
- Deficient Knowledge
- Noncompliance
- Anxiety

Because these nursing diagnoses are commonly used for the administration of all types of drugs, they will not be repeated for each chapter. The nurse should keep these nursing diagnoses in mind when administering any drug.

Planning   Game Plan

After the nursing diagnoses are formulated, the nurse determines a goal and develops expected outcomes, which are patient oriented. An **expected outcome** is a direct statement of patient goals to be achieved. The expected outcome describes the maximum level of wellness that is reasonably attainable for the patient. For example, common expected patient outcomes related to drug administration, in general, include:

- The patient will effectively manage the therapeutic regimen.
- The patient will understand the drug regimen.
- The patient will comply with the drug regimen.

The expected outcomes define the expected behavior of the patient or family that indicates the problem is being resolved or that progress toward resolution is occurring.

The nurse selects the appropriate interventions on the basis of expected outcomes to develop a plan of action or patient care plan. Planning for nursing actions specific to the drug to be administered can result in greater accuracy in drug administration, enhanced patient understanding of the drug regimen, and improved patient compliance with the prescribed drug therapy after discharge from the hospital. For example, during the initial assessment interview, the patient may report an allergy to penicillin. This information is important, and the nurse must now plan the best methods of informing all members of the health care team of the patient's allergy to penicillin.

The planning phase describes the steps for carrying out nursing activities or interventions that are specific and that will meet the expected outcomes. Planning anticipates the implementation phase or the carrying out of nursing actions that are specific to the drug being administered. If, for example, the patient is to receive a drug by the intravenous route, the nurse must plan the materials needed and the patient instruction for administration of the drug by this route. In this instance, the planning phase occurs immediately before the implementation phase and is necessary to carry out the technique of intravenous administration correctly. Failing to plan effectively may result in forgetting to obtain all of the materials necessary for drug administration.

Implementation   Doing it

Implementation is the carrying out of a plan of action and is a natural outgrowth of the assessment and planning phases of the nursing process. When related to the administration of drugs, implementation refers to the preparation and administration of one or more drugs to a specific patient. Before administering a drug, the nurse reviews the subjective and objective data obtained on assessment and considers any additional data, such as blood pressure, pulse, or statements made by the patient. The decision of whether to administer the drug is based on an analysis of all information. For example, a patient is hypertensive and is supposed to receive a drug to lower the blood pressure. Objective data obtained at the time of admission included a blood pressure of 188/110. Additional objective data obtained immediately before the administration of the drug included a blood pressure of 182/110. A decision was made by the nurse to administer the drug because the change in the patient's blood pressure was minimal. However, if the patient's blood pressure was 132/84, and this was only the second dose of the drug, the nurse could decide to withhold the drug and contact the prescribing health care provider. Giving or withholding a drug or contacting the patient's health care provider are nursing activities related to the implementation phase of the nursing process.

The more common nursing diagnoses used when administering drugs are Effective Therapeutic Regimen Management, Ineffective Therapeutic Regimen Management, Deficient Knowledge, and Noncompliance. Nursing interventions applicable to each of these nursing diagnoses are discussed in the following sections. However, each patient is an individual, and nursing care must be planned on an individual basis after a careful collection and analysis of the data. In addition, each drug is different and may have various effects in the body. (For drugs discussed in subsequent chapters, some possible nursing diagnoses related to that specific drug are discussed.)

Effective Therapeutic Regimen Management

This nursing diagnosis takes into consideration that the patient is willing to regulate and integrate into daily living the treatment regimen such as the self-administration of medications. For this nursing diagnosis to be used, the patient verbalizes the desire to manage the medication regimen. When the patient is willing and able to manage the treatment regimen, he or she may simply need information concerning the drug, method of administration, what type of reactions to expect, and what to report to the primary health care provider. A patient willing to take responsibility may need the nurse to develop a teaching plan that gives the patient the information needed to manage the therapeutic regimen properly (see Chapter 5 for more information on educating patients).

Ineffective Therapeutic Regimen Management

NANDA defines Ineffective Therapeutic Regimen Management as "a pattern of regulating and integrating into daily living a program for treatment of illness and the sequelae of illness that is unsatisfactory for meeting specific health goals." In the case of medication administration, the patient may not be taking the medication correctly or following the medication regimen prescribed by the primary health care provider.

The reasons for not following the drug regimen vary (Display 4.1). For example, some people do not fill their prescriptions because they do not have enough money to pay for them. Other patients skip doses, take the drug at the wrong times, or take an incorrect dose. Some may simply forget to take the drug; others take a drug for a few days, see no therapeutic effect, and quit.

When working with a patient who is not managing the drug regimen correctly, the nurse must ensure that the patient understands the drug regimen. It is essential to provide written instructions. The nurse must first assess the patient's ability to read English and his or her reading level. Some resources, such as Medline Plus (www.nlm.nih.gov/medline plus/druginformation.html) offer information in other languages, such as Spanish. If possible, the nurse should allow the patient to administer the drug before he or she is dismissed from the health care facility. The nurse should determine if adequate funds are available to obtain the drug and any necessary supplies. For example, when a bronchodilator is administered by inhalation, a spacer or extender may be required for proper administration. This device is an additional expense. A referral to the social services department of the institution may help the patient when finances are a problem.

DISPLAY 4.1 Possible Causes of Ineffective Therapeutic Regimen Management

Extended therapy for chronic illness causes patient to become discouraged
Troublesome adverse reactions
Lack of understanding of the purpose for the drug
Forgetfulness
Misunderstanding of oral or written instructions on how to take the drug
Weak nurse–patient relationships
Lack of funds to obtain drug
Mobility problems
Lack of family support
Cognitive deficits
Visual or hearing defects

Reprinted with permission from Carpenito-Moyet, L. J. (2006). *Nursing diagnosis: Application to clinical practice* (11th ed., pp. 473–480). Philadelphia: Lippincott Williams & Wilkins.

Figure 4.2 Various types of drug containers may be used to help individuals remember to take their medication at the correct time.

For those who forget to take the drug, the nurse may suggest the use of small compartmentalized boxes marked with the day of the week or time the drug is to be taken (Fig. 4.2). These containers can be obtained from the local pharmacy.

It is important to discuss the drug regimen with the patient, including the reason the drug is to be taken, the times, the amount, adverse reactions to expect, and reactions that should be reported. The patient needs a thorough understanding of the desired or expected therapeutic effect and the approximate time expected to attain that effect. For example, a patient may become discouraged after taking an antidepressant for 5 to 7 days and seeing no response. An explanation that 2 to 3 weeks is required before the depression begins to lift will, in many cases, promote compliance.

It is important to provide ways to minimize adverse reactions if possible. For example, many anticholinergic drugs cause dry mouth. The nurse instructs the patient to take frequent sips of water or suck on hard candy to help minimize the discomfort of a dry mouth.

Frequent follow-up sessions are needed to determine compliance with the drug regimen. If a follow-up visit is not feasible, the nurse considers a telephone call or home visit. It is vital that the nurse strive to develop a caring and nurturing relationship with the patient. Compliance is enhanced when a patient trusts the nurse and feels comfortable confiding any problem encountered during drug therapy.

Deficient Knowledge

Deficient Knowledge is the absence or deficiency of cognitive information on a specific subject. In the case of self-administration of drugs, the patient lacks sufficient knowledge to administer the drug regimen correctly. It may also relate to a lack of interest in learning, cognitive limitation, or inability to remember.

Most patients, at least in the initial treatment stages, lack knowledge about the drug, its possible adverse reactions, and the times and method of administration. At times, the patient may lack knowledge about the disease condition. In these situations, the nurse addresses the specific knowledge deficit (e.g., adverse reactions, disease process, method of administration) in words that the patient can understand. It is important for the nurse to determine first what information the patient is lacking and then plan a teaching session that directly pertains to the specific area of need (see Chapter 5 for more information on patient education). If the patient lacks the cognitive ability to understand the information concerning self-administration of drugs, then one or more of the caregivers should be taught to administer the proper treatment regimen.

Noncompliance

Noncompliance is behavior of the patient or caregiver that fails to coincide with the therapeutic plan agreed on by the patient and the prescribing health care provider. Patients are noncompliant for various reasons, such as a lack of information about the drug, the reason the drug is prescribed, or the expected or therapeutic results. Some patients find the adverse effects so bothersome that they discontinue taking the drug without notifying the prescribing health care provider. Display 4.1 identifies some reasons for this.

Noncompliance also can be the result of anxiety or bothersome side effects. The nurse can relieve anxiety by allowing the patient to express feelings or concerns, by actively listening as the patient verbalizes feelings, and by providing information so that the patient can be fully informed about the drug. Many patients have a tendency to discontinue use of the drug once the symptoms have been relieved. It is important to emphasize the importance of completing the prescribed course of therapy. For example, failure to complete a course of antibiotic therapy may result in recurrence of the infection. To combat noncompliance the nurse finds out the exact reason for the noncompliance, if possible. Factors related to noncompliance are similar to those listed in Display 4.1.

Anxiety

Anxiety is a vague uneasiness or apprehension that manifests itself in varying degrees, from expressions of concern regarding drug regimen to total lack of compliance with the drug regimen. When anxiety is high, the ability to focus on details is reduced. If the patient or caregiver is given information concerning the medication regimen during a high-anxiety state, the patient may not remember the information. This could lead to noncompliance. The anxiety experienced during drug administration depends on the severity of the illness, the occurrence of adverse reactions, and the knowledge level of the patient. Anxiety usually decreases with understanding of the therapeutic regimen. To decrease anxiety before discussing the treatment regimen with the patient, the nurse takes time to talk with and actively listen to the patient. This helps to build a caring relationship and decrease patient anxiety. It is critical for the nurse to allow time for a thorough explanation and to answer all questions and concerns in language the patient can understand.

It is important to identify and address the specific fear and, if possible, reassure the patient that the drug will alleviate the symptoms or, if possible, cure the disorder. The nurse thoroughly explains any procedure. The nurse actively listens and provides encouragement as the patient expresses fears and concerns. Reassurance and understanding on the part of the nurse are required; the amount of reassurance and understanding depends on the individual patient.

Evaluation

Evaluation is a decision-making process that involves determining the effectiveness of the nursing interventions in meeting the expected outcomes. When related to the administration of a drug, this phase of the nursing process is used to evaluate the patient's response to drug therapy. Expected outcomes define the expected behavior of the patient or family that indicates that the problem is being resolved or that progress toward resolution is occurring. Expected outcomes serve as a basis for evaluating the effectiveness of nursing interventions. For example, if the nursing intervention is to "monitor the blood pressure every hour," the expected outcome is that "the patient experiences no further elevation in blood pressure."

The evaluation is complete if the expected outcomes have been accomplished or if progress has occurred. If the outcomes have not been accomplished, different interventions are needed. During the administration of the drug the expected response is alleviation of specific symptoms or the presence of a therapeutic effect. Evaluation also may be used to determine if the patient or family member understands the drug regimen.

To evaluate the patient's response to therapy, and depending on the drug administered, the nurse may check the patient's blood pressure every hour, inquire whether pain has been relieved, or monitor the patient's pulse every 15 minutes. After evaluation, certain other decisions may need to be made and plans of action implemented. For example, the nurse may need to notify the primary health care provider of a marked change in a patient's pulse and respiratory rate after a drug was administered, or the nurse may need to change the bed linen because sweating occurred after a drug used to lower the patient's elevated temperature was administered.

The nurse can evaluate the patient's or family's understanding of the drug regimen by noting if one or both appear to understand the material that has been presented. Facial expression may indicate that one or both do or do not understand what has been explained. The nurse also may ask questions about the information that has been given to evaluate further the patient's or family's understanding.

THINK CRITICALLY: PHARMACOLOGY IN PRACTICE

1. Mr. Phillip, aged 72 years, confides to you that he is not taking the drug prescribed by his primary health care provider. He states he took the drug for a while and then quit. Explain some possible reasons Mr. Phillip could have for not taking his drug. Discuss questions you could ask to assess the reason for Mr. Phillip's noncompliance.

2. Mrs. Moore is 85 years of age and lives alone. She is prescribed several drugs by the primary health care

provider but is worried about taking the drugs and the side effects that might occur. She comes to the outpatient clinic after 1 week, and you learn that she has not filled her prescription and is not taking the drugs. Your nursing diagnosis is Ineffective Therapeutic Regimen Management related to anxiety about taking the prescribed drugs. Determine what information you would seek to obtain from Mrs. Moore. Identify important nursing interventions for this diagnosis.

3. Ms. Chase is receiving three drugs for the treatment of difficulty breathing and swelling of her legs. You are giving these drugs for the first time. Discuss what questions you would ask Ms. Chase to obtain subjective data.

● Test Your Knowledge

1. The nurse greets the new clinic patient, asking "tell me about the pain you are having." This is an example of gathering data. Describe the type of data; select all that apply.

- A. Baseline Assessment
- B. Objective Data
- C. Ongoing Assessment
- D. Subjective Data

2. A patient states that he does not understand why he has to take a specific medication. The most accurate nursing diagnosis for this man would be _____.

- A. Therapeutic regimen management
- B. Anxiety
- C. Noncompliance
- D. Deficient knowledge

3. When the nurse enters subjective data in the patient's record, this information is obtained from _____.

- A. the primary health care provider
- B. other members of the health care team
- C. the patient or family
- D. laboratory and x-ray reports

4. During the evaluation phase of the nursing process, the nurse makes _____.

- A. decisions regarding the effectiveness of nursing interventions based on the outcome
- B. sure nursing procedures have been performed correctly
- C. notations regarding the patient's response to medical treatment
- D. a list of all adverse reactions the patient may experience while taking the drug

● Prepare for the NCLEX

1. The nurse makes a note in the chart that the patient's pain has lessened following a 14-day course of antibiotics. This is an example of which phase of the nursing process?

- A. Assessment
- B. Analysis
- C. Implementation
- D. Evaluation

To check your answers, see Appendix E.

the**Point** *For more NCLEX questions, log on to http://thepoint.lww.com to access more than 1000 questions.*

5

Patient and Family Teaching

LEARNING OBJECTIVES

On completion of this chapter, the student will:

1. Identify important aspects of the teaching/learning process.
2. Discuss the three domains of learning.
3. Discuss important aspects of adult learning.
4. Explain how the nursing process can be used to develop a teaching plan.
5. Identify basic information to consider when developing a teaching plan.
6. Discuss suggestions the nurse can make to the patient to adapt drug administration in the home.

Patient **teaching** is an integral part of nursing. Why are we as nurses concerned about patient teaching? It improves the patient outcome of being able to manage drug therapy in the home or outpatient setting. When a drug is prescribed, the patient and the family must be made aware of all information concerning the drug. The nurse is responsible for supplying the patient with accurate and up-to-date information about the drugs prescribed. The patient must be educated about the drugs he or she has taken while in the hospital and any drugs to be taken after being discharge. Therefore, patient teaching is an ongoing process both while the patient is an inpatient and as the patient prepares for discharge. The teaching/learning process is the means through which the patient is made aware of the drug regimen.

Teaching/Learning Process

Teaching is an interactive process that promotes **learning**. Both the patient and the nurse must be actively involved if teaching is to be effective. Learning is acquiring new knowledge or skills. When learning occurs, the patient's behavior, thinking, or both can change.

A patient must have **motivation** (having a desire or seeing a need) to learn. Motivation depends on the patient's perception of the need to learn. Educating the patient about the disease process improves the patient's motivation to learn. Encouraging patient participation in planning realistic and attainable goals also promotes motivation. If the patient has no motivation, he or she is likely to be noncompliant.

Creating an accepting and positive atmosphere also enhances learning. Physical discomfort negatively affects the patient's concentration and, thus, the ability to learn. Making sure the patient is not in pain is vital to the teaching/learning process.

Three Domains of Learning

Learning occurs in three domains: cognitive, affective, and psychomotor. When developing a teaching plan for the patient, the nurse must consider each domain.

Cognitive Domain

The **cognitive domain** refers to intellectual activities such as thought, recall, decision making, and drawing conclusions. In this domain, the patient uses previous experiences, prior knowledge, and perceptions to give meaning to new information or to modify previous thinking. The nurse makes use of the patient's cognitive abilities when information is given to the patient or caregivers about the disease process, medication regimen, and adverse reactions. The patient uses the cognitive domain to process the information, ask questions, and make decisions.

Affective Domain

The **affective domain** includes the attitudes, feelings, beliefs, trust and opinions of the patient or caregiver. Health care providers often ignore these aspects of patient teaching. It is easy to pull a preprinted teaching outline off the computer or obtain preprinted material. This type of material is often used as a checklist to teach the patient about a drug and the therapeutic regimen. These checklists are useful in helping the nurse remember important aspects to be covered when teaching the patient about the drug and important information to give to the patient for future reference. However, the use of checklists does not take into account the affective domain.

Figure 5.1 The nurse uses skills to build a therapeutic relationship to enhance learning.

Perhaps the most important prerequisite to learning about the patient's affective behavior is to develop a therapeutic relationship with the patient (a relationship that is based on trust and caring). When the nurse takes the time to develop a therapeutic relationship, the patient/family has confidence in the nurse and more confidence in the information conveyed. As shown in Figure 5.1, the nurse approaches the patient and caregivers with respect and encourages the expression of thoughts and feelings. Exploring the patient's beliefs about health and illness enhances the nurse's understanding of the patient's affective behavior.

Psychomotor Domain

The **psychomotor domain** involves learning physical skills (such as injection of insulin) or tasks (such as performing a dressing change). The nurse teaches a task or skill using a step-by-step method. The patient is allowed hands-on practice supervised by the nurse. Mastery of the skill is assessed by having the patient or caregiver perform a return demonstration under the watchful eye of the nurse.

NURSING PROCESS
As a Framework for Patient Teaching

The nursing process is a systematic method of identifying patient health needs, devising a plan of care to meet the identified needs, initiating the plan, and evaluating its effectiveness. This process provides the necessary framework to develop an effective teaching plan. However, the teaching plan differs from the nursing process in that the nursing process encompasses all of the patient's health care needs, whereas the teaching plan focuses primarily on the patient's learning needs. Nurses must be actively involved in teaching if they are to educate their patients about the proper way to take drugs, the possibility of adverse reactions, and the signs and symptoms of toxicity (if applicable).

ASSESSMENT

Assessment is the data-gathering phase of the nursing process. Assessment assists the nurse in choosing the best teaching methods and individualizing the teaching plan. To develop an effective teaching plan, the nurse must first determine the patient's needs. Needs stem from three areas: (1) information the patient or family needs to know about a particular drug; (2) patient's or family member's ability to learn, accept, and use information; and (3) any barriers or obstacles to learning.

Some drugs have simple uses and, therefore, relatively little patient teaching is needed. For example, applying a nonprescription ointment to the skin requires only minimal teaching. Other drugs, such as insulin, require detailed information that may need to be given over several days.

Assessing an individual's ability to learn may be difficult. Not all adults have the same literacy level. The information to be taught should be geared to the patient's educational and reading level. When assessing language and literacy skills, it is important to remember that some patients do not read well. The nurse must carefully assess the patient's ability to communicate. Without accurate communication, learning will not occur. If the patient has a learning impairment, a family member or friend should be included in the teaching process. Most people readily understand what is being taught, but some cannot. For example, a visually impaired patient may be unable to read a label or printed directions supplied by the primary health care provider, pharmacist, or nurse. Another means of teaching will need to be used.

Through assessment, the nurse determines what barriers or obstacles (if any) may prevent the patient or family member from fully understanding the material being presented. Taking into consideration the patient's cultural background is helpful when planning a teaching session. For example, for some patients, an interpreter is needed. In other cultures, a certain individual (e.g., mother or grandmother) is the decision maker in the family. In such cases, it is important for the nurse to include the decision maker and the patient in the teaching session.

NURSING DIAGNOSES (ANALYSIS)

The nursing diagnosis is formulated after analyzing the information obtained during the assessment phase. Examples of nursing diagnoses related to the administration of drugs are listed in the Nursing Diagnosis Checklist.

Nursing Diagnosis Checklist

❏ **Effective Therapeutic Regimen Management**
❏ **Ineffective Therapeutic Regimen Management** related to lack of knowledge
❏ **Deficient Knowledge** related to the drug regimen, possible adverse reactions, disease process, or other factors

The nursing diagnosis *Effective Therapeutic Regimen Management* generally describes a patient who is successfully managing the medication regimen. The nurse uses this nursing diagnosis to enhance the patient's management by teaching the patient possible adverse reactions that could affect his or her health and how to manage them or reduce the potential harmful effects.

The nursing diagnosis *Ineffective Therapeutic Regimen Management* is useful for discharge teaching, especially when the nurse must teach the client how to manage the medication regimen. Often, chronic illness or a variety of health problems may mean that the patient is taking as many as eight or more medications and may have difficulty managing a complicated medication regimen. This diagnosis describes individuals who are having difficulty achieving positive results.

Deficient Knowledge is a nursing diagnosis that may be used when the patient has a deficit in cognitive knowledge or psychomotor skills necessary to administer a medication properly. The defining characteristic would be that the patient would report deficient knowledge or request information, or the patient does not correctly perform a prescribed skill necessary to the medication regimen. It is sometimes difficult to know exactly when to use the nursing diagnosis of Deficient Knowledge because all nursing diagnoses have related patient teaching as part of their nursing interventions. If teaching is related directly to a nursing diagnosis, then incorporate the teaching into the plan.

PLANNING

Planning is the development of strategies to be used in the teaching plan and the selection of information to be taught. Planning begins with the development of a goal and the expected outcomes that the nurse will use to measure attainment of the goal. The nurse then develops a teaching plan based on the expected outcomes using the information gained during the assessment. Display 5.1 identifies important information to include in the teaching plan. Display 5.2 identifies basic information to consider when developing a teaching plan.

Developing an Individualized Teaching Plan

Teaching plans are individualized because patients' needs are not identical. Areas covered in an individualized teaching plan vary depending on the drug prescribed, the primary health care provider's preference for including or excluding specific facts about the drug, and what the patient needs to know to take the drug correctly. Teaching strategies must reflect individual learning needs and ability. For example, a patient who speaks and reads only Spanish will not benefit from discharge instructions given or written in English. Different strategies must be implemented, such as providing instructions written in Spanish or communicating through another nurse who is fluent in the Spanish language.

Selecting Relevant Information

When developing an individualized teaching plan for patients and their families, the nurse must select information relevant to a specific drug, adapt teaching to the individual's level of understanding, and avoid medical terminology unless terms are explained or defined. It is important to remember that repetition enhances learning. Several teaching sessions help the nurse to assess better what the patient is actually learning and provide time for clarification. The patient should be encouraged to ask questions and express feelings.

IMPLEMENTATION

Implementation is the actual performance of the interventions identified in the teaching plan—putting the plan into action. Teaching at an appropriate time for each patient fosters learning. For example, patient teaching is not performed when there are visitors (unless they are to be involved in the administration of the patient's drugs), immediately before discharge from the hospital, or if the patient is sedated or in pain.

Plans for teaching should begin when a patient comes to the hospital, and sessions can begin at a time when the patient is alone, alert, and free of distractions. Teaching continues each day until discharge. The nurse gears teaching to the patient's level of understanding and, when necessary, provides written as well as oral instructions. If a lot of information is given, it is often best to present the material in two or more sessions. Drug administration modifications may be necessary once the patient is at home (see Patient Teaching to Improve Patient Outcomes: Preparing the Patient and Family for Drug Administration in the Home). The nurse keeps these modifications in mind when teaching the patient.

EVALUATION

To determine the effectiveness of patient teaching, the nurse evaluates the patient's knowledge of the material presented. Evaluation can occur in several ways, depending on the nature of the information. For example, if the patient is being taught to administer insulin, a return demonstration by the patient with the nurse observing the patient's technique is an evaluation method.

Questions such as "Do you understand?" or "Is there anything you don't understand?" should be avoided because the patient may feel uncomfortable admitting a lack of understanding. Or, the patient may not feel well enough to be aware of what they don't know. When factual material is being evaluated, the nurse should periodically ask the patient to list or repeat some of the information presented.

DISPLAY 5.1 Important Information to Include in the Teaching Plan

1. Therapeutic response expected from the drug
2. Adverse reactions to expect when taking the drug
3. Adverse reactions to report to the nurse or primary health care provider
4. Dosage and route
5. Any special considerations or precautions associated with the particular drug prescribed
6. Additional education regarding special considerations for certain drugs, such as techniques for giving injections, applying topical patches, or instilling eye drops

DISPLAY 5.2 Basic Considerations When Developing a Drug Teaching Plan

General material to consider when developing a teaching plan includes information on the dosage regimen and adverse reactions, issues relating to family members, and basic information about drugs, drug containers, and drug storage.

Dosage Regimen
The nurse must consider the following general points when teaching about the dosage regimen:

- Capsules or tablets should be taken with water unless the primary health care provider or pharmacist directs otherwise (e.g., take with food, milk, or an antacid). Some liquids, such as coffee, tea, fruit juice, and carbonated beverages, may interfere with the action of certain drugs.
- It is important not to chew capsules before swallowing; they must be swallowed whole. The patient also should not chew tablets unless they are labeled "chewable." This is because some tablets have special coatings that are required for specific purposes, such as proper absorption of the drug or prevention of irritation of the lining of the stomach.
- The dose (amount) of a drug or the time between doses is never increased or decreased unless directed by the primary health care provider.
- A prescription drug or nonprescription drug course of therapy recommended by a primary health care provider is not stopped or omitted except on the advice of the primary health care provider.
- If the symptoms for which a drug was prescribed do not improve, or become worse, the primary health care provider must be contacted as soon as possible, because a change in dosage or a different drug may be necessary.
- If a dose of a drug is omitted or forgotten, the next dose must not be doubled or the drug taken at more frequent intervals unless advised to do so by the primary health care provider.
- All health care workers, including physicians, dentists, nurses, and health personnel, must always be informed of all drugs (prescription and nonprescription) currently being taken on a regular or occasional basis.
- The exact names of all prescription and nonprescription drugs currently being taken should be kept in a wallet or purse for instant reference when seeing a physician, dentist, or other health care provider.
- Check prescriptions carefully when obtaining refills from the pharmacy and report any changes in the prescribed drug (e.g., changes in color, size, shape) to the pharmacist or primary health care provider before taking the drug, because an error may have occurred.
- Wear a MedicAlert bracelet or other type of medical identification when taking a drug for a long time. This is especially important for drugs such as anticoagulants, steroids, oral hypoglycemic agents, insulin, or digitalis. In case of an emergency, the bracelet ensures that medical personnel are aware of health problems and current drug therapy.

Adverse Drug Effects
Information about adverse drug effects of the prescribed drug must be included when the nurse develops a teaching plan for the patient. The nurse should teach the patient the following general points about adverse drug effects:

- All drugs cause adverse reactions (side effects). Examples of some of the more common adverse reactions are nausea, vomiting, diarrhea, constipation, skin rash, dizziness, drowsiness, and dry mouth. Some effects may be mild and subside with time or when the primary health care provider adjusts the dosage. In some instances, mild reactions, such as dry mouth, may have to be tolerated. Some adverse reactions, however, are potentially serious and even life-threatening.
- Adverse reactions are always reported to the primary health care provider as soon as possible.
- Medical personnel must be informed of all drug allergies before any treatment or drug is given.

Family Members
The nurse considers the following points concerning family members when developing a teaching plan:

- A drug prescribed for one family member is never given to another family member, relative, or friend unless directed to do so by the primary health care provider.
- The nurse makes sure that all family members or relatives are aware of all drugs, prescription and nonprescription, that are currently being taken by the patient.

Drugs, Drug Containers, and Drug Storage
The following are important facts about drugs, drug containers, and the storage of drugs that the nurse must consider when developing a teaching plan:

- The term *drug* applies to both nonprescription and prescription drugs.
- A drug must be kept in the container in which it was dispensed or purchased. Some drugs require special containers, such as light-resistant (brown) bottles, to prevent deterioration that may occur on exposure to light.
- The original label on the drug container must not be removed while it is used to hold the drug. All directions on the label (e.g., "shake well before using," "keep refrigerated," "take before meals") must be followed to ensure drug effectiveness.
- Two or more different drugs must never be mixed in one container, even for a brief time, because one drug may chemically affect another. Mixing drugs can also lead to mistaking one drug for another, especially when the size and color are similar.
- All drugs must be kept out of the reach of children and pets.
- Do not expose a drug to excessive sunlight, heat, cold, or moisture, because deterioration may occur.
- When traveling, always carry drugs in their original containers with proper labeling.
- A prescription must never be saved for later use unless the primary health care provider so advises.

Patient Teaching for Improved Patient Outcomes

Preparing the Patient and Family for Drug Administration in the Home

Once the patient is at home, some modifications may be necessary to ensure safe drug administration. The nurse provides written instructions using words that the patient and caregiver can understand. It is important to modify your teaching by using the following suggestions:

✓ For patients taking more than one drug, develop a clear, easy-to-read drug schedule for the patient or caregiver to consult.
✓ Try using a daily calendar as an inexpensive, yet effective, means for scheduling.
✓ If the patient or caregiver has a problem with drug names, refer to the drug by shape or color if appropriate. Another idea is to number bottles and use this number on the drug chart.
✓ Suggest the use of commercially available drug organizers.
✓ If your patient finds it helpful to keep all drugs together, suggest using a small box to hold all the containers and keep it away from children and pets.
✓ If temporary refrigeration is necessary, suggest the use of a small cooler or insulated bag.
✓ If equipment items, such as needles and syringes, are used, suggest keeping all the supplies in one area. If the supplies came in a delivery box, suggest that the patient use it for storage.
✓ Advise the patient to use an approved container with a properly fitting lid for safe disposal of needles and syringes. Return used supplies to the hospital, pharmacy, or local health facility.
✓ Explain the importance of disposing any unused medication in the proper facility and not to flush items into the water supply through a toilet.

Adult Learning

Generally, adults learn only what they feel they need to learn. Adults learn best when they have a strong inner motivation to acquire a new skill or new knowledge. They will learn less if they are passive recipients of "canned" educational content. Adults have a vast array of experiences and knowledge to bring to a new learning experience. Teachers who use this experience will bring about the greatest behavior change. Whereas 83% of adults are visual learners, only 11% learn by listening. Most adults retain the information taught if they are able to "do" something with that new knowledge immediately. For example, in teaching a patient how to administer his or her own insulin, the nurse would demonstrate the technique, allow time for supervised practice, and, as soon as the patient appears ready, allow the patient to prepare and inject the insulin. Most adults prefer an informal learning environ-

ment in which mutual exchange and freedom of expression prevail.

Pharmacology in Practice: A Case Study Approach

Because adults learn best by applying concepts they already know, this book uses a case study approach to help nurses learn about drug information. Throughout the various units, nurses will be introduced to pharmacology concepts by a group of patients from Any Ambulatory Clinic.

Meet the Patients

Lillian Chase is a 36-year-old woman who has had asthma for most of her childhood and adult life. After an accident, she suffered seizures and injuries to both her head and her leg; she now needs knee replacement surgery. Additionally, she is a smoker who has hypertension.

Alfredo Garcia speaks little English. He is seen for an upper respiratory infection, and, upon examination, we discover he lives with hypertension.

Mrs. Moore is 85 years of age and seems forgetful and confused at times. She was able to manage her heart failure until she had a urinary tract infection. Her chest pain is now worse, and she has lots of medications to manage.

Mr. Park, aged 77 years, is staying in a long-term care facility following hip replacement surgery. The stress of the procedure has caused an outbreak of *Herpes zoster* (shingles).

Betty Peterson lives in an apartment. She suffers from aches, pains, and depression.

Mr. Phillip is a 72–year-old widower, and he lives alone. He has both diabetes and early-stage chronic kidney disease. His children do not live close; therefore, in addition to managing his own health care issues, he must learn to live alone and manage a household.

Janna Wong is a 16-year-old high school gymnast. We learn from Janna's mother that she was recovering from mononucleosis before the school year. They both attribute her increased fatigue level to Janna's busy extracurricular schedule.

In each unit, information related to specific types of drugs is discussed and these patients present with both acute and chronic medical problems. The aforementioned patients throughout the units challenge the nurse to think critically about each case to achieve the best management approach. In the Think Critically: Pharmacology in Practice sections of each chapter, different patient scenarios are presented for discussion and reflection to explore the best way to meet patient needs.

THINK CRITICALLY: PHARMACOLOGY IN PRACTICE

1. Typically, patients are seen in the order of their appointment times, if no urgent need presents. As the nurse obtains vital signs in the clinic, information about the urgency of the visit can often be assessed.

Review the list of patients you will learn about in this textbook and prepare a list of questions you would want to ask to help you determine who the primary health care provider should see first in the clinic.

● Test Your Knowledge

1. An interactive process that promotes learning is defined as:
   A. motivation
   B. cognitive ability
   C. psychomotor domain
   – D. teaching

2. When developing a teaching plan, the nurse assesses the affective learning domain, which means that the nurse considers the patient's:
   – A. attitudes, feelings, beliefs, and opinions
   B. ability to perform a return demonstration
   C. intellectual ability
   D. home environment

3. Actual development of the strategies to be used in the teaching plan and selection of the information to be taught occur in this phase of the nursing process:
   A. assessment
   – B. planning
   C. implementation
   D. evaluation

4. A patient is preparing for discharge from the hospital tomorrow. She tells you that she has some questions about the medications that she will be taking at home. She explains that the regimen is complicated, and she is afraid she will not be able to remember when to take her medications. Which of the following nursing diagnoses would be most appropriate for this patient?
   A. Effective Individual Therapeutic Regimen Management
   – B. Ineffective Therapeutic Regimen Management
   C. Deficient Knowledge
   D. Risk for Ineffective Home Management

● Prepare for the NCLEX

1. Unless the primary health care provider or clinical pharmacist directs otherwise, the nurse informs the patient to take oral medications with:
   A. fruit juice
   B. milk
   – C. water
   D. food

To check your answers, see Appendix E.

the**Point**. *For more NCLEX questions, log on to http://thepoint.lww.com to access more than 1000 questions.*

Anti-Infectives

The body is equipped with a natural defense system, our skin and bodily secretions. Infections occur when a pathogenic microorganism (which can cause a disease) breaches the defense system. Microbes enter the body in different ways, such as through a break in the skin, or by ingestion, breathing, or contact with the mucous membranes of the body.

This unit discusses drugs used to kill or retard the growth of microorganisms that invade the body. These are classed together as anti-infective drugs. They include drugs used to treat infections from bacteria, viruses, fungi, and protozoans. Those that work to destroy bacteria are categorized according to the chemical classification of the drug and presented in separate chapters (6 to 10). These drugs include the sulfonamides, penicillins, cephalosporins, tetracycline/aminoglycoside/macrolide/lincosamide group, fluoroquinolone, and miscellaneous anti-infectives.

Drugs that are used against bacteria are either bacteriostatic (they slow or retard the multiplication of bacteria) or bactericidal (they destroy the bacteria). Some drugs are considered *broad spectrum*, meaning they destroy a large number of different types of bacteria from the same strain, such as gram-negative bacteria. Other drugs are specific to particular bacteria and are called *narrow-spectrum* antibiotics.

Bacterial resistance is the ability of bacteria to produce substances that inactivate or destroy the antibiotic. Because bacteria have this ability, many more drugs have been developed in addition to the sulfonamides and penicillins to fight bacterial infections. They include cephalosporins, the tetracycline group, and various other drugs.

To determine if a specific type of bacteria is sensitive to an antibiotic drug, culture and sensitivity tests are performed. A culture is performed by placing infectious material obtained from areas such as the skin, respiratory tract, and blood on a culture plate that contains a special growing medium. This growing medium is "food" for the bacteria. After a specified time, the bacteria are examined under a microscope and identified. The sensitivity test involves placing the infectious material on a separate culture plate and then placing small disks impregnated with various antibiotics over the area. After a specified time, the culture plate is examined. If there is little or no growth around a disk, the bacteria are considered sensitive to that particular antibiotic. Therefore, the infection will be controlled by this antibiotic. If there is considerable growth around the disk, then the bacteria are considered resistant to that particular antibiotic, and the infection will not be controlled by this antibiotic.

Antibiotics can disrupt the normal flora (nonpathogenic microorganisms in the body), causing a secondary infection or superinfection. This new infection is "superimposed" on the original infection. The destruction of large numbers of nonpathogenic bacteria (normal flora) by the antibiotic alters the chemical environment. This allows uncontrolled growth of bacteria or fungal microorganisms that are not affected by the antibiotic being administered. A superinfection may occur with the use of any antibiotic, especially when these drugs are given for a long time or when repeated courses of therapy are necessary. Therefore, patient teaching is essential to ensure the proper course of therapy to reduce these other infections.

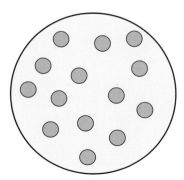

A. Culture plate with small disks containing various antibiotics.

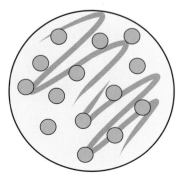

B. Infectious material is spread on the culture plate.

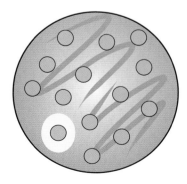

C. After a specific time, the culture plate is inspected. If there is little or no growth around a disk, the bacteria is said to be sensitive to that antibiotic.

Sensitivity testing

Viruses are organisms that do not have a typical cell structure and use host cells to grow and divide. Because viruses use the DNA or RNA of other cells, their ability to change has posed a problem in making drugs to treat viral infections. Recent scientific discoveries have led to the production of more effective antiviral drugs. Chapter 12 covers those drugs that are used to treat viral infections.

Fungal and protozoal infections have played a more prominent role in health issues in recent years because of advances in medical treatments that cause immunosuppression (a reduction in white blood cells). Infections that were minor at one time have become life-threatening in immunosuppressed patients because low numbers of infection-fighting white blood cells leave the body unable to resist the infection. These drugs are covered in Chapter 13.

PHARMACOLOGY IN PRACTICE

Each unit in this book features a specific case study which corresponds to the drug therapy in a selected chapter. In this unit, our patient focus is on Janna Wong, who is a 16-year-old high school gymnast. Janna was brought to the clinic by her mother with complaints of a persistent cough that now is producing slight blood-tinged sputum. When the clinic nurse took her vital signs, they were recorded as a temperature of 101.5° F, pulse = 95, respiration rate of 18 breaths per minute. Janna's mother notes that she was recovering from mononucleosis before the school year started. They both attribute her increased fatigue level to Janna's busy extracurricular schedule. The primary health care provider ordered a chest x-ray which demonstrates fluid accumulation in her right lung base.

After reading the chapters in this unit, you will be reviewing additional medical orders to help in the selection of medications by the primary health care provider. You will formulate a plan with the patient and her family to administer medications properly and help return her to her optimal state of wellness.

Sulfonamides

anorexia
antibacterial
aplastic anemia
bacteriostatic
crystalluria
hypersensitivity
leukopenia

pruritus
Stevens-Johnson syndrome
stomatitis
thrombocytopenia
toxic epidermal necrolysis
urticaria

LEARNING OBJECTIVES

On completion of this chapter, the student will:

1. Discuss the uses, general drug actions, and general adverse reactions, contraindications, precautions, and interactions for the sulfonamides.
2. Discuss important preadministration and ongoing assessment activities the nurse should perform on the patient taking sulfonamides.
3. List nursing diagnoses particular to a patient taking sulfonamides.
4. Discuss ways to promote an optimal response to therapy, how to manage adverse reactions, and important points to keep in mind when educating patients about the use of the sulfonamides.
5. Identify the rationale for increasing fluid intake when taking sulfonamides.
6. Describe the objective signs indicating that a severe skin reaction, such as Stevens-Johnson syndrome, is present.

• SULFONAMIDES

The sulfonamides (sulfa drugs) were the first antibiotic drugs developed that effectively treated infections. Sulfonamides are **antibacterial** agents, meaning they are active against bacteria. Sulfadiazine, sulfisoxazoll, and sulfamethizole are examples of sulfonamide preparations. Although the use of sulfonamides began to decline after the introduction of more effective anti-infectives such as the penicillins and other antibiotics, these drugs remain important for the treatment of certain types of infections.

Actions

The sulfonamides are primarily **bacteriostatic** because of their ability to inhibit the activity of folic acid in bacterial cell metabolism. The sulfonamides are well absorbed by the gastrointestinal (GI) system and excreted by the kidneys (see Chapter 49). They are often used to control infections caused by both gram-positive or -negative bacteria, such as *Escherichia coli*, *Staphylococcus aureus*, and *Klebsiella* and *Enterobacter* species. Once the rate of bacterial multiplication is slowed, the body's own defense mechanisms (white blood cells) are able to rid the body of the invading microorganisms and therefore control the infection.

When sulfasalazine interacts with intestinal bacteria it helps to inhibit the inflammatory process, which is how the drug works to treat ulcerative colitis.

Uses

The sulfonamides are often used according in the treatment of infections such as:

- Urinary tract infections (UTIs) and acute otitis media
- Ulcerative colitis
- Mafenyde (Sulfamylon) and silver sulfadiazine (Silvadene) are topical sulfonamides used in the treatment and prevention of infections in second- and third-degree burns.

Additional uses of the sulfonamides are given in the Summary Drug Table: Sulfonamides.

Adverse Reactions

The sulfonamides are capable of causing a variety of adverse reactions. Some of these are serious or potentially serious; others are mild. **Anorexia** (loss of appetite) is an example of a mild adverse reaction.

Gastrointestinal System Reactions

- Nausea, vomiting, anorexia
- Diarrhea, abdominal pain
- **Stomatitis** (inflammation of the mouth)

In some instances, these may be mild. At other times they may cause serious problems, such as pronounced weight loss, requiring discontinuation of the drug.

Summary Drug Table SULFONAMIDES

Generic Name	Trade Name	Uses	Adverse Reactions	Dosage Ranges
Single Agents				
® sulfadiazine *sul-fah-dye'-ah-zeen*		UTIs, chancroid, acute otitis media, *Hemophilus influenzae* and meningococcal meningitis, rheumatic fever	Vomiting, headache, diarrhea, chills, fever, anorexia, crystalluria, stomatitis, urticaria, pruritus, hematologic changes, Stevens-Johnson syndrome, nausea	Loading dose: 2–4 g orally; maintenance dose: 2–4 g/day orally in 4–6 divided doses
sulfasalazine *sul-fah-sal'-ah-zeen*	Azulfidine, Azulfidine EN-tabs	UTI, acute otitis media, *Hemophilus influenzae*, and meningococcal meningitis	Same as sulfadiazine; may cause skin and urine to turn orange-yellow	Initial therapy: 1–4 g/day orally in divided doses; maintenance dose: 2 g/day orally in evenly spaced doses (500 mg QID)
® sulfisoxazole *sul-fih-sox'-ah-zoll*		Same as sulfadiazine	Same as sulfadiazine	Loading dose: 2–4 g orally; maintenance dose: 4–8 g/day orally in 4–6 divided doses
Urinary Anti-Infective Combinations				
trimethoprim (TMP) and sulfamethoxazole (SMZ) *trye-meth'-oh-prim; sul-fah-meth-ox'-ah-zoll*	Bactrim, Bactrim DS, Septra, Septra DS	Acute bacterial UTI, acute otitis media, traveler's diarrhea due to *Escherichia coli*	Headache, GI disturbances, allergic skin reactions, hematologic changes, Stevens-Johnson syndrome, anorexia, glossitis	160 mg TMP/800 mg SMZ orally q 12 hr; 8–10 mg/kg/day (based on TMP) IV in 2–4 divided doses
Topical Sulfonamide Preparations				
mafenide *maf'-eh-nyde*	Sulfamylon	Second- and third-degree burns	Pain or burning sensation, rash, itching, facial edema	Apply to burned area 1–2 times/day
silver sulfadiazine *sil'-ver sul-fah-dye'-ah-zeen*	Silvadene, Thermazene, SSD (cream)	Same as mafenyde	Leukopenia, skin necrosis, skin discoloration, burning sensation	Same as mafenyde

® This drug should be administered at least 1 hour before or 2 hours after a meal.

Other Reactions

- Chills, fever
- **Crystalluria** (crystals in the urine) Drink lots of water
- Photosensitivity

Various types of **hypersensitivity** (allergic) reaction may be seen during sulfonamide therapy, including **urticaria** (hives), **pruritus** (itching), generalized skin eruptions, or severe reactions leading to potentially lethal conditions such as **toxic epidermal necrolysis** (TEN) or **Stevens-Johnson syndrome** (SJS).

! NURSING ALERT
TEN and SJS are serious and sometimes fatal hypersensitivity reactions. Widespread sloughing of both the skin and mucous membranes can occur. Internal organ involvement can cause death. Patients with SJS may complain of fever, cough, muscular aches and pains, and headache, all of which are signs and symptoms of many other disorders. The nurse must be alert for the additional signs of lesions on the skin and mucous membranes, eyes, and other organs, a diagnostically important indicator of these problems. The lesions appear as red wheals or blisters, often starting on the face, in the mouth, or on the lips, neck, and extremities. These conditions may occur with the administration of other types of drugs. The nurse must notify the primary health care provider and withhold the next dose of the drug. In addition, the nurse must exercise care to prevent injury to the involved areas.

The most frequent adverse reaction seen with the topical application of a sulfonamide is a burning sensation or pain when the drug is applied to the skin. Other possible allergic reactions include rash, itching, edema, and urticaria. Burning, rash, and itching may also be seen with the use of silver sulfadiazine. It may be difficult to distinguish between adverse reactions due to the use of mafenyde or silver sulfadiazine and those that occur from a severe burn injury or from other agents used for the management of burns.

The following hematologic changes may occur during prolonged sulfonamide therapy:

- **Leukopenia**—decrease in the number of white blood cells
- **Thrombocytopenia**—decrease in the number of platelets
- **Aplastic anemia**—anemia due to deficient red blood cell production in the bone marrow

These changes are examples of serious adverse reactions. If any of these occur, discontinuation of sulfonamide therapy may be required.

Contraindications

The sulfonamides are contraindicated in patients with hypersensitivity to the sulfonamides, during lactation, and in children younger than 2 years of age. The sulfonamides are not used near the end (at term) of pregnancy (pregnancy category D). If the sulfonamides are given near the end of pregnancy, significantly high blood levels of the drug may occur, causing jaundice or hemolytic anemia in the neonate. In addition, the sulfonamides are not used for infections caused by group A beta-hemolytic streptococci because the sulfonamides have *not* been shown to be effective in preventing the complications of rheumatic fever or glomerulonephritis.

Precautions

The sulfonamides are used with caution in patients with renal impairment, hepatic impairment, or bronchial asthma.

These drugs are given with caution to patients with allergies. Safety for use during pregnancy has not been established (pregnancy category C, except at term; see above).

Interactions

The following interactions may occur when a sulfonamide is administered with another agent:

Interacting Drug	Common Use	Effect of Interaction
oral anticoagulants	Blood thinner; prevent clot formation	Increased action of the anticoagulant
methotrexate	Immunosuppression and chemotherapy	Increased bone marrow suppression
hydantoins	Anticonvulsants	Increased serum hydantoin level

CHRONIC CARE ALERT

When diabetic patients are prescribed sulfonamides, assess for a possible hypoglycemic reaction. Sulfonamides may inhibit the (hepatic) metabolism of the oral hypoglycemic drugs tolbutamide (Orinase) and chlorpropamide (Diabinese).

HERBAL ALERT

Cranberries and cranberry juice are commonly used remedies for preventing and relieving symptoms of UTIs. The use of cranberries in combination with antibiotics has been recommended by physicians for the long-term suppression of UTIs. Cranberries are thought to prevent bacteria from attaching to the walls of the urinary tract. The suggested dose is 6 ounces of juice twice daily. Extremely large doses can produce GI disturbances, such as diarrhea or abdominal cramping. Although cranberries may relieve symptoms or prevent the occurrence of a UTI, their use will not cure a UTI. If an individual suspects a UTI, medical attention is necessary.

NURSING PROCESS
PATIENT RECEIVING A SULFONAMIDE

ASSESSMENT

Preadministration Assessment
Before the initial administration of the drug, it is important to assess the patient's general appearance and take and record the vital signs. The nurse obtains information regarding the symptoms experienced by the patient and the length of time these symptoms have been present. Many infections are diagnosed and treated in ambulatory settings; therefore it is important for the nurse to ask about self-remedies the patient may have tried before seeing a primary health care provider. Depending on the type and location of the infection or disease, the nurse reviews the results of tests such as a urine culture, urinalysis, complete blood count, intravenous pyelogram, renal function tests, and examination of the stool.

Ongoing Assessment
During the course of therapy, the nurse evaluates the patient at periodic intervals for response to the drug—that is, a relief of symptoms and a decrease in temperature (if it was elevated before therapy started), as well as the occurrence of any adverse reactions.

If fever is present and the patient's temperature suddenly increases or if the temperature was normal and suddenly increases, the nurse instructs the patient to contact the primary health care provider immediately.

The ongoing assessment for patients receiving sulfasalazine for ulcerative colitis includes observation for evidence of the relief or intensification of the symptoms of the disease. The nurse asks the patient to inspect all stool samples and to contact the primary health care provider regarding changes in their number and appearance.

When administering a sulfonamide for a burn, the nurse inspects the burned areas every 1 to 2 hours, because some treatment regimens require keeping the affected areas covered with the mafenyde or silver sulfadiazine ointment at all times. Any adverse reactions should be reported immediately to the primary health care provider.

NURSING DIAGNOSES

Drug-specific nursing diagnoses include the following:

- ❏ **Impaired Urinary Elimination** related to effect on the bladder from sulfonamides
- ❏ **Impaired Skin Integrity** related to burns
- ❏ **Impaired Skin Integrity** related to photosensitivity or severe allergic reaction to the sulfonamides
- ❏ **Risks for (Secondary) Infection** related to lowered white blood cell count resulting from sulfonamide therapy

Nursing diagnoses related to drug administration are discussed in Chapter 4.

PLANNING

The expected patient outcomes depend on the reason for administration of the sulfonamide but may include an optimal response to drug therapy, meeting patient needs related to the management of adverse drug reactions, and an understanding of the therapeutic regimen.

IMPLEMENTATION

Promoting an Optimal Response to Therapy

The patient receiving a sulfonamide drug almost always has an active infection. Some patients may be receiving one of these drugs to prevent an infection (prophylaxis) or as part of the management of a disease such as ulcerative colitis.

Unless the primary health care provider orders otherwise, the nurse gives sulfonamides to the patient whose stomach is empty—that is, 1 hour before or 2 hours after meals. If GI irritation occurs, the nurse may give sulfasalazine with food or immediately after meals.

Sulfasalazine may cause the urine and skin to take on an orange-yellow color; this is not abnormal. Crystalluria may occur during administration of a sulfonamide, although this problem occurs less frequently with some of the newer sulfonamide preparations. Often, this potentially serious problem can be prevented by increasing fluid intake during sulfonamide therapy. It is important to instruct the patient to drink a full glass (8 ounces) of water when taking an oral sulfonamide and to drink at least eight large glasses of water each day until therapy is finished.

Monitoring and Managing Patient Needs

The nurse must observe the patient for adverse reactions, especially an allergic reaction (see Chapter 1). If one or more adverse reactions should occur, the nurse withholds the next dose of the drug and notifies the primary health care provider.

IMPAIRED URINARY ELIMINATION. Because one adverse effect of the sulfonamide drugs is altered elimination patterns, it is important that the nurse help the patient maintain adequate fluid intake and output. The nurse can encourage patients to increase fluid intake to 2000 mL or more per day to prevent crystalluria and stones (calculi) forming in the genitourinary tract, as well as to aid in

removing microorganisms from the urinary tract. It is important to measure and record the patient's intake and output every 8 hours and notify the primary health care provider if the urinary output decreases or the patient fails to increase his or her oral intake.

LIFESPAN ALERT – Gerontology

Because renal impairment is common in older adults, the nurse should administer the sulfonamides with great caution. There is an increased danger of the sulfonamides causing additional renal damage when renal impairment is already present. An increase of fluid intake up to 2000 mL (if the older adult can tolerate this amount) decreases the risk of crystals and stones forming in the urinary tract. The older adult may be hesitant to increase oral fluid intake because of fear of incontinence. It is important for the nurse to assess for this fear and teach the patient when to take fluids to maintain continence and reduce the risk of crystal formation.

IMPAIRED SKIN INTEGRITY: BURN INJURY. When mafenyde or silver sulfadiazine is used in treating burns, the treatment regimen is outlined by the primary health care provider or the personnel in the burn treatment unit. There are various burn treatment regimens, such as debridement (removal of burned or dead tissue from the burned site), special dressings, and cleansing of the burned area. The use of a specific treatment regimen often depends on the extent of the burned area, the degree of the burns, and the physical condition and age of the patient. Other concurrent problems, such as lung damage from smoke or heat or physical injuries that occurred at the time of the burn injury, also may influence the treatment regimen. When instructed to do so, the nurse cleans and removes debris present on the surface of the skin before each application of mafenyde or silver sulfadiazine and applies these drugs with a sterile gloved hand. The drug is applied in a layer approximately 1/16 inch thick; thicker application is not recommended. The patient is kept away from any draft of air because even the slightest movement of air across the burned area can cause pain. It is important to warn the patient that stinging or burning may be felt during, and for a short time after, application of mafenyde. Some burning also may be noted with the application of silver sulfadiazine.

IMPAIRED SKIN INTEGRITY: PHOTOSENSITIVITY. The skin can become more sensitive to sunlight during sulfonamide therapy. Patients should be cautioned to wear protective clothing and sunscreen when outside. In areas where the climate is overcast, solar glare and indirect sunshine can cause a sunburn reaction. The skin should be inspected each shift when treatment is started for signs of sores or blisters indicating the possibility of a severe allergic reaction. The skin and mucous membranes should be inspected for up to 14 days after the end of therapy, the period of time during which reactions can still occur.

RISK FOR SECONDARY INFECTION. The nurse monitors the patient for leukopenia and thrombocytopenia. Leukopenia may result in signs and symptoms of an infection, such as fever, sore throat, and cough. The nurse protects the patient with leukopenia from individuals who have an infection.

Thrombocytopenia is manifested by easy bruising and unusual bleeding after moderate to slight trauma to the skin or mucous membranes. The extremities of the patient with thrombocytopenia are handled with care to prevent bruising. Care is taken to prevent trauma when moving the patient. The nurse inspects the skin daily for the extent of bruising and evidence of exacerbation of existing ecchymotic areas. It is important to encourage the patient to use a soft-bristled toothbrush to prevent any trauma to the mucous membranes of the oral cavity. The nurse reports any signs of leukopenia or thrombocytopenia immediately, because these are indications to stop drug therapy.

Educating the Patient and Family

When a sulfonamide is prescribed for an infection, some outpatients have a tendency to discontinue the drug once symptoms are gone. When teaching the patient and family, the nurse emphasizes the importance of completing the prescribed course of therapy to ensure all microorganisms causing the infection are eradicated. Failure to complete a course of therapy may result in a recurrence of the infection. The nurse should develop a teaching plan to include the following information:

- Take the drug as prescribed.
- Take the drug on an empty stomach either 1 hour before or 2 hours after a meal (exception: sulfasalazine [Azulfidine] is taken with food or immediately after a meal).
- Take the drug with a full glass of water. Do not increase or decrease the time between doses unless directed to do so by the primary health care provider.
- Drink *at least* eight to ten 8-ounce glasses of fluid every day.
- When taking sulfasalazine, the skin or urine may turn orange-yellow; this is not abnormal. Soft contact lenses may acquire a permanent yellow stain. It is a good idea to seek the advice of an ophthalmologist regarding corrective lenses while taking this drug.
- Prolonged exposure to sunlight may result in skin reactions similar to a severe sunburn (photosensitivity reactions). When going outside, cover exposed areas of the skin or apply a protective sunscreen to exposed areas.
- Notify the primary health care provider immediately if the following should occur: fever, skin rash or other skin problems, nausea, vomiting, unusual bleeding or bruising, sore throat, or extreme fatigue.
- Complete the full course of therapy. Do not discontinue this drug (unless advised to do so by the primary health care provider) even though the symptoms of the infection have disappeared.
- Keep all follow-up appointments to ensure the infection is controlled.

EVALUATION

- Therapeutic response is achieved, and there is no evidence of infection.

- Adverse reactions are identified, reported to the primary health care provider, and managed successfully with appropriate nursing interventions:
  - ☑ Patient maintains an adequate fluid intake for proper urinary elimination.
  - ☑ Skin is intact and free of inflammation, irritation, infection, or ulcerations.
- Patient and family demonstrate an understanding of the drug regimen.

THINK CRITICALLY: PHARMACOLOGY IN PRACTICE

1. Mrs. Moore, aged 85 years, has been prescribed a sulfonamide for a UTI and is to take the drug for 10 days. You note that Mrs. Moore seems forgetful and at times confused. Determine what problems might be associated with Mrs. Moore's mental state and her possible noncompliance with her prescribed treatment regimen.

● Test Your Knowledge

1. A nurse working in the clinic asks how the sulfonamides control an infection. The most accurate answer is that these drugs _____.

   A. encourage the production of antibodies
   B. inhibit folic acid metabolism
   C. reduce urine output
   D. make the urine alkaline, which eliminates bacteria

2. Patients receiving sulfasalazine for ulcerative colitis are told that the drug _____.

   A. is not to be taken with food
   B. rarely causes adverse effects
   C. may cause hair loss
   D. may turn the urine an orange-yellow color

3. On an overcast day, the nurse instructs the patient taking sulfonamides to _____.

   A. wear sunscreen
   B. sunbathe without fear of skin reaction
   C. stay indoors with blinds shut
   D. protect feet from harm

4. The nurse can evaluate the patient's response to therapy by asking him if _____.

   A. he completed the entire course of therapy
   B. his symptoms have been relieved
   C. he has seen any evidence of blood in the urine
   D. has experienced any constipation

● Prepare for the NCLEX

1. When mafenyde (Sulfamylon) is applied to a burned area, the nurse _____.

   A. first covers the burned area with a sterile compress
   B. irrigates the area with normal saline solution

C. warns the patient that stinging or burning may be felt

D. instructs the patient to drink two to three extra glasses of water each day

● Calculate Medication Dosages

1. The primary health care provider prescribed sulfasalazine oral suspension 500 mg every 8 hours. The nurse has sulfasalazine oral suspension 250 mg/5 mL on hand. What dosage would the nurse give? 10 mL

2. The primary health care provider orders sulfamethoxazoll 2 g orally initially, followed by 1 g orally two times a day. The nurse has 1000-mg tablets on hand. How many tablets would the nurse give for the initial dose? 2 tabs

To check your answers, see Appendix E.

the**Point** *For more NCLEX questions, log on to http://thepoint.lww.com to access more than 1000 questions.*

Penicillins

anaphylactic shock
angioedema
bactericidal
bacterial resistance
beta-lactam ring
cross-allergenicity
cross-sensitivity
culture and sensitivity test
glossitis

methicillin-resistant *Staphylococcus aureus* (MRSA)
pathogens
penicillinase
phlebitis
prophylaxis
pseudomembranous colitis
superinfection

LEARNING OBJECTIVES

On completion of this chapter, the student will:

1. Identify the uses, general drug actions, and general adverse reactions, contraindications, precautions, and interactions of the penicillins.
2. Identify important preadministration and ongoing assessment activities the nurse should perform on the patient taking penicillin.
3. List nursing diagnoses particular to a patient taking penicillin.
4. Discuss hypersensitivity reactions and pseudomembranous colitis as they relate to antibiotic therapy.
5. Discuss ways to promote optimal response to therapy, nursing actions to minimize adverse effects, and important points to keep in mind when educating patients about the use of penicillins.

• PENICILLINS

The antibacterial properties of natural penicillins were discovered in 1928 by Sir Arthur Fleming while he was performing research on influenza. Ten years later, British scientists studied the effects of natural penicillins on disease-causing microorganisms. However, it was not until 1941 that natural penicillins were used clinically for the treatment of infections. Although used for more than 50 years, the penicillins are still an important and effective group of antibiotics for the treatment of susceptible **pathogens** (disease-causing microorganisms).

Actions

Bacterial cells have select components that differ from human cells, such as specific enzymes and a cell wall. Antibiotics target these differences (Fig. 7.1). The mechanisms of action of the penicillins inhibit the following bacterial cell activities:

• Cell wall synthesis
• DNA or RNA synthesis
• Protein synthesis

There are four groups of penicillins: natural penicillins, penicillinase-resistant penicillins, aminopenicillins, and extended-spectrum penicillins. See the Summary Drug Table: Penicillins for a more complete listing of the penicillins.

Natural Penicillins

Although the sulfonamides were used before the penicillins, the natural penicillins were the first large-scale antibiotics used to combat infection. Enzymes known as penicillin-binding proteins (PBPs) are involved in bacterial cell wall synthesis and cell division. Interference with these processes inhibits cell wall synthesis, causing rapid destruction of the cell. These drugs worked very well because bacteria have a receptor on the cell wall that attracts the penicillin molecule. When the drug attaches to the cell, a portion of the drug molecule (the **beta-lactam ring**) breaks the cell wall and the cell dies (**bactericidal** action). Because the natural penicillins have been used for many years, drug-resistant strains of microorganisms have developed, making the natural penicillins less effective than some of the new antibiotics in treating a broad range of infections. Various types of **bacterial resistance** have developed against the penicillins.

Penicillinase-Resistant Penicillins

One example of bacterial resistance is the ability of certain bacteria to produce **penicillinase**, an enzyme that inactivates penicillin. The penicillinase-resistant penicillins were developed to combat this problem.

Aminopenicillins

The natural penicillins have a fairly narrow spectrum of activity, which means that they are effective against only a few strains of bacteria. Newer, chemically modified aminopenicillins were developed to combat this problem. These

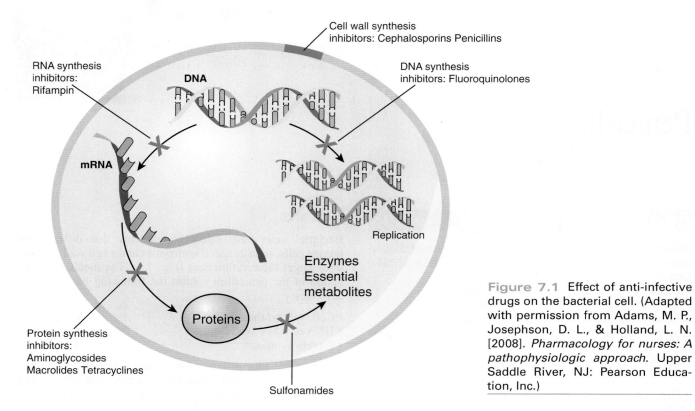

RNA synthesis inhibitors: Rifampin

Cell wall synthesis inhibitors: Cephalosporins Penicillins

DNA synthesis inhibitors: Fluoroquinolones

DNA

mRNA

Replication

Protein synthesis inhibitors: Aminoglycosides Macrolides Tetracyclines

Proteins

Enzymes Essential metabolites

Sulfonamides

Figure 7.1 Effect of anti-infective drugs on the bacterial cell. (Adapted with permission from Adams, M. P., Josephson, D. L., & Holland, L. N. [2008]. *Pharmacology for nurses: A pathophysiologic approach.* Upper Saddle River, NJ: Pearson Education, Inc.)

Summary Drug Table PENICILLINS

Generic Name	Trade Name	Uses	Adverse Reactions	Dosage Ranges
Natural Penicillins (Narrow Spectrum)				
® penicillin G (aqueous) *pen-ih-sill'-in*	Pfizerpen	Infections due to susceptible microorganisms; meningococcal meningitis, septicemia	Glossitis, stomatitis, gastritis, furry tongue, nausea, vomiting, diarrhea, rash, fever, pain at injection site, hypersensitivity reactions, hematopoietic changes	Up to 20–30 million Units/day IV or IM; dosage may also be based on weight
® penicillin G benzathine *ben-zah-theen*	Bicillin C-R, Bicillin L-A, Permapen	Infections due to susceptible microorganisms, syphilis; prophylaxis of rheumatic fever or chorea	Same as penicillin G	Up to 2.4 million Units/day IM
® penicillin G procaine		Moderate to severe infections due to susceptible organisms	Same as penicillin G	600,000–2.4 million Units/day IM
penicillin V	Veetids	Infections due to susceptible organisms	Same as penicillin G	125–500 mg orally q 6 hr or q 8 hr
Semisynthetic Penicillins				
Penicillinase-Resistant Penicillins (Narrow Spectrum) ® dicloxacillin *dye-klox-ah-sill'-in*		Same as penicillin G	Same as penicillin G	125–250 mg orally q 6 hr

(table continues on page 67)

Summary Drug Table PENICILLINS (continued)

Generic Name	Trade Name	Uses	Adverse Reactions	Dosage Ranges
℞ nafcillin *naf-sill'-in*		Same as penicillin G	Same as penicillin G	500 mg IV q 4 hr
℞ oxacillin *ox-ah-sill'-in*	Bactocill	Same as penicillin G	Same as penicillin G	500 mg–1 g orally q 4–6 hr; 250 mg–1 g q 4–6 hr IM, IV
Aminopenicillins (Broad Spectrum) amoxicillin *ah-mox-ih-sill'-in*	Amoxil, Trimox	Same as penicillin G	Same as penicillin G	500–875 mg orally q 12 hr or 250 mg orally q 8 hr
℞ ampicillin *am-pih-sill'-in*	Principen	Same as penicillin G	Same as penicillin G	250–500 mg orally q 6 hr; 1–12 g/day IM, IV in divided doses q 4–6 hr
Penicillin/Beta–Lactamase Inhibitor Combinations ℞ amoxicillin and clavulanate *ah-mox-ih-sill'-in/ klah-vew-lan'-ate*	Augmentin	Same as penicillin G	Same as penicillin G	250 mg orally q 8 hr or 500 mg orally q 12 hr For severe infections: up to 875 mg q 12 hr
℞ ampicillin/sulbactam *am-pih-sill'-in/ sull-bak'-tam*	Unasyn	Same as penicillin G	Same as penicillin G	1.5 g–3 g q 6 hr IM or IV
℞ piperacillin and tazobactam *pih-per-ah-sill'-in/ tay-zoe-bak'-tam*	Zosyn	Same as penicillin G	Same as penicillin G	3.375 g–4.5 g q 6 hr IV
℞ ticarcillin and clavulanate *tye-kar-sill'-in klah-vew-lan'-ate*	Timentin	Same as penicillin G	Same as penicillin G	Up to 3.1 g IV q 4–6 hr or 200–300 mg/kg/day IV in divided doses q 4–6 hr
Extended-Spectrum Penicillins				
℞ carbenicillin indanyl *in-dah-nill*	Geocillin	UTIs caused by *E. coli*, *Proteus*, *Enterobacter*	Same as penicillin G	382–764 mg orally QID
℞ piperacillin *pih-per-ah-sill'-in*		Same as penicillin G	Same as penicillin G	3–4 g q 4–6 hr IV or IM; maximum dosage, 24 g/ day
℞ ticarcillin *tye-kar-sill'-in*	Ticar	Same as penicillin G	Same as penicillin G	150–300 mg/kg/day IV every 3, 4, or 6 hours; maximum dosage IM, 2–g injection

℞ This drug should be administered at least 1 hour before or two hours after a meal.

Penicillins

y

penicillins are a result of chemical treatment of a biological precursor to penicillin. Because of their chemical modifications, they are more slowly excreted by the kidneys and thus have a somewhat wider spectrum of antibacterial activity.

Certain bacteria have developed the ability to produce enzymes called *beta-lactamases*, which are able to destroy the beta-lactam ring of the drug. Fortunately, chemicals were discovered that inhibit the activity of these enzymes. Penicillin–beta-lactamase inhibitor combinations are a type of penicillin with a wider spectrum of antibacterial activity. Examples of these beta-lactamase inhibitors are clavulanic acid, sulbactam, and tazobactam. When these chemicals are used alone, they have little antimicrobial activity. However, when combined with certain penicillins, they extend the spectrum of the penicillin's antibacterial activity. The beta-lactamase inhibitors bind with the penicillin and protect the penicillin from destruction. Examples of combinations of penicillins with beta-lactamase inhibitors are given in Display 7.1; also see the Summary Drug Table: Penicillins for more information on these combinations.

Extended-Spectrum Penicillins

Extended-spectrum penicillins are effective against an even wider range of bacteria than the broad-spectrum penicillins. These penicillins are used to destroy bacteria such as *Pseudomonas*.

Identifying the Appropriate Penicillin: Sensitivity and Resistance

After a culture and sensitivity report is received, the strain of microorganisms causing the infection is known, and the antibiotics to which these microorganisms are sensitive and resistant are identified (see Unit 2 introduction). The primary health care provider then selects the antibiotic to which the microorganism is sensitive, because that is the antibiotic that will be effective in the treatment of the infection.

Penicillins are bactericidal against sensitive microorganisms (i.e., those microorganisms that are affected by a drug) provided there is an adequate concentration of penicillin in the body. The concentration of any drug in the body is referred to as the *blood level*. An inadequate concentration (or inadequate blood level) of penicillin may produce bacteriostatic activity, which may or may not control the infection.

Uses

Infectious Disease
The natural and semisynthetic penicillins are used in the treatment of moderate to mildly severe bacterial infections. Penicillins may be used to treat infections such as:

- Urinary tract infections (UTIs)
- Septicemia
- Meningitis
- Intra-abdominal infections
- Sexually transmitted infections (syphilis)
- Pneumonia and other respiratory infections

Examples of infectious microorganisms (bacteria) that may respond to penicillin therapy include pneumococci

---

DISPLAY 7.1 Penicillin–Beta-Lactamase Inhibitor Combinations

- Augmentin—combination of amoxicillin and clavulanic acid
- Timentin—combination of ticarcillin and clavulanic acid
- Unasyn—combination of ampicillin and sulbactam
- Zosyn—combination of piperacillin and tazobactam

and group A beta-hemolytic streptococci. Because of the increasing resistance of staphylococci to penicillin G, the penicillinase-resistant penicillins are used as initial therapy for any suspected staphylococcal infection until culture and sensitivity results are known.

Prophylaxis

Because penicillin targets bacterial cells, it is of no value in treating viral or fungal infections. However, the primary health care provider occasionally prescribes penicillin as **prophylaxis (prevention)** against a potential secondary bacterial infection that can occur in a patient with a viral infection. In these situations the viral infection has weakened the body's defenses and the person is susceptible to other infections, particularly a bacterial infection. Penicillin also may be prescribed as prophylaxis for a potential infection in high-risk individuals, such as those with a history of rheumatic fever. Penicillin is taken several hours or in some instances days before and after an operative procedure, such as dental, oral, or upper respiratory tract procedures, that can result in bacteria entering the bloodstream. Taking penicillin before and after the procedure will usually prevent a bacterial infection in high-risk patients. Penicillin also may be given prophylactically on a continuing basis to those with rheumatic fever or chronic ear infections.

Resistance to Drugs

When antibiotics are used by one person for a while, or by a group of people that live in close proximity (as in a long-term care facility), drug resistance becomes an issue. Some bacteria may be naturally resistant to an antibiotic, or they may acquire a resistance to the drug. When the susceptible bacteria are destroyed, what remains are the resistant bacteria. As a result, strains of drug-resistant bacteria multiply. These can range from the penicillinase enzyme–producing bacteria to **methicillin-resistant *Staphylococcus aureus* (MRSA)**.

MRSA is a type of bacteria that is resistant to certain antibiotics. These antibiotics include methicillin and other, more common antibiotics, such as oxacillin, penicillin, and amoxicillin. According to the Centers for Disease Control and Prevention in 2008, staphylococcal infections, including MRSA, occur most frequently among persons who are in hospitals and health care facilities (such as skilled nursing facilities and dialysis centers) and who have weakened immune systems. In recent years, outbreaks in the community have heightened the public's awareness of MRSA. Also emerging is a new resistance associated with bacteria that have both natural and acquired resistance. An example is vancomycin-resistant enterococci (VRE). This drug resistance is affecting severely ill, immunocompromised patients in intensive care, transplant, and some cancer treatment units.

Adverse Reactions

Gastrointestinal System Reactions

- **Glossitis** (inflammation of the tongue) when given orally
- Stomatitis (inflammation of the mouth), dry mouth
- Gastritis
- Nausea, vomiting
- Diarrhea, abdominal pain

Administration route reactions include pain at the injection site when given intramuscularly (IM) and irritation of the vein and **phlebitis** (inflammation of a vein) when given intravenously (IV).

Hypersensitivity Reactions

A hypersensitivity (or allergic) reaction to a drug occurs in some individuals, especially those with a history of allergy to many substances. Signs and symptoms of a hypersensitivity to penicillin are highlighted in Display 7.2.

Anaphylactic shock, which is a severe form of hypersensitivity reaction, also can occur (see Chapter 1). Anaphylactic shock occurs more frequently after parenteral administration but can occur with oral use. This reaction is likely to be immediate and severe in susceptible individuals. Signs of anaphylactic shock include severe hypotension, loss of consciousness, and acute respiratory distress. If not immediately treated, anaphylactic shock can be fatal.

Once an individual is allergic to one penicillin, he or she is usually allergic to all of the penicillins. Those allergic to penicillin also have a higher incidence of allergy to the cephalosporins (see Chapter 8). Allergy to drugs in the same or related groups is called **cross-sensitivity** or **cross-allergenicity**.

Superinfections

A **superinfection** can develop rapidly and is potentially serious and even life-threatening. Bacterial superinfections are seen with administration of the oral penicillins and occur in the bowel. Symptoms of bacterial superinfection of the bowel include diarrhea or bloody diarrhea, rectal bleeding, fever, and abdominal cramping. **Pseudomembranous colitis** is a commonly occurring bacterial superinfection.

DISPLAY 7.2 Signs and Symptoms of Hypersensitivity to Penicillin

> Skin rash
> Urticaria (hives)
> Sneezing
> Wheezing
> Pruritus (itching)
> Bronchospasm (spasm of the bronchi)
> Laryngospasm (spasm of the larynx)
> Angioedema (also called angioneurotic edema)—swelling of the skin and mucous membranes, especially around and in the mouth and throat
> Hypotension—can progress to shock
> Signs and symptoms resembling serum sickness—chills, fever, edema, joint and muscle pain, and malaise

NURSING ALERT

Pseudomembranous colitis may occur after 4 to 9 days of treatment with penicillin or as long as 6 weeks after the drug is discontinued.

LIFESPAN ALERT – Gerontology

Older adults who are debilitated, chronically ill, or taking penicillin for an extended period are more likely to develop a superinfection. Pseudomembranous colitis is one type of a bacterial superinfection. This potentially life-threatening problem develops because of an overgrowth of the microorganism *Clostridium difficile*. This organism produces a toxin that affects the lining of the colon. Signs and symptoms include severe diarrhea with visible blood and mucus, fever, and abdominal cramps. This adverse reaction usually requires immediate discontinuation of the antibiotic. Mild cases may respond to drug discontinuation. Moderate to severe cases may require treatment with IV fluids and electrolytes, protein supplementation, and oral vancomycin.

[handwritten margin notes: everything slows down; Normal T maybe 97.5; polypharmacy]

Candidiasis or moniliasis is a common type of fungal superinfection. Fungal superinfections commonly occur in the gastrointestinal (GI) and reproductive systems. Symptoms include lesions of the mouth or tongue, vaginal discharge, and anal or vaginal itching.

Vaginal yeast infections are frequent because a yeast-like fungus normally exists in small numbers in the vagina. The multiplication rate of these microorganisms is normally slowed and kept under control by a strain of bacteria (Döderlein's bacillus) in the vagina. If penicillin therapy destroys these normal microorganisms of the vagina, the fungi become uncontrolled, multiply at a rapid rate, and cause symptoms of the fungal infection candidiasis (or moniliasis).

Other Reactions

Other adverse reactions associated with penicillin include hematopoietic (blood cell) changes:

- Anemia (low red blood cell count)
- Thrombocytopenia (low platelet count)
- Leukopenia (low white blood cell count)
- Bone marrow depression

Contraindications and Precautions

Penicillins are contraindicated in patients with a history of hypersensitivity to penicillin or the cephalosporins.

Penicillins should be used cautiously in patients with renal disease, asthma, bleeding disorders, GI disease, pregnancy (Pregnancy Category C) or lactation (may cause diarrhea or candidiasis in the infant), and history of allergies. Any indication of sensitivity is reason for caution.

Interactions *VIP*

The following interactions may occur when a penicillin is administered with another agent.

*[vertical side tab: Penicillins]*

Interacting Agent	Common Use	Effect of Interaction
oral contraceptives (with estrogen)	Contraception	Decreased effectiveness of contraceptive agent (with ampicillin, penicillin V).
tetracyclines	Anti-infective	Decreased effectiveness of penicillins
anticoagulants	Prevent blood clots	Increased bleeding risks (with large doses of penicillins)
beta-adrenergic blocking drugs	Blood pressure control and heart problems	May increase the risk for an anaphylactic reaction

[handwritten: Use Back up plan]

HERBAL ALERT

Goldenseal (*Hydrastis canadensis*) is an herb found growing in certain areas of the northeastern United States, particularly the Ohio River valley. Goldenseal has been used to wash inflamed or infected eyes and in making yellow dye. There are many more traditional uses of the herb, including as an antiseptic for the skin, mouthwash for canker sores, and the treatment of sinus infections and digestive problems such as peptic ulcers and gastritis. In the 19th century, goldenseal was touted as an "herbal antibiotic" for treating gonorrhea and UTIs. Though used over time by American Indian tribes as an insect repellent, stimulant, and diuretic, there is no scientific evidence to support its benefit for these purposes. Another myth surrounding goldenseal's use is that taking the herb masks the presence of illicit drugs in the urine. Evidence does support the use of goldenseal to treat diarrhea caused by bacteria or intestinal parasites, such as *Giardia*. The herb is contraindicated during pregnancy and in patients with hypertension. Adverse reactions are rare when the herb is used as directed. However, this herb should not be taken for more than a few days to 1 week.

NURSING PROCESS
PATIENT RECEIVING PENICILLIN

ASSESSMENT

Preadministration Assessment
Before administering the first dose of penicillin, the nurse obtains or reviews the patient's general health history. The health history includes an allergy history, a history of all medical and surgical treatments, a drug history, and the current symptoms of the infection. If the patient has a history of allergy—particularly a drug allergy—the nurse must explore this area to ensure the patient is not allergic to penicillin or a cephalosporin.

The nurse should take and record vital signs. When appropriate, it is important to obtain a description of the signs and symptoms of the infection from the patient or family. The nurse assesses the infected area (when possible) and records findings on the patient's chart. It is important to describe accurately any signs and symp-toms related to the patient's infection, such as color and type of drainage from a wound, pain, redness and inflammation, color of sputum, or presence of an odor. In addition, the nurse should note the patient's general appearance. A **culture and sensitivity test** is almost always ordered, and the nurse should obtain the results before giving the first dose of penicillin.

Ongoing Assessment
The nurse evaluates the patient daily for a response to therapy, such as a decrease in temperature, the relief of symptoms caused by the infection (such as pain or discomfort), an increase in appetite, and a change in the appearance or amount of drainage (when originally present). Once an infection is controlled, patients often look better and even state that they feel better. It is important to record these evaluations on the patient's chart. The nurse notifies the primary health care provider if signs and symptoms of the infection appear to worsen.

Additional culture and sensitivity tests may be performed during therapy because microorganisms causing the infection may become resistant to penicillin, or a superinfection may occur. A urinalysis, complete blood count, and renal and hepatic function tests also may be performed at intervals during therapy.

NURSING ALERT

The nurse should observe the patient closely for a hypersensitivity reaction, which may occur any time during therapy with the penicillins. If it should occur, it is important to contact the primary health care provider immediately and withhold the drug until the patient is seen by the primary health care provider.

NURSING DIAGNOSES

Drug-specific nursing diagnoses include the following:

- ❏ **Impaired Skin Integrity** related to hypersensitivity to penicillin
- ❏ **Risk for Ineffective Respiratory Function** related to an allergic reaction to penicillin
- ❏ **Diarrhea** related to a bacterial secondary infection or superinfection
- ❏ **Impaired Oral Mucous Membranes** related to a secondary bacterial or fungal infection
- ❏ **Impaired Comfort: Increased Fever** related to ineffectiveness of penicillin against the infection

Nursing diagnoses related to drug administration are discussed in Chapter 4.

PLANNING

The expected outcomes for the patient depend on the reason for administering penicillin but may include an optimal response to drug therapy, meeting patient needs related to management of common adverse reactions, and an understanding of the therapeutic regimen.

IMPLEMENTATION

Promoting Optimal Response to Therapy: Proper Administration

The results of a culture and sensitivity test take several days, because time must be allowed for the bacteria to grow on the culture media. However, infections are treated as soon as possible. In a few instances, the primary health care provider may determine that a penicillin is the treatment of choice until the results of the culture and sensitivity tests are known. In many instances, the primary health care provider selects a broad-spectrum antibiotic for initial treatment because of the many penicillin-resistant strains of microorganisms.

Adequate blood levels of the drug must be maintained for the agent to be effective. Accidental omission or delay of a dose results in decreased blood levels, which will reduce the effectiveness of the antibiotic. It is best to give oral penicillins on an empty stomach, 1 hour before or 2 hours after a meal. Penicillin V and amoxicillin may be given without regard to meals.

Penicillin is ordered in units or milligrams. The exact equivalency usually is stated on the container or package insert. In most health care facilities, the drug is prepared in the pharmacy and delivered to the nurse for administration. When this service is not available in preparing a parenteral form of penicillin, the nurse should shake the vial thoroughly before withdrawing the drug to ensure even distribution of the drug in the solution. Some forms of penicillin are in powder or crystalline form and must be made into a liquid (reconstituted) before being withdrawn from the vial. The manufacturer's directions regarding reconstitution are printed on the label or package insert. The manufacturer indicates the type of diluent (a solution compatible with the drug) to be used when reconstituting a specific drug. Some powdered or crystalline drugs, when reconstituted with a given amount of diluent, may yield slightly more or less than the amount of the diluent added to the vial. If there is any question regarding the reconstitution of any drug, the nurse consults with a clinical pharmacist.

When administering penicillin IM, the nurse warns the patient that there may be a stinging or burning sensation at the time the drug is injected into the muscle. Penicillin solutions are often thick or viscous. Discomfort at the time of injection occurs because the drug is irritating to the tissues. The nurse inspects previous areas used for injection for continued redness, soreness, or other problems. It is important to inform the primary health care provider if previously used areas for injection appear red or the patient reports pain in the area.

> **⚠ NURSING ALERT**
>
> The nurse questions the patient about allergy to penicillin before administering the first dose, even when an accurate drug history has been taken. It is important to tell patients that the drug they are receiving is penicillin, because information regarding a drug allergy may have been forgotten at the time the initial drug history was obtained. If a patient states he or she is allergic to penicillin or a cephalosporin, the nurse withholds the drug and contacts the primary health care provider.

Monitoring and Managing Patient Needs

IMPAIRED SKIN INTEGRITY. Dermatologic reactions such as hives, rashes, and skin lesions can occur with the administration of penicillin. Treatment of minor hypersensitivity reactions may include administration of an antihistamine such as diphenhydramine (Benadryl) for a rash or itching. In mild cases, or where the benefit of the drug outweighs the discomfort of skin lesions, the nurse administers frequent skin care. Emollients, antipyretic creams, or a topical corticosteroid may be prescribed to promote comfort. Harsh soaps and perfumed lotions are avoided. The nurse instructs the patient to avoid rubbing the area and not to wear rough or irritating clothing. It is important to report a rash or hives to the primary health care provider because this may be a precursor to a severe anaphylactic reaction (see section on Hypersensitivity Reactions). In severe cases, the primary health care provider may discontinue the penicillin therapy.

RISK FOR INEFFECTIVE RESPIRATORY FUNCTION. Major hypersensitivity reactions, such as bronchospasm, laryngospasm, hypotension, and **angioedema**, require immediate treatment with drugs such as epinephrine, cortisone, or an IV antihistamine. When respiratory difficulty occurs, a tracheostomy may need to be performed.

> **⚠ NURSING ALERT**
>
> After administering penicillin IM in the outpatient setting, the nurse asks the client to wait in the area for at least 30 minutes. Anaphylactic reactions are most likely to occur within 30 minutes after injection.

DIARRHEA. Diarrhea may be an indication of a superinfection of the GI tract or pseudomembranous colitis. The nurse inspects all stools and notifies the primary health care provider if diarrhea occurs, because it may be necessary to stop the drug. If diarrhea does occur and there appears to be blood and mucus in the stool, it is important to save a sample of the stool and test for occult blood using a test such as Hemoccult. If the stool tests positive for blood, the nurse saves the sample for possible further laboratory analysis.

The nurse observes the patient for other symptoms of a bacterial or fungal superinfection in the vaginal or anal area, such as pain or itching. It is important to report any signs and symptoms of a superinfection to the primary health care provider before administering the next dose of the drug. When symptoms are severe, additional treatment measures may be necessary, such as administration of an antipyretic drug for fever or an antifungal drug.

IMPAIRED ORAL MUCOUS MEMBRANES. The administration of oral penicillin may result in a fungal superinfection in the oral cavity. This condition is characterized by varying degrees of oral mucous membrane inflammation, swollen and red tongue, swollen gums, and pain in the mouth and throat. To detect this problem early, the nurse inspects the patient's mouth daily for evidence of glossitis, sore tongue, ulceration, or a black, furry tongue. The nurse can explain that, if the diet permits, yogurt, buttermilk, or *Acidophilus* capsules may be taken to reduce the risk of fungal superinfection.

The nurse inspects the mouth and gums often and gives frequent mouth care with a nonirritating solution. A soft-bristled toothbrush is used when brushing is needed. A nonirritating soft diet may be required. The nurse monitors the dietary intake to ensure the patient is receiving adequate nutrition. Antifungal agents or local anesthetics are sometimes recommended to soothe the irritated membranes.

IMPAIRED COMFORT: INCREASED FEVER. The nurse takes vital signs every 4 hours, or more often if necessary. It is important to report any increase in temperature to the primary health care provider, because additional treatment measures, such as administration of an antipyretic drug or change in the drug or dosage, may be necessary. An increase in body temperature several days after the start of therapy may indicate a secondary bacterial infection or failure of the drug to control the original infection. On occasion, the fever may be caused by an adverse reaction to the penicillin. In these cases, the fever can usually be managed by using an antipyretic drug.

Educating the Patient and Family

Any time a drug is prescribed for a patient, the nurse is responsible for ensuring that the patient has a thorough understanding of the drug, the treatment regimen, and adverse reactions. Some patients do not adhere to the prescribed drug regimen for a variety of reasons, such as failure to comprehend the prescribed regimen or failure to understand the importance of continued and uninterrupted therapy. The nurse describes the drug regimen and stresses the importance of continued and uninterrupted therapy when teaching the patient who is prescribed an antibiotic.

The nurse provides the following information to patients prescribed an antibiotic:

- Prophylaxis—Take the drug as prescribed until the primary health care provider discontinues therapy.
- Infection—Complete the full course of therapy. Do not stop taking the drug, even if the symptoms have disappeared, unless directed to do so by the primary health care provider.
- Take the drug at the prescribed times of day because it is important to keep an adequate amount of drug in the body throughout the entire 24 hours of each day.
- Penicillin (oral)—Take the drug on an empty stomach either 1 hour before or 2 hours after meals (exceptions: penicillin V and amoxicillin).
- Take each dose with a full 8-ounce glass of water.
- Oral suspensions—Keep the container refrigerated (if so labeled), shake the drug well before pouring (if so labeled), and return the drug to the refrigerator immediately after pouring the dose. Drugs that require refrigeration lose their potency when kept at room temperature. A small amount of the drug may be left

after the last dose is taken. Discard any remaining drug, because the drug (in suspension form) begins to lose its potency after a few weeks (7 to 14 days).
- To reduce the risk of superinfection during antibiotic therapy, take yogurt, buttermilk, or *Acidophilus* capsules.
- If you are a woman who has been prescribed ampicillin and penicillin V and who takes birth control pills containing estrogen, use additional contraception measures.
- Notify the primary health care provider immediately should one or more of the following occur: skin rash; hives (urticaria); severe diarrhea; vaginal or anal itching; black, furry tongue; sores in the mouth; swelling around the mouth or eyes; breathing difficulty; or GI disturbances such as nausea, vomiting, and diarrhea. Do not take the next dose of the drug until the problem has been discussed with the primary health care provider.
- Notify the primary health care provider if the symptoms of the infection do not improve or if the condition becomes worse.
- Never skip doses or stop therapy unless told to do so by the primary health care provider (see Patient Teaching for Improved Patient Outcomes: Preventing Anti-Infective Resistance). When a penicillin is to be taken for a long time for prophylaxis, you may feel well despite the need for long-term antibiotic therapy. There may be a tendency to omit one or more doses or even neglect to take the drug for an extended time.

Patient Teaching for Improved Patient Outcomes

Preventing Anti-Infective Resistance

The nurse:

✓ Reviews the reason for the drug and the prescribed drug regimen, including drug name, correct dose, and frequency of administration.

✓ Stresses the importance of continued and uninterrupted therapy, even if the patient feels better after a few doses and symptoms have disappeared.

✓ Instructs the patient to continue taking the drug until the drug is finished or the prescriber discontinues therapy.

✓ Urges the patient and family to discard any unused drug once therapy is discontinued or completed.

✓ Warns the patient not to use any leftover antibiotic or to take another family member's antibiotic as self-treatment for a suspected infection.

✓ Reviews the possible adverse reactions and the signs and symptoms of a new infection or of a worsening infection, both verbally and in writing.

✓ Instructs the patient and family to notify the health care provider at once should the patient experience any adverse reactions or signs and symptoms of infection.

EVALUATION

- Therapeutic response is achieved, and there is no evidence of infection.
- Adverse reactions are identified, reported to the primary health care provider, and managed successfully with appropriate nursing interventions:
  ☑ Skin is intact and free of infection.
  ☑ Lungs function effectively.
  ☑ Patient reports adequate bowel movements.
  ☑ Mucous membranes are moist and intact.
  ☑ Patient reports comfort without fever.
- Patient and family demonstrate understanding of the drug regimen.

THINK CRITICALLY: PHARMACOLOGY IN PRACTICE

1. Janna Wong's chest x-ray indicates an infection is present in her lungs, and the primary health care provider has diagnosed pneumococcal pneumonia. As the nurse, what other diagnostic tests do you anticipate the primary health care provider would typically order on this patient before determining the type of anti-infective to order?

   She is started on a course of oral amoxicillin. Her mother states that when she had to take penicillin she could not eat afterward, so she asks if a special note can be written to get her out of class to take her medications between meals. What should the nurse's response be?

   Discuss the importance of taking the entire course of the medication no matter whether Janna feels better before it is complete.

2. After administering IM penicillin to a patient in the ambulatory care clinic, you request that the patient wait about 30 minutes before leaving. The patient is reluctant to stay, saying that she has a busy schedule. Discuss how you would handle this situation.

● Test Your Knowledge

1. Bacterial cells are different from human cells because they

   A. have a cell wall
   B. synthesize DNA and RNA
   C. contain a beta-lactam ring
   D. contain proteins

2. A patient taking oral penicillin reports he has a sore mouth. On inspection, the nurse notes a black, furry tongue and bright red oral mucous membranes. The primary care provider is notified immediately, because these symptoms may be caused by

   A. a vitamin C deficiency
   B. a superinfection
   C. dehydration
   D. poor oral hygiene

3. The nurse correctly administers penicillin V

   A. 1 hour before or 2 hours after meals
   B. without regard to meals
   C. with meals to prevent GI upset
   D. every 3 hours around the clock

4. After administering penicillin in an outpatient setting, the nurse

   A. asks the patient to wait 10 to 15 minutes before leaving the clinic
   B. instructs the patient to report any numbness or tingling of the extremities
   C. keeps pressure on the injection site for 10 minutes
   D. asks the patient to wait in the area for at least 30 minutes

● Prepare for the NCLEX

1. When reviewing a patient's culture and sensitivity test results, the nurse learns that the bacteria causing the infection are sensitive to penicillin. The nurse interprets this result to mean that

   A. the patient is allergic to penicillin
   B. penicillin will be effective in treating the infection
   C. penicillin will not be effective in treating the infection
   D. the test must be repeated to obtain accurate results

● Calculate Medication Dosages

1. A patient is prescribed amoxicillin for oral suspension. The drug is reconstituted to a solution of 250 mg/5 mL. The caregiver insists on using a spoon to administer the drug. Answer the following questions: How much amoxicillin will 1 teaspoon contain? The primary health care provider prescribes 500 mg. How many milliliters (mL) will the nurse administer?

2. The primary care provider orders 500 mg of Augmentin oral suspension. Read the label below to answer the following questions:

   A. How much water will be required for reconstitution?
   B. Describe the process you would go through to reconstitute this drug.
   C. When reconstituted, what will be the strength of the solution?

To check your answers, see Appendix E.

the**Point** *For more NCLEX questions, log on to http://thepoint.lww.com to access more than 1000 questions.*

Penicillins

Cephalosporins

disulfiram-like reaction   otitis media
malaise   perioperative period
nephrotoxicity   thrombophlebitis

LEARNING OBJECTIVES

On completion of this chapter, the student will:

1. Explain the difference between the first-, second-, third-, and fourth-generation cephalosporins.
2. Discuss uses, general drug action, adverse reactions, contraindications, precautions, and interactions associated with cephalosporins.
3. Discuss important preadministration and ongoing assessment activities the nurse should perform on the patient taking cephalosporins.
4. List nursing diagnoses particular to a patient taking cephalosporins.
5. Discuss ways to promote an optimal response to therapy, how to manage common adverse reactions, special considerations related to administration, and important points to keep in mind when educating patients about the use of the cephalosporins.

• CEPHALOSPORINS

The cephalosporins are a valuable group of drugs that are effective in the treatment of infection with almost all of the strains of bacteria affected by the penicillins, as well as some strains of bacteria that have become resistant to penicillin. Cephalosporins are structurally and chemically related to penicillin.

The cephalosporins are divided into first-, second-, third-, and fourth-generation drugs. Particular cephalosporins also may be differentiated within each group according to the microorganisms that are sensitive to the drug. In general, progression from the first-generation to the fourth-generation drugs shows an increase in the sensitivity of gram-negative microorganisms and a decrease in the sensitivity of gram-positive microorganisms. For example, a first-generation cephalosporin would be more useful against gram-positive microorganisms than would a third-generation cephalospo-

rin. This scheme of classification is becoming less clearly defined as newer drugs are introduced. The fourth generation of cephalosporins has a broader spectrum and longer duration of resistance to beta-lactamase (see Chapter 7). These drugs are used to treat urinary tract and skin infections and hospital-acquired pneumonias. Examples of first-, second-, third-, and fourth-generation cephalosporins are listed in Display 8.1. For a more complete listing, see the Summary Drug Table: Cephalosporins.

Actions

Cephalosporins have a beta-lactam ring and target the bacterial cell wall, making it defective and unstable. This action is similar to the action of penicillin. The cephalosporins are usually bactericidal.

Uses

The cephalosporins are used in the treatment of infections caused by bacteria, including:

- Respiratory infections   Pheumonia
- **Otitis media** (ear infection)
- Bone/joint infections
- Genitourinary tract and other infections caused by bacteria
  Pre-op, Intra OP, Post op

Culture and sensitivity tests (see Chapter 7) are performed whenever possible to determine which antibiotic, including a cephalosporin, will best control an infection caused by a specific strain of bacteria.

Cephalosporins also may be used throughout the **perioperative period**—that is, during the preoperative, intraoperative, and postoperative periods—to prevent infection in patients having surgery on a contaminated or potentially contaminated area, such as the gastrointestinal (GI) tract or

DISPLAY 8.1 Examples of First-, Second-, Third-, and Fourth-Generation Cephalosporins

- First generation—cephalexin (Keflex), cefazolin (Ancef)
- Second generation—cefaclor (Raniclor), cefoxitin (Mefoxin), cefuroxime (Zinacef)
- Third generation—cefoperazone (Cefobid), cefotaxime (Claforan), ceftriaxone (Rocephin)
- Fourth generation—cefepime (Maxipime)

Generic Name	Trade Name	Uses	Adverse Reactions	Dosage Ranges
First-Generation Cephalosporins				
cefadroxil *sef-ah-drox'-ill*	Duricef	Infections due to susceptible microorganisms	Nausea, vomiting, diarrhea, hypersensitivity reactions, superinfection, nephrotoxicity, headache, Stevens-Johnson syndrome, pseudomembranous colitis	1–2 g/day orally in divided doses
cefazolin *she-fah'-zoe-lin*	Ancef, Kefzol	Same as cefadroxil; perioperative prophylaxis	Same as cefadroxil	250 mg–1 g IM, IV q 6–12 hr Perioperative: 0.5–1 g IM, IV
cephalexin *sef'-ah-lex-in*	Keflex	Same as cefadroxil	Same as cefadroxil	1–4 g/day orally in divided doses
Second-Generation Cephalosporins				
cefaclor *sef'-ah-klor*	Raniclor	Infections due to susceptible microorganisms	Nausea, vomiting, diarrhea, hypersensitivity reactions, nephrotoxicity, headache, hematologic reactions	250 mg orally q 8 hr
cefotetan *sef-oh-tee'-tan*		Same as cefaclor; perioperative prophylaxis	Same as cefaclor	1–2 g IM, IV q 12 hr for 5–10 days; perioperative; 1–2 g in a single dose IV
cefoxitin *sef-ox'-ih-tin*	Mefoxin	Same as cefaclor; perioperative prophylaxis	Same as cefaclor	1–2 g IV q 6–8 hr
cefprozil *sef-proe'-zil*	Cefzil	Same as cefaclor	Same as cefaclor	250–500 mg orally q 12 hr
cefuroxime *sef-yoor-ox'-eem*	Ceftin, Zinacef	Same as cefaclor; preoperative prophylaxis	Same as cefaclor	250 mg orally BID; 750 mg–1.5 g IM or IV q 8 hr
Third-Generation Cephalosporins				
cefdinir *sef'-din-eer*	Omnicef	Same as cefaclor	Same as cefaclor	300 mg orally q 12 hr or 600 mg orally q 24 hr orally
cefditoren *sef'-dih-tore-en*	Spectracef	Same as cefaclor	Same as cefaclor	200–400 mg orally BID
cefixime *she-fix'-eem*	Suprax	Same as cefaclor	Same as cefaclor	400 mg/day orally
cefoperazone *sef-oh-per'-ah-zone*	Cefobid	Same as cefaclor	Same as cefaclor	2–4 g/day IM, IV in equally divided doses
cefotaxime *sef-oh-taks'-eem*	Claforan	Same as cefaclor; perioperative prophylaxis	Same as cefaclor	2–8 g/d IM, IV in equally divided doses q 6–8 hr; maximum 12 g/day
cefpodoxime *sef-poe-dox'-eem*	Vantin	Same as cefaclor; sexually transmitted infection treatment	Same as cefaclor	100–400 mg/day orally in equally divided doses
ceftazidime *sef-taz'-ih-deem*	Fortaz	Same as cefaclor	Same as cefaclor	250 mg–2g IV, IM q 8–12 hr
® ceftibuten *sef-tah-byoo'-ten*	Cedax	Same as cefaclor	Same as cefaclor	400 mg/daily orally
ceftriaxone *sef-try-ax'-on*	Rocephin	Same as cefaclor; perioperative prophylaxis; gonorrhea	Same as cefaclor	1–2 g/d IM, IV q 12 hr maximum 4 g/day; perioperative, 1 g IV; gonorrhea, 250 mg IM as a single dose
Fourth-Generation Cephalosporins				
cefepime *sef'-ah-pime*	Maxipime	Same as cefaclor; febrile neutropenia	Same as cefaclor	0.5–2 g IV, IM q 12 hr

® This drug should be administered at least 1 hour before or 2 hours after a meal.

vagina. In some instances, a specific drug may be recommended for postoperative prophylactic use only.

Adverse Reactions

Gastrointestinal System Reactions

- Nausea
- Vomiting
- Diarrhea

Other Reactions

- Headache
- Dizziness
- **Malaise**   *discomfort, un easiness*
- Heartburn
- Fever
- **Nephrotoxicity** (damage to the kidneys by a toxic substance)   *poison*
- Hypersensitivity (allergic) reactions—may occur with administration of the cephalosporins and may range from mild to life-threatening. Mild hypersensitivity reactions include pruritus, urticaria, and skin rashes; the more serious reactions include Stevens-Johnson syndrome and hepatic and renal dysfunction.
- Aplastic anemia (anemia due to deficient red blood cell production)
- Toxic epidermal necrolysis (death of the epidermal layer of the skin)

> **NURSING ALERT**
> Because of the close relationship of the cephalosporins to penicillin, a patient who is allergic to penicillin also may be allergic to the cephalosporins. Approximately 10% of the people allergic to a penicillin drug are also allergic to a cephalosporin drug.

Administration route reactions include pain, tenderness, and inflammation at the injection site when given intramuscularly (IM), and phlebitis or **thrombophlebitis** (inflammation of a vein with formation of a clot in the vein) along the vein when given intravenously (IV). Therapy with cephalosporins may result in a bacterial or fungal superinfection. Diarrhea may be an indication of pseudomembranous colitis, which is one type of bacterial superinfection (see Chapter 7).

Contraindications and Precautions

The nurse should not administer cephalosporins if the patient has a history of allergies to cephalosporins or penicillins.

Cephalosporins should be used cautiously in patients with renal disease, hepatic impairment, bleeding disorder, pregnancy (pregnancy category B), and known penicillin allergy.

Interactions

The following interactions may occur when a cephalosporin is administered with another agent:

Interacting Drug	Common Use	Effect of Interaction
aminoglycosides	Anti-infective	Increased risk for nephrotoxicity
oral anticoagulants	Blood thinner	Increased risk for bleeding
loop diuretics	Hypertension, reduce edema	Increased cephalosporin blood level

probenecid (Benemid, used for gout pain) will increase the levels of most cephalosporins (*except* cefoperazone, ceftazidime, and ceftriaxone).

> **NURSING ALERT**
> A **disulfiram-like reaction** may occur if alcohol is consumed within 72 hours after administration of certain cephalosporins (i.e., cefamandole, cefoperazone, and cefotetan). Symptoms of a disulfiram-like reaction (associated with the use of disulfiram [Antabuse], a drug used to treat alcoholism) include flushing, throbbing in the head and neck, respiratory difficulty, vomiting, sweating, chest pain, and hypotension. Severe reactions may cause arrhythmias and unconsciousness.

NURSING PROCESS
PATIENT RECEIVING A CEPHALOSPORIN

ASSESSMENT

Preadministration Assessment
Before the administration of the first dose of a cephalosporin, it is important to obtain a general health history. The health history includes an allergy history, a history of all medical and surgical treatments, a drug history, and the current symptoms of the infection. If the patient has a history of allergy, particularly a drug allergy, the nurse explores this area to ensure that the patient is not allergic to a cephalosporin. Patients with a history of an allergy to penicillin may also be allergic to a cephalosporin. If an allergy to either of these drug groups is suspected, the nurse informs the primary health care provider of this before the first dose of the drug is given. The nurse should check to be sure any culture and sensitivity tests are done before the first dose of the drug is administered. Liver and kidney function tests may be ordered by the primary health care provider.

Ongoing Assessment
An ongoing assessment is important in evaluating the patient's response to therapy, such as a decrease in temperature, the relief of symptoms caused by the infection (e.g., pain or discomfort), an increase in appetite, and a change in the appearance or amount of drainage (when originally present). The nurse notifies the primary health care provider if signs of the infection appear to worsen. The nurse checks the patient's skin regularly for rash and is alert for any loose stools or diarrhea.

NURSING DIAGNOSES

Drug-specific nursing diagnoses include the following:

❏ **Risk for Impaired Skin Integrity** related to hypersensitivity to cephalosporin therapy
❏ **Risk for Impaired Comfort: Increased Fever** related to ineffectiveness of cephalosporin against the infection
❏ **Impaired Urinary Elimination** related to nephrotoxic effects
❏ **Diarrhea** related to superinfection

Nursing diagnoses related to drug administration are discussed in Chapter 4.

PLANNING

The expected outcomes for the patient depend on the reason for administration but may include an optimal response to therapy (infectious process controlled), meeting patient needs related to the management of adverse drug reactions, and an understanding of the therapeutic regimen.

IMPLEMENTATION

Promoting an Optimal Response to Therapy

ORAL ADMINISTRATION. The nurse must question the patient about allergy to cephalosporins or the penicillins before administering the first dose, even when an accurate drug history has been taken. Information regarding a drug allergy may have been forgotten or not documented at the time the initial drug history was obtained. If a patient gives a history of possible cephalosporin or penicillin allergy, the nurse withholds the drug and contacts the primary health care provider.

The nurse administers cephalosporins around the clock to the patient to provide adequate blood levels. Most cephalosporins may be taken with food to prevent gastric upset. Ceftibuten (Cedax) should not be taken with food. The nurse should administer these oral medications at least 1 hour before or 2 hours after meals. However, if the patient experiences GI upset, the nurse can administer the drug with food. The absorption of oral cefuroxime and cefpodoxime is increased when given with food.

Some cephalosporins are available as powder for a suspension and are reconstituted by a pharmacist or a nurse. The nurse should shake oral suspensions well before administering them. It is important to keep this form of the drug refrigerated until it is used.

CHRONIC CARE ALERT
People with phenylketonuria (PKU) need to be aware that the oral suspension cefprozil (Cefzil) contains phenylalanine, a substance that people with PKU cannot process. In addition, diabetic patients who use urine testing for determining diabetic medicine dosing and who are prescribed cephalosporins need to be aware that this drug may interfere with accurate test results. The primary care provider should be consulted before diet and drug changes are made.

PARENTERAL ADMINISTRATION. The nurse should read the manufacturer's package insert for each drug for instructions regarding reconstitution of powder for injection, storage of unused portions, life of the drug after it is reconstituted, methods of IV administration, and precautions to be taken when the drug is administered.

LIFESPAN ALERT – Gerontology
When a cephalosporin is given IM, the nurse injects the drug into a large muscle mass, such as the gluteus muscle or lateral aspect of the thigh. If the patient has been nonambulatory for any length of time or has paralysis, the nurse assesses the muscle carefully because the large muscle may be atrophied. It is important to rotate injection sites. The nurse warns the patient that at the time the drug is injected into the muscle, there may be a stinging or burning sensation and the area may be sore for a short time. The nurse informs the primary health care provider if previously used areas for injection appear red or if the patient reports continued pain in the area

Monitoring and Managing Patient Needs
The nurse observes the patient closely for any adverse drug reactions, particularly signs and symptoms of a hypersensitivity reaction.

IMPAIRED SKIN INTEGRITY. The nurse inspects the skin every 4 hours for redness, rash, or lesions that appear as red wheals or blisters. It is important to report a rash or hives to the primary health care provider because this may be a precursor to a severe, possibly fatal syndrome (Stevens-Johnson) or anaphylactic reaction (see Chapters 6 and 7). When a rash or irritation is present, the nurse administers frequent skin care. Emollients, antipyretic creams, or a topical corticosteroid may be prescribed. An antihistamine may be prescribed. Harsh soaps and perfumed lotions are avoided. The nurse instructs the patient to avoid rubbing the area and not to wear rough or irritating clothing. In severe cases of skin impairment, the primary health care provider may discontinue the cephalosporin therapy. The nurse closely observes the patient for signs and symptoms of a bacterial or fungal superinfection (see Chapter 7). If a superinfection occurs, the nurse contacts the primary health care provider before the next dose of the drug is due.

IMPAIRED COMFORT: INCREASED FEVER. The nurse takes vital signs every 4 hours or as ordered by the primary health care provider. It is important to report any increase in temperature to the primary health care provider, because additional treatment measures, such as administration of an antipyretic drug or change in the drug or dosage, may be necessary.

IMPAIRED URINARY ELIMINATION. Nephrotoxicity may occur with the administration of cephalosporins. An early sign of this adverse reaction may be a decrease in urine output. The nurse should measure and record the fluid intake and output and notify the primary health care provider if the output is less than 500 mL daily (Fig. 8.1). Any changes in the fluid intake–output ratio or in the appearance of the urine also may indicate

Figure 8.1 The nurse monitors for decreased urinary output in the patient receiving cephalosporins.

nephrotoxicity. It is important that the nurse report these findings to the primary health care provider promptly.

LIFESPAN ALERT – Gerontology

The older adult is more susceptible to the nephrotoxic effects of the cephalosporins, particularly if renal function is already diminished because of aging or disease. If renal impairment is present, a lower dosage and monitoring of blood creatinine levels are indicated. Blood creatinine levels greater than 4 mg/dL indicate serious renal impairment. In elderly patients with decreased renal function, a dosage adjustment may be necessary.

DIARRHEA. Frequent liquid stools may be an indication of a superinfection or pseudomembranous colitis. If pseudomembranous colitis occurs, it is usually seen 4 to 10 days after treatment is started.

The nurse inspects each bowel movement and immediately reports to the primary health care provider the occurrence of diarrhea or loose stools containing blood and mucus, because it may be necessary to discontinue drug therapy and institute treatment for diarrhea, a superinfection, or pseudomembranous colitis.

If blood and mucus appear to be in the stool, the nurse saves a sample of the stool and tests for occult blood using a test such as Hemoccult. If the stool tests positive for blood, the sample is saved for possible additional laboratory testing for blood.

Educating the Patient and Family

The nurse carefully reviews the dosage regimen with the patient and family and provides the following information:

- Complete the full course of therapy. Do not stop the drug, even if the symptoms have disappeared, unless directed to do so by the primary health care provider.
- Take the drug at the prescribed times of day, because it is important to keep an adequate amount of drug in the body throughout the entire 24 hours of each day.
- Consider taking each dose with food or milk if GI upset occurs after administration.

- Oral suspensions—keep the container refrigerated (if so labeled), shake the drug well before pouring (if so labeled), and return the drug to the refrigerator immediately after pouring the dose. Drugs that require refrigeration lose their potency when kept at room temperature. If a small amount of the drug is left after the last dose is taken, discard it, because the drug (in suspension form) begins to lose potency after a few weeks.
- Avoid drinking alcoholic beverages when taking the cephalosporins and for 3 days after completing the course of therapy, because severe reactions may occur.
- Notify the primary health care provider immediately if any one or more of the following occurs: vomiting, skin rash, hives (urticaria), severe diarrhea, vaginal or anal itching, sores in the mouth, swelling around the mouth or eyes, breathing difficulty, or GI disturbances such as nausea, vomiting, and diarrhea. Do not take the next dose of the drug until the problem is discussed with the primary health care provider (see Patient Teaching for Improved Patient Outcomes: Superinfections).
- Never give this drug to another individual even though his or her symptoms appear to be the same as yours.
- Notify the primary health care provider if the symptoms of the infection do not improve or if the condition becomes worse.

EVALUATION

- Therapeutic response is achieved, and there is no evidence of infection.
- Adverse reactions are identified, reported to the primary health care provider, and managed successfully with appropriate nursing interventions:
  - ☑ Skin is intact and free of inflammation, irritation, infection, or ulcerations.
  - ☑ Patient reports comfort without fever.
  - ☑ Patient maintains an adequate fluid intake for proper urinary elimination.
  - ☑ Patient does not experience diarrhea.
- Patient and family demonstrate an understanding of the drug regimen.

Patient Teaching for Improved Patient Outcomes

Superinfections

Antibiotics are one of the most commonly administered types of drug therapy in the home. Any patient taking antibiotics, especially cephalosporins, is susceptible to superinfection. The nurse makes sure the patient knows the signs and symptoms of superinfection.

A bacterial superinfection commonly occurs in the bowel. The nurse teaches the patient to report any of the following:

✓ Fever
✓ Burning sensation in the mouth or throat
✓ Localized redness, inflammation, and excoriation, particularly inside the mouth, in the groin, or in skin folds of the anogenital area
✓ Abdominal cramps
✓ Scaly, reddened, papular rash commonly in the breast folds, axillae, groin, or umbilicus
✓ Diarrhea, possibly severe with visible blood and mucus

A fungal superinfection commonly occurs in the mouth, vagina, and anogenital areas. The nurse teaches the patient to report any of the following:

✓ Creamy white, lacelike patches on the tongue, mouth, or throat
✓ White or yellow vaginal discharge
✓ Anal or vaginal itching

THINK CRITICALLY: PHARMACOLOGY IN PRACTICE

1. Alfredo Garcia is seen in the outpatient clinic for a severe upper respiratory infection. The primary health care provider prescribes a cephalosporin and asks you to give the patient instructions for taking the drug. You note that the patient appears to understand very little English. Discuss how you would solve this problem. Determine what information you would include in a teaching plan and how you would evaluate the effectiveness of the teaching plan for this patient.

● Test Your Knowledge

1. Cephalosporins are divided into "generations" according to:
   A. when they were discovered
   B. their administration method
   C. manufacturer's preference
   D. sensitivity to microorganisms

2. The nurse observes a patient taking a cephalosporin for common adverse reactions, which include _____.

A. hypotension, dizziness, urticaria
B. nausea, vomiting, diarrhea
C. skin rash, constipation, headache
D. bradycardia, pruritus, insomnia

3. When giving a cephalosporin by the IM route, the nurse tells the patient that _____.
   A. a stinging or burning sensation and soreness at the site may be experienced
   B. the injection site will be red for several days
   C. all injections will be given in the same area
   D. the injection will not cause any discomfort

4. The nurse observes a patient receiving a cephalosporin for Stevens-Johnson syndrome. The signs and symptoms that might indicate this syndrome include _____.
   A. swelling of the extremities
   B. increased blood pressure and pulse rate
   C. lesions on the skin or mucous membranes
   D. pain in the joints

● Prepare for the NCLEX

1. A nurse asks if the patient is allergic to penicillin before the first dose of the cephalosporin is given. The rationale for this question is that persons allergic to penicillin _____.
   A. are usually allergic to most antibiotics
   B. respond poorly to antibiotic therapy
   C. require higher doses of other antibiotics
   D. have a higher incidence of allergy to the cephalosporins

● Calculate Medication Dosages

1. The physician prescribes 1 g of cefoxitin (Mefoxin) for parenteral administration. Cefoxitin is available in a solution of 250 mg/1 mL. What amount of cefoxitin would the nurse prepare? _____

To check your answers, see Appendix E.

the**Point**. *For more NCLEX questions, log on to http://thepoint.lww.com to access more than 1000 questions.*

Tetracyclines, Aminoglycosides, Macrolides, and Lincosamides

adjunctive treatment
blood dyscrasias
bowel preparation
enteric-coated
Helicobacter pylori
hematuria

hepatic coma
myasthenia gravis
neuromuscular blockade
neurotoxicity
ototoxicity
proteinuria

LEARNING OBJECTIVES

On completion of this chapter, the student will:

1. Discuss the uses, general drug action, adverse reactions, contraindications, precautions, and interactions of the tetracyclines, aminoglycosides, macrolides, and lincosamides.
2. Discuss important preadministration and ongoing assessment activities the nurse should perform on the patient taking a tetracycline, aminoglycoside, macrolide, or lincosamide.
3. List nursing diagnoses particular to a patient taking a tetracycline, aminoglycoside, macrolide, or lincosamide.
4. Discuss ways to promote an optimal response to therapy, how to manage adverse reactions, and important points to keep in mind when educating patients about the use of a tetracycline, aminoglycoside, macrolide, or lincosamide.

This chapter discusses four groups of broad-spectrum antibiotics: the tetracyclines, the aminoglycosides, the macrolides, and the lincosamides. The drugs in these categories all interfere with the protein synthesis portion of cell growth in the bacterial cell. The Summary Drug Table: Tetracyclines, Aminoglycosides, Macrolides, and Lincosamides describe the types of broad-spectrum antibiotics discussed in this chapter.

•TETRACYCLINES

The tetracyclines are a group of anti-infectives composed of natural and semisynthetic compounds. They are useful in select infections when the organism shows sensitivity (see Chapter 7) to the tetracyclines, such as cholera, Rocky Mountain spotted fever, and typhus. These drugs are also useful when a patient is allergic to the penicillins or cephalosporins.

Actions   *bacterialstatic–slowdown*

The tetracyclines exert their effect by inhibiting bacterial protein synthesis, which is a process necessary for reproduction of the microorganism.

Uses

These antibiotics are effective in the treatment of infections caused by a wide range of gram-negative and gram-positive microorganisms. Tetracyclines are used as broad-spectrum antibiotics when penicillin is contraindicated, and also to treat the following infections:

- Rickettsial diseases (Rocky Mountain spotted fever, typhus fever, and tick fevers)
- Intestinal amebiasis
- Some skin and soft tissue infections
- Uncomplicated urethral, endocervical, or rectal infections caused by *Chlamydia trachomatis*
- Severe acne as an **adjunctive treatment** (therapy used in addition to a primary treatment)
- Infection with ***Helicobacter pylori*** (a bacterium in the stomach that can cause peptic ulcer) in combination with metronidazole and bismuth subsalicylate.

Growing resistance to the drugs is a problem with the tetracyclines.

Adverse Reactions

Gastrointestinal System Reactions

- Nausea or vomiting
- Diarrhea
- Epigastric distress
- Stomatitis
- Sore throat

Other Reactions

- Skin rashes
- Photosensitivity reaction (demeclocycline seems to cause the most serious photosensitivity reaction, whereas minocycline is least likely to cause this type of reaction)

Summary Drug Table TETRACYCLINES, AMINOGLYCOSIDES, MACROLIDES, AND LINCOSAMIDES

Generic Name	Trade Name	Uses	Adverse Reactions	Dosage Ranges
Tetracyclines				
℞ demeclocycline *deh-meh-kloe-sye'-kleen*	Declomycin	Treatment of infections due to susceptible microorganisms	Nausea, vomiting, diarrhea, dizziness, headache, hypersensitivity reactions, photosensitivity reactions, pseudomembranous colitis, hematologic changes, discoloration of teeth in fetus and young children	150 mg orally QID or 300 mg orally BID; gonorrhea: 600 mg orally initially then 300 mg orally q 12 hr for 4 days
doxycycline *dox-ih-sye'-kleen*	Atridox, Doryx, Monodox, Periostat, Oracea, Vibra-Tabs, Vibramycin	Same as demeclocycline	Same as demeclocycline	100 mg orally q 12 hr first day then 100 mg/day orally Severe infections: 100 mg q 12 hr
minocycline *min-oh-sye'-kleen*	Arestin, Dynacin, Minocin, Solodyn	Same as demeclocycline	Same as demeclocycline	200 mg orally initially then 100 mg orally q 12 hr
℞ tetracycline *tet-rah-sye'-kleen*	Sumycin	Same as demeclocycline	Same as demeclocycline	1–2 g/day orally in 2–4 divided doses
tigecycline *tih-geh-sye'-kleen* (glycylcycline similar to tetracycline)	Tygacil	Complicated skin structures and complicated intra-abdominal infections	Nausea, vomiting, diarrhea	100 mg IV initially then 50 mg IV q 12 hr
Aminoglycosides				
amikacin *am-ih-kay'-sin*	Amikin	Treatment of serious infections caused by susceptible strains of microorganisms	Nausea, vomiting, diarrhea, rash, ototoxicity, nephrotoxicity, hypersensitivity reactions, neurotoxicity, superinfections, neuromuscular blockade	15 mg/kg IM, IV, in divided doses, not to exceed 1.5 g/day
gentamicin *jen-tah-mye'-sin*		Same as amikacin	Same as amikacin	3 mg/kg/day in 3 divided doses IM or IV For life-threatening infection: 5 mg/kg/day in divided doses
kanamycin *kan-ah-mye'-sin*	Kantrex	Same as amikacin; for hepatic coma and for suppression of intestinal bacteria	Same as amikacin	7.5–15 mg/kg/day in divided doses IM, not to exceed 15 mg/kg/day in divided doses IV; not to exceed 1.5 g/day
neomycin *nee-oh-mye'-sin*		Same as amikacin, same as kanamycin	Same as amikacin	Preoperative prophylaxis: 1 g/day orally for 3 days Hepatic coma: 4–12 g/day in divided doses
paramycin *pa-rah-mye'-sin*	Humatin	Hepatic coma, intestinal amebiasis	Same as amikacin	25–35 mg/kg/day
streptomycin *strep-toe-mye'-sin*		Same as amikacin, treatment of tuberculosis	Same as amikacin	15 mg/kg/day IM or 25–30 mg/kg IM 2–3 times per week

(table continues on page 82)

Summary Drug Table TETRACYCLINES, AMINOGLYCOSIDES, MACROLIDES, AND LINCOSAMIDES (continued)

Generic Name	Trade Name	Uses	Adverse Reactions	Dosage Ranges
tobramycin *toe-bra-mye'-sin*		Same as amikacin	Same as amikacin	3–5 mg/kg/day IM, IV in 3 equal doses
Macrolides				
℞ azithromycin *ay-zith-roe-mye'-sin*	Zithromax, Zmax	Same as demeclocycline	Nausea, vomiting, diarrhea, abdominal pains, hypersensitivity reactions, pseudomembranous colitis	500 mg orally first day then 250 mg/day orally
clarithromycin *klar-ith-roe-mye'-sin*	Biaxin	Same as demeclocycline, *H. pylori* therapy	Same as azithromycin	250–500 mg orally q 12 hr
dirithromycin *dir-ith-roe-mye'-sin*		Same as demeclocycline	Anorexia, constipation, dry mouth, hypersensitivity reactions, photosensitivity reactions, pseudomembranous colitis, electrolyte imbalance	500 mg orally
℞ erythromycin base *er-ith-roe-mye'-sin*	E-Mycin, Eryc, EryPed, E.E.S.	Same as demeclocycline	Same as azithromycin	250 mg orally q 6 hr or 333 mg q 8 hr up to 4 g /day
telithromycin *tell-ith-roe-mye'-sin*	Ketek	Same as demeclocycline	Visual disturbance, nausea, diarrhea, vomiting, headache, dizziness	800 mg orally q 24 hr
Lincosamides				
clindamycin *klin-dah-mye'-sin*	Cleocin	Same as demeclocycline MRSA	Abdominal pain, esophagitis, nausea, vomiting, diarrhea, skin rash, pseudomembranous colitis, hypersensitivity reactions	Serious infection: 150–450 mg orally q 6 hr; severe infection: 600–2700 mg/day in 2–4 equal doses; life-threatening infection: up to 4.8 g/day IV, IM
℞ lincomycin *lin-koe-mye'-sin*	Lincocin	Same as demeclocycline	Same as clindamycin	500 mg orally q 6–8 hr; 600 mg IM q 12–24 hr; up to 8 g/day IV in life-threatening situations

℞ This drug should be administered at least 1 hour before or 2 hours after a meal.

Contraindications

Tetracyclines are contraindicated in the patient known to be hypersensitive to any of the tetracyclines; during pregnancy, because of the possibility of toxic effects to the developing fetus (pregnancy category D), and during lactation and in children younger than 9 years of age.

LIFESPAN ALERT – PEDIATRIC

Tetracyclines are not given to children younger than 9 years of age unless their use is absolutely necessary, because these drugs may cause permanent yellow-gray-brown discoloration of the teeth. The use of tetracyclines, especially prolonged or repeated therapy, may result in overgrowth of nonsusceptible bacterial or fungal organisms.

Precautions

Tetracyclines should be used cautiously in patients with impaired renal function (when degradation of the tetracyclines occurs, the agents are highly toxic to the kidneys) and those with liver impairment (doses greater that 2 g/day can be extremely damaging to the liver).

CHRONIC CARE ALERT

Tetracyclines may increase the risk of toxicity in patients who take digitalis drugs for heart disease. The effects of toxicity could last for months after tetracycline administration discontinues. Caution the patient and family to inform the primary care provider about the tetracycline drug therapy should digitalis toxicity symptoms appear.

Interactions

The following interactions may occur when a tetracycline is administered with another agent:

Interacting Drug or Agent	Common Use	Effect of Interaction
antacids containing aluminum, zinc, magnesium, or bismuth salts	Relief of heartburn and GI upset	Decreased effectiveness of tetracycline
oral anticoagulants	Blood thinner	Increased risk for bleeding
oral contraceptives	Contraception *Back up plan*	Decreased effectiveness of contraceptive agent (breakthrough bleeding or pregnancy)
digoxin	Management of heart disease	Increased risk for digitalis toxicity (see Chapter 38)

CHRONIC CARE ALERT
Tetracyclines may reduce insulin requirements in patients with diabetes. Blood glucose levels should be monitored frequently during tetracycline therapy.

• AMINOGLYCOSIDES *bacterial cide*

The aminoglycosides include amikacin (Amikin), gentamicin, kanamycin (Kantrex), neomycin, streptomycin, and tobramycin.

Actions

The aminoglycosides exert their bactericidal effect by blocking a step in protein synthesis necessary for bacterial multiplication. They disrupt the functional ability of the bacterial cell wall, causing cell death.

Uses

Aminoglycosides are used primarily in the treatment of infections caused by gram-negative microorganisms. In addition, the drugs may be used to reduce bacteria (normal flora) in the bowel when patients are having abdominal surgery or when a patient is in a **hepatic coma**. Because the oral aminoglycosides are poorly absorbed, they are useful in suppressing GI bacteria. For example, kanamycin (Kantrex) and neomycin are used before surgery to reduce intestinal bacteria. It is thought this reduces the possibility of abdominal infection that may occur after surgery on the bowel. This drug treatment protocol is called a **bowel preparation** (bowel prep).

Kanamycin, neomycin, and paromomycin are used orally in the management of hepatic coma. In this disorder, liver failure results in an elevation of blood ammonia levels. By reducing the number of ammonia-forming bacteria in the intestines, blood ammonia levels may be lowered, thereby temporarily reducing some of the symptoms associated with this disorder.

respiratory infection w influenza

Adverse Reactions

General system reactions include the following:

• Nausea
• Vomiting
• Anorexia
• Rash
• Urticaria – *hives*

More serious adverse reactions may lead to discontinuation of the drug. These reactions include:

• Nephrotoxicity (damage to the kidneys by a toxic substance)
• **Ototoxicity** (damage to the hearing organs by a toxic substance) *ringing or buzzing*
• **Neurotoxicity** (damage to the nervous system by a toxic substance)

Signs and symptoms of nephrotoxicity may include **proteinuria** (protein in the urine), **hematuria** (blood in the urine), increase in the blood urea nitrogen (BUN) level, decrease in urine output, and an increase in the serum creatinine concentration. Nephrotoxicity is usually reversible once the drug is discontinued.

Signs and symptoms of ototoxicity include tinnitus (ringing in the ears), dizziness, roaring in the ears, vertigo, and a mild to severe loss of hearing. If hearing loss occurs, it is usually permanent. Ototoxicity may occur during drug therapy or even after therapy is discontinued. The short-term administration of kanamycin and neomycin as a preparation for bowel surgery rarely causes these two adverse reactions.

Signs and symptoms of neurotoxicity include numbness, skin tingling, circumoral (around the mouth) paresthesia, peripheral paresthesia, tremors, muscle twitching, convulsions, muscle weakness, and **neuromuscular blockade** (acute muscular paralysis and apnea).

The administration of the aminoglycosides may result in a hypersensitivity reaction, which can range from mild to severe and, in some cases, be life threatening. Mild hypersensitivity reactions may require only discontinuing the drug, whereas the more serious reactions require immediate treatment. When aminoglycosides are given, individual drug references, such as the package insert, should be consulted for more specific adverse reactions. As with other anti-infectives, bacterial or fungal superinfections and pseudomembranous colitis (see Chapter 7) may occur with the use of these drugs.

Contraindications

The aminoglycosides are contraindicated in patients with hypersensitivity to aminoglycosides, preexisting hearing loss, **myasthenia gravis**, and parkinsonism. They are also contraindicated during lactation or pregnancy (pregnancy category C, except for neomycin, amikacin, gentamicin, kanamycin, netilmicin, and tobramycin, which are in pregnancy category D). Aminoglycosides are also contraindicated for long-term therapy, because of the potential for ototoxicity and nephrotoxicity.

muscle exhaustion / mind to ground

Precautions

The aminoglycosides are used cautiously in elderly patients and patients with renal failure (dosage adjustments may be necessary) and neuromuscular disorders.

Interactions

The following interactions may occur when an aminoglycoside is administered with another agent:

Interacting Drug	Common Use	Effect of Interaction
cephalosporins	Anti-infective agent	Increased risk of nephrotoxicity
loop diuretics (water pills)	Management of edema and water retention	Increased risk of ototoxicity
Pavulon or Anectine (general anesthetics)	Anesthesia (e.g., for surgery)	Increased risk of neuromuscular blockade

• MACROLIDES

The macrolides are effective against a variety of pathogenic organisms, particularly infections of the respiratory and genitourinary tract.

Actions

The macrolides are bacteriostatic or bactericidal in susceptible bacteria. The drugs act by causing changes in protein function and synthesis.

Uses

These antibiotics are effective as prophylaxis before dental or other procedures in patients allergic to penicillin and in the treatment of:

• A wide range of gram-negative and gram-positive infections
• Acne vulgaris and skin infections
• Upper respiratory infections caused by *Hemophilus influenzae* (with sulfonamides)

Adverse Reactions

Gastrointestinal (GI) reactions include the following:

• Nausea
• Vomiting
• Diarrhea
• Abdominal pain or cramping

As with almost all antibacterial drugs, pseudomembranous colitis may occur, ranging in severity from mild to life-threatening. Visual disturbances (associated with telithromycin) may also occur.

Contraindications

These drugs are contraindicated in patients with hypersensitivity to the macrolides and in patients with preexisting liver disease. Telithromycin (Ketek) should not be ordered if a patient is taking cisapride (Propulsid) or pimozide (Orap).

Precautions

Macrolides should be used cautiously in patients who have liver dysfunction or myasthenia gravis (a disease that affects the myoneural junction in nerves and is manifested by extreme weakness and exhaustion of the muscles), or who are pregnant or lactating (azithromycin and erythromycin are in pregnancy category B; clarithromycin, dirithromycin, troleandomycin, and telithromycin are in pregnancy category C).

Interactions

The following interactions may occur when a macrolide is administered with another agent:

Interacting Drug	Common Use	Effect of Interaction
antacids (kaolin, aluminum salts, or magaldrate)	Relief of GI upset, such as diarrhea	Decreased absorption and effectiveness of the macrolides
digoxin	Management of cardiac and respiratory disorders	Increased serum levels
anticoagulants	Blood thinner	Increased risk of bleeding
clindamycin, lincomycin, or chloramphenicol	Anti-infective agent	Decreased therapeutic activity of the macrolides
theophylline	Management of respiratory problems, such as asthma	Increased serum theophylline level

• LINCOSAMIDES

The lincosamides, another group of anti-infectives with a high potential for toxicity, are usually used only for treating serious infections in which penicillin or erythromycin (a macrolide) is not effective.

Actions

The lincosamides act by inhibiting protein synthesis in susceptible bacteria, causing cell death.

Uses

These antibiotics are effective in the treatment of infections caused by a range of gram-negative and gram-positive microorganisms. Lincosamides are used for the more serious infections and may be used in conjunction with other antibiotics.

Adverse Reactions

Gastrointestinal System Reactions

- Abdominal pain
- Esophagitis
- Nausea
- Vomiting
- Diarrhea

Other Reactions

- Skin rash
- Blood dyscrasias (an abnormality of the blood cell structure or function) *imbalance components of blood / nose bleeds*

These drugs also can cause pseudomembranous colitis, which may range from mild to very severe. Discontinuing the drug may relieve mild symptoms of pseudomembranous colitis.

Contraindications

The lincosamides are contraindicated in infants younger than 1 month of age and in patients:

- Hypersensitive to the lincosamides
- Taking cisapride (Propulsid) or the antipsychotic drug pimozide (Orap) *not on market / not seen very often*
- With minor bacterial or viral infections

Precautions

These drugs should be used cautiously in patients with a history of GI disorders, renal disease, liver impairment, or myasthenia gravis (lincosamides have neuromuscular blocking action).

Interactions

The following interactions may occur when a lincosamide is administered with another agent:

Interacting Drug	Common Use	Effect of Interaction
kaolin- or aluminum-based antacids	Relief of stomach upset	Decreased absorption of the lincosamides
neuromuscular blocking drugs	Anesthesia	Increased action of neuromuscular blocking drug, possibly leading to severe and profound respiratory depression

NURSING PROCESS

PATIENT RECEIVING A TETRACYCLINE, AMINOGLYCOSIDE, MACROLIDE, OR LINCOSAMIDE

ASSESSMENT

Preadministration Assessment

It is important to establish an accurate database before the administration of any antibiotic. The nurse should identify and record signs and symptoms of the infection. Signs and symptoms may vary and often depend on the organ or system involved and whether the infection is external or internal. Examples of some of the signs and symptoms of an infection in various areas of the body are pain, drainage, redness, changes in the appearance of sputum, general malaise, chills and fever, cough, and swelling.

The nurse obtains a thorough allergy history, especially a history of drug allergies. Some antibiotics have a higher incidence of hypersensitivity reactions in those with a history of allergy to drugs or other substances. If the patient has a history of allergies and has not told the primary health care provider, the nurse should not administer the first dose of the drug until the problem is discussed with the primary health care provider.

The primary health care provider may order culture and sensitivity tests, and these should also be performed before the first dose of the drug is given. Other laboratory tests such as renal and hepatic function tests, complete blood count, and urinalysis may also be ordered by the primary health care provider. In persons with impaired hearing or at risk for hearing loss, a hearing test may be recommended.

When kanamycin or neomycin is given for hepatic coma, the nurse must evaluate the patient's level of consciousness and ability to swallow.

Ongoing Assessment

An ongoing assessment is important during therapy with the tetracyclines, macrolides, and lincosamides. The nurse should take vital signs every 4 hours or as ordered by the primary health care provider. The nurse must notify the primary health care provider if there are changes in the vital signs, such as a significant drop in blood pressure, an increase in the pulse or respiratory rate, or a sudden increase in temperature. When an aminoglycoside is being administered, it is important to monitor the patient's respiratory rate because neuromuscular blockade has been reported with the administration of these drugs. The nurse reports any changes in the respiratory rate or rhythm to the primary health care provider because immediate treatment may be necessary. When kanamycin or neomycin is given for hepatic coma, the nurse evaluates and records the patient's general condition and changes in mentation daily.

Each day, the nurse compares current signs and symptoms of the infection against the initial signs and symptoms and records any specific findings in the patient's chart.

When an antibiotic is ordered for prevention of a secondary infection (prophylaxis), the nurse observes the patient for signs and symptoms that may indicate the beginning of an infection despite the prophylactic use of the antibiotic. If signs and symptoms of an infection occur, the nurse must report them to the primary health care provider.

NURSING DIAGNOSES

Drug-specific nursing diagnoses include the following:

- ❑ **Impaired Comfort: Increased Fever** related to ineffectiveness of anti-infective therapy
- ❑ **Altered Thought Process** related to increased ammonia blood levels
- ❑ **Ineffective Tissue Perfusion: Renal** related to adverse drug reactions to aminoglycosides
- ❑ **Disturbed Sensory Perception: Auditory** related to adverse drug reactions to aminoglycosides
- ❑ **Risk for Injury** related to visual disturbances from telithromycin treatment or paresthesia secondary to neurotoxicity
- ❑ **Diarrhea** related to superinfection secondary to anti-infective therapy, adverse drug reaction

Nursing diagnoses related to drug administration are discussed in Chapter 4.

PLANNING

The expected outcomes for the patient may include an optimal response to therapy, which includes control of the infectious process or prophylaxis of bacterial infection, meeting of patient needs related to the management of adverse drug effects, and an understanding of the therapeutic regimen.

IMPLEMENTATION

Promoting an Optimal Response to Therapy

These drugs are of no value in the treatment of infections caused by a virus or fungus. There may be times when a secondary bacterial infection has occurred or may occur when the patient has a fungal or viral infection. The primary health care provider may then order one of the broad-spectrum antibiotics, but its purpose is for preventing (prophylaxis) or treating a secondary bacterial infection that could potentially develop after the primary fungal or viral infection.

ORAL ADMINISTRATION. Adverse reactions to most anti-infective drugs include nausea, vomiting, or abdominal pain. Patients may want to eat foods when these drugs are administered to reduce GI problems. It is important for the nurse to know how medications will be affected if taken with foods.

Tetracyclines. It is important to give tetracyclines on an empty stomach. The exceptions are minocycline (Minocin) and tigecycline (Tygacil), which may be taken with food. All tetracyclines should be given with a full glass of water (8 oz).

❗ NURSING ALERT

The nurse should not give tetracyclines along with dairy products (milk or cheese), antacids, laxatives, or products containing iron. When the aforementioned drugs are prescribed, the nurse makes sure they are given 2 hours before or after the administration of a tetracycline. Food or drugs containing calcium, magnesium, aluminum, or iron prevent the absorption of the tetracyclines if ingested concurrently.

Aminoglycosides. When kanamycin or neomycin is given to suppress intestinal bacteria before surgery, the primary health care provider's orders regarding the timing of the administration of the drug are extremely important. Omission of a dose or failure to give the drug at the specified time may result in inadequate suppression of intestinal bacteria. When neomycin is given, **enteric-coated** erythromycin may be given at the same time as part of bowel preparation. Enteric-coated tablets have a special coating that prevents the drug from being absorbed in the stomach. Absorption takes place lower in the GI tract after the coating has dissolved.

Macrolides. The nurse gives clarithromycin and telithromycin without regard to meals, and clarithromycin may be taken with milk if desired. Dirithromycin is given with food or within 1 hour of eating. Azithromycin is given 1 hour or more before a meal or 2 hours or more after a meal. Erythromycin is given on an empty stomach (1 hour before or 2 hours after meals) and with 180 to 240 mL of water.

Lincosamides. Food impairs the absorption of lincomycin. The patient should take nothing by mouth (except water) for 1 to 2 hours before and after taking lincomycin. The nurse should give clindamycin with food or a full glass of water.

PARENTERAL ADMINISTRATION. When these drugs are given intramuscularly, the nurse inspects previous injection sites for signs of pain or tenderness, redness, and swelling. Some antibiotics may cause temporary local reactions, but persistence of a localized reaction should be reported to the primary health care provider. It is important to rotate injection sites and record the site used for injection in the patient's chart.

When these drugs are given intravenously (IV), the nurse should inspect the needle site and area around the needle for signs of extravasation of the IV fluid or signs of tenderness, pain, and redness (which may indicate phlebitis or thrombophlebitis). If these symptoms are apparent, the nurse should restart the IV in another vein and bring the problem to the attention of the primary health care provider.

Monitoring and Managing Patient Needs

The nurse observes the patient at frequent intervals, especially during the first 48 hours of therapy. It is important to report to the primary health care provider the occurrence of any adverse reaction before the next dose of the drug is due. The nurse should report serious adverse reactions, such as a severe hypersensitivity reaction, respiratory difficulty, severe diarrhea, or a decided drop in blood pressure, to the primary health care provider immediately, because a serious adverse reaction may require emergency intervention.

IMPAIRED COMFORT: INCREASED FEVER. The nurse monitors the temperature at frequent intervals, usually every 4 hours unless the patient has an elevated temperature. When the patient has an elevated temperature the nurse checks the temperature, pulse, and respirations every hour until the temperature returns to normal, and administers an antipyretic medication if prescribed by the primary care provider.

ALTERED THOUGHT PROCESS: HEPATIC COMA. When the aminoglycosides kanamycin and neomycin are administered orally as treatment for hepatic coma, the nurse exercises care. During the early stages of this disorder, various changes in the level of consciousness may be seen. At times, the patient may appear lethargic and respond poorly to commands. Because of these changes in the level of consciousness, the patient may have difficulty swallowing, and a danger of aspiration is present. If the patient appears to have difficulty taking an oral drug, the nurse withholds the drug and contacts the primary health care provider.

INEFFECTIVE TISSUE PERFUSION: RENAL. The patient taking an aminoglycoside is at risk for nephrotoxicity. The nurse measures and records the intake and output and notifies the primary health care provider if the output is less than 750 mL/day. It is important to keep a record of the fluid intake and output as well as the patient's daily weight to assess hydration and renal function. The nurse encourages fluid intake to 2000 mL/day (if the patient's condition permits). Any changes in the intake–output ratio or in the appearance of the urine may indicate nephrotoxicity. The nurse reports these types of changes to the primary health care provider promptly. In turn, the primary health care provider may order daily laboratory tests (e.g., serum creatinine and BUN) to monitor renal function. The nurse reports elevations in the creatinine or BUN level to the primary health care provider because elevation may indicate renal dysfunction.

🛇 **NURSING ALERT**
Neuromuscular blockade or respiratory paralysis may occur after administration of the aminoglycosides. Therefore, it is extremely important that any symptoms of respiratory difficulty be reported immediately. If neuromuscular blockade occurs, it may be reversed by the administration of calcium salts, but mechanical ventilation may be required.

DISTURBED SENSORY PERCEPTION: AUDITORY. The patient taking aminoglycosides is at risk for ototoxicity. Auditory changes are irreversible, usually bilateral, and may be partial or total. The risk is greater in patients with renal impairment or those with preexisting hearing loss. It is important for the nurse to detect any problems with hearing and report them to the primary health care provider because continued drug administration could lead to permanent hearing loss.

RISK FOR INJURY. Telithromycin (Ketek) is a drug related to the macrolides. It can cause the patient's eyes to have difficulty focusing and accommodating to light. Patients should be cautioned regarding the potential for accidents and injury when driving, operating machinery, or engaging in other hazardous activities.

The nurse should be alert for symptoms such as numbness or tingling of the skin, circumoral paresthesia,

peripheral paresthesia (numbness or tingling in the extremities), tremors, and muscle twitching or weakness. The nurse reports any symptom of neurotoxicity immediately to the primary health care provider. Convulsions can occur if the drug is not discontinued.

🛇 **NURSING ALERT**
To detect ototoxicity, the nurse carefully evaluates the patient's complaints or comments related to hearing, such as a ringing or buzzing in the ears or difficulty hearing. If hearing problems do occur, the nurse reports this problem to the primary health care provider immediately. To monitor for damage to the eighth cranial nerve, an evaluation of hearing may be done by audiometry before and throughout the course of therapy.

DIARRHEA. Diarrhea may be an indication of a superinfection or pseudomembranous colitis, both of which can be serious. The nurse should inspect all stools for blood or mucus. If diarrhea does occur and blood and mucus appear to be in the stool, the nurse saves a sample of the stool and tests for occult blood using a test such as Hemoccult. If the stool tests positive for blood, the nurse saves the stool for possible further laboratory analysis.

The nurse should encourage the patient with diarrhea to drink fluids to replace those lost with the diarrhea. It is also important to maintain an accurate intake and output record to help determine fluid balance.

The nurse observes the patient for other signs and symptoms of a bacterial or fungal superinfection, such as vaginal or anal itching, sores in the mouth, diarrhea, fever, chills, and sore throat. It is important to report any new signs and symptoms occurring during antibiotic therapy to the primary health care provider, who must then decide if these problems are part of the original infection or if a superinfection has occurred.

Educating the Patient and Family

The patient and family must understand the prescribed therapeutic regimen. It is not uncommon for patients to stop taking a prescribed drug because they feel better. A detailed plan of teaching helps to reduce the incidence of this problem.

The nurse should explain, in easy-to-understand terms, the adverse reactions associated with the specific prescribed antibiotic. The nurse advises the patient to contact the primary health care provider if any potentially serious adverse reactions, such as hypersensitivity reactions, moderate to severe diarrhea, sudden onset of chills and fever, sore throat, or sores in the mouth, occur.

The nurse develops a teaching plan that includes the following information:

- Take the drug at the prescribed time intervals. These intervals are important because a certain amount of the drug must be in the body at all times for the infection to be controlled.
- Do not increase or omit the dose unless advised to do so by the primary health care provider.

- Complete the entire course of treatment. Never stop the drug, except on the advice of a primary health care provider, before the course of treatment is completed even if symptoms improve or disappear. Failure to complete the prescribed course of treatment may result in a return of the infection.
- Take each dose with a full (8-ounce) glass of water. Follow the directions given by the pharmacist regarding taking the drug on an empty stomach or with food (see Patient Teaching for Improved Patient Outcomes: Avoiding Drug–Food Interactions).
- Notify the primary health care provider if symptoms of the infection become worse or there is no improvement in the original symptoms after about 5 days.
- When a tetracycline has been prescribed, avoid exposure to the sun or any type of tanning lamp or bed. When exposure to direct sunlight is unavoidable, completely cover the arms and legs and wear a wide-brimmed hat to protect the face and neck. Application of a sunscreen may or may not be effective. Therefore, consult the primary health care provider before using a sunscreen to prevent a photosensitivity reaction.

EVALUATION

- Therapeutic response is achieved, and there is no evidence of infection.
- Adverse reactions are identified, reported to the primary health care provider, and managed successfully with appropriate nursing interventions:
  - ☑ Patient reports comfort without fever.
  - ☑ Orientation and mentation remain intact.
  - ☑ Patient has adequate renal tissue perfusion.
  - ☑ Patient has intact auditory sensory perception.
  - ☑ No evidence of injury is seen due to visual disturbances.
  - ☑ Patient does not experience diarrhea.
- Patient and family demonstrate an understanding of the drug regimen.

Patient Teaching for Improved Patient Outcomes

Avoiding Drug–Food Interactions

✓ In some instances, drugs may be taken with food or milk to minimize the risk for GI upset. However, most tetracyclines, when given with foods containing calcium, such as dairy products, are not absorbed as well as when they are taken on an empty stomach. So, if the patient is to receive tetracycline at home, it is important to be sure he or she knows to take the drug on an empty stomach, 1 hour before or 2 hours after a meal.

✓ Be sure to teach the patient to read labels in the grocery store and beware of items (e.g., cereals) that may be fortified with calcium.

✓ In addition, teach the patient to avoid the following dairy products before or after taking tetracycline:
  - Milk (whole, low-fat, skim, condensed, or evaporated) and milkshakes
  - Cream (half-and-half, heavy, light), sour cream, coffee creamers, and creamy salad dressings
  - Eggnog
  - Cheese (natural and processed) and cottage cheese
  - Yogurt and frozen yogurt
  - Ice cream, ice milk, and frozen custard

THINK CRITICALLY: PHARMACOLOGY IN PRACTICE

1. Mr. Park, aged 77 years, a patient in a skilled nursing facility, has been receiving clarithromycin (Biaxin) for an upper respiratory infection for 9 days. The nurse assistant reports that he has had fecal incontinence for the past 2 days. Analyze whether this matter should be investigated.
2. When taking the drug history of Mrs. Moore, aged 85 years, a patient in the outpatient clinic, you note that she has been taking 0.25 mg digoxin, one baby aspirin, and the tetracycline minocycline (Minocin). Based on your knowledge of the tetracyclines, determine whether there is any reason to be concerned about Mrs. Moore's drug regimen. Explain your answer.

● Test Your Knowledge

1. A patient asks the nurse why the primary health care provider prescribed an anti-infective when she was told that she has a viral infection. The correct response by the nurse is that the antibiotic may be used to prevent a _____.

   A. primary fungal infection
   B. repeat viral infection
   C. secondary bacterial infection
   D. breakdown of the immune system

2. A patient is receiving erythromycin for an infection. The patient's response to therapy is best evaluated by _____.

   A. monitoring vital signs every 4 hours
   B. comparing initial and current signs and symptoms
   C. monitoring fluid intake and output
   D. asking the patient if he is feeling better

3. When asked to describe a photosensitivity reaction, the nurse correctly states that this reaction may be described as a(n) _____.

   A. tearing of the eyes on exposure to bright light
   B. aversion to bright lights and sunlight
   C. sensitivity to products in the environment
   D. exaggerated sunburn reaction when the skin is exposed to sunlight

● Prepare for the NCLEX

1. When giving one of the macrolide antibiotics, the nurse assesses the patient for the most common adverse reactions, which are _____.

   A. related to the GI tract
   B. skin rash and urinary retention
   C. sores in the mouth and hypertension
   D. related to the nervous system

● Calculate Medication Dosages

1. Mr. Baker is prescribed azithromycin for a lower respiratory tract infection. The nurse tells Mr. Baker to take the drug on an empty stomach. Azithromycin is available in 250-mg tablets. The primary health care provider has ordered 500 mg on the first day, followed by 250 mg on days 2 to 5. How many tablets would Mr. Baker take on the first day? _____ On the last day of therapy? _____

2. A patient is prescribed 600 mg of lincomycin every 12 hours IM. The drug is available as 300 mg/mL. How many milliliters would the nurse administer?

3. A patient is prescribed 200 mg of minocycline oral suspension initially, followed by 100 mg orally every 12 hours. The minocycline is available as an oral suspension of 50 mg/5 mL. How many milliliters would the nurse administer as the initial dose? _____

To check your answers, see Appendix E.

the**Point** *For more NCLEX questions, log on to http://thepoint.lww.com to access more than 1000 questions.*

Fluoroquinolones and Miscellaneous Anti-Infectives

As antibiotics became resistant to various microorganisms, researchers sought to develop more powerful drugs that would be effective against these resistant pathogens. The anti-infectives discussed in this chapter are such drugs; they have minor similarity to each other and do not belong to any one of the drug groups discussed in Chapters 6 through 9. Some of these drugs are used to treat a broad spectrum of infections, others only for the treatment of one type of infection; still others may be limited to the treatment of serious infections not treatable by other anti-infectives. The Summary Drug Table: Fluoroquinolones and Miscellaneous Anti-Infectives lists the drugs discussed in this chapter.

• FLUOROQUINOLONES

The fluoroquinolones include ciprofloxacin (Cipro), gatifloxacin (Tequin), lomefloxacin (Maxaquin), moxifloxacin (Avelox), and ofloxacin (Floxin). *no longer on the market*

Actions

The fluoroquinolones exert their bactericidal effect by interfering with the synthesis of bacterial DNA. This interference prevents cell reproduction, leading to death of the bacteria.

Uses

The fluoroquinolones are effective in treating infections caused by gram-positive and gram-negative microorganisms. They are primarily used in the treatment of the following:

- Lower respiratory infections
- Bone and joint infections
- Urinary tract infections
- Infections of the skin
- Sexually transmitted infections

Ciprofloxacin, norfloxacin, and ofloxacin are available in ophthalmic forms for infections in the eyes.

Adverse Reactions

Common adverse effects include the following:

- Nausea
- Diarrhea
- Headache
- Abdominal pain or discomfort
- Dizziness
- **Photosensitivity**, which is a more serious adverse reaction seen with the administration of the fluoroquinolones, especially lomefloxacin and sparfloxacin

The administration of any drug may result in a hypersensitivity reaction, which can range from mild to severe and, in some cases, be life-threatening. Mild hypersensitivity reactions may require only discontinuing the drug, whereas the more serious reactions require immediate treatment (see Chapters 1 and 7). Bacterial or fungal superinfections and pseudomembranous colitis (see Chapter 7) may occur with the use of both of these drugs. See the Summary Drug Table: Fluoroquinolones and Misc. Anti-Infectives for more information.

Contraindications and Precautions

Fluoroquinolones are contraindicated in patients with a history of hypersensitivity to the fluoroquinolones, in children

Summary Drug Table FLUOROQUINOLONES AND MISCELLANEOUS ANTI-INFECTIVES

Generic Name	Trade Name	Uses	Adverse Reactions	Dosage Ranges
Fluoroquinolones				
ciprofloxacin *sih-proe'-flox-ah-sin*	Cipro, Proquin	Treatment of infections due to susceptible microorganisms	Nausea, diarrhea, headache, abdominal discomfort, photosensitivity, superinfections, hypersensitivity reactions	250–750 mg orally q 12 hr; 200–400 mg IV q 12 hr
gemifloxacin *jem-ah-flox'-ah-sin*	Factive	Bronchitis and community acquired pneumonia	Vomiting, diarrhea, stomach pain, restlessness, dizziness, confusion, taste changes, sleep disturbances	320 mg/day orally
levofloxacin *lee-voe-flox'-ah-sin*	Levaquin	Same as ciprofloxacin	Same as ciprofloxacin	250–750 mg/day orally, IV
moxifloxacin *mocks-ah-flox'-ah-sin*	Avelox	Same as ciprofloxacin	Same as ciprofloxacin	400 mg/day orally
℞ norfloxacin *nor-flox'-ah-sin*	Noroxin	Urinary tract infections, STIs, prostatitis	Same as ciprofloxacin	400 mg orally q 12 hr; 800 mg as single dose for STI
ofloxacin *oh-flox'-ah-sin*	Floxin	Same as ciprofloxacin	Same as ciprofloxacin	200–400 mg orally, IV q 12 hr
Miscellaneous Drugs Inhibiting RNA/DNA Synthesis				
daptomycin *dap-toe-mye'-sin*	Cubicin	Complicated skin and skin structure infections, *S. aureus* blood infections	Nausea, diarrhea, constipation, rash, vein irritation	4 mg/kg IV daily for 7–14 day
linezolid *lih-nez'-oh-lid*	Zyvox	Infections with vancomycin–resistant *Enterococcus faecium*; pneumonia from *Staphylococcus aureus* and penicillin-susceptible *Streptococcus pneumoniae*; skin and skin structure infections	Nausea, diarrhea, headache, insomnia, pseudomembranous colitis	600 mg orally or IV q 12 hr
Miscellaneous Drugs Inhibiting Bacterial Cell Wall Synthesis				
aztreonam *az'-tree-oh-nam*	Azactam	Gram-negative bacterial infections	Nausea, diarrhea, hypotension, rash and headache	500 mg–1 g q 8–12 hr
doripenem *dor-ih-pen'-em*	Doribax	Complicated intra-abdominal or urinary tract infections	Headache, nausea, diarrhea, and anemia	500 mg IV q 8 hr
imipenem-cilastatin *ih-mih-pen'-em/* *sye-lah-stat'-in*	Primaxin	Serious infections caused by *Staphylococcus* spp, *Streptococcus* spp, and *Escherichia coli*	Nausea, diarrhea	250 mg–1 g q 6 hr, not to exceed 4 g/day
meropenem *meh-row-pen'-em*	Merrem IV	Intra-abdominal and soft tissue infections caused by multiresistant gram-negative organisms	Headache, diarrhea, abdominal pain, nausea, pain and inflammation at injection site, pseudo-membranous colitis	500 mg–1 g IV q 8 hr
vancomycin *van-koe-mye'-sin*	Vancocin	Serious susceptible gram-positive infections not responding to treatment with other antibiotics	Nausea, chills, fever, urticaria, sudden fall in blood pressure, with redness on face, neck, arms, and back, nephrotoxicity, ototoxicity	500 mg–2 g/day orally in divided doses; 500 mg IV q 6 hr or 1 g IV q 12 hr

(table continues on page 92)

Fluoroquinolones and Miscellaneous
Anti-Infectives

Summary Drug Table FLUOROQUINOLONES AND MISCELLANEOUS ANTI-INFECTIVES (continued)

Generic Name	Trade Name	Uses	Adverse Reactions	Dosage Ranges
Miscellaneous Anti-infectives				
quinupristin-dalfopristin *kwin-yoo'-pris-tin*	Synercid	VREF	Vein inflammation, nausea, vomiting, diarrhea	7.5 mg/kg IV q 8 hr
spectinomycin *spek-tin-oh-mye'-sin*	Trobincin	Gonorrhea	Soreness at injection site, urticaria, dizziness, rash, chills, fever, hypersensitivity reactions	2 g IM as single dose; up to 4 g IM

Ⓕ This drug should be administered at least 1 hour before or 2 hours after a meal.

younger than 18 years of age, and in pregnancy (category C). These drugs also are contraindicated in patients whose life-styles do not allow for adherence to the precautions regarding photosensitivity.

Fluoroquinolones are used cautiously in patients with diabetes, renal impairment, patients with a history of seizures, older patients, and patients on dialysis.

Interactions

The following interactions may occur when a fluoroquinolone is administered with another agent:

Interacting Drug	Common Use	Effect of Interaction
theophylline	Management of respiratory problems, such as asthma	Increased serum theophylline level
cimetidine *Tagamet*	Management of gastrointestinal (GI) upset	Interferes with elimination of the antibiotic
oral anticoagulants	Blood thinner	Increased risk of bleeding
antacids, iron salts, or zinc	Relief of heartburn and GI upset	Decreased absorption of the antibiotic
nonsteroidal anti-inflammatory drugs (NSAIDs)	Relief of pain and inflammation	Risk of seizure activity

There is also a risk of severe cardiac arrhythmias when the fluoroquinolones gatifloxacin and moxifloxacin are administered with drugs that increase the QT interval (e.g., quinidine, procainamide, amiodarone, sotalol).

● MISCELLANEOUS DRUGS INHIBITING RNA/DNA SYNTHESIS

The daptomycin and oxazolidinone drugs are new classes of anti-infectives that interfere with RNA and DNA synthesis — *cell production* within the bacterial cell. *Slow down or stop*

Actions

Linezolid (Zyvox) is the first drug in a new drug class, the oxazolidinones. This drug acts by binding to a site on a specific ribosomal RNA and preventing the formation of a component necessary for the bacteria to replicate. It is both bacteriostatic (e.g., to enterococci and staphylococci) and bactericidal (e.g., against streptococci). Daptomycin is a member of a new category of antibacterial agents called *cyclic lipopeptides*. This drug binds to the cell membrane, depolarizing the wall and inhibiting protein DNA and RNA synthesis, which causes the bacterial cell to die.

Uses

Linezolid is used in the treatment of **vancomycin-resistant** *Enterococcus faecium* **(VREF),** health care and community-acquired pneumonias, and skin and skin structure infections, including those caused by methicillin-resistant *Staphylococcus aureus* (MRSA). Daptomycin is used to treat complicated skin and skin structure bacterial infections as well as *S. aureus* infections of the blood.

Adverse Reactions

The most common adverse reactions include the following:

- Nausea
- Vomiting
- Diarrhea or constipation
- Headache and dizziness
- Insomnia
- Rash

Less common adverse reactions include:

- Fatigue
- Depression
- Nervousness
- Photosensitivity

Pseudomembranous colitis and thrombocytopenia are the most serious adverse reactions caused by linezolid.

Contraindications and Precautions

Linezolid is contraindicated in patients who are allergic to the drug or who are pregnant (category C) or lactating and in patients with **phenylketonuria**. Daptomycin is contraindicated in patients with a known hypersensitivity to daptomycin, and it should not be used during pregnancy (category B) or lactation.

Linezolid is used cautiously in patients with bone marrow depression, hepatic dysfunction, renal impairment, hypertension, and hyperthyroidism. Daptomycin should be used cautiously in patients taking warfarin (Coumadin).

Interactions

The following interactions may occur when linezolid is administered with another agent:

- Antiplatelet drugs (aspirin or the nonsteroidal anti-inflammatory drugs [NSAIDs])—increased risk of bleeding and thrombocytopenia
- Monamine oxidase inhibitor (MAOI) antidepressants—decreased effectiveness
- Large amounts of food containing tyramine (e.g., aged cheese, caffeinated beverages, yogurt, chocolate, red wine, beer, pepperoni)—risk of severe hypertension

The following interactions may occur when daptomycin is administered with another agent:

- Statin drugs (cholesterol reduction)—myopathy with elevated CPK levels

• MISCELLANEOUS DRUGS INHIBITING CELL WALL SYNTHESIS

The carbapenems, vancomycin, and monobactams drugs all play a role in the inhibition of the bacterial cell wall synthesis.

Actions

Carbapenems inhibit synthesis of the bacterial cell wall and cause the death of susceptible cells. Vancomycin acts against susceptible gram-positive bacteria by inhibiting bacterial cell wall synthesis and increasing cell wall permeability. Aztreonam has a beta-lactam nucleus and therefore is called a *monobactam*. This is structurally different from the beta-lactam ring of the penicillins, yet it still functions to inhibit bacterial cell wall synthesis.

Uses

Meropenem (Merrem IV) is used for intra-abdominal infections and bacterial meningitis. Imipenem-cilastatin (Primaxin) is used to treat serious infections, endocarditis, and septicemia. Doripenem (Doribax) is used to treat intra-abdominal and complicated urinary tract infections caused by bacteria. Vancomycin (Vancocin) is used in the treatment of serious gram-positive infections that do not respond to treatment with other anti-infectives. It also may be used in treating anti-infective–associated pseudomembranous colitis

caused by *Clostridium difficile*. The monobactams have bactericidal action and are used to treat gram-negative microorganisms.

Adverse Reactions

The most common adverse reactions with these drugs include nausea, vomiting, diarrhea, and rash. As with many other anti-infectives, there is a risk of pseudomembranous colitis. The nurse needs to assess stools for blood when the patient has diarrhea.

Carbapenems also can cause an abscess or phlebitis at the injection site. An abscess is suspected if the injection site appears red or is tender and warm to the touch. Tissue sloughing at the injection site also may occur.

Nephrotoxicity (damage to the kidneys) and ototoxicity (damage to the organs of hearing) may be seen with the administration of vancomycin especially in patients with pre-existing kidney disease. Additional adverse reactions include chills, fever, urticaria, and sudden fall in blood pressure with parenteral administration. For more information, see Summary Drug Table: Fluoroquinolones and Misc. Anti-Infectives.

Contraindications, Precautions, and Interactions

Carbapenems and aztreonam are contraindicated in patients who are allergic to cephalosporins and penicillins and in patients with renal failure. These drugs are not recommended in children younger than 3 months or for women during pregnancy (category B) or lactation. Carbapenems are used cautiously in patients with central nervous system (CNS) disorders, seizure disorders, or renal or hepatic failure. The excretion of carbapenems is inhibited when the drug is administered to a patient also taking probenecid (Benemid). Aztreonam should be used cautiously in patients with renal or hepatic impairment.

Vancomycin should not be used in patients with a known hypersensitivity to the drug and is used cautiously in patients with renal or hearing impairment and during pregnancy (category C) and lactation. When administered with other ototoxic and nephrotoxic drugs, additive effects may occur. In other words, one drug alone may not cause the hearing or kidney problem, but when another drug with similar adverse effects is given with vancomycin; the patient is more likely to experience a problem.

• SPECTINOMYCIN

Actions and Uses

Spectinomycin (Trobicin) is chemically related to but different from the aminoglycosides (see Chapter 9). This drug exerts its action by interfering with bacterial protein synthesis. Spectinomycin is used for treating gonorrhea in patients who are allergic to penicillins, cephalosporins, or probenecid (Benemid).

Adverse Reactions

Soreness at the injection site, urticaria, dizziness, rash, chills, fever, and hypersensitivity reactions may occur as side effects of this drug.

Contraindications, Precautions, and Interactions

Spectinomycin is contraindicated in patients with known hypersensitivity to the drug. In addition, the drug should not be given to infants. If another sexually transmitted infection (STI) is present with gonorrhea, additional anti-infectives may be needed to eradicate the infectious processes. Safe use during pregnancy (category B) or lactation or in children has not been established. No significant drug or food interactions for spectinomycin are known.

● QUINUPRISTIN/DALFOPRISTIN

Actions and Uses

Quinupristin/dalfopristin is a bacteriostatic agent used in the treatment of VREF. It has bactericidal action against both methicillin-susceptible and methicillin-resistant staphylococci.

Adverse Reactions

This drug is irritating to the vein. After peripheral infusion of quinupristin/dalfopristin, the vein should be flushed with 5% dextrose in water (D_5W), because the drug is incompatible with saline or heparin flush solutions. Other adverse reactions include nausea, vomiting, and diarrhea.

Contraindications, Precautions, and Interactions

This drug is contraindicated in patients with a known hypersensitivity to quinupristin/dalfopristin. Because prolonged use of anti-infectives can disrupt normal flora, the patient should be monitored for secondary bacterial or fungal infections. This drug should not be used during pregnancy (category B) and lactation. When taking quinupristin/dalfopristin, the serum levels of the following drugs may increase: antiretrovirals, antineoplastic and immunosuppressant agents, calcium channel blockers, benzodiazepines, and cisapride.

NURSING PROCESS
PATIENT RECEIVING A FLUOROQUINOLONE OR MISCELLANEOUS ANTI-INFECTIVE

ASSESSMENT

Preadministration Assessment
Before administering a fluoroquinolone or miscellaneous anti-infective, the nurse identifies and records the signs and symptoms of the infection. It is particularly important for the nurse to obtain a thorough allergy history, especially a history of drug allergies. The nurse should take and record vital signs as well. The primary health care provider may order culture and sensitivity tests, and the culture is obtained before the first dose of the drug is given. Other laboratory tests, such as renal and hepatic function tests, complete blood count, and urinalysis, also may be ordered before and during drug therapy for early detection of toxic reactions.

Ongoing Assessment
During drug therapy with the miscellaneous anti-infectives or fluoroquinolones, it is important for the nurse to perform an ongoing assessment. In general, the nurse compares the initial signs and symptoms of the infection, which were recorded during the initial assessment, with the current signs and symptoms. The nurse then records these findings in the patient's chart. The nurse monitors the patient's vital signs every 4 hours or as ordered by the primary health care provider. The nurse should notify the primary health care provider if there are changes in the vital signs, such as a significant drop in blood pressure, an increase in the pulse or respiratory rate, or a sudden increase in temperature.

NURSING DIAGNOSES

Drug-specific nursing diagnoses include the following:

❏ **Anxiety** related to feelings about seriousness of illness, route of administration, other factors
❏ **Risk for Impaired Comfort** related to fever
❏ **Risk for Impaired Skin Integrity** related to photosensitivity
❏ **Acute Pain** related to tissue injury during drug therapy
❏ **Diarrhea** related to superinfection secondary to antibiotic therapy adverse drug reaction
❏ **Risk for Impaired Urinary Elimination** related to adverse drug effects (nephrotoxicity)
❏ **Risk for Disturbed Sensory Perception: Auditory** related to adverse drug effects (ototoxicity)

Nursing diagnoses related to drug administration are discussed in Chapter 4.

PLANNING

The expected outcomes for the patient may include an optimal response to therapy, which includes control of the infectious process, meeting of patient needs related to the management of adverse drug reactions, and an understanding of the therapeutic regimen.

IMPLEMENTATION

Promoting an Optimal Response to Therapy
A variety of adverse reactions can be seen with the administration of the fluoroquinolones or aminoglycosides. The nurse observes the patient, especially during the first 48 hours of therapy. It is important to report the occurrence of any adverse reaction to the primary health care provider before the next dose of the drug is due. If a serious adverse reaction, such as a hypersensitivity

reaction, respiratory difficulty, severe diarrhea, or a decided drop in blood pressure, occurs the nurse contacts the primary health care provider immediately.

The nurse always listens to, evaluates, and reports any complaints the patient may have; certain complaints may be an early sign of an adverse drug reaction. The nurse should report all changes in the patient's condition and any new problems that occur (e.g., nausea or diarrhea) as soon as possible. It is then up to the primary health care provider to decide if these changes or problems are a part of the patient's infectious process or the result of an adverse drug reaction.

The nurse encourages patients who receive the fluoroquinolones to increase their fluid intake. Norfloxacin is given on an empty stomach (e.g., 1 hour before or 2 hours after meals). Some drugs are made so that they release the drug over time in the body; these formulations are known as **extended-release** (XR), sustained-release (SR), or controlled-release (CR) drugs. Because the amount of drug would be too great if released in the body at once, it is important to swallow these medications whole. Patients should not crush, chew, or break extended-release medications. If the patient is taking an antacid, ciprofloxacin and moxifloxacin should be administered 2 to 4 hours before or 6 to 8 hours after the antacid.

INTRAMUSCULAR ADMINISTRATION. To promote an optimal response to therapy when giving spectinomycin intramuscularly (IM), the nurse inspects for previous injection sites and signs of pain or tenderness, redness, and swelling. In addition, the nurse reports any persistent local reaction to the primary health care provider.

> **! NURSING ALERT**
>
> The nurse should administer each IV dose of vancomycin over 60 minutes. Too rapid an infusion may result in a sudden and profound fall in blood pressure and shock. When giving the drug IV, the nurse closely monitors the infusion rate and the patient's blood pressure. The nurse reports any decrease in blood pressure or occurrence of throbbing neck or back pain. These symptoms could indicate a severe adverse reaction referred to as red-neck or **red-man syndrome**.
>
> Other symptoms of this syndrome include fever, chills, paresthesias, and erythema (redness) of the neck and back.
>
> The nurse reports patient complaints of difficulty hearing or tinnitus (ringing in the ears) to the primary health care provider before the next dose is due. In addition, the nurse monitors the fluid intake and output and brings any decrease in the urinary output to the attention of the primary health care provider.

INTRAVENOUS ADMINISTRATION. When these drugs are administered intravenously (IV), the nurse inspects the needle site and area around the needle at frequent intervals for signs of **extravasation**, or leakage into the soft tissue, of the IV fluid. More frequent assessments are performed if the patient is restless or uncooperative. Many of the miscellaneous anti-infectives irritate the vein when administered by the IV route.

The rate of infusion is checked every 15 minutes and adjusted as needed. This is especially important when administering vancomycin, because rapid infusion of the drug can result in severe hypotension and shock. The nurse inspects the vein used for the IV infusion every 4 to 8 hours for signs of tenderness, pain, and redness (which may indicate phlebitis or thrombophlebitis). If these symptoms are apparent, the IV infusion is restarted in another vein and the problem brought to the attention of the primary health care provider.

Monitoring and Managing Patient Needs
Although the drugs in this chapter are different, many of the patient problems are similar. The nurse should consider the commonalities of the drugs to look for common problems.

ANXIETY. Patients may exhibit varying degrees of anxiety related to their illness and infection and the necessary drug therapy. When these drugs are given by the parenteral route, patients may experience anxiety because of the discomfort or pain that accompanies an IM injection or IV administration. The nurse reassures the patient that every effort will be made to reduce pain and discomfort, although complete pain relief may not always be possible.

IMPAIRED COMFORT: INCREASED FEVER. The infectious process is accompanied by an elevation in temperature. When the patient is being treated for the infection, the nurse must monitor the vital signs, particularly the body temperature. As the anti-infective works to rid the body of the infectious organism, the body temperature should return to normal. The nurse monitors the vital signs (temperature, pulse, and respiration) frequently to assess the drug's effectiveness in eradicating the infection. The nurse checks the vital signs every 4 hours, or more frequently if the temperature is elevated. The primary health care provider is notified if a temperature rises over 101°F.

IMPAIRED SKIN INTEGRITY. The fluoroquinolone drugs cause dangerous photosensitivity reactions. Patients have experienced severe reactions even when they used sunscreen or sunblock products. Patients should be cautioned to wear cover-up clothing with long sleeves and wide-brimmed hats when outside in addition to sunblock preparations. Patients should be aware that glare during hazy or cloudy days can cause skin reactions as readily as direct sunlight on a clear day.

ACUTE PAIN: TISSUE INJURY. Pain at the injection site may occur when these drugs are given IM. The nurse warns the patient that discomfort may be felt when it is injected and that additional discomfort may be experienced for a brief time afterward. The nurse places a warm, moist compress over the injection site to help alleviate the discomfort.

Many of these anti-infectives are irritating to the vein when administered IV. The nurse should read instructions carefully for infusion rates. For intravenously administered fluoroquinolones, as with other caustic drugs, the nurse inspects the needle site and the area around the needle every hour for signs of extravasation of the IV fluid. The nurse performs these assessments more frequently if the patient is restless or uncooperative. It is important to check the rate of infusion every 15 minutes and adjust it as needed. The proper flush solution is used after the infusion to keep the vein open and minimize irritation. The nurse should inspect the vein used for the IV infusion every 4 hours for signs of tenderness, pain, and redness (which may indicate phlebitis or thrombophlebitis). If these are apparent, the nurse must restart the IV in another vein and bring the problem to the attention of the primary health care provider.

All fluoroquinolone drugs can cause pain, inflammation, or rupture of a tendon. The Achilles tendon is particularly vulnerable. This problem can be so severe that prolonged disability results, and, at times, surgical intervention may be necessary to correct the problem.

DIARRHEA. Because superinfections and pseudomembranous colitis can occur during therapy with these drugs, the nurse checks the patient's stools and reports any incidence of diarrhea immediately because this may indicate a superinfection or pseudomembranous colitis. If diarrhea does occur and blood and mucus appear in the stool, the nurse should save a sample of the stool and test it for occult blood using a test such as Hemoccult. If the stool tests positive for blood, it is important to save the sample for possible additional laboratory tests.

IMPAIRED URINARY ELIMINATION. It is important for the nurse to monitor for nephrotoxicity. The nurse measures and records intake and output while the patient is receiving these drugs. Any changes in the intake–output ratio or in the appearance of the urine must be reported immediately, because these may indicate nephrotoxicity.

DISTURBED SENSORY PERCEPTION: AUDITORY. The nurse also closely monitors for ototoxicity in all patients receiving an anti-infective. It is important to report any ringing in the ears, difficulty hearing, or dizziness to the primary health care provider. Changes in hearing may not be noticed initially by the patient, but when changes occur they usually progress from difficulty in hearing high-pitched sounds to problems hearing low-pitched sounds.

Educating the Patient and Family

Carefully planned patient and family education is important to foster compliance, relieve anxiety, and promote therapeutic effect. The nurse explains all adverse reactions associated with the specific prescribed antibiotic to the patient. The nurse advises the patient of the signs and symptoms of potentially serious adverse reactions, such as hypersensitivity reactions, moderate to severe diarrhea, and sudden onset of chills and fever. The nurse should explain to the patient the necessity of contacting the primary health care provider immediately if such symptoms occur. To reduce the incidence of noncompliance with the treatment regimen, a teaching plan is developed to include the information that appears in the Patient Teaching for Improved Patient Outcomes: Taking Anti-Infectives.

EVALUATION

- Therapeutic response is achieved, and there is no evidence of infection.
- Adverse reactions are identified, reported to the primary health care provider, and managed successfully with appropriate nursing interventions:
  - ☑ Anxiety is managed successfully.
  - ☑ Patient reports comfort without fever.
  - ☑ Skin is intact and free of inflammation, irritation, infection, or ulcerations.
  - ☑ Patient reports no pain or injury.
  - ☑ Patient does not experience diarrhea.
  - ☑ Patient maintains an adequate fluid intake for proper urinary elimination.
  - ☑ Patient's hearing is intact.
- Patient and family demonstrate an understanding of the drug regimen.

Patient Teaching for Improved Patient Outcomes

Taking Anti-Infectives

✓ Take the drug at the prescribed time intervals. These time intervals are important because a certain amount of the drug must be in the body at all times for the infection to be controlled.

✓ Drink six to eight 8-ounce glasses of fluid while taking these drugs, and take each dose with a full glass of water.

✓ Do not increase or omit the dose unless advised to do so by the primary health care provider.

✓ Complete the entire course of treatment. Do not stop the drug, except on the advice of a primary health care provider, before the course of treatment is completed, even if symptoms improve or disappear. Failure to complete the prescribed course of treatment may result in a return of the infection.

✓ Follow the directions supplied with the prescription regarding taking the drugs with meals or on an empty stomach. Take drugs that must be taken on an empty stomach, 1 hour before or 2 hours after a meal.

✓ Distinguish between immediate- and extended-release medications. Do not break, chew, or crush extended-release medications.

✓ Notify the primary health care provider if symptoms of the infection become worse or if original symptoms do not improve after 5 to 7 days of drug therapy.

✓ Avoid any exposure to sunlight or ultraviolet light (tanning beds, sunlamps) while taking these drugs and for several weeks after completing the course of therapy. Wear sunblock, sunglasses, and protective clothing when exposed to sunlight.

✓ Avoid tasks requiring mental alertness until response to the drug is known.

Specific Instructions Regarding Fluoroquinolone Therapy

✓ When taking the fluoroquinolones, report any signs of tendinitis, such as pain or soreness in the leg, shoulder, or back of the heel. Periodic applications of ice may help relieve the pain. Until tendinitis or tendon rupture can be excluded, rest the involved area and avoid exercise.

✓ Do not take antacids or drugs containing iron or zinc, because these drugs will decrease absorption of the fluoroquinolone.

THINK CRITICALLY: PHARMACOLOGY IN PRACTICE

1. The charge nurse asks you to discuss the drug quinupristin/dalfopristin (Synercid) and VREF at a team conference. Determine what specific points about preventing transmission of this condition you would discuss at the conference.

● Test Your Knowledge

1. Patients taking a fluoroquinolone are encouraged to _____.

   A. nap 1 to 2 hours daily while taking the drug
   B. eat a high-protein diet
   C. increase their fluid intake
   D. avoid foods high in carbohydrate

2. Which of the following complaints by a man taking vancomycin would be most indicative that he is experiencing ototoxicity?

   A. Tingling of the extremities
   B. Complaints that he is unable to hear the television
   C. Changes in mental status
   D. Short periods of dizziness

3. When giving spectinomycin for gonorrhea, the nurse advises the patient to _____.

   A. return for a follow-up examination
   B. limit fluid intake to 1200 mL/day while taking the drug
   C. return the next day for a second injection
   D. avoid drinking alcohol for the next 10 days

4. When monitoring the IV infusion of vancomycin, the nurse makes sure the drug infuses over a period of 60 minutes because rapid infusion can result in _____.

   A. fluid overload and respiratory distress
   B. a sudden and profound fall in blood pressure
   C. fluid deficit and dehydration
   D. a sudden and severe rise in blood pressure

● Prepare for the NCLEX

1. A patient is prescribed moxifloxacin. The nurse notes that the patient is also taking an antacid. The nurse correctly administers moxifloxacin _____.

   A. once daily orally, 4 hours before the antacid
   B. twice daily orally, immediately after the antacid
   C. once daily IM without regard to the administration of the antacid
   D. every 12 hours IV without regard to the administration of the antacid

● Calculate Medication Dosages

1. A patient is prescribed 500 mg of vancomycin orally every 6 hours. The drug is available in 500-mg tablets. The nurse administers _____.

2. Aztreonam 500 mg IV is ordered. The drug is available in a vial with 500 mg/15 mL. The nurse administers _____.

3. The primary health care provider prescribes linezolid 400 mg orally. The drug is available as an oral suspension in strength of 100 mg/5 mL. The nurse administers _____.

To check your answers, see Appendix E.

the**Point**: *For more NCLEX questions, log on to http://thepoint.lww.com to access more than 1000 questions.*

Antitubercular Drugs

LEARNING OBJECTIVES

On completion of this chapter, the student will:

1. Discuss the drugs used in the treatment of mycobacteria for tuberculosis and leprosy.
2. Discuss the uses, general drug actions, contraindications, precautions, interactions, and general adverse reactions associated with the administration of the antitubercular drugs.
3. Discuss important preadministration and ongoing assessment activities the nurse should perform on the patient taking an antitubercular drug.
4. List nursing diagnoses particular to a patient taking an antitubercular drug.
5. Describe directly observed therapy (DOT).
6. Discuss ways to promote an optimal response to therapy, how to manage adverse reactions, and important points to keep in mind when educating patients about the use of the antitubercular drugs.

Tuberculosis (TB) is a major health problem throughout the world, especially in Asia and Africa; almost 2 million deaths each year are caused by TB. The World Health Organization (WHO) predicts that 9.2 million people worldwide will contract this disease each year. Individuals living in crowded conditions, those with compromised immune systems, and those with debilitative conditions are especially susceptible to TB. People with human immunodeficiency virus (HIV) infection are especially at risk for TB because of their compromised immune systems.

Tuberculosis is an infectious disease caused by the *Mycobacterium tuberculosis* bacterium. The pathogen is also referred to as the *tubercle bacillus*. The disease is transmitted from one person to another by droplets dispersed in the air when an infected person coughs or sneezes. These droplet nuclei are then inhaled by noninfected persons. Although TB primarily affects the lungs, other organs may be affected also. For example, if the immune system is inadequate, the infection can spread from the lungs to other organs of the body.

Extrapulmonary (outside of the lungs) tuberculosis is the term used to distinguish TB affecting the lungs from infection with the *M. tuberculosis* bacillus in other organs of the body. Organs that can be affected include the liver, kidneys, spleen, and uterus. Tuberculosis responds well to long-term treatment with a combination of three or more antitubercular drugs.

Antitubercular drugs are used to treat active cases of TB. They are also used as **prophylactic (preventative)** therapy to prevent the spreading of TB. The drugs used to treat TB do not "cure" the disease, but they do render the patient noninfectious to others. Antitubercular drugs are classified as primary (first-line) and secondary (second-line) drugs. Primary drugs provide the foundation for treatment. Secondary drugs are less effective and more toxic than primary drugs. These drugs are used in various combinations to treat TB. Sensitivity testing may be done to determine the most effective combination treatment, especially in areas of the country where patients may become resistant to therapy.

> **NURSING ALERT**
>
> Active TB in patients infected with HIV can be difficult to diagnose. Because the patients' immune systems are deficient, TB skin tests may not show a reaction even when the disease is present. X-ray studies, sputum analyses, or physical examinations may be needed to diagnose *M. tuberculosis* infection accurately in patients with HIV infection.

Secondary drugs are used to treat extrapulmonary TB or drug-resistant microorganisms. The primary antitubercular drugs are discussed in this chapter. Both primary and secondary antitubercular drugs are listed in the Summary Drug Table: Antitubercular Drugs. Certain fluoroquinolones such as ciprofloxacin, ofloxacin, and levofloxacin have proven effective against TB and are considered secondary drugs (see Chapter 10).

Actions

Most antitubercular drugs are bacteriostatic against the *M. tuberculosis* bacillus. These drugs usually act to inhibit bacterial cell wall synthesis, which slows the multiplication rate of the bacteria. Only isoniazid is bactericidal, with rifampin and streptomycin having some bactericidal activity.

Uses

Antitubercular drugs are used with other drugs to treat active TB. Isoniazid (INH), however, may be used alone in preventive therapy (prophylaxis). For example, when a person is diagnosed with TB, family members of the infected individual must be given prophylactic treatment with isoniazid for 6 months to 1 year. Display 11.1 identifies prophylactic uses for isoniazid.

Standard Treatment

Standard treatment for TB is divided into two phases: the initial phase, followed by a continuing phase. During the initial phase, drugs are used to kill the rapidly multiplying *M. tuberculosis* and to prevent drug resistance. The initial phase lasts approximately 2 months and the continuing phase approximately 4 months, with the total treatment regimen lasting for 6 to 9 months, depending on the patient's response to therapy.

The initial phase involves using the following drugs: isoniazid, rifampin (Rifadin), and pyrazinamide, along with ethambutol (Myambutol). The Centers for Disease Control and Prevention (CDC) recommends that treatment begin as soon as possible after the diagnosis of TB. The recommended treatment regimen is for the administration of rifampin, isoniazid, pyrazinamide, and ethambutol for a minimum of 2 months. The second or continuation phase includes only the drugs rifampin and isoniazid. The CDC recommends this phase for 4 months or up to 7 months in special populations. These special circumstances include the following:

- Positive sputum culture after completion of initial treatment
- Cavitary (hole or pocket of) disease and positive sputum culture after initial treatment
- Noninclusion of pyrazinamide in the initial treatment
- Positive sputum culture after initial treatment in a patient with previously diagnosed HIV infection

DISPLAY 11.1 Prophylactic Uses for Isoniazid (INH)

Isoniazid may be used in the following situations:
- Household members and other close associates of those recently diagnosed as having tuberculosis
- Those whose tuberculin skin test has become positive in the last 2 years
- Those with positive skin tests whose radiographic (x-ray) findings indicate nonprogressive, healed, or **quiescent** (causing no symptoms) tubercular lesions
- Those at risk of developing tuberculosis (e.g., those with Hodgkin's disease, severe diabetes mellitus, leukemia, and other serious illnesses and those receiving corticosteroids or drug therapy for a malignancy)
- All patients younger than 35 years (primarily children to age 7) who have a positive skin test
- Persons with acquired immunodeficiency syndrome (AIDS) or those who are positive for HIV and have a positive tuberculosis skin test *or* a negative tuberculosis skin test but have a history of a prior significant reaction to purified protein derivative (a skin test for tuberculosis)

Retreatment

At times, treatment fails because of inadequate initial drug treatment or noncompliance with the therapeutic regimen. When treatment fails, retreatment is necessary. Retreatment generally includes the use of four or more antitubercular drugs. Retreatment drug regimens most often consist of the secondary drugs ethionamide (Trecator), aminosalicylic acid (Paser), cycloserine (Seromycin), and capreomycin (Capastat). Ofloxacin (Floxin) and ciprofloxacin (Cipro) may also be used in retreatment. Sometimes during retreatment, seven or more drugs may be used, with the ineffective drugs discontinued when susceptibility test results are available. Treatment is individualized based on the susceptibility of the microorganism. Up to 24 months of continued treatment after sputum cultures are no longer positive for TB can be part of the plan.

Resistance to the Antitubercular Drugs

Of increasing concern is the development of mutant strains of TB that are resistant to many of the antitubercular drugs currently in use. Bacterial resistance develops, sometimes rapidly, with the use of antitubercular drugs. Treatment is individualized and based on laboratory studies that identify the drugs to which the organism is susceptible. The CDC recommends using three or more drugs with initial therapy, as well as in retreatment, because using a combination of drugs slows the development of bacterial resistance. Tuberculosis caused by drug-resistant organisms should be considered in patients who have no response to therapy and in patients who have been treated in the past.

This chapter discusses the following primary antitubercular drugs: ethambutol, isoniazid, pyrazinamide, and rifampin. Other primary and secondary drugs are listed in the Summary Drug Table: Antitubercular Drugs.

● ETHAMBUTOL

Adverse Reactions

Generalized Reactions

- Dermatitis and pruritus
- Joint pain
- Anorexia
- Nausea and vomiting

Severe Reactions

- Anaphylactoid reactions (unusual or exaggerated allergic reactions)
- **Optic neuritis** (a decrease in visual acuity and changes in color perception); optic neuritis is dose related

Contraindications, Precautions, and Interactions

Ethambutol is not recommended for patients with a history of hypersensitivity to the drug or children younger than

Summary Drug Table ANTITUBERCULAR DRUGS

Generic Name	Trade Name	Uses	Adverse Reactions	Dosage Ranges
Primary (First-Line) Drugs				
ethambutol *eth-am'-byoo-toll*	Myambutol	Pulmonary TB	Optic neuritis, fever, pruritus, headache, nausea, anorexia, dermatitis, hypersensitivity, psychic disturbances	15–25 mg/kg/day orally
isoniazid (INH) *eye-soe-nye'-ah-zid*	Nydrazid	Active TB; prophylaxis for TB	Peripheral neuropathy, nausea, vomiting, epigastric distress, jaundice, hepatitis, pyridoxine deficiency, skin eruptions, hypersensitivity	*Active TB*: 5 mg/kg (up to 300 mg/d) orally or 15 mg/kg 2–3 times weekly *TB prophylaxis*: 300 mg/day orally
pyrazinamide *peer-ah-zin'-ah-mide*		Active TB	Hepatotoxicity, nausea, vomiting, diarrhea, myalgia, rashes	15–30 mg/kg/day orally maximum 3 g/day orally; 50–70 mg/kg twice weekly orally
rifabutin *rif-ah-byoo'-tin*	Mycobutin	*Mycobacterium avium*	Nausea, vomiting, diarrhea, rash, discolored urine	300 mg/day orally or 150 mg orally BID
rifampin *rif-am'-pin*	Rifadin, Rimactane	Active TB, Hansen's disease	Heartburn, drowsiness, fatigue, dizziness, epigastric distress, hematologic changes, renal insufficiency, rash, body fluid discoloration	10 mg/kg (up to 600 mg/day) orally, IV
rifapentine *rif-ah-pen'-teen*	Priftin	Active TB	Hyperuricemia, proteinuria, hematuria, rash, lymphopenia	600 mg twice weekly orally
Combination Drugs				
isoniazid 150 mg and rifampin 300 mg	Rifamate	TB	See individual drugs	1–2 tablets daily orally
isoniazid 50 mg, rifampin 120 mg, and pyrazinamide 300 mg	Rifater	TB	See individual drugs	1–2 tablets daily orally
Secondary (Second-Line) Drugs				
aminosalicylate *ah-meen-oh-sal'-sah-late* (*p*-aminosalicylic acid; 4-aminosalicylic acid)	Paser	TB	Nausea, vomiting, diarrhea, abdominal pain, hypersensitivity reactions	4 g (1 packet) orally TID
capreomycin *kap-ree-oh-mye'-sin*	Capastat	TB	Hypersensitivity reactions, nephrotoxicity, hepatic impairment, pain and in duration at injection site, ototoxicity	1 g/day (maximum 20 mg/kg/day) IM
cycloserine *sye-kloe-ser'-een*	Seromycin	TB	Convulsions, somnolence, confusion, renal impairment, sudden development of congestive heart failure, psychoses	500 mg–1 g orally in divided doses
ethionamide *eh-thye-on-am'-ide*	Trecator	TB, Hansen's disease	Nausea, vomiting, diarrhea, headache	15–20 mg/kg/day orally

(table continues on page 101)

Summary Drug Table ANTITUBERCULAR DRUGS (continued)

Generic Name	Trade Name	Uses	Adverse Reactions	Dosage Ranges
streptomycin *strep-toe-mye'-sin* (although still available, this drug is seldom used)		TB; infections due to susceptible microorganisms	Nephrotoxicity, ototoxicity, numbness, tingling, paresthesia of the face, nausea, dizziness	15 mg/kg but no more than 1 g IM daily (120 g therapeutic maximum)
Drugs to treat *M. leprae*				
clofazimine *kloe-fazz'-ih-meen*	Lamprene	Hansen's disease	Skin pigmentation (pink to brown), skin dryness, rash, abdominal/epigastric pain, nausea, vomiting, burning or itching of the eyes, dizziness, headache	100 mg/day orally
dapsone *dap'-sone*		Hansen's disease, dermatitis herpetiformis; *pneumocystis carinii* pneumonia; pneumonia prophylaxis	Hemolytic anemia, headache, insomnia, phototoxicity, nausea, vomiting, anorexia, rash, fever, jaundice, toxic epidermal necrolysis	50–300 mg/day orally

Ⓡ This drug should be administered at least 1 hour before or 2 hours after a meal.

13 years. The drug is used with caution during pregnancy (category B), in patients with hepatic or renal impairment, and in patients with diabetic retinopathy or cataracts.

• ISONIAZID

Adverse Reactions

The incidence of adverse reactions appears to be higher when larger doses of isoniazid are prescribed.

Generalized Reactions

- Nausea and vomiting
- Epigastric distress
- Fever
- Skin eruptions
- Hematologic changes
- Jaundice
- Hypersensitivity

Toxicity

- **Peripheral neuropathy** (numbness and tingling of the extremities) is the most common symptom of toxicity.
- Severe, and sometimes fatal, hepatitis has been associated with isoniazid therapy and may appear after many months of treatment.

Contraindications and Precautions

Isoniazid is contraindicated in patients with a history of hypersensitivity to the drug. The drug is used with caution during pregnancy (category C) or lactation and in patients with hepatic and renal impairment.

Interactions

The following interactions may occur when isoniazid is administered with another agent:

Interacting Drug	Common Use	Effect of Interaction
antacids containing aluminum salts	Relief of heartburn and gastrointestinal upset	Reduced absorption of isoniazid
anticoagulants	Blood thinner	Increased risk for bleeding
phenytoin	Antiseizure drug	Increased serum levels of phenytoin
alcohol (in beverages)	Social situations	Higher incidence of drug-related hepatitis

When isoniazid is taken with foods containing tyramine, such as aged cheese and meats, bananas, yeast products, and alcohol, an exaggerated sympathetic-type response can occur (i.e., hypertension, increased heart rate, and palpitations).

compliance goes way down

• PYRAZINAMIDE

Adverse Reactions

Generalized Reactions

- Nausea and vomiting
- Diarrhea
- Myalgia (aches)
- Rashes

Hepatotoxicity

Hepatotoxicity is the principal adverse reaction seen with pyrazinamide use. Symptoms of hepatotoxicity may range from none (except for slightly abnormal hepatic function test results) to a more severe reaction such as jaundice.

Contraindications and Precautions

Pyrazinamide is contraindicated in patients with a history of hypersensitivity to the drug, acute **gout** (a metabolic disorder resulting in increased levels of uric acid and causing severe joint pain), or severe hepatic damage.

Pyrazinamide should be used cautiously in patients during pregnancy (category C) and lactation and in patients with hepatic and renal impairment, HIV infection, and diabetes mellitus.

Interactions

When pyrazinamide is administered with the antigout medications allopurinol (Zyloprim), colchicine, or probenecid (Benemid), its effectiveness decreases.

• RIFAMPIN

Adverse Reactions

Generalized reactions include the following:

- Nausea and vomiting
- Epigastric distress, heartburn, fatigue
- **Vertigo** (dizziness)
- Rash
- Reddish-orange discoloration of body fluids (urine, tears, saliva, sweat, and sputum)
- Hematologic changes, renal insufficiency

Contraindications and Precautions

Rifampin is contraindicated in patients with a history of hypersensitivity to the drug. The drug is used with caution during pregnancy (category C) and lactation and in patients with hepatic or renal impairment.

Interactions

The following interactions may occur when rifampin is administered with another agent:

Interacting Drug	Common Use	Effect of Interaction
antiretrovirals (efavirenz, nevirapine)	HIV infection	Decreased serum levels of antiretrovirals
Digoxin	Management of cardiac problems	Decreased serum levels of digoxin
oral contraceptives	Contraception	Decreased contraceptive effectiveness

Interacting Drug	Common Use	Effect of Interaction
Isoniazid	Antitubercular agent	Higher risk of hepatotoxicity
oral anticoagulants	Blood thinner	Increased risk for bleeding
oral hypoglycemics	Antidiabetic agent	Decreased effectiveness of oral hypoglycemic agent
chloramphenicol		Increased risk for seizures
Phenytoin	Anti-infective agent / Antiseizure agent	Decreased effectiveness of phenytoin
Verapamil		Decreased effectiveness of verapamil

Note: **Leprosy**, also referred to as *Hansen's disease*, is caused by the bacterium ***Mycobacterium leprae***. Leprosy is a chronic, communicable disease that is not easily spread and has a long incubation period. Since 1985, the prevalence of leprosy has dropped by 90%. About 100 new cases are diagnosed yearly in the United States (primarily the southern states, Hawaii, and U.S. possessions).

Peripheral nerves are affected, causing sensory loss and muscle weakness. The traditional fear of leprosy relates to skin involvement, which may present with lesions confined to a few isolated areas or may be fairly widespread over the entire body. Dapsone, clofazimine (Lamprene), rifampin (Rifadin), and ethionamide (Trecator) are drugs currently used to treat leprosy. The leprostatic drugs are listed in the Summary Drug Table: Antitubercular Drugs.

NURSING PROCESS
PATIENT RECEIVING AN ANTITUBERCULAR DRUG

ASSESSMENT

Preadministration Assessment
Once the diagnosis of TB is confirmed, the primary health care provider selects the drug that will best control the spread of the disease and make the patient noninfectious to others. Many laboratory and diagnostic tests may be necessary before starting antitubercular therapy, including radiographic studies, culture and sensitivity tests, and various types of laboratory tests, such as a complete blood count. It also is important to assess the family history and a history of contacts if the patient has active TB.

Depending on the severity of the disease, patients may be treated initially in the hospital and then discharged for supervised follow-up care, or they may have all treatment instituted on an outpatient basis.

Ongoing Assessment
When performing the ongoing assessment, the nurse observes the patient daily for the appearance of adverse reactions. These observations are especially important when a drug is known to be nephrotoxic or ototoxic.

It is important to report any adverse reactions to the primary health care provider. In addition, the nurse carefully monitors vital signs daily or as frequently as every 4 hours when the patient is hospitalized.

NURSING DIAGNOSES

Drug administration specific nursing diagnoses are the following:

❏ **Acute Pain** related to frequent injection of antitubercular drug
❏ **Imbalanced Nutrition: Less than Body Requirements** related to gastric upset and general poor health status
❏ **Risk of Ineffective Therapeutic Regimen Management** related to indifference, lack of knowledge, long-term treatment regimen, other factors

The nursing diagnosis of Ineffective Therapeutic Regimen Management may be especially important with patients considering the long-term therapy required to treat TB. Refer to interventions discussed in Chapter 4 to deal with those patient needs.

PLANNING

The expected outcomes for the patient may include an optimal response to antitubercular therapy, meeting patient needs related to the management of common adverse reactions, and an understanding of and compliance with the prescribed treatment regimen.

IMPLEMENTATION

Promoting an Optimal Response to Therapy

The diagnosis of TB, along with the necessity of long-term treatment and follow-up, is often distressing to the patient. Patients with a diagnosis of TB may have many questions about the disease and its treatment. As such, the nurse allows time for the patient and family members to ask questions. In some instances, it may be necessary to refer the patient to other health care workers, such as a social service worker or a dietitian.

MONITORING AND MANAGING PATIENT NEEDS.   Managing adverse reactions in patients taking antitubercular drugs is an important responsibility of the nurse. The nurse must continuously observe for signs of adverse reactions and immediately report them to the primary health care provider

ACUTE PAIN: FREQUENT PARENTERAL INJECTIONS.   When administering the antitubercular drug by the parenteral route, the nurse is careful to rotate the injection sites. At the time of each injection, the nurse inspects previous injection sites for signs of swelling, redness, and tenderness. If a localized reaction persists or if the area appears to be infected, it is important to notify the primary health care provider.

IMBALANCED NUTRITION: LESS THAN BODY REQUIREMENTS.   When TB affects patients who live in crowded and impoverished conditions, malnutrition may be prevalent. In some cases alcoholism may compound the patient's difficulties.

This complicates the administration of drugs and compromises the general condition of the patient's gastrointestinal tract. Ethambutol should be given at the same time daily and may be given without regard to food. Pyrazinamide may also be given with food. The nurse should give other antitubercular drugs by the oral route and on an empty stomach, unless epigastric upset occurs. If gastric upset occurs, it is important to notify the primary health care provider before the next dose is given. If a dose is missed, the nurse should tell the patient not to double the dose the next day. An alternative, twice-weekly dosing regimen has been developed to promote compliance on an outpatient basis. This may improve patient nutrition by decreasing the gastric upset of frequent dosing. Combination drugs (e.g., Rifater, which contains isoniazid, rifampin, and pyrazinamide) are being manufactured to promote compliance and reduce the need to take multiple drugs that produce gastric upset.

The nurse teaches the patient to minimize alcohol consumption because of the increased risk of hepatitis. Frequently, the inclusion of pyridoxine (vitamin B_6) is recommended to promote nutrition and prevent neuropathy.

It is helpful to explain to patients that their bodily fluids (urine, feces, saliva, sputum, sweat, and tears) may be colored reddish-orange from the different drugs and that this is normal. It is even more important to teach the patient that this is different from the skin and eye color changes that could indicate hepatic dysfunction (jaundice). The nurse must carefully monitor all patients at least monthly for any evidence of liver dysfunction. It is important to instruct patients to report any of the following symptoms: anorexia, nausea, vomiting, fatigue, weakness, yellowing of the skin or eyes, darkening of the urine, or numbness in the hands and feet

LIFESPAN ALERT – Gerontology
Older adults are particularly susceptible to a potentially fatal hepatitis when taking isoniazid, especially if they consume alcohol on a regular basis. Two other antitubercular drugs, rifampin and pyrazinamide, can cause liver dysfunction in the older adult as well. Careful observation and monitoring for signs of liver impairment are necessary (e.g., increased serum aspartate aminotransferase [AST], alanine aminotransferase [ALT], and bilirubin levels, and jaundice).

INEFFECTIVE THERAPEUTIC REGIMEN MANAGEMENT.   Because the antitubercular drugs must be taken for prolonged periods, compliance with the treatment regimen becomes a problem and increases the risk of development of resistant strains of TB. To help prevent the problem of noncompliance, **directly observed therapy (DOT)** is used to administer these drugs. With DOT, the patient makes periodic visits to the office of the primary care provider or the health clinic, where the drug is taken in the presence of the nurse. The nurse watches the patient swallow each dose of the medication regimen. In some cases, the nurse uses DOT to administer the antitubercular drug in the patient's home, place of employment, or school. DOT may occur daily or two to three times weekly, depending on the patient's health care regimen. Studies indicate that taking the drugs intermittently does not cause a drop in the therapeutic blood levels of antitubercular drugs, even if the drugs are given only two or three times a week.

Educating the Patient and Family

Antitubercular drugs are given for a long time, and careful patient and family education and close medical supervision are necessary. Noncompliance can be a problem whenever a disease or disorder requires long-term treatment. For this reason, the DOT method of administration is preferred. The patient and family must understand that short-term therapy is of no value in treating this disease. The nurse remains alert for statements made by the patient or family that may indicate future noncompliance with the drug regimen necessary in controlling the disease. See Patient Teaching for Improve Patient Outcomes: Increasing Compliance in Tubercular Drug Treatment Program for more information.

EVALUATION

- Therapeutic response is achieved, and there is no evidence of infection.
- Adverse reactions are identified, reported to the primary health care provider, and managed successfully with appropriate nursing interventions:
  ☑ Patient manages injection pain.
  ☑ Patient maintains an adequate nutritional status.
  ☑ Patient manages the therapeutic regimen effectively.
- Patient and family demonstrate an understanding of the drug regimen.

Patient Teaching for Improved Patient Outcomes

Increasing Compliance in Tubercular Drug Treatment Program

The nurse:
✓ Discusses tuberculosis, its causes and communicability, and the need for long-term therapy for disease control.
✓ Reinforces that short-term treatment is ineffective.
✓ Reviews the drug therapy regimen, including the prescribed drugs, doses, and frequency of administration.
✓ Reassures the patient that various combinations of drugs are effective in treating tuberculosis.
✓ Urges the patient to take the drugs exactly as prescribed and not to omit, increase, or decrease the dosage unless directed to do so by the health care provider.
✓ Instructs the patient about possible adverse reactions and the need to notify prescriber should any occur.

✓ Arranges for direct observation therapy with the patient and family.
✓ Instructs the patient in measures to minimize gastrointestinal upset.
✓ Advises the patient to avoid alcohol and the use of nonprescription drugs, especially those containing aspirin, unless use is approved by the health care provider.
✓ Reassures the patient and family that the results of therapy will be monitored by periodic laboratory and diagnostic tests and follow-up visits with the health care provider.

THINK CRITICALLY: PHARMACOLOGY IN PRACTICE

1. Betty Peterson has come into the clinic with complaints of a chronic cough. Ms. Peterson requests that a TB skin test be performed as well as a chest x-ray. She is concerned that she will be diagnosed with TB, telling the nurse that she watched a TV show about the rise in TB in crowded areas. When the nurse questions Betty, she states that "a lot of people" live in the apartment next door. Determine what rationales the nurse would use in teaching Ms. Peterson about risks for TB.

● Test Your Knowledge

1. Which of the following drugs is the only antitubercular drug to be prescribed alone?

   A. rifampin
   B. pyrazinamide
   C. streptomycin
   D. isoniazid

2. The nurse monitors the patient taking isoniazid for toxicity. The most common symptom of toxicity is _____.

   A. peripheral edema
   B. circumoral edema
   C. peripheral neuropathy
   D. jaundice

3. Which of the following is a dose-related adverse reaction to ethambutol?

   A. peripheral neuropathy
   B. optic neuritis
   C. hyperglycemia
   D. fatal hepatitis

4. Which of the following antitubercular drugs is contraindicated in patients with gout?

   A. rifampin
   B. streptomycin
   C. isoniazid
   D. pyrazinamide

● Prepare for the NCLEX

1. The nurse explains to the patient that to slow bacterial resistance to an antitubercular drug, the primary health care provider may prescribe _____.

   A. at least three antitubercular drugs
   B. an antibiotic to be given with the drug
   C. vitamin B_6
   D. that the drug be given only once a week

● Calculate Medication Dosages

1. A patient is prescribed isoniazid syrup 300 mg. The isoniazid is available as 50 mg/mL. The nurse should administer _____.

2. Oral rifampin 600 mg is prescribed. The drug is available in 150-mg tablets. The nurse should administer _____.

To check your answers, see Appendix E.

the**Point** *For more NCLEX questions, log on to http://thepoint.lww.com to access more than 1000 questions.*

Antiviral Drugs

LEARNING OBJECTIVES

On completion of this chapter, the student will:

1. Discuss the uses, general drug actions, adverse reactions, contraindications, precautions, and interactions of antiviral drugs.
2. Discuss important preadministration and ongoing assessment activities the nurse should perform on the patient receiving an antiviral/antiretroviral drug.
3. List nursing diagnoses particular to a patient taking an antiviral drug.
4. List possible goals for a patient taking an antiviral/ antiretroviral drug.
5. Discuss ways to promote an optimal response to therapy and manage adverse reactions, and special considerations to keep in mind when educating the patient and the family about the antiviral/antiretroviral drugs.

Compared with a fungus or bacterium, a virus is a very tiny infectious organism. A virus enters the body through various routes. It can be swallowed, inhaled, injected with a contaminated needle, or transmitted through the bite of an insect. To reproduce, the virus needs the cellular material of another living cell (the host cell). The virus attaches to a cell, enters it, and releases its DNA or RNA inside the cell. The viral material takes control of the cell and forces it to replicate the virus. The cell releases new viruses, which go on to infect other cells (Fig. 12.1). The infected cell usually dies, because the virus keeps it from performing its normal functions.

More than 200 viruses have been identified as capable of producing disease. Common viral infections are those of the nose, throat, and respiratory system. An example is the common cold or influenza. A wart comes from a common virus that infects the skin. Other common viral infections are caused by the herpes viruses. Eight different herpes viruses infect people. Systemic viral infections occur when a virus attacks the nervous system (West Nile), liver (hepatitis C), or white blood cells (immunodeficiency diseases). The drugs used to treat viral infection can be split into two categories: antiviral and antiretroviral agents. For a more complete listing, see the Summary Drug Table: Antiviral Drugs.

• ANTIVIRALS

Actions

Drugs that combat viral infections are called *antiviral drugs*. Antiviral drugs work by interfering with the virus's ability to reproduce in a cell. Antiviral medications are limited in their ability to treat viral infections because viruses are tiny and replicate inside cells, changing how the cell works depending on the type of cell they invade. In comparison, a bacterial organism is relatively large and commonly reproduces outside of cells (e.g., in the bloodstream). This makes antiviral drugs more difficult to develop. Antiviral drugs can be toxic to human cells, and viruses can develop resistance to antiviral drugs. Antibiotics are not effective against viral infections, but if a person has a bacterial infection in addition to a viral infection, an antibiotic is often necessary.

Uses

Labeled Uses

Although infections caused by viruses are common, antiviral drugs have limited use because they are effective against only a small number of specific viral infections (Display 12.1). Antiviral drugs are used in the treatment or prevention of infections caused by:

- Cytomegalovirus (CMV) in transplant recipients
- Herpes simplex virus (HSV) 1 and 2 (genital) and herpes zoster
- Human immunodeficiency virus (HIV)
- Influenza A and B (respiratory tract illness)
- Respiratory syncytial virus (RSV; severe lower respiratory tract infection primarily affecting children)
- Hepatitis B and C

Unlabeled Uses

Because there are a limited number of antiviral drugs and more than 200 viral diseases, the primary health care provider

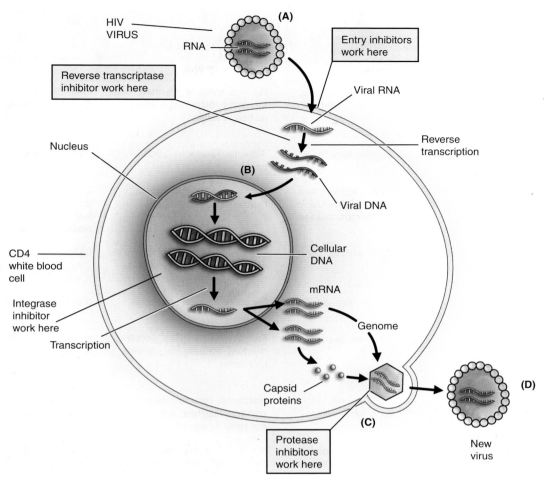

Figure 12.1 Example of viral infection—HIV replication and drug targeting. (**A**) HIV enters a CD4 cell, sheds its protective coating, and inserts its genetic material into the cell. (**B**) HIV DNA enters the nucleus of the CD4 cell and transmits instructions to duplicate HIV DNA. (**C**) The viral RNA and viral proteins assemble at the cell membrane into a new virus. (**D**) The newly assembled HIV leaves the cell to infect other CD4 cells.

may decide to prescribe an antiviral drug for an **unlabeled use** even though its effectiveness for that use is not documented. Approval by the U.S. Food and Drug Administration (FDA) is necessary for a drug to be prescribed. On occasion, the use of a drug for a specific disorder or condition may be under investigation, or it may be approved for use in another country. In this instance, the drug may be prescribed by the primary health care provider for the condition under investigation. The use of the drug for a specific disorder or condition that is not officially approved by the FDA is called an unlabeled use. Examples of unlabeled uses of the antiviral drugs include treatment of CMV and HSV infections after transplantation procedures and varicella pneumonia; the treatment of CMV retinitis in immunocompromised patients; and the use of ribavirin (in aerosol form) for influenza A and B, acute and chronic hepatitis, herpes genitalis, and measles (in oral form).

Adverse Reactions

Gastrointestinal System Reactions

• Nausea, vomiting
• Diarrhea

Other Reactions

• Headache
• Rash
• Fever
• Insomnia

Contraindications

The nurse should not administer antivirals if the patient has a history of allergies to the drug or other antivirals. Cidofovir

(text continues on page 110)

Summary Drug Table ANTIVIRAL DRUGS

Generic Name	Trade Name	Uses	Adverse Reactions	Dosage Ranges
Antivirals				
acyclovir ay-sye'-kloe-veer	Zovirax	HSV herpes zoster, varicella zoster	Nausea, vomiting, diarrhea, fever, headache, dizziness, confusion, rashes, myalgia	Oral: 200–800 mg q 4 hr for 5 doses per day, treat for 5–10 d; IV: 5–10 mg/kg q 8 hr; Topical: apply to lesions q 3 hr
adefovir dipivoxil ah-def'-oh-veer	Hepsera	Chronic hepatitis B	Asthenia, headache, abdominal pain	10 mg/day orally
amantadine ah-man'-tah-deen	Symmetrel	Prevention and treatment of influenza A; Parkinson's disease	Nausea, diarrhea, dizziness, hypotension, insomnia	200 mg/day orally or 100 mg daily for patient over age 65; begin before flu exposure and continue 10 day postexposure
cidofovir sih-doe'-foe-veer	Vistide	CMV retinitis	Headache, nausea, vomiting, diarrhea, anorexia, dyspnea, alopecia, rash, neutropenia, fever, chills	5 mg/kg IV once a week for 2 wk, then once every 2 wk for maintenance
℞ entecavir en-teh'-kah-veer	Baraclude	Chronic hepatitis B	Dizziness, fatigue, headache	0.5–1 mg/day orally
famciclovir fam-sih'-kloe-veer	Famvir	Acute herpes zoster, HSV-2	Fatigue, fever, nausea, vomiting, diarrhea, sinusitis, constipation, headache	Herpes zoster: 500 mg orally q 8 hr for 7 days; HSV-2: 125 mg orally BID for 5 days
foscarnet foss-kar'-net	Foscavir	CMV retinitis; acyclovir-resistant HSV-1 and 2	Headache, seizures, nausea, vomiting, diarrhea, anemia, abnormal renal function test results	CMV retinitis: 90–120 mg/kg/d IV; HSV: 40 mg/kg IV q 8–12 hr
ganciclovir gan-sih'-kloe-veer		CMV prevention in transplant recipients	Anorexia, vomiting, diarrhea, fever, sweats, anemia, leukopenia	5 mg/kg IV q 12 hr for 14–21 d, then daily
oseltamivir oh-sell-tam'-ih-veer	Tamiflu	Prevention and treatment of influenza A and B	Nausea, vomiting, diarrhea	75 mg orally BID for 5 days
ribavirin (inhalation) rye-bah-vye'-rin	Virazole	RSV, chronic hepatitis C	Worsening of pulmonary status, bacterial pneumonia, hypotension	Administered by aerosol with special aerosol generator
ribavirin/interferon combination	Copegus, Rebetol, Ribaspheres	In combination with interferon for hepatitis C	Fatigue, headache, myalgia, anorexia, nausea, vomiting, insomnia, nervousness	800–1200 mg orally BID
rimantadine rih-man'-tah-deen	Flumadine	Influenza A	Lightheadedness, dizziness, insomnia, nausea, anorexia	100 mg/day orally BID
valacyclovir val-ah-sye'-kloe-veer	Valtrex	Herpes zoster; HSV1-2	Nausea, headache	HSV-1:2 g q 12 hr for 1 day HSV-2 initial: 1 g BID for 10 days Recurrent infection: 500 mg orally BID for 5 days Herpes zoster: 1 g orally TID for 7 days
valganciclovir val-gan-sih'-kloe-veer	Valcyte	CMV retinitis, CMV prevention in transplant recipients	Headache, insomnia, diarrhea, nausea, vomiting, pancytopenia, fever	900 mg orally BID; Transplant recipient start 10 days before transplantation and continue 100 days after transplantation
zanamivir zah-nam'-ah-veer	Relenza	Prevention and treatment of influenza A, B	Nausea, headache, rhinitis	5 mg inhalation q 12 hr

(table continues on page 109)

Summary Drug Table ANTIVIRAL DRUGS (continued)

Generic Name	Trade Name	Uses	Adverse Reactions	Dosage Ranges
Antiretrovirals				
abacavir ah-bak'-ah-veer	Ziagen	HIV infection	Nausea, vomiting, diarrhea, anorexia, liver dysfunction	300 mg orally BID or 600 mg once daily
amprenavir am-pren'-ah-veer	Agenerase	HIV infection	Peripheral and circumoral paresthesias, nausea, vomiting, diarrhea, abdominal pain, rash, pruritus	1200 mg orally BID
atazanavir ah-taz'-ah-nah-veer	Reyataz	HIV infection	Nausea, rash	300–400 mg/day
darunavir dah-roon'-ah-veer	Prezista	HIV infection	Headache, diarrhea, constipation, and pain	600 mg orally BID
delavirdine dell-ah-veer'-deen	Rescriptor	HIV infection	Headache, nausea, diarrhea	400 mg orally TID
® didanosine (ddl) dye-dan'-oh-seen	Videx	HIV infection	Headache, nausea, rash, vomiting, peripheral neuropathy, abdominal pain, diarrhea	Oral: 400 mg/day or 200 mg BID; for patients weighing less than 60 kg, 250 mg/day or 125 mg BID
efavirenz ef-ah-veer'-enz	Sustiva	HIV infection	Rash, pruritus, dizziness, insomnia, fatigue, nausea, vomiting	600 mg/day orally
emtricitabine em-trih-sih'-tah-been	Emtriva	HIV infection	Headache, nausea, vomiting, diarrhea, rash	200 mg/day orally
enfuvirtide en-foo-veer'-tide	Fuzeon	HIV infection	Injection site discomfort, in duration, erythema	90 mg subcutaneous injection BID
etravirine eh"-trah-veer'-een	Intelence	HIV infection	Rash, nausea, diarrhea	200 mg orally BID
fosamprenavir foss-am-pren'-ah-veer	Lexiva	HIV infection	Headache, nausea, vomiting, diarrhea, rash	1400 mg/day orally
indinavir in-din'-ah-veer	Crixivan	HIV infection	Headache, nausea, vomiting, diarrhea, kidney/bladder stones	800 mg orally q 8 hr
lamivudine (3TC) lam-ih-vew'-deen	Epivir, Epivir-HB	HIV infection, chronic hepatitis B infection	Headache, nausea, diarrhea, nasal congestion, cough, fatigue	HIV: 150 mg orally BID HBV: 100 mg/day orally daily
maraviroc mah-rah'-veer-ock	Selzentry	HIV infection	Dizziness, cough, rash, abdominal and muscle pains	150–600 mg/day depending upon other antiviral medications
nelfinavir nell-fin'-ah-veer	Viracept	HIV infection	Diarrhea	750 mg orally TID or 1250 mg orally BID
nevirapine neh-veer'-ah-peen	Viramune	HIV infection	Rash, fever, headache, nausea, stomatitis, liver dysfunction	200 mg orally BID
raltegravir ral-teg'-rah-veer	Isentress	HIV infection	Headache, nausea, diarrhea, fever	400 mg orally BID
ritonavir rih-tonn'-ah-veer	Norvir	HIV infection	Peripheral and circumoral paresthesias, nausea, vomiting, diarrhea, anorexia	600 mg orally BID

(table continues on page 110)

Summary Drug Table ANTIVIRAL DRUGS (continued)

Generic Name	Trade Name	Uses	Adverse Reactions	Dosage Ranges
saquinavir *sah-kwin'-a-veer*	Fortovase, Invirase	HIV infection	Headache, nausea, diarrhea, heartburn, flatulence	Fortovase: Six 200-mg capsules orally TID Invirase: Three 200-mg capsules orally TID
stavudine *stay-vew'-den*	Zerit	HIV infection	Headache, nausea, diarrhea, fever, rash, peripheral neuropathy	40 mg orally q 12 hr
telbivudine *tel-biv'-yew-deen*	Tyzeka	Chronic hepatitis B	Headache, abdominal pain, flu-like syndrome, fatigue, URI symptoms	600 mg/day orally
tenofovir disoproxil *teh-noe'-foe-veer*	Viread	HIV infection	Nausea, vomiting, diarrhea, flatulence	300 mg/day orally
tipranavir *tih-pran'-ah-veer*	Aptivus	HIV infection	Nausea, diarrhea	500 mg orally BID
zalcitabine *zal-sit'-tah-been*	Hivid	HIV infection	Peripheral neuropathy, abnormal liver function	0.75 mg orally q 8 hr
zidovudine (AZT) *zye-doe'-vew-deen*	Retrovir	HIV infection, prevention of maternal-fetal HIV transmission	Asthenia, malaise, weakness, headache, anorexia, diarrhea, nausea, abdominal pain, dizziness, insomnia, anemia, agranulocytosis	600 mg/day orally in divided doses; 1 mg/kg IV q 4 hr
Antiretroviral Combinations				
abacavir/lamivudine	Epzicom	See individual drugs above	See individual drugs above	One tablet daily (600 mg/300 mg dose)
abacavir/lamivudine/zidovudine	Trizivir	See individual drugs above	See individual drugs above	One tablet orally twice daily (300mg/150 mg/300 mg dose)
efavirenz/emtricitabine/tenofovir disoproxil	Atripla	See individual drugs above	See individual drugs above	One tablet orally daily (600 mg/200 mg/300 mg)
emtricitabine/tenofovir disoproxil	Truvada	See individual drugs above	See individual drugs above	One tablet orally BID (200 mg/300 mg dose)
lamivudine/zidovudine	Combivir	See individual drugs above	See individual drugs above	One tablet orally BID (150 mg/300 mg dose)
lopinavir/ritonavir *low-pin'-ah-veer/ rih-tonn'-ah-veer*	Kaletra	See individual drugs above	See individual drugs above	One tablet orally BID (400 mg/100 mg dose)

Ⓡ This drug should be administered at least 1 hour before or 2 hours after a meal.

(Vistide) should not be given to patients who have renal impairment or in combination with medications that are nephrotoxic, such as aminoglycosides. Ribavirin should not be used in patients with unstable cardiac disease. These drugs should be used during pregnancy (pregnancy categories B and C) and lactation only when the benefit outweighs the risk to the fetus or child (ribavirin is in pregnancy category X).

Precautions

Antivirals should be used cautiously in patients with renal impairment, low blood cell counts, history of epilepsy (rimantadine), and history of respiratory disease (zanamivir).

DISPLAY 12.1 Description of Viral Infections

Cytomegalovirus

CMV, a virus of the herpes family, is a common viral infection. Healthy individuals may become infected, yet have no symptoms. However, immunocompromised patients (such as those with HIV or cancer) may have the infection. Symptoms include malaise, fever, pneumonia, and superinfection. Infants may acquire the virus from the mother while in the uterus, resulting in learning disabilities and mental retardation. CMV can infect the eye, causing retinitis. Symptoms of CMV retinitis are blurred vision and decreased visual acuity. Visual impairment is irreversible and can lead to blindness if untreated.

Herpes simplex virus

HSV is divided into HSV-1, which causes oral, ocular, or facial infections, and HSV-2, which causes genital infection. However, either type can cause disease at either body site. HSV-1 causes painful vesicular lesions in the oral mucosa, face, or around the eyes. HSV-2 or genital herpes is usually transmitted by sexual contact and causes painful vesicular lesions on the mucous membranes of the genitalia. Vaginal lesions may appear as mucous patches with grayish ulcerations. The patient may appear irritable, lethargic, and jaundiced, and may have difficulty breathing or experience seizures. The lesions usually heal within 2 weeks. Immunosuppressed patients may develop a severe systemic disease.

Herpes zoster

Herpes zoster (shingles) is caused by the varicella (chickenpox) virus. It is highly contagious. The virus causes chickenpox in the child and is easily spread via the respiratory system. Recovery from childhood chickenpox results in the infection lying dormant in the nerve cells. The virus may become reactivated later in life as the older adult's immune system weakens or the individual

becomes ill with other disorders. The lesions of herpes zoster appear as pustules along a sensory nerve route. Pain often continues for several months after the lesions have healed.

Human immunodeficiency virus

HIV or AIDS is a type of viral infection transmitted through an infected person's bodily secretions, such as blood or semen. HIV destroys the immune system, causing the body to develop opportunistic infections such as Kaposi's sarcoma, *Pneumocystis carinii* pneumonia, or tuberculosis. Symptoms include chills and fever, night sweats, dry productive cough, dyspnea, lethargy, malaise, fatigue, weight loss, and diarrhea.

Influenza

Influenza, commonly called the "flu," is an acute respiratory illness caused by influenza viruses A and B. Symptoms include fever, cough, sore throat, runny or stuffy nose, headache, muscle aches, and extreme fatigue. Most people recover within 1 to 2 weeks. Influenza may cause severe complications such as pneumonia in children, the elderly, and other vulnerable groups. The viruses causing influenza continually change over time, which enables them to evade the immune system of the host. These rapid changes in the most commonly circulating types of influenza virus necessitate annual changes in the composition of the "flu" vaccine.

Respiratory syncytial virus

RSV infection is highly contagious and affects mostly children, causing bronchiolitis and pneumonia. Infants younger than 6 months are the most severely affected. In adults, RSV causes colds and bronchitis, with fever, cough, and nasal congestion. When RSV affects immunocompromised patients, the consequences can be severe and sometimes fatal.

Interactions

The following interactions may occur when an antiviral is administered with another agent:

Interacting Drug	Common Use	Effect of Interaction
probenecid	Gout treatment	Increased serum levels of the antivirals
cimetidine	Gastric upset, heartburn	Increased serum level of the antiviral valacyclovir
ibuprofen	Pain relief	Increased serum level of the antiviral adefovir
imipenem-cilastatin	Anti-infective agent	With ganciclovir only, increased risk of seizures
anticholinergic agents	Management of bladder spasms	With amantadine only, increased adverse reactions of anticholinergic agent
theophylline	Management of respiratory problems	With acyclovir only, increased serum level of theophylline

• ANTIRETROVIRALS

Actions

HIV, the virus that causes acquired immunodeficiency syndrome (AIDS) is a **retrovirus**. Retroviruses attack the host cell just like a virus; the difference is that RNA is the primary component of the virus instead of DNA. Retroviruses also contain an enzyme called *reverse transcriptase* that is used to turn the RNA of the virus into DNA, helping to reproduce more of the virus. To control the disease effectively, a number of drugs are used that work at different portions of the life cycle of the virus. This multidrug therapy is called **highly active antiretroviral therapy (HAART)**. The following types of drugs are used in HAART (for more information see the Summary Drug Table: Antiviral Drugs):

- Protease inhibitors, which block the protease enzyme so the new viral particles cannot mature
- Reverse transcriptase inhibitors, which block the reverse transcriptase enzyme so the HIV material can not change into DNA in the new cell
- Entry inhibitors, which prevent the attachment or fusion of HIV to a cell such as CCR5 inhibitors

Antiviral Drugs

• Integrase inhibitors, which prevent enzymes from integrating HIV genetic material into the cell's DNA

Uses

Antiretroviral drugs are used in the treatment of HIV infection and AIDS.

Adverse Reactions

Gastrointestinal System Reactions

• Nausea, vomiting
• Diarrhea
• Altered taste

Other Reactions

• Headache, fever, and chills
• Rash
• Numbness and tingling in the **circumoral** area (around the mouth) or peripherally, or both

Contraindications

The nurse should not administer antiretrovirals if the patient has a history of allergies to the drug or other antiretrovirals. Women who are lactating should not use antiretroviral drugs. Antiretrovirals should not be prescribed to the patient who is using cisapride, pimozide, triazolam, midazolam, or an ergot derivative. Ritonavir is contraindicated if the patient is taking bupropion (Wellbutrin), zolpidem (Ambien), or an antiarrhythmic drug.

Precautions

Antiretrovirals should be used cautiously in patients with diabetes mellitus, impaired hepatic function, pregnancy (pregnancy categories B and C), or hemophilia. Caution should be used for the patient taking indinavir who has a history of kidney or bladder stone formation. If a patient has a sulfonamide allergy, the drugs fosamprenavir and amprenavir should be used cautiously.

Interactions

The following interactions may occur when an antiretroviral is administered with another agent:

Interacting Drug	Common Use	Effect of Interaction
antifungals	Eliminate or manage fungal infections	Increased serum level of the antiretroviral
clarithromycin	Treat bacterial infection	Increased serum level of both drugs
sildenafil	Treat erectile dysfunction	Increased adverse reactions of sildenafil
opioid analgesics	Pain relief	Risk of toxicity with ritonavir

Interacting Drug	Common Use	Effect of Interaction
anticoagulant, anticonvulsant, antiparasitic agents	Prevent blood clots, seizures, parasitic infections, respectively	Decreased effectiveness when taking ritonavir
interleukins	Prevent severely low platelet counts usually related to chemotherapy	Risk of antiretroviral toxicity
fentanyl	Analgesia, used typically with procedures requiring anesthesia	Increased serum level of fentanyl
oral contraceptives	Birth control	Decreased effectiveness of the birth control agent
rifampin	Pulmonary tuberculosis	With afavirenz, nevirapine only; decreased serum levels of antivirals

HERBAL ALERT

Individuals have tried St. John's wort for both the antidepressive and antiviral effects of the supplement. Researchers have found that in patients with HIV infection who receive prescribed protease inhibitors, the effectiveness of drug therapy is reduced if the patient also takes St. John's wort. Patients need to be instructed to disclose the use of all over-the-counter medications and supplements to their primary health care provider to prevent potentially harmful interactions.

NURSING PROCESS
PATIENT RECEIVING AN ANTIVIRAL/ ANTIRETROVIRAL DRUG

ASSESSMENT

Preadministration Assessment
Preadministration assessment of the patient receiving an antiviral drug depends on the patient's symptoms or diagnosis. These patients may have a serious infection that weakens their natural defenses against disease. Before administering the antiviral drug, the nurse determines the patient's general state of health and resistance to infection. The nurse then records the patient's symptoms and complaints. In addition, the nurse takes and records the patient's vital signs. Additional assessments may be necessary in certain types of viral infections or in patients who are acutely ill. For example, before treatment of patients with HSV-1 or HSV-2 infection, the nurse inspects the areas of the body affected with the lesions (e.g., the mouth, face, eyes, or genitalia) as a baseline for comparison during therapy.

Ongoing Assessment
The ongoing assessment depends on the reason for giving the antiviral drug. It is important to make a daily assessment for improvement of the signs and symptoms

identified in the initial assessment. The nurse monitors for and reports any adverse reactions from the antiviral drug. In addition, the nurse inspects the intravenous (IV) infusion site several times a day for redness, inflammation, or pain and reports any signs of phlebitis.

NURSING DIAGNOSES

Drug-specific nursing diagnoses include the following:

❏ **Risk for Imbalanced Nutrition: Less Than Body Requirements** related to adverse reaction of antiviral drugs
❏ **Risk for Impaired Skin Integrity** related to initial infection, adverse drug reactions, administration of the antiviral drug
❏ **Risk for Injury** related to patient's mental status, peripheral neuropathy, and generalized weakness
❏ **Body Image Disturbance** related to body fat redistribution
❏ **Acute Pain** related to kidney or bladder stones or inflammation caused by antiviral drugs

Nursing diagnoses that are related to drug administration are discussed in Chapter 4.

PLANNING

The expected outcomes for the patient depend on the reason for administration of the antiviral drug, but may include an optimal response to therapy, meeting of patient needs related to the management of adverse reactions, and an understanding of the therapeutic regimen.

IMPLEMENTATION

Promoting an Optimal Response to Therapy
Because these drugs may be used in the treatment of certain types of severe and sometimes life-threatening viral infections, the patient may be concerned about the diagnosis and prognosis. The nurse should allow the patient and family members time to talk and ask questions about treatment methods, especially when the drug is given IV. It is important to prepare the antiviral drugs according to the manufacturer's directions. The administration rate is ordered by the primary health care provider.

AMANTADINE. The nurse administers this drug for the prevention or treatment of respiratory tract illness caused by influenza A virus. Some patients are prescribed this drug to manage extrapyramidal effects caused by drugs used to treat Parkinsonism. The nurse should observe the patient for adverse effects similar to those associated with cholinergic blocking drugs (see Chapter 27).

RIBAVIRIN. The nurse gives ribavirin by inhalation using a small particle aerosol generator (called a *SPAG-2 aerosol generator*). It is important to discard and replace the solution every 24 hours. This drug can worsen respiratory status. Sudden deterioration of respiratory status can occur in infants receiving ribavirin, and it is important to monitor respiratory function closely throughout

therapy. The nurse should immediately report any worsening of respiratory function to the primary health care provider. Female caregivers should know that the drug is a pregnancy category X drug, and women of childbearing age should take care not to inhale the drug. In patients requiring mechanical ventilation, treatment should be provided only by health care providers familiar with the specific ventilator.

IV ADMINISTRATION. Rapid infusion or bolus administration of the antivirals has created toxicity in patients due to excessive plasma levels of the drug. The nurse should always check the recommended infusion rate of the drug and not exceed the rate.

Monitoring and Managing Patient Needs
RISK FOR IMBALANCED NUTRITION: LESS THAN BODY REQUIREMENTS. The metabolic needs of patients with HIV infection are demanding. Because the antiviral drugs may cause anorexia, nausea, or vomiting, providing adequate nutrition becomes a real challenge. The gastrointestinal (GI) effects range from mild to severe. Many of the drugs can be given without regard to food. Two exceptions are didanosine (Videx) and entecavir (Baraclude). These drugs are provided in a buffered or enteric-coated form. The nurse mixes the buffered powder with 4 ounces of water (not juice), stirs until it is dissolved, and gives it to the patient to drink immediately. The nurse avoids generating dust when preparing the medication.

The patient may be able to tolerate small, frequent meals with soft, nonirritating foods if nausea is mild. Frequent sips of carbonated beverages or hot tea may be helpful for others. It is important to keep the atmosphere clean and free of odors. The nurse provides good oral care before and after meals. Sometimes daily-dose drugs can be given at bedtime to reduce the nausea. If nausea is severe or the patient is vomiting, the nurse notifies the primary health care provider.

RISK FOR IMPAIRED SKIN INTEGRITY. The nurse monitors any skin lesions carefully for worsening or improvement. Should the lesions not improve, the nurse informs the primary health care provider. Accurate observation and documentation are essential. If an antiviral drug is administered topically, the nurse uses gloves when applying to avoid spreading the infection. These drugs may also cause a rash as an adverse reaction. The nurse notes and reports any rash to the primary health care provider.

When administering the drug by the IV route, the nurse must closely observe the injection site for signs of phlebitis. The nurse takes care to prevent trauma because even slight trauma can result in bruising if the platelet count is low. If injections are given, pressure is applied at the injection site to prevent bleeding. Occasionally, headache or a slight fever may occur in patients taking antiviral drugs. An analgesic may be prescribed to manage these effects. Depending on the patient's symptoms, the nurse monitors vital signs every 4 hours or as ordered by the primary health care provider.

RISK FOR INJURY. Some patients with a viral infection are acutely ill. Others may experience fatigue, lethargy, dizziness, or weakness as an adverse reaction to the antiviral/antiretroviral agent. The nurse monitors these patients carefully. Call lights are placed in a convenient place for the patient and are answered promptly by the nurse. If fatigue, dizziness, confusion, or weakness is present, the patient may require assistance with ambulation or activities of daily living. The nurse plans activities so as to provide adequate rest periods. Other drugs can damage the peripheral nerves, especially when used with other neurotoxic agents. The nurse watches for signs of peripheral neuropathy (numbness, tingling, or pain in the feet or hands). It is important to report these signs immediately to the primary health care provider.

DISTURBED BODY IMAGE. Patients taking the protease inhibitors (saquinavir, ritonavir, indinavir, nelfinavir, fosamprenavir, amprenavir, and atazanavir) have experienced redistribution of body fat. Movement is to the center of the body, so patients appear to have thinner arms and legs with a rounder abdomen or enlarged breasts. Sometimes body fat relocates to the area behind the neck (sometimes called a *buffalo hump*). The nurse should spend time with these patients, encouraging them to verbalize their feelings regarding this change in appearance. It is also important for the nurse to acknowledge these feelings as being both valid and important to the patient.

ACUTE PAIN. The drug indinavir (Crixivan) has been known to cause kidney or bladder stones in patients. Antiretroviral drugs have been known to cause acute pancreatitis. Patients should be assessed for pain when the nurse performs a routine vital signs check. Any pain should be explored for location and intensity. When assessing the patient for GI problems such as nausea, vomiting, abdominal pain, and jaundice, the nurse should be alert because these are symptoms of pancreatitis, and particular care should be taken in assessment of pain. Acute, sudden-onset pain should be reported to the primary health care provider for both treatment and further assessment for more involved disease.

❗ NURSING ALERT

Patients receiving antiretroviral drugs for HIV infection may continue to contract opportunistic infections and other complications of HIV disease. The nurse monitors all patients closely for signs of infection such as fever (even low-grade fever), malaise, sore throat, or lethargy. All caregivers are reminded to use good handwashing technique.

Educating the Patient and Family

When an antiviral drug is given orally, the nurse explains the dosage regimen to the patient and family and instructs the patient to take the drug exactly as directed for the full course of therapy. If a dose is missed, the patient should take it as soon as remembered but should not double the dose at the next dosage time. Any adverse reactions should be reported to the primary health care provider or the nurse. The patient must

understand that these drugs do not cure viral infections, but they can decrease symptoms and increase feelings of well-being.

The nurse instructs patients to report any symptoms of infection, such as an elevated temperature (even a slight elevation), sore throat, difficulty breathing, weakness, or lethargy. Again, the nurse reviews possible signs of pancreatitis (nausea, vomiting, abdominal pain, jaundice) and peripheral neuropathy (tingling, burning, numbness, or pain in the hands or feet). Any indication of pancreatitis or peripheral neuropathy must be reported at once.

The nurse includes the following information in the teaching plan for antiviral drugs:

- Antiviral drugs are not a cure for viral infections, but they will shorten the course of disease outbreaks and promote healing of the lesions. The drugs will not prevent the spread of the disease to others. Topical drugs should not be applied more frequently than prescribed but should be applied with a finger cot or gloves. All lesions should be covered. There should be no sexual contact while lesions are present. Notify the primary health care provider if burning, stinging, itching, or rash worsens or becomes pronounced.
- Some drugs cause photosensitivity, so precautions should be taken when going outdoors, such as wearing sunscreen, head coverings, and protective clothing. Patients should also refrain from using tanning beds.
- Some patients have experienced an acute exacerbation of the disease when medications used to treat hepatitis B are stopped. Hepatic function should be closely monitored in these patients.
- Those taking antiretrovirals should be cautioned that there is an increased risk of adverse reactions (hypotension, visual disturbances, prolonged penile erection) when the drug sildenafil (Viagra) is used. Symptoms should be reported promptly to the primary health care provider.
- Some drugs affect mental status. Activities requiring mental alertness, such as driving a car, should be delayed until the effect of the drug is apparent because vision and coordination can be affected. Patients should rise slowly from a prone to a sitting position to decrease the possibility of lightheadedness caused by orthostatic hypotension. Changes, such as nervousness, tremors, slurred speech, or depression, should be reported.
- Some patients are on an alternate dosage schedule. In this case, it is important to mark the calendar to designate the days the drug is to be taken.
- Patients taking saquinavir need to know that the two brand name drugs (Invirase and Fortovase) are not interchangeable.
- Zanamivir (Relenza) is taken every 12 hours for 5 days using a "Diskhaler" delivery system. If a bronchodilator is also prescribed for use at the same time, the bronchodilator is used before the zanamivir. The drug may cause dizziness. The patient should use caution when driving an automobile or operating dangerous

machinery. Treatment with this drug does not decrease the risk of transmission of influenza to others.

EVALUATION

- Therapeutic response is achieved and there is management of the infection and viral load.
- Adverse reactions are identified, reported to the primary health care provider, and managed successfully with appropriate nursing interventions:
  - ☑ Patient maintains an adequate nutritional status.
  - ☑ Skin is intact and free of inflammation, irritation, infection, or ulcerations.
  - ☑ No evidence of injury is seen.
  - ☑ Perceptions of body changes are managed successfully.
  - ☑ Patient is free of pain.
- Patient and family demonstrate an understanding of the drug regimen.

THINK CRITICALLY: PHARMACOLOGY IN PRACTICE

1. Mr. Park, aged 77 years, has herpes zoster. The primary health care provider prescribes acyclovir 200 mg every 4 hours during Mr. Park's waking hours. Discuss what information you would give the skilled nursing facility staff concerning herpes zoster, the drug regimen, and the possible adverse reactions.

● Test Your Knowledge

1. Which of the following adverse reactions would the nurse expect in a patient receiving acyclovir by the oral route?

- A. Nausea and vomiting
- B. Constipation and urinary frequency
- C. Conjunctivitis and blurred vision
- D. Nephrotoxicity

2. Which of the following would the nurse report immediately in a 3-month-old patient receiving ribavirin?

- A. Any worsening of the respiratory status
- B. Refusal to take foods or fluids
- C. Drowsiness
- D. Constipation

3. The nurse is administering didanosine properly when _____.

- A. tablets are crushed and mixed thoroughly with 1 oz of water
- B. the drug is prepared for subcutaneous injection
- C. the drug is given with meals
- D. the drug is given mixed with orange juice or apple juice

4. Administration of antiretrovirals can result in _____.

- A. abnormal hair growth
- B. body fat redistribution
- C. cardiac arrest
- D. discoloration of the skin

● Prepare for the NCLEX

1. As a nurse on a pediatric unit, you are making the assignment to care for an infant receiving aerosol ribavirin for RSV. Which of the following nurses should be assigned to care for this patient?

- A. Doris, a 22-year-old registered nurse
- B. Ariel, a female respiratory therapist
- C. Brad, a 26-year-old licensed practical nurse
- D. Vanessa, a 45-year-old pediatric certified nurse

● Calculate Medication Dosages

1. The patient is prescribed amantadine 200 mg. The drug is available in 100-mg tablets. The nurse administers _____.

2. A patient is prescribed 2 inhalations of zanamivir. The drug is available as one 5-mg blister per inhalation and is to be given with a "Diskhaler" device. How many milligrams will the nurse administer with 2 inhalations?

3. The nurse is to administer 100 mg of zidovudine orally. The drug is available as syrup 50 mg/5 mL. The nurse administers _____.

To check your answers, see Appendix E.

the**Point**. *For more NCLEX questions, log on to http://thepoint.lww.com to access more than 1000 questions.*

Antifungal and Antiparasitic Drugs

LEARNING OBJECTIVES

On completion of this chapter, the student will:

1. Distinguish between superficial and systemic fungal infections.
2. Distinguish between helminthic infections, protozoal infections, and amebiasis.
3. Discuss the uses, general drug action, adverse reactions, contraindications, precautions, and interactions of antifungal and antiparasitic drugs.
4. Discuss important preadministration and ongoing assessment activities the nurse should perform on the patient receiving an antifungal and antiparasitic drug.
5. List nursing diagnoses particular to a patient taking an antifungal and antiparasitic drug.
6. List possible goals for a patient taking an antifungal and antiparasitic drug.
7. Discuss ways to promote an optimal response to therapy, how to manage adverse reactions, and important points to keep in mind when educating the patient and the family about the antifungal and antiparasitic drugs.

• ANTIFUNGAL DRUGS

A **fungus** is a single-celled, colorless plant that lacks chlorophyll (Fig. 13.1). Fungi that cause disease in humans may be yeastlike or moldlike; the resulting infections are called fungal or **mycotic infections**.

Fungal infections range from superficial skin infections to life-threatening systemic infections. The superficial mycotic infections occur on the surface of, or just below, the skin or nails (see Chapter 53). Systemic fungal infections are serious infections that occur when fungi gain entrance into the interior of the body. These deep mycotic infections develop inside the body in sites such as in the lungs, brain, or gas-

trointestinal (GI) tract. Treatment for deep mycotic infections is often difficult and prolonged.

Yeast infections, such as those caused by *Candida albicans*, are known as **candidiasis**. Candidiasis affects women in the vulvovaginal area and immunocompromised patients with chronic conditions in the perineum or the oral cavity, or systemically. Infection of the mouth by the microorganism *C. albicans* is commonly called **thrush**. Patients who are at increased risk for candidal infections are those who have diabetes, are pregnant, or are taking oral contraceptives, antibiotics, or corticosteroids such as posttransplant or surgical patients. The Summary Drug Table: Antifungal Drugs identifies drugs that are used to combat fungal infections.

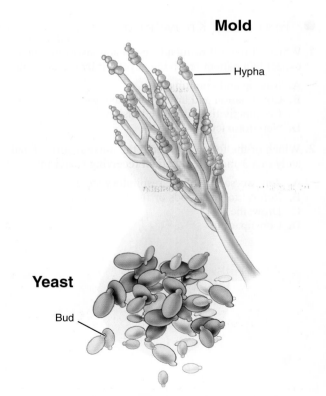

Mold

— Hypha

Yeast

Bud

Figure 13.1 Examples of infection-causing fungi.

Summary Drug Table ANTIFUNGAL DRUGS

Generic Name	Trade Name	Uses	Adverse Reactions	Dosage Ranges
amphotericin B *am-foe-ter'-ih-sin*	Abelcet, AmBisome, Amphotec, Fungizone	Systemic fungal infections, cryptococcal meningitis in patients with HIV infection	Headache, hypotension, fever, shaking, chills, malaise, nausea, vomiting, diarrhea, abnormal renal function, joint and muscle pain	Desoxycholate: 1–1.5 mg/kg/day IV; Lipid-based: 3–6 mg/kg/day IV
anidulafungin *an"-ih-doo-la-fun'-jin*	Eraxis	Abdominal and esophageal candidiasis	Headache, rash, nausea, vomiting	100–200 mg loading dose IV, followed by 50–100 mg/day IV for at least 14 days
caspofungin *kass-poe-fun'-jin*	Cancidas	Invasive aspergillosis, hepatic insufficiency	Headache, rash, nausea, vomiting, abdominal pain, hematologic changes, fever	70 mg loading dose IV, followed by 50 mg/day IV for at least 14 days
fluconazole *floo-kon'-ah-zole*	Diflucan	Oropharyngeal and esophageal candidiasis, vaginal candidiasis, cryptococcal meningitis	Headache, nausea, vomiting, diarrhea, skin rash	50–400 mg/day orally, IV
flucytosine (5-FC) *floo-sye'-toe-seen*	Ancobon	Systemic fungal infections	Nausea, diarrhea, rash, anemia, leukopenia, thrombocytopenia, renal insufficiency	50–150 mg/kg/day orally q 6 hr
griseofulvin *griz-ee-oh-full'-vin*	Grifulvin V, Gris-PEG	Ringworm infections of the skin, hair, nails	Nausea, vomiting, diarrhea, oral thrush, headache, rash, urticaria	For ringworm and jock itch: 330–375 mg orally in a single or divided dose. For athlete's foot: 660–750 mg/day orally in divided doses; take for 2–6 wk until the infection is completely gone
itraconazole *eye-trah-kon'-ah-zole*	Sporanox	Systemic fungal infections, may be used for nail infections	Nausea, vomiting, diarrhea, rash, abdominal pain, edema, hypokalemia in dosages over 600 mg/d	200–400 mg/day orally; IV as a single or divided dose Nail infections: 200 mg BID for 1 wk, then repeat in 3 wk
ketoconazole *kee-toe-kon'-ah-zole*	Nizoral	Treatment of systemic fungal infections	Nausea, vomiting, abdominal pain, headache, pruritus	200 mg/day orally; may increase to 400 mg/day orally
micafungin *mye-ka-fun'-jin*	Mycamine	Esophageal candidiasis, candidal infection prevention in stem cell transplantation	Rash, pruritus, facial swelling, vasodilation, flushing, headache, dizziness, anorexia, nausea, vomiting	150 mg/day IV
nystatin, oral *nye-stat'-in*	Mycostatin	Nonesophageal GI membrane candidiasis	Rash, diarrhea, nausea, vomiting	500,000–1 million units TID
posaconazole *poe"-sa-kon'-ah-zole*	Noxafil	Oral/pharyngeal candidiasis, prophylaxis of fungal infections	Headache, fever, abdominal pain, diarrhea, low potassium, red, white cells and platelets	100–200 mg orally, 1–3 times daily
terbinafine *ter-bin'-ah-feen*	Lamisil	Nail fungal infections	Headache, nausea, flatulence, diarrhea, rash	250 mg/day for 6–12 wk
voriconazole *vor-ih-kon'-ah-zole*	Vfend	Aspergillus systemic fungal infections	Visual disturbances, fever, rash, headache, anorexia, nausea, vomiting, diarrhea, peripheral edema, photosensitivity	Loading dose: 6 mg/kg q 12 hr for the first day Maintenance: If tolerated orally: 200 mg q 12 hr; if unable to take orally: 4 mg/kg q 12 hr IV until able to switch to oral drug

Actions

Antifungal drugs may be **fungicidal** (able to destroy fungi) or **fungistatic** (able to slow or retard the multiplication of fungi). Amphotericin B (Fungizone IV), miconazole (Monistat), nystatin (Mycostatin), voriconazole (Vfend), micafungin (Mycamine), and ketoconazole (Nizoral) are thought to have an effect on the cell membrane of the fungus. The fungicidal or fungistatic effect of these drugs appears to be related to their concentration in body tissues. Fluconazole (Diflucan) has fungistatic activity that appears to result from the depletion of sterols (a group of substances related to fats) in the fungus cells.

Griseofulvin (Grisactin) exerts its effect by being deposited in keratin precursor cells, which are then gradually lost (because of the constant shedding of top skin cells) and replaced by new, noninfected cells. The mode of action of flucytosine (Ancobon) is to inhibit DNA and RNA synthesis in the fungus. Clotrimazole (Lotrimin, Mycelex) binds with phospholipids in the fungal cell membrane, increasing permeability of the cell and resulting in loss of intracellular components. See Table 13.1 for names of topical antifungals.

Uses

Antifungal drugs are used prophylactically to prevent fungal infection in immunocompromised patients. They are also used to treat the following:

- Superficial and deep fungal infections
- Systemic infections such as aspergillosis, candidiasis, and cryptococcal meningitis
- Superficial infections of nailbeds and oral, anal, and vaginal areas

The specific uses of antifungal drugs appear in the Summary Drug Table: Antifungal Drugs. Miconazole is an antifungal drug used to treat vulvovaginal "yeast" infections and is representative of all the vaginal antifungal agents. Fungal infections of the skin or mucous membranes may be treated with topical or vaginal preparations. A listing of the topical antifungal drugs appears in Table 13.1, and the vulvovaginal antifungal agents are listed in Table 13.2.

HERBAL ALERT

Researchers have identified several antifungal herbs that are effective against skin infections, such as **tea tree oil** (*Melaleuca alternifolia*) and **garlic** (*Allium sativum*). Tea tree oil comes from an evergreen tree native to Australia. The herb has been used as a nonirritating antimicrobial for cuts, stings, wounds, burns, and acne. It can be found in shampoos, soaps, and lotions. Tea tree oil should not be ingested orally but is effective when used topically for minor cuts and stings. Topical application is most effective when used in a cream with at least 10% tea tree oil. Several commercially prepared ointments are available. The cream is applied to affected areas twice daily for several weeks.

Garlic is also used as an antifungal. A cream of 0.4% ajoene (the antifungal component of garlic) was found to relieve symptoms of athlete's foot and, like tea tree oil, is applied twice daily.

Table 13.1 Topical Antifungal Drugs

Generic Name (Form)	Trade names
amphotericin B (cream or lotion)	Fungizone
butenafine HCl (cream)	Mentax
ciclopirox (cream, lotion)	Loprox, Penlac Nail Lacquer
clioquinol (cream)	
clotrimazole (cream, solution, lotion)	Lotrimin
econazole (cream)	Spectazole
gentian violet (solution)	
haloprogin	Halotex
miconazole nitrate (cream, solution, spray)	Fungoid Tincture, Lotrimin, Micatin, Monistat
naftifine (cream, gel)	Naftin
oxiconazole nitrate (cream, lotion)	Oxistat
sulconazole nitrate (cream, solution)	Exelderm
tolnaftate (cream, solution, gel, spray)	Aftate, Genaspor, Tinactin, Ting
triacetin (solution, cream, spray)	Fungoid, Ony-Clear Nail
undecylenic acid (ointment, cream, powder)	Cruex, Desenex

Table 13.2 Vaginal Antifungal Drugs

Generic Name	Select Trade Name(s)
butoconazole *byoo-toe-koe'-nuh-zoll*	Femstat 3, Gynazole-1, Mycelex-3
clotrimazole *kloe-trye'-mah-zoll*	Lotrimin 3, Mycelex-7,
miconazole *mih-kon'-ah-zoll*	Monistat 3, Monistat 7, Monistat Dual Pak, M-Zole 3 Combination Pack
nystatin *nye-stat'-in*	
terconazole *tare-kon'-ah-zoll*	Terazol 7, Terazol 3
tioconazole *tee-oh-kon'-ah-zoll*	Monistat 1, Vagistat-1

Adverse Reactions

Systemic Administration

- Headache
- Rash
- Anorexia and malaise
- Abdominal, joint, or muscle pain
- Nausea, vomiting, diarrhea

Contraindications

Antifungal drugs are contraindicated in patients with a history of allergy to the drug. Most of the systemic antifungal medications are contraindicated during pregnancy and lactation, and are used only when the situation is life-threatening and outweighs the risk to the fetus.

Griseofulvin is not recommended for those with severe liver disease. Voriconazole is contraindicated when patients are taking the following medications: terfenadine, astemizole, sirolimus, rifampin, rifabutin, carbamazepine, ritonavir, ergot alkaloids, or long-acting barbiturates.

Both voriconazole and itraconazole are contraindicated in patients taking cisapride, pimozide, or quinidine. The systemic agent itraconazole should not be used to treat fungal nail infections in patients with a history of heart failure.

Precautions

Antifungals should be used cautiously in patients with renal dysfunction or hepatic impairment. Specific precautions include

- Use amphotericin B cautiously in patients who have electrolyte imbalances or who currently use antineoplastic drugs (because severe bone marrow suppression can result).
- Administer griseofulvin cautiously with penicillin because of possible cross-sensitivity.
- Itraconazole should be used with caution in patients with human immunodeficiency virus (HIV) infection or hypochlorhydria (low levels of stomach acid).

Interactions

Possible interactions depend on the individual drugs, and many interactions can occur. See Table 13.3 for more drug interaction information.

Table 13.3 Possible Interactions Between Antifungal and Other Drugs

Interacting Drug	Common Use	Effect of Interaction
Amphotericin B corticosteroids	Reduce Inflammation	Risk for severe hypokelemia
digoxin	Management of cardiac problems	Increased risk of digitalis toxicity
aminoglycosides	Anti-infective agent	Increased risk of nephrotoxicity
cyclosporine	Immunosuppressant (particularly for transplant recipients)	Increased risk of nephrotoxicity
flucytosine	Antifungal	Drug toxicity
miconazole	Antifungal for vaginal infections	Decreased effectiveness of amphotericin B
Fluconazole oral hypoglycemics	Diabetes control	Increased effect of oral hypoglycemic
phenytoin	Seizure control	Decreased effectiveness of phenytoin
Griseofulvin barbiturates	Sedation	Decreased effectiveness of sedative
oral contraceptives	Birth control	Decreased effectiveness of birth control (breakthrough bleeding, pregnancy, or amenorrhea)
salicylates	Analgesia, pain relief	Decreased serum level of pain reliever
Itraconazole digoxin and cyclosporine	See above	Elevated blood levels of itraconazole
phenytoin, histamine antagonists	Antiseizure drug and GI acid suppressant, respectively	Decreased blood levels of itraconazole
isoniazid and rifampin	Antitubercular drugs	Decreased blood levels of itraconazole

(table continues on page 120)

Table 13.3 **Possible Interactions Between Antifungal and Other Drugs** (continued)

Interacting Drug	Common Use	Effect of Interaction
Ketoconazole		
histamine antagonists and antacids	Control of GI upset	Decreased absorption of Ketoconazole
rifampin or isoniazid	Antitubercular drugs	May decrease the blood levels of ketoconazole
Posaconazole		
cimetadine	GI acid suppressant	May decrease the blood levels of posaconazole
phenytoin	Seizure control	Increased effectiveness of phenytoin
rifabutin	Antitubercular drugs	May decrease the blood levels of posaconazole
statins	Reduce cholesterol	Increased effectiveness of statins
Voriconazole		
methadone, tacrolimus, the statins, benzodiazepines, calcium channel blockers	Addiction control and pain relief, immunosuppressant, lipid-lowering agents, sedative hypnotics, and blood pressure or angina control, respectively	Increased effectiveness of voriconazole
sulfonylureas	Diabetes control	Hypoglycemia
vinca alkaloids	Antineoplastic (chemotherapy) agents	Increased risk of neurotoxicity
Micafungin		
sirolimus	Immunosuppression	Risk of greater immunosuppression
nifedipine	Management of angina (chest pain)	Risk of nifedipine toxicity
Terbinafine		
beta blockers and antidepressants	Cardiac problems and depression, respectively	Increased effectiveness of the beta blocker and antidepressant
Fluconazole, ketoconazole, itraconazole, vorixonazole, or griseofulvin		
warfarin	Blood thinner	Increased risk of bleeding

NURSING PROCESS
PATIENT RECEIVING AN ANTIFUNGAL DRUG

ASSESSMENT

Preadministration Assessment
The nurse assesses the patient for signs of infection before giving the first dose of an antifungal drug. It also is important to ask about pain and to describe white plaques or sore areas on mucous membranes of the oral or perineal areas, as well as any vaginal discharge. The nurse takes and records vital signs. The nurse weighs the patient scheduled to receive amphotericin or flucytosine because the dosage of the drug is determined according to the patient's weight.

Ongoing Assessment
The ongoing assessment involves careful observation of the patient every 2 to 4 hours for adverse drug reactions when the antifungal drug is given by the oral or parenteral route. When these drugs are administered topically or on an outpatient basis, the nurse must instruct the patient what to look for when gathering ongoing assessment data. This should include signs of improvement and adverse reactions, both minor and severe (requiring immediate notification of the primary health care provider).

NURSING DIAGNOSES

Drug-specific nursing diagnoses are the following:

❑ **Impaired Comfort** related to intravenous (IV) administration of amphotericin B
❑ **Risk for Ineffective Tissue Perfusion: Renal** related to adverse reactions of the antifungal drug

Nursing diagnoses related to drug administration are discussed in Chapter 4.

PLANNING

The expected outcomes for the patient depend on the reason for administering the antifungal drug, but may include a therapeutic response to the antifungal drug, patient needs related to the management of adverse reactions, and an understanding of the therapeutic regimen.

IMPLEMENTATION

Promoting an Optimal Response to Therapy: Administering Specific Antifungal Drugs

AMPHOTERICIN B. Amphotericin B is given only under close supervision in the hospital setting. Its use is reserved for serious and potentially life-threatening fungal infections. The nurse administers this drug daily or every other day over several days or months.

The IV solution of amphotericin B is light sensitive and should be protected from exposure to light. If the solution is used within 8 hours, there is negligible loss of drug activity. Therefore, once the drug is reconstituted, the nurse should administer the medication immediately, because the typical IV infusion is for a period of 6 hours or more. The nurse should consult the primary health care provider or hospital pharmacist regarding whether to use a protective covering for the infusion container.

! NURSING ALERT

Renal damage is the most serious adverse reaction to the use of amphotericin B. Renal impairment usually improves with a modification of the dosage regimen (reduced dosage or increased time between doses). Serum creatinine levels and blood urea nitrogen (BUN) levels are checked frequently during the course of therapy to monitor kidney function. If the BUN exceeds 40 mg/dL or the serum creatinine level exceeds 3 mg/dL, the primary health care provider may discontinue the drug or reduce the dosage until renal function improves.

NON–SYSTEMIC ANTIFUNGAL INFECTION PREPARATIONS. When a vaginal fungal infection is treated with miconazole during pregnancy, a vaginal applicator may be contraindicated. Manual insertion of the vaginal tablets may be preferred. Because small amounts of these drugs may be absorbed from the vagina, they are used only when essential during the first trimester.

Oral thrush infections (candidiasis) may be treated with oral solutions. The patient is instructed to swish and hold the solution in the mouth for several seconds (or as long as possible), gargle, then swallow the solution. Oral infections also may be treated with medication lozenges. Sometimes the vaginal troche preparation of an antifungal medication is prescribed for oral use. The patient needs specific instructions on how to use the medication to prevent confusion and improper use.

Monitoring and Managing Patient Needs

IMPAIRED COMFORT: MEDICATION ADMINISTRATION. When the nurse administers amphotericin B by IV infusion, immediate adverse reactions can occur. Nausea, vomiting, hypotension, tachypnea, fever, and chills (sometimes called *rigors*) may occur within 15 to 20 minutes of beginning the IV infusion. To prevent these adverse reactions, patients may be premedicated with antipyretics, antihistamines, or antiemetics. It is important to monitor the patient's temperature, pulse, respirations, and blood pressure carefully during the first 30 minutes to 1 hour

of treatment. The nurse should monitor vital signs every 2 to 4 hours during therapy, depending on the patient's condition. The nurse also checks the IV infusion rate and the infusion site frequently during administration of the drug. This is especially important if the patient is restless or confused.

Patients should be taught before the drug is given that the side effects can be uncomfortable. Warm blankets should be provided for patient comfort. Reassurance is given to the patient that the medications administered before the antifungal are to help ease the adverse reactions. Instruction should include that the reactions decrease with ongoing therapy.

RISK FOR INEFFECTIVE TISSUE PERFUSION: RENAL. When the patient is taking a drug that is potentially toxic to the kidneys, the nurse must carefully monitor fluid intake and output. In some instances, the nurse may need to perform hourly measurements of urine output. Periodic laboratory tests are usually ordered to monitor the patient's response to therapy and detect toxic reactions. Serum creatinine and BUN levels are checked frequently during the course of therapy to monitor kidney function. If the BUN exceeds 40 mg/dL or if the serum creatinine level exceeds 3 mg/dL, the primary health care provider may discontinue the drug therapy or reduce the dosage until renal function improves.

LIFESPAN ALERT – Gerontology

Before administering fluconazole to an elderly patient or a patient with renal impairment, the primary health care provider may order a creatinine clearance test. The nurse reports the laboratory results to the primary health care provider because the dosage may be adjusted based on the test results.

Educating the Patient and Family

If the patient is being treated in the ambulatory care setting, the nurse includes the following points in the teaching plan:

- Clean the involved area and apply the ointment or cream to the skin as directed by the primary health care provider.
- Do not increase or decrease the amount used or the number of times the ointment or cream should be applied unless directed to do so by the primary health care provider.
- During treatment for a ringworm infection, keep towels and facecloths for bathing separate from those of other family members to avoid the spread of the infection. It is important to keep the affected area clean and dry.

Drug-specific teaching points include:

- Flucytosine—Nausea and vomiting may occur with this drug. Reduce or eliminate these effects by taking a few capsules at a time during a 15-minute period. If nausea, vomiting, or diarrhea persists, notify the primary health care provider as soon as possible.

- Griseofulvin—Beneficial effects may not be noticed for some time; therefore, take the drug for the full course of therapy. Avoid exposure to sunlight and sunlamps because an exaggerated skin reaction (which is similar to severe sunburn) may occur even after a brief exposure to ultraviolet light. Notify the primary health care provider if fever, sore throat, or skin rash occurs.
- Ketoconazole—Complete the full course of therapy as prescribed by the primary health care provider. Do not take this drug with an antacid. In addition, avoid the use of nonprescription drugs unless use of a specific drug is approved by the primary health care provider. This drug may produce headache, dizziness, and drowsiness. If drowsiness or dizziness occur, use caution while driving or performing other hazardous tasks. Notify the primary health care provider if pronounced abdominal pain, fever, or diarrhea occurs.
- Itraconazole—The drug is taken with food. Therapy continues for at least 3 months until infection is controlled. Report unusual fatigue, yellow skin, darkened urine, anorexia, nausea, and vomiting.
- Miconazole—If the drug (cream or tablet) is administered vaginally, insert the drug high in the vagina using the applicator provided with the product. Wear a sanitary napkin after insertion of the drug to prevent staining of the clothing and bed linen. Continue taking the drug during the menstrual period if vaginal route is being used. Do not have intercourse while taking this drug, or advise the partner to use a condom to avoid reinfection. To prevent recurrent infections, avoid nylon and tight-fitting garments. If there is no improvement in 5 to 7 days, stop using the drug and consult a primary care provider, because a more serious infection may be present. If abdominal pain, pelvic pain, rash, fever, or offensive-smelling vaginal discharge is present, do not use the drug, but notify the primary health care provider.

EVALUATION

- Therapeutic response is achieved and there is no evidence of infection.
- Adverse reactions are identified, reported to the primary health care provider, and managed successfully with appropriate nursing interventions:
  - ☑ Patient reports comfort, without fever or chills.
  - ☑ Kidney perfusion is maintained.
- Patient and family demonstrate understanding of the drug regimen.

●ANTIPARASITICS

A **parasite** is an organism that lives in or on another organism (the host) without contributing to the survival or well-being of the host. These infections are infrequent in most populations in the United States except the immunocompromised. Helminthiasis (invasion of the body by parasitic worms) and protozoal infections (invasion of the body by single-celled parasites or malaria) are worldwide health problems. What makes these diseases especially worthy of concern is the frequency of global air travel in modern society. Conditions once confined to specific parts of the world can now be spread in hours or days by air travel.

●ANTHELMINTIC DRUGS

Roundworms, pinworms, whipworms, hookworms, and tapeworms are examples of helminths. The most common parasitic worm across the world is the roundworm. In the United States, the most common worm seen is the pinworm. *Anthelmintic* (against helminths) drugs are used to treat helminthiasis.

Actions and Uses

Although the actions of anthelmintic drugs vary, their primary purpose is to kill parasites.

Albendazole (Albenza) interferes with the synthesis of the parasite's microtubules, resulting in death of susceptible larvae. This drug is used to treat larval forms of pork tapeworm and to treat liver, lung, and peritoneum disease caused by the dog tapeworm.

Mebendazole (Vermox) blocks the uptake of glucose by the helminth, resulting in depletion of the helminth's own glycogen. This drug is used to treat whipworm, pinworm, roundworm, American hookworm, and the common hookworm.

The activity of pyrantel (Antiminth) is probably due to its ability to paralyze the helminth. Paralysis causes the helminth to release its grip on the intestinal wall, after which it can be excreted in the feces. Pyrantel is used to treat roundworm and pinworm.

The exact mechanism of action of thiabendazole (Mintezol) is unknown. This drug appears to suppress egg or larval production and therefore may interrupt the life cycle of the helminth. Thiabendazole is used to treat threadworm.

Adverse Reactions

Generalized adverse reactions include the following:

- Drowsiness, dizziness
- Nausea, vomiting
- Abdominal pain and cramps, diarrhea

Adverse reactions associated with the anthelmintic drugs, if they do occur, are usually mild when the drug is used in the recommended dosage. Rash is a serious adverse reaction to pyrantel, which is sold **over the counter** (without a prescription). As such, patients may begin self-treatment before notifying their primary health provider. Therefore, it is important for the nurse to instruct the patient to notify the primary health care provider if this skin reaction occurs. For more information, see the Summary Drug Table: Antiparasitic Drugs.

Contraindications and Precautions

The anthelmintic drugs are contraindicated in patients with known hypersensitivity to the drugs and during pregnancy (category C). They should be used cautiously in lactating patients and patients with hepatic or renal impairment, and malnutrition or anemia.

Summary Drug Table ANTIPARASITIC DRUGS

Generic Name	Trade Name	Uses	Adverse Reactions	Dosage Ranges
Anthelmintic Drugs				
albendazole al-ben'-dah-zoll	Albenza	Parenchymal neurocys-ticercosis due to pork tapeworms, hydatid disease (caused by the larval form of the dog tapeworm)	Abnormal liver function test results, abdominal pain, nausea, vomiting, headache, dizziness	Weight greater than or equal to 60 kg: 400 mg Weight less than 60 kg: 15 mg/kg/day
ivermectin eye-ver-mek'-tin	Stromectol	Treatment of thread-worm	Pruritus, rash, lymph node tenderness	Single dose of 200 mcg/kg
mebendazole meh-ben'-dah-zoll		Treatment of whipworm, pinworm, roundworm, common and American hookworm	Transient abdominal pain, diarrhea	100 mg orally morning and evening for 3 consecutive days; Pinworm: 100 mg orally as a single dose
pyrantel pye-ran'-tel	Antiminth, Reese's Pin-worm	Treatment of pinworm and roundworm	Anorexia, nausea, vomiting, abdominal cramps, diar-rhea, rash (serious)	11 mg/kg orally as a single dose; maximum dose, 1000 mg
thiabendazole thye-ah-ben'-da-zoll	Mintezol	Treatment of threadworm	Hypersensitivity reactions, drowsiness, dizziness, rash (serious)	Weight less than 150 lb: 10 mg/lb per dose orally Weight greater than 150 lb: 1.5 g/dose orally Maximum daily dose, 3 g
Antiprotozoal Drugs				
Primary Antimalarial Drugs				
chloroquine klor'-oh-kween	Aralen	Treatment and preven-tion of malaria, extrain-testinal amebiasis	Hypotension, electrocardio-graphic changes, headache, nausea, vomiting, anorexia, diarrhea, abdominal cramps, visual disturbances	Treatment: 160–200 mg IM and repeat in 6 hr if necessary Prevention: 300 mg orally weekly; begin 1–2 wk before travel and continue for 4 wk after return from endemic area
doxycycline dox-ih-sye'-kleen	Monodox, Vibramycin, Vibra-Tabs	Short-term prevention of malaria	Photosensitivity, anorexia, nausea, vomiting, diarrhea, superinfection, rash	100 mg orally daily, 1–2 days before travel and for 4 wk after return from endemic area
quinine kwi'-nine		Treatment of malaria	Nausea, vomiting, cinchon-ism, skin rash, visual disturbances	260–650 mg TID for 6–12 days
Other Antiprotozoal Drugs				
atovaquone ah-toe'-vah-kwone	Mepron	Prevention and treat-ment of PCP	Nausea, vomiting, diarrhea, headache, rash	750 mg orally BID for 21 days
atovaquone and proguanil ah-toe'-vah-kwone and pro-gwa'-nill	Malarone	Prevention and treat-ment of malaria	Headache, fever, myalgia, abdominal pain, diarrhea	Prevention: 1–2 days before travel, 1 tablet orally per day during period of exposure and for 7 d after exposure Treatment: 4 tablets orally daily for 3 days
hydroxychloroquine hye-drox-ee-klor'-oh-kwin	Plaquenil	Prevention and treat-ment of malaria, SLE, and rheumatoid arthritis	Nausea, vomiting, diarrhea, headache	Prevention: begin 1–2 wk before travel, 310 mg/wk orally, con-tinue for 4 wk after return from endemic area Treatment: 620 mg orally in 2 doses

(table continues on page 124)

Summary Drug Table ANTIPARASITIC DRUGS (continued)

Generic Name	Trade Name	Uses	Adverse Reactions	Dosage Ranges
mefloquine *meh'-flow-kwin*	Lariam	Prevention and treatment of malaria	Vomiting, dizziness, disturbed sense of balance, nausea, fever, headache, visual disturbances	Prevention: begin 1 wk before travel, 250 mg/wk orally, continue for 4 wk after return from endemic area Treatment: 5 tablets orally as a single dose
metronidazole *meh-troe-nye'-dah-zoll*	Flagyl	Treatment of intestinal amebiasis, trichomoniasis, anaerobic microorganisms	Headache, nausea, peripheral neuropathy, disulfiram-like interaction with alcohol	750 mg orally TID for 5–10 days
nitazoxanide *nye-tah-zocks'-ah-nide*	Alinia	Diarrhea caused by *Giardia lamblia*	Abdominal pain, nausea, vomiting, diarrhea, headache	500 mg orally q 12 hr with food
paromomycin *par-oh-moe-mye'-sin*	Humatin	Treatment of intestinal amebiasis	Nausea, vomiting, diarrhea	25–35 mg/kg/day in 3 divided doses with meals for 5–10 days
pentamidine *pen-tah'-mih-deen*	Pentam, Nebupent	PCP	IM: pain at injection site Fatigue, metallic taste, anorexia, shortness of breath, dizziness, rash, cough	Injection: 4 mg/kg IM or IV daily, for 14 days Aerosol (preventative): 300 mg/wk for 4 wk by nebulizer
primaquine *prim'-ah-kween*		Treatment of malaria	Nausea, vomiting, epigastric distress, abdominal cramps	26.3. mg/d orally for 14 days
pyrimethamine *peer-ih-meth'-ah-meen*	Daraprim	Prevention and treatment of malaria	Nausea, vomiting, hematologic changes, anorexia	Prevention: 25 mg orally once weekly Treatment: 50 mg/day for 2 days
sulfadoxine and pyrimethamine *sul-fah-dox'-een* and *peer-ih-meth'-ah-meen*	Fansidar	Prevention and treatment of malaria	Hematologic changes, nausea, emesis, headache, hypersensitivity reactions, Stevens-Johnson syndrome	Prevention: 1 tablet orally weekly Treatment: 2–3 tablets orally as a single dose
tinidazole *tih-nye'-dah-zoll*	Tindamax	*Giardia lamblia*, trichomoniasis	Nausea, vomiting, metallic taste	Single dose of 2 g orally

Interactions

The following interactions may occur when an anthelmintic is administered with another agent:

Interacting Drug	Common Use	Effect of Interaction
albendazole (Albenza)		
dexamethasone	Inflammation or immunosuppression	Increased effectiveness of albendazole
cimetidine	Relief of GI problems, such as heartburn	Increased effectiveness of albendazole
mebendazole (Vermox)		
hydantoins and carbamazepine	Seizure control	Lower levels of mebendazole
thiabendazole (Mintezol)		
xanthine derivatives	Management of respiratory problems	Increased serum level, possible toxic effects of the xanthines

•ANTIPROTOZOAL DRUGS

One of the greatest protozoal problems worldwide is the treatment and prevention of malaria. Although rare in the United States, with global travel, more people may be at risk depending on where they go. The protozoal infections seen in the United States include giardiasis (contracted from contaminated food or water), trichomoniasis, toxoplasmosis, and opportunistic infections (such as pneumonia seen in immunocompromised patients). Examples of antiprotozoal drugs in use today are listed in the Summary Drug Table: Antiparasitics Drugs.

Actions

Protozoa are single-celled animals. The protozoan that causes malaria is *Plasmodium falciparum*. Malaria is transmitted from person to person by certain species of the *Anopheles* mosquito. Figure 13.2 illustrates the life cycle of malaria transmission and the drugs used in treatment. Transmission

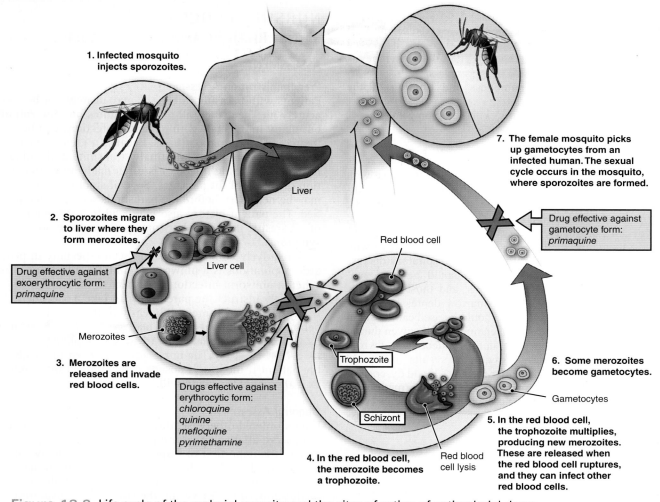

1. Infected mosquito injects sporozoites.

7. The female mosquito picks up gametocytes from an infected human. The sexual cycle occurs in the mosquito, where sporozoites are formed.

Liver

Drug effective against gametocyte form: *primaquine*

2. Sporozoites migrate to liver where they form merozoites.

Red blood cell

Drug effective against exoerythrocytic form: *primaquine*

Liver cell

Merozoites

Trophozoite

3. Merozoites are released and invade red blood cells.

6. Some merozoites become gametocytes.

Drugs effective against erythrocytic form:
chloroquine
quinine
mefloquine
pyrimethamine

Schizont

Gametocytes

5. In the red blood cell, the trophozoite multiplies, producing new merozoites. These are released when the red blood cell ruptures, and they can infect other red blood cells.

4. In the red blood cell, the merozoite becomes a trophozoite.

Red blood cell lysis

Figure 13.2 Life cycle of the malarial parasite and the sites of action of antimalarial drugs.

of the more common protozoans (*Giardia, Trichomonas,* and *Toxoplasma* spp). occurs through contaminated food or water, by fecal matter, or sexual intercourse. In immunocompromised patients, the organism *Pneumocystis jiroveci* causes pneumonia.

Drugs interfere with, or are active against, the life cycle of the protozoan. Antiprotozoal drugs work to inhibit DNA synthesis, killing the organism.

Uses

Infectious Disease

Antiprotozoal drugs may be used to treat infections such as:

- Malaria
- Giardiasis
- Toxoplasmosis
- Intestinal amebiasis

- Sexually transmitted infections (trichomoniasis)
- *Pneumocystis* pneumonia (PCP)

Prophylaxis

Antimalarial drugs are used for suppressing (i.e., preventing) malaria.

Adverse Reactions

GI reactions include the following:

- Anorexia
- Nausea, vomiting
- Abdominal cramping and diarrhea

Other Reactions

- Headache and dizziness
- Visual disturbances or tinnitus

- Hypotension or changes detected on an electrocardiogram (ECG; associated with chloroquine)
- **Cinchonism**—a group of symptoms associated with quinine administration, including tinnitus, dizziness, headache, GI disturbances, and visual disturbances. These symptoms usually disappear when the dosage is reduced.
- Peripheral neuropathy (numbness and tingling of the extremities), with metronidazole
- Nephrotoxicity and ototoxicity, with paromomycin

Contraindications and Precautions

Antiprotozoal drugs are contraindicated in patients with known hypersensitivity. Many of the drugs are contraindicated during pregnancy (most are pregnancy category C; except metronidazole, nitazoxanide, pregnancy category B; doxycycline, pregnancy category D; quinine, pregnancy category X). Quinine should not be prescribed for patients with myasthenia gravis, because it may cause respiratory distress and dysphagia. Antiprotozoal drugs should be used cautiously in children, lactating patients, and those who have hepatic or renal disease or bone marrow depression. Pregnancy category B antiprotozoals should be used cautiously in patients during pregnancy and lactation (can be given during the second and third trimesters) and in patients with thyroid disease (iodoquinol interferes with the results of thyroid function tests up to 6 months after therapy), blood dyscrasias, seizure disorders, severe hepatic impairment (metronidazole), bowel disease (paromomycin use interferes with absorption causing ototoxicity and renal impairment), or history of alcohol dependency.

Interactions

Foods that acidify the urine (cranberries, plums, prunes, meats, cheeses, eggs, fish, and grains) may interact with chloroquine and increase its excretion, thereby decreasing the effectiveness of the antimalarial drug. The following interactions may also occur when an antiprotozoal is administered with another agent:

Interacting Drug	Common Use	Effect of Interaction
antacids	GI upset	Decreased absorption of the antimalarial
iron	Treat anemia	Decreased absorption of the antimalarial
digoxin	Treat cardiac disease	Increased risk of digoxin toxicity
cimetidine	Management of GI upset or heartburn	Decreased metabolism of metronidazole
phenobarbital	Sedative	Increased metabolism of metronidazole
Quinine		
warfarin	Blood thinner, prevents blood clots	Increased risk of bleeding

NURSING PROCESS
PATIENT RECEIVING AN ANTIPARASITIC DRUG

ASSESSMENT

Preadministration Assessment

Patients with parasitic infections may or may not be acutely ill. The acutely ill patient requires hospitalization, but many individuals with parasitic infections can be treated on an outpatient basis. Because a great number of infections are gastrointestinally transmitted, the diagnosis of a parasitic infection is often made by examination of the stool for parasites. Several stool specimens may be necessary before the parasite is seen and identified. The patient history also may lead to a suspicion of a parasitic infection, but some patients have no symptoms.

A relatively common infection seen especially in pediatric populations is a pinworm (helminth) infection. When a pinworm infection is suspected, the nurse will frequently instruct the parent how to take a specimen from the anal area, preferably early in the morning before the patient gets out of bed. Specimens are taken by swabbing the perianal area with a cellophane tape–covered swab. The nurse also may need to weigh the patient if the drug's dosage is determined by weight or if the patient is acutely ill.

Ongoing Assessment

Unless ordered otherwise, the nurse instructs the parent to observe all stools that are passed after the drug is given. It is important to inspect each stool visually for passage of the helminth. If stool specimens are to be saved for laboratory examination, the nurse follows facility procedure for saving the stool and transporting it to the laboratory. If the patient is acutely ill or has a massive infection, it is important to monitor vital signs every 4 hours and measure and record fluid intake and output. The nurse observes the patient for adverse drug reactions, as well as severe episodes of diarrhea. It is important to notify the primary health care provider if these occur.

NURSING DIAGNOSES

The nursing diagnoses depend on the patient and the type of parasitic infection. Drug-specific nursing diagnoses are the following:

- ❏ **Diarrhea** related to parasitic invasion of body
- ❏ **Risk for Deficient Fluid Volume** related to parasitic invasion of body
- ❏ **Imbalanced Nutrition: Less Than Body Requirements** related to adverse effects of drug therapy
- ❏ **Risk for Impaired Respiratory Function** related to adverse effects of drug therapy

Nursing diagnoses related to drug administration are discussed in Chapter 4.

PLANNING

The expected outcomes for the patient depend on the reason for administering the antiparasitic but may include an optimal response to drug therapy, meeting patient needs related to management of common adverse reactions, and an understanding of the therapeutic regimen.

IMPLEMENTATION

Promoting an Optimal Response to Therapy: Proper Administration

When treating a patient for a parasitic infection, the nurse must instruct the family on methods to prevent reinfection or passing the infection on to other persons. The nurse instructs the family in frequent changing and washing of bed linens and undergarments. Caregivers need to also take care in obtaining or handling stool specimens. The nurse instructs the patient to wash his or her hands thoroughly after personal care and before meals.

When taking the drug pentamidine, patients should be placed in a reclining or supine position to prevent adverse effects should a sudden decrease in blood pressure occur. The patient should be monitored for hypotension over a number of doses to be sure the patient remains stable during treatments.

When administering an antimalarial drug, such as chloroquine, for prophylaxis (prevention), therapy should begin 2 weeks before exposure and continue for 6 to 8 weeks after the client leaves the area where malaria is prevalent.

Monitoring and Managing Patient Needs

DIARRHEA AND RISK FOR FLUID VOLUME DEFICIT. Daily stool specimens may be ordered to be sent to the laboratory for examination. The nurse keeps a record of the number, consistency, color, and frequency of stools. The nurse immediately delivers all stool specimens saved for examination to the laboratory because the organisms may die (and therefore cannot be seen microscopically). The nurse should inform laboratory personnel that the patient has a parasite, because the specimen must be kept at or near body temperature until examined under a microscope.

The nurse also monitors fluid intake and output, symptoms of a fluid volume deficit, and makes sure the patient is clean and the room free of odor. If dehydration is apparent, the nurse notifies the primary health care provider. If the patient is or becomes dehydrated, oral or IV fluid and electrolyte replacement may be necessary.

IMBALANCED NUTRITION: LESS THAN BODY REQUIREMENTS. GI upset may occur, causing nausea, vomiting, abdominal pain, and diarrhea. Taking the drug with food often helps to alleviate the nausea. The patient may require frequent, small meals of easily digested food. A discussion of eating habits, food preferences, and food aversions assists in meal planning. The nurse monitors body weight daily to identify any changes (increase or decrease). The nurse should make sure that meals are well balanced nutrition-ally, appetizing, and attractively served. The nurse may consult the dietitian if necessary.

RISK FOR IMPAIRED RESPIRATORY FUNCTION. Bronchospasm or cough is more likely to occur when inhaled treatments of pentamidine are given. The primary health care provider may prescribe a bronchodilator to be given before the pentamidine treatment. The nurse should instruct the patient and caregivers in the proper methods of administration and care of the respiratory equipment used at home with pentamidine (see Patient Teaching for Improved Patient Outcomes: Administering Pentamidine at Home).

Educating the Patient and Family

When an antiparasitic is prescribed on an outpatient basis, the nurse gives the patient or family member complete instructions about taking the drug, as well as household precautions that should be followed until the parasite is eliminated from the intestine. The nurse develops a patient education plan to include the following:

- Follow the dosage schedule exactly as printed on the prescription container. It is absolutely necessary to follow the directions for taking the drug to eradicate the parasite.
- Follow-up stool specimens will be necessary because this is the only way to determine the success of drug therapy.
- When an infection is diagnosed, multiple members of the family may be infected, and all household members may need to be treated. Playmates of the infected child may also need to be treated.
- It is important to wash all bedding and bed clothes once treatment has started.
- Daily bathing (showering is best) is recommended. Disinfect toilet facilities daily, and disinfect the bathtub or shower stall immediately after bathing. Use the disinfectant recommended by the primary health care provider or use chlorine bleach. Scrub the surfaces thoroughly and allow the disinfectant to remain in contact with the surfaces for several minutes.
- Wash the hands thoroughly after urinating or defecating and before preparing and eating food. Clean under the fingernails daily and avoid putting fingers in the mouth or biting the nails.
- Food handlers should not resume work until a full course of treatment is completed and stools do not contain the parasite.
- Child care workers should be especially careful of diaper disposal and proper handwashing to prevent the spread of infections.
- Report any symptoms of infection (low-grade fever or sore throat) or thrombocytopenia (easy bruising or bleeding).
- Albendazole can cause serious harm to a developing fetus. Inform women of childbearing age of this. Explain that a barrier contraceptive is recommended during the course of therapy and for 1 month after discontinuing the therapy.

When an antimalarial drug is used for preventing malaria and taken once a week, the patient also must take the drug on the same day each week. The prevention program is usually started 1 week before the individual departs to an area where malaria is prevalent.

EVALUATION

- Therapeutic response is achieved, and there is no evidence of infection.
- Adverse reactions are identified, reported to the primary health care provider, and managed successfully with appropriate nursing interventions:
  ☑ Patient reports adequate bowel movements.
  ☑ Adequate fluid volume is maintained.
  ☑ Patient maintains an adequate nutritional status.
  ☑ Lungs function effectively.
- Patient and family demonstrate understanding of the drug regimen.

Patient Teaching for Improved Patient Outcomes

Administering Pentamidine at Home
The patient may be required to receive aerosol pentamidine at home. Before discharge, the nurse checks to make sure that arrangements have been made to deliver the specialized equipment and supplies, such as nebulizer and diluent, to the home. The nurse also instructs the patient and caregiver on how to administer the drug, for example:

✓ Prepare the solution immediately before its use.
✓ Dissolve the contents of one vial in 6 mL sterile water and protect the solution from light.
✓ Place the entire solution in the prebulizer's reservoir. Do not put any other drugs into the reservoir.
✓ Attach the tubing to the nebulizer and reservoir.
✓ Place the mouthpiece in your mouth and turn on the nebulizer.
✓ Breathe in and out deeply and slowly. The entire treatment should last 30 to 45 minutes.
✓ Tap the reservoir periodically to ensure that all of the drug is aerosolized.
✓ When the treatment is finished, turn off the nebulizer.
✓ Clean the equipment according to the manufacturer's instructions.
✓ Allow tubing, reservoir, and mouthpiece to air dry.
✓ Store the equipment in a clean plastic bag and put it away for the next dose.
✓ Use a calendar to mark the days you are to receive the drug and check off each time you've done the treatment.

THINK CRITICALLY: PHARMACOLOGY IN PRACTICE

1. A nurse is preparing to administer amphotericin B to a patient with a systemic mycotic infection. This is the first time the nurse has administered amphotericin B. Determine what information the nurse should be aware of concerning the administration of this drug.
2. A child in a family of four children is found to have pinworms. Determine what you would include in a teaching plan to prevent the spread of pinworms to other family members.

● Test Your Knowledge

1. Mycotic infections are caused by:
   A. bacteria
   B. fungi
   C. parasites
   D. viruses

2. A patient asks how antimalarial drugs prevent or treat malaria. The nurse correctly responds that this group of drugs:
   A. kills the mosquito that carries the protozoa
   B. interferes with the life cycle of the protozoa causing the malaria
   C. ruptures the red blood cells that contain merozoites
   D. increases the body's natural immune response to the protozoa

3. Which of the following laboratory tests would the nurse monitor in patients receiving flucytosine?
   A. Liver function tests
   B. Complete blood count
   C. Renal functions tests
   D. Prothrombin levels

4. When discussing the adverse reactions of an anthelmintic, the nurse correctly states that:
   A. Patients must be closely observed for 2 hours after the drug is given.
   B. Adverse reactions are usually mild when recommended doses are used.
   C. Most patients experience severe adverse reaction and must be monitored closely.
   D. No adverse reactions are associated with these drugs.

● Prepare for the NCLEX

1. Mr. Carr is receiving amphotericin B for a systemic fungal infection. Which of the following would most likely indicate to the nurse that Mr. Carr is experiencing an adverse reaction to amphotericin B?
   A. Fever and chills
   B. Abdominal pain
   C. Drowsiness
   D. Flushing of the skin

● Calculate Medication Dosages

1. A patient weighs 140 pounds. If amphotericin B 1.5 mg/kg/d is prescribed, what is the total daily dosage of amphotericin B for this patient?

2. The primary care provider has prescribed fluconazole 200 mg orally initially, followed by 100 mg orally daily. On hand are fluconazole 100-mg tablets. What would the nurse administer as the initial dose?

3. Pyrantel 360 mg is prescribed. The drug is available in 180-mg capsules. The nurse administers _____.

To check your answers, see Appendix E.

the**Point**. *For more NCLEX questions, log on to http://thepoint.lww.com to access more than 1000 questions.*

Drugs Used to Manage Pain

How do people protect their bodies from harm? Typically, they sense danger and pull away or remove themselves from the harmful object or situation. The body uses pain to warn about potential or actual danger to body tissues. The danger can be something outside the body, such as heat, or inside the body, such as a blood clot. Pain is the unpleasant sensory and emotional perceptions associated with actual or potential tissue damage.

The nervous system is the agent involved in the recognition and perception of pain. Essentially, nerve fibers in the tissue are stimulated by stretching (an example would be the swelling of a blood clot that would force the nerve to stretch) or a noxious substance, such as a flame or a pin prick. In the peripheral (outside or distal) tissues, the nerve endings (or receptors) are activated and send a message to the spinal cord. Here, the nerve impulses are transferred across different nerve pathways in the central nervous system and sent to the brainstem. From this area, the message goes to the brain cortex, where the perception of pain occurs.

• ACUTE VERSUS CHRONIC PAIN

The two basic types of pain are acute pain and chronic pain. *Acute pain* is brief and lasts less than 3 to 6 months. Causes range from a sunburn to postoperative, procedural, or traumatic pain. Acute pain usually subsides when the injury heals. *Chronic pain* lasts more than 6 months and is often associated with specific diseases, such as cancer, sickle cell anemia, and end-stage organ or system failure. Various neuropathic and musculoskeletal disorders, such as headaches, fibromyalgia, rheumatoid arthritis, and osteoarthritis, are also causes of chronic pain.

Pain is treated with medications that correct or help to heal the site of tissue and nerve damage or stimulation (peripherally) or that change or modulate the brain's perception of the pain signal (centrally). When patients recover more slowly than expected from injury and illness, pain may be the key factor.

• ANALGESICS AND PAIN RELIEF

Analgesics are drugs used to relieve pain. The chapters in this unit deal with drugs used in managing pain. *Opioid* is the general term used for the opium-derived or synthetic analgesics used in pain control. *Narcotic* is a term referring to the properties of a drug to produce numbness or a stupor-like state. Although the terms *opioid* and *narcotic* were once interchangeable, law enforcement agencies have generalized the term narcotic to mean a drug that is addictive and abused or used illegally. Health care providers use the term opioid to describe drugs used in pain relief.

The nonopioid analgesics are a group of drugs used to relieve mild to moderate pain. They can be divided into three categories: salicylates, nonsalicylates (acetaminophen), and nonsteroidal anti-inflammatory drugs (NSAIDs). These drugs are discussed in Chapters 14 and 15. A number of combination nonopioid analgesics are available over the counter and by prescription as well. The NSAIDs have emerged as important drugs in the treatment of the chronic pain and inflammation associated with dis-

Pain perceived

Message transferred to brain stem

Message to spinal cord

Activation of nerve

Noxious stimuli (heat)

Pain Perception Pathway

orders such as rheumatoid arthritis and osteoarthritis. Drugs used to treat migraine headaches are also covered in Chapter 15; these drugs impact the nerve impulses controlling blood vessels in the brain.

Chapter 16 discusses the major uses of the opioid analgesics in the relief or management of moderate to severe acute and chronic pain. The ability of an opioid analgesic to relieve pain depends on several factors, such as the drug, the dose, the route of administration, the type of pain, the patient, and the length of time the drug has been administered. Treatment of moderate to severe pain may include both an opioid and a nonopioid analgesic. Manufacturers make products containing a combination of these drugs for ease of administration and standard selection of dosage combinations so the primary health care provider can prescribe the most effective pain relief. These combination products are listed in Chapter 16. If too much of an opioid is taken, opioid antagonists may be used; these drugs are discussed in Chapter 17. To complete this unit's discussion of pain management, Chapter 18 reviews the use of drugs for anesthesia—the elimination of sensation and the perception of pain.

• PAIN ASSESSMENT AND MANAGEMENT

The key nursing role in administering nonopioid and opioid drug therapy is careful assessment of pain and monitoring of the patient's response to the medications. To prescribe effective analgesics for pain management, the primary health care provider needs two key assessments about pain from the nurse: location and intensity.

Assessment of location helps the primary health care provider prescribe drugs that target the pain peripherally or centrally. The strength of the analgesic is determined by the patient's report of the pain intensity. The World Health Organization (WHO) uses a three-step analgesic ladder based on intensity as a guideline for treating pain (see Chapter 16 for detailed information).

Pain management in acute and chronic illness is an important responsibility of the nurse. In managing pain, the nurse needs to overcome the three main barriers to proper pain management, which have to do with assessment, intervention, and evaluation:

- Primary health care providers do not prescribe proper pain medicine doses.
- Nurses do not administer adequate medication for relief of pain.
- Patients do not report accurate levels of pain.

The factors associated with these barriers to successful pain management are too numerous to be examined in detail in this unit, but nurses should be sensitive to patient needs and to their role in providing adequate pain control.

After reading the chapters in this unit, you will be asked to determine which patients are at risk for complications associated with opioid administration and what actions should be taken for proper assessment and administration of medications in the treatment of pain.

PHARMACOLOGY IN PRACTICE

Mr. Park, aged 77 years, lived alone at home. One day, as he was working in the garden, he fell. He lay in the garden with a fractured hip for about 2 hours before he was found. This event, compounded with other stressors of living alone, initiated an outbreak of herpes zoster (shingles). In the haste of Mr. Park's admission, the nurse's assessment of pain did not differentiate the neuralgic pain of the shingles outbreak from that of the acute fracture pain.

Nonopioid Analgesics: Salicylates and Nonsalicylates

LEARNING OBJECTIVES

On completion of this chapter, the student will:

1. Discuss the types, uses, general drug actions, common adverse reactions, contraindications, precautions, and interactions of the salicylates and acetaminophen.
2. Discuss important preadministration and ongoing assessment activities the nurse should perform for the patient taking salicylates or acetaminophen.
3. List nursing diagnoses particular to a patient taking salicylates or acetaminophen.
4. Discuss the ways to promote an optimal response to therapy, how to manage common adverse reactions, and important points to keep in mind when educating patients about the use of salicylates or acetaminophen.

This chapter deals with the nonopioid analgesics: the salicylates and acetaminophen. Subsequent chapters cover the nonsteroidal anti-inflammatory drugs (NSAIDs) and the opioid analgesics. Both opioid and nonopioid analgesics are used to treat pain. Pain can be described as "the unpleasant sensory and emotional perception associated with actual or potential tissue damage" (International Association for the Study of Pain, 1979).*

Understanding Pain

Important tasks for the nurse caring for a patient with pain include early and ongoing assessment and intervention to promote healing. To treat pain effectively, the nurse needs a good understanding of the patient's pain experience. This is

---

*International Association for the study of Pain (1979). Subcommittee on Toxonomy: Pain terms: A list with definitions and notes on usage. *Pain, 6,* 249.

challenging, because sometimes patients feel the provider is too busy to worry about the pain, or a previous bad pain management situation will make the patient think providers do not want or know how to treat the pain. In addition, patients sometimes offer only a vague or poor description of their pain experience. Therefore, it is essential that the nurse conduct a thorough pain assessment. The nurse needs to know what the pain is like initially and how the pain changes after medications are administered. Guidelines for the initial pain assessment are listed in Display 14.1.

Pain Assessment

The intensity of pain is subjective, because the sensation of pain is a complex phenomenon that is uniquely experienced

DISPLAY 14.1 Guidelines for the Initial Pain Assessment

Many nurses think of pain as the fifth vital sign, with assessment of pain just as important as the assessment of pulse, respiration, blood pressure, and temperature. The following subject areas may help to guide the pain assessment.

Assessment Guidelines
- Patient's subjective description of the pain (What does the pain feel like?)
- Location(s) of the pain
- Intensity, severity, and duration
- Any factors that influence the pain
- Quality of the pain
- Patterns of coping
- Effects of previous therapy (if applicable)
- Nurses' observations of patient's behavior

Sample Assessment Questions
Questions to include in the assessment of pain may include the following:
- Does the pain keep you awake at night? Prevent you from falling asleep or staying asleep?
- What makes your pain worse? What makes it better?
- Can you describe what your pain feels like? Sharp, stabbing, burning, or throbbing?
- Does the pain affect your mood? Are you depressed? Irritable? Anxious?
- What over-the-counter or herbal remedies have you used for the pain?
- Does the pain affect your activity level? Are you able to walk? Perform self-care activities?

by each individual. Nurses may find it difficult to measure objectively signs of pain that match the level of distress reported by the patient. Therefore, the patient's report of pain should always be taken seriously. Failure to assess pain adequately is a major factor in the undertreatment of pain.

To understand the patient's pain level, the nurse asks the patient to describe the pain using a standardized pain scale measurement tool. The patient is taught to rate the pain on a scale of 0 to 10, with 0 being "no pain" and 10 being the "most severe pain imagined" by the patient. Sometimes it is hard for patients to think about their pain experience in a quantitative manner, like assigning a number to it. For those who find it difficult to quantify pain numerically, other methods to describe pain have been developed. Many of these are visual and may be useful, such as scales of colors or facial expressions. The Wong-Baker FACES Pain Rating Scale (Fig. 14.1) is an example of a visual tool to measure pain. This is especially helpful with children or populations that have trouble understanding or cannot tell the nurse about their pain using numbers.

Many nurses consider pain as the fifth vital sign and assessment of pain just as important as the assessment of temperature, pulse, respirations, and blood pressure. Accurate assessment of pain is necessary if pain management is to be effective. Patients with pain are often undertreated because of an inadequate nursing assessment.

• SALICYLATES

The salicylates are drugs derived from salicylic acid. Salicylates are useful in pain management because of their **analgesic** (pain-relieving), **antipyretic** (fever-reducing), and anti-inflammatory effects. Examples include aspirin (acetylsalicylic acid) and magnesium salicylate. Specific salicylates are listed in the Summary Drug Table: Nonopioid Analgesics: Salicylates and Nonsalicylates.

thinning blood- aggregation

Actions

Salicylates lower body temperature by dilating peripheral blood vessels. The blood flows out to the extremities, resulting in the dissipation of the heat of fever, which in turn cools the body. The analgesic action of the salicylates is due to the inhibition of **prostaglandins**. Prostaglandins are fatty acid derivatives found in almost every tissue of the body and body fluid. When prostaglandins are released, the sensitivity of pain receptors in the tissue increases, making the patient more likely to feel pain. Salicylates inhibit the production of prostaglandins, making pain receptors less likely to send the pain message to the brain. The reduction in prostaglandins is also thought to account for the anti-inflammatory activity of salicylates.

Aspirin more potently inhibits prostaglandin synthesis and has greater anti-inflammatory effects than other salicylates. In addition, aspirin prolongs the bleeding time by inhibiting the **aggregation** (clumping) of platelets. When bleeding time is prolonged, it takes a longer time for the blood to clot after a cut, surgery, or other injury to the skin or mucous membranes. Other salicylates do not have as great an effect on platelets as aspirin. This effect of aspirin on platelets is irreversible and lasts for the life of the platelet (7 to 10 days).

HERBAL ALERT

Willow bark has a long history of use as an analgesic. Willows are trees or shrubs that grow in moist places, often along river banks in temperate or cold climates. When used as a medicinal herb, willow bark is collected in early spring from young branches. In addition to its use as a pain reliever, the bark and leaves of various willow species have been used to lower fever and reduce inflammation. The salicylates were isolated from willow bark and identified as the most likely source of the bark's anti-inflammatory effects. The chemical structure was replicated in the laboratory and mass produced as synthetic salicylic acid. Years later, a modified version (acetylsalicylic acid) was first sold as aspirin. Aspirin became the most widely used pain reliever, fever reducer, and anti-inflammatory agent, leaving willow bark to be cast aside. The synthetic anti-inflammatory drugs work quickly and have a higher potency than willow bark. Willow bark takes longer to work and fairly high doses may be needed to achieve a noticeable effect. However, fewer adverse reactions are associated with willow bark than with the salicylates. Although adverse reactions are rare with willow bark, it should be used with caution in patients with peptic ulcers and medical conditions in which aspirin is contraindicated.

Uses

Salicylate nonopioid analgesics are used for:

• Relieving mild to moderate pain
• Reducing elevated body temperature (exception: diflunisal which is not used as an antipyretic)

Summary Drug Table NONOPIOID ANALGESICS: SALICYLATES AND NONSALICYLATES

Generic Name	Trade Name	Uses	Adverse Reactions	Dosage Ranges
Salicylates				
aspirin (acetylsalicylic acid) *ass'-purr-in*	Bayer, Ecotrin, Ecotrin (enteric coated), Empirin Buffered: Ascriptin, Asprimox, Bufferin, Alka-Seltzer with Aspirin	Analgesic, antipyretic, anti-inflammatory, stroke prevention in men	Nausea, vomiting, epigastric distress, gastrointestinal bleeding, tinnitus, allergic and anaphylactic reactions; salicylism with overuse	325–650 mg orally or rectally q 4 hr, up to 8 g/day
diflunisal *dye-floo'-ni-sal*	Dolobid	Same as aspirin	Same as aspirin	250–500 mg q 8–12 hr (maximum dose, 1.5 g/day)
magnesium salicylate *mag-nee'-see-um sal-ih'-sah-late*	Bufferin, Ecotrin	Same as aspirin	Same as aspirin	650 mg orally q 4 hr or 1090 mg TID
salsalate *sal-sa'-late*	Amigesic, Disalcid	Anti-inflammatory	Same as aspirin	3000 mg/day orally in divided doses
Nonsalicylate				
acetaminophen (APAP) *a-sea-tah-min'-oh-fen*	Tempra, Tylenol (multiple trade names)	Analgesic, antipyretic	Rare when used as directed; skin eruptions, urticaria, hemolytic anemia, pancytopenia, jaundice, hepatotoxicity	325–650 mg/day orally q 4–6 hr; maximum dose, 4 g/day

- Treating inflammatory conditions, such as rheumatoid arthritis, osteoarthritis, and rheumatic fever
- Decreasing the risk of myocardial infarction in those with unstable angina or previous myocardial infarction (aspirin only)
- Reducing the risk of transient ischemic attacks or strokes in men who have had transient ischemia of the brain due to fibrin platelet emboli (aspirin only). This use has been found to be effective only in men (not women).
- Helping maintain pregnancy in special at-risk populations (low-dose aspirin therapy). For example, it may be used to prevent or treat inadequate uterine–placental blood flow.

Adverse Reactions

Gastrointestinal (GI) system reactions include:

- Gastric upset, heartburn, nausea, vomiting
- Anorexia
- GI bleeding

Although salicylates are relatively safe when taken as recommended on the label or by the primary health care provider, their use can occasionally result in more serious reactions. Loss of blood through the GI tract may occur with salicylate use. The amount of blood lost is insignificant when one normal dose is taken. However, use of these drugs over a long period, even in normal doses, can result in significant blood loss. Some individuals are allergic to aspirin and other salicylates. Allergy to salicylates may be manifested by hives, rash, angioedema, bronchospasm with asthma-like symptoms, and anaphylactoid reactions.

Contraindications

Salicylates are contraindicated in patients with known hypersensitivity to salicylates or NSAIDs. Because salicylates prolong bleeding time, they are contraindicated in those with bleeding disorders or tendencies. These include patients with GI bleeding (from any cause), blood dyscrasias (abnormalities), and those receiving anticoagulant or antineoplastic drugs. Salicylates are classified as pregnancy category D (aspirin) and C drugs and should be used cautiously during pregnancy and lactation. Children or teenagers with influenza or chickenpox should not take salicylates, particularly aspirin, because their use appears to be associated with **Reye's syndrome** (a life-threatening condition characterized by vomiting and lethargy progressing to coma).

Precautions

Salicylates should be used cautiously in patients during lactation and in those with hepatic or renal disease, preexisting hypoprothrombinemia, and vitamin K deficiency. The drugs are also used with caution in patients with GI irritation, such as peptic ulcers, and in patients with mild diabetes or gout.

CHRONIC CARE ALERT

Aspirin is an over-the-counter (OTC) medication that patients may use to self-treat for pain. Some may take more aspirin than the recommended dosage, and toxicity can then result in a condition called **salicylism**. Signs and symptoms of salicylism include dizziness, **tinnitus** (a ringing sound in the ear), impaired hearing, nausea, vomiting, flushing, sweating, rapid, deep breathing, tachycardia, diarrhea, mental confusion, lassitude, drowsiness, respiratory depression, and coma (from large doses). Mild salicylism usually occurs with repeated administration of large doses of a salicylate. This condition is reversible with reduction of the drug dosage.

Interactions

Know

Foods containing salicylates (e.g., curry powder, paprika, licorice, prunes, raisins, and tea) may increase the risk of adverse reactions. The following interactions may occur when a salicylate is administered with another agent:

Interacting Drug	Common Use	Effect of Interaction
anticoagulant	Blood thinner	Increased risk for bleeding
NSAIDs	Pain relief	Increased serum levels of the NSAID
activated charcoal	Antidote (usually to poisons)	Decreased absorption of the salicylates
antacids	Relief of gastric upset, heartburn	Decreased effects of the salicylates
carbonic anhydrase inhibitors	Reduction of intraocular pressure; also used as diuretic	Increased risk for salicylism

• NONSALICYLATES

The major drug classified as a nonsalicylate analgesic is acetaminophen (APAP). It is the most widely used aspirin substitute for patients who are allergic to aspirin or who experience extreme gastric upset when taking aspirin. Acetaminophen is also the drug of choice for treating children with fever and flulike symptoms.

Actions

Acetaminophen is a nonsalicylate, nonopioid analgesic whose mechanism of action is unknown. The analgesic and antipyretic activity of acetaminophen is the same as salicylates. However, acetaminophen does not possess anti-inflammatory action and is of no value in the treatment of inflammation or inflammatory disorders. Acetaminophen does not inhibit platelet aggregation; therefore, it is the analgesic of choice when bleeding tendencies are an issue.

Uses

Acetaminophen is used for:

- Treating mild to moderate pain
- Reducing elevated body temperature (fever).
- Managing pain and discomfort associated with arthritic disorders

Tylenol's antedote is Mucomyst - Acetylcysteine

The drug is particularly useful for those with aspirin allergy and bleeding disorders, such as bleeding ulcer or hemophilia, those receiving anticoagulant therapy, and those who have recently had minor surgical procedures.

Adverse Reactions

Adverse reactions to acetaminophen are rare when the drug is used as directed. Adverse reactions associated with acetaminophen usually occur with chronic use or when the recommended dosage is exceeded. They include the following:

- Skin eruptions, urticaria (hives)
- Hemolytic anemia
- **Pancytopenia** (a reduction in all cellular components of the blood)
- Hypoglycemia
- **Jaundice** (yellow discoloration of the skin), hepatotoxicity (damage to the liver), and hepatic failure

Acute acetaminophen poisoning or toxicity can occur after a single 10- to 15-g dose of acetaminophen. Doses of 20 to 25 g may be fatal. With excessive doses, the liver cells undergo necrosis (die), and death can result from liver failure. The risk of liver failure increases in patients who drink alcohol habitually. Signs of acute acetaminophen toxicity include nausea, vomiting, confusion, liver tenderness, hypotension, cardiac arrhythmias, jaundice, and acute hepatic and renal failure.

Contraindications and Precautions

Hypersensitivity to acetaminophen is a contraindication to its use. Hepatotoxicity has occurred in habitual alcohol users after therapeutic dosages. The individual taking acetaminophen should avoid alcohol if taking more than an occasional dose of acetaminophen and avoid taking acetaminophen concurrently with the salicylates or the NSAIDs. Acetaminophen is classified as a pregnancy category B drug and is used cautiously during pregnancy and lactation. If an analgesic is necessary, it appears safe for short-term use. The drug is used cautiously in patients with severe or recurrent pain or high or continued fever because this may indicate a serious untreated illness. If pain persists for more than 5 days or if redness or swelling is present, the primary health care provider should be consulted.

 LIFESPAN ALERT – Gerontology

If liver damage is present in an older adult, acetaminophen should be used with caution.

Interactions *Know*

The following interactions may occur when acetaminophen is administered with another agent:

Interacting Drug	Common Use	Effect of Interaction
barbiturates	Sedation, central nervous system depressants	Increased possibility of toxicity and decreased effect of acetaminophen
hydantoins	Anticonvulsants	Increased possibility of toxicity and decreased effect of acetaminophen

Interacting Drug	Common Use	Effect of Interaction
isoniazid and rifampin	Tuberculosis medications	Increased possibility of toxicity and decreased effect of acetaminophen
loop diuretics	Control of fluid imbalance	Decreased effectiveness of the diuretic

CHRONIC CARE ALERT

Polypharmacy interactions: When administering acetaminophen to diabetic patients, care needs to be taken when blood glucose testing is done. Acetaminophen may alter blood glucose test results, resulting in falsely lower blood glucose values. As a result, inaccurate and lower doses of antidiabetic medications may be given to the patient taking acetaminophen.

NURSING PROCESS

PATIENT RECEIVING A SALICYLATE OR A NONSALICYLATE

ASSESSMENT

Preadministration Assessment

The patient's pain scale rating and location of the pain are the two key data items of every pain assessment (see Fig. 14.1). Before giving a nonopioid analgesic to a patient, the nurse assesses the type, onset, intensity, and location of the pain (see Display 14.1). It is important to determine if this problem is different in any way from previous episodes of pain or discomfort. If the patient is receiving a nonopioid analgesic for an arthritic, musculoskeletal disorder or soft tissue inflammation, the nurse should examine the joints or areas involved. The appearance of the skin over the joint or affected area or any limitation of motion is documented. The nurse evaluates the patient's ability to carry out activities of daily living. This important information is used to develop a care plan, as well as to evaluate the response to drug therapy.

NURSING ALERT

Before administering acetaminophen, the nurse assesses the overall health and alcohol usage of the patient. Patients who are malnourished or who consume alcohol habitually are at greater risk for developing hepatotoxicity (damage to the liver) with the use of acetaminophen.

Ongoing Assessment

During the ongoing assessment, the nurse monitors the patient for relief of pain and reassesses the patient's pain rating 30 to 60 minutes after administration of the drug. If pain persists, it is important to assess and document its severity, location, and intensity. (Examples of questions to ask the patient appear in Display 14.1.) The nurse monitors the vital signs every 4 hours or more frequently if necessary. Hot, dry, flushed skin and a decrease in urinary output may develop. If temperature elevation is prolonged, dehydration can occur. The nurse also assesses the joints for decreased inflammation and greater mobility. Any adverse reactions, such as unusual

or prolonged bleeding or dark stools, are reported to the primary care provider.

NURSING DIAGNOSES

Drug-specific nursing diagnoses are the following:

❑ **Impaired Comfort** related to fever of the disease process (e.g., infection or surgery)
❑ **Chronic** or **Acute Pain** related to peripheral nerve damage and/or tissue inflammation due to aspirin therapy
❑ **Impaired Physical Mobility** related to muscle and joint stiffness
❑ **Disturbed Sensory Perception: Auditory** related to impaired hearing

Nursing diagnoses related to drug administration are discussed in Chapter 4.

PLANNING

The expected outcomes of the patient depend on the reason for administering a nonopioid analgesic, but may include an optimal response to drug therapy, which includes relief of pain and fever, supporting patient needs related to the management of adverse drug reactions, and an understanding of the therapeutic regimen.

IMPLEMENTATION

Promoting an Optimal Response to Therapy

SALICYLATES. The patient should avoid salicylates for at least 1 week before any type of major or minor surgery, including dental surgery, because of the possibility of postoperative bleeding. In addition, the patient should not use salicylates after any type of surgery until complete healing has occurred because of the effects of salicylates on platelets. The patient may use acetaminophen or an NSAID after surgery or a dental procedure, when relief of mild pain is necessary.

The nurse observes the patient for adverse drug reactions. When high doses of salicylates are administered (e.g., to those with severe arthritic disorders), the nurse observes the patient for signs of salicylism. Should signs of salicylism occur, the nurse should notify the primary health care provider before the next dose is given because a reduction in dose or determination of the plasma salicylate level may be necessary. Therapeutic salicylate levels are between 100 and 300 mcg/mL. The following are the symptoms associated with increasing levels of salicylates:

• Levels greater than 150 mcg/mL may result in symptoms of mild salicylism, namely tinnitus (ringing sound in the ear), difficulty hearing, dizziness, nausea, vomiting, diarrhea, mental confusion, central nervous system depression, headache, sweating, and hyperventilation (rapid, deep breathing).
• Levels greater than 250 mcg/mL may result in symptoms of mild salicylism plus headache, diarrhea, thirst, and flushing.

• Levels greater than 400 mcg/mL may result in respiratory alkalosis, hemorrhage, excitement, confusion, asterixis (involuntary jerking movements especially of the hands), pulmonary edema, convulsions, tetany (muscle spasms), fever, coma, shock, and renal and respiratory failure.

> ### ▮ NURSING ALERT
> Serious GI toxicity can cause bleeding, ulceration, and perforation and can occur at any time during therapy, with or without symptoms. Although minor GI problems are common, the nurse should remain alert for ulceration and bleeding in patients receiving long-term therapy, even if no previous gastric symptoms have been experienced.

The nurse monitors the patient for signs and symptoms of acute salicylate toxicity or salicylism. Initial treatment includes induction of emesis or gastric lavage to remove any unabsorbed drug from the stomach. Activated charcoal diminishes salicylate absorption if given within 2 hours of ingestion. Further therapy is supportive (reduce hyperthermia and treat severe convulsions with diazepam). Hemodialysis is effective in removing the salicylate but is used only in patients with severe salicylism.

ACETAMINOPHEN. The nurse administers acetaminophen with a full glass of water. The patient may take this drug with meals or on an empty stomach. Symptoms of overdosage include nausea, vomiting, diaphoresis, and generalized malaise. Acute overdosage may be treated with administration of the drug acetylcysteine (Mucomyst) to prevent liver damage.

> ### ▮ NURSING ALERT
> The nurse immediately reports any signs of acetaminophen toxicity, such as nausea, vomiting, anorexia, malaise, diaphoresis, abdominal pain, confusion, liver tenderness, hypotension, arrhythmias, jaundice, and any other indication of acute hepatic or renal failure. Early diagnosis is important because liver failure may be reversible. Toxicity is treated with gastric lavage, preferably within 4 hours of ingestion of the acetaminophen. Liver function studies are performed frequently. Acetylcysteine (Mucomyst) is an antidote to acetaminophen toxicity and acts by protecting liver cells and destroying acetaminophen metabolites. It is administered by nebulizer within 24 hours after ingestion of the drug and after the gastric lavage.

Monitoring and Managing Patient Needs

IMPAIRED COMFORT. If the patient is receiving the analgesic for reduction of elevated body temperature, the nurse checks the temperature immediately before and 45 to 60 minutes after administration of the drug. If a suppository form of the drug is used, it is important to check the patient after 30 minutes for retention of the suppository. If the drug fails to lower an elevated temperature, the nurse notifies the primary health care provider because other means of temperature control, such as a cooling blanket, may be necessary. Patients can be made more comfortable by changing the clothing and bedding when it becomes damp because of the fluid loss during fever.

However, some health care providers may not prescribe an antipyretic for the patient with an elevated temperature because evidence suggests that fever is the result of the immune system's production of disease-fighting antibodies. The decision to treat an elevated temperature with an antipyretic is an individual one, based on the cause of the fever, the amount of discomfort to the patient, and the patient's physical condition.

PAIN. The nurse notifies the primary health care provider if the salicylate or acetaminophen fails to relieve the patient's pain or discomfort. The nurse gives the salicylate with food, milk, or a full glass of water to prevent gastric upset. The nurse checks to see if a new pain experience may be caused by gastric bleeding or inflammation. If gastric distress occurs, the nurse notifies the primary health care provider because other drug therapy may be necessary. An antacid may be prescribed to minimize GI distress. The nurse also checks the color of the stools. Black or dark stools or bright red blood in the stool may indicate GI bleeding. The nurse reports to the primary care provider any change in the color of the stool.

IMPAIRED PHYSICAL MOBILITY. The patient may have an acute or chronic disorder with varying degrees of mobility. The patient may be in acute pain or have long-standing mild to moderate pain. Along with the pain there may be skeletal deformities, such as the joint deformities seen with advanced rheumatoid arthritis. Considering the nature of the patient's condition, the nurse's assistance with ambulation may be required. The nurse determines the degree of immobility of the patient and assists the patient as needed.

> ### ▮ LIFESPAN ALERT – Gerontology
> Salicylates are prescribed for the pain and inflammation associated with arthritis. Because older adults have a higher incidence of both rheumatoid arthritis and osteoarthritis and may use the nonopioid analgesics on a long-term basis, they are particularly vulnerable to GI bleeding. The nurse should encourage the patient to take the drug with a full glass of water or with food because this may decrease the GI effects.

DISTURBED SENSORY PERCEPTION: AUDITORY. The nurse also should assess the patient for tinnitus or impaired hearing. Tinnitus or impaired hearing probably indicates high blood salicylate levels. If this is suspected, the nurse should withhold the drug and report any sensory alterations immediately. It is a good idea to explain to the patient that hearing loss disappears gradually after the drug therapy is discontinued.

> ### ▮ NURSING ALERT
> Studies suggest that the use of salicylates (especially aspirin) may be involved in the development of Reye's syndrome in children with chickenpox or influenza. This rare but life-threatening disorder is characterized by vomiting and lethargy, progressing to coma. Therefore, use of salicylates in children with chickenpox, fever, or flulike symptoms is not recommended. Acetaminophen is recommended for managing symptoms associated with these disorders.

EDUCATING THE PATIENT AND FAMILY

In some instances, a nonopioid analgesic may be prescribed for a prolonged period, such as when the patient has arthritis. Some patients may discontinue use of the drug, fail to take the drug at the prescribed or recommended intervals, increase the dose, or decrease the time interval between doses, especially if there is an increase or decrease in their symptoms. The patient and family must understand that the drug is to be taken even though symptoms have been relieved. The nurse develops a teaching plan to include the following general points:

- Take the drug exactly as prescribed by the primary health care provider. Do not increase or decrease the dosage, and do not take any OTC drugs without first consulting the primary health care provider. Notify the primary health care provider or dentist if the pain is not relieved.
- Take the drug with food or a full glass of water unless indicated otherwise by the primary health care provider. If gastric upset occurs, take the drug with food or milk. If the problem persists, contact the primary health care provider.
- Inform all health care providers, including dentists, when these drugs are taken on a regular or occasional basis.
- If the drug is used to reduce fever, contact the primary health care provider if the temperature continues to remain elevated for more than 24 hours.
- Do not consistently use an OTC nonopioid analgesic to treat chronic pain without first consulting the primary health care provider.
- Severe or recurrent pain or high or continued fever may indicate serious illness. If pain persists more than 10 days in adults, or if fever persists more than 3 days, consult the primary health care provider.

SALICYLATES. Advise patients taking a salicylate to notify the primary health care provider if any of the following symptoms occur: ringing in the ears, GI pain, nausea, vomiting, flushing, sweating, thirst, headache, diarrhea, episodes of unusual bleeding or bruising, or dark stools (see Patient Teaching for Improved Patient Outcomes: Detecting Gastrointestinal Bleeding). When teaching about salicylates, also include the following information:

- All drugs deteriorate with age. Salicylates often deteriorate more rapidly than many other drugs. If there is a vinegar odor to the salicylate, discard the entire contents of the container. Purchase salicylates in small amounts when used on an occasional basis. Keep the container tightly closed at all times because salicylates deteriorate rapidly when exposed to air, moisture, and heat.
- The ingredients of some OTC drugs include aspirin. The name of the salicylate may not appear in the name of the drug, but it is listed on the label. Do not use these products while taking a salicylate, especially during high-dose or long-term salicylate therapy. Consult the pharmacist about the product's ingredients if in doubt.

- If surgery or a dental procedure, such as tooth extraction or gum surgery, is anticipated, notify the primary health care provider or dentist. Salicylates may be discontinued 1 week before the procedure because of the possibility of postoperative bleeding.

ACETAMINOPHEN. When teaching patients and families about acetaminophen, include the following information:

- If taking medication for arthritis, do not change from aspirin to acetaminophen without consulting the primary

---

Patient Teaching for Improved Patient Outcomes

Detecting Gastrointestinal Bleeding

The patient with pain and inflammation from a musculoskeletal disorder commonly receives salicylates or NSAIDs (see Chapter 15). These drugs are readily available OTC, so a patient who is prescribed one drug, such as an NSAID, may also take an OTC salicylate, such as aspirin, for headaches or additional pain relief. When taken alone, these drugs may cause GI irritation, possibly leading to GI bleeding. If taken in combination or with high doses, or for long periods, the patient's risk for GI bleeding increases dramatically. Be sure to teach your patient how to look for signs and symptoms of GI bleeding. Instruct the patient to report any of the following:

✓ Abdominal pain or distention, especially any sudden increases
✓ Vomiting that appears:
  - bright red or blood streaked (indicates fresh or recent bleeding)
  - dark red, brown, or black, similar to the consistency of coffee grounds (indicates partial digestion of retained blood)
✓ Stools that appear:
  - black, loose, and tarry
  - bright red, red streaked, maroon, or dark mahogany colored

Also instruct your patient how to check the stools for occult blood (guaiac) by doing the following:

1. Gather necessary supplies, including chemical testing solution, testing card, and applicator.
2. After passing stool and opening the flap of the testing card, obtain a sample of stool and place a thin smear on the first window or slot marked as "1" or "A."
3. Then, obtain a second sample from another area of the same stool and place a thin smear on the second window or slot marked as "2" or "B."
4. Close the flap of the test card and place the card in the proper packaging material for transfer to the health care provider for analysis.

health care provider. Acetaminophen lacks the anti-inflammatory properties of aspirin.

- Notify the primary health care provider if any of the following adverse reactions occur: dyspnea, weakness, dizziness, bluish discoloration of the nailbeds, unexplained bleeding, bruising, or sore throat.
- Avoid the use of alcoholic beverages.

EVALUATION

- Therapeutic response is achieved, and pain is relieved.
- Adverse reactions are identified, reported to the primary health care provider, and managed successfully with appropriate nursing interventions:
  ❏ Patient reports comfort without fever.
  ❏ Discomfort is reduced or eliminated.
  ❏ Patient maintains adequate mobility.
  ❏ Hearing remains intact.
- Patient and family demonstrate an understanding of the drug regimen.

THINK CRITICALLY: PHARMACOLOGY IN PRACTICE

1. Betty Peterson is at the outpatient clinic with complaints of muscular aches and pain. She is currently taking a nonprescription aspirin product. She states she is experiencing some gastric upset. She tells you that she plans to begin taking Tylenol because she has heard that it does not cause upset stomach. What assessments would be important for the nurse to make? What information would you give Betty concerning Tylenol?

● Test Your Knowledge

1. At a team conference, the nurse explains that the anti-inflammatory actions of the salicylates are most likely due to:
   A. a decrease in the prothrombin time
   B. a decrease in the productions of endorphins
   C. the inhibition of prostaglandins
   D. vasodilation of the blood vessels

2. Which of the following symptoms would the nurse expect in a patient experiencing salicylism?
   A. Dizziness, tinnitus, mental confusion
   B. Diarrhea, nausea, weight loss
   C. Constipation, anorexia, rash
   D. Weight gain, hyperglycemia, urinary frequency

3. When administering a salicylate, the nurse correctly administers the drug:
   A. between meals
   B. with a carbonated beverage
   C. with food or milk
   D. dissolved in juice

4. While taking acetaminophen, patients who consume alcohol habitually are monitored by the nurse for symptoms of toxicity, which include:
   A. hypertension
   B. visual disturbances
   C. liver tenderness
   D. skin lesions

5. Which of the following drugs would the nurse most likely administer to a child with an elevated temperature?
   A. Baby aspirin
   B. Acetaminophen
   C. Fenoprofen
   D. Diflunisal

● Prepare for the NCLEX

1. A nurse instructs the patient taking aspirin to avoid foods containing salicylates because this increases the risk of adverse reactions. Which foods should the patient avoid?
   A. Salt, soft drinks
   B. Broccoli, milk
   C. Prunes, tea
   D. Liver, pepper

● Calculate Medication Dosages

1. The physician orders acetaminophen elixir 180 mg orally. Acetaminophen elixir is available in a 120-mg/mL solution. The nurse administers _____.

2. Aspirin 650 mg orally is prescribed. On hand is aspirin in 325-mg tablets. The nurse administers _____.

To check your answers, see Appendix E.

the**Point** *For more NCLEX questions, log on to http://thepoint.lww.com to access more than 1000 questions.*

Nonopioid Analgesics: Nonsteroidal Anti-Inflammatory Drugs (NSAIDs) and Migraine Headache Medications

KEY TERMS

cyclooxygenase
cyclooxygenase-1 (COX-1)

cyclooxygenase-2 (COX-2)
transient ischemic attack

LEARNING OBJECTIVES

On completion of this chapter, the student will:

1. Discuss the types, uses, general drug actions, common adverse reactions, contraindications, precautions, and interactions of the NSAIDs.
2. Describe the types, general drug actions, common adverse reactions, contraindications, precautions, and interactions of drugs used to treat migraine headaches.
3. Discuss important preadministration and ongoing assessment activities the nurse should perform on the patient taking the NSAIDs.
4. List nursing diagnoses particular to a patient taking an NSAID.
5. Discuss the ways to promote an optimal response to therapy, how to manage common adverse reactions, and important points to keep in mind when educating patients about the use of NSAIDs.

Because of the mode of action of nonsteroidal anti-inflammatory drugs (NSAIDs), some texts include the salicylates in the NSAID group. Although the chemical and physiologic effects are similar, this text discusses the salicylates in a separate chapter (see Chapter 14). The NSAIDs are nonopioid analgesics. This chapter covers general information on the NSAIDs, which are listed in the Summary Drug Table: Nonsteroidal Anti-Inflammatory Drugs and Migraine Medications. Like the salicylates, the NSAIDs have anti-inflammatory, antipyretic, and analgesic effects.

● NONSTEROIDAL ANTI-INFLAMMATORY DRUGS

Actions

The NSAIDs are so named because they have anti-inflammatory effects, but they do not belong to the steroidal group of substances and thus do not possess the adverse reactions associated with the steroids (see Chapter 44). In addition, NSAIDs have analgesic and antipyretic properties. Although their exact mechanisms of actions are not known, the NSAIDs are thought to inhibit prostaglandin synthesis by blocking the action of the enzyme **cyclooxygenase**, an enzyme responsible for prostaglandin synthesis. The NSAIDs also inhibit the activity of two related enzymes:

- **cyclooxygenase-1 (COX-1)**, an enzyme that helps to maintain the stomach lining
- **cyclooxygenase-2 (COX-2)**, an enzyme that triggers pain and inflammation

The traditional NSAIDs, such as ibuprofen and naproxen, are thought to regulate pain and inflammation by blocking COX-2. However, these drugs also inhibit COX-1, the enzyme that helps maintain the lining of the stomach. Therefore, blocking the effects of COX-2 produces pain relief, and blocking the effects of COX-1 produces adverse reactions. This inhibition of COX-1 causes unwanted gastrointestinal (GI) reactions such as stomach irritation and ulcers. The NSAID celecoxib (Celebrex) appears to work by specifically inhibiting the COX-2 enzyme without inhibiting the COX-1 enzyme. Celecoxib relieves pain and inflammation with less potential for GI adverse reactions.

Uses

The NSAIDs are used for the treatment of the following:

- Pain associated with osteoarthritis, rheumatoid arthritis, and other musculoskeletal disorders
- Mild to moderate pain
- Primary dysmenorrhea (menstrual cramps)
- Fever (reduction)

Adverse Reactions

Gastrointestinal System Reactions

- Nausea, vomiting, dyspepsia
- Anorexia, dry mouth
- Diarrhea, constipation
- Epigastric pain, indigestion, abdominal distress or discomfort, bloating

(text continues on page 144)

Summary Drug Table NONSTEROIDAL ANTI-INFLAMMATORY DRUGS AND MIGRAINE HEADACHE MEDICATIONS

Generic Name	Trade Name	Uses	Adverse Reactions	Dosage Ranges
diclofenac *dye-kloe'-fen-ak*	Cataflam, Flector (transdermal), Voltaren	Acute or chronic pain of rheumatoid arthritis, osteoarthritis, ankylosing spondylitis, and dysmenorrhea	Nausea, gastric or duodenal ulcer formation, GI bleeding	50–200 mg orally divided into 2 or 3 doses
etodolac *ee-toe-doe'-lak*		Osteoarthritis, rheumatoid arthritis, and acute pain	Dizziness, nausea, dyspepsia, rash, constipation, bleeding, diarrhea, tinnitus	300–500 mg BID; maximum daily dose 1200 mg
fenoprofen *fen-oh-proe'-fen*	Nalfon 200	Same as etodolac	Same as etodolac	300–600 mg orally 3 or 4 times daily; maximum daily dose 3.2 g
flurbiprofen *flure-bih'-proe-fen*	Ansaid	Same as etodolac	Same as etodolac	Up to 300 mg/day orally in divided doses
ibuprofen *eye-byoo'-proe-fen*	Advil, Motrin, Nuprin	Mild to moderate pain, rheumatoid disorders, dysmenorrhea, fever	Nausea, dizziness, dyspepsia, gastric or duodenal ulcer, GI bleeding, headache	400 mg orally q 4–6 hr; maximum daily dose 3.2 g
indomethacin *in-doe-meth'-ah-sin*	Indocin	Rheumatoid disorders	Nausea, constipation, gastric or duodenal ulcer, GI bleeding, hematologic changes	25–50 mg orally, 3 to 4 times daily
ketoprofen *kee-toe-proe'-fen*		Mild to moderate pain, rheumatoid disorders, dysmenorrhea, aches and fever	Dizziness, visual disturbances, nausea, constipation, vomiting, diarrhea, gastric or duodenal ulcer formation, GI bleeding	12.5–75 mg orally, TID
ketorolac *kee'-toe-roll-ak*		Moderate to severe acute pain	Dyspepsia, nausea, GI pain and bleeding	Single dose: 60 mg IM or 30 mg IV Multiple dosing: 10 mg q 4–6 hr; maximum daily dose 40 mg
meclofenamate *meh-kloe-fen-am'-ate*		Rheumatoid arthritis, mild to moderate pain, dysmenorrhea with heavy menstrual flow	Headache, dizziness, tiredness, insomnia, nausea, dyspepsia, constipation, rash, bleeding	50–400 mg orally q 4–6 hr, maximum dose 400 mg/day
mefenamic *meh-feh-nam'-ick*	Ponstel	Episodic acute mild to moderate pain (less than 1 wk duration)	Dizziness, tiredness, nausea, dyspepsias, rash, constipation, bleeding, diarrhea	250–500 mg q 6 hr
meloxicam *mel-ox'-ih-kam*	Mobic	Osteoarthritis	Nausea, dyspepsia, GI pain, headache, dizziness, somnolence, insomnia, rash	7.5–15 mg/day orally
nabumetone *nah-byoo'-meh-tone*		Rheumatoid arthritis and osteoarthritis	Dizziness, tiredness, nausea, dyspepsia, rash, constipation, bleeding, diarrhea	1000–2000 mg/day orally
naproxen *nah-prox'-en*	Aleve, Anaprox, Naprosyn, Naprelan	Rheumatoid, juvenile and osteoarthritis, mild to moderate pain, dysmenorrhea, general aches and fever	Dizziness, headache, nausea, vomiting, gastric or duodenal ulcer, GI bleeding	250–500 mg q 6–8 hr orally; maximum daily dose 1.25 g
oxaprozin *ox-ah-proe'-zin*	Daypro	Rheumatoid arthritis and osteoarthritis	Dizziness, nausea, dyspepsia, rash, constipation, GI bleeding, diarrhea	1200 mg/day orally

(table continues on page 143)

Summary Drug Table — NONSTEROIDAL ANTI-INFLAMMATORY DRUGS AND MIGRAINE HEADACHE MEDICATIONS (continued)

Generic Name	Trade Name	Uses	Adverse Reactions	Dosage Ranges
piroxicam *peer-ox'-ih-kam*	Feldene	Mild to moderate pain, rheumatoid arthritis and osteoarthritis	Nausea, vomiting, diarrhea, gastric or duodenal ulcer, GI bleeding	20 mg/day orally as a single dose or 10 mg orally BID
sulindac *soo-lin'-dak*	Clinoril	Mild to moderate pain, rheumatoid arthritis, ankylosing spondylitis, osteoarthritis, gouty arthritis	Nausea, vomiting, diarrhea, constipation, gastric or duodenal ulcer, GI bleeding	150–200 mg orally BID
tolmetin *toll'-meh-tin*	Tolectin	Rheumatoid, juvenile and osteoarthritis	Nausea, vomiting, diarrhea, constipation, gastric or duodenal ulcer, GI bleeding	400 mg orally TID or BID; maximum daily dose 1800 mg
Primarily COX-2 Inhibitor				
celecoxib *sell-ah-cok'-sib*	Celebrex	Acute pain, rheumatoid arthritis, ankylosing spondylitis, primary dysmenorrhea, and osteoarthritis; reduction of colorectal polyps in familial adenomatous polyposis	Headache, dyspepsia, rash See cardiovascular precautions	100–200 mg orally BID
Agents for Migraines – Serotonin 5-HT Receptor Agonists				
almotriptan *al-moe-trip'-tan*	Axert	Acute migraine headache pain	Headache, dizziness, fatigue, somnolence, nausea, dry mouth, flushing, hot/cold sensations, pain in chest, neck or paresthesia.	6.25–12.5 mg orally, may be repeated in 2 hr
eletriptan *el-ih-trip'-tan*	Relpax	Acute migraine headache pain	Same as almotriptan	20–40 mg orally at onset of symptoms, may be repeated in 2 hr, not to exceed 80 mg/day
frovatriptan *froe-vah-trip'-tan*	Frova	Acute migraine headache pain	Same as almotriptan	2.5 mg orally, at onset of symptoms, may be repeated in 2 hr, not to exceed 7.5 mg/day
naratriptan *nar'-ah-trip-tan*	Amerge	Acute migraine headache pain	Same as almotriptan	1–2.5 mg orally, at onset of symptoms, may be repeated in 4 hr, not to exceed 5 mg/day
rizatriptan *rye-zah-trip'-tan*	Maxalt	Acute migraine headache pain	Same as almotriptan	5–10 mg orally at onset of symptoms, may be repeated in 4 hr, not to exceed 30 mg/day
sumatriptan *soo-mah-trip'-tan*	Imitrex	Acute migraine and cluster headache pain	Same as almotriptan	25–100 mg orally; 20 mg nasally; 6 mg subcut; 25 mg rectally; may be repeated in 2 hr, not to exceed 100 mg/day
zolmitriptan *zoll-mih-trip'-tan*	Zomig	Acute migraine headache pain	Same as almotriptan	2.5–5 mg orally; 5 mg nasally; may be repeated in 2 hr, not to exceed 10 mg/day

(table continues on page 144)

Nonopioid Analgesics

⬤ *Summary Drug Table*	NONSTEROIDAL ANTI-INFLAMMATORY DRUGS AND MIGRAINE HEADACHE MEDICATIONS (continued)				
Generic Name	**Trade Name**	**Uses**	**Adverse Reactions**	**Dosage Ranges**	
Ergotamine derivatives					
dihydroergotamine *dye-hye-droe-er-got'-ah-meen*	DHE 45, Migranal	Acute migraine and cluster headache pain	Nausea, rhinitis, altered taste	Nasally: total dose of 2 mg; parenteral: no more than 3 mg injected in 24 hr	
ergotamine *er-got'-ah-meen*	Ergomar	Vascular headaches	Nausea, rhinitis, altered taste	2 mg sublingual; may be repeated in 30 min, not to exceed 6 mg/day	

- Intestinal ulceration, stomatitis
- Jaundice

Central Nervous System Reactions

- Dizziness, anxiety, lightheadedness, vertigo
- Headache
- Drowsiness, somnolence (sleepiness), insomnia
- Confusion, depression
- Stroke, psychic disturbances

Cardiovascular System Reactions

- Decrease or increase in blood pressure
- Congestive heart failure, cardiac arrhythmias
- Myocardial infarction

Renal System Reactions

- Polyuria (excessive urination), dysuria (painful urination), oliguria (reduced urine output)
- Hematuria (blood in the urine), cystitis
- Elevated blood urea nitrogen (BUN)
- Acute renal failure in those with impaired renal function

Hematologic System Reactions

- Pancytopenia (reduction in blood cell components), thrombocytopenia (reduced platelet count)
- Neutropenia (abnormally few neutrophils), eosinophilia (low eosinophil count), leukopenia (reduced white blood cell count), agranulocytosis (reduced granulocyte count)
- Aplastic anemia

Integumentary System Reactions

- Rash, erythema (redness), irritation, skin eruptions
- Ecchymosis (subcutaneous hemorrhage), purpura (excessive skin hemorrhage causing red-purple patches under the skin)
- Exfoliative dermatitis, Stevens-Johnson syndrome

Metabolic/Endocrine System Reactions

- Decreased appetite, weight increase or decrease
- Flushing, sweating
- Menstrual disorders, vaginal bleeding
- Hyperglycemia or hypoglycemia (high or low blood sugar)

Sensory and Other Reactions

- Taste change
- Rhinitis (runny nose)
- Tinnitus (ringing in the ears)
- Visual disturbances, blurred or diminished vision, diplopia (double vision), swollen or irritated eyes, photophobia (sensitivity to light), reversible loss of color vision
- Thirst, fever, chills
- Vaginitis

Contraindications   *Know PG, HTN*

The NSAIDs are contraindicated in patients with known hypersensitivity. There is a cross-sensitivity to other NSAIDs. Therefore, if a patient is allergic to one NSAID, there is an increased risk of an allergic reaction with any other NSAID. Hypersensitivity to aspirin is a contraindication for all NSAIDs. In general, NSAIDs are contraindicated during the third trimester of pregnancy and during lactation. Some NSAIDs are not used to treat rheumatoid or osteoarthritis; these include ketorolac, mefenamic, and meloxicam. Celecoxib is contraindicated in patients who are allergic to sulfonamides or have a history of cardiac disease or stroke. Ibuprofen is contraindicated in those who have hypertension, peptic ulceration, or GI bleeding.

> **❗ NURSING ALERT**
>
> Celecoxib is associated with an increased risk of serious cardiovascular thrombosis, myocardial infarction, and stroke, all of which can be fatal. All NSAIDs may carry a similar risk. The nurse should always question the patient regarding a history of risk for or actual cardiovascular disease before administering NSAIDs. Because of this risk, celecoxib should not be used to relieve postoperative pain from coronary artery bypass graft (CABG).

Precautions

The NSAIDs should be used cautiously during pregnancy (category B), by elderly patients (increased risk of ulcer formation in patients older than 65 years), and by patients with bleeding disorders, renal disease, cardiovascular disease, or hepatic impairment.

Interactions _Know_

The following interactions may occur when an NSAID is administered with another agent:

Interacting Drug	Common Use	Effect of Interaction
anticoagulants	Blood thinner	Increased risk of bleeding
lithium	Antipsychotic drug used for bipolar disorder	Increased effectiveness and possible toxicity of lithium
cyclosporine	Antirejection agent (immunosuppressant)	Increased effectiveness of cyclosporine
hydantoins	Anticonvulsant	Increased effectiveness of anticonvulsant
diuretics	Excretion of extra body fluid	Decreased effectiveness of diuretic
antihypertensive drugs	Blood pressure control	Decreased effectiveness of antihypertensive drug
acetaminophen in long-term use	Pain relief	Increased risk of renal impairment

HERBAL ALERT

Capsicum (hot pepper) has been cultivated in almost every society. Peppers are valued as a spice and flavoring for food. Capsaicin is the substance in peppers that, when applied topically, produces sensations varying from warmth to burning. For years, herbalists assumed that capsaicin worked by simply dilating blood vessels and increasing the supply of nutrients to injured joints. That may be a factor, but capsaicin actually works in a very different way.

People suffering from osteoarthritis have elevated levels of decapeptide substance P (DSP) in their blood and in the synovial fluid that bathes their joints. DSP has two undesirable functions. First, it breaks down the cartilage cushions in joints, contributing to osteoarthritis. Second, it serves as a pain neurotransmitter in both osteoarthritis and rheumatoid arthritis.

Researchers have discovered that capsaicin inhibits the activity of DSP. A cream containing capsaicin, when rubbed on the skin, penetrates to arthritic joints, where it stops the destruction of cartilage, relieves pain, and increases flexibility. Side effects include a localized burning sensation during the first few weeks of use, which diminishes with continued application.

People suffering from ulcers are usually warned to avoid spicy foods. But new research suggests that capsaicin produces the opposite effect—that capsaicin might actually protect against peptic ulcers. A number of experiments over the years have found that capsaicin protects the gastric mucosal membrane against damage from alcohol and aspirin.

• DRUGS USED IN THE TREATMENT OF MIGRAINE HEADACHES

Pain associated with migraine headaches is believed to be caused by vascular spasms. Drugs used to treat migraine headaches are given (1) prophylactically to prevent the

Saratonin released

spasms or (2) to treat the acute pain when a migraine occurs. The mechanism of action and classification of the drugs to prevent migraine headaches are different from those used to treat the acute pain of the migraine attack. Prophylactic treatment may include drugs from the following categories: beta blockers (see Chapter 25), calcium channel blockers (see Chapter 36), antidepressant medications (see Chapter 22), or anticonvulsant drugs (see Chapter 30). The selective serotonin (5-HT) agonists used to relieve the acute pain are covered in this chapter and are listed in the Summary Drug Table: Nonsteroidal Anti-Inflammatory Drugs and Migraine Medications.

Actions and Uses

The symptoms of migraine headaches are believed to be caused by local cranial vasodilation and stimulation of trigeminal nerves. Activation of the 5-HT receptors causes vasoconstriction and reduces the neurotransmission which in turn produces pain relief. Selective serotonin drugs are used for the relief of moderate to severe pain and inflammation related to migraine headaches. Because reduced GI motility can happen during a migraine event, delayed absorption of oral drugs may occur and alternative routes of administration are needed: rectal, internasal, or subcutaneous injection. _SL nasal spray_

Adverse Reactions

These agents are generally well tolerated, with most adverse reactions mild and transient. The most common are dizziness, nausea, fatigue, pain, dry mouth, and flushing.

Cardiovascular System Reactions

- Coronary artery vasospasm
- Cardiac arrhythmias and tachycardia
- Myocardial infarction

Contraindications and Precautions

These drugs are contraindicated in patients with a known hypersensitivity to selective serotonin agonists and should only be used when a clear diagnosis of migraine headache has been established. 5-HT agonists should not be used in patients with ischemic heart disease (such as angina or myocardial infarction), **transient ischemic attacks** (TIA), uncontrolled hypertension, or those patients taking monoamine oxidase inhibitor (MAOI) antidepressants. These drugs should be used cautiously in patients with hepatic or renal function impairment, such as the elderly or patients requiring dialysis. Because these are pregnancy category C drugs, they should only be used during pregnancy when the benefit outweighs the risk to the fetus. Caution should be exercised when administering them to lactating mothers.

Interactions

The following interactions may occur when a selective serotonin drug is administered with another agent:

Sympathetic Fight or Flight - Stomach ↓ emptying

Interacting Drug	Common Use	Effect of Interaction
cimetidine	Decrease gastric secretions	Increased effectiveness of the 5-HT agonist
oral contraceptives	Birth control	Increased effectiveness of the 5-HT agonist
sibutramine	Appetite suppressant	Central nervous system irritability

NURSING PROCESS

PATIENT RECEIVING A NONSTEROIDAL ANTI-INFLAMMATORY DRUG OR MIGRAINE MEDICATION

ASSESSMENT

Preadministration Assessment

Before administering an NSAID, the nurse needs to determine if the patient has any history of allergy to aspirin or any other NSAID. The nurse determines if the patient has a history of GI bleeding, cardiovascular disease, stroke, hypertension, peptic ulceration, or impaired hepatic or renal function. If so, the nurse notifies the primary health care provider before administering an NSAID.

In addition, before giving an NSAID to a patient, the nurse assesses and documents the type, onset, intensity, and location of the pain. It is important to determine if this problem is different in any way from previous episodes of pain or discomfort. If the patient is receiving an NSAID for arthritis, a musculoskeletal disorder, or soft tissue inflammation, the nurse should examine the joints or areas involved. The appearance of the skin over the joint or affected area or any limitation of motion is documented. The nurse evaluates the patient's ability to carry out activities of daily living. This important information is used to develop a care plan, as well as to evaluate the response to drug therapy.

> **❗ NURSING ALERT**
>
> Ibuprofen is available to individuals as an over-the-counter (OTC) drug that may be purchased without a prescription. When assessing patients with pain, the nurse should ask what medications the patient is currently taking or has tried for pain relief already. Because of the risk of Reye's syndrome from aspirin, ibuprofen is used in treatment of children with juvenile arthritis and for fever reduction in children 6 months to 12 years of age.

Ongoing Assessment

Drugs used for mild to moderate pain are primarily administered at home or in long-term care settings. The responsibility of monitoring the relief of pain falls upon the patient or caregiver in these settings with follow up made by the nurse. The nurse instructs the patient or caregiver to reassess the patient's pain rating 30 to 60 minutes after administration of the drug. If pain persists, it is important to note its severity, location, and intensity, and relay this information to the nurse. Hot, dry, flushed skin and a decrease in urinary output may develop if temperature elevation is prolonged; consequently, dehydration can occur. The nurse asks the patient or caregiver to make note if these problems arise and the patient is at risk for dehydration. The nurse also instructs in the monitoring of joints for a decrease in inflammation and greater mobility. The nurse instructs the patient and caregiver about adverse reactions, such as unusual or prolonged bleeding or dark-colored stools, and to report these observations to the primary health care provider.

NURSING DIAGNOSES

Drug-specific nursing diagnoses are the following:

- ❑ **Acute or Chronic Pain** related to peripheral tissue damage caused by the disease process or GI bleeding or inflammation from NSAID therapy
- ❑ **Impaired Physical Mobility** related to muscle and joint stiffness
- ❑ **Disturbed Sensory Perception: Visual** related to damage to optical field
- ❑ **Impaired Skin Integrity** related to photosensitivity when using 5-HT agonists

Nursing diagnoses related to drug administration are discussed in Chapter 4.

PLANNING

The expected outcomes for the patient depend on the reason for administration of the NSAID, but may include an optimal response to drug therapy, which includes relief of pain and fever, supporting the patient's needs related to the management of adverse reactions, and an understanding of the therapeutic regimen.

IMPLEMENTATION

Promoting an Optimal Response to Therapy

The nurse should give the NSAID with food, milk, or antacids. Patients who do not experience adequate pain relief using one NSAID may have success using another NSAID. However, several weeks of treatment may be necessary to achieve full therapeutic response.

> **◼ CHRONIC CARE ALERT**
>
> Migraine headache sufferers with phenylketonuria should be informed that rizatriptan (Maxalt) and zolmitriptan (Zomig) contains phenylalanine and should be avoided.

SUMATRIPTAN INJECTION FOR MIGRAINE HEADACHE PAIN. Administration of sumatriptan should be just below the skin in the subcutaneous tissue. This drug should be given at the onset of the headache, but can be administered any time during the attack. A second injection can be delivered after one hour if pain has not been relieved. The drug is dispensed in prefilled syringes, and should be used for only one injection and disposed of properly, even if the entire amount in the syringe is not used.

No more than two injections should be given in any 24-hour period. The nurse should observe the patient administering his or her first dose of sumatriptan by subcutaneous injection to be sure proper technique is used.

Monitoring and Managing Patient Needs

PAIN. NSAIDs are prescribed for the pain and inflammation associated with arthritis. Because older adults have a higher incidence of both rheumatoid arthritis and osteoarthritis and may use the NSAID on a long-term basis, they are particularly vulnerable to GI bleeding. The nurse should encourage the patient to take the drug with a full (8-ounce) glass of water or with food, because this may decrease adverse GI effects. The nurse checks whether a new pain experience may be caused by gastric bleeding or inflammation.

> **LIFESPAN ALERT – Gerontology**
> Age appears to increase the possibility of adverse reactions to the NSAIDs. The risk of serious ulcer disease in adults older than 65 years is increased with higher doses of the NSAIDs. Use greater care and begin with reduced dosages in the elderly, increasing the dosage slowly.

IMPAIRED PHYSICAL MOBILITY. The nurse provides comfort measures to the patient with pain from the limbs or joints affected by the various musculoskeletal disorders. Limbs are supported by proper positioning; applications of heat or cold, joint rest, and avoidance of joint overuse are additional comfort measures. Various orthopedic devices, such as splints and braces, may be used to support inflamed joints. The use of assistive mobility devices, such as canes, crutches, and walkers, eases pain by limiting movement or stress from weight bearing on painful joints. The nurse assists the patient while ambulating or using assistive devices to walk (Fig. 15.1). Patients with osteoarthritis should exhibit an increased range of motion and a reduction in tenderness, pain, stiffness, and swelling.

Figure 15.1 The nurse can assess the effects of pain medication while assisting the elderly patient with ambulation.

It is important to observe the patient receiving an NSAID for adverse drug reactions throughout therapy. GI reactions are the most common and can be severe, especially in those prone to upper GI tract disease. Cardiovascular reactions can be severe and even lead to death. Because of the severity of some of these adverse drug reactions, the nurse notifies the primary health care provider of any complaints the patient may have.

> **NURSING ALERT**
> The nurse withholds the next dose and notifies the primary health care provider immediately if any gastric or cardiac symptoms occur.

DISTURBED SENSORY PERCEPTION: VISUAL. NSAIDs may cause visual disturbances. The nurse reports any complaints of blurred or diminished vision or changes in color vision to the primary health care provider. Corneal deposits and retinal disturbances may also occur. The primary health care provider may discontinue therapy if ocular changes are noted. Blurred vision may be significant and warrants thorough examination. Because visual changes may be asymptomatic, patients on long-term therapy require periodic eye examinations.

IMPAIRED SKIN INTEGRITY: PHOTOSENSITIVITY. The skin can become more sensitive to sunlight when a patient takes 5-HT agonists for migraine headache pain relief. Patients should be cautioned to wear protective clothing and sunscreen when outside. The nurse should teach patients that exposure to ultraviolet light in tanning salons can also cause a reaction; therefore, tanning should be discouraged when using these drugs until tolerance is determined.

Educating the Patient and Family
In many instances, an NSAID may be prescribed for a prolonged period, such as when the patient has arthritis. Some patients may discontinue their drug use, fail to take the drug at the prescribed or recommended intervals, increase the dose, or decrease the time interval between doses, especially if there is an increase or decrease in their symptoms. The patient and family must understand that the drug is to be taken even though symptoms have been relieved. The nurse develops a teaching plan to include the following information:

- Take the drug exactly as prescribed by the primary health care provider. Do not increase or decrease the dosage, and do not take any OTC drugs without first consulting the primary health care provider. Notify the primary health care provider or dentist if pain is not relieved.
- Take the drug with food or a full glass of water unless indicated otherwise by the primary health care provider. If gastric upset occurs, take the drug with food or milk. If the problem persists, contact the primary health care provider.
- Whether taking an NSAID on a regular or occasional basis, inform all health care providers, including dentists, that you are taking it.

Nonopioid Analgesics

- If the drug is used to reduce fever, contact the primary health care provider if the temperature remains elevated for more than 24 hours after beginning therapy.
- Do not consistently use an OTC nonopioid analgesic to treat chronic pain without first consulting the primary health care provider.
- Severe or recurrent pain or high or continued fever may indicate serious illness. If pain persists more than 10 days in adults, or if fever persists more than 3 days, consult the primary health care provider.
- Avoid using aspirin or other salicylates when taking an NSAID.
- The drug may take several days to produce an effect (relief of pain and tenderness). If some or all of the symptoms are not relieved after 2 weeks of therapy, continue taking the drug, but notify the primary health care provider.
- These drugs may cause drowsiness, dizziness, or blurred vision. Use caution while driving or performing tasks that require alertness.
- Notify the primary health care provider if any of the following adverse reactions occur: skin rash, itching, visual disturbances, weight gain, edema, diarrhea, black stools, nausea, vomiting, chest/leg pain, numbness or persistent headache. See the Patient Teaching for Improved Patient Outcomes: Using Over-the-Counter Nonsteroidal Anti-Inflammatory Drugs.

Instructions for using selective serotonin agonists for migraine headache pain:

- These drugs are used to treat actual migraine headache pain; they will not prevent or reduce the number of migraine headaches.
- Administer the drug at the onset of migraine symptoms. Doses can be repeated one time after one hour (2 hours for nasal spray).
- Never take more than 2 doses in a 24-hour period. Notify the primary health care provider when the headache is not relieved.

EVALUATION

- Therapeutic response is achieved and discomfort is reduced.
- Adverse reactions are identified, reported to the primary health care provider, and managed successfully with appropriate nursing interventions:
  - ☑ Patient reports reduced or eliminated pain.
  - ☑ Patient reports improved mobility.
  - ☑ Patient's sight is intact.
  - ☑ Skin is intact and free of inflammation, irritation, or ulcerations.
- Patient and family demonstrate an understanding of the drug regimen.

Patient Teaching for Improved Patient Outcomes

Using Over-the-Counter Nonsteroidal Anti-Inflammatory Drugs

Quite a few NSAIDs are available as OTC products. OTC formulations such as ibuprofen (Advil, Motrin, and Nuprin), ketoprofen, and naproxen sodium (Aleve) are available to any consumer. The potential for misuse is high, especially when one is confronted by the large number of advertisements on television and in print heralding the wonderful benefits of these products.

Now, more than ever, patients need to be educated about these products. A thorough drug history and knowledge of the consumer's underlying disorder are essential to setting up an effective teaching program. In addition to the topics that are normally addressed with any drug teaching plan, the nurse stresses the following:

✓ Indications for using the drug (the reason the patient might take it)
✓ Dosage information, including frequency and maximum daily amounts
✓ Possible drug–drug and drug–food interactions
✓ Possible adverse effects, including life-threatening ones such as bleeding, cardiovascular, and stroke risk
✓ Need to read and heed all manufacturer's instructions, including the number of days that the patient should use the drug and when to notify the physician (e.g., if fever is not resolved within 3 days or pain persists)

Although this is not a foolproof remedy for eliminating possible misuse, thorough patient education can help minimize the risk of problems associated with OTC NSAIDs.

THINK CRITICALLY: PHARMACOLOGY IN PRACTICE

1. Mr. Park, aged 77 years, is prescribed celecoxib for osteoarthritis. He is confused at times and has difficulty hearing. In developing a teaching plan for Mr. Park, discuss what assessments would be important. Identify points to include in his teaching plan.

● Test Your Knowledge

1. The nurse monitors for which of the common adverse reactions when administering naproxen to a patient?

    A. Headache, dyspepsia
    B. Blurred vision, constipation
    C. Anorexia, tinnitus
    D. Stomatitis, confusion

2. An elderly patient is receiving sulindac. The nurse is aware that older adults taking NSAIDs are at increased risk for _____.

    A. ulcer disease
    B. stroke
    C. myocardial infarction
    D. gout

3. When a patient is receiving an NSAID, the nurse must monitor the patient for _____.

    A. agitation, which indicates nervous system involvement
    B. urinary retention, which indicates renal insufficiency
    C. decrease in white blood cell count, which increases the risk for infection
    D. GI symptoms, which can be serious and sometimes fatal

4. Which of the following statements would the nurse be certain to include in a teaching plan for the patient taking an NSAID?

    A. If GI upset occurs, take this drug on an empty stomach.
    B. Avoid the use of aspirin or other salicylates when taking these drugs.
    C. These drugs can cause extreme confusion and should be used with caution.
    D. Relief from pain and inflammation should occur within 30 minutes after the first dose.

● Prepare for the NCLEX

1. The nurse teaches a patient to self administer sumatriptan; when is this injection contraindicated?

    A. at the onset of a migraine headache
    B. when a visual aura is seen
    C. 2 hours following a previous dose
    D. weekly prophylactic use

● Calculate Medication Dosages

1. Naproxen (Naprosyn) oral suspension 250 mg is prescribed. The dosage on hand is oral suspension 125 mg/5 mL. The nurse administers _____.

2. The physician orders celecoxib (Celebrex) 200 mg orally. The nurse has celecoxib 100-mg tablets on hand. The nurse administers _____.

To check your answers, see Appendix E.

thePoint *For more NCLEX questions, log on to http://thepoint.lww.com to access more than 1000 questions.*

Nonopioid Analgesics

Opioid Analgesics

adjuvant
agonist
agonist-antagonist
cachectic

miosis
partial agonist
patient-controlled
   analgesia

LEARNING OBJECTIVES

On completion of this chapter, the student will:

1. Discuss the uses, general drug action, general adverse reactions, contraindications, precautions, and interactions of the opioid analgesics.
2. Discuss important preadministration and ongoing assessment activities the nurse should perform on the patient taking the opioid analgesics.
3. List nursing diagnoses particular to a patient taking an opioid analgesic.
4. Discuss ways to promote optimal response to therapy, how to manage adverse reactions, and important points to keep in mind when educating patients about the use of opioid analgesics.

Pain is universal. The World Health Organization (WHO) has addressed the problem of pain by developing a "pain ladder" that directs treatment for pain in three steps (Fig. 16.1). For mild pain, a Step 1 nonopioid analgesic may be prescribed. If necessary, an **adjuvant** (extra helping) agent may be used to promote the pain-relieving effect. If pain persists or worsens even with appropriate dosage increases, a Step 2 or Step 3 analgesic is indicated. Step 2 and Step 3 analgesics contain opioid substances. Most patients with severe pain require a Step 2 or Step 3 analgesic.

Opioid analgesics are the analgesics obtained from the opium plant. More than 20 different alkaloids are obtained from the unripe seed of the opium poppy. The analgesic properties of opium have been known for hundreds of years. The opioid analgesics are controlled substances (see Chapter 1) used to treat moderate to severe pain. These drugs do not change the tissues where the pain sensation originates; instead, they change how the patient perceives the pain sensation.

• OPIOID ANALGESICS

The opiates are natural substances obtained from raw opium. They include morphine sulfate, codeine, hydrochlorides of opium alkaloids, and camphorated tincture of opium. Morphine sulfate, when extracted from raw opium and treated chemically, yields the semisynthetic opioids hydromorphone, oxymorphone, oxycodone, and heroin. Heroin is an illegal narcotic substance in the United States and is not used in medicine. Synthetic opioids are those manufactured analgesics with properties and actions similar to the natural opioids. Examples of synthetic opioid analgesics are methadone, levorphanol, remifentanil, and meperidine. Additional analgesics are listed in the Summary Drug Table: Opioid Analgesics.

Actions

Cells in the central nervous system (CNS) have receptor sites called *opiate receptors*. Although opiates are attracted to many different receptor sites, the mu and kappa receptors

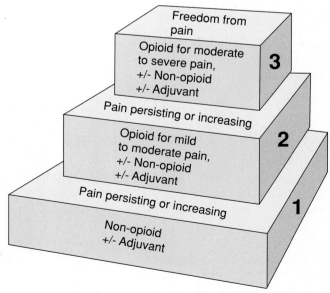

Figure 16.1 World Health Organization pain relief ladder. (Adapted with permission from WHO [2008].)

(text continues on page 152)

Summary Drug Table OPIOID ANALGESICS

Generic Name	Trade Name	Uses	Adverse Reactions*	Dosage Ranges
Agonists				
alfentanil *al-fen'-tah-nil*	Alfenta	Anesthetic adjunct	Respiratory depression, skeletal muscle rigidity, constipation, nausea, vomiting	Individualize dosage and titrate to obtain desired effect
codeine *koe'-deen*		Moderate to severe pain, antitussive, anesthetic adjunct	Sedation, sweating, headache, dizziness, lethargy, confusion, lightheadedness	Analgesic: 15–60 mg q 4–6 hr orally, subcut, IM
fentanyl *fen'-tah-nil*	Actiq Fentora Sublimaze	Severe pain, anesthetic adjunct, management of breakthrough cancer pain	Sweating, headache, vertigo, lethargy, confusion, nausea, vomiting, respiratory depression	Same as alfentanil 200–1600 mcg/dose, depending on pain severity
fentanyl transdermal systems	Duragesic	Chronic pain unmanaged by other opioids	Sedation, sweating, headache, vertigo, lethargy, confusion, lightheadedness, nausea, vomiting	Individualized dosage: 25–175-mcg transdermal patch (dose is amount absorbed per hour)
hydromorphone *hye-droe-mor'-fone*	Dilaudid	Moderate to severe pain	Sedation, vertigo, lethargy, confusion, lightheadedness, nausea, vomiting	2–4 mg orally, q 4–6 hr; 3 mg q 6–8 hr rectally; 1–2 mg IM or subcut q 4–6 hr
levorphanol tartrate *lee-vor'-fah-noll*	Levo-Dromoran	Moderate to severe pain, preoperative sedation	Dizziness, nausea, vomiting, dry mouth, sweating, respiratory depression	2 mg orally, q 3–6 hr; 1 mg IV q 3–8 hr
meperidine *meh-per'-ih-deen*	Demerol	Acute moderate to severe pain, preoperative sedation, anesthetic adjunct	Lightheadedness, constipation, dizziness, nausea, vomiting, respiratory depression	50–150 mg orally, IM, subcut, q 3–4 hr
methadone *meth'-ah-doan*	Dolophine	Severe pain; treatment of opioid dependence	Lightheadedness, dizziness, sedation, nausea, vomiting, constipation	Analgesic: 2.5–10 mg orally, IM, subcut q 4 hr; detoxification: 10–40 mg orally, IV
morphine *mor'-feen*	Avinza, Kadian, Duramorph; timed release: MS Contin, Oramorph SR	Acute/chronic pain, preoperative sedation, anesthetic adjunct, dyspnea	Sedation, hypotension, increased sweating, constipation, dizziness, drowsiness, nausea, vomiting, dry mouth, somnolence, respiratory depression	Acute pain relief: 10–30 mg q 4 hr; chronic pain relief: individualized
oxycodone *ok-see-koe'-doan*	Roxicodone; timed release: OxyContin	Moderate to severe pain	Lightheadedness, sedation, constipation, dizziness, nausea, vomiting, sweating, respiratory depression	10–30 mg orally q 4 hr
oxymorphone *ok-see-mor'-fone*	Opana	Moderate to severe pain, preoperative sedation, obstetric analgesia	Lightheadedness, sedation, constipation, dizziness, nausea, vomiting, respiratory depression	1–1.5 mg subcut or IM q 4–6 hr
propoxyphene *proe-pox'-ih-feen*	Darvon, Darvon-N	Moderate to severe pain	Lightheadedness, sedation, constipation, dizziness, nausea, vomiting, respiratory depression	65–100 mg orally q 4 hr; maximum dose 600 mg/day

(table continues on page 152)

Opioid Analgesics

Summary Drug Table OPIOID ANALGESICS (continued)

Generic Name	Trade Name	Uses	Adverse Reactions*	Dosage Ranges
remifentanil HCl *reh-mih-fen'-tah-nill*	Ultiva	Anesthetic adjunct	Lightheadedness, skeletal muscle rigidity, nausea, vomiting, respiratory depression, sweating	Same as alfentanil
sufentanil *suh-fen'-tah-nill*	Sufenta	Anesthetic adjunct	Same as alfentanil	Same as alfentanil
tramadol *tram'-ah-doll*	Ultram	Moderate to severe chronic pain	Same as morphine sulfate	Titrate individual dose starting at 25 mg up to 100 mg/day

Agonists-Antagonists

Generic Name	Trade Name	Uses	Adverse Reactions*	Dosage Ranges
buprenorphine *byoo-preh-nor'-feen*	Buprenex, Suboxone, Subutex	Moderate to severe chronic pain, treatment of opioid dependence	Lightheadedness, sedation, dizziness, nausea, vomiting, respiratory depression	Parenteral: 0.03 mg q 6 hr IV or IM Sublingual: 12–16 mg/day
butorphanol *byoo-tor'-fah-noll*	Stadol,	Acute pain, anesthetic adjunct	Lightheadedness, sedation, constipation, dizziness, nausea, vomiting, respiratory depression	1–4 mg IM, 0.5–2 mg IV; Nasal spray (NS): 1 mg (spray), repeat in 60–90 min; may repeat q 3–4 hr
nalbuphine *nal'-byoo-feen*	Nubain	Moderate to severe chronic pain, anesthetic adjunct	Lightheadedness, sedation, constipation, dizziness, nausea, vomiting, respiratory depression	10 mg/70 kg subcut, IM, or IV q 3–6 hr
pentazocine *pen-taz'-oh-seen*	Talwin	Same as nalbuphine	Same as nalbuphine	30–60 mg IM, subcut, IV q 3–4 hr; maximum daily dose 360 mg

*Adverse reactions of opioid analgesics are discussed extensively in the chapter. Some of the reactions may be less severe or intense than others.

produce the analgesic, sedative, and euphoric effects associated with analgesic drugs.

Drugs that bind well to a receptor are called **agonist** agents. An opioid analgesic may be classified as an agonist, partial agonist, or mixed agonist-antagonist. The agonist binds to a receptor and causes a response. A **partial agonist** binds to a receptor, but the response is limited (i.e., is not as great as with the agonist). An **agonist-antagonist** has properties of both the agonist and antagonist. These drugs have some agonist activity at the receptor sites and some antagonist activity at the receptor sites. Antagonists bind to a receptor and cause no response. An antagonist can reverse the effects of the agonist. This reversal is possible because the antagonist competes with the agonist for a receptor site. Drugs that act as opioid antagonists are discussed in Chapter 17.

In addition to the pain-relieving effects, other, nonintended responses occur when the opiate receptor sites are stimulated. These include respiratory depression, decreased gastrointestinal (GI) motility, and **miosis** (pinpoint pupils). Table 16.1 identifies the responses in the body associated with three of the opiate receptors. The actions of the opioid analgesics on the various organs and structures of the body (also called *secondary pharmacologic effects*) are shown in Display 16.1. With long-term use, the patient's body adapts to these secondary effects. The only bodily system that does not adapt and compensate is the GI system. Slow GI

Table 16.1 Bodily Responses Associated With Opioid Receptor Sites

Receptor	Bodily Response
Mu	Morphine-like supraspinal analgesia, respiratory and physical depression, miosis, reduced GI motility
Delta	Dysphoria, psychotomimetic effects (e.g., hallucinations), respiratory and vasomotor stimulations caused by drugs with antagonist activity
Kappa	Sedation and miosis

DISPLAY 16.1 Secondary Pharmacologic Effects of the Opioid Analgesics

- **Cardiovascular**—peripheral vasodilation, decreased peripheral resistance, inhibition of baroreceptors (pressure receptors located in the aortic arch and carotid sinus that regulate blood pressure), orthostatic hypotension, and fainting
- **Central nervous system**—euphoria, drowsiness, apathy, mental confusion, alterations in mood, reduction in body temperature, feelings of relaxation, dysphoria (depression accompanied by anxiety); nausea and vomiting are caused by direct stimulation of the emetic chemoreceptors located in the medulla. The degree to which these occur usually depends on the drug and the dose.
- **Dermatologic**—histamine release, pruritus, flushing, and red eyes
- **Gastrointestinal**—decrease in gastric motility (prolonged emptying time); decrease in biliary, pancreatic, and intestinal secretions; delay in digestion of food in the small intestine; increase in resting tone, with the potential for spasms, epigastric distress, or biliary colic (caused by constriction of the sphincter of Oddi). These drugs can cause constipation and anorexia.
- **Genitourinary**—urinary urgency and difficulty with urination, caused by spasms of the ureter. Urinary urgency also may occur because of the action of the drugs on the detrusor muscle of the bladder. Some patients may experience difficulty voiding because of contraction of the bladder sphincter.
- **Respiratory**—depressant effects on respiratory rate (caused by a reduced sensitivity of the respiratory center to carbon dioxide)
- **Cough**—suppression of the cough reflex (antitussive effect) by exerting a direct effect on the cough center in the medulla. Codeine has the most noticeable effect on the cough reflex.
- **Medulla**—Nausea and vomiting can occur when the chemoreceptor trigger zone located in the medulla is stimulated. To a varying degree, opioid analgesics also depress the chemoreceptor trigger zone. Therefore, nausea and vomiting may or may not occur when these drugs are given.

motility and the resulting constipation are always a problem in opioid therapy.

The most widely used opioid, morphine sulfate, is an effective drug for moderately severe to severe pain. Morphine sulfate is considered the prototype (model) opioid. Morphine sulfate also is considered the gold standard in pain management—morphine sulfate's actions, uses, and ability to relieve pain are the standards against which other opioid analgesics are often compared. Charts called *equal-analgesic conversions* compare other opioid doses with the doses of morphine sulfate that would be used for the same level of pain control.

Other opioids, such as meperidine and levorphanol, are effective for the treatment of moderate to severe pain. For mild to moderate pain, the primary health care provider may order an opioid such as codeine or pentazocine.

Uses

The opioid analgesics are used primarily for the treatment of moderate to severe acute and chronic pain and in the treatment and management of opiate dependence. In addition, the opioid analgesics may be used for the following reasons:

- To decrease anxiety and sedate the patient before surgery. Patients who are relaxed and sedated when an anesthetic agent is given are easier to anesthetize (requiring a smaller dose of an induction anesthetic), as well as easier to maintain under anesthesia.
- To support anesthesia (i.e., as an adjunct during anesthesia)
- To promote obstetric analgesia
- To relieve anxiety in patients with dyspnea (breathing difficulty) associated with pulmonary edema
- Administered intrathecally or epidurally, to control pain for extended periods without apparent loss of motor, sensory, or sympathetic nerve function
- To relieve pain associated with a myocardial infarction (morphine sulfate is the agent of choice)
- To manage opiate dependence
- To induce conscious sedation before a diagnostic or therapeutic procedure in the hospital setting
- To treat severe diarrhea and intestinal cramping (camphorated tincture of opium may be used)
- To relieve severe, persistent cough (codeine may be helpful, although the drug's use has declined)

Adverse Reactions

[handwritten: ABC Breathing]

Central Nervous System Reactions

- Euphoria, weakness, headache
- Lightheadedness, dizziness, sedation
- Miosis, insomnia, agitation, tremor
- Increased intercranial pressure, impairment of mental and physical tasks

Respiratory System Reactions

- Depression of rate and depth of breathing

Gastrointestinal System Reactions

- Nausea, vomiting
- Dry mouth, biliary tract spasms
- Constipation, anorexia

Cardiovascular System Reactions

- Facial flushing
- Tachycardia, bradycardia, palpitations
- Peripheral circulatory collapse

Genitourinary System Reactions

- Urinary retention or hesitancy
- Spasms of the ureters and bladder sphincter

Allergic and Other Reactions

- Pruritus, rash, and urticaria
- Sweating, pain at injection site, and local tissue irritation

Contraindications

All opioid analgesics are contraindicated in patients with known hypersensitivity to the drugs. These drugs are contraindicated in patients with acute bronchial asthma, emphysema, or upper airway obstruction and in patients with head

[handwritten: Asthma, Emphysema]

injury or increased intracranial pressure. The drugs are also contraindicated in patients with convulsive disorders, severe renal or hepatic dysfunction, and acute ulcerative colitis. The opioid analgesics are pregnancy category C drugs (oxycodone is in pregnancy category B) and are not recommended for use during pregnancy or labor because they may prolong labor or cause respiratory depression in the neonate. The use of opioid analgesics is recommended during pregnancy only if the benefit to the mother outweighs the potential harm to the fetus.

Precautions

Opioid analgesics should be used cautiously in elderly patients and in patients considered *opioid naive*, that is, who have not been medicated with opioid drugs before and who are consequently at greatest risk for respiratory depression. The drugs should be administered cautiously in patients undergoing biliary surgery (because of the risk for spasm of the sphincter of Oddi; in these patients, meperidine is the drug of choice). Patients who are lactating should wait at least 4 to 6 hours after taking the drug to breast-feed the infant. Additional precautions apply to patients with undiagnosed abdominal pain, hypoxia, supraventricular tachycardia, prostatic hypertrophy, and renal or hepatic impairment.

Interactions

The following interactions may occur when an opioid analgesic is administered with another agent:

Interacting Drug	Common Use	Effect of Interaction
alcohol	Social occasions	Increased risk for CNS depression
antihistamines	Prevent or relieve allergic reactions	Increased risk for CNS depression
antidepressants	Alleviate depression	Increased risk for CNS depression
sedatives	Sedation	Increased risk for CNS depression
phenothiazines	Relief of agitation, anxiety, vomiting	Increased risk for CNS depression
opioid agonist-antagonist	Gynecologic or obstetric pain relief	Opioid withdrawal symptoms (if long-term opioid use)
barbiturates	Used in general anesthesia	Respiratory depression, hypotension, or sedation

HERBAL ALERT

The name *passionflower* denotes many of the approximately 400 species of herb in the genus *Passiflora*. Passionflower has been used in medicine to treat pain, anxiety, and insomnia. Some herbalists use it to treat symptoms of parkinsonism. Passionflower is often used in combination with other natural substances, such valerian, chamomile, and hops, for promoting relaxation, rest, and sleep. Although no adverse reactions have been reported, large doses may cause CNS depression. The use of passionflower is contraindicated in pregnancy and in patients taking the monoamine oxidase inhibitors (MAOIs). Passionflower contains coumarin; the risk of bleeding may be increased in patients taking warfarin (Coumadin) and passionflower. The following are recommended dosages for passionflower:

- Tea: 1–4 cups per day (made with 1 tablespoon of the crude herb per cup)
- Tincture (2 g/5 mL): 2 teaspoons (10 mL) 3–4 times daily
- Dried herb: 2 g 3–4 times daily.

NURSING PROCESS
PATIENT RECEIVING AN OPIOID ANALGESIC FOR PAIN

ASSESSMENT

Preadministration Assessment

As part of the preadministration assessment, the nurse assesses and documents the type, onset, intensity, and location of the pain. The nurse documents a description of the pain (e.g., sharp, dull, stabbing, throbbing) and an estimate of when the pain began. Further questioning and more detailed information about the pain are necessary if the pain is of a different type than the patient had been experiencing previously or if it is in a different area.

The nurse reviews the patient's health history, allergy history, and past and current drug therapies. This is especially important when an opioid is given for the first time because data may be obtained during the initial history and physical assessment that require the nurse to contact the primary health care provider. For example, the patient may state that nausea and vomiting occurred when he or she was given a drug for pain several years ago. Further questioning of the patient is necessary because this information may influence the primary health care provider's decision to administer a specific opioid drug.

If promethazine (Phenergan) is used with an opioid to enhance the effects and reduce the dosage of the opioid, the nurse should take the patient's blood pressure, pulse, and respiratory rate before giving the drug.

Ongoing Assessment

The nurse obtains the blood pressure, pulse and respiratory rate, and pain rating in 5 to 10 minutes if the drug is given intravenously (IV), 20 to 30 minutes if the drug is administered intramuscularly (IM) or subcutaneously (subcut), and 30 or more minutes if the drug is given orally. It is important to notify the primary health care provider if the analgesic is ineffective, because a higher dose or a different opioid analgesic may be required.

During the ongoing assessment, it is important for the nurse to ask about the pain regularly and to believe the patient and family in their reports of pain. Nursing judgment must be exercised, because not all instances of a change in pain type, location, or intensity require notifying the primary health care provider. For example, if a patient recovering from recent abdominal surgery experiences pain in the calf of the leg (suggesting venous thrombosis), the nurse should immediately notify the primary health care provider. However, it is not important to contact the primary health care provider for pain that is slightly worse because the patient has been moving in bed.

The opioid-naive patient who does not use opioids routinely and is being given an opioid drug for acute pain relief or a surgical procedure is at greatest risk for respiratory depression after opioid administration. Respiratory depression may occur in patients receiving a normal dose if the patient is vulnerable (e.g., in a weakened or debilitated state). Elderly, **cachectic (malnourished/in general poor health),** or debilitated patients may receive a reduced initial dose until their response to the drug is known. If the patient's respiratory rate is 10 breaths/min or less, the nurse monitors the patient at more frequent intervals and notifies the primary health care provider immediately. Patients involved in long-term opioid therapy for pain relief build tolerance to the physical adverse effects of the drugs; respiratory depression is typically not seen in these patients.

When an opiate is used as an antidiarrheal drug, the nurse records each bowel movement, as well as its appearance, color, and consistency. The nurse should notify the primary health care provider immediately if diarrhea is not relieved or becomes worse, if the patient has severe abdominal pain, or if blood in the stool is noted.

NURSING DIAGNOSES

Drug-specific nursing diagnoses are the following:

- **Ineffective Breathing Pattern** related to pain and effects on breathing center by opioids
- **Risk for Injury** related to dizziness or lightheadedness from opioid administration
- **Constipation** related to the decreased GI motility caused by opioids
- **Imbalanced Nutrition: Less Than Body Requirements** related to anorexia caused by opioids

Nursing diagnoses related to drug administration are discussed in Chapter 4.

PLANNING

The expected outcomes of the patient may include relief of pain, supporting the patient needs related to the management of adverse reactions, an understanding of **patient-controlled analgesia** (PCA; when applicable), absence of injury, adequate nutrition intake, and understanding of and compliance with the prescribed treatment regimen.

IMPLEMENTATION

Relieving Acute Pain

PCA allows postsurgical patients to administer their own analgesic by means of an IV pump system (Fig. 16.2). The patient does not have to wait for the nurse to administer the medicine. Pumps are preset with small amounts of the opioid medication that the patient can administer by pushing a button on the pump. The medication can be delivered, for example, when the patient begins to feel pain or when the patient wishes to ambulate but wants some medication to prevent pain on getting out of bed. Many postoperative patients require less opioid when they can self-administer the medicine for pain. When patients take less opioid, they also experience fewer unpleasant adverse reactions, such as nausea and constipation. Because the self-administration system is under the control of the nurse, who adds the drug to the infusion pump and sets the time interval (or lockout interval) between doses, the patient cannot receive an overdose of the drug.

Relieving Chronic Severe Pain

Morphine sulfate is the most widely used drug in the management of chronic severe pain. The fact that this drug can be given orally, subcut, IM, IV, and rectally in the form of a suppository makes it tremendously versatile. Medication for chronic pain should be scheduled around the clock and not given on a PRN (as-needed) basis. With any chronic pain medication, the oral route

Figure 16.2 PCA allows the client to self-administer medication as necessary to control pain.

is preferred as long as the patient can swallow or can tolerate sublingual administration.

Using the concept of the WHO pain ladder for chronic pain, medications that work to relieve pain both peripherally and centrally will be ordered. To provide good pain relief based on the pain ladder, drugs that combine a nonopioid and an opioid analgesic are available. These drugs work well at dealing with the inflammation at the peripheral site, as well as modifying the pain perception centrally in the brain. Table 16.2 lists many of these drugs and their combination ingredients.

Controlled-released forms of opioids are indicated for the management of moderate to severe pain when a continuous, around-the-clock analgesic is needed for an extended time. Examples of these drugs include oxycodone (OxyContin) and morphine sulfate (Oramorph SR). The medication is given once every 8 to 12 hours; the actual drug is slowly released over time so the patient does not get all the medication at once. Controlled-released drugs are not intended for use as a PRN analgesic. The patient may experience fewer adverse reactions with oxycodone products than with morphine sulfate, and the drug is effective and safe for elderly patients. Controlled-release tablets should be swallowed whole and are not to be broken, chewed, or crushed.

When long-acting forms of the opioids are used, a fast-acting form may be given for breakthrough pain. These are typically ordered on a PRN basis to be used between the long-acting doses for acute pain episodes. Morphine sulfate in oral or sublingual tablets is commonly used. Oral transmucosal fentanyl (Actiq) is also used to treat breakthrough pain.

Fentanyl transdermal is a transdermal system that is effective in the management of severe pain associated with diseases like cancer. The transdermal system allows for a timed-release patch containing the drug fentanyl to be activated over a 72-hour period. A small number of patients may require systems applied every 48 hours. The nurse monitors for adverse effects in the same manner as for other opioid analgesics.

LIFESPAN ALERT – Gerontology
The transdermal route should be used with caution in the elderly, because the amount of subcutaneous tissue is reduced in the aging process. The transdermal route of drug administration is used because it treats severe pain most effectively, and should not be used simply for the convenience of administration.

When pain is best relieved by a combination of drugs and not just the opioid analgesics alone, a mixture of an oral opioid and other drugs may be used to obtain relief. Brompton's mixture is one of the most commonly used solutions. In addition to the opioid, such as morphine sulfate or methadone, other drugs may be used in the solution, including antidepressants, stimulants, aspirin, acetaminophen, and tranquilizers. The pharmacist prepares the solution according to the primary health care provider's instructions. It is necessary to monitor for the adverse reactions of each drug contained in the solution. The time interval for administration varies. Some primary health care providers may order the mixture on a PRN basis; others may order it given at regular intervals.

Over time, the patient taking an opioid analgesic develops tolerance to it. The rate at which tolerance develops varies according to the dosage, the route of administration, and the individual. Patients taking oral medications develop tolerance more slowly than those taking the drugs parenterally. Some patients develop tolerance quickly and need larger doses every few weeks, whereas others are maintained on the same dosage schedule throughout the course of the illness.

The fear of respiratory depression is a concern for many nurses administering an opioid, and some nurses may hesitate to administer the drug. However, respiratory

Table 16.2 **Opioid/Nonopioid Combination Oral Analgesics**		
Brand Name	**Opioid**	**Nonopioid**
Tylenol #3	codeine 30 mg	acetaminophen 300 mg
Lortab	hydrocodone 2.5 mg	acetaminophen 167 mg
Vicodin	hydrocodone 5 mg	acetaminophen 500 mg
Vicodin ES	hydrocodone 7.5 mg	acetaminophen 750 mg
Percodan	oxycodone 5 mg	aspirin 325 mg
Percocet	oxycodone 5 mg	acetaminophen 325 mg
Roxicet	oxycodone 5 mg	acetaminophen 325 mg
Darvon-Compound 65	propoxyphene 65 mg	aspirin 389 mg; caffeine 32.4 mg
Darvocet-N 50	propoxyphene 50 mg	acetaminophen 325 mg
Darvocet-N 100	propoxyphene 100 mg	acetaminophen 650 mg

depression rarely occurs in patients using an opioid for chronic pain. In fact, these patients usually develop tolerance to the respiratory depressant effects of the drug very quickly. Nurses should be more concerned about adverse effects on the GI system. The decrease in GI motility causes constipation, nausea, acute abdominal pain, and anorexia. It is important to provide a thorough, aggressive bowel program to patients when they are taking opioid medications.

NURSING ALERT

When patients experience a drop in respiratory rate, the nurse should attempt to increase the rate by coaching the patient to breathe. Should an antidote be needed, naloxone (Narcan) should be administered with great caution and only when necessary in patients receiving an opioid for severe pain. Naloxone removes all of the pain-relieving effects of the opioid and may lead to withdrawal symptoms or the return of intense pain.

Using Transdermal System Pain Management

When using a transdermal system, it is important to ensure that only one patch is on at a time to prevent additive effects of the drug. The nurse finds and removes the old patch before replacing it with a new one. Before the new transdermal patch is applied, the nurse dates and initials the patch with a water resistant pen. Use only water to cleanse the site before application, because soaps, oils, and other substances may irritate the skin. Rotate site of application and do not apply over hair. To ensure complete contact with the skin surface, press for 10 to 20 seconds (Fig. 16.3). After 72 hours, remove the system and, if continuous therapy is prescribed, apply a new system. The used patch should be folded carefully so the system adheres to itself for proper disposal.

Using Epidural Pain Management

Administration of morphine sulfate and fentanyl by the epidural route has provided an alternative to the IM or oral route. This approach was introduced with the idea

Figure 16.3 The nurse applies the transdermal patch securely.

that very small doses of opioid would provide long-lasting pain relief with significantly fewer systemic adverse reactions.

Epidural administration offers several advantages over other routes, including lower total dosages of the drug used, fewer adverse reactions, and greater patient comfort. This type of pain management is used for postoperative pain, labor pain, and intractable chronic pain. The administration of the opioid is either by bolus or by continuous infusion pump.

Patients experience pain relief with fewer adverse reactions; the adverse reactions experienced are those related to processes under direct CNS control. The most serious adverse reaction associated with the epidurally administered opioids is respiratory depression. Patients using epidural analgesics for chronic pain are monitored for respiratory problems with an apnea monitor. The patient may also experience sedation, confusion, nausea, pruritus, or urinary retention. Fentanyl is increasingly used as an alternative to morphine sulfate because patients experience fewer adverse reactions.

NURSING ALERT

Epidural analgesia should be administered only by those specifically trained in the use of IV and epidural anesthetics. Oxygen, resuscitative, and intubation equipment should be readily available.

Nursing care includes close monitoring of the patient for respiratory depression immediately after insertion of the epidural catheter and throughout therapy. Vital signs are taken every 30 minutes, apnea monitors are used, and an opioid antagonist, such as naloxone, is readily available.

Policies and procedures for administering, monitoring, and documenting drugs given through the epidural route must be specific to the nurse practice act in each state and in accordance with federal and state regulations. This type of analgesia is most often managed by registered nurses with special training in the care and management of epidural catheters.

Monitoring and Managing Patient Needs

The nurse should contact the primary health care provider immediately if any of the following are present:

- Significant decrease in the respiratory rate or a respiratory rate of 10 breaths/min or less
- Significant increase or decrease in the pulse rate or a change in the pulse quality
- Significant decrease in blood pressure (systolic or diastolic) or a systolic pressure below 100 mm Hg

INEFFECTIVE BREATHING PATTERN. Opioids may depress the cough reflex. The nurse should encourage patients receiving an opioid, even for a few days, to cough and breathe deeply every 2 hours. This task prevents the pooling of secretions in the lungs, which can lead to hypostatic pneumonia and other lung problems. The patient may be fearful that exercise will cause even greater pain. The nurse should perform tasks, such as getting the patient out of bed, and encourage therapeutic activities, such as deep breathing, coughing, and leg exercises (when ordered), when the drug is producing its greatest analgesic effect, usually 1 to 2 hours after the nurse administers the opioid. If the patient experiences nausea and vomiting, the nurse should notify the primary health care provider. A different analgesic or an antiemetic may be necessary.

RISK FOR INJURY. Opioids may produce orthostatic hypotension, which in turn results in dizziness. The nurse immediately reports to the primary health care provider any significant change in the patient's vital signs. Particularly vulnerable are postoperative patients and individuals whose ability to maintain blood pressure has been compromised. The nurse should assist the patient with ambulatory activities and with rising slowly from a sitting or lying position. Miosis (pinpoint pupils) may occur with the administration of some opioids and is most pronounced with morphine sulfate, hydromorphone, and hydrochlorides of opium alkaloids. Miosis decreases the ability to see in dim light. The nurse keeps the room well lit during daytime hours and advises the patient to seek assistance when getting out of bed at night.

CONSTIPATION. Most patients should begin taking a stool softener or laxative with the initial dose of an opioid analgesic. Decreased GI motility due to the opioids, in addition to lower food and water intake and decreased mobility, cause the constipation. The nurse keeps a daily record of bowel movements and informs the primary health care provider if constipation appears to be a problem. Many patients need to continue taking a laxative for as long as they take an opioid analgesic. If the patient is constipated despite the use of a stool softener or laxative, the primary health care provider may prescribe an enema or other means of relieving constipation.

IMBALANCED NUTRITION: LESS THAN BODY REQUIREMENTS. When an opioid is prescribed for a prolonged time, anorexia (loss of appetite) may occur. Those receiving an opioid for pain relief caused by a terminal illness often have severe anorexia from the disease and the opioid. The nurse assesses food intake after each meal. When anorexia is prolonged, the nurse weighs the patient as ordered by the primary health care provider. It is important for the nurse to notify the primary health care provider of continued weight loss and anorexia. Supplements may be ordered and administered orally, enterally, or parenterally.

OPIOID DRUG DEPENDENCE. Patients receiving the opioid analgesics for acute pain do not develop physical dependence. Delays in medication administration cause patients to ask repeatedly for pain medication. This behavior is sometimes interpreted as drug-seeking behavior or it may be associated with the fear of making a patient drug dependent. Nurses are also fearful that patients with a history of psychologic dependence might become dependent again when given pain medication.

These individuals experience pain, too. They need to be provided adequate pain relief to *prevent* returning to dependency behaviors. Typically it is the behavior of the nurses and primary health care providers in delaying administration of opioids for good pain control that causes the problems associated with appearances of dependence.

Drug dependence can, however, occur in a newborn whose mother was dependent on opiates during pregnancy. Withdrawal symptoms in the newborn usually appear during the first few days of life. Symptoms include irritability, excessive crying, yawning, sneezing, increased respiratory rate, tremors, fever, vomiting, and diarrhea.

MANAGEMENT OF OPIOID DEPENDENCE. Two opioids are used in the treatment and management of opiate dependence: levomethadyl and methadone. Levomethadyl is given in an opiate dependency clinic to maintain control over the delivery of the drug. Because of its potential for serious and life-threatening prearrhythmic effects, levomethadyl is reserved for treating addicted patients who have had no response to other treatments. Levomethadyl is not taken daily; the drug is administered three times a week (Monday/Wednesday/Friday or Tuesday/Thursday/Saturday). Daily use of the usual dose will cause serious overdose.

! NURSING ALERT

If transferring from levomethadyl to methadone, the nurse should wait 48 hours after the last dose of levomethadyl before administering the first dose of methadone or other opioid.

Methadone, a synthetic opioid, may be used for the relief of pain, but it also is used in the detoxification and maintenance treatment of those dependent on opioids. Detoxification involves withdrawing the patient from the opioid while preventing withdrawal symptoms. Maintenance therapy is designed to reduce the patient's desire to return to the drug that caused dependence, as well as to prevent withdrawal symptoms. Dosages vary with the patient, the length of time the individual has been dependent, and the average amount of drug used each day. Patients enrolled in an outpatient methadone program for detoxification or maintenance therapy on

DISPLAY 16.2 Symptoms of the Abstinence Syndrome

Early Symptoms
Yawning, lacrimation, rhinorrhea, sweating

Intermediate Symptoms
Mydriasis, tachycardia, twitching, tremor, restlessness, irritability, anxiety, anorexia

Late Symptoms
Muscle spasm, fever, nausea, vomiting, kicking movements, weakness, depression, body aches, weight loss, severe backache, abdominal and leg pains, hot and cold flashes, insomnia, repetitive sneezing, increased blood pressure, respiratory rate, and heart rate

methadone must continue to receive methadone when hospitalized. In adults, withdrawal symptoms are known as the *abstinence syndrome* (see Display 16.2 for more information).

Educating the Patient and Family

The nurse informs the patient that the drug he or she is receiving is for pain. It also is a good idea to include additional information, such as how often the drug can be given and the name of the drug being given.

If a patient is to receive drugs through a PCA infusion pump, the nurse teaches the patient how to use the machine during the preoperative period rather than waiting until the patient is in pain in the postoperative unit (see Patient Teaching for Improved Patient Outcomes: Using Patient Controlled Analgesia for Postoperative Pain). The nurse notifies the primary health care provider if the patient does not understand the PCA procedure so that an alternative method of pain relief can be ordered.

Opioids for outpatient use may be prescribed in the oral form or as a timed-release transdermal patch. In certain cases, such as when terminally ill patients are being cared for at home, the nurse may give the family instruction in the parenteral administration of the drug or use of an IV pump.

When an opioid has been prescribed, the nurse includes the following points in the teaching plan:

- This drug may cause drowsiness, dizziness, and blurring of vision. Use caution when driving or performing tasks requiring alertness.
- Avoid the use of alcoholic beverages unless use has been approved by the primary health care provider. Alcohol may intensify the action of the drug and cause extreme drowsiness or dizziness. In some instances, the use of alcohol and an opioid can have extremely serious and even life-threatening consequences that may require emergency medical treatment.
- Take the drug as directed on the container label and do not exceed the prescribed dose. Contact the primary health care provider if the drug is not effective.
- If GI upset occurs, take the drug with food.
- Notify the primary health care provider if nausea, vomiting, and constipation become severe.

EVALUATION

- Therapeutic response is achieved and discomfort is reduced. If ordered, the patient demonstrates the ability to use PCA effectively.
- Adverse reactions are identified, reported to the primary health care provider, and managed successfully with appropriate nursing interventions:
  ☑ An adequate breathing pattern is maintained.
  ☑ No evidence of injury is seen.
  ☑ Patient reports adequate bowel movements.
  ☑ Patient maintains an adequate nutritional status.
- Patient and family demonstrate an understanding of the drug regimen.

Know

Patient Teaching for Improved Patient Outcomes

Using Patient Controlled Analgesia for Postoperative Pain

In some situations, IV opioid analgesics may be ordered for pain relief following a surgical procedure. If the patient is able to participate the primary health care provider may offer PCA. The purpose of this is to allow the patient to manage pain to recuperate faster and return to daily activities of life sooner. During preoperative teaching, the nurse makes sure to review the following steps with the patient:

✓ How the pump works; the machine regulates the dose of the drug as well as the time interval between doses.
✓ The location of the control button that activates the administration of the drug; the difference between the control button and the button to call the nurse (when both are similar in appearance and feel).
✓ Use the machine to prevent pain, such as when the patient feels the need for pain relief or is about to engage in an activity that might cause pain (e.g., coughing, exercises, or getting out of bed).
✓ Push the button once; the button does not need to be depressed to keep the drug flowing in the IV.
✓ The dose of drug is ordered by the primary health care provider and set by the nurse. If the control button is used too soon after the last dose, the machine will not deliver the drug until the correct time; therefore the patient does not need to worry about taking too much drug.

THINK CRITICALLY: PHARMACOLOGY IN PRACTICE

1. Betty Peterson is prescribed meperidine (Demerol) for gallbladder pain. You discover in her health history on the chart that she has a history of alcohol and drug use. Determine how to ensure that all the nursing staff will provide her with adequate pain management during her hospital stay.

2. Mrs. Moore, aged 85 years, is taking morphine sulfate to manage severe pain occurring as the result of heart failure. The primary health care provider has prescribed an around-the-clock dosage regimen. Mrs. Moore tells the nurse that she is taking the pain drug 1 to 2 hours before the next dose is due. What strategies would you use to determine if this is the correct dosing of opioid analgesic?

● Test Your Knowledge

1. The nurse explains to the patient that some opioids may be used as part of the preoperative medication regimen to _____.

   A. increase intestinal motility
   B. facilitate passage of an endotracheal tube
   C. enhance the effects of the skeletal muscle relaxant
   D. lessen anxiety and sedate the patient

2. Each time the patient requests an opioid analgesic, the nurse must _____.

   A. check the patient's diagnosis
   B. talk to the patient to see if he is awake
   C. determine the exact location and intensity of the pain
   D. administer the drug with food to prevent gastric upset

3. When administering opioid analgesics to an elderly patient, the nurse monitors the patient closely for _____.

   A. an increased heart rate
   B. euphoria
   C. confusion
   D. a synergistic reaction

4. When administering a timed-release medication to a patient, the nurse must be aware that _____.

   A. it should not be crushed
   B. the medication is stronger
   C. serious cardiac arrhythmias may develop
   D. CNS stimulation is possible

● Prepare for the NCLEX

1. Which of the following findings requires that the nurse immediately contact the primary health care provider?

   A. Pulse rate of 80 bpm
   B. Complaint of breakthrough pain
   C. Respiratory rate of 20 breaths/min
   D. Systolic blood pressure of 140 mm Hg

● Calculate Medication Dosages

1. A patient is prescribed oral morphine sulfate 12 mg. The dosage available is 10 mg/mL. The nurse administers _____.

2. A patient is prescribed fentanyl (Sublimaze) 50 mcg IM 30 minutes before surgery. The nurse has available a vial with a dosage strength of 0.05 mg/1 mL. The nurse calculates the dosage and administers _____.

To check your answers, see Appendix E.

the**Point**. *For more NCLEX questions, log on to http://thepoint.lww.com to access more than 1000 questions.*

Opioid Antagonists

antagonist   opioid naive

LEARNING OBJECTIVES

On completion of this chapter, the student will:

1. Discuss the uses, general drug action, general adverse reactions, contraindications, precautions, and interactions of the opioid antagonists.
2. Discuss important preadministration and ongoing assessment activities the nurse should perform on the patient receiving the opioid antagonists.
3. List nursing diagnoses particular to a patient taking an opioid antagonist.
4. Discuss ways to promote optimal response to therapy, how to manage adverse reactions, and important points to keep in mind when educating patients about the use of opioid antagonists.

An **antagonist** is a substance that counteracts the action of something else. A drug that is an opioid antagonist has a greater affinity for a cell receptor than an opioid drug (agonist), and by binding to the cell it prevents a response to the opioid. Thus, an opioid antagonist reverses the actions of an opioid. One of the most severe adverse reactions to opioid treatment is respiratory depression. Specific antagonists have been developed to reverse the respiratory depression associated with the opioids. The two opioid antagonists in use today are naloxone (Narcan) and nalmefene (Revex). Naloxone is capable of restoring respiratory function within 1 to 2 minutes after administration. Naltrexone (another antagonist) is used primarily to treat alcohol dependence and to block the effects of suspected opioids if they are being used by a person undergoing treatment for alcohol dependence.

• OPIOID ANTAGONISTS

Actions

Administration of an antagonist prevents or reverses the effects of opioid drugs. The antagonist reverses the opioid effects by competing for the opiate receptor sites and dis-

placing the opioid drug (see Chapter 16). If the individual has taken or received an opioid, the effects of the opioid are reversed. An antagonist drug is not selective for specific adverse reactions. When an antagonist is given to reverse a specific adverse reaction, such as respiratory depression, it is important to remember the antagonist reverses *all* effects. Therefore, a patient who receives an antagonist to reverse respiratory effects will also experience a reversal of pain relief—that is, the pain will return. If the individual has not taken or received an opioid, an antagonist has no drug effect.

Uses

Opioid antagonists are used for the treatment of the following:

• Postoperative acute respiratory depression
• Opioid adverse effects (reversal)
• Suspected acute opioid overdosage

Adverse Reactions

Generalized reactions include:

• Nausea and vomiting
• Sweating
• Tachycardia
• Increased blood pressure
• Tremors

See the Summary Drug Table: Opioid Antagonists for more information.

Contraindications, Precautions, and Interactions

Antagonists are contraindicated in those with a hypersensitivity to the opioid antagonists. Antagonists are used cautiously in those who are pregnant (pregnancy category B), in infants of opioid-dependent mothers, and in patients with an opioid dependency or cardiovascular disease. These drugs also are used cautiously during lactation.

These drugs may produce withdrawal symptoms in individuals who are physically dependent on the opioid. Antagonists may prevent the action or intended use of opioid antidiarrheals, antitussives, and analgesics.

161

Summary Drug Table OPIOID ANTAGONISTS

Generic Name	Trade Name	Uses	Adverse Reactions	Dosage Ranges
nalmefene *nal'-meh-feen*	Revex	Complete or partial reversal of opioid effects after surgery or overdose	Nausea, vomiting, tachycardia, hypertension, return of postoperative pain, fever, dizziness	Postoperative opioid reversal: 0.25 mcg/kg; may be repeated in 2–5-min increments
naloxone *nah-lox'-own*	Narcan	Same as nalmefene	Same as nalmefene	Postoperative opioid reversal: 0.1–0.2 mg IV at 2–3 min intervals Suspected opioid overdose: 0.4–2 mg IV at 2–3-min intervals

NURSING PROCESS
PATIENT RECEIVING AN OPIOID ANTAGONIST FOR RESPIRATORY DEPRESSION

ASSESSMENT

Preadministration Assessment
Patients involved in long-term opioid therapy for pain relief build tolerance to the physical adverse effects of the drugs. It is the patient who does not use opioids routinely and who is being given an opioid drug for acute pain relief or a surgical procedure who is at most risk for respiratory depression after opioid administration. These patients are described as **opioid naive**.

Sometimes the somnolence and pain relief produced by the opioid drug will slow the patient's breathing pattern. This can be alarming to the nurse if the respiratory rate has been rapid because of anxiety and pain. The nurse should make efforts to arouse the patient and coach his or her breathing pattern if possible. Before administration of the antagonist, the nurse obtains the blood pressure, pulse, and respiratory rate and reviews the record for the drug suspected of causing the symptoms of respiratory depression. If there is sufficient time, the nurse also should review the initial health history, allergy history, and current treatment modalities.

Ongoing Assessment
As part of the ongoing assessment during the administration of the antagonist, the nurse monitors the blood pressure, pulse, and respiratory rate at frequent intervals, usually every 5 minutes, until the patient responds. This monitoring is more frequent if respiratory depression occurs in the immediate postoperative setting. After the patient has shown a response to the drug, the nurse monitors vital signs every 5 to 15 minutes. The nurse should notify the primary health care provider if any adverse drug reactions occur because additional medical treatment may be needed. The nurse monitors the respiratory rate, rhythm, and depth; pulse; blood pressure; and level of consciousness until the effects of the opioid wear off.

❗ NURSING ALERT
The effects of some opioids may last longer than the effects of naloxone (Narcan). A repeat dose of naloxone may be ordered by the primary health care provider if results obtained from the initial dose are unsatisfactory. The duration of close patient observation depends on the patient's response to the administration of the opioid antagonist.

NURSING DIAGNOSES

Drug-specific nursing diagnoses are the following:

❏ **Impaired Spontaneous Ventilation** related to brain response to slow breathing induced by the opioid drug
❏ **Acute Pain** related to antagonist drug displacing opioid drug at cell receptor sites

Nursing diagnoses related to drug administration are discussed in Chapter 4.

PLANNING

The expected outcome for the patient with respiratory depression is an optimal response to therapy and support of patient needs related to the management of adverse drug effects. This is essentially a return to normal respiratory rate, rhythm, and depth. The nurse meets the patient's needs by providing adequate ventilation of the body as well as continued pain relief.

IMPLEMENTATION

Promoting an Optimal Response to Therapy
Frequently, the use of naloxone is in the controlled setting of the postanesthesia recovery unit (also called the *postanesthesia care unit* [PACU] or *surgical recovery room*). As the patient awakens from the deep operative sleep, the nurse balances the need for continued pain relief against the person's ability to breathe independently after the procedure.

Monitoring and Managing Patient Needs
IMPAIRED SPONTANEOUS VENTILATION. Depending on the patient's condition, the nurse may use cardiac monitoring, artificial ventilation (respirator), and other drugs during and after the administration of naloxone. It is important to keep suction equipment readily available

Opioid Antagonists

because abrupt reversal of opioid-induced respiratory depression may cause vomiting. The nurse must maintain a patent airway and should turn and suction the patient as needed.

If naloxone is given by intravenous (IV) infusion, the primary health care provider orders the IV fluid and amount, the drug dosage, and the infusion rate. Giving the drug by IV infusion requires use of a secondary line, an IV piggyback or an IV push.

NURSING ALERT

When naloxone is used to reverse respiratory depression and the resulting somnolence, the drug is given by slow IV push until the respiratory rate begins to increase and somnolence abates. Keep in mind that giving a rapid bolus will cause withdrawal and return of intense pain.

ACUTE PAIN. When the antagonist drug is given to patients, they experience pain abruptly, because the opioid no longer works in the body. The nurse assesses the pain level and begins to treat the pain again. The nurse needs to review the circumstances that led to the use of the antagonist as an opioid reversal drug. Steps can then be taken to resume pain relief without the adverse reaction.

If the patient is in a setting where family members may be present, it is the nurse's responsibility to educate the family about the action of the drug and what they will see happen. It can be distressing for others to see a person experience intense pain when the antagonist begins to work if they do not understand the reason for the intervention.

The nurse monitors fluid intake and output and notifies the primary health care provider of any change in the fluid intake–output ratio. Of course, the nurse should notify the primary health care provider if there is any sudden change in the patient's condition.

EVALUATION

- Therapeutic response is achieved and drug toxicity is reversed.
- Adverse reactions are identified, reported to the primary health care provider, and managed successfully with appropriate nursing interventions:
  - ☑ Patient's respiratory rate, rhythm, and depth are normal.
  - ☑ Pain relief is resumed.
- Patient and family demonstrate an understanding of the drug regimen.

THINK CRITICALLY: PHARMACOLOGY IN PRACTICE

1. When Mr. Park came to the preoperative unit, he complained that the pain on his back (where the shingles rash was erupting) was greater than the pain in his broken hip. On rounds before the surgical procedure to repair his hip, the primary health care provider

assured him that the acyclovir would begin to alleviate some of the pain from the rash. Following the surgical procedure, the surgeon ordered meperidine (Demerol) for postoperative pain management. In assessing Mr. Park, he reports his pain is "8 out of 10" on a 0-10 pain scale. The nurse promptly gives the drug, and approximately 20 minutes after receiving an injection of meperidine, the nurse discovers Mr. Park's vital signs are blood pressure 80/50 mm Hg, pulse rate 120 bpm, and respiratory rate 8 breaths/min. Determine what action, if any, the nurse should take.

2. Explain the term *opiate naive* and describe which patients are more likely to experience respiratory depression and which patients are not as likely to experience this adverse reaction to opioid therapy. Discuss important preadministration and ongoing nursing assessments you would make when giving a patient naloxone for severe respiratory depression caused by meperidine.

● Test Your Knowledge

1. Which opioid antagonist would most likely be prescribed for treatment of a patient who is experiencing an opioid overdose?
   - **A.** naltrexone
   - **B.** naloxone
   - **C.** naproxen
   - **D.** nifedipine

● Prepare for the NCLEX

1. Which patient, given an opioid analgesic for acute pain, should the nurse monitor most closely for respiratory distress?
   - **A.** Patient with cancer taking morphine sulfate regularly
   - **B.** Athlete who is taking Percocet for a leg injury
   - **C.** Man who has never used an opioid pain medication
   - **D.** Methadone client with a broken arm

● Calculate Medication Dosages

1. A patient is prescribed 0.8 mg naloxone IV for postoperative respiratory depression caused by morphine. Available is a vial with 1 mg/mL. The nurse administers _____.

2. In the recovery room, the physician prescribes naloxone 0.4 mg by injection as the initial dose for opioid-induced respiratory depression; it may be followed in 5 minutes with 0.2 mg. Orders read that the nurse should contact the primary health care provider when a total of 1 mg is given. How many times can the nurse give the drug before contacting the primary health care provider?

To check your answers, see Appendix E.

thePoint. *For more NCLEX questions, log on to http://thepoint.lww.com to access more than 1000 questions.*

Anesthetic Drugs

LEARNING OBJECTIVES

On completion of this chapter, the student will:

1. State the uses of local anesthesia, methods of administration, and nursing responsibilities when administering a local anesthetic.
2. Describe the purpose of a preanesthetic drug and the nursing responsibilities associated with the administration of a preanesthetic drug.
3. Identify several drugs used for local and general anesthesia.
4. List and briefly describe the four stages of general anesthesia.
5. Discuss important nursing responsibilities associated with caring for a patient receiving a preanesthetic drug and during the postanesthesia care (recovery room) period.

A nesthesia is a loss of feeling or sensation. Anesthesia may be induced by various drugs that can bring about partial or complete loss of sensation. There are two types of anesthesia: local anesthesia and general anesthesia. **Local anesthesia**, as the term implies, is the provision of a sensation-free state in a specific area (or region). With a local anesthetic, the patient is fully awake but does not feel pain in the area that has been anesthetized. However, some procedures performed under local anesthesia may require the patient to be sedated. Although not fully awake, sedated patients may still hear what is going on around them. **General anesthesia** is the provision of a sensation-free state for the entire body. When a general anesthetic is given, the patient loses consciousness and feels no pain. Reflexes, such as the swallowing and gag reflexes, are lost during deep general anesthesia (Fig. 18.1).

Both physicians and nurses administer anesthesia. An **anesthesiologist** is a physician with special training in administering anesthesia. A nurse **anesthetist** is a nurse with a master's degree and special training who is qualified to administer anesthetics.

• LOCAL ANESTHESIA

The various methods of administering a local anesthetic include topical application, local infiltration, and regional anesthesia.

Topical Anesthesia

Topical anesthesia involves the application of the anesthetic to the surface of the skin, open area, or mucous membrane. The anesthetic may be applied with a cotton swab or sprayed on the area. This type of anesthesia may be used to desensitize the skin or mucous membrane to the injection of a deeper local anesthetic. In some instances, topical anesthetics may be applied by the nurse.

Local Infiltration Anesthesia

Local infiltration anesthesia is the injection of a local anesthetic drug into tissues. This type of anesthesia may be used for dental procedures, the suturing of small wounds, or making an incision into a small area, such as that required for removing a superficial piece of tissue for biopsy.

Regional Anesthesia

Regional anesthesia is the injection of a local anesthetic around nerves so that the area supplied by these nerves will not send pain signals to the brain. The anesthetized area is usually larger than the area affected by local infiltration anesthesia. Spinal anesthesia and conduction blocks are two types of regional anesthesia.

Spinal Anesthesia

Spinal anesthesia is a type of regional anesthesia that involves the injection of a local anesthetic drug into the subarachnoid space of the spinal cord, usually at the level of the second lumbar vertebra. There is a loss of feeling (anesthesia) and movement in the lower extremities, lower abdomen, and perineum.

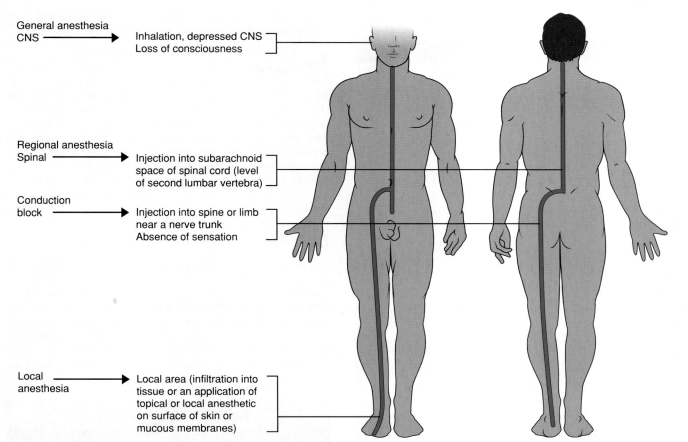

General anesthesia
CNS ⟶ Inhalation, depressed CNS
Loss of consciousness

Regional anesthesia
Spinal ⟶ Injection into subarachnoid
space of spinal cord (level
of second lumbar vertebra)

Conduction
block ⟶ Injection into spine or limb
near a nerve trunk
Absence of sensation

Local ⟶ Local area (infiltration into
anesthesia tissue or an application of
topical or local anesthetic
on surface of skin or
mucous membranes)

Figure 18.1 Sites and mechanisms of action of drugs used for anesthesia.

Conduction Blocks

A **conduction block** is a type of regional anesthesia produced by injection of a local anesthetic drug into or near a nerve trunk. Examples of a conduction block include an **epidural block** (injection of a local anesthetic into the space surrounding the dura of the spinal cord); a **transsacral** (caudal) **block** (injection of a local anesthetic into the epidural space at the level of the sacrococcygeal notch); and **brachial plexus block** (injection of a local anesthetic into the brachial plexus). Epidural—especially—and transsacral blocks are often used in obstetrics. A brachial plexus block may be used for surgery of the arm or hand.

The placement of the needle or a catheter requires strict aseptic technique by a skilled physician. Drug injected through the catheter spreads freely throughout the tissues in the space, interrupting pain conduction at the points where sensory nerve fibers exit from the spinal cord.

A catheter may be placed to give intermittent injections to maintain anesthesia over time such as the immediate postoperative period.

Preparing the Patient for Local Anesthesia

Depending on the procedure performed, preparing the patient for local anesthesia may or may not be similar to preparing the patient for general anesthesia. For example, administering a local anesthetic for dental surgery or for suturing a small wound may require that the nurse explain to the patient how the anesthetic will be administered, take the patient's allergy history, and, when applicable, prepare the area to be anesthetized, which may involve cleaning the area with an antiseptic or shaving the area. Other local anesthetic procedures may require the patient to be fasting (taking in nothing by mouth), because a sedative may also be administered. The nurse may administer an intravenous (IV) sedative, such as the central nervous system (CNS) depressant drug midazolam (Versed), during some local anesthetic procedures, such as cataract surgery or a colonoscopy.

Administering Local Anesthesia

The physician or dentist administers a local injectable anesthetic. These drugs may be mixed with epinephrine to cause local vasoconstriction. The drug stays in the tissue longer when epinephrine is used. This is contraindicated, however, when the local anesthetic is used on an extremity. When preparing these medications, the nurse should proceed cautiously and be aware of when epinephrine is to be used and when it should not be used. Table 18.1 lists the more commonly used local anesthetics.

Table 18.1 Example of Local Anesthetics

Generic Name	Trade Name
articaine	Septocaine
bupivacaine	Marcaine
chloroprocaine	Nesacaine, Nesacaine-MPF
lidocaine	Xylocaine
mepivacaine	Carbocaine, Isocaine
prilocaine	Citanest
procaine	Novocain
ropivacaine	Naropin

Nursing Responsibilities

When caring for a patient receiving local anesthesia, the nurse may be responsible for applying a dressing to the surgical area if appropriate. Depending on the reason for using local anesthesia, the nurse also may be responsible for observing the area for bleeding, oozing, or other problems after the administration of the anesthetic.

• PREANESTHETIC DRUGS

A **preanesthetic drug** is one given before the administration of anesthesia. The nurse usually gives a preanesthetic drug before the administration of general anesthesia, but occasionally may give it before injection of the local anesthetic to sedate the patient. The preanesthetic agent may consist of one drug or a combination of drugs.

Uses of Preanesthetic Drugs

The general purpose, or use, of the preanesthetic drug is to prepare the patient for anesthesia. The more specific purposes of these drugs include the following:

- Opioid or antianxiety drug—to decrease anxiety and apprehension immediately before surgery. The patient who is calm and relaxed can be anesthetized more quickly, usually requires a smaller dose of an induction drug, may require less anesthesia during surgery, and may have a smoother recovery from the anesthesia period (awakening from anesthesia).
- Cholinergic blocking drug—to decrease secretions of the upper respiratory tract. Some anesthetic gases and volatile liquids are irritating to the lining of the respiratory tract and thereby increase mucous secretions. The cough and swallowing reflexes are lost during general anesthesia, and excessive secretions can pool in the lungs, resulting in pneumonia or atelectasis (lung collapse) during the postoperative period. The administration of a cholinergic blocking drug, such as glycopyrrolate (Robinul), dries up secretions of the upper respiratory tract and decreases the possibility of excessive mucus production.

- Antiemetic—to decrease the incidence of nausea and vomiting during the immediate postoperative recovery period.

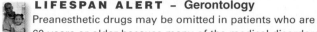
LIFESPAN ALERT – Gerontology
Preanesthetic drugs may be omitted in patients who are 60 years or older because many of the medical disorders for which these drugs are contraindicated are seen in older individuals. For example, atropine and glycopyrrolate, drugs that can be used to decrease secretions of the upper respiratory tract, are contraindicated in certain medical disorders, such as prostatic hypertrophy, glaucoma, and myocardial ischemia. Other preanesthetic drugs that depress the CNS, such as opioids, barbiturates, and antianxiety drugs, with or without antiemetic properties, may be contraindicated in the older individual.

Selection of Preanesthetic Drugs

The preanesthetic drug is usually selected by the anesthesiologist and may consist of one or more drugs (Table 18.2). An opioid (see Chapter 17), antianxiety drug (see Chapter 20), or barbiturate (see Chapter 21) may be given to relax or sedate the patient. Barbiturates are used only occasionally; opioids are usually preferred for sedation. A cholinergic blocking drug (see Chapter 27) is given to dry secretions in the upper respiratory tract. Scopolamine and glycopyrrolate also have

Table 18.2 Examples of Preanesthetic Drugs

Generic Name	Trade Name
Opioids	
fentanyl	Sublimaze
meperidine	Demerol
morphine	
Barbiturates	
pentobarbital	Nembutal
secobarbital	Seconal
Cholinergic Blocking Drugs	
atropine	
glycopyrrolate	Robinul
scopolamine	
Antianxiety Drugs With Antiemetic Properties	
hydroxyzine	Atarax, Vistaril
Antianxiety Drugs	
chlordiazepoxide	Librium
diazepam	Valium
lorazepam	Ativan
midazolam	Versed
Sedative Drugs	
droperidol	Inapsine

atropine dries out mouth
Phenagan

pre an
relieves anxiety

mild sedative properties, and atropine may or may not produce some sedation. Antianxiety drugs have sedative action; when combined with an opioid, they allow a lowering of the opioid dosage because they also have the ability to potentiate (increase the effect of) the sedative action of the opioid. Diazepam (Valium), an antianxiety drug, is one of the more commonly used drugs for preoperative sedation.

Nursing Responsibilities

When caring for a patient receiving a preanesthetic drug, the nurse assesses the patient's physical status and gives an explanation of the anesthesia. In some hospitals, the anesthesiologist examines the patient the day or evening before surgery, although this may not be possible in emergency situations. Some hospitals use operating room or postanesthesia care unit (PACU) staff members to visit the patient before surgery to explain certain facts, such as the time of surgery, the effects of the preanesthetic drug, preparations for surgery, and the PACU. Proper explanation of anesthesia, the surgery itself, and the events that may occur in preparation for surgery, as well as care after surgery, requires a team approach. The nurse's responsibilities include the following:

- Describes or explains the preparations for surgery ordered by the physician. Examples of preoperative preparations include fasting from midnight (or the time specified by the physician), enema, shaving of the operative site, use of a hypnotic for sleep the night before, and the preoperative injection about 30 minutes before surgery.
- Describes or explains immediate postoperative care, such as that given in the PACU (also called the *recovery room*) or a special postoperative surgical unit, and the activities of the health care team during this period. The nurse explains that the patient's vital signs will be monitored frequently and that other equipment, such as IV lines and fluids and hemodynamic (cardiac) monitors, may be used.
- Demonstrates, describes, and explains postoperative patient activities, such as deep breathing, coughing, and leg exercises.
- Emphasizes the importance of pain control, and makes sure the patient understands that relieving pain early on is better than trying to hold out, not take the medicine, and later attempt to relieve the pain. The nurse teaches the patient how to use the patient-controlled analgesia (PCA) pump.
- Tailors the preoperative explanations to fit the type of surgery scheduled. Not all of these teaching points may require inclusion in every explanation.

● GENERAL ANESTHESIA

The administration of general anesthesia requires the use of one or more drugs. The choice of anesthetic drug depends on many factors, including:

- General physical condition of the patient
- Area, organ, or system being operated on
- Anticipated length of the surgical procedure

The anesthesiologist selects the anesthetic drugs that will produce safe anesthesia, analgesia (absence of pain), and, in some surgeries, effective skeletal muscle relaxation. General anesthesia is most commonly achieved when the anesthetic vapors are inhaled or administered IV. Volatile liquid anesthetics produce anesthesia when their vapors are inhaled. Volatile liquids are liquids that evaporate on exposure to air. Examples of volatile liquids include halothane, desflurane, and enflurane. Gas anesthetics are combined with oxygen and administered by inhalation. Examples of gas anesthetics are nitrous oxide and cyclopropane.

Drugs Used for General Anesthesia

Barbiturates and Similar Agents

Methohexital (Brevital), which is an ultrashort-acting barbiturate, is used for the following:

- Induction of anesthesia
- Short surgical procedures with minimal painful stimuli
- In conjunction with or as a supplement to other anesthetics

These types of drugs have a rapid onset and a short duration of action. They depress the CNS to produce hypnosis and anesthesia but do not produce analgesia. Recovery after a small dose is rapid.

Etomidate (Amidate), a nonbarbiturate, is used for induction of anesthesia. Etomidate also may be used to supplement other anesthetics, such as nitrous oxide, for short surgical procedures. It is a hypnotic without analgesic activity.

Propofol (Diprivan) is used for induction and maintenance of anesthesia. It also may be used for sedation during diagnostic procedures and procedures that use a local anesthetic. This drug also is used for continuous sedation of intubated or respiratory-controlled patients in intensive care units.

Benzodiazepines

Midazolam, a short-acting benzodiazepine CNS depressant, is used as a preanesthetic drug to relieve anxiety; for induction of anesthesia; for conscious sedation before minor procedures, such as endoscopy; and to supplement nitrous oxide and oxygen for short surgical procedures. When the drug is used for induction anesthesia, the patient gradually loses consciousness over a period of 1 to 2 minutes.

Ketamine

Ketamine (Ketalar) is a rapid-acting general anesthetic. It produces an anesthetic state characterized by profound analgesia, cardiovascular and respiratory stimulation, normal or enhanced skeletal muscle tone, and occasionally mild respiratory depression. Ketamine is used for diagnostic and surgical procedures that do not require relaxation of skeletal muscles, for induction of anesthesia before the administration of other anesthetic drugs, and as a supplement to other anesthetic drugs.

Gases and Volatile Liquids

Nitrous oxide is the most commonly used anesthetic gas. It is a weak anesthetic and is usually used in combination with other anesthetic drugs. It does not cause skeletal muscle relaxation. The chief danger in the use of nitrous oxide is

Anesthetic Drugs

hypoxemia. Nitrous oxide is nonexplosive and is supplied in blue cylinders (oxygen tanks are green).

Enflurane (Ethrane) is a volatile liquid anesthetic that is delivered by inhalation. Induction and recovery from anesthesia are rapid. Muscle relaxation for abdominal surgery is adequate, but greater relaxation may be necessary and may require the use of a skeletal muscle relaxant. Enflurane may produce mild stimulation of respiratory and bronchial secretions when used alone. Hypotension may occur when anesthesia deepens.

Halothane (Fluothane) is a volatile liquid given by inhalation for induction and maintenance of anesthesia. Induction and recovery from anesthesia are rapid, and the depth of anesthesia can be rapidly altered. Halothane does not irritate the respiratory tract, and an increase in tracheobronchial secretions usually does not occur. Halothane produces moderate muscle relaxation, but skeletal muscle relaxants may be used in certain types of surgeries. This anesthetic may be given with a mixture of nitrous oxide and oxygen.

Isoflurane (Forane) is a volatile liquid given by inhalation. It is used for induction and maintenance of anesthesia.

Methoxyflurane (Penthrane), a volatile liquid, provides analgesia and anesthesia. It is usually used with nitrous oxide but may also be used alone. Methoxyflurane does not produce good muscle relaxation, and a skeletal muscle relaxant may be required.

Desflurane (Suprane), a volatile liquid, is used for induction and maintenance of anesthesia. A special vaporizer is used to deliver this anesthetic, because delivery by mask results in irritation of the respiratory tract.

Sevoflurane (Ultane) is an inhalational analgesic. It is used for induction and maintenance of general anesthesia in adult and pediatric patients for both inpatient and outpatient surgical procedures.

Opioids

The opioid analgesic fentanyl (Sublimaze) and the neuroleptic drug (major tranquilizer) droperidol (Inapsine) may be used together as a single drug called Innovar. The combination of these two drugs results in **neuroleptanalgesia**, which is characterized by general quietness, reduced motor activity, and profound analgesia. Complete loss of consciousness may not occur unless other anesthetic drugs are used. A combination of fentanyl and droperidol may be used for the tranquilizing effect and analgesia for surgical and diagnostic procedures. It may also be used as a preanesthetic for the induction of anesthesia and in the maintenance of general anesthesia.

The use of droperidol as a tranquilizer, as an antiemetic to reduce nausea and vomiting during the immediate postanesthesia period, as an induction drug, and as an adjunct to general anesthesia has decreased because of its association with fatal cardiac arrhythmias. Fentanyl may be used alone as a supplement to general or regional anesthesia. It may also be administered alone or with other drugs as a preoperative drug and as an analgesic during the immediate postoperative period.

Remifentanil (Ultiva) is used for induction and maintenance of general anesthesia and for continued analgesia

Table 18.3	Examples of Muscle Relaxants Used During General Anesthesia	
Generic Name	**Trade Name**
atracurium	Tracrium
cisatracurium	Nimbex
doxacurium	Nuromax
mivacurium	Mivacron
pancuronium	Pavulon
succinylcholine	Anectine

during the immediate postoperative period. This drug is used cautiously in patients with a history of hypersensitivity to fentanyl.

Skeletal Muscle Relaxants

The various skeletal muscle relaxants that may be used during general anesthesia are listed in Table 18.3. These drugs are administered to produce relaxation of the skeletal muscles during certain types of surgeries, such as those involving the chest or abdomen. They may also be used to facilitate the insertion of an endotracheal tube. Their onset of action is usually rapid (45 seconds to a few minutes), and their duration of action is 30 minutes or more.

Stages of General Anesthesia

General surgical anesthesia is divided into the following stages:

- Stage I—analgesia
- Stage II—delirium
- Stage III—surgical analgesia
- Stage IV—respiratory paralysis

Display 18.1 describes the stages of general anesthesia more completely. With newer drugs and techniques, the stages of anesthesia may not be as prominent as those described in Display 18.1. In addition, movement through the first two stages is usually very rapid.

Anesthesia begins with a loss of consciousness. This is part of the induction phase (stage I). The patient is now relaxed and can no longer comprehend what is happening. After consciousness is lost, additional anesthetic drugs are administered. Some of these drugs are also used as part of the induction phase, as well as for deepening anesthesia. Depending on the type of surgery, an endotracheal tube also may be inserted to provide an adequate airway and to assist in administering oxygen and other anesthetic drugs. The endotracheal tube is removed during the postanesthesia period once the gag and swallowing reflexes have resumed. If an IV line was not inserted before the patient's arrival in surgery, it is inserted by the anesthesiologist before the administration of an induction drug.

DISPLAY 18.1 Stages of General Anesthesia

Stage I
Induction is a part of stage I anesthesia. It begins with the administration of an anesthetic drug and lasts until consciousness is lost. With some induction drugs, such as the short-acting barbiturates, this stage may last only 5 to 10 seconds.

Stage II
Stage II is the stage of delirium and excitement. This stage is also brief. During this stage, the patient may move about and mumble incoherently. The muscles are somewhat rigid, and the patient is unconscious and cannot feel pain. During this stage, noises are exaggerated and even quiet sounds may seem extremely loud to the patient. If surgery were attempted at this stage, there would be a physical reaction to painful stimuli, yet the patient would not remember sensing pain. During these first two stages of anesthesia, the nurse and other health care professionals avoid any unnecessary noise or motion.

Stage III
Stage III is the stage of surgical analgesia and is divided into four parts, planes, or substages. The anesthesiologist differentiates these planes by the character of the respirations, eye movements, certain reflexes, pupil size, and other factors. The levels of the planes range from plane 1 (light) to plane 4 (deep). At plane 2 or 3, the patient is usually ready for the surgical procedure.

Stage IV
Stage IV is the stage of respiratory paralysis and is a rare and dangerous stage of anesthesia. At this stage, respiratory arrest and cessation of all vital signs may occur.

Nursing Responsibilities

Preanesthesia

Before surgery, and during the administration of general anesthesia, the nurse has the following responsibilities:

- Performing the required tasks and procedures as prescribed by the physician and hospital policy before surgery and recording these tasks on the patient's chart. Examples of these tasks include administering a hypnotic agent before surgery, shaving the operative area, taking vital signs, seeing that the operative consent form is signed, checking that all jewelry or metal objects are removed from the patient, administering enemas, inserting a catheter, inserting a nasogastric tube, and teaching.
- Checking the chart for any recent abnormal laboratory test results. If a recent abnormal laboratory test finding was included in the patient's chart shortly before surgery, the nurse must make sure that the surgeon and the anesthesiologist are aware of the abnormality. The nurse attaches a note to the front of the chart and may also contact the surgeon or anesthesiologist by telephone.
- Placing a list of known or suspected drug allergies or idiosyncrasies on the front of the chart.
- Administering the preanesthetic (preoperative) drug.
- Instructing the patient to remain in bed and placing the bed's side rails up once the preanesthetic drug has been given.

Preanesthetic drugs must be administered on time to produce their intended effects. Failure to give the preanesthetic drug on time may result in such events as increased respiratory secretions caused by the irritating effect of anesthetic gases and the need for an increased dose of the induction drug because the preanesthetic drug has not had time to sedate the patient.

Postanesthesia: Post-Anesthesia Care Unit

After surgery, the nurse has the following responsibilities, which vary according to where the nurse first sees the postoperative patient:

- Admitting the patient to the unit according to hospital procedure or policy.
- Checking the airway for patency, assessing the respiratory status, and giving oxygen as needed.
- Positioning the patient to prevent aspiration of vomitus and secretions.
- Checking blood pressure and pulse, IV lines, catheters, drainage tubes, surgical dressings, and casts.
- Reviewing the patient's surgical and anesthesia records.
- Monitoring the blood pressure, pulse, and respiratory rate every 5 to 15 minutes until the patient is discharged from the area.
- Checking the patient every 5 to 15 minutes for emergence from anesthesia. Suctioning is provided as needed.
- Exercising caution in administering opioids. The nurse must check the patient's respiratory rate, blood pressure, and pulse before these drugs are given and 20 to 30 minutes after administration (see Chapter 17). The physician is contacted if the respiratory rate is below 10 breaths/min before the drug is given or if the respiratory rate falls below 10 breaths/min after the drug is given.
- Discharging the patient from the area to his or her room or other specified area. The nurse must record all drugs administered and nursing tasks performed before the patient leaves the PACU.

THINK CRITICALLY: PHARMACOLOGY IN PRACTICE

1. A nurse with whom you are working complains she was reprimanded and asked to fill out an incident report for not giving a preanesthetic drug on time. She states that she is being unfairly accused of an error because the drug was given 10 minutes before the patient was taken to surgery. Explain why this is a potentially serious error.

● Test Your Knowledge

1. When planning preoperative care, the nurse expects that a preanesthetic medication is given _____ before the patient is transported to surgery.

   A. 20 minutes
   B. 30 minutes
   C. 40 minutes
   D. 60 minutes

Anesthetic Drugs

2. Which of the following drugs is the most commonly used gas for general anesthesia?

    A. Ethylene
    B. Enflurane
    C. Nitrous oxide
    D. Sevoflurane

3. Neuroleptanalgesia is used to promote general quietness, reduce motor activity, and induce profound analgesia. Which of the following two drugs are used in combination to accomplish neuroleptanalgesia?

    A. Fentanyl and droperidol
    B. Morphine and glycopyrrolate
    C. Atropine and meperidine
    D. Fentanyl and midazolam

4. One use of skeletal muscle relaxants as part of general anesthesia is to:

    A. prevent movement during surgery
    B. facilitate insertion of the endotracheal tube
    C. allow for deeper anesthesia
    D. produce additional anesthesia

● Calculate Medication Dosages

1. As a preoperative medication for a patient going to surgery, the anesthesiologist prescribes meperidine (Demerol) 50 mg IM. Meperidine is available in solution of 50 mg/mL. The nurse prepares to administer _____.

2. Glycopyrrolate (Robinul) is prescribed for a patient as part of the preoperative preparation for surgery. The drug dose recommendation is 0.002 mg/lb. The patient weighs 150 lb. The nurse expects the primary care provider to prescribe _____.

To check your answers, see Appendix E.

the**Point**. *For more NCLEX questions, log on to http://thepoint.lww.com to access more than 1000 questions.*

Drugs That Affect the Central Nervous System

The nervous system is a complex part of the human body concerned with the regulation and coordination of body activities such as movement, behavior, digestion, and sleep. The nervous system has two main divisions: the central nervous system (CNS) and the peripheral nervous system (PNS). The CNS consists of the brain and the spinal cord. The PNS connects all parts of the body with the CNS.

The CNS receives, integrates, and interprets nerve impulses. Drugs that affect the CNS alter mood, sensation, and the interpretation of information in the brain. These drugs are featured in Unit IV.

This unit begins with drugs that stimulate the CNS. Chapter 19 discusses the CNS stimulants used to reverse respiratory depression or to treat children with attention deficit hyperactivity disorder (ADHD). Drugs that have a depressing effect on neurotransmission in the CNS are used to treat anxiety (Chapter 20). The sedative/hypnotic drugs (Chapter 21) are used to treat insomnia or are used to produce a calming effect when patients are about to undergo a surgical or diagnostic procedure.

Drugs that act on the CNS are used to change mood or behavior. These drugs may take many days or even weeks to produce a therapeutic response. Chapter 22 discusses drugs used to treat depression, which is one of the most common mental health disorders. Depression is characterized by impaired functioning and feelings of intense sadness, helplessness, and worthlessness. People experiencing major depressive episodes exhibit physical and psychological symptoms, such as appetite disturbances, sleep disturbances, and loss of interest in job, family, and other activities usually enjoyed.

A psychotic disorder is characterized by extreme personality disorganization and the loss of contact with reality. Drugs given to patients with a psychotic disorder, such as schizophrenia, are called *antipsychotic drugs* or *neuroleptics*. The antipsychotic drugs are discussed in Chapter 23.

PHARMACOLOGY IN PRACTICE

Our patient focus in this unit is Mr. Phillip, a 72-year-old man with both diabetes and early-stage chronic kidney disease. His own medical problems are compounded by the fact that his wife of 47 years has recently died. His children do not live close by; therefore, in addition to managing his own health care issues, he must learn to live alone and manage a household. After reading the chapters in this unit, you will be asked to evaluate his inability to sleep, enjoy daily activities, and deal with his loss issues. Additionally, we will examine the impact when two drugs have the potential to compound adverse reactions.

Central Nervous System Stimulants

analeptics
anorexiants

attention deficit
 hyperactivity disorder
narcolepsy

LEARNING OBJECTIVES

On completion of this chapter, the student will:

1. List the three types of central nervous system (CNS) stimulants.
2. Discuss the uses, general drug actions, general adverse reactions, contraindications, precautions, and interactions of the CNS stimulants.
3. Discuss important preadministration and ongoing assessment activities the nurse should perform on the patient taking a CNS stimulant.
4. List nursing diagnoses particular to a patient taking a CNS stimulant.
5. Discuss ways to promote an optimal response to drug therapy, how to manage common adverse drug reactions, and important points to keep in mind when educating patients about the use of CNS stimulants.

This chapter discusses the drugs that stimulate the central nervous system (CNS) and the nursing implications related to their administration. The CNS stimulants include the **analeptics**, drugs that stimulate the respiratory center of the brain and cardiovascular system; the amphetamines, used to treat children with **attention deficit hyperactivity disorder** (ADHD). Drugs being developed for the treatment of children include fewer amphetamines because of their high abuse potential and their ability to produce euphoria and wakefulness. The drug class of **anorexiants**, drugs used to suppress the appetite, is also covered in this chapter.

Actions

Analeptics increase the depth of respirations by stimulating special receptors located in the carotid arteries and upper aorta. These special receptors (called *chemoreceptors*) are sensitive to the amount of oxygen in arterial blood.

Stimulation of these receptors results in an increase in the depth of respirations. In larger doses, drugs like doxapram (Dopram) increase the respiratory rate by stimulating the medulla.

One of the most widely used CNS stimulants is caffeine. It is a mild-to-potent analeptic CNS stimulant. The degree of its stimulating effect depends on the dose administered. Caffeine stimulates the CNS at all levels, including the cerebral cortex, the medulla, and the spinal cord. Caffeine has mild analeptic (respiratory-stimulating) activity. Other actions include cardiac stimulation (which may produce tachycardia), dilation of coronary and peripheral blood vessels, constriction of cerebral blood vessels, and skeletal muscle stimulation. Caffeine also has mild diuretic activity. People take caffeine on their own in the form of coffee, tea, or even chocolate, yet caffeine's use as a therapeutic drug for stimulation in the neonatal setting is growing.

Modafinil (Provigil), another analeptic, is used to treat **narcolepsy** (a disorder that causes an uncontrollable desire to sleep during normal waking hours even though the individual has a normal nighttime sleeping pattern). The exact mechanism of action is not known, but the drug is thought to bind to dopamine, thereby reducing the number of episodes. It does not cause cardiac and other systemic stimulatory effects like other CNS stimulants.

The amphetamines are sympathomimetic (i.e., adrenergic) drugs that stimulate the CNS (see Chapter 24). Their drug action results in an elevation of blood pressure, wakefulness, and an increase or decrease in pulse rate. Amphetamines also produce a euphoric state that increases their dependency potential, making their prescription less frequent.

One condition successfully treated by amphetamines is ADHD in children. ADHD is a condition of both children and adults and is characterized by inattention, hyperactivity, and impulsivity. Symptoms appear early in a child's life. Because these behaviors, when independently present, can be normal in any individual, it is important that the child receive a thorough examination and appropriate diagnosis by a well-qualified professional before drug therapy is initiated. How amphetamines, which are CNS stimulants, work on ADHD is unknown.

The anorexiants are nonamphetamine drugs pharmacologically similar to the amphetamines. Their ability to suppress the appetite is thought to be due to their action on the appetite center in the hypothalamus.

Summary Drug Table — CENTRAL NERVOUS SYSTEM STIMULANTS

Generic Name	Trade Name	Uses	Adverse Reactions	Dosage Ranges
Analeptics				
armodafinil ar-moe-daf'-ih-nil	Nuvigil	Narcolepsy, obstructive sleep apnea, sleepiness due to shift work	Headache, nausea, insomnia	150–250 mg/day orally in a single morning dose
caffeine kah-feen'	Cafcit, Stay Awake, Vivarin	Fatigue, drowsiness, as adjunct in analgesic formulation, respiratory depression	Palpitations, nausea, vomiting, insomnia, tachycardia, restlessness	100–200 mg orally q 3–4 hr Respiratory depression: 500 mg/1 g IM, IV
doxapram dox'-ah-pram	Dopram	Respiratory depression: postanesthesia, drug-induced, acute respiratory insufficiency superimposed on COPD	Dizziness, headache, apprehension, disorientation, nausea, cough, dyspnea, urinary retention	0.5–1 mg/kg IV
modafinil moe-daf'-in-ill	Provigil	Narcolepsy, obstructive sleep apnea	Headache, nausea	200–400 mg/day orally
Amphetamines				
amphetamine am-fet'-ah-meen		Narcolepsy, ADHD, exogenous obesity	Insomnia, nervousness, headache, tachycardia, anorexia, dizziness, excitement	Narcolepsy: 5–60 mg/day orally in divided doses ADHD: 5 mg BID, increase by 10 mg/wk until desired effect
amphetamine/ dextroamphetamine	Adderall	Narcolepsy, ADHD	Same as amphetamine	Same as amphetamine
dexmethylphenidate dex-meh-thill-fen'-ih-date	Focalin	ADHD	Nervousness, insomnia, loss of appetite, abdominal pain, weight loss, tachycardia, skin rash	2.5 mg orally BID; maximum dosage, 20 mg/day
dextroamphetamine dex-troe-am-fet'-ah-meen	Dexedrine, DextroStat	Narcolepsy, ADHD	Same as amphetamine	Narcolepsy: 5–60 mg/day orally in divided doses ADHD: up to 40 mg/day orally
lisdexamfetamine lis-dex'-am-fet-ah-meen	Vyvanse	ADHD	Same as amphetamine	30–70 mg/day orally in one morning dose
methamphetamine meth-am-fet'-ah-meen	Desoxyn	ADHD, exogenous obesity	Same as amphetamine	ADHD: Up to 25 mg/day orally Obesity: 5 mg orally 30 min before meals
methylphenidate meh-thill-fen'-ih-date	Concerta, Metadate, Ritalin, Methylin, Daytrana (transdermal patch)	ADHD, narcolepsy	Insomnia, anorexia, dizziness, headache, abdominal pain	5–60 mg/day orally
Anorexiants				
benzphetamine benz-fet'-ah-meen	Didrex	Obesity	Insomnia, nervousness, headache, dry mouth, palpitations, tachycardia, dizziness, excitement	25–50 mg orally 1–3 times/day
diethylpropion dye-eth'-ill-proe-pee-on	Tenuate, Tenuate Dospan	Obesity	Same as benzphetamine	Immediate release: 25 mg orally TID Sustained release: 75 mg once daily

Short term use

(table continues on page 175)

Summary Drug Table CENTRAL NERVOUS SYSTEM STIMULANTS (continued)

Generic Name	Trade Name	Uses	Adverse Reactions	Dosage Ranges
phendimetrazine	Bontril	Obesity	Same as benzphetamine	35 mg orally 2–3 times/day
phentermine *fen-ter'-meen*	Ionamin, Adipex-P	Obesity	Same as benzphetamine	8 mg orally TID or 15–37.5 mg orally as a single daily dose
sibutramine *sih-byoo'-trah-meen*	Meridia	Obesity	Insomnia, headache, dry mouth, constipation, rhinitis, pharyngitis	5–15 mg orally once daily
Miscellaneous Drugs				
atomoxetine *at'-oh-mox-eh-teen*	Strattera	ADHD (acts like antidepressant rather than stimulant)	Headache, decreased appetite, abdominal pain, vomiting, cough	Initial dose: 40 mg/day orally, may increase up to 100 mg/day orally
sodium oxybate *ox'-ih-bate*	Xyrem	Narcolepsy, excessive daytime sleepiness	Headache, dizziness, somnolence	4.5–9 g/ night taken in 2 doses at least 2 1/2 hrs apart

Uses

The CNS stimulants are used in the treatment of the following:

- ADHD
- Drug-induced respiratory depression
- Postanesthesia respiratory depression, without reduction of analgesia
- Narcolepsy
- Sleep apnea
- Exogenous obesity
- Fatigue (caffeine)

Adverse Reactions

Neuromuscular System Reactions

- Excessive CNS stimulation, headache, dizziness
- Apprehension, disorientation, and hyperactivity

Other Reactions

- Nausea, vomiting, cough, dyspnea
- Urinary retention, tachycardia, and palpitations

For more information on adverse reactions, see the Summary Drug Table: Central Nervous System Stimulants.

Contraindications

The CNS stimulants are contraindicated in patients with known hypersensitivity or convulsive disorders, and in those with ventilation disorders (e.g., chronic obstructive pulmonary disease [COPD]). The nurse should not administer CNS stimulants to patients with cardiac problems, severe hypertension, or hyperthyroidism. CNS stimulants are not recommended as treatment for depression. Amphetamines and anorexiants should not be taken concurrently or within 14 days of antidepressant medications. In addition, amphetamines are contraindicated in patients with glaucoma. Most anorexiants are classified as pregnancy category X and should not be used during pregnancy. Although sibutramine and armodafinil are pregnancy category C drugs, safety has not been proven.

⬛ NURSING ALERT

Amphetamines and anorexiants have abuse and addiction potential. These drugs are recommended only for short-term use in selected patients for treatment of obesity. Long-term use of amphetamines for obesity may result in tolerance to the drug and a tendency to increase the dose. Extreme psychological dependency may also occur.

Precautions

The CNS stimulants should be used cautiously in patients with respiratory illness, renal or hepatic impairment, and history of substance abuse. The CNS stimulants should be used cautiously in pregnant or lactating women.

Interactions

The following interactions may occur when a CNS stimulant is administered with another agent:

Interacting Drug	Common Use
anesthetics	Anesthesia during surgical procedures
theophylline	Respiratory problems, such as asthma
oral contraceptives	Birth control

Central Nervous System Stimulants

NURSING PROCESS
PATIENT RECEIVING A CENTRAL NERVOUS SYSTEM STIMULANT

ASSESSMENT

Assessment of the patient receiving a CNS stimulant depends on the drug, the patient, and the reason for administration.

Preadministration Assessment
RESPIRATORY DEPRESSION. When a CNS stimulant is prescribed for respiratory depression, initial patient assessments include the blood pressure, pulse, and respiratory rate. It is important to note the depth of the respirations and any pattern to the respiratory rate, such as shallow respirations or alternating deep and shallow respirations. The nurse reviews recent laboratory test results (if any), such as arterial blood gas studies. It is important to review the chart to identify the drugs given that caused the respiratory depression.

ATTENTION DEFICIT HYPERACTIVITY DISORDER. When an amphetamine is prescribed for any reason, the nurse weighs the patient and takes the blood pressure, pulse, and respiratory rate before starting drug therapy. The nurse should initially observe the child with ADHD for the various patterns of abnormal behavior. The nurse records a summary of the behavior pattern in the patient's chart to provide a comparison with future changes that may occur during therapy. If the child is hospitalized, the nurse enters a daily summary of the child's behavior in the patient's record. This provides a record of the results of therapy.

LIFESPAN ALERT – Pediatric
An increased risk of suicidal ideation in children and adolescents has been found when using the drug atomoxetine (Strattera). Patients with ADHD started on atomoxetine should be monitored carefully for suicidal thoughts or behaviors. The nurse should teach the family about specific behaviors to observe for that would indicate a need to contact the primary health care provider.

OBESITY. When an anorexiant or amphetamine is used as part of obesity treatment, the drug is usually prescribed for outpatient use. The nurse obtains and records the blood pressure, pulse, respiratory rate, and weight before therapy is started and at each outpatient visit.

Ongoing Assessment
RESPIRATORY DEPRESSION. After administering an analeptic, the nurse carefully monitors the patient's respiratory rate and pattern until the respirations return to normal. The nurse also monitors the level of consciousness, the blood pressure, and pulse rate at 5- to 15-minute intervals or as ordered by the primary health care provider. The nurse may draw blood for arterial blood gas analysis

at intervals to determine the effectiveness of the analeptic, as well as the need for additional drug therapy. It is important to observe the patient for adverse drug reactions and to report their occurrence immediately to the primary health care provider.

NURSING DIAGNOSES

Drug-specific nursing diagnoses are the following:

- ❏ **Disturbed Sleep Pattern** related to CNS stimulation and hyperactivity, nervousness, insomnia, other (specify)
- ❏ **Ineffective Breathing Pattern** related to respiratory depression
- ❏ **Imbalanced Nutrition: Less Than Body Requirements** related to diminished appetite

Nursing diagnoses related to drug administration are discussed in Chapter 4.

PLANNING

The expected outcomes for the patient depend on the reason for administration of a CNS stimulant, but may include an optimal response to therapy, support of patient needs related to management of adverse drug reactions, and an understanding of the therapeutic regimen.

IMPLEMENTATION

Promoting an Optimal Response to Therapy
Amphetamines may be used in the short-term treatment of exogenous obesity (obesity caused by a persistent calorie intake that is greater than needed by the body). However, their use in treating exogenous obesity has declined, because the long-term use of the amphetamines for obesity carries the potential for dependence and abuse.

Monitoring and Managing Patient Needs
DISTURBED SLEEP PATTERN. When CNS stimulant therapy causes insomnia, the nurse administers the drug early in the day (when possible) to diminish sleep disturbances. The patient is provided with distracting activities and encouraged not to nap during the day.

Other stimulants, such as coffee, tea, or cola drinks, are avoided. In some patients, nervousness, restlessness, and palpitations may occur. The vital signs are checked every 6 to 8 hours or more often if tachycardia, hypertension, or palpitations occur. The adverse drug reactions that may occur with amphetamine use may be serious enough to require discontinuation of the drug. In some instances, the adverse drug effects are mild and may even disappear during therapy. In many cases, these adverse reactions diminish with continued use as physical tolerance develops. The nurse informs the primary care provider of all adverse reactions. If tolerance does develop, the dosage is not increased.

LABS - ABGs - gives bicarbs ↑ CO_2

Central Nervous System Stimulants

LIFESPAN ALERT – Gerontology

Older adults are especially sensitive to the effects of the CNS stimulants and may exhibit excessive anxiety, nervousness, insomnia, and mental confusion. Cardiovascular disorders, common in the older adult, may be worsened by the CNS stimulants. Careful monitoring is important because these reactions may result in the need to discontinue use of the drug. *nutrition, confusion, sleep, toxicity, tachycardia*

These drugs may also be helpful in managing narcolepsy, a disorder manifested by an uncontrollable desire to sleep during normal waking hours even though the individual has a normal nighttime sleeping pattern. The individual with narcolepsy may fall asleep from a few minutes to a few hours many times in one day. The disorder begins in adolescence or young adulthood and persists throughout life.

INEFFECTIVE BREATHING PATTERN. Respiratory depression can be a serious event requiring administration of a respiratory stimulant. When an analeptic drug is administered, the nurse notes and records the rate, depth, and character of the respirations before the drug is given. This provides a baseline for evaluating the effectiveness of drug therapy. Also before administering the drug, the nurse ensures that the patient has a patent airway. Oxygen is usually administered before, during, and after drug administration. After administration, the nurse monitors respirations closely and records the effects of therapy.

When respiratory depression occurs in the postsurgical setting, the nurse should assess carefully the patient's level of pain. Respiratory depression can occur after a surgical procedure from the combination of drugs used to produce anesthesia. Opioid reversal drugs, such as naloxone (Narcan), that reverse the effects of opioid agents replace the pain relief drug at the receptor site of the cell. This means that the patient can experience a sudden and severe return of pain because the pain relief effect of the drug is eliminated along with the reversal of respiratory depression. Use of analeptic drugs for respiratory stimulation can enhance the breathing pattern without changing the effect of the opioid drug. Therefore, breathing improves and pain relief continues for the patient.

Nausea and vomiting may occur with the administration of an analeptic; therefore, the nurse should keep a suction machine nearby in case the patient vomits. Urinary retention may result from doxapram administration; therefore, the nurse measures intake and output and notifies the primary health care provider if the patient cannot void or the bladder appears to be distended on palpation.

IMBALANCED NUTRITION: LESS THAN BODY REQUIREMENTS. One of the adverse reactions to the use of CNS stimulants for the child with ADHD is decreased appetite. Although decreased appetite is a desired effect when treating a patient with weight problems, it is not desirable when treating ADHD. Long-term treatment with the CNS stim-

ulants is also thought to retard growth in children. Therefore it is important to monitor weight and growth patterns of children on long-term treatment with the CNS stimulant drugs.

The nurse instructs parents to monitor the eating patterns of the child while he or she is taking CNS stimulants. Parents should be taught to prepare nutritious meals and snacks. A good breakfast is important to provide, because the child in school may not feel hungry at lunch time. The child should be checked frequently with height and weight measurements to monitor growth. When a CNS stimulant, such as dextroamphetamine, is administered to treat a child with ADHD, the drug regimen may be interrupted periodically under direction of the primary health provider to evaluate the effectiveness of drug management.

Educating the Patient and Family

The nurse explains the therapeutic regimen and adverse drug reactions to the patient and family. The type of information included in the teaching plan depends on the drug and the reason for its use. It is important to emphasize the need to follow the recommended dosage schedule. The nurse may include the following additional teaching points:

infl. sleep appetite

- ADHD: Give the drug in the morning 30 to 45 minutes before breakfast and before lunch. Do not give the drug in the late afternoon. Keep a journal of the child's behavior, including the general pattern of behavior, socialization with others, and attention span. Bring this record to each primary health care provider or clinic visit, because this record may help the primary health care provider determine future drug dosages or additional treatment modalities. The primary health care provider may prescribe drug therapy only on school days, when high levels of attention and performance are necessary.
- Narcolepsy: Keep a record of the number of times per day that periods of sleepiness occur, and bring this record to each visit to the primary health care provider or clinic.
- Amphetamines and anorexiants: These drugs are taken early in the day to avoid insomnia. Do not increase the dose or take the drug more frequently, except on the advice of the primary health care provider. These drugs may impair the ability to drive or perform hazardous tasks and may mask extreme fatigue. If dizziness, lightheadedness, anxiety, nervousness, or tremors occur, contact the primary care provider. Avoid or decrease the use of coffee, tea, and carbonated beverages containing caffeine (see Patient Teaching for Improved Patient Outcomes: Using Anorexiants for Weight Loss).
- Caffeine (oral, nonprescription): Over-the-counter caffeine preparations should be avoided if the individual has a history of heart disease, high blood pressure, or stomach ulcers. These products are intended for occa-

sional use and should not be used if heart palpitations, dizziness, or lightheadedness occur.

EVALUATION

- Therapeutic response is achieved and respiratory depression is reversed; the child's behavior and school performance are improved; or the desired weight loss is achieved.
- Adverse reactions are identified, reported to the primary health care provider, and managed successfully with appropriate nursing interventions:
  - ☑ Patient reports fewer episodes of inappropriate sleep patterns.
  - ☑ Breathing pattern is maintained.
  - ☑ Patient maintains an adequate nutritional status.
- Patient and family demonstrate an understanding of the drug regimen.

Patient Teaching for Improved Patient Outcomes

Using Anorexiants for Weight Loss

The nurse:
- ✓ Reviews reasons for the drug and prescribed drug regimen, including drug name, dosage, and frequency of administration.
- ✓ Stresses the importance of taking the drug exactly as prescribed, including not to increase the dose or take more frequently unless instructed to do so by the prescriber.
- ✓ Reinforces use of drug for short-term therapy only.
- ✓ Warns about possible abuse, drug tolerance, and psychological dependency.
- ✓ Reviews possible adverse reactions, especially CNS overstimulation, with instructions to notify the health care provider immediately should any occur.
- ✓ Instructs to take drug early in the day to minimize insomnia.
- ✓ Cautions about safety measures because of possible impairment in ability to drive or perform hazardous tasks.
- ✓ Advises to avoid other stimulants, including those containing caffeine such as coffee, tea, and cola drinks; provides a written list of foods to avoid.
- ✓ Urges to read labels of foods and nonprescription drugs for possible stimulant content.
- ✓ Reinforces prescribed dietary and exercise program for weight reduction, both verbally and in writing.
- ✓ Reassures that results of therapy will be monitored by continued follow-up visits with health care provider.
- ✓ Arranges for follow-up visits as necessary.

THINK CRITICALLY: PHARMACOLOGY IN PRACTICE

1. Mrs. Chase is given a special diet and prescribed an anorexiant to help her lose 20 lb before she has reconstructive knee surgery. Determine what instructions you would include in a teaching plan for this patient.

● Test Your Knowledge

1. Initial assessment of the child with ADHD includes _____.

    A. assessing to which stimuli the child responds the most
    B. determining the child's intelligence
    C. obtaining a summary of the child's behavior pattern
    D. obtaining vital signs

2. When assessing the patient receiving doxapram for chronic pulmonary disease, the nurse observes the patient for adverse drug reactions, which may include _____.

    A. headache, dizziness, variations in heart rate
    B. diarrhea, drowsiness, hypotension
    C. decreased respiratory rate, weight gain, bradycardia
    D. fever, dysuria, constipation

3. When teaching a patient with narcolepsy who is receiving an amphetamine, the nurse instructs the patient to _____.

    A. record the times of the day the medication is taken
    B. take the medication at bedtime as well as in the morning
    C. take the drug with meals
    D. keep a record of how often periods of sleepiness occur

4. When administering an amphetamine, the nurse first checks to see if the patient is taking or has taken a monoamine oxidase inhibitor (MAOI) because _____.

    A. a lower dosage of the amphetamine may be needed
    B. a higher dosage of the amphetamine may be needed
    C. the amphetamine can be substituted as the antidepressant drug
    D. the amphetamine is not given within 14 days of the MAOI

● Prepare for the NCLEX

1. A child with ADHD is admitted to the pediatric unit for a fractured tibia. Dexmethylphenidate is prescribed 7.5 mg BID; when should these doses be given?

    A. 7 AM and 11 AM
    B. 7 AM and 5 PM
    C. 9 AM and 5 PM
    D. 9 AM and 9 PM

● Calculate Medication Dosages

1. Phentermine hydrochloride 8 mg three times a day orally is prescribed as an adjunct for weight loss. The total amount of drug the patient will receive daily is _____. Is this an appropriate dose for this drug?

2. Modafinil 400 mg is prescribed. The drug is available in 200-mg tablets. The nurse administers _____.

To check your answers, see Appendix E.

the**Point** *For more NCLEX questions, log on to http://thepoint.lww.com to access more than 1000 questions.*

Antianxiety Drugs

LEARNING OBJECTIVES

On completion of this chapter, the student will:

1. Discuss the uses, general drug actions, general adverse reactions, contraindications, precautions, and interactions associated with the administration of the antianxiety drugs.
2. Discuss important preadministration and ongoing assessment activities the nurse should perform on the patient taking antianxiety drugs.
3. List nursing diagnoses particular to a patient taking antianxiety drugs.
4. Discuss ways to promote an optimal response to therapy, how to manage common adverse reactions, and important points to keep in mind when educating patients about the use of antianxiety drugs.

Anxiety is a feeling of apprehension, worry, or uneasiness that may or may not be based on reality. Anxiety may be seen in many types of situations, ranging from the "jitters" and excitement of a new job to the acute panic that may be seen during withdrawal from alcohol. Although a certain amount of anxiety is normal, excess anxiety interferes with day-to-day functioning and can cause undue stress in the lives of some individuals. Drugs used to treat anxiety are called *antianxiety drugs*. Another term that refers to the antianxiety drugs is **anxiolytics**.

Antianxiety drugs include the benzodiazepines and the nonbenzodiazepines. Examples of the benzodiazepines include alprazolam (Xanax), chlordiazepoxide (Librium), diazepam (Valium), and lorazepam (Ativan). Long-term use of benzodiazepines can result in **physical** or **psychological dependence**. Therefore, these drugs are classified as schedule IV in the Controlled Substances Act by the Drug Enforcement Agency (DEA) regulations (see Chapter 1). Nonbenzodiazepines useful as antianxiety drugs include buspirone (BuSpar), doxepin (Sinequan), and hydroxyzine (Atarax).

Actions

Anxiolytic drugs exert their tranquilizing effect by blocking certain neurotransmitter receptor sites. In turn, this prevents the neurotransmission of the anxious perception and the body's physical reaction to the anxiety. Benzodiazepines exert their tranquilizing effect by potentiating the effects of gamma-aminobutyric acid (GABA), an inhibitory transmitter. Nonbenzodiazepines exert their action in various ways. For example, buspirone is thought to act on the brain's serotonin receptors. Hydroxyzine (Atarax or Vistaril) produces its antianxiety effect by acting on the hypothalamus and brainstem reticular formation.

Uses

Antianxiety drugs are used in the management of the following:

• Anxiety disorders and panic attacks
• Preanesthetic sedation and muscle relaxation
• Convulsions or seizures
• Alcohol withdrawal

Adverse Reactions

Frequent, early reactions include:

• Mild drowsiness or sedation
• Lightheadedness or dizziness
• Headache

Other adverse body system reactions include:

• Lethargy, apathy, fatigue
• Disorientation
• Anger
• Restlessness
• Nausea, constipation or diarrhea, dry mouth
• Visual disturbances

See the Summary Drug Table: Antianxiety Drugs for more information.

Dependence

Long-term use of antianxiety drugs may result in physical dependence and **tolerance** (increasingly larger dosages required to obtain the desired effect). Withdrawal symptoms

Sch 4 (handwritten)

Summary Drug Table ANTIANXIETY DRUGS

CNS depression, hard to wake up, anger (handwritten)

Generic name	Trade Name	Uses	Adverse Reactions	Dosage Ranges
Benzodiazepines				
alprazolam *al-prah'-zoe-lam*	Niravam, Xanax *PRN.T* (handwritten)	Anxiety disorders, short-term relief of anxiety, panic attacks	Transient mild drowsiness, lightheadedness, headache, depression, constipation, diarrhea, dry mouth	0.25–0.5 mg orally TID, may be increased to 4 mg/day in divided doses
chlordiazepoxide *klor-dye-az-eh-pox'-ide*	Librium	Anxiety disorders, short-term relief of anxiety, acute alcohol withdrawal	Same as alprazolam	Anxiety: 5–25 mg orally 3 or 4 times daily Acute alcohol withdrawal: 50–100 mg IM, then 25–50 mg IM
clonazepam *klon-az'-eh-pam*	Klonopin	Panic disorder, anticonvulsant	Same as alprazolam	0.25 mg orally BID
clorazepate *klor-az'-eh-pate*	Tranxene	Anxiety disorders, short-term relief of anxiety, acute alcohol withdrawal, anticonvulsant	Same as alprazolam	Anxiety: 15–60 mg/day orally in divided doses Acute alcohol withdrawal: Up to 90 mg/day with taper-off schedule
diazepam *dye-az'-eh-pam*	Valium	Anxiety disorders, short-term relief of anxiety, acute alcohol withdrawal, anticonvulsant, preoperative muscle relaxant	Same as alprazolam	Individualize dosage: 2–10 mg IM, IV, or orally 2–4 times daily
lorazepam *lor-az'-eh-pam*	Ativan	Anxiety disorders, short-term relief of anxiety, preanesthetic	Same as alprazolam	1–10 mg/day orally in divided doses; when used as preanesthetic: up to 4 mg IM, IV
oxazepam *ox-az'-eh-pam*		Anxiety disorders, short-term relief of anxiety	Same as alprazolam	10–30 mg orally 3–4 times daily
Nonbenzodiazepines				
buspirone *byoo-spye'-rone*	BuSpar	Anxiety disorders, short-term relief of anxiety	Dizziness, drowsiness	15–60 mg/day orally in divided doses
doxepin *dox'-eh-pin*	Sinequan	Anxiety and depression	Same as buspirone	75–150 mg/day, up to 300 mg/day for those severely ill
hydroxyzine *hye-drox'-ih-zeen*	Atarax, Vistaril	Anxiety and tension associated with psychoneurosis, pruritus, preanesthetic sedative	Dry mouth, transitory drowsiness, involuntary motor activity	25–100 mg orally QID Preanesthetic: 50–100 mg orally or 25–100 mg IM
meprobamate *meh-proe-bah'-mate*		Anxiety disorders, short-term relief of anxiety	Drowsiness, ataxia, nausea, dizziness, slurred speech, headache, weakness, vomiting, diarrhea	1.2–1.6 g/day orally in 3–4 doses, not to exceed 2.4 g/day

have occurred when the drug is stopped after as few as 4 to 6 weeks of therapy with a benzodiazepine.

NURSING ALERT

Symptoms of benzodiazepine withdrawal include increased anxiety, concentration difficulties, tremor, and sensory disturbances, such as paresthesias, photophobia, hypersomnia, and metallic taste.

Typically, withdrawal symptoms are more likely to occur when the benzodiazepine is taken for 3 months or more and

is abruptly discontinued. Therefore, antianxiety drugs must never be discontinued abruptly. Instead, a gradually decreasing dosage schedule (known as *tapering*) should be used when the drug is to be stopped. The onset of withdrawal symptoms usually occurs within 1 to 10 days after discontinuing the drug, with the duration of withdrawal symptoms from 5 days to 1 month. Symptoms of withdrawal are identified in Display 20.1.

Some antianxiety drugs, such as buspirone, are associated with less physical dependence potential and less effect on motor ability and cognition.

Antianxiety Drugs

DISPLAY 20.1 Symptoms of Withdrawal

- Increased anxiety
- Fatigue
- Hypersomnia
- Metallic taste
- Concentration difficulties
- Headache
- Tremors
- Numbness in the extremities
- Nausea
- Sweating
- Muscle tension and cramps
- Psychoses
- Hallucinations
- Memory impairment
- Convulsions (possible)

Contraindications

[handwritten margin notes: Elderly, Toxicity, Narrow angled Glaucoma, PG, Lactation]

The nurse should not administer antianxiety drugs to patients with known hypersensitivity, psychoses, and acute narrow-angle glaucoma. The benzodiazepines are contraindicated during pregnancy (category D drugs) and labor because of reports of floppy infant syndrome manifested by sucking difficulties, lethargy, and hypotonia seen in the newborn. Lactating women should also avoid the benzodiazepines because of the effect on the infant, who becomes lethargic and loses weight.

Buspirone is a pregnancy category B drug and hydroxyzine is a pregnancy category C drug. Their safety is still questionable because adequate studies have not been performed in pregnant women. All of these drugs are also contraindicated when patients are in a coma or shock, and if the vital signs of the patient in acute alcoholic intoxication are low.

Precautions

Antianxiety drugs are used cautiously in elderly patients and in patients with impaired liver function, impaired kidney function, or debilitation.

Interactions

The following interactions may occur when an anxiolytic is administered with another agent:

Interacting Drug	Common Use	Effect of Interaction
alcohol	Relaxation and enjoyment in social situations	Increased risk for CNS depression or convulsions
analgesics	Pain relief	Increased risk for CNS depression
tricyclic antidepressants	Management of depression	Increased risk for sedation and respiratory depression
antipsychotics	Control of psychotic symptoms	Increased risk for sedation and respiratory depression
digoxin	Management of cardiac problems	Increased risk for digitalis toxicity

NURSING PROCESS
PATIENT RECEIVING AN ANTIANXIETY DRUG

ASSESSMENT

Preadministration Assessment
A patient receiving an antianxiety drug may be treated in the hospital or in an outpatient setting (Fig. 20.1). Before starting therapy for the hospitalized patient, the nurse obtains a complete medical history, including mental status and anxiety level. In the case of mild anxiety, patients may (but sometimes may not) give a reliable history of their illness.

When severe anxiety is present, the patient may be unable to communicate effectively. Therefore, it is important to obtain portions of the history from a family member or friend. During the intake history, the nurse observes the patient for behavioral signs indicating anxiety (e.g., inability to focus, extreme restlessness, facial grimaces, tense posture).

Figure 20.1 Hospitalization can be an anxious experience for patients. Anxiolytic medications can help the patient focus on patient teaching and activities of daily living to improve patient outcomes.

[handwritten notes at bottom: VS, Mental Status ~w,w,w,w,w; Hyperventilation; Family, History of Abuse]

Physical assessment should include the blood pressure, pulse, respiratory rate, and weight. Physiologic manifestations of anxiety can include increased blood pressure and pulse rate, increased rate and depth of respiration, and increased muscle tension. An anxious patient may have cool and pale skin.

The nurse makes sure to obtain a history of any past drug or alcohol use. This information can help establish what the patient has used in the past as coping mechanisms. Individuals with mild anxiety or depression do not necessarily require inpatient care. These patients are usually seen at periodic intervals in the primary health care provider's office or in a mental health outpatient setting. The preadministration assessments of the outpatient are the same as those for the hospitalized patient.

Ongoing Assessment

An ongoing assessment is important for the patient taking an antianxiety drug. The nurse checks the patient's blood pressure before drug administration. If systolic pressure has dropped 20 mm Hg, the nurse withholds the drug and notifies the primary health care provider. The nurse periodically monitors the patient's mental status and anxiety level during therapy and assesses for improvement or worsening of behavioral and physical signs identified in the preadministration assessment.

The nurse can ask the patient or a family member about adverse drug reactions or any other problems occurring during therapy. The nurse then brings these reactions or problems to the attention of the primary health care provider. The nurse documents a general summary of the patient's outward behavior and any complaints or problems in the patient's record. The nurse then compares new information with previous notations and observations.

NURSING DIAGNOSES

Drug-specific nursing diagnoses are the following:

- ❏ **Risk for Injury** related to dizziness or hypotension and gait problems
- ❏ **Impaired Comfort** related to dryness in GI tract from medications
- ❏ **Ineffective Individual Coping** related to situation causing anxiety

Nursing diagnoses related to drug administration are discussed in Chapter 4.

PLANNING

The expected patient outcomes may include an optimal response to drug therapy, support of patient needs in relation to managing adverse drug reactions, and an understanding of the therapeutic regimen.

IMPLEMENTATION

Promoting an Optimal Response to Therapy

During initial therapy, the nurse observes the patient closely for adverse drug reactions. Some adverse reac-

tions, such as episodes of postural hypotension and drowsiness or dry mouth, may need to be tolerated because drug therapy must continue. The antianxiety drugs are not recommended for long-term use. When the antianxiety drugs are used for short periods (1 to 2 weeks), tolerance, dependence, or withdrawal symptoms usually do not develop. The nurse reports any signs of tolerance or dependence, such as the patient needing larger doses of drug or complaints of increased anxiety and agitation (see Display 20.1).

Monitoring and Managing Patient Needs

RISK FOR INJURY. When these drugs are given in the outpatient setting, the nurse should instruct both the patient and family about adverse reactions (dizziness, lightheadedness, or ataxia) that can cause a patient to fall and become injured. This is very important when the drugs are administered to elderly patients in an outpatient setting.

LIFESPAN ALERT – Gerontology

Benzodiazepines are excreted more slowly in older adults, causing a prolonged drug effect. The drugs may accumulate in the blood, resulting in an increase in adverse reactions or toxicity. For this reason, the initial dose should be small, and the dose increased gradually until a therapeutic response is obtained.

However, lorazepam and oxazepam are relatively safe for older adults when given in normal dosages. Buspirone also is a safe choice for older adults with anxiety, because it does not cause excessive sedation, and the risk of falling is not as great.

When the patient is hospitalized, the nurse develops a nursing care plan to meet the patient's individual needs. Vital signs can be monitored at frequent intervals, usually three or four times daily. Patients can be monitored for symptoms such as dizziness or lightheadedness. Patients can be instructed to stay in bed and call for assistance to get up out of the bed or chair, and may need to be supervised for all ambulatory activities. The nurse should provide total assistance with activities of daily living to the patient experiencing extreme sedation. This includes help with eating, dressing, and ambulating. In some instances, such as when a hypotensive episode occurs, the vital signs are taken more often. Then the nurse reports any significant change in the vital signs to the primary health care provider. The sedation and drowsiness that sometimes occur with the use of an antianxiety drug may decrease as therapy continues.

Parenteral administration is indicated primarily in acute states when it is difficult for the patient to take the medication by mouth. When these drugs are given intramuscularly (IM), the nurse gives them in a large muscle mass, such as the gluteus muscle. The nurse observes the patient closely for at least 3 hours after parenteral administration. The patient is kept lying down (when possible) for 30 minutes to 3 hours after the drug is given.

[handwritten margin note: Toxicit. Smaller doses]

[handwritten note at bottom: P- Monitor closely - 30 min. p.t. after meds.]

[vertical text right margin: Antianxiety Drugs]

Don't take w/alcohol

LIFESPAN ALERT – Gerontology

Parenteral (intravenous [IV] or IM) administration to older adults, the debilitated, and those with limited pulmonary reserve requires that the nurse exert extreme care because the patient may experience apnea and cardiac arrest. Resuscitative equipment should be readily available during parenteral (particularly IV) administration.

IMPAIRED COMFORT. Antianxiety drugs can cause both dryness of the mucous membranes and slower transit in the intestines, leading to constipation. Nursing interventions to relieve some of these reactions may include offering frequent sips of water to relieve dry mouth and provide adequate hydration. The patient may also chew sugarless gum or suck on hard candy to reduce discomfort from dry mouth. The nurse may administer oral antianxiety drugs with food or meals to decrease the possibility of gastrointestinal (GI) upset. Meals should include fiber, fruits, and vegetables to aid in preventing constipation. However, the nurse should use great care when administering these drugs orally, because some patients have difficulty swallowing (because of a dry mouth or other causes).

INEFFECTIVE INDIVIDUAL COPING. When the patient is an outpatient, the nurse observes the patient for a response to therapy at the time of each clinic visit. In some instances, the nurse may question the patient or a family member about the response to therapy. The type of questions asked depends on the patient and the diagnosis, and may include open-ended questions such as "How are you feeling?" "Do you feel less nervous?" or "Would you like to tell me how everything is going?" Many times the nurse may need to rephrase questions or direct the conversation toward other subjects until these patients feel comfortable enough to discuss their therapy.

Once the patient has reduced the anxious behavior, the nurse may be able to help the patient identify what is precipitating the panic attacks or causing anxiety. It is important for the nurse to help patients understand that there are health care providers who can help them gain skills to cope with situations before the anxious behavior returns.

Although rare, benzodiazepine toxicity may occur from an overdose of the drug. Benzodiazepine toxicity causes sedation, respiratory depression, and coma. Flumazenil (Romazicon) is an antidote (antagonist) for benzodiazepine toxicity and acts to reverse the sedation, respiratory depression, and coma within 6 to 10 minutes after IV administration. Adverse reactions to flumazenil include agitation, confusion, seizures, and, in some cases, symptoms of benzodiazepine withdrawal. Adverse reactions to flumazenil, related to the symptoms of benzodiazepine withdrawal, are relieved by the administration of the benzodiazepine.

Educating the Patient and Family

The nurse evaluates the patient's ability to assume responsibility for taking drugs at home. The nurse explains any adverse reactions that may occur with a specific antianxiety drug and encourages the patient or family members to contact the primary health care provider immediately if a serious adverse reaction occurs. The nurse should include the following points in a teaching plan for the patient or family member:

- Take the drug exactly as directed. Do not increase, decrease, or omit a dose or discontinue use of this drug unless directed to do so by the primary health care provider.
- Do not discontinue use of the drug abruptly because withdrawal symptoms may occur.
- Avoid driving or performing other hazardous tasks if drowsiness occurs.
- Do not take any nonprescription drug unless the specific drug has been approved by the primary health care provider.
- Inform physicians, dentists, and other health care providers of therapy with this drug.
- Do not drink alcoholic beverages unless approval is obtained from the primary health care provider.
- If dizziness occurs when changing position, rise slowly when getting out of bed or a chair. If dizziness is severe, always have help when changing positions.
- If dryness of the mouth occurs, relieve it by taking frequent sips of water, sucking on hard candy, or chewing gum (preferably sugarless).
- Prevent constipation by eating foods high in fiber, increasing fluid intake, and exercising if condition permits.
- Keep all appointments with the primary health care provider because close monitoring of therapy is essential.
- Report any unusual changes or physical effects to the primary health care provider.

Interactions, only as needed at first

EVALUATION *sign, constipation - drink fluids*

- Therapeutic response is achieved and patient reports a decrease in feelings of anxiety.
- Adverse reactions are identified, reported to the primary health care provider, and managed successfully with appropriate nursing interventions:
  - ☑ No evidence of injury is seen.
  - ☑ Patient reports comfort without increased GI distress.
  - ☑ Patient manages coping effectively.
- Patient and family demonstrate an understanding of the drug regimen.

THINK CRITICALLY: PHARMACOLOGY IN PRACTICE

1. Mrs. Moore, aged 85 years, is hospitalized for congestive heart failure. She is improving, but has been complaining of feelings of anxiety. Her respirations are 32 breaths/min, heart rate 88 beats/min, and blood pressure 118/60 mm Hg. The primary health care provider prescribes alprazolam (Xanax) 0.25 mg orally three times a day. As part of the discharge

IM glutuous maximas vastus lateralus

planning, what precautions would the nurse relay to her caregivers about this medication given Mrs. Moore's age? Discuss what assessment findings would indicate increased anxiety.

● Test Your Knowledge

1. Alprazolam (Xanax) is contraindicated in patients with _____.

   A. a psychotic disorder
   B. congestive heart failure
   C. diabetes
   D. hypertension

2. Which of the following drugs is a schedule IV controlled substance?

   A. hydroxyzine (Vistaril)
   B. doxepin (Sinequan)
   C. buspirone (BuSpar)
   D. chlordiazepoxide (Librium)

3. Which of the following is a sign of drug withdrawal and not an adverse reaction?

   A. Dizziness
   B. Metallic taste
   C. Constipation
   D. Sedation

4. The benzodiazepines are pregnancy category D drugs that should not be taken while lactating because the newborn may become _____.

   A. depressed
   B. excited and irritable
   C. lethargic and lose weight
   D. hypoglycemic

● Prepare for the NCLEX

1. A family member calls the nurse to report that the patient taking an antianxiety medication is hypotensive. The nurse instructs the family member to:

   A. give oral fluids to increase the blood pressure
   B. have the patient rise slower from a lying or sitting position
   C. take the patient to a local fire station three times a week to check blood pressure
   D. stop the medication until the nurse checks with the primary health care provider

● Calculate Medication Dosages

1. Hydroxyzine (Vistaril) 100 mg IM is prescribed. Available is a vial with 100 mg hydroxyzine per milliliter. The nurse administers _____.

2. The patient is prescribed 30 mg oxazepam three times a day orally. The drug is available in 15-mg tablets. The nurse administers _____.

To check your answers, see Appendix E.

the**Point**. *For more NCLEX questions, log on to http://thepoint.lww.com to access more than 1000 questions.*

Sedatives and Hypnotics

Sedatives and hypnotics are primarily used to treat insomnia. According to the National Sleep Foundation, insomnia affects nearly 70 million people in the United States. It may be caused by lifestyle changes, such as a new job, moving to a new town, returning to school, jet lag, chronic pain, headaches, stress, or anxiety.

In many cases, insomnia occurs during hospitalization. Patients are in unfamiliar surroundings that are unlike the home situation. Noises and lights at night often interfere with or interrupt sleep. An important part of meeting patient needs during illness is to help the patient gain rest and sleep. Sleep deprivation may interfere with the healing process; therefore, a **hypnotic** may be given. These drugs also may be prescribed for short-term use to promote sleep after discharge from the hospital.

A hypnotic is a drug that induces drowsiness or sleep, that is, it allows the patient to fall asleep and stay asleep. Hypnotics are given at night or bedtime. A **sedative** is a drug that produces a relaxing, calming effect. Sedatives are usually given during daytime hours, and although they may make the patient drowsy, they usually do not produce sleep.

Sedatives and hypnotics may be divided into two classes: barbiturates and nonbarbiturates. The nonbarbiturates are classified into two groups: benzodiazepines and nonbenzodiazepines. Barbiturates were once the drugs of choice to treat insomnia and anxiety. The nonbarbiturates are now used as sedatives more frequently than the barbiturates, because the benzodiazepines are more effective in treating insomnia, and the adverse reactions of barbiturates are more severe. The benzodiazepines are also used as antianxiety drugs (see Chapter 20). Examples of the benzodiazepines discussed in this chapter include temazepam (Restoril) and triazolam (Halcion).

The nonbenzodiazepines are a group of unrelated drugs. Examples include eszopiclone (Lunesta), and zolpidem (Ambien). Barbiturates, benzodiazepines, and nonbenzodiazepines are listed in the Summary Drug Table: Sedatives and Hypnotics.

Actions

Barbiturates

All barbiturates have essentially the same mode of action. Depending on the dose given, these drugs are capable of producing central nervous system (CNS) depression and mood alteration ranging from mild excitation to mild sedation, hypnosis (sleep), and deep coma. These drugs also are respiratory depressants; the degree of depression usually depends on the dose given. When these drugs are used as hypnotics, their respiratory depressant effect is usually similar to that occurring during sleep.

Benzodiazepines and Nonbenzodiazepines

Nonbarbiturate sedatives and hypnotics have essentially the same mode of action as the barbiturates—that is, they depress the CNS. The benzodiazepine effect on GABA (gamma-aminobutyric acid) to potentiate neural inhibition is discussed in Chapter 20. However, these drugs have a lesser effect on the respiratory rate—another reason why they are chosen over barbiturates for insomnia.

Like the barbiturates, the nonbenzodiazepines effects diminish after approximately 2 weeks. Persons taking these drugs for longer than 2 weeks may have a tendency to increase the dose to produce the desired effects (e.g., sleep, sedation). Physical tolerance and psychological dependence may occur, especially after prolonged use of high doses.

Sedatives and Hypnotics

Summary Drug Table SEDATIVES AND HYPNOTICS

Generic Name	Trade Name	Uses	Adverse Reactions	Dosage Ranges
Benzodiazepines				
estazolam *es-taz'-eh-lam*		Hypnotic	Headache, heartburn, nausea, palpitations, rash, somnolence, vomiting, weakness, body and joint pain	1–2 mg orally
flurazepam *flur-az'-eh-pam*	Dalmane	Hypnotic	Same as estazolam	15–30 mg orally
quazepam *kwa'-zeh-pam*	Doral	Hypnotic	Same as estazolam	7.5–15 mg orally
temazepam *teh-maz'-eh-pam*	Restoril	Hypnotic	Same as estazolam	15–30 mg orally
triazolam *trye-ay'-zoe-lam*	Halcion	Sedative, hypnotic	Same as estazolam	0.125–0.5 mg orally at bedtime
Nonbenzodiazepines				
dexmedetomidine *dex-med-eh-toe'-meh-deen*	Precedex	Sedation during intubation	Hypotension, nausea, bradycardia	1 mcg/kg over 10 minutes IV
eszopiclone *es-zoe'-pih-kloan*	Lunesta	Chronic insomnia	Headache, somnolence, taste changes, chest pain, migraine, edema	1–3 mg orally at bedtime
ramelteon *ram-el'-tee-on*	Rozerem	Insomnia	Dizziness, headache	8 mg orally at bedtime
zaleplon *zal'-ah-plon*	Sonata	Transient insomnia	Dizziness, headache, rebound insomnia, nausea, myalgia	10 mg orally at bedtime
ⓕ zolpidem *zoll'-pih-dem*	Ambien, Ambien CR (*controlled release*)	Transient insomnia	Drowsiness, headache, myalgia, nausea	10 mg orally at bedtime
Barbiturates				
pentobarbital *pen-toe-bar'-bih-tall*	Nembutal	Sedative, hypnotic, preoperative sedation	Respiratory and CNS depression, nausea, vomiting, constipation, diarrhea, bradycardia, hypotension, syncope, hypersensitivity reactions, headache	Available only in parenteral form: 100 mg deep IM or IV, may titrate up to 200–500 mg
secobarbital *see-koe-bar'-bih-tall*	Seconal	Hypnotic, preoperative sedation	Same as pentobarbital sodium	Hypnotic: 100 mg orally at bedtime Sedation: 200–300 mg orally 1–2 hr before procedure

ⓕ This drug should not be administered with food (especially high-fat meals).

However, their addictive potential appears to be less than that of the barbiturates. Discontinuing use of a sedative or hypnotic after prolonged use may result in mild to severe withdrawal symptoms.

Uses

The sedative and hypnotic drugs are used in the treatment of:

• Insomnia

• Convulsions or seizures

They are also used as adjuncts for anesthesia and for:

• Preoperative sedation
• Conscious sedation

 LIFESPAN ALERT — Gerontology
Elderly patients may require a smaller hypnotic dose, and in some instances, a sedative dose produces sleep.

Adverse Reactions

- Nervous system reactions include dizziness, drowsiness, and headache.
- A common gastrointestinal reaction is nausea.

drug hangover, grossy

Contraindications

These drugs are contraindicated in patients with known hypersensitivity to sedatives or hypnotics. The nurse should not administer these drugs to comatose patients, those with severe respiratory problems, those with a history of drug and alcohol habitual use, or pregnant or lactating women. The barbiturates are classified as pregnancy category D drugs.

Benzodiazepines (e.g., estazolam, quazepam, temazepam, triazolam) used for sedation are classified as pregnancy category X drugs. Most nonbenzodiazepines are pregnancy category B or C drugs.

 LIFESPAN ALERT – Childbearing Women
Women taking barbiturates or benzodiazepines should be warned of the potential risk to the fetus so that contraceptive methods may be instituted, if necessary. A child born to a mother taking benzodiazepines may experience withdrawal symptoms during the postnatal period.

Precautions

Sedatives and hypnotics should be used cautiously in lactating patients and in patients with hepatic or renal impairment, habitual alcohol use, and mental health problems.

 LIFESPAN ALERT – Gerontology
The nurse uses these drugs cautiously in older adults or in those who are debilitated because these patients are more sensitive to the effects of the sedatives or hypnotics.

Interactions

The following interactions may occur when a sedative or hypnotic is administered with another agent:

Interacting Drug	Common Use	Effect of Interaction
antidepressants	Management of depression	Increased sedative effect
opioid analgesics antihistamines	Pain relief, relief of allergy symptoms (runny nose and itching)	Increased sedative effect
phenothiazines (e.g., Thorazine)	Management of agitation and psychotic symptoms	Increased sedative effect
cimetidine	Management of gastric upset	Increased sedative effect
alcohol	Relaxation and enjoyment in social situations	Increased sedative effect

Patients may not volunteer information regarding their use of alternative or complementary remedies. The nurse should always inquire about use of herbal products. Although lab testing is not conclusive, medical reports indicate a pos-

sible interaction with eucalyptus products causing increased sedation.

 HEALTH SUPPLEMENT ALERT
Melatonin is a hormone produced by the pineal gland in the brain. Melatonin has been used in treating insomnia, overcoming jet lag, and improving the effectiveness of the immune system, and as an antioxidant. The most significant use—at low doses—is the short-term treatment of insomnia. Melatonin obtained from animal pineal tissue is not recommended for use because of the risk of contamination. The synthetic form of melatonin does not carry this risk. Supplements should be purchased from a reliable source to minimize the risk of contamination. Drowsiness may occur within 30 minutes after taking the supplement. The drowsiness may persist for an hour or more, affecting any activity that requires mental alertness, such as driving. Possible adverse reactions include headache and depression. Although uncommon, allergic reactions (difficulty breathing, hives, or swelling of lips, tongue, or face) to melatonin have been reported.

NURSING PROCESS
PATIENT RECEIVING A SEDATIVE OR HYPNOTIC

ASSESSMENT

Preadministration Assessment
Before administering a sedative or hypnotic, the nurse notes the patient's blood pressure, pulse, and respiratory rate. Changes in vital signs (especially hypotension) may occur after drug administration, so having baseline values is important for comparison. In addition to the vital signs, the nurse assesses the patient's status by asking the following questions:

Hypnotic Drug (for sleep disturbances) Administration:

- Is the patient uncomfortable? If the reason for discomfort is pain, an analgesic, rather than a hypnotic, may be required.
- Is it too early for the patient to receive the drug? Is a later hour preferred?
- Does the patient receive an opioid analgesic every 4 to 6 hours? A hypnotic may not be necessary because an opioid analgesic can also induce drowsiness and sleep.
- Are there disturbances in the environment that may keep the patient awake and decrease the effectiveness of the drug?

Sedative Drug (for relaxing and calming) Administration:

- Is the sedative for a surgical procedure, and is its administration correctly timed?
- Has a consent form for the procedure been signed before the medication is given? Informed consent cannot be established if the patient has medication in his or her system.

 NURSING ALERT
Barbiturates have little or no analgesic action, so the nurse does not give these drugs if the patient has pain

and cannot sleep. Barbiturates, when given in the presence of pain, may cause restlessness, excitement, and delirium.

If the patient is receiving one of these drugs for daytime sedation, the nurse assesses the patient's general mental state and level of consciousness. If the patient appears sedated and difficult to awaken, the nurse withholds the drug and contacts the primary health care provider as soon as possible.

❧ HERBAL ALERT

Valerian was originally used in Europe and was brought to North America on the *Mayflower* (Fig. 21.1). The herb is widely used for its sedative effects in conditions of mild anxiety or restlessness. It is particularly useful in individuals with insomnia. Valerian improves overall sleep quality by shortening the length of time it takes to fall asleep and decreasing the number of nighttime awakenings.

Formulated as a tea, tablet, capsule, or tincture, valerian is classified as "generally recognized as safe" (GRAS) for use in the United States. When used as an aid to sleep, valerian is taken approximately 1 hour before bedtime; less is used for anxiety. Valerian can be used in combination with other calming herbs, such as lemon balm or chamomile. It may take 2 to 4 weeks before the full therapeutic effect (i.e., improvement of

Figure 21.1 The root of the herb valerian is used medicinally. (From Facts and Comparisons [2003]. *Guide to popular natural products* [3rd ed., p. I-16]. St. Louis: Facts and Comparisons.)

mood and sleep patterns) occurs. Individuals have been known to experience withdrawal symptoms when they stop taking valerian abruptly.

Ongoing Assessment

Before administering the drug each time, the nurse should perform an assessment that includes the patient's vital signs (temperature, pulse, respiration, and blood pressure) and level of consciousness (e.g., alert, confused, or lethargic). This is especially important when the drug is to be given as needed (PRN). After assessing the patient, the nurse makes a decision regarding administration of the drug.

The nurse checks to see if the drug helped the patient sleep on previous nights. If not, a different drug or dose may be needed, and the nurse should consult the primary health care provider regarding the drug's ineffectiveness.

If the patient has a PRN order for an opioid analgesic or other CNS depressant and a hypnotic, the nurse should consult the primary health care provider regarding the time interval between administrations of these drugs. Usually, at least 2 hours should elapse between administration of a hypnotic and any other CNS depressant, but this interval may vary, depending on factors such as the patient's age and diagnosis.

▮ NURSING ALERT

The nurse withholds the drug and notifies the primary health care provider if one or more vital signs significantly vary from the database, if the respiratory rate is 10 breaths/min or below, or if the patient appears lethargic.

NURSING DIAGNOSES

Drug-specific nursing diagnoses are the following:

- ❑ **Risk for Injury** related to drowsiness or impaired memory
- ❑ **Ineffective Breathing Pattern** related to respiratory depression
- ❑ **Ineffective Individual Coping** related to excessive use of medication

Nursing diagnoses related to drug administration are discussed in Chapter 4.

PLANNING

The expected outcomes for the patient depend on the reason for administration of a sedative or hypnotic but may include an optimal response to drug therapy (e.g., sedation or sleep), support of patient needs related to management of adverse drug reactions, and an understanding of the therapeutic regimen.

IMPLEMENTATION

Promoting an Optimal Response to Therapy

To promote the effects of the sedative or hypnotic drug, the nurse provides supportive care, such as back rubs, night lights or a darkened room, and a quiet atmosphere. The patient is discouraged from drinking beverages containing caffeine, such as coffee, cola, or energy drinks, which can contribute to wakefulness.

The nurse never leaves hypnotics and sedatives at the patient's bedside to be taken at a later hour; hypnotics and sedatives are controlled substances (see Chapter 1). In addition, the nurse never leaves these drugs unattended in the nurses' station, hallway, or other areas to which patients, visitors, or hospital personnel have direct access.

❗ NURSING ALERT

Some sleep medicines (zolpidem) may cause memory loss or amnesia. A person may not remember getting up out of bed, driving, or eating. These drugs only should be taken when a person plans for 7 to 8 hours of sleep.

Monitoring and Managing Patient Needs

RISK FOR INJURY. It is important that the nurse observe the patient for adverse drug reactions. During periods when the patient is excited or confused, the nurse protects the patient from harm and provides supportive care and a safe environment. The nurse assesses the patient receiving a sedative dose and determines what safety measures must be taken. After administration of a hypnotic, the nurse may raise the side rails of the bed and advise the patient to remain in bed and to call for assistance if it is necessary to get out of bed. Patients receiving sedative doses may or may not require this safety measure, depending on the patient's response to the drug. The nurse observes the patient receiving a hypnotic 1 to 2 hours after the drug is given to evaluate the effect of the drug. The nurse notifies the primary health care provider if the patient fails to sleep, awakens one or more times during the night, or experiences an adverse drug reaction. In some instances, supplemental doses of a hypnotic may be ordered if the patient awakens during the night.

Excessive drowsiness and headache the morning after a hypnotic has been given (drug hangover) may occur in some patients. The nurse reports this problem to the primary health care provider because a smaller dose or a different drug may be necessary. The nurse assists the patient with ambulation, if necessary. When getting out of bed, the patient is encouraged to rise to a sitting position first, wait a few minutes, and then rise to a standing position.

Patients using these drugs in an outpatient setting are taught about the hazards of operating machinery or involvement in other potentially hazardous tasks until they are sure that concentration and focus are not affected.

👤 LIFESPAN ALERT – Gerontology

The older adult is at greater risk for oversedation, dizziness, confusion, or **ataxia** (unsteady gait) when taking a sedative or hypnotic. The nurse checks elderly and debilitated patients for a **paradoxical reaction**, such as marked excitement, or confusion. If excitement or confusion occurs, the nurse observes the patient at frequent intervals (as often as every 5 to 10 minutes may be necessary) for the duration of this occurrence and institutes safety measures to prevent injury. If oversedation, extreme dizziness, or ataxia occurs, the nurse notifies the primary health care provider.

INEFFECTIVE BREATHING PATTERN. Sedatives and hypnotics depress the CNS and can cause respiratory depression. The nurse carefully assesses respiratory function (rate, depth, and quality) before administering a sedative, 30 minutes to 1 hour after administering the drug, and frequently thereafter. When administering barbiturates, the nurse needs to be aware that the possibility of adverse reactions is greater than that from other sedatives and hypnotics.

The nurse should instruct the patient not to drink alcohol when taking sedatives or hypnotics. Alcohol is a CNS depressant, as are the sedatives and hypnotics. When alcohol and a sedative or hypnotic are taken together, there is an additive effect and an increase in CNS depression, which has, on occasion, resulted in death. The nurse must emphasize the importance of abstaining from alcohol use while taking this drug and stress that the use of alcohol and any one of these drugs can result in serious effects.

INEFFECTIVE INDIVIDUAL COPING. Sedatives and hypnotics are best given for no more than 2 weeks and preferably for a shorter time. Sedatives and hypnotics can become less effective after they are taken for a prolonged period. Thus, there may be a tendency to increase the dose without consulting the primary health care provider. To ensure compliance with the treatment regimen, the nurse emphasizes the importance of not increasing or decreasing the dose unless a change in dosage is recommended by the primary health care provider. In addition, the nurse stresses the importance of not repeating the dose during the night if sleep is interrupted or sleep lasts only a few hours, unless the primary health care provider has approved taking the drug more than once per night.

Although the practice is not recommended, a patient with sleep disturbances may be taking one of these drugs for an extended period of time. A sedative or hypnotic can cause drug dependency. The nurse must never suddenly discontinue use of these drugs when there is a question of possible dependency. Patients who have been taking a sedative or hypnotic for several weeks should gradually withdraw from taking the drug to prevent withdrawal symptoms (see Chapter 20). Symptoms of withdrawal include restlessness, excitement, euphoria, and confusion. Withdrawal can result in serious consequences, especially in those with existing diseases or disorders.

Educating the Patient and Family

In educating the patient and family about sedatives and hypnotics, several general points must be considered. The nurse gives the patient and family an explanation of the prescribed drug and dosage regimen, as well as situations that should be avoided. The nurse develops a teaching

Don't eat high fat meal - interrupts w absorption

plan to include one or more of the following items of information:

- The primary health care provider usually prescribes these drugs for short-term use only.
- If the drug appears to be ineffective, contact the primary health care provider. Do not increase the dose unless advised to do so by the primary health care provider.
- Notify the primary health care provider if any adverse drug reactions occur.
- Do not drink any alcoholic beverage 2 hours before, with, or 8 hours after taking the drug.
- When taking the drug as a sedative, be aware that the drug can impair the mental and physical abilities required for performing potentially dangerous tasks, such as driving a car or operating machinery.
- After taking a drug to sleep, observe caution when getting out of bed at night. Keep the room dimly lit and remove any obstacles that may result in injury when getting out of bed. Never attempt to drive or perform any hazardous task after taking a drug intended to produce sleep.
- Do not use these drugs if you are pregnant, considering becoming pregnant, or breast-feeding.
- Do not use over-the-counter cold, cough, or allergy drugs while taking this drug unless their use has been approved by the primary health care provider. Some of these products contain antihistamines or other drugs that also may cause mild to extreme drowsiness. Others may contain an adrenergic drug, which is a mild stimulant, and therefore will defeat the purpose of the sedative or hypnotic.
- Do not take zolpidem with food. A high-fat meal or snack can interfere with the absorption of the following drugs: eszopiclone, ramelteon or zaleplon.

EVALUATION

- Therapeutic response is achieved and sleep pattern is improved or the patient is calm and relaxed for a procedure.
- Adverse reactions are identified, reported to the primary health care provider, and managed successfully with appropriate nursing interventions:
  - ☑ No evidence of injury is seen.
  - ☑ An adequate breathing pattern is maintained.
  - ☑ Patient manages coping effectively.
- Patient and family demonstrate an understanding of the drug regimen.

THINK CRITICALLY: PHARMACOLOGY IN PRACTICE

1. Mr. Phillip's wife was killed in an automobile accident, and he has had trouble coping with the loss. He complains of being unable to sleep for more than an hour before he wakes. The primary health care provider prescribes a hypnotic, 1 capsule per night for use

during the next 3 weeks. In 2 weeks, he calls the primary health care provider's office and asks for a refill of his prescription. Determine what questions you would ask Mr. Phillip. Explain why you would ask them.

● Test Your Knowledge

1. Which of these of these assessments should the nurse report immediately to the primary health provider?
   - **A.** Dizziness when arising from the chair
   - **B.** Heart rate of 80 beats/min
   - **C.** Respiration rate of 8 breaths/min
   - **D.** Joint pain

2. When giving a hypnotic to an elderly patient, the nurse is aware that _____.
   - **A.** smaller doses of the drug are usually given to older patients
   - **B.** elderly patients usually require larger doses of a hypnotic
   - **C.** older adults excrete the drug faster than younger adults
   - **D.** dosages of the hypnotic may be increased each night until the desired effect is achieved

3. Which of the following points should be included in a teaching plan for a patient taking a sedative or hypnotic?
   - **A.** An alcoholic beverage may be served 1 to 2 hours before a sedative is taken without any ill effects.
   - **B.** Dosage of the sedative may be increased if sleep is not restful.
   - **C.** These drugs may safely be used for 6 months to 1 year when given for insomnia.
   - **D.** Do not use any over-the-counter cold, cough, or allergy medications while taking a sedative or hypnotic.

4. Which of the following sedatives/hypnotics is a pregnancy category X drug?
   - **A.** zolpidem (Ambien)
   - **B.** amobarbital (Amytal)
   - **C.** temazepam (Restoril)
   - **D.** eszopiclone (Lunesta)

● Prepare for the NCLEX

1. An elderly woman has arthritis in her lower back, and the pain keeps her awake at night. She asks if she can have a "sleeping pill." In considering her request, the nurse must take into account that hypnotic medications might _____.
   - **A.** not be the drug of choice when pain causes insomnia
   - **B.** be given instead of an analgesic to relieve her pain
   - **C.** often increase the pain threshold
   - **D.** be added to an analgesic to improve this situation

p.t. assessment
other drugs taking + herbs
Dont drink or drive

● Calculate Medication Dosages

1. Halcion 0.125 mg is prescribed. The drug is available in 0.125-mg tablets. The nurse administers _____.

2. Eszopiclone (Lunesta) 2 mg is prescribed for insomnia. The drug is available in 1-mg tablets. The nurse administers _____.

To check your answers, see Appendix E.

the**Point**⁕ *For more NCLEX questions, log on to http://thepoint.lww.com to access more than 1000 questions.*

Antidepressant Drugs

depression
dysphoric
endogenous
neurohormones

orthostatic hypotension
priapism
tardive dyskinesia
tyramine

LEARNING OBJECTIVES

On completion of this chapter, the student will:

1. Define depression and identify symptoms of a major depressive episode.
2. Name the different types of antidepressant drugs.
3. Discuss the uses, general drug actions, general adverse reactions, contraindications, precautions, and interactions of the antidepressant drugs.
4. Discuss important preadministration and ongoing assessment activities that the nurse should perform on the patient taking antidepressant drugs.
5. List nursing diagnoses particular to a patient taking antidepressant drugs.
6. Discuss ways to promote an optimal response to therapy, how to manage common adverse reactions, and important points to keep in mind when educating patients about the use of antidepressant drugs.

Depression may be described as feeling sad, unhappy, or "down in the dumps." Most of us feel this way at one time or another for short periods. A major depressive episode is a depressed or **dysphoric** (extreme or exaggerated sadness, anxiety, or unhappiness) mood that interferes with daily functioning. For a classification of clinical depression, five or more of the symptoms listed in Display 22.1 need to occur daily or nearly every day for a period of 2 weeks or more. The symptoms of clinical depression are not the result of normal bereavement, such as the loss of a loved one, or another disease, such as hypothyroidism.

Clinical depression is treated with antidepressant drugs, and psychotherapy is used with the antidepressants in treating major depressive episodes. The four types of antidepressants are

• Tricyclic antidepressants (TCAs)
• Selective serotonin reuptake inhibitors (SSRIs)

• Monoamine oxidase inhibitors (MAOIs)
• Atypical antidepressants

● TRICYCLIC ANTIDEPRESSANTS

Actions

For several years it was thought that antidepressants blocked the reuptake of the **endogenous** (produced by the body) neurotransmitters norepinephrine and serotonin. This action resulted in stimulation of the central nervous system (CNS) and alleviation of the depressed mood. This theory is now being questioned. New research indicates that the effects of antidepressants are related to slow adaptive changes in norepinephrine and serotonin receptor systems. Treatment with antidepressants is thought to produce complex changes in the sensitivities of both presynaptic and postsynaptic receptor sites. Antidepressants increase the sensitivity of postsynaptic alpha-adrenergic and serotonin receptors and decrease the sensitivity of the presynaptic receptor sites. This enhances recovery from the depressive episode by making neurotransmission activity more effective, as visualized in Figure 22.1. The TCAs, such as amitriptyline and doxepin (Sinequan), inhibit reuptake of norepinephrine or serotonin in the brain.

Uses

Tricyclic antidepressant drugs are used in the treatment of the following:

• Depressive episodes
• Bipolar disorder
• Obsessive-compulsive disorders

DISPLAY 22.1 Symptoms of Depression   *Review*

• Feelings of hopelessness or helplessness
• Diminished interest in activities of life
• Significant weight loss or gain (without dieting)
• Insomnia (inability to sleep) or hypersomnia (excessive sleeping)
• Agitation, restlessness, or irritability
• Fatigue or loss of energy
• Feelings of worthlessness
• Excessive or inappropriate guilt
• Diminished ability to think or concentrate, or indecisiveness
• Recurrent thoughts of death or suicide (or suicide attempt)

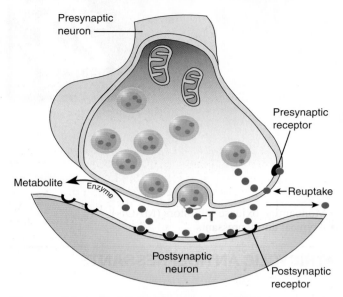

Figure 22.1 Antidepressant drugs inhibit the reuptake of the neurotransmitter (T), thus making it available to the postsynaptic neuron.

- Chronic neuropathic pain
- Depression accompanied by anxiety disorders
- Enuresis

Unlabeled uses include peptic ulcer disease, sleep apnea, panic disorder, bulimia nervosa, premenstrual symptoms, and some dermatologic problems. These drugs may be used with psychotherapy in severe cases.

Adverse Reactions

Generalized reactions include:

- Anticholinergic effects (e.g., sedation, dry mouth, visual disturbances, urinary retention)
- Constipation and photosensitivity

⚠ NURSING ALERT
Although the TCAs are not considered antipsychotic agents, the drug amoxapine has been associated with **tardive dyskinesia** and neuroleptic malignant syndrome (NMS). Tardive dyskinesia is a syndrome of involuntary movement that may be irreversible. Symptoms of NMS are similar and include muscle rigidity, altered mental status, and autonomic system problems, such as tachycardia or sweating. These syndromes tend to occur more readily in elderly women; the drug should be discontinued, the primary health care provider notified immediately, and treatment of adverse effects begun quickly.

Contraindications

The TCAs are contraindicated in patients with known hypersensitivity to the drugs. The TCAs are not given within 14 days of the MAOI antidepressants, to patients with a recent myocardial infarction, or to children or lactating mothers. These drugs are in pregnancy categories C and D, and the safety of their use during pregnancy has not been established. Doxepin is contraindicated in patients with glaucoma or in those with a tendency for urinary retention.

Precautions

The TCAs should be used cautiously in patients with cardiac disease, hepatic or renal impairment, hyperthyroid disease, history of seizure activity, narrow-angle glaucoma or increased intraocular pressure, urinary retention, and risk of suicidal ideation or behavior.

⚠ NURSING ALERT
The TCAs can cause cardiac-related adverse reactions, such as tachycardia and heart block. The nurse therefore gives these drugs with caution to the person with preexisting cardiac disease, and to the elderly.

Interactions

The following interactions may occur when a TCA is administered with another agent:

Interacting Drugs	Effect of Common Use	Interaction
sedatives, hypnotics, and analgesics	Sedation and pain relief, respectively	Increased risk of respiratory and nervous system depression
dicumarol	Blood thinner	Increased risk for bleeding
cimetidine	Treatment of gastric upset	Increased anticholinergic symptoms (dry mouth, urinary retention, blurred vision)
MAOIs	Antidepressant agents	Increased risk for hypertensive episodes, severe convulsions, and hyperpyretic episodes
adrenergic agents	Neuromuscular agents	Increased risk for arrhythmias and hypertension

● SELECTIVE SEROTONIN REUPTAKE INHIBITORS

Actions

The SSRIs inhibit CNS uptake of serotonin (a CNS neurotransmitter). The increase in serotonin levels is thought to act as a stimulant to reverse depression.

Uses

The SSRIs are used in the treatment of the following:

- Depressive episodes
- Obsessive-compulsive disorders
- Bulimia nervosa

Unlabeled uses include panic disorders; premenstrual syndrome and post-traumatic stress disorders; generalized anxiety and social phobias; Raynaud's disease; migraine headaches; diabetic neuropathy; and hot flashes. These drugs may be used with psychotherapy in severe cases.

Adverse Reactions

Neuromuscular System Reactions

- Somnolence, dizziness
- Headache, insomnia
- Tremor, weakness

Gastrointestinal and Genitourinary System Reactions

- Constipation, dry mouth, nausea
- Pharyngitis, runny nose, and abnormal ejaculation

Contraindications

The SSRIs are contraindicated in patients with a hypersensitivity to the drugs and during pregnancy (category C). Patients taking cisapride (Propulsid), pimozide (Orap), or carbamazepine (Tegretol) should not take fluoxetine (Prozac).

Precautions

The SSRI antidepressants should be used cautiously in patients with diabetes mellitus, cardiac disease, impaired liver or kidney function, and risk for suicidal ideation or behavior. Patients should not be switched to an SSRI antidepressant drug within 2 weeks of stopping an MAOI antidepressant.

Interactions

The following interactions may occur when an SSRI is administered with another agent:

Interacting Drugs	Common Use	Effect of Interaction
other antidepressants	Treatment of depression	Increased risk of toxic effects
cimetidine	Relief of gastric upset	Increased anticholinergic symptoms (dry mouth, urinary retention, blurred vision)
nonsteroidal anti-inflammatory drugs	Relief of inflammation and pain	Increased risk for GI bleeding
lithium (interaction with fluoxetine)	Treatment of bipolar disorder	Increased risk of lithium toxicity

Note that the effectiveness of fluoxetine is decreased in patients who smoke cigarettes during administration of the drug.

HERBAL ALERT

The SSRIs should not be administered with preparations containing St. John's wort because there is an increased risk for a severe sedative effect.

• MONOAMINE OXIDASE INHIBITORS

Actions

Drugs classified as MAOIs inhibit the activity of monoamine oxidase, a complex enzyme system responsible for inactivating certain neurotransmitters. Blocking monoamine oxidase results in an increase in endogenous epinephrine, norepinephrine, dopamine, and serotonin in the nervous system. An increase in these **neurohormones** (secreted rather than transmitted neurosubstances) stimulates the CNS. New drugs have been developed and MAOIs are typically not the first drugs chosen for treating depression.

Uses

The MAOI antidepressants are used in the treatment of depressive episodes, and may be used in conjunction with psychotherapy in severe cases. Unlabeled uses include bulimia, night terrors, migraine headaches, seasonal affective disorder, and multiple sclerosis.

Adverse Reactions

- Neuromuscular reactions include **orthostatic hypotension**, dizziness, vertigo, headache, and blurred vision.
- Gastrointestinal (GI) and genitourinary system reactions include constipation, dry mouth, nausea, diarrhea, and impotence.
- A serious adverse reaction associated with MAOIs is hypertensive crisis (extremely high blood pressure), which may occur when foods containing **tyramine** (an amino acid) are eaten (see Patient Teaching for Improved Patient Outcomes: Avoiding Drug–Food Interactions With MAOIs).

NURSING ALERT

One of the earliest symptoms of hypertensive crisis is headache (usually occipital), followed by a stiff or sore neck, nausea, vomiting, sweating, fever, chest pain, dilated pupils, and bradycardia or tachycardia. If a hypertensive crisis occurs, immediate medical intervention is necessary to reduce the blood pressure. Strokes (cerebrovascular accidents) and death have been reported.

occipital headache ... med emerg

Contraindications and Precautions

The MAOI antidepressants are contraindicated in the elderly and in patients with known hypersensitivity to the drugs, pheochromocytoma, liver and kidney disease, cerebrovascular disease, hypertension, history of headaches, or congestive heart failure. Safety has not been established for use in patients younger than 16 years or during pregnancy (category C) or lactation.

The MAOIs should be used cautiously in patients with impaired liver function, history of seizures, parkinsonian symptoms, diabetes, hyperthyroidism, or risk of suicidal

Peptic ulcer (handwritten)

Summary Drug Table ANTIDEPRESSANTS

Generic name	Trade Name	Uses	Adverse Reactions	Dosage Ranges
Tricyclic Antidepressants *TCA Bipolor, OCD, neuropathic pain, enurisis* (handwritten)				
amitriptyline am-ee-trip'-tih-leen		Depression, neuropathic pain, eating disorders	Sedation, anticholinergic effects (dry mouth, dry eyes, urinary retention), constipation	Up to 150 mg/day orally in divided doses; 20–30 mg IM QID; severely depressed hospitalized patient: up to 300 mg/day orally. Do not administer IV
amoxapine ah-mox'-ah-peen		Depression accompanied by anxiety	Same as amitriptyline	50 mg orally 2–3 times daily up to 300 mg/day, if poor response may go up to 600 mg/day
clomipramine kloe-mip'-rah-meen	Anafranil	Obsessive-compulsive disorder (OCD)	Same as amitriptyline, sexual dysfunction	25–250 mg/day orally in divided doses
desipramine de—sip'-rah-meen	Norpramin	Depression, eating disorders	Same as amitriptyline	100–200 mg/day orally, not to exceed 300 mg/day
doxepin dox'-eh-pin	Sinequan	Anxiety or depression, emotional symptoms accompanying organic disease	Same as amitriptyline	25–150 mg/day orally in divided doses
imipramine ih-mip'-rah-meen	Tofranil, Tofranil PM	Depression, enuresis, eating disorders	Same as amitriptyline	100–200 mg/day orally in divided doses Childhood enuresis (older than 6 yr): 25 mg/day, 1 hr before bedtime, not to exceed 2.5 mg/kg/day
mirtazapine mer-tah'-zah-peen	Remeron	Depression	Sedation, dry mouth, constipation, orthostatic hypotension	15–45 mg/day orally
nortriptyline nor-trip'-tih-leen	Aventyl, Pamelor	Depression, premenstrual symptoms	Same as amitriptyline	25 mg orally 3–4 times/day; not to exceed 150 mg/day
protriptyline proe-trip'-tih-leen	Vivactil	Depression, sleep apnea	Same as amitriptyline	15–40 mg/day orally in 3–4 doses, not to exceed 60 mg/day
trimipramine trye-mip'-rah-meen	Surmontil	Depression, peptic ulcer disease	Same as amitriptyline	75–150 mg/day orally in divided doses, not to exceed 300 mg/day
Selective Serotonin Reuptake Inhibitors *SSRI, OCD, Bulemia, with Migranes, PMS, Neoopath* (handwritten)				
citalopram sih-tal'-oh-pram	Celexa	Depression, panic disorder, posttraumatic stress disorder (PTSD), premenstrual disorder	Nausea, dry mouth, sweating, somnolence, insomnia, anorexia, diarrhea	20–40 mg/day orally
escitalopram es-sih-tal'-oh-pram	Lexapro	Depression, generalized anxiety disorder, panic disorder	Headache, insomnia, somnolence, nausea	10–20 mg/day orally
fluoxetine floo-ox'-eh-teen	Prozac, Prozac Weekly, Sarafem	Depression, bulimia, OCD, panic disorder, premenstrual dysphoric disorder (Sarafem only)	Anxiety, nervousness, somnolence, insomnia, drowsiness, asthenia, tremor, headache, nausea, diarrhea, constipation, dry mouth, anorexia	20 mg/day orally in the morning or up to 80 mg/day (dose split between morning and at noon)

diabetic (handwritten)

(table continues on page 197)

Summary Drug Table ANTIDEPRESSANTS (continued)

Generic name	Trade Name	Uses	Adverse Reactions	Dosage Ranges
fluvoxamine *floo-vox'-ah-meen*		OCD, depression	Headache, nervousness, somnolence, insomnia, nausea, diarrhea, dry mouth, constipation, dyspepsia, ejaculatory disturbances	50–300 mg/day orally in divided doses
paroxetine *par-ox'-eh-teen*	Paxil	Depression, OCD, panic disorder, general anxiety disorder, social anxiety disorder, PTSD	Headache, tremors, somnolence, nervousness, dizziness, insomnia, nausea, diarrhea, constipation, dry mouth, sweating, weakness, sexual dysfunction	20–50 mg/day orally
sertraline *sir'-trah-leen*	Zoloft	Depression, OCD, panic disorders, PTSD	Headache, drowsiness, anxiety, dizziness, insomnia, fatigue, nausea, diarrhea, dry mouth, ejaculatory disturbances, sweating	50–200 mg/day orally
Monoamine Oxidase Inhibitors				
phenelzine *fen'-el-zeen*	Nardil	Atypical depression	Orthostatic hypotension, vertigo, dizziness, nausea, constipation, dry mouth, diarrhea, headache, restlessness, blurred vision, hypertensive crisis	45–90 mg/day orally in divided doses
tranylcypromine *tran-ill-sip'-roe-meen*	Parnate	Atypical depression	Same as phenelzine	30–60 mg/day orally in divided doses
isocarboxazid *eye-so-car-box'-ah-zid*	Marplan	Depression	Same as phenelzine	10–40 mg/day orally
Atypical Antidepressant Drugs				
bupropion *byoo-proe'-pee-on*	Wellbutrin, Wellbutrin SR, Zyban (smoking cessation)	Depression, neuropathic pain, attention deficit hyperactivity disorder (ADHD), smoking cessation	Agitation, dizziness, dry mouth, insomnia, sedation, headache, nausea, vomiting, tremor, constipation, weight loss, anorexia, excess sweating	100–300 mg/day orally in divided doses; sustained release, 1 tablet BID orally
duloxetine *doo-lox'-eh-teen*	Cymbalta	Depression, diabetic peripheral neuropathy, fibromyalgia, stress incontinence	Insomnia, dry mouth, nausea, constipation	40–60 mg/day orally
maprotiline *mah-proe'-tih-leen*		Depression, anxiety associated with depression	Sedation, dry mouth, constipation, orthostatic hypotension	75–150 mg/day orally; for severe depression, dosage may increase to 225 mg/day orally
nefazodone *neh-faz'-oh-doan*		Depression	Somnolence, insomnia, dizziness, nausea, dry mouth, constipation, headache, weakness	200–600 mg/day orally in divided doses
trazodone *traz'-oh-doan*		Depression, alcohol craving	Drowsiness, dizziness, priapism, dry mouth, nausea, vomiting, constipation, fatigue, nervousness	150–400 mg/day orally in divided doses, not to exceed 600 mg/day
venlafaxine *ven-lah-fax'-een*	Effexor, Effexor XR	Depression, anxiety disorders, premenstrual disorder	Headache, insomnia, dizziness, nervousness, weakness, anorexia, nausea, constipation, dry mouth, somnolence, sweating	75–225 mg/day orally in divided doses

[handwritten margin note, left side: "Bad one"]

[handwritten note across Monoamine Oxidase Inhibitors row: "MAOI – Interact. ↓ MAOI   stop use 14 days"]

[vertical text, right margin: Antidepressant Drugs]

Patient Teaching for Improved Patient Outcomes

Avoiding Drug–Food Interactions With MAOIs

If your patients are taking MAOIs, they need to avoid foods containing tyramine. Otherwise they may experience a life-threatening reaction, hypertensive crisis. Be sure to instruct your patients to avoid the following foods:

✓ Aged cheese (e.g., blue, Camembert, cheddar, Emmenthaler, mozzarella, parmesan, Romano, Stilton, Swiss)
✓ Sour cream
✓ Yogurt
✓ Beef or chicken livers
✓ Pickled herring
✓ Fermented meats (e.g., bologna, pepperoni, salami, dried fish)
✓ Undistilled alcoholic beverages (e.g., imported beer, ale, red wine, especially Chianti and sherry)
✓ Caffeinated beverages (e.g., coffee, tea, colas)
✓ Chocolate
✓ Certain fruits and vegetables (e.g., avocado, bananas, fava beans, figs, raisins, sauerkraut)
✓ Yeast extracts
✓ Soy sauce

ideation or behavior. Individuals on MAOIs should not take decongestants without permission of their primary healthcare provider.

Interactions

The following interactions may occur when an MAOI antidepressant is administered with another agent (see Patient Teaching for Improved Patient Outcomes: Avoiding Drug–Food Interactions With MAOIs):

Interacting Drugs or Agent	Common Use	Effect of Interaction
sedatives, hypnotics, and analgesics	Sedation and pain relief, respectively	Increased risk for adverse reactions during surgery
thiazide diuretic	Relief of fluid retention	Increased hypotensive effects of the MAOI
meperidine	Pain relief	Increased risk for hypertensive episodes, severe convulsions, and hyperpyretic episodes
adrenergic agents	Neuromuscular agent	Increased risk for cardiac arrhythmias and hypertension
tyramine or tryptophan	Amino acids found in some foods	Hypertensive crisis, which may occur up to 2 weeks after the MAOI is discontinued
antitussives	Relieve cough	Hypotension, fever, nausea, jerking motions to the leg, and coma

• ATYPICAL ANTIDEPRESSANTS

Actions

The mechanism of action of most of the atypical antidepressants is not clearly understood. It is thought that they affect neurotransmission of serotonin, norepinephrine, and dopamine. Examples of this group of drugs include venlafaxine (Effexor) and bupropion (Wellbutrin).

Uses

Atypical antidepressant drugs may be used in conjunction with psychotherapy in severe cases or alone in the treatment of the following:
• Depressive episodes
• Depression accompanied by anxiety disorders
• Diabetic peripheral neuropathic pain
    Unlabeled uses include enhancing weight loss and treating aggressive behaviors, neuropathic pain, menstrual disorders, cocaine withdrawal and alcohol cravings, fibromyalgia, and stress incontinence.

Adverse Reactions

Neuromuscular System Reactions

• Somnolence, migraine headache
• Hypotension, dizziness, lightheadedness, and vertigo
• Blurred vision, photosensitivity, insomnia, nervousness or agitation, and tremor

Gastrointestinal System Reactions

• Nausea, dry mouth, anorexia, thirst
• Diarrhea, constipation, bitter taste

Other System Reactions

• Fatigue, tachycardia, and palpitations
• Change in libido, impotence
• Skin rash, itching, vasodilation resulting in flushing and excessive sweating

    Additional adverse reactions and adverse reactions associated with the use of all the antidepressant drugs are listed in the Summary Drug Table: Antidepressants.

Contraindications

The atypical antidepressant drugs are contraindicated in patients with known hypersensitivity to the drugs. Among the atypical antidepressants, bupropion and maprotiline are pregnancy category B drugs. Other miscellaneous antidepressants discussed in this chapter are in pregnancy category C. Safe use of the antidepressants during pregnancy has not been established. They should be used during pregnancy only when the potential benefits outweigh the potential hazards to the developing fetus. Maprotiline should not be used with patients who have a seizure disorder or during the acute phase of a myocardial infarction. Patients taking cisapride, pimozide, or carbamazepine should not take nefazodone because of risk for hepatic failure.

> **NURSING ALERT**
> The smoking cessation product Zyban is a form of the antidepressant drug bupropion. Smokers should not use Zyban if they are currently taking bupropion for management of depression, because of the possibility of bupropion overdose.

Precautions

Atypical antidepressants should be used cautiously in patients with cardiac disease, renal or hepatic impairment, hyperthyroid disease, or risk of suicidal ideation or behavior.

Interactions

The following interactions may occur when an atypical antidepressant is administered with another agent:

Interacting Drug	Common Use	Effect of Interaction
sedatives, hypnotics, and analgesics	Sedation and pain relief, respectively	Increased risk of respiratory and nervous system depression
warfarin	Anticoagulation (blood thinner)	Increased risk for bleeding
cimetidine	GI upset	Increased anticholinergic symptoms (dry mouth, urinary retention, blurred vision)
antihypertensive agents	Treatment of high blood pressure	Increased risk for hypotension
MAOIs	Antidepressant	Increased risk for hypertensive episodes, severe convulsions, and hyperpyretic episodes

> **HERBAL ALERT**
> Patients should be assessed for use of herbal preparations containing St. John's wort because of the potential for adverse reactions when taken with antidepressants.

NURSING PROCESS
PATIENT RECEIVING AN ANTIDEPRESSANT DRUG

ASSESSMENT

Preadministration Assessment
A patient receiving an antidepressant drug may be treated in the hospital or in an outpatient setting. Before starting therapy for the hospitalized patient, the nurse obtains a complete medical history. The nurse assesses the patient's mental status to determine the degree of depression and obtain a baseline for comparison with future assessments. The patient may report feelings of anxiety, worthlessness, guilt, helplessness, and hopeless-

ness. The nurse documents any subjective feelings as well as slowness to answer questions, a monotone speech pattern, and any sadness or crying.

The preadministration assessments of the outpatient are basically the same as those for the hospitalized patient. The nurse obtains a complete medical history and a history of the symptoms of depression from the patient, a family member, or the patient's hospital records. The nurse performs a physical assessment, which includes obtaining blood pressure measurements on both arms with the patient in a sitting position, pulse and respiratory rate, and weight.

During the initial interview, the nurse observes the patient for symptoms of depression and the potential for suicide. It is important for the nurse to note the presence of suicidal thoughts. The nurse accurately documents in the patient's record and reports to the primary health care provider any statements concerning suicide and the ability of the patient to carry out any suicidal intentions. If the patient does make statements about suicide, the nurse must ask about intent using simple, straightforward questions.

Ongoing Assessment
The nurse monitors vital signs at least daily as part of the ongoing assessment. The vital signs are monitored more frequently if the drug used is one that carries the risk for a hypertensive or hypotensive adverse reaction. The nurse reports any significant change in the vital signs to the primary health care provider.

OUTPATIENT ASSESSMENT. Ultimately, the hospitalized patient may be discharged from the acute care setting. Some patients, such as those with mild depression, do not require inpatient care. These patients are usually seen at periodic intervals in the primary health care provider's office or in a mental health outpatient setting.

At the time of each visit to the primary health care provider or clinic, the nurse observes the patient for a response to therapy. In some instances, the nurse may question the patient or a family member about the response to therapy. The type of questions asked depends on the patient and the diagnosis and may include questions such as:

- How are you feeling?
- How would you describe your depressed feelings?
- How would you rate your depression?
- Would you like to tell me how everything is going?

The nurse may need to rephrase questions or direct conversation toward other subjects until the patient feels comfortable and can discuss therapy. The nurse should ask the patient or a family member about adverse drug reactions or any other problems occurring during therapy, because it is important to bring these reactions or problems to the attention of the primary health care provider. The nurse documents in the patient's record a general summary of the patient's outward behavior and any complaints or problems and compares these notations with previous notations and observations.

NURSING DIAGNOSES

Drug-specific nursing diagnoses are the following:

❏ **Self-Care Deficit Syndrome** related to inability to participate in activities of daily living secondary to somnolence, drowsiness, and depressive state

❏ **Disturbed Sleep Pattern** related to depression, and excessive drowsiness

❏ **Imbalanced Nutrition: Less Than Body Requirements** related to anorexia, constipation, and depression

❏ **Risk for Suicide** related to suicidal ideation and adverse reaction to antidepressive drug

❏ **Acute Pain** related to **priapism**

Nursing diagnoses related to drug administration are discussed in Chapter 4.

PLANNING

The expected outcomes of the patient depend on the reason for administration of an antidepressant, but may include an optimal response to drug therapy, support of patient needs related to the management of adverse drug reactions, and an understanding the therapeutic regimen.

IMPLEMENTATION

Promoting an Optimal Response to Therapy

Response to antidepressant medications is not rapid. It can take a number of weeks for the drugs to take effect. Fluoxetine is an example of a drug that may take as long as 4 weeks to attain a full therapeutic effect. Some adverse reactions, such as dry mouth, episodes of orthostatic hypotension, and drowsiness, appear long before the intended effect of the antidepressant. The inability to deal with the unpleasantness of these adverse reactions is one of the greatest reasons patients stop taking antidepressants. The two adverse reactions that patients have the most trouble tolerating are somnolence and dry mouth. During initial therapy or whenever the dosage is increased or decreased, the nurse observes the patient closely for adverse drug reactions and any behavioral changes. The nurse reports to the primary health care provider any change in behavior or the appearance of adverse reactions because a further increase or decrease in dosage may be necessary or use of the drug may need to be discontinued.

When caring for hospitalized patients with depression, the nurse must develop a nursing care plan to meet the patient's individual needs. When the antidepressants are given parenterally, the nurse gives these drugs intramuscularly (IM) in a large muscle mass, such as the gluteus muscle. The nurse keeps the patient lying down (when possible) for about 30 minutes after administering the drug.

Monitoring and Managing Patient Needs

SELF-CARE DEFICIT SYNDROME. Initially, the patient may need assistance with self-care, because patients with depression often do not have the physical or emotional energy to perform self-care activities. This is complicated by the fact that many antidepressants cause excessive drowsiness during the initial stages of treatment, and patients may need assistance with ambulation and self-care activities. These problems usually subside as the depression lifts and tolerance to the adverse reactions builds with continued use of the antidepressant. To minimize the risk for injury, the nurse assists the patient when necessary and makes the environment as safe as possible. When orthostatic hypotension is an effect of drug therapy, the nurse instructs the patient to rise from a lying position to a sitting position. The patient remains in a sitting position for a few minutes before rising to a standing position. Position changes are made slowly, with the nurse at the bedside to offer assistance if necessary.

If the patient has a difficult time with self-care because of the depression or sedative effects of the antidepressants, the nurse provides total assistance with activities of daily living, including help with eating, dressing, and ambulating. However, the nurse encourages self-care, whenever possible, allowing sufficient time for the patient to accomplish tasks to the fullest extent of his or her ability. It is important for the nurse to provide positive feedback when appropriate. As a therapeutic effect of the drug is attained, the patient will be able to resume self-care (if no other physical conditions interfere).

The nurse writes behavioral records at periodic intervals, the frequency of which depends on hospital or unit guidelines. An accurate assessment of the patient's behavior aids the primary health care provider in planning therapy and thus becomes an important part of nursing management. Patients with a poor response to drug therapy may require dosage changes, a change to another antidepressant drug, or the addition of other therapies to the treatment regimen.

DISTURBED SLEEP PATTERN. Many of the antidepressant drugs cause somnolence. This adverse reaction is one of the greatest reasons patients stop taking the medication. When the nurse administers the drug at night, the sedative effects promote sleep, and the adverse reactions appear less troublesome. An exception to this is the SSRIs; it is best to administer those medications in the morning.

The nurse should assess the environment to help promote sleep at night and wakefulness during the day. Drapes should be shut at night and opened in the day to let in light, and clocks should be available for the patient to see the time of day. These activities will help the patient to reorient to daytime and nighttime, thereby promoting an effective sleep pattern.

IMBALANCED NUTRITION: LESS THAN BODY REQUIREMENTS. Depressed patients may not feel like eating; therefore, they lose weight. This can be potentiated by the adverse reactions of anorexia and constipation. The nurse monitors dietary intake and helps the dietitian in providing nutritious meals, taking into consideration foods that the patient likes and dislikes. Fluid intake and foods high in fiber are important for the patient to prevent constipation. Weighing the patient weekly is important for monitoring weight loss or gain. To minimize the dry mouth that frequently accompanies administration of antidepressants, the nurse provides good oral hygiene, frequent sips of fluids, and sugarless gum or hard candy.

Patients receiving MAOIs require strict dietary control because foods containing tyramine should not be eaten. The nurse asks family members and visitors not to bring food to the patient and explains why this is important. When an MAOI is prescribed, it is critical that the nurse give the patient a list of foods containing tyramine and to emphasize the importance of not eating foods on the list. If the patient has trouble understanding this dietary restriction, it may be necessary to observe the patient closely when eating in a community setting to be sure food is not taken or accepted from other patients.

LIFESPAN ALERT – Pediatric
Studies show that children and adolescents with major depressive disorders have an increased risk of suicidal ideation when prescribed antidepressant medications.

RISK FOR SUICIDE. Patients with a high suicide potential require a well-supervised environment and protection from suicidal acts. For patients with severe depression, suicide precautions are important until a therapeutic effect is achieved. When the patient is hospitalized, policies of observation must be strictly followed for the patient's protection.

Of greatest concern to the nurse is the depressed patient who has suicidal ideation, but has not been identified as such. Patients in a depressive state may lack the energy to carry out plans for ending their own life. Because the full therapeutic effect of the antidepressant may not be attained for 10 days to 4 weeks, patients have time to gain enough energy to carry out an injurious act upon themselves. Patients with suicidal tendencies must be monitored closely. Report any expressions of guilt, hopelessness, or helplessness, insomnia, weight loss, and direct or indirect threats of suicide.

Oral administration requires great care because some patients have difficulty swallowing (e.g., because of a dry mouth). After administration of an oral drug, the nurse inspects the patient's oral cavity to be sure the drug has been swallowed. If the patient resists having his or her oral cavity checked, the nurse reports this refusal to the primary health care provider. Patients planning suicide may try to keep the drug on the side of the mouth or under the tongue and not swallow in an effort to hoard or save enough of the drug to commit suicide at a later time. Other patients may refuse to take the drug. If the patient refuses to take the drug, the nurse contacts the primary health care provider regarding this problem because parenteral administration of the drug may be necessary.

LIFESPAN ALERT – Gerontology
Older men with prostatic enlargement are at increased risk for urinary retention when they take tricyclic antidepressants.

ACUTE PAIN. An uncommon but potentially serious adverse reaction of trazodone is priapism (a persistent erection of the penis). This can be very painful and if not treated within a few hours, priapism can result in impotence. Because this can be an embarrassing adverse reaction, the nurse needs to instruct the patient to report any prolonged or inappropriate penile erection. The drug is discontinued immediately and the primary care provider notified. Injection of alpha-adrenergic stimulants (e.g., norepinephrine) may be helpful in treating priapism. In some cases, surgical intervention may be required.

Educating the Patient and Family
Once some patients are discharged to the home setting, noncompliance with drug therapy is a problem, because of unpleasant adverse drug effects. It is very important that the nurse educate the patient or family members thoroughly about the importance of managing the reactions so that the patient will continue the proper drug regimen. The nurse evaluates the patient's ability to assume responsibility for taking drugs at home (see Patient Teaching for Improved Patient Outcomes: Empowering Patient Responsibility for Antidepressant Drug Therapy). The administration of antidepressant drugs becomes a family responsibility if the outpatient appears to be unable to manage his or her own drug therapy.

The nurse explains any adverse reactions that may occur with a specific antidepressant drug and encourages the patient or family member to contact the primary health care provider immediately if a serious drug reaction occurs. The nurse includes the following points in a teaching plan for the patient or family member:

- Inform the primary health care provider, dentist, and other medical personnel of therapy with this drug.
- If dizziness occurs when changing position, rise slowly when getting out of bed or a chair. If dizziness is severe, always have help when changing positions.
- Relieve dry mouth by taking frequent sips of water, sucking on hard candy, or chewing gum (preferably sugarless gum).
- Keep all clinic appointments or appointments with the primary health care provider because close monitoring of therapy is essential.
- Do not take the antidepressants during pregnancy. Notify the primary health care provider if you are pregnant or wish to become pregnant.
- Report any unusual changes or physical effects to the primary health care provider.
- Avoid prolonged exposure to sunlight or sunlamps because an exaggerated reaction to the ultraviolet light may occur (photosensitivity), resulting in a burn.
- For male patients who take trazodone and who experience prolonged, inappropriate, and painful erections, stop taking the drug and notify the primary care provider.

EVALUATION

- Therapeutic response is achieved and the depressive mood is improved.
- Adverse reactions are identified, reported to the primary health care provider, and managed successfully through appropriate nursing interventions:
  - ☑ Patient resumes ability to care for self.
  - ☑ Patient reports fewer episodes of inappropriate sleep patterns.
  - ☑ Patient maintains an adequate nutritional status.
  - ☑ Patient does not attempt suicide.
  - ☑ Patient is free of pain.
- Patient and family demonstrate an understanding of the drug regimen.

Patient Teaching for Improved Patient Outcomes

Empowering Patient Responsibility for Antidepressant Drug Therapy

The nurse:

✓ Explains the reason for drug therapy, including the type of antidepressant prescribed, drug name, dosage, and frequency of administration.

✓ Enlists the aid of family members to ensure compliance with therapy, including checking patient's oral cavity to be sure drug has been swallowed.

✓ Urges the patient to take the drug exactly as prescribed and not to increase or decrease dosage, omit doses, or discontinue use of the drug unless directed to do so by health care provider.

✓ Advises that full therapeutic effect may not occur for several weeks.

✓ Instructs in signs and symptoms of behavioral changes indicative of therapeutic effectiveness or increasing depression and suicidal tendencies.

✓ Reviews measures to reduce the risk for suicide.

✓ Instructs about possible adverse reactions with instructions to notify health care provider should any occur.

✓ Reinforces safety measures such as changing positions slowly and avoiding driving or hazardous tasks.

✓ Advises avoidance of alcohol and use of nonprescription drugs unless use is approved by health care provider.

✓ Encourages patient to inform other health care providers and medical personnel about drug therapy regimen.

✓ Instructs in measures to minimize dry mouth.

✓ Emphasizes importance of avoiding foods containing tyramine (if MAOIs are prescribed) and provides written list of foods to avoid.

✓ Reassures results of therapy will be monitored by periodic laboratory tests and follow-up visits with the health care provider.

✓ Assists with arrangements for follow-up visits.

THINK CRITICALLY: PHARMACOLOGY IN PRACTICE

1. Mr. Phillip has been severely depressed for about 2 months, following the death of his wife in a car accident. Two weeks ago, the primary care provider prescribed amitriptyline 30 mg orally daily. His family is concerned because he is still depressed. Mr. Phillip's daughter is concerned because he feels drowsy and can't seem to get up until 11 AM or noon on most days. They are requesting that the dosage be increased. Discuss what information you will give Mr. Phillip and his family and what assessments you can make. How might this drug be interacting with other drugs prescribed in earlier chapters of this unit?

● Test Your Knowledge

1. When administering an antidepressant to a patient contemplating suicide, it is most important for the nurse to _____.

   A. have the patient remain upright for at least 30 minutes after taking the antidepressant
   B. assess the patient in 30 minutes for a therapeutic response to the drug
   C. monitor the patient for an occipital headache
   D. inspect the patient's oral cavity to be sure the drug was swallowed

2. Which of the following adverse reactions would the nurse expect to find in a patient taking amitriptyline?

   A. Constipation and abdominal cramps
   B. Bradycardia and double vision
   C. Sedation and dry mouth
   D. Polyuria and hypotension

3. Clinical depression is suspected in which of the following patients?

   A. Woman who is crying about her mastectomy performed yesterday
   B. Line worker who lost his job in a manufacturing plant 3 months ago
   C. Person diagnosed with hypothyroidism
   D. Child who had a parent commit suicide

4. Which of the following antidepressants would be most likely to cause the patient to have a seizure?

   A. amitriptyline
   B. bupropion
   C. sertraline
   D. venlafaxine

● Prepare for the NCLEX

1. The nurse instructs the patient taking a MAOI not to eat foods containing _____.

   A. glutamine
   B. sugar
   C. tyramine
   D. large amounts of iron

● Calculate Medication Dosages

1. The primary care provider prescribes trazodone 150 mg orally. Available are 50-mg tablets. The nurse administers _____.

2. The primary care provider prescribes oral paroxetine (Paxil) 50 mg/day. The drug is available as oral suspension with a strength of 10 mg/5 mL. The nurse administers _____.

To check your answers, see Appendix E.

the**Point** *For more NCLEX questions, log on to http://thepoint.lww.com to access more than 1000 questions.*

Antipsychotic Drugs

A
ntipsychotic drugs are administered to patients experiencing a psychotic disorder. The term *psychosis* refers to a group of symptoms that affect mood and behavior. **Hallucinations** (false sensations or perceptions having no basis in reality) or **delusions** (false beliefs that cannot be changed with reason) are usually present. Other symptoms include disorganized speech, behavior disturbance, social withdrawal, **flattened affect** (absence of an emotional response to any situation or condition), and **anhedonia** (finding no pleasure in activities that are normally pleasurable).

Although lithium is not a true antipsychotic drug, it is grouped with the antipsychotics because of its use in regulating the severe fluctuations of the manic phase of **bipolar disorder** (a psychiatric disorder characterized by severe mood swings from extreme hyperactivity to depression). During the manic phase, the person experiences altered thought processes, which can lead to bizarre delusions. The drug

diminishes the frequency and intensity of hyperactive (manic) episodes.

Actions

Antipsychotic drugs are thought to act by inhibiting or blocking the release of the neurotransmitter dopamine in the brain and possibly increasing the firing of nerve cells in certain areas of the brain. These effects may be responsible for the ability of these drugs to suppress the symptoms of certain psychotic disorders. Because these drugs block dopamine transmission, they also produce unpleasant extrapyramidal effects (see Adverse Reactions). Examples of antipsychotic drugs include chlorpromazine (Thorazine), haloperidol (Haldol), and fluphenazine (Prolixin).

Another group of antipsychotic drugs is classified as atypical antipsychotics. It is believed they act on serotonin receptors as well as on the dopamine receptors in the brain. They are termed *atypical* because the typical extrapyramidal side effects are lessened. Examples of the atypical antipsychotic drugs include clozapine (Clozaril) and aripiprazole (Abilify). The Summary Drug Table: Antipsychotic Drugs gives a more complete listing of the antipsychotic drugs.

Uses

The antipsychotic drugs are used in the treatment of the following:

- Acute and chronic psychoses, such as schizophrenia
- Bipolar (manic-depressive) illness
- Agitated behaviors associated with dementia

Selected drugs may be used for their adverse effects to treat minor conditions; for example, chlorpromazine may be used to treat uncontrollable hiccoughs, and chlorpromazine and prochlorperazine (Compazine) are used as antiemetics.

Special Considerations: Lithium

Lithium carbonate is rapidly absorbed after oral administration. The most common adverse reactions include tremors, nausea, vomiting, thirst, and polyuria. Toxic reactions may occur when serum lithium levels are greater than 1.5 mEq/L (Table 23.1). Because some of these toxic reactions are potentially serious, lithium blood level measurements are usually obtained during therapy, and the dosage of lithium is adjusted accordingly.

EPS - group of Adv. Reac.

Summary Drug Table ANTIPSYCHOTIC DRUGS

Generic Name	Trade Name	Uses	Adverse Reactions	Dosage Ranges
Manic drugs				
lithium *lith'-ee-um* have to get labs 1.5 is toxic	Eskalith, Lithobid	Manic episodes of bipolar disorder	Headache, drowsiness, tremors, nausea, polyuria (see Table 23.1) ↑ intensity of Pyshocot	Based on lithium serum levels; average dose range is 900–1800 mg/day orally in divided doses
Typical Antipsychotics				
chlorpromazine *klor-proe'-mah-zeen*	Thorazine	Psychotic disorders, nausea, vomiting, intractable hiccups	Hypotension, drowsiness, TD, nasal congestion, dry mouth, dystonia, EPS, behavioral changes, photosensitivity	Psychiatric disorders: up to 400 mg/day orally in divided doses Nausea and vomiting: 10–25 mg orally, 25–50 mg IM, 50–100 mg rectally
fluphenazine *floo-fen'-ah-zeen*	Prolixin	Psychotic disorders	Drowsiness, tachycardia, EPS, dystonia, akathisia, hypotension	0.5–10 mg/day orally in divided doses, up to 20 mg/day; 1.25–10 mg/day IM in divided doses
haloperidol *hay-loe-per'-ih-dole*	Haldol	Psychotic disorders; Tourette's syndrome, hyperactivity, behavior problems in children	EPS, akathisia, dystonia, TD, drowsiness, headache, dry mouth, orthostatic hypotension	0.5–5 mg orally BID or TID with dosage up to 100 mg/day in divided doses; 2–5 mg IM Children 0.05–0.075 mg/kg/day orally
loxapine *lox'-ah-peen*	Loxitane	Psychotic disorders	EPS, akathisia, dystonia, TD, drowsiness, headache, dry mouth, orthostatic hypotension	10–100 mg/day orally, not to exceed 250 mg/day
molindone *moe-lin'-doan*	Moban	Schizophrenia	EPS, drowsiness, increased libido, TD, rash, nausea, dry mouth, constipation	50–100 mg/day orally in divided doses
perphenazine *per-fen'-ah-zeen*		Psychotic disorders	Hypotension, postural hypotension, TD, photophobia, urticaria, nasal congestion, dry mouth, akathisia, dystonia, pseudoparkinsonism, behavioral changes, headache, photosensitivity	4–16 mg orally 2–4 times/day
pimozide *pih'-moe-zyde*	Orap	Tourette's syndrome	Parkinson-like symptoms, motor restlessness, dystonia, oculogyric crisis, TD, dry mouth, diarrhea, headache, rash, drowsiness	Initial dose: 1–2 mg/day orally Maintenance dose: up to 10 mg/day orally
prochlorperazine *proe-klor-per'-ah-zeen*	Compazine	Psychotic disorders, nausea, vomiting, anxiety	EPS, sedation, TD, dry eyes, blurred vision, constipation, dry mouth, photosensitivity	Psychotic disorders: up to 150 mg orally, 10–20 mg IM Nausea, vomiting: 15–40 mg/day orally in divided doses Anxiety: 5 mg orally TID
promazine *proe'-mah-zeen*	Sparine	Psychotic disorders	Drowsiness, EPS, dystonia, akathisia, hypotension	10–200 mg orally, IM q 4–6 hr
thioridazine *thee-oh-rid'-ah-zeen*		Schizophrenia	Cardiac arrhythmias, drowsiness, TD, nausea, dry mouth, constipation, diarrhea	50–100 mg orally TID, not to exceed 800 mg/day

(table continues on page 206)

Antipsychotic Drugs

Dementia

Summary Drug Table ANTIPSYCHOTIC DRUGS (continued)

Generic Name	Trade Name	Uses	Adverse Reactions	Dosage Ranges
thiothixene *thye-oh-thick'-seen*	Navane	Schizophrenia	EPS, drowsiness, nausea, diarrhea, TD	6–30 mg/day orally, not to exceed 60 mg/day
trifluoperazine *trye-floo-oh-per'-ah-zeen*		Psychotic disorders, anxiety	Drowsiness, pseudoparkinsonism, dystonia, akathisia, TD, photophobia, blurred vision, dry mouth, salivation, nasal congestion, nausea, discolored urine (pink to red-brown)	Psychosis: 4–20 mg/day orally in divided doses; Anxiety: 1–2 mg orally BID
Atypical Antipsychotics				
aripiprazole *ay-ri-pip'-rah-zoll*	Abilify	Psychotic disorders	Agitation, akathisia, anxiety, drowsiness, headache, constipation, dry mouth, nausea	10–30 mg/day orally
clozapine *kloe'-zah-peen*	Clozaril, Fazaclo	Severely ill schizophrenic patients with no response to other therapies	Drowsiness, sedation, akathisia, tachycardia, nausea, agranulocytosis	Initial dose: 25–50 mg/day, titrate up to 300–400 mg/day orally, not to exceed 900 mg/day
olanzapine *oh-lan'-zah-peen*	Zyprexa	Schizophrenia, short-term treatment of manic episodes of bipolar disorder	Agitation, dizziness, nervousness, akathisia, constipation, fever, weight gain	5–20 mg/day orally
olanzapine/fluoxetine *oh-lan'-zah-peen* *floo-ox'-eh-teen*	Symbyax	Bipolar depressive episodes	Same as olanzapine	6-mg/25-mg combination tablet taken in the evening orally
paliperidone *pal-ee-per'-ih-doan*	Invega	Psychotic disorders	Dizziness, weakness, headache, dry mouth, increased saliva, weight gain, stomach pain	6–12 mg/day orally
quetiapine *kweh-tye'-ah-pyne*	Seroquel	Psychotic disorders, manic episodes of bipolar disorder	Orthostatic hypotension, dizziness, vertigo, nausea, constipation, dry mouth diarrhea, headache, restlessness, blurred vision	150–750 mg/day orally in divided doses
risperidone *ris-per'-ih-doan*	Risperdal	Psychotic disorders; adolescent schizophrenia and mania	Agitation, dizziness, nervousness, akathisia, constipation, fever, weight gain	1–3 mg orally BID; adolescents: 0.5 – 6 mg orally once daily
ziprasidone *zih-pray'-sih-doan*	Geodon	Schizophrenia, bipolar mania, acute agitation	Somnolence, drowsiness, sedation, headache, arrhythmias, dyspepsia, fever, constipation, EPS	80 mg orally BID

Adverse Reactions

Generalized System Reactions

- Sedation, headache, hypotension
- Dry mouth, nasal congestion
- Urticaria, **photophobia** (intolerance to light), **photosensitivity** (abnormal sensitivity when exposed to light). Photosensitivity can result in severe sunburn when patients taking antipsychotic drugs are exposed to the sun or ultraviolet light, such as a tanning bed.

Behavioral Changes

- Possible increase in the intensity of the psychotic symptoms
- Lethargy, hyperactivity, paranoid reactions, agitation, and confusion

A decrease in dosage may eliminate some of these symptoms, but it also may be necessary to try another drug. Changes in psychotic behaviors may not be seen for days or weeks, although adverse reactions affecting the patient's ability to feel or move may occur before then. Patients may independently stop using the drug because of the unpleasantness

Table 23.1 Lithium Toxicity	
Serum Lithium Level	**Signs of Toxicity**
1.5–2 mEq/L	Diarrhea, vomiting, nausea, drowsiness, muscular weakness, lack of coordination (early signs of toxicity)
2–3 mEq/L	Giddiness, ataxia, blurred vision, tinnitus, vertigo, increasing confusion, slurred speech, blackouts, myoclonic twitching or movement of entire limbs, choreoathetoid movements, urinary or fecal incontinence, agitation or manic-like behavior, hyperreflexia, hypertonia, dysarthria
More than 3 mEq/L	May produce a complex clinical picture involving multiple organs and organ systems, including seizures (generalized and focal), arrhythmias, hypotension, peripheral vascular collapse, stupor, muscle group twitching, spasticity, coma

of the reactions, thus causing the psychotic symptoms to return. It is important for the nurse to monitor for these conditions and notify the primary health care provider immediately. Three of the more serious motor syndromes are described in the following sections.

Extrapyramidal Syndrome

Among the most significant adverse reactions associated with the antipsychotic drugs are the extrapyramidal effects. The term **extrapyramidal syndrome** (EPS) refers to a group of adverse reactions affecting the extrapyramidal portion of the nervous system as a result of antipsychotic drugs. This part of the nervous system affects body posture and promotes smooth and uninterrupted movement of various muscle groups. Antipsychotics disturb the function of the extrapyramidal portion of the nervous system, causing abnormal muscle movement. Extrapyramidal effects include Parkinson-like symptoms, **akathisia**, and **dystonia** (Display 23.1). Extrapyramidal effects usually diminish with a reduction in the dosage of the antipsychotic drug. Typically, the primary health care provider prescribes an antiparkinsonism drug, such as benztropine (see Chapter 29), to reduce the incidence of Parkinson-like symptoms.

Tardive Dyskinesia

Tardive dyskinesia (TD) is a syndrome consisting of irreversible, involuntary dyskinetic movements. TD is characterized by rhythmic, involuntary movements of the tongue, face, mouth, or jaw and sometimes the extremities. The tongue may protrude, and there may be chewing movements, puckering of the mouth, and facial grimacing. TD is a late-appearing reaction and may be observed in patients receiving an antipsychotic drug or after discontinuation of antipsychotic drug therapy. Because TD is nonreversible, drug

DISPLAY 23.1 Extrapyramidal Syndrome

- Parkinson-like symptoms—fine tremors, muscle rigidity, masklike appearance of the face, slowness of movement, slurred speech, and unsteady gait
- Akathisia—extreme restlessness and increased motor activity
- Dystonia—facial grimacing and twisting of the neck into unnatural positions

therapy must be discontinued when symptoms occur during the course of therapy. Because of the risk of TD, it is best to use the smallest dose and the shortest duration of treatment that produces a satisfactory clinical response. The use of atypical antipsychotic drugs has increased because they are less likely to cause TD effects.

Neuroleptic Malignant Syndrome

Neuroleptic malignant syndrome (NMS) is a rare reaction characterized by a combination of extrapyramidal effects, hyperthermia, and autonomic disturbance. It typically occurs within 1 month after the antipsychotic drug regimen is begun. NMS is potentially fatal and requires intensive symptomatic treatment and immediate discontinuation of the drug causing the syndrome. Once the antipsychotic drug is discontinued, recovery occurs within 7 to 10 days.

Contraindications

Antipsychotics are contraindicated in patients with known hypersensitivity to the drugs, in comatose patients, and in those who are severely depressed, have bone marrow depression, blood dyscrasias, Parkinson's disease (specifically, haloperidol), liver impairment, coronary artery disease, or severe hypotension or hypertension.

Antipsychotic drugs are classified as pregnancy category C drugs (except for clozapine, which is pregnancy category B). Safe use of these drugs during pregnancy and lactation has not been clearly established. Antipsychotics should be used only when clearly needed and when the potential benefit outweighs any potential harm to the fetus.

Lithium is contraindicated in patients with hypersensitivity to tartrazine, renal or cardiovascular disease, sodium depletion, and dehydration, and in patients receiving diuretics. Lithium is a pregnancy category D drug and is contraindicated during pregnancy and lactation. For women of childbearing age, contraceptives may be prescribed while they are taking lithium.

Precautions

Antipsychotic drugs are used cautiously in patients with respiratory disorders, glaucoma, prostatic hypertrophy, epilepsy, decreased renal function, and peptic ulcer disease.

Antipsychotic Drugs

LIFESPAN ALERT – Gerontology

Because drug metabolism and excretion are altered in elderly or debilitated patients, doses may be instituted at one-half to one-third the recommended dose for younger adults and increased more gradually than in younger adults.

Lithium is monitored carefully in patients who sweat profusely, experience diarrhea or vomiting, or who have an infection or fever causing fluid loss.

Interactions

The following interactions may occur when an antipsychotic is administered with another agent:

Interacting Drug	Common Use	Effect of Interaction
anticholinergic drugs	Management of gastrointestinal (GI) problems such as peptic ulcer disease	Increased risk for TD and psychotic symptoms
immunologic drugs	Treatment of chronic illness such as cancer, arthritis, human immunodeficiency virus (HIV) infection	Increased severity of bone marrow suppression
antacids	Relief of GI upset, heartburn	Decreased effectiveness of lithium
loop diuretics	Management of cardiac problems	Increased risk for lithium toxicity
lithium combined with other antipsychotics	Management of psychotic symptoms	Increased risk for lithium toxicity
alcohol	Relaxation and enjoyment in social situations	Increased risk for central nervous system depression

NURSING PROCESS

PATIENT RECEIVING AN ANTIPSYCHOTIC DRUG

ASSESSMENT

Preadministration Assessment

A patient receiving an antipsychotic drug may be treated in the hospital or in an outpatient setting. The nurse assesses the patient's mental status before and periodically throughout therapy. The nurse must note the presence of hallucinations or delusions and document them accurately in the patient's record.

Before starting therapy for the hospitalized patient, the nurse obtains a complete mental health, social, and medical history. In the case of psychosis, patients often are unable to give a reliable history of their illness. When available, the nurse obtains the mental health history from a family member or friend. As the history is taken, the nurse observes the patient for any behavior patterns that appear to be deviations from normal. Examples of deviations include poor eye contact, failure to answer questions completely, inappropriate answers to questions, a monotone speech pattern, and inappropriate laughter, sadness, or crying.

During the initial assessment, the nurse may need to rely more on observation of the patient than actual physical assessment. Ideally, assessment should include obtaining blood pressure, pulse, respiratory rate, and weight. The patient may react violently due to fear caused by the psychosis; therefore, touching can be perceived by the patient as a threatening gesture and should be avoided.

Some patients, such as those with mild schizophrenia, do not require inpatient care. The nurse usually sees these patients at periodic intervals in the mental health outpatient setting. The initial assessments of the outpatient are basically the same as those for the hospitalized patient. The nurse obtains a complete medical history and a history of the symptoms of the mental disorder from the patient, a family member, or the patient's hospital records. During the initial interview, the nurse observes the patient for what appear to be deviations from a normal behavior pattern. The nurse also should assess the patient's vital signs and body weight.

Ongoing Assessment

Many antipsychotic drugs are administered for a long time, which makes the ongoing assessment an important part of determining therapeutic drug effects and monitoring for adverse reactions, particularly EPS (see Display 23.1) and TD. The role of the nurse is important in the administration of these drugs both in the inpatient and clinic settings for the following reasons:

- The patient's response to drug therapy on an inpatient basis requires around-the-clock assessments, because frequent dosage adjustments may be necessary during therapy.
- Accurate assessments for the appearance of adverse drug effects assume a greater importance when the patient may be unable to verbalize physical changes to the primary health care provider or nurse.

NURSING DIAGNOSES

Drug-specific nursing diagnoses are the following:

- ❏ **Risk for Injury** related to hypotension or sedation
- ❏ **Impaired Physical Mobility** related to impaired motor ability
- ❏ **Risk for Infection** related to **agranulocytosis**
- ❏ **Imbalanced Fluid Volume** related to lithium toxicity

Nursing diagnoses related to drug administration are discussed in Chapter 4.

PLANNING

The expected outcomes for the patient depend on the reason for drug administration, but may include an optimal response to drug therapy, meeting of patient needs related

Baselines on every thing
LABS
Family History = involvement - vi for compliance

to management of adverse drug reactions, an absence of injury, and understanding of the therapeutic regimen.

IMPLEMENTATION

Promoting an Optimal Response to Therapy

The nurse develops a nursing care plan to meet the patient's individual needs.

MANAGING CARE OF THE INPATIENT. Behavioral records should be written at periodic intervals (frequency depends on hospital or unit guidelines). An accurate description of the patient's behavior aids the primary health care provider in planning therapy and thus becomes an important part of nursing management. Patients with a poor response to drug therapy may require dosage changes, a change to another psychotherapeutic drug, or the addition of other therapies to the treatment regimen. However, it is important for the nurse to know that full response to antipsychotic drugs takes several weeks.

If the patient's behavior is violent or aggressive, antipsychotic drugs may have to be given parenterally. The nurse may require assistance in securing the patient and should give the drugs intramuscularly (IM) in a large muscle mass, such as the gluteus muscle. The nurse keeps the patient lying down (when possible) for about 30 minutes after administering the drug.

NURSING ALERT

In combative patients or those who have serious manifestations of acute psychosis (e.g., hallucinations or loss of contact with reality), parenteral administration may be repeated every 1 to 4 hours until the desired effects are obtained. The nurse monitors the patient closely for cardiac arrhythmias or rhythm changes, or hypotension.

The nurse may give antipsychotic drugs orally as a single daily dose or in divided doses several times a day. Oral administration, especially in the long-term care setting, requires great care, because some patients have difficulty swallowing (because of a dry mouth or other causes). After administration of an oral drug, the nurse inspects the patient's oral cavity to be sure the drug has been swallowed. If the patient resists having his or her oral cavity checked, the nurse reports this refusal to the primary health care provider.

Other patients may refuse to take the drug altogether. The nurse should never force a patient to take an oral drug. If the patient refuses the drug, the nurse contacts the primary health care provider regarding this problem because parenteral administration of the medication may be necessary.

Oral liquid concentrates are available for patients who can more easily swallow a liquid. To aid in administration to debilitated or elderly patients, oral drugs can be mixed in liquids such as fruit juices, tomato juice, milk, or carbonated beverages. Semisolid foods, such as soups or puddings, may also be used.

MANAGING CARE OF THE OUTPATIENT. At the time of each visit of the patient to the primary health care provider's office or clinic, the nurse observes the patient for a response to therapy. In some instances, the nurse may question the patient or a family member about the response to therapy. The questions asked depend on the patient and the diagnosis, and may include questions such as:

• Are you feeling nervous or restless?
• Do you hear voices that others can not hear?
• Tell me how everything is going?

The nurse may need to rephrase questions or direct conversation toward other subjects until these patients feel comfortable and are able to discuss their therapy.

The nurse asks the patient or a family member about adverse drug reactions or any other problems occurring during therapy. The nurse brings these reactions or problems to the attention of the primary health care provider. The nurse should document in the patient's record a general summary of the patient's outward behavior and any complaints or problems. The nurse then compares these notations with previous notations and observations.

Monitoring and Managing Patient Needs

The patient may need to tolerate some adverse reactions, such as dry mouth, episodes of orthostatic hypotension, and drowsiness during drug therapy. Nursing interventions to relieve some of these reactions may include offering frequent sips of water, assisting the patient out of the bed or chair, and supervising all ambulatory activities.

RISK FOR INJURY. Antipsychotic drugs may cause extreme drowsiness and sedation, especially during the first or second weeks of therapy. This reaction may impair mental or physical abilities. The nurse provides total assistance with activities of daily living to the patient experiencing extreme sedation, including help with eating, dressing, and ambulating. If hypotension or sedation occurs with these drugs, administration at bedtime helps to minimize the risk of injury. During hypotensive episodes, it is important to monitor vital signs at least daily; depending on the patient's behavior, the nurse may monitor vital signs more frequently. The nurse should report any significant change in vital signs to the primary health care provider.

Drowsiness usually diminishes after 2 or 3 weeks of therapy. However, if the patient continues to be troubled by drowsiness and sedation, the primary health care provider may decide to prescribe a lower dosage.

IMPAIRED PHYSICAL MOBILITY. During initial therapy or whenever the dosage is increased or decreased, the nurse observes the patient closely for adverse drug reactions, including TD. The nurse may use the Abnormal Involuntary Movement Scale (AIMS) to screen the patient for symptoms (Display 23.2) and any behavioral changes. Because these adverse effects are considered "late stage," the nurse needs to be alert to their presence. The nurse reports to the primary health care provider any change in behavior or the appearance of adverse reactions. An immediate decrease in dosage will not change the condition, but may prevent further deterioration of the patient.

Antipsychotic Drugs

DISPLAY 23.2 Abnormal Involuntary Movement Scale Screening Tool

Client identification:_____Date:_____

Rated by: _____

Either before or after completing the examination procedure, observe the client unobtrusively at rest (e.g., in waiting room).

The chair to be used in this examination should be a hard, firm one without arms.

After observing the client, he or she may be rated on a scale of 0 (none), 1 (minimal), 2 (mild), 3 (moderate), and 4 (severe) according to the severity of symptoms.

Ask the client whether there is anything in his/her teeth (i.e., gum, candy, etc.) and, if there is, to remove it.

Ask client about the current condition of his/her teeth. Ask client if he/she wears dentures. Do teeth or dentures bother client now?

Ask client whether he/she notices any movement in mouth, face, hands, or feet. If yes, ask to describe and to what extent the movements currently bother patient or interfere with his/her activities.

0 1 2 3 4	Ask client to tap thumb with each finger as rapidly as possible for 10–15 seconds; separately with right hand, then with left hand. (Observe facial and leg movements.)
0 1 2 3 4	Flex and extend client's left and right arms (one at a time).
0 1 2 3 4	*Ask client to stand up. (Observe in profile. Observe all body areas again, hips included.)
0 1 2 3 4	Have client sit in chair with hands on knees, legs slightly apart, and feet flat on floor (look at entire body for movements while in this position)
0 1 2 3 4	Ask client to sit with hands hanging unsupported. If male, hands between legs; if female and wearing a dress, hands hanging over knees. (Observe hands and other body areas.)
0 1 2 3 4	Ask client to open mouth. (Observe tongue at rest within mouth.) Do this twice.
0 1 2 3 4	Ask client to protrude tongue. (Observe abnormalities of tongue movement.) Do this twice.
0 1 2 3 4	Ask client to extend both arms outstretched in front with palms down. (Observe trunk, legs, and mouth.)
0 1 2 3 4	*Have client walk a few paces, turn, and walk back to chair. (Observe hands and gait.) Do this twice.

* Activated movements.

! NURSING ALERT

Because there is no known treatment for TD and because it is irreversible in patients, the nurse must immediately report symptoms. These include rhythmic, involuntary movements of the tongue, face, mouth, jaw, or the extremities.

Patients can experience mobility problems if EPS occurs while taking the antipsychotic drugs. The nurse observes the patient for extrapyramidal effects, which include muscular spasms of the face and neck, the inability to sleep or sit still, tremors, rigidity, or involuntary rhythmic movements. The nurse also assists with ambulation and reassures the patient that symptoms will decline when the dosage of the antipsychotic is decreased. In addition, the nurse notifies the primary health care provider of the occurrence of these symptoms because they may indicate a need for dosage adjustment.

RISK FOR INFECTION. The use of the drug clozapine has been associated with severe agranulocytosis, or decreased white blood cell (WBC) count. This bone marrow suppression can make the patient more susceptible to illness and infection. To ensure close monitoring of this adverse reaction, clozapine is available only through a patient management system (a program that combines WBC testing, patient monitoring, and pharmacy and drug distribution services). Only a 1-week supply of this drug is dispensed at a time. A weekly WBC count is done throughout therapy and for 4 weeks after therapy is discontinued. In addition, the nurse monitors the patient for adverse reactions that indicate bone marrow suppression:

lethargy, weakness, fever, sore throat, malaise, mucous membrane ulceration, or "flulike" complaints.

IMBALANCED FLUID VOLUME. Fluid volume determines the concentration of lithium in the blood. The dosage of lithium is individualized according to serum levels and clinical response to the drug. The desirable serum lithium level is between 0.6 and 1.2 mEq/L. Blood samples are drawn immediately before the next dose of lithium (8 to 12 hours after the last dose) when lithium levels are relatively stable. During the acute phase, the nurse monitors serum lithium levels twice weekly or until the patient's manic phase is under control. During maintenance therapy, the serum lithium levels are monitored every 2 to 4 months.

Lithium toxicity is closely related to serum lithium levels and can occur even when the drug is administered at therapeutic doses. Adverse reactions are seldom observed at serum lithium levels of less than l.5 mEq/L, except in the patient who is especially sensitive to lithium. Toxic symptoms may occur with serum lithium levels of 1.5 mEq/L or greater. Levels should not exceed 2 mEq/L (see Table 23.1). Therefore, the nurse must continually monitor patients taking lithium for signs of toxicity, such as diarrhea, vomiting, nausea, drowsiness, muscular weakness, and lack of coordination. For early symptoms, the primary health care provider may order a dosage reduction or discontinue the drug for 24 to 48 hours and then gradually restart the drug therapy at a lower dosage.

LIFESPAN ALERT – Gerontology
Older adults are at increased risk for lithium toxicity because of a decreased rate of excretion. Lower dosages may be necessary to decrease the risk of toxicity.

For patients receiving lithium therapy, the nurse increases the oral fluid intake to about 3000 mL/day. It is important to keep fluids readily available and to offer extra fluids throughout waking hours. If there is any question regarding the oral fluid intake, the nurse monitors intake and output.

Educating the Patient and Family
Noncompliance is a problem with some patients once they are discharged to the home setting. It is important for the nurse to evaluate accurately the patient's ability to assume responsibility for taking drugs at home. The administration of antipsychotic drugs becomes a family responsibility if the outpatient appears to be unable to manage his or her own drug therapy.

The nurse explains any adverse reactions that may occur with a specific antipsychotic drug and encourages the patient or family members to contact the primary health care provider immediately if a serious drug reaction occurs. The nurse includes the following points in a teaching plan for the patient or family member:

- Keep all primary care provider and clinic appointments, because close monitoring of therapy is essential.
- Report any unusual changes or physical effects to the primary health care provider.
- Take the drug exactly as directed. Do not increase, decrease, or omit a dose or discontinue use of this drug unless directed to do so by the primary health care provider.
- Do not drive or perform other hazardous tasks if drowsiness occurs.
- Do not take any nonprescription drug unless use of a specific drug has been approved by the primary health care provider.
- Inform physicians, dentists, and other medical personnel of therapy with this drug.
- Do not drink alcoholic beverages unless approval is obtained from the primary health care provider.
- If dizziness occurs when changing position, rise slowly when getting out of bed or a chair. If dizziness is severe, always have help when changing positions.
- To relieve dry mouth, take frequent sips of water, suck on hard candy, or chew gum (preferably sugarless).
- Notify your primary care provider if you become pregnant or intend to become pregnant during therapy.
- Immediately report the occurrence of the following adverse reactions: restlessness, inability to sit still, muscle spasms, masklike expression, rigidity, tremors, drooling, or involuntary rhythmic movements of the mouth, face, or extremities.
- Avoid exposure to the sun. If exposure is unavoidable, wear sunblock, keep arms and legs covered, and wear a sun hat.

- Note that only a 1-week supply of clozapine is dispensed at a time. The drug is obtained through a special program designed to ensure the required blood monitoring. Weekly WBC laboratory tests are required. Immediately report any signs of weakness, fever, sore throat, malaise, or flulike symptoms to the primary health care provider.
- Note that olanzapine is available as a tablet to swallow or as an orally disintegrating tablet. When using the orally disintegrating tablet, peel back the foil on the blister packaging. Using dry hands, remove the tablet, and place the entire tablet in the mouth. The tablet will disintegrate immediately with or without liquid.
- Remember to take lithium with food or immediately after meals to avoid stomach upset. Drink at least 10 large glasses of fluid each day and add extra salt to food. Prolonged exposure to the sun may lead to dehydration. If any of the following occurs, do not take the next dose and immediately notify the primary health care provider: diarrhea, vomiting, fever, tremors, drowsiness, lack of muscle coordination, or muscle weakness.

EVALUATION

- Therapeutic effect is achieved and psychotic behavior is decreased.
- Adverse reactions are identified, reported to the primary health care provider, and managed successfully through appropriate nursing interventions:
  ☑ No evidence of injury is seen.
  ☑ Patient maintains adequate mobility.
  ☑ No evidence of infection is seen.
  ☑ Adequate fluid volume is maintained.
- Patient and family demonstrate an understanding of the drug regimen.

THINK CRITICALLY: PHARMACOLOGY IN PRACTICE

1. As a nurse on the mental health unit, you are assigned to discuss extrapyramidal effects at a medical-surgical unit's team conference. Identify which patients and drugs are most likely to cause these adverse reactions. Discuss how you would present and explain this topic to the nurses on the medical-surgical unit. Describe the points you would stress.

● Test Your Knowledge

1. A patient taking fluphenazine (Prolixin) for schizophrenia is also prescribed the antiparkinsonism drug benztropine. What is the best explanation for adding an antiparkinsonism drug to the drug regimen?

   A. prevents severe allergic reaction from sun exposure
   B. promotes the effects of fluphenazine
   C. reduces fine tremors, muscle rigidity, and slow movement
   D. decreases hallucinations and delusions

2. Which of the following behaviors would the nurse expect to see in a patient experiencing TD?

   A. Muscle rigidity, dry mouth, insomnia
   B. Rhythmic, involuntary movements of the tongue, face, mouth, or jaw
   C. Muscle weakness, paralysis of the eyelids, diarrhea
   D. Dyspnea, somnolence, muscle spasms

3. Which of the following symptoms would indicate to the nurse that a patient taking lithium is experiencing toxicity?

   A. Constipation, abdominal cramps, rash
   B. Stupor, oliguria, hypertension
   C. Nausea, vomiting, diarrhea
   D. Dry mouth, blurred vision, difficulty swallowing

4. Which of the following drugs is least likely to produce extrapyramidal effects?

   A. chlorpromazine
   B. haloperidol
   C. molindone
   D. risperidone

● Prepare for the NCLEX

1. In giving discharge instructions to a patient taking lithium, the nurse stresses that the patient should.

   A. eat a diet high in carbohydrates and low in proteins
   B. increase oral fluid intake to approximately 3000 mL/day
   C. have blood drawn before each dose of lithium is administered
   D. avoid eating foods high in amines

● Calculate Medication Dosages

1. A patient is prescribed quetiapine (Seroquel) 100 mg BID. The drug is available in 50 mg tablets. The nurse would administer _____.

2. Lithium 600 mg is prescribed. Use the drug label below to determine the correct dosage. The nurse administers.

To check your answers, see Appendix E.

the**Point**. *For more NCLEX questions, log on to http://thepoint.lww.com to access more than 1000 questions.*

Drugs That Affect the Peripheral Nervous System

Chapters 24 through 27 focus on drugs that affect the peripheral nerves in the body. The peripheral nervous system (PNS) comprises all nerves outside of the brain and spinal cord. Because the nerves extend throughout the body, these drugs affect many different body systems. The PNS is divided into the somatic nervous system and the autonomic nervous system. The somatic branch of the PNS is concerned with sensation and voluntary movement. The sensory part of the somatic nervous system sends messages to the brain concerning the internal and external environment, such as sensations of heat, pain, cold, and pressure. The movement part of the somatic nervoussystem is concerned with the voluntary movement of skeletal muscles, such as those used in walking, talking, or writing a letter.

The autonomic branch of the PNS is concerned with functions essential to the survival of the organism. Functional activity of the autonomic nervous system is not controlled consciously (i.e., the activity is automatic). This system controls blood pressure, heart rate, gastrointestinal activity, and glandular secretions.

The autonomic branch is further divided into the sympathetic and the parasympathetic nervous systems. The sympathetic nervous system tends to regulate the expenditure of energy and is operative when the organism is confronted with stressful situations. The sympathetic system is also called the *adrenergic branch*. Chapter 24 discusses drugs that mimic the effects of the sympathetic system—the adrenergic drugs. Again, these drugs impact many different body systems and organs; therefore, the concept of

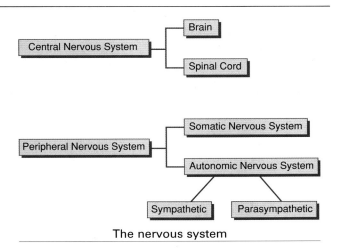

The nervous system

shock is the major focus of Chapter 24. Drugs that block or inhibit the system are called *antiadrenergic drugs, adrenergic blocking drugs, or sympatholytics.* One of the major body systems impacted by adrenergic blocking drugs is the heart and vascular system. Some of the drugs used to treat hypertension are featured in Chapter 25.

The parasympathetic nervous system helps conserve body energy and is partly responsible for such activities as slowing the heart rate, digesting food, and eliminating bodily wastes. The parasympathetic nervous system is known as the *cholinergic branch.* Drugs that enhance neurotransmission are discussed in Chapter 26; those that block transmission are covered in Chapter 27.

PHARMACOLOGY IN PRACTICE

Our patient focus in this unit is Mr. Park, a 77-year-old man who has been given his preoperative medications for hip surgery. He is very concerned about the function of his bowels, having experienced diarrhea with incontinence when on a course of antibiotics. Mr. Park is fearful of another loss of bowel control and repeatedly wants to be up out of the bed. After reading the chapters in this unit, you will be asked to explain and reassure him that the drugs used during the operative period will not cause loose stools. Additionally, we will examine the impact on many organ systems when adrenergic or cholinergic drugs are used.

Adrenergic Drugs

24

KEY TERMS

adrenergic
autonomic nervous system
neurotransmitter
parasympathetic
peripheral nervous system

shock
sympathetic
sympathomimetic
vasopressors

LEARNING OBJECTIVES

On completion of this chapter, the student will:

1. Discuss the activity of the autonomic nervous system, specifically the sympathetic branch.
2. Discuss the types of shock, physiologic responses of shock, and the use of adrenergic drugs in the treatment of shock.
3. Discuss the uses, general drug actions, contraindications, precautions, interactions, and adverse reactions associated with the administration of adrenergic vasopressor drugs.
4. Discuss important preadministration and ongoing assessment activities the nurse should perform on the patient taking adrenergic drugs.
5. List nursing diagnoses particular to a patient taking adrenergic drugs.
6. Discuss ways to promote an optimal response to therapy, how to manage common adverse reactions, and important points to keep in mind when educating patients about the use of adrenergic drugs.

One component of the **peripheral nervous system** (PNS) is a system of nerves that automatically regulates bodily functions—the **autonomic nervous system**. This system is further divided into the **sympathetic** and the **parasympathetic** nervous system branches (Table 24.1). The sympathetic branch is regulated by involuntary control. In other words, a person does not have control over what this system does. Activation of this branch is often called the *fight-or-flight response*. These nerves are activated when the body is confronted with stressful situations, such as danger, intense emotion, or severe illness. The sympathetic branch has control over a person's heart rate, breathing rate, and ability to divert blood to the skeletal muscles—to enable a person to run, for example. Another term for the sympathetic branch

is the **adrenergic** branch because the system is based on the neurohormone adrenalin (epinephrine).

Norepinephrine is a **neurotransmitter** produced naturally by the body. It is the primary neurotransmitter in the sympathetic branch of the autonomic nervous system.

In the sympathetic branch of the autonomic nervous system, adrenergic drugs produce activity similar to the neurotransmitter norepinephrine. Another name for these drugs is **sympathomimetic** (i.e., mimicking the actions of the sympathetic nervous system) drugs. The adrenergic drugs produce pharmacologic effects similar to the effects that occur in the body when the sympathetic nerves (norepinephrine) and the medulla (epinephrine) are stimulated. The primary effects of these drugs occur on the heart, the blood vessels, and the smooth muscles, such as the bronchi of the lung. Metaraminol and isoproterenol (Isuprel) are examples of adrenergic drugs.

Actions ~~What is shock~~

The purpose of stimulating the sympathetic (adrenergic) nerves is to divert blood flow to the vital organs so that the body can deal with a stressful situation. In general, adrenergic drugs produce one or more of the following responses in varying degrees:

- Central nervous system—wakefulness, quick reaction to stimuli, quickened reflexes
- Autonomic nervous system—relaxation of the smooth muscles of the bronchi; constriction of blood vessels, sphincters of the stomach; dilation of coronary blood vessels; decrease in gastric motility
- Heart—increase in the heart rate
- Metabolism—increased use of glucose (sugar) and liberation of fatty acids from adipose tissue

Adrenergic Nerve Receptors

The degree to which any organ is affected by the sympathetic nervous system depends on which postsynaptic nerve receptor sites are activated (Fig. 24.1). Adrenergic nerves have either alpha (α) or beta (β) receptors. Drugs that act on the receptors are called *selective* or *nonselective*. Adrenergic drugs may be selective (act on α receptors or β receptors only) or nonselective (act on both α and β receptors). For example, isoproterenol acts chiefly on β receptors; it is considered a selective drug. Epinephrine is a nonselective drug and acts on both α and β receptors.

A works on own—↑ pulse, ↑ sweating, ↓ bowels. <u>Pupils</u>
S—fight or flight
P   digest

Table 24.1 Action of the Autonomic Nervous System on Body Organs and Structures

Organs or Structures	Types of Sympathetic (Adrenergic) Receptor	Sympathetic (Adrenergic) Effects	Parasympathetic (Cholinergic) Effects
Heart	β	Increase in heart rate, heart muscle contractility, increase in speed of atrioventricular conduction	Decrease in heart rate, decrease in heart muscle contractility
Blood vessels 1. Skin, mucous membranes 2. Skeletal muscle	α Cholinergic,* β	Constriction Usually dilation	—
Bronchial muscles	β	Relaxation	Contraction
Gastrointestinal 1. Muscle motility, tone 2. Sphincters 3. Gallbladder	β α	Decrease Usually contraction Relaxation	Increase Usually relaxation Contraction
Urinary bladder 1. Detrusor muscle 2. Trigone, sphincter muscles	β α	Relaxation Contraction	Contraction Relaxation
Eye 1. Radial muscle of iris 2. Sphincter muscle of iris 3. Ciliary muscle	α	Contraction (pupil dilates)	Contraction (pupil constricts) Contraction
Skin 1. Sweat glands 2. Pilomotor muscles	Cholinergic* α	Increased activity in localized areas Contraction (gooseflesh)	—
Uterus	β	Relaxation	—
Salivary glands	α	Thickened secretions	Copious, watery secretions
Liver	β	Glycogenolysis	—
Lacrimal and nasopharyngeal glands		—	Increased secretion
***Male sex organs**	α	Emission	Erection

*See Chapter 26.

Whether an adrenergic drug acts on α, β, or α and β receptors accounts for the variation of responses to this group of drugs. Table 24.2 lists the type of adrenergic nerve receptor that corresponds with each action of the autonomic nervous system on the body. The α and β receptors can be further grouped as α_1- and α_2-adrenergic receptors and β_1- and β_2-adrenergic receptors.

Uses

Adrenergic drugs have a variety of uses and may be given for the treatment of the following:

- Hypovolemic and septic **shock**   *inadequate tissue perfussion*
- Moderately severe to severe episodes of hypotension
- Control of superficial bleeding during surgical and dental procedures of the mouth, nose, throat, and skin
- Cardiac decompensation and arrest
- Allergic reactions (anaphylactic shock, angioneurotic edema)
- Temporary treatment of heart block

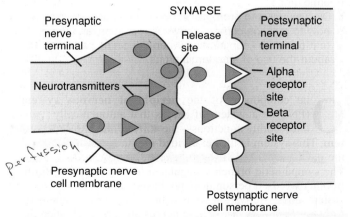

Figure 24.1 Neurotransmission in the PNS. Neurotransmitter molecules (e.g., norepinephrine), released by the presynaptic nerve, cross the synapse and bind with α and β receptors in the cell membrane of the postsynaptic nerve, resulting in the transmission of the nerve impulse.

Table 24.2 Effects of the Adrenergic Receptors

Receptor	Site	Effect
α_1	Peripheral blood vessels	Vasoconstriction of peripheral blood vessels
α_2	Presynaptic neuron	Regulates release of neurotransmitters; decreases tone, motility, and secretions of gastrointestinal tract
β_1	Myocardium	Increased heart rate, increased force of myocardial contraction
β_2	Peripheral blood vessels	Vasodilation of peripheral vessels
	Bronchial smooth muscles	Bronchodilation

- Ventricular arrhythmias (under certain conditions)
- Respiratory distress (as bronchodilators)
- Nasal congestion and glaucoma (topical formulation)

Adrenergic drugs may also be used as a vasoconstricting adjunct to local anesthetics to prolong anesthetic action in the tissues. The adrenergic drugs used primarily as **vasopressors** (drugs that raise the blood pressure because of their ability to constrict blood vessels) are listed in the Summary Drug Table: Adrenergic Drugs. Sympathomimetics are also used as bronchodilators in the treatment of respiratory problems (see Chapter 34) or topically in the treatment of glaucoma (see Chapter 54). These drugs are listed in the Summary Drug Table: Adrenergic Drugs by name only; more information is provided in the noted respective chapters.

Shock

Adrenergic drugs are important in the care and treatment of patients in shock. Shock is a state of inadequate tissue perfusion. In shock, the supply of arterial blood and oxygen flowing to the cells and tissues is inadequate. To counteract the symptoms of shock, the body initiates physiologic mechanisms (e.g., the release of epinephrine and norepinephrine). In some situations, the body is able to compensate, and blood pressure is maintained. However, if shock is untreated and compensatory mechanisms of the body fail, irreversible shock occurs and death follows. There are three types of shock: hypovolemic shock, cardiogenic shock, and distributive shock. Table 24.3 describes the various types of shock.

Various clinical manifestations may be present in a patient in shock. For example, in the early stages of shock, the extremities may be warm because vasodilation is initiated, and blood flow to the skin and extremities is maintained. If the condition is untreated, blood flow to vital organs, skin, and extremities is compromised. The patient becomes cool and clammy, which is referred to as "cool" or "cold" shock. Regardless of the type, shock results in a decrease in cardiac output, decrease in arterial blood pressure (hypotension), reabsorption of water by the kidneys (causing a decrease in urinary output), decrease in the exchange of oxygen and carbon dioxide in the lungs, increase in carbon dioxide and decrease in oxygen in the blood, hypoxia (decreased oxygen reaching the cells), and increased concentration of intravascular fluid. This scenario compromises the functioning of vital organs such as the heart, brain, and kidneys. The

various physiologic responses caused by shock are listed in Table 24.4.

Adrenergic drugs improve hemodynamic status by improving myocardial contractility and increasing heart rate, which results in increased cardiac output. Peripheral resistance is increased by vasoconstriction. In cardiogenic shock or advanced shock associated with low cardiac output, an adrenergic drug may be used with a vasodilating drug. A vasodilator, such as nitroprusside (see Chapter 36) or nitroglycerin (see Chapter 37), improves myocardial performance because the adrenergic drug maintains blood pressure.

Adverse Reactions

Adverse reactions associated with the administration of adrenergic drugs depend on the drug used, the dose administered, and individualized patient response. Some common adverse reactions include:

- Cardiac arrhythmias (bradycardia and tachycardia)
- Headache
- Nausea and vomiting
- Increased blood pressure (which may reach dangerously high levels)

Additional adverse reactions for specific adrenergic drugs are listed in the Summary Drug Table: Adrenergic Drugs.

LIFESPAN ALERT – Gerontology
The older adult is especially vulnerable to adverse reactions of adrenergic drugs, particularly epinephrine. In addition, older adults are more likely to have preexisting cardiovascular disease that predisposes them to potentially serious cardiac arrhythmias. The nurse closely monitors all elderly patients taking an adrenergic drug. It is important to report any changes in the pulse rate or rhythm immediately. In addition, epinephrine may temporarily increase tremor and rigidity in older adults with Parkinson's disease.

Contraindications

Adrenergic drugs are contraindicated in patients with known hypersensitivity. Isoproterenol is contraindicated in patients with tachyarrhythmias, tachycardia, or heart block caused by digitalis toxicity, ventricular arrhythmias, and angina pectoris. Dopamine is contraindicated in those with pheochro-

Summary Drug Table ADRENERGIC DRUGS

Generic Name	Trade Name	Uses	Adverse Reactions	Dosage Ranges
Adrenergic (Sympathomimetic) Drugs Used Primarily for Vasopressor Effects				
dobutamine *doe-byoo'-tah-meen*		Cardiac decompensation due to depressed contractility caused by organic heart disease or cardiac surgical procedures	Headache, nausea, increased heart rate, increase in systolic blood pressure, palpitations, anginal and nonspecific chest pain	2.5–10 mcg/kg/min IV (up to 40 mcg/kg/min); titrate to patient's hemodynamic and renal status
dopamine *doe'-pah-meen*		Shock due to myocardial infarction, trauma, open heart surgery, renal failure, and chronic cardiac decompensation in congestive heart failure	Nausea, vomiting, ectopic beats, tachycardia, anginal pain, palpitations, hypotension, dyspnea	2–50 mcg/kg/min IV (infusion rate determined by patient's response)
epinephrine *eh-pih-neh'-frin*	EpiPen	Ventricular standstill; treatment and prophylaxis of cardiac arrest, heart block; mucosal congestion and acute sinusitis; prolong regional/local anesthetics; anaphylactic reactions	Anxiety, restlessness, headache, lightheadedness, dizziness, nausea, dysuria, pallor	Cardiac arrest: 0.5–1.0 mg IV Respiratory distress (e.g., anaphylaxis): 0.1–0.25 mg of hay fever, rhinitis
isoproterenol *eye-soe-proe-tare'-eh-noll*	Isuprel	Shock, bronchospasm during anesthesia, cardiac standstill and arrhythmias	Anxiety, sweating, flushing, headache, lightheadedness, dizziness, nausea, vomiting, tachycardia	Shock: 4 mcg/mL diluted solution IV Cardiac arrhythmias, cardiac standstill: 0.02–0.06 mg of diluted solution IV, or 1:5000 solution intracardiac injection
metaraminol *meh-tah-ram'-ih-noll*		Hypotension with spinal anesthesia, hypotension due to hemorrhage, drug reactions, surgical complication, shock associated with brain damage	Headache, apprehension, palpitations, nausea, projectile vomiting, urinary urgency	2–10 mg IM, subcut; 15–100 mg in 250- or 500-mL solution IV
midodrine *mid'-oh-dryne*	ProAmatine	Orthostatic hypotension, only when patient is considerably impaired	Paresthesias, headache, pain, dizziness, supine hypertension, bradycardia, piloerection, pruritus, dysuria, chills	10 mg orally TID during daylight hours when patient is upright
norepinephrine (levarterenol) *nor-ep-ih-nef'-rin*	Levophed	Shock, hypotension, cardiac arrest	Restlessness, headache, dizziness, bradycardia, hypertension	2–4 mcg/min, rate adjusted to maintain desired blood pressure
Short-Acting β₂ Agonists (SABA — Adrenergic or Sympathomimetics Used for Acute Respiratory Symptom Relief)*				
albuterol	Proventil, Ventolin			
ephedrine				
epinephrine	Adrenalin, Epinephrine Mist, Primatene Mist			
bitolterol	Tornalate			
levalbuterol	Xopenex			
metaproterenol	Alupent			

(table continues on page 219)

Summary Drug Table ADRENERGIC DRUGS (continued)

Generic Name	Trade Name	Uses	Adverse Reactions	Dosage Ranges
pirbuterol	Maxair Autohaler			
terbutaline	Brethine			

Long-Acting β₂ Agonists (LABA — Adrenergic or Sympathomimetics Used for Long-Term Respiratory Management)*

arformoterol	Brovana			
formoterol	Foradil			
salmeterol	Serevent Diskus			

α₂-Adrenergic Agonists (Optic Agents)**

brimonidine tartrate	Alphagan			

Sympathomimetics**

apraclonidine	Iopidine			
dipivefrin (**dipivalyl epinephrine**)	Propine, AKPro			
epinephrine	Epifrin, Glaucon Solution			

*See Chapter 34 for detailed information.
**See Chapter 54 for detailed information.

mocytoma (adrenal gland tumor), unmanaged arrhythmias, and ventricular fibrillation. Epinephrine is contraindicated in patients with narrow-angle glaucoma, and as a local anesthetic adjunct in fingers and toes. Norepinephrine is contraindicated in patients who are hypotensive from blood volume deficits. Midodrine causes severe hypertension in the patient who is lying down (supine); therefore, it is used

for orthostatic hypotension only when the patient is considerably impaired.

NURSING ALERT

Supine hypertension is a potentially dangerous adverse reaction in the patient taking midodrine. The drug should be given only to patients whose lives are impaired despite stan-

Table 24.3 Types of Shock

Type*	Description
Hypovolemic	Occurs when the blood volume is significantly diminished. *Examples*: hemorrhage; fluid loss caused by burns, dehydration, or excess diuresis.
Cardiogenic-obstructive shock	Occurs when cardiac output is insufficient and perfusion to the vital organs cannot be maintained. *Examples*: a result of acute myocardial infarction, ventricular arrhythmias, congestive heart failure, or severe cardiomyopathy. Obstructive shock is categorized with cardiogenic shock. It occurs when obstruction of blood flow results in inadequate tissue perfusion. *Examples*: pericardial tamponade, restrictive pericarditis, and severe cardiac valve dysfunction.
Distributive (vasogenic) shock	Occurs when there are changes to the blood vessels causing dilation, but no additional blood volume. The blood is redistributed within the body. This category is further differentiated: • Septic shock—circulatory insufficiency resulting from overwhelming infection (e.g., central line infection) • Anaphylactic shock—hypersensitivity resulting in massive systemic vasodilation (e.g., drug allergic reaction) • Neurogenic shock—interference with PNS control of blood vessels (e.g., spinal cord injury)

*Other causes of shock include hypoglycemia, hypothyroidism, and Addison's disease.

Adrenergic Drugs

give IV, O2, V/S (low) 80 palp
ck extremities, elevate
call dr

Table 24.4 Physiologic Manifestations of Shock

Bodily System	Possible Signs and Symptoms
Integumentary (skin)	Pallor, cyanosis, cold and clammy, sweating
Central nervous system	Agitation, confusion, disorientation, coma
Cardiovascular	Hypotension, tachycardia, arrhythmias, wide pulse pressure, gallop rhythm
Respiratory	Tachypnea, pulmonary edema
Renal	Urinary output less than 20 mL/h
Metabolic (endocrine)	Acidosis

dard treatment offered. The nurse can minimize this reaction by administering midodrine during the day while the patient is in an upright position. The following is a suggested dosing schedule for the administration of midodrine: shortly before arising in the morning, midday, and late afternoon (not after 6:00 PM). Drug therapy should continue only in the patient whose orthostatic hypotension improves during the initial treatment.

Precautions

These drugs are used cautiously in patients with coronary insufficiency, cardiac arrhythmias, angina pectoris, diabetes, hyperthyroidism, occlusive vascular disease, or prostatic hypertrophy. Patients with diabetes may require an increased dosage of insulin. Adrenergic drugs are classified as pregnancy category C and are used with extreme caution during pregnancy.

Interactions

The following interactions may occur when an adrenergic drug is administered with another agent:

Interacting Drug	Common Use	Effect of Interaction
antidepressants	Treatment of depression	Increased sympathomimetic effect
oxytocin	Induction of uterine contractions	Increased risk of hypertension
bretylium	Treatment of severe cardiac problems	Increased risk of arrhythmias

There is an increased risk of seizures, hypotension, and bradycardia when dopamine is administered with phenytoin (Dilantin). Metaraminol is used cautiously in patients taking digoxin because of an increased risk for cardiac arrhythmias. There is an increased risk of hypertension when dobutamine is administered with the β-adrenergic blocking drugs.

Code status-? DNR

NURSING PROCESS
PATIENT RECEIVING AN ADRENERGIC DRUG

ASSESSMENT

Assessment of the patient receiving an adrenergic drug differs depending on the drug, the patient, and the reason for administration. For example, assessment of the patient in shock who is to be treated with norepinephrine is different from that for the patient receiving epinephrine with a local anesthetic while having a tooth cavity repaired. Both are receiving adrenergic drugs, but the circumstances are much different.

HERBAL ALERT

Ephedra (Ma Huang) and the many substances of the *Ephedra* genus have been used medicinally (e.g., *E. sinica* and *E. intermedia*). Ephedra (ephedrine) preparations have traditionally been used to relieve cold symptoms and improve respiratory function, and as an adjunct in weight loss. Large doses may cause a variety of adverse reactions, such as hypertension and irregular heart rate. The use of ephedra has shifted from relief of respiratory problems to an aid to weight loss and enhanced athletic performance. Before taking this herb, the patient should consult a primary health care provider. Ephedra should not be used with the cardiac glycosides, halothane, guanethidine, monoamine oxidase inhibitors (MAOIs) antidepressants, or oxytocin, or by patients taking St. John's wort. The U.S. Food and Drug Administration (FDA) warns the public not to take ephedrine-containing dietary supplements. Stroke and heart attack have resulted from taking these products. Many producers of weight loss supplements are removing the ephedra component because of potential legal liability.

Preadministration Assessment

When a patient is to receive an adrenergic agent for shock, the nurse obtains the blood pressure, pulse rate and quality, and respiratory rate and rhythm. The nurse assesses the patient's symptoms, problems, or needs before administering the drug and records any subjective or objective data on the patient's chart. In emergencies, the nurse must make assessments quickly and accurately. This information provides an important database that is used during treatment.

A general survey of the patient also is necessary. It is important to look for additional symptoms of shock, such as cool skin, cyanosis, diaphoresis, and a change in the level of consciousness. Other assessments may be necessary if the hypotensive episode is due to trauma, severe infection, or blood loss.

Ongoing Assessment

During the ongoing assessment, the nurse observes the patient for the effect of the drug, such as improved breathing of the patient with asthma, or response of blood pressure to the administration of the vasopressor. During therapy, the nurse evaluates and documents the drug effect. The nurse also takes and documents the vital signs. Comparison of assessments made before and after administration may help the primary health care provider determine future use of the drug for this patient. It is important to report adverse drug reactions to the primary health care provider as soon as possible.

NURSING DIAGNOSES

Drug-specific nursing diagnoses are the following:

❑ **Ineffective Tissue Perfusion** related to hypovolemia, blood loss, impaired distribution of fluid, impaired circulation, impaired transport of oxygen across alveolar and capillary bed, other (specify)
❑ **Decreased Cardiac Output** related to altered heart rate and/or rhythm
❑ **Disturbed Sleep Pattern** related to adverse reactions (nervousness) to the drug and the environment

Nursing diagnoses related to drug administration are discussed in Chapter 4.

PLANNING

The expected outcomes of the patient depend on the reason for administering an adrenergic agent, but may include an optimal response to drug therapy, meeting patient needs related to management of adverse drug reactions, and an understanding of the therapeutic regimen.

IMPLEMENTATION

Promoting an Optimal Response to Therapy

Management of the patient receiving an adrenergic agent varies and depends on the drug used, the reason for administration, and the patient's response to the drug. In most instances, adrenergic drugs are potent and potentially dangerous. The nurse must exercise great care in the calculation and preparation of these drugs for administration. Although adrenergic drugs are potentially dangerous, proper supervision and management before, during, and after administration will minimize the occurrence of any serious problems. The nurse reports and documents any complaint the patient may have while taking an adrenergic drug. However, nursing judgment is necessary when reporting adverse reactions. The nurse must report some adverse effects, such as the development of cardiac arrhythmias, immediately, regardless of the time of day or night. The nurse also should report other adverse effects, such as anorexia, but this is usually not an emergency.

Management of shock is aimed at providing basic life support (airway, breathing, and circulation) while attempting to correct the underlying cause. Antibiotics, inotropes, hormones (e.g., insulin, thyroid), and other drugs may be used to treat the underlying disease. However, the initial pharmacologic intervention is aimed at supporting the circulation with vasopressors.

Monitoring and Managing Patient Needs

INEFFECTIVE TISSUE PERFUSION. If the patient is being given an adrenergic drug for hypotension, there is already a problem with tissue perfusion. Administration of the adrenergic drug may correct the problem or, if the blood pressure becomes too high, tissue perfusion may again be a problem. By maintaining the blood pressure at the systolic rate prescribed by the primary health care provider, tissue perfusion will be maintained.

When a patient is in shock and experiencing ineffective tissue perfusion, there is a decrease in oxygen, resulting in an inability of the body to nourish its cells at the capillary level. If the patient has marked hypotension, the administration of a vasopressor is required. The primary health care provider determines the cause of the hypotension and then selects the best method of treatment. Some hypotensive episodes require the use of a less potent vasopressor, such as metaraminol; at other times, a more potent vasopressor, such as dobutamine, dopamine, or norepinephrine, is necessary.

The nurse considers the following points when administering the potent vasopressors dopamine and norepinephrine:

• Use an electronic infusion pump to administer these drugs.
• Do not mix dopamine with other drugs, especially sodium bicarbonate or other alkaline intravenous (IV) solutions. Check with the hospital pharmacist before adding a second drug to an IV solution containing this drug.
• Administer norepinephrine and dopamine only by the IV route. Do not dilute these drugs in an IV solution before administration. The primary health care provider orders the IV solution, the amount of drug added to the solution, and the initial rate of infusion.
• Monitor blood pressure every 2 minutes from the beginning of therapy until the desired blood pressure is achieved, then monitor the blood pressure and pulse rate at frequent intervals, usually every 5 to 15 minutes, during the administration of these drugs.
• Adjust the rate of administration according to the patient's blood pressure. The rate of administration of the IV solution is increased or decreased to maintain the patient's blood pressure at the systolic pressure ordered by the primary health care provider.
• Readjustment of the rate of flow of the IV solution is often necessary. The frequency of adjustment depends on the patient's response to the vasopressor.
• Inspect the needle site and surrounding tissues at frequent intervals for leakage (extravasation, infiltration) of the solution into the subcutaneous tissues surrounding the needle site. If leakage occurs, establish another IV line immediately, discontinue the IV containing the vasopressor, and notify the primary health care provider. These drugs are particularly damaging when they leak into surrounding tissues. The nurse should know the

Adrenergic Drugs

extravasation protocol and have orders signed by the primary health provider to implement the protocol.
- Never leave the patient receiving these drugs unattended.

Monitoring the patient in shock requires vigilance on the part of the nurse. The patient's heart rate, blood pressure, and electrocardiogram are monitored continuously. Urine output is measured often (usually hourly), and accurate intake and output measurements are taken. Monitoring of central venous pressure by a central venous catheter provides an estimate of the patient's fluid status. Sometimes additional hemodynamic monitoring is necessary with a pulmonary artery catheter. The use of a pulmonary artery catheter allows the nurse to monitor a number of parameters, such as cardiac output and peripheral vascular resistance. The nurse adjusts therapy according to the primary health care provider's instructions.

The less potent vasopressors, such as metaraminol, also require close patient supervision during administration. The nurse follows the same procedure as for norepinephrine and dopamine, but may take blood pressure and pulse determinations at less frequent intervals, usually every 15 to 30 minutes. The nurse needs sound clinical judgment to determine the frequency because there is no absolute minimum or maximum time limit between determinations.

DECREASED CARDIAC OUTPUT. The heart rate and stroke volume determine cardiac output. The stroke volume is determined in part by the contractile state of the heart and the amount of blood in the ventricle available to be pumped out. The interventions listed to support tissue perfusion also help to support cardiac output of the patient in shock.

When the patient is in shock, it is important for the nurse to monitor vital signs (heart rate and rhythm, respiratory rate, and blood pressure) carefully and often (every 15 to 30 minutes) to determine the severity of shock. For example, as cardiac output decreases, compensatory tachycardia develops to increase cardiac output. As shock deepens, the pulse volume becomes progressively weaker and assumes a "thready" feel. The heart rate increases and the heart rhythm may become irregular. Initially, the respiratory rate is rapid, as the patient experiences air hunger, but in profound shock, the respiratory rate decreases. Blood pressure decreases as shock progresses.

NURSING ALERT

Regardless of the actual numeric reading of the blood pressure, a progressive decrease in blood pressure is serious. The nurse reports to the primary health care provider any progressive decrease in blood pressure, a decrease in systolic blood pressure below 100 mm Hg, or any decrease of 20 mm Hg or more of the patient's normal blood pressure.

DISTURBED SLEEP PATTERN. Often adrenergic drugs are used in the critical care setting. These units can be as busy in the middle of the night as they are in the middle of the day. Patients can easily get confused regarding the time

of day. This can cause a great deal of stress in the patient. It is helpful to identify circumstances that disturb sleep, such as the nurse taking vital signs during the night or turning the overhead light on during the night. The nurse plans care with as few interruptions as possible or makes modifications. For example, to filter light, curtains can be drawn over windows and between patients in critical care units. The nurse has to weigh the importance of monitoring patient status and vital signs or providing comfort interventions when administering the adrenergic drugs. A thorough explanation of the reason for close monitoring of the vital signs by the nurse is necessary. In addition, caffeinated beverages are avoided, especially after 5:00 PM. Other sleep aids may be used (e.g., warm milk, back rub, progressive relaxation, or bedtime snack).

Educating the Patient and Family

Only medical personnel give some adrenergic drugs, such as the vasopressors. The nurse's responsibility for teaching involves explaining the drug to the patient or family. Depending on the situation, the nurse may include facts such as how the drug will be given (e.g., the route of administration) and what results are expected. The nurse must use judgment regarding some of the information given to the patient or family regarding administration of an adrenergic drug in life-threatening situations, because certain facts, such as the seriousness of the patient's condition, are usually best explained by the primary health care provider.

EDUCATING THE PATIENT RECEIVING MIDODRINE. When midodrine is given to patients with severe orthostatic hypotension, the nurse explains the importance of taking the drug during daytime hours when the patient is upright. The patient can take doses in 3-hour intervals if needed to control symptoms. The drug should not be taken within 4 hours of bedtime. In addition, to control supine hypertension, a potentially fatal adverse reaction, the patient should not become fully supine. The nurse explains to the patient that he or she may need to sleep with the head of the bed elevated. If urinary retention is a problem, the patient is instructed to urinate before taking the drug. The nurse stresses the importance of returning for regular medical evaluation. The patient is instructed to report any changes in vision, pounding in the head when lying down, slow heart rate, or difficulty urinating.

Evaluation

- Therapeutic effect is achieved and perfusion is maintained.
- Adverse reactions are identified, reported to the primary health care provider, and managed successfully through appropriate nursing interventions.
  - ☑ Adequate tissue perfusion is maintained.
  - ☑ Adequate cardiac output is maintained.
  - ☑ Patient reports fewer episodes of inappropriate sleep patterns.
- Patient (if able) and family demonstrate an understanding of the drug regimen.

THINK CRITICALLY: PHARMACOLOGY IN PRACTICE

1. Plan a teaching program to explain the autonomic nervous system to a group of nurses at a staff education meeting.

● Test Your Knowledge

1. The physician prescribes norepinephrine, a potent vasopressor, to be administered to a patient in shock. The rate of the administration of the IV fluid containing the norepinephrine is:

A. maintained at a set rate of infusion
B. adjusted per protocol to maintain the patient's blood pressure
C. given at a rate not to exceed 5 mg/min
D. discontinued when the blood pressure is 100 mm Hg systolic

2. At what intervals would the nurse monitor the blood pressure of a patient administered norepinephrine?

A. Every 5 to 15 minutes
B. Every 30 minutes
C. Every hour
D. Every 4 hours

3. Which of the following are the common adverse reactions the nurse would expect with the administration of the adrenergic drugs?

A. Bradycardia, lethargy, bronchial constriction
B. Increase in appetite, nervousness, drowsiness
C. Anorexia, vomiting, hypotension
D. Headache, nervousness, nausea

4. When dobutamine is administered with the β-adrenergic blocking drugs, the nurse is aware of an increased risk for_____.

A. Seizures
B. Arrhythmias
C. Hypotension
D. Hypertension

● Prepare for the NCLEX

1. An adult with a honeybee allergy was stung and calls the nurse at the clinic. The patient has two EpiPens at home. The solution is 1 mg/mL and each EpiPen contains 0.3 mL.

What drug dose has the patient taken if two injections were already given? _____

● Calculate Medication Dosages

1. The physician orders 0.5 mg of 1:1000 epinephrine solution IV. The drug is available in 1:1000 solution 1 mg/mL. The nurse administers _____.

To check your answers, see Appendix E.

the**Point** *For more NCLEX questions, log on to http://thepoint.lww.com to access more than 1000 questions.*

Adrenergic Blocking Drugs

α-adrenergic blocking
α/β-adrenergic blocking
antiadrenergic
β-adrenergic blocking
cardiac arrhythmia
first-dose effect

glaucoma
orthostatic hypotension
pheochromocytoma
postural hypotension
sympatholytic

LEARNING OBJECTIVES

On completion of this chapter, the student will:

1. List the four types of adrenergic blocking drugs.
2. Discuss the uses, general drug actions, general adverse reactions, contraindications, precautions, and interactions of the adrenergic blocking drugs.
3. Discuss important preadministration and ongoing assessment activities the nurse should perform on the patient taking adrenergic blocking drugs.
4. List nursing diagnoses particular to a patient taking adrenergic blocking drugs.
5. Discuss ways to promote an optimal response to therapy, how to manage common adverse reactions, nursing actions that may be taken to minimize orthostatic or postural hypotension, and important points to keep in mind when educating patients about the use of adrenergic blocking drugs.

Norepinephrine is a substance that transmits nerve impulses across the sympathetic branch of the autonomic nervous system (see figure in the Unit V introduction). Activation of these nerves is sometimes called our *fight-or-flight response*. Drugs that facilitate transmission are called *adrenergic* drugs and were covered in Chapter 24. Drugs that reverse the response are called *adrenergic blocking* drugs. Also called **sympatholytic** drugs, these agents block the transmission of norepinephrine in the sympathetic system. Drugs blocking neurotransmission in the sympathetic nervous system work *directly* by blocking the receptor, or *indirectly* by preventing release of norepinephrine. They may be divided into four groups:

- **Alpha (α)-adrenergic blocking** drugs—drugs that block α-adrenergic receptors. These drugs produce their greatest effect on the α-receptors of the adrenergic nerves that control the vascular system.
- **Beta (β)-adrenergic blocking** drugs—drugs that block β-adrenergic receptors. These drugs produce their greatest effect on the β receptors of adrenergic nerves, primarily the β receptors of the heart.
- **α/β-Adrenergic blocking** drugs—drugs that block both α- and β-adrenergic receptors. These drugs act on both α and β nerve fibers.
- Centrally- and peripherally-acting **antiadrenergic** drugs—drugs that prevent the release of the neurotransmitter. These drugs block the adrenergic nerve impulse in both the central and peripheral nervous systems.

Each of these groups is discussed individually, followed by an example of the Nursing Process for the group as a whole. The focal group of drugs in this chapter is the β-adrenergic blocking drugs. See the Summary Drug Table: Adrenergic Blocking Drugs for a more complete listing of these drugs.

α-ADRENERGIC BLOCKING DRUGS

Actions

Stimulation of α-adrenergic nerves results in vasoconstriction (see Table 24.1 in Chapter 24). If stimulation of α-adrenergic nerves is interrupted or blocked, the result is vasodilation. This is the direct opposite of the effect of an adrenergic drug with α activity. The primary drugs used in this category cause vasodilation by relaxing the smooth muscle of blood vessels. They are also used in ophthalmic preparations to constrict the pupil. Phentolamine (Regitine) is an example of an α-adrenergic blocking drug.

Uses

α-Adrenergic blocking drugs are used in the treatment of the following:

- Hypertension caused by **pheochromocytoma** (a tumor of the adrenal gland that produces excessive amounts of epinephrine and norepinephrine)
- Hypertension during preoperative preparation

They are also used to prevent or treat tissue damage caused by extravasation of dopamine.

Suppresses or decreases

Summary Drug Table ADRENERGIC BLOCKING DRUGS

Generic Name	Trade Name	Uses	Adverse Reactions	Dosage Ranges
α-Adrenergic Blocking Drugs				
phentolamine *fen-toll'-ah-meen*	Regitine	Diagnosis of pheochromocytoma, hypertensive episodes before and during surgery, prevention/treatment of dermal necrosis after IV administration of norepinephrine or dopamine	Weakness, dizziness, flushing, nausea, vomiting, orthostatic hypotension	5 mg IV, IM Tissue necrosis: 5–10 mg in 10 mL saline solution infiltrated into affected area
β-Adrenergic Blocking Drugs (Beta Blockers)				
acebutolol *ay-seh-byoo'-toe-loll*	Sectral	Hypertension, ventricular arrhythmias	Bradycardia, dizziness, weakness, hypotension, nausea, vomiting, diarrhea, nervousness	Hypertension: 400 mg orally in 1–2 doses Arrhythmias: 400–1200 mg/day orally in divided doses
atenolol *ay-ten'-oh-loll*	Tenormin, Tenoretic	Hypertension, angina, acute MI	Bradycardia, dizziness, fatigue, weakness, hypotension, nausea, vomiting, diarrhea, nervousness	Hypertension/angina:50–200 mg/day orally Acute MI: 5 mg IV over 5 min, may be repeated
betaxolol *beh-tax'-oh-loll*	Kerlone	Hypertension	Bradycardia, dizziness, hypotension, bronchospasm, nausea, vomiting, diarrhea, nervousness	10–20 mg/day orally, consider starting dose of 5 mg daily for elders
bisoprolol *bye-soe'-proe-loll*	Zebeta	Hypertension	Same as acebutolol	2.5–10 mg orally daily; maximum dose, 20 mg orally daily
carteolol *kar'-tee-oh-loll*		Hypertension	Same as acebutolol	2.5–10 mg/day orally
esmolol *ess'-moe-loll*	Brevibloc	Supraventricular tachycardia, noncompensatory tachycardia	Hypotension, weakness, lightheadedness, urinary retention	50–200 mcg/kg/min IV, loading dose may be as high as 500 mcg/kg over 1 minute
metoprolol *meh-toe'-proe-loll*	Lopressor, Toprol-XL	Hypertension, angina, MI, HF	Dizziness, hypotension, HF, cardiac arrhythmia, nausea, vomiting, diarrhea	Hypertension/angina: 100–450 mg/day orally; Extended release 50–100 mg/day orally; HF: 25 mg–200 mg/day orally; Acute MI: 3 bolus doses of 5 mg IV
nadolol *nay-doe'-loll*	Corgard	Hypertension, angina	Dizziness, hypotension nausea, vomiting, diarrhea, HF, cardiac arrhythmia	Hypertension: 40–80 mg/day orally; angina: 40–80, may go to 240 mg/day orally
nebivolol *neh-biv'-oh-loll*	Bystolic	Hypertension	Dizziness, headache, nausea, diarrhea, tingling extremities	5–40 mg/daily
penbutolol *pen-byoo'-toe-loll*	Levatol	Hypertension	Bradycardia, dizziness, hypotension, nausea, vomiting, diarrhea	20 mg orally daily

(table continues on page 226)

Summary Drug Table ADRENERGIC BLOCKING DRUGS (continued)

Generic Name	Trade Name	Uses	Adverse Reactions	Dosage Ranges
pindolol *pin'-doe-loll*	Visken	Hypertension	Bradycardia, dizziness, hypotension, nausea, vomiting, diarrhea	5–60 mg/day orally BID
propranolol *proe-pran'-oh-loll*	Inderal	Cardiac arrhythmias, MI, angina, hypertension, migraine prophylaxis, hypertrophic subaortic stenosis, pheochromocytoma, essential tremor	Bradycardia, dizziness, hypotension, nausea, vomiting, diarrhea, bronchospasm, hyperglycemia, pulmonary edema	Arrhythmias: 10–30 mg orally TID, QID; Hypertension: 120–240 mg/day orally in divided doses; Angina: 80–320 mg/day orally in divided doses; Migraine: 160–240 mg/day orally in divided doses
® sotalol *soh'-tah-loll*	Betapace, Betapace AF	Ventricular arrhythmias (maintain normal sinus rhythm— Betapace AF only)	Dizziness, hypotension, nausea, vomiting, diarrhea, respiratory distress	160–320 mg/day orally in divided doses
timolol *tih'-moe-loll*	Blocadren	Hypertension, MI, migraine prophylaxis	Dizziness, hypotension, nausea, vomiting, diarrhea, pulmonary edema	Hypertension: 10–40 mg/day orally in divided doses; MI: 10 mg orally BID; Migraine: 20 mg/d orally
Topical Preparations				
betaxolol (ophthalmic) *beh-tax'-oh-loll*	Betoptic	Glaucoma	Brief ocular discomfort, tearing	1 gtt BID
timolol (ophthalmic)	Timoptic	Glaucoma	Ocular irritation, tearing	1 gtt BID
α/β-Adrenergic Blocking Drugs				
carvedilol *car-veh'-dih-loll*	Coreg	Hypertension, HF, left ventricular dysfunction	Bradycardia, hypotension, cardiac insufficiency, fatigue, dizziness, diarrhea	6.25–25 mg orally BID
labetalol *lah-bet'-ah-loll*	Trandate	Hypertension Crisis	Fatigue, drowsiness, insomnia, hypotension, impotence, diarrhea	200–400 mg/day orally in divided doses IV: 20 mg over 2 min with blood pressure monitoring, may repeat
Antiadrenergic Drugs: Centrally Acting				
clonidine *klon'-nih-deen*	Catapres, Catapres-TTS (transdermal)	Hypertension, Severe pain in patients with cancer	Drowsiness, dizziness, sedation, dry mouth, constipation, syncope, dreams, rash	100–600 mcg/day orally Transdermal: release rate 0.1-0.3 mg/24 hr
guanabenz *gwah'-nah-benz*		Hypertension	Dry mouth, sedation, dizziness, headache, weakness, arrhythmias	4–32 mg orally BID
guanfacine *gwan'-fah-sine*	Tenex	Hypertension	Dry mouth, somnolence, asthenia, dizziness, headache, constipation, fatigue	1–3 mg/day orally at bedtime
methyldopa or methyldopate *meh'-thill-doe-pah, meh'-thill-doe-pate*		Hypertension, hypertensive crisis	Bradycardia, aggravation of angina pectoris, heart failure, sedation, headache, rash, nausea, vomiting, nasal congestion	250 mg orally BID or TID; maintenance dose, 2 g/day; 250–500 mg q 6 hr IV

NCLEX

(table continues on page 227)

Summary Drug Table ADRENERGIC BLOCKING DRUGS (continued)

Generic Name	Trade Name	Uses	Adverse Reactions	Dosage Ranges
Antiadrenergic Drugs: Peripherally Acting				
alfuzosin *al-foo-zoe'-sin*	Uroxatral	BPH	Headache, dizziness	10 mg orally daily
doxazosin *dok-say-zoe'-sin*	Cardura	Hypertension, BPH	Headache, dizziness, fatigue	Hypertension: 1–8 mg orally daily; BPH: 1–16 mg orally daily
mecamylamine *mek-ah-mill'-ah-meen*	Inversine	Hypertension	Dizziness, syncope, dry mouth, nausea, constipation, urinary retention	2.5 mg orally BID
prazosin *pray-zoe'-sin*	Minipress	Hypertension	Dizziness, postural hypotension, drowsiness, headache, loss of strength, palpitation, nausea	1–20 mg orally daily in divided doses
reserpine *reh–sir'–pyne*	Serpalan	Hypertension, psychosis	Bradycardia, dizziness, nausea, vomiting, diarrhea, nasal congestion	Hypertension: 0.1–0.5 mg orally daily; psychosis: 0.1–1 mg orally daily
tamsulosin *tam–soo–loe' sin*	Flomax	BPH	Headache, ejaculatory dysfunction, dizziness, rhinitis	0.4 mg orally daily
terazosin *tare–ah'–zoe–sin*	Hytrin	Hypertension, BPH	Dizziness, postural hypotension, headache, dyspnea, nasal congestion	Hypertension: 1–20 mg orally daily; BPH: 1–10 mg orally daily

Ⓡ This drug should be administered at least 1 hour before or 2 hours after a meal.
*See Chapter 54 for detailed information.

Adverse Reactions

Administration of an α-adrenergic blocking drug may result in weakness, orthostatic hypotension, cardiac arrhythmias, hypotension, and tachycardia. See the Summary Drug Table: Adrenergic Blocking Drugs for more information

Contraindications, Precautions, and Interactions

α-Adrenergic blocking drugs are contraindicated in patients who are hypersensitive to the drugs and in patients with coronary artery disease. These drugs are used cautiously during pregnancy (category C) and lactation, after a recent myocardial infarction (MI), and in patients with renal failure or Raynaud's disease. When phentolamine (Regitine) is administered with epinephrine, there is decreased vasoconstrictor and hypertensive action.

• β-ADRENERGIC BLOCKING DRUGS

Actions

β-Adrenergic blocking drugs are also called *β blockers*. These drugs decrease the stimulation of the sympathetic nervous system on certain tissues. β-Adrenergic receptors are found mainly in the heart. Stimulation of β receptors of the heart results in an increase in the heart rate. Blocking the nerve impulse of β-adrenergic nerves decreases the heart rate and dilates the blood vessels (Fig. 25.1). These drugs decrease the heart's excitability, decrease cardiac workload and oxygen consumption, and provide membrane-stabilizing effects that contribute to the antiarrhythmic activity of the β-adrenergic blocking drugs. Examples of β-adrenergic blocking drugs used for cardiac purposes are esmolol (Brevibloc) and propranolol (Inderal).

β-Adrenergic blocking drugs such as betaxolol (Betoptic) and timolol (Timoptic) are used to treat glaucoma. **Glaucoma** is a narrowing or blockage of the drainage channels (canals of Schlemm) between the anterior and posterior chambers of the eye. This results in a buildup of pressure (increased intraocular pressure) in the eye. Blindness may occur if glaucoma is left untreated. When the aforementioned drugs are used topically as ophthalmic drops, they appear to reduce the production of aqueous humor in the anterior chamber of the eye, lessening the effects of glaucoma.

Uses

β-Adrenergic blocking drugs are used in the treatment of the following:

Figure 25.1 β-Adrenergic blocking drugs prevent epinephrine and norepinephrine from occupying receptor sites on cell membranes. This action alters cell functions normally stimulated by epinephrine and norepinephrine, according to the number of receptor sites occupied by the β-blocking drugs. (Adapted by J. Harley from *Encyclopedia Britannica Medical and Health Annual* [1983]. Chicago: Encyclopedia Britannica.)

- Hypertension (first choice drug for patients with stable angina)
- **Cardiac arrhythmia** (abnormal rhythm of the heart), such as ventricular or supraventricular tachycardia
- Migraine headaches
- Heart failure
- Angina pectoris
- Glaucoma (topical ophthalmic eye drops)

β-Adrenergic blockers are also used to prevent reinfarction in patients with a recent MI (1 to 4 weeks after the MI).

CHRONIC CARE ALERT
Hypertension research studies demonstrate better patient outcomes for African Americans when β blockers are used in combination with diuretics than other drugs to treat hypertension, such as angiotensin-converting enzyme (ACE) inhibitors.

Adverse Reactions

- Cardiac reactions that affect the body in a generalized manner include orthostatic hypotension, bradycardia, dizziness, vertigo, and headache.
- Gastrointestinal (GI) reactions include hyperglycemia, nausea, vomiting, and diarrhea.

- Another bodily system reaction is bronchospasm (especially in those with a history of asthma).

Many of these reactions are mild and may disappear with therapy. More serious adverse reactions include symptoms of congestive heart failure (HF; i.e., dyspnea, weight gain, peripheral edema).

LIFESPAN ALERT – Gerontology
Older adults are at increased risk for adverse reactions when taking β-adrenergic blocking drugs. The nurse should monitor the older adult closely for confusion, heart failure, worsening of angina, shortness of breath, and peripheral vascular insufficiency (e.g., cold extremities, paresthesia of the hands, weak peripheral pulses).

Contraindications, Precautions, and Interactions

These drugs are contraindicated in patients with an allergy to β blockers, in patients with sinus bradycardia, second- or third-degree heart block, or heart failure, and in those with asthma, emphysema, or hypotension. The drugs are used cautiously in patients with diabetes, thyrotoxicosis, or peptic ulcer. COPD

LIFESPAN ALERT – Pregnancy
β Blockers are recommended for pregnant women over other hypertensive drugs because the risk to the fetus is less with these drugs.

The following interactions may occur when a β-adrenergic blocker is administered with another agent:

Interacting Drug	Common Use	Effect of Interaction
antidepressants (monoamine oxidase inhibitors [MAOIs], selective serotonin reuptake inhibitors [SSRIs])	Management of depression	Increased effect of the β blocker, bradycardia
nonsteroidal anti-inflammatory drugs (NSAIDs), salicylates	Pain relief	Decreased effect of the β blocker
loop diuretics	Management of cardiovascular problems	Increased risk of hypotension
clonidine	Management of cardiovascular problems	Increased risk of paradoxical hypertensive effect
cimetidine	Management of GI problems	Increased serum level of the β blocker and higher risk of β blocker toxicity
lidocaine	Management of cardiac problems	Increased serum level of the β blocker and higher risk of β blocker toxicity

• α/β-ADRENERGIC BLOCKING DRUGS

Actions

α/β-Adrenergic blocking drugs block the stimulation of both the α- and β-adrenergic receptors, resulting in peripheral vasodilation. The two drugs in this category are carvedilol (Coreg) and labetalol (Trandate).

Uses

Carvedilol is used to treat essential hypertension and in HF to reduce progression of the disease. Labetalol is used in the treatment of hypertension, either alone or in combination with another drug, such as a diuretic.

Adverse Reactions

Most adverse effects of α/β-adrenergic blocking drugs are mild and do not require discontinuation of therapy. General body system adverse reactions include fatigue, dizziness, hypotension, drowsiness, insomnia, weakness, diarrhea, dyspnea, chest pain, bradycardia, and skin rash.

Contraindications, Precautions, and Interactions

α/β-Adrenergic blockers are contraindicated in patients with hypersensitivity to the drugs, bronchial asthma, decompensated heart failure, and severe bradycardia. The drugs are used cautiously in patients with drug-controlled HF, chronic bronchitis, or impaired hepatic or cardiac function, in those with diabetes, and during pregnancy (category C) and lactation.

The following interactions may occur when an α/β-adrenergic blocker is administered with another agent:

Interacting Drug	Common Use	Effect of Interaction
antidepressants (tricyclics and SSRIs)	Management of depression	Increased risk of tremors
cimetidine	Management of GI problems	Increased effect of the adrenergic blocker
halothane	Anesthetic for surgery	Increased effect of the adrenergic blocker
clonidine	Management of cardiovascular problems	Increased effect of the clonidine
digoxin	Management of cardiac problems	Increased serum level of the digoxin and higher risk of digoxin toxicity

• CENTRALLY- AND PERIPHERALLY-ACTING ANTIADRENERGIC DRUGS

Actions

One group of antiadrenergic drugs inhibits the release of norepinephrine from certain adrenergic nerve endings in the peripheral nervous system. This group is composed of *peripherally-acting* (i.e., acting on peripheral structures) antiadrenergic drugs. An example of a peripherally-acting antiadrenergic drug for treating hypertension is prazosin (Minipress). These drugs are also used to treat benign prostatic hypertrophy (BPH). Another group of antiadrenergic drugs are called *centrally-acting* antiadrenergic drugs because they act on the central nervous system (CNS) rather than on the peripheral nervous system. This group affects specific CNS centers, thereby decreasing some of the activity of the sympathetic nervous system. Although the action of both types of antiadrenergic drugs is somewhat different, the results are basically the same. An example of a centrally-acting antiadrenergic drug is clonidine (Catapres).

Uses

Antiadrenergic drugs are used mainly for the treatment of certain cardiac arrhythmias, hypertension, and BPH (see the Summary Drug Table: Adrenergic Blocking Drugs).

Adverse Reactions

• Dry mouth, drowsiness, sedation, anorexia, rash, malaise, and weakness are generalized reactions to antiadrenergic drugs that work on the CNS.
• Hypotension, weakness, lightheadedness, and bradycardia are adverse reactions associated with the administration of peripherally acting antiadrenergic drugs.

Contraindications, Precautions, and Interactions

Centrally acting antiadrenergic drugs are contraindicated in active hepatic disease, antidepressant therapy using monoamine oxidase inhibitors (MAOIs), and in patients with a history of hypersensitivity to these drugs. The centrally-acting antiadrenergic drugs are used cautiously in patients with a history of liver disease or renal impairment, and during pregnancy and lactation.

The peripherally-acting antiadrenergic drugs are contraindicated in patients with a hypersensitivity to any of the drugs. Reserpine (Serpasil) is contraindicated in patients who have an active peptic ulcer or ulcerative colitis and in patients who are mentally depressed. Reserpine is used cautiously in patients with a history of depression, in those with renal impairment or cardiovascular disease, and during pregnancy and lactation.

The following interactions may occur when an antiadrenergic drug is administered with another agent:

Interacting Drug	Common Use	Effect of Interaction
adrenergic drugs	Management of cardiovascular problems	Increased risk of hypertension
levodopa	Management of Parkinson's disease	Decreased effect of the levodopa, hypotension
anesthetic agents	Surgical anesthesia	Increased effect of the anesthetic
β blockers	Management of cardiovascular problems	Increased risk of hypertension
lithium	Treatment of psychosis	Increased risk of lithium toxicity
haloperidol	Treatment of psychosis	Increased risk of psychotic behavior

NURSING PROCESS
PATIENT RECEIVING AN ADRENERGIC BLOCKING DRUG

ASSESSMENT

Assessment depends on the drug, the patient, and the reason for administration.

Preadministration Assessment

The nurse establishes an accurate database before any adrenergic blocking drug is administered for the first time. If, for example, the patient has hypertensive disease, the nurse notes the subjective and objective symptoms as well as vital signs during the initial assessment. Patients with hypertension must have their blood pressure and pulse taken on both arms in sitting, standing, and supine positions before therapy is begun. If the patient has a cardiac arrhythmia, the initial assessment includes taking the pulse rate, determining the pulse rhythm, and noting the patient's general appearance.

If the drug is given for anginal pain, the nurse records the onset, type (e.g., sharp, dull, squeezing), radiation, location, intensity, and duration of anginal pain. The nurse also questions the patient regarding any precipitating factors of the anginal pain, such as exertion or emotional stress. Once drug therapy is started, evaluation of the effects of therapy can be made by comparing the patient's current symptoms with the symptoms experienced before therapy was initiated.

Subjective data (i.e., the patient's complaints or description of symptoms) also are obtained at this time, and the primary health care provider usually orders an electrocardiogram. Additional diagnostic studies and laboratory tests also may be ordered.

If the drug is given to treat HF, the patient is assessed for evidence of the disease, such as dyspnea (especially on exertion), peripheral edema, distended neck veins, and cough.

Ongoing Assessment

It is important for the nurse to perform ongoing assessment of the patient receiving adrenergic blocking drug therapy. This assessment often depends on the reason the drug is administered. For all adrenergic blocking drugs, it is important for the nurse to observe these patients continually for the appearance of adverse reactions. Some adverse reactions are mild, whereas others, such as diarrhea, may cause a problem, especially if the patient is elderly or debilitated.

Typically hypertensive patients will be asked to monitor their own blood pressures between clinic visits. This can be accomplished by obtaining equipment for the home or periodic visits to a local fire station or pharmacy. More in-depth information regarding care of the patient with hypertension is provided in Chapter 36.

NURSING DIAGNOSES.

Drug-specific nursing diagnoses are the following:

❑ **Impaired Comfort** related to drying of secretions secondary to medication
❑ **Ineffective Tissue Perfusion: Peripheral** related to hypotension
❑ **Risk for Injury** related to vertigo, dizziness, weakness, and syncope secondary to hypotension

Nursing diagnoses related to drug administration are discussed in Chapter 4.

PLANNING

The expected outcomes for the patient depend on the reason for administration of an adrenergic blocking drug, but may include an optimal response to drug therapy, meeting of patient needs related to the management of adverse reactions, and an understanding of the therapeutic regimen.

IMPLEMENTATION

Promoting an Optimal Response to Therapy

Most adrenergic blocking drugs may be given without regard to food. However, the nurse should administer drugs preventing release of neurotransmitters (antiadrenergics) at the same time each day because the fluctuation in blood level can affect blood pressure. Sotalol (Betapace) is given on an empty stomach because food may reduce absorption of the drug.

When adrenergic blocking drugs are given to patients to control hypertension, angina, or cardiac arrhythmias, it is important to communicate with the primary health care provider about the patient's response to therapy. When given for a cardiac arrhythmia, these drugs can provoke new or worsen existing ventricular arrhythmias. If angina worsens or does not appear to be controlled by the drug, the nurse should contact the primary health care provider immediately.

When the drug is administered for hypertension, the nurse monitors the patient for a decrease in blood pressure. If there is a significant increase in blood pressure, the nurse administers the dose and notifies the primary health care provider immediately because additional drug therapy may be necessary.

When a β-adrenergic blocking ophthalmic preparation, such as timolol, is administered to patients with glaucoma, it is important to insist that they have periodic follow-up examinations by an ophthalmologist. At these examinations, the intraocular pressure should be measured to determine the effectiveness of drug therapy.

Monitoring and Managing Patient Needs

IMPAIRED COMFORT. Some patients may experience one or more adverse drug reactions during treatment with adrenergic blocking drugs. As with any drug, the nurse must report adverse reactions to the primary health care provider and record the reactions on the patient's chart. Nursing judgment in this matter is necessary, because some adverse reactions are serious or potentially serious. In these cases, the nurse should withhold the next dose of the drug and contact the primary health care provider immediately. The nurse also reports to the primary health care provider any adverse reactions that pose no serious threat. Adverse reactions that pose no serious threat to the patient's well-being, such as dry mouth or mild constipation, may have to be tolerated by the patient. It is important to assure the patient that, in some instances, these less serious reactions disappear or lessen in intensity over time.

! NURSING ALERT

When administering a sympatholytic drug, such as propranolol (Inderal), the nurse should take an apical pulse rate and blood pressure before giving the drug. If pulse is below 60 beats/min, if there is any irregularity in the patient's heart rate or rhythm, or if systolic blood pressure is less than 90 mm Hg, the nurse should withhold the drug and contact the primary health care provider.

However, even minor adverse drug reactions can be distressing to the patient, especially when they persist for a long time. Therefore, when possible, the nurse should relieve minor adverse reactions with simple nursing measures. For example, the nurse can assist the patient with dry mouth by giving frequent sips of water or by allowing the patient to suck on a piece of hard candy (provided that the patient does not have diabetes or is not on a special diet that limits sugar intake) to relieve a dry mouth. The nurse can help relieve a patient's constipation by encouraging increased fluid intake, unless extra fluids are contraindicated. The primary health care provider also may order a laxative or stool softener. It is important for the nurse to maintain a daily record of bowel elimination. The nurse can help the patient minimize certain GI side effects, such as anorexia, diarrhea, and constipation, by administering drugs at a specific time in relation to meals, with food, or with antacids.

INEFFECTIVE TISSUE PERFUSION: PERIPHERAL. During therapy with an adrenergic blocking drug for hypertension, the nurse should take the patient's blood pressure before each dose is given. Some patients have an unusual

response to the drugs. In addition, some drugs may, in some individuals, decrease the blood pressure at a more rapid rate than other drugs. It is important to monitor the patient's blood pressure on both arms and in the sitting, standing, and supine positions for the first week or more of therapy. Once the patient's blood pressure has stabilized, the nurse should take the blood pressure before each drug administration using the same arm and position for each reading. It is a good idea to make a notation on the medication administration record or care plan about the position and arm used for blood pressure determinations. Measuring the blood pressure near the end of the dosing interval or near the end of the day after the last dose of the day helps to determine if the blood pressure is controlled throughout the day.

The patient with a life-threatening arrhythmia may receive an adrenergic blocking drug, such as propranolol, by the intravenous (IV) route. When these drugs are administered IV, cardiac monitoring is necessary. Patients not in a specialized unit, such as a coronary care unit, are usually transferred to one as soon as possible. When administering these drugs for a life-threatening arrhythmia, it is important for the nurse to supervise the patient continually, monitor the blood pressure and respiratory rate frequently, and perform cardiac monitoring.

When propranolol is administered orally for a less serious cardiac arrhythmia, cardiac monitoring is usually not necessary. The nurse should monitor the patient's blood pressure and pulse rate and rhythm at varying intervals, depending on the length of treatment and the patient's response to the drug.

RISK FOR INJURY. Administration of the adrenergic blocking drugs may cause hypotension. If the drug is administered for hypertension, then a decrease in blood pressure is expected.

! NURSING ALERT

If a significant decrease in blood pressure (a drop of 20 mm Hg systolic or a systolic pressure below 90 mm Hg) occurs after a dose of an adrenergic blocking drug, the nurse should withhold the drug and notify the primary health care provider immediately. A dosage reduction or discontinuation of the drug may be necessary. Some adrenergic blocking drugs (e.g., prazosin or terazosin) may cause a **first-dose effect**. A first-dose effect occurs when the patient experiences marked hypotension (or postural hypotension) and syncope with sudden loss of consciousness with the first few doses of the drug.

The first-dose effect may be minimized by decreasing the initial dose and administering the dose at bedtime. The dosage can then be slowly increased every 2 weeks until a full therapeutic effect is achieved. If the patient experiences syncope, the nurse places the patient in a recumbent position and treats supportively. This effect is self-limiting and in most cases does not recur after the initial period of therapy. Lightheadedness and dizziness are more common than loss of consciousness. The following paragraphs discuss these effects and provide interventions for management.

DISPLAY 25.1 Minimizing the Effects of Adrenergic Blocking Drugs

Assisting patients to minimize the uncomfortable effects of adrenergic blocking drugs can be challenging. The following measures may be useful:

• Instruct patients to rise slowly from a sitting or lying position.
• Provide assistance for the patient getting out of bed or a chair if symptoms of postural hypotension are severe. Place the call light nearby and instruct patients to ask for assistance each time they get in and out of bed or a chair.
• Assist the patient in bed to a sitting position and have the patient sit on the edge of the bed for about 1 minute before ambulating.
• Help seated patients to a standing position and instruct them to stand in one place for about 1 minute before ambulating.
• Remain with the patient while he or she is standing in one place, as well as during ambulation.
• Instruct the patient to avoid standing in one place for prolonged periods. This is rarely a problem in the hospital but should be included in the patient and family discharge teaching plan.
• Teach the patient to avoid taking hot showers or baths, which tend to increase vasodilation.

On occasion, patients receiving an adrenergic blocking drug may experience postural or orthostatic hypotension. **Postural hypotension** is characterized by a feeling of lightheadedness and dizziness when the patient suddenly changes from a lying to a sitting or standing position, or from a sitting to a standing position. **Orthostatic hypotension** is characterized by similar symptoms and occurs when the patient changes or shifts position after standing in one place for a long period. See Display 25.1 for tips on how to minimize these adverse reactions.

Symptoms of postural or orthostatic hypotension often lessen with time, and the patient may be allowed to get out of bed or a chair slowly without assistance. The nurse must exercise good judgment in this matter. Allowing the patient to rise from a lying or sitting position without help is done only when the determination has been made that the symptoms have lessened and ambulation poses no danger of falling.

Educating the Patient and Family

Some patients do not adhere to the prescribed drug regimen for a variety of reasons, such as failure to comprehend the prescribed regimen, the cost of drug therapy, and failure to understand the importance of continued and uninterrupted therapy. If the nurse detects failure to adhere to the prescribed drug regimen, he or she should investigate the possible cause of the problem. In some instances, financial assistance may be necessary; in other instances, patients need to know why they are taking a drug and why therapy must be continuous to attain and maintain an optimal state of health and well-being.

The nurse should describe the drug regimen and stress the importance of continued and uninterrupted therapy when teaching the patient who is prescribed an adrenergic blocking drug. Patient education will differ according to the reason the adrenergic blocking drug was prescribed.

EDUCATING THE PATIENT WITH HYPERTENSION, CARDIAC ARRHYTHMIA, OR ANGINA. If a β-adrenergic blocking drug has been prescribed for hypertension, cardiac arrhythmia, angina, or other cardiac disorders, the patient must have a full understanding of the treatment regimen. In some instances, the primary health care provider may advise the hypertensive patient to lose weight or eat a special diet, such as the DASH (Dietary Approaches to Stop Hypertension) diet. A special diet also may be recommended for the patient with angina or a cardiac arrhythmia. When appropriate, the nurse should stress the importance of diet and weight loss in the therapy of hypertension.

It is important to include the following additional points in the teaching plan for the patient with hypertension, angina, or a cardiac arrhythmia:

• Do not stop taking the drug abruptly, except on the advice of the primary health care provider. Most of these drugs require that the dosage be gradually decreased to prevent precipitation or worsening of adverse effects.
• Notify the primary health care provider promptly if adverse drug reactions occur.
• Observe caution while driving or performing other hazardous tasks because these drugs (β-adrenergic blockers) may cause drowsiness, dizziness, or lightheadedness.
• Immediately report any signs of HF (weight gain, difficulty breathing, or edema of the extremities).
• Do not use any nonprescription drug (e.g., cold or flu preparations or nasal decongestants) unless use of a specific drug has been approved by the primary health care provider.
• Inform dentists and other primary health care providers of therapy with this drug.
• Keep all primary health care provider appointments because close monitoring of therapy is essential.
• Check with a primary health care provider or pharmacist to determine if the drug is to be taken with food or on an empty stomach.

In addition, when an adrenergic blocking drug is prescribed for hypertension, the primary health care provider may want the patient to monitor his or her own blood pressure between office visits (see Patient Teaching for Improved Patient Outcomes: Monitoring Blood Pressure at Home).

EVALUATION

• Therapeutic effect is achieved and hypertension or other disease is controlled.
• Adverse reactions are identified, reported to the primary health care provider, and managed successfully through appropriate nursing interventions.

☑ Dryness is managed and comfort maintained.
☑ Peripheral tissue perfusion is maintained.
☑ No evidence of injury is seen.
• Patient and family demonstrate an understanding of the drug regimen.

Patient Teaching for Improved Patient Outcomes

Monitoring Blood Pressure at Home

The nurse:

✓ Teaches the patient and a family member how to take an accurate blood pressure reading. This involves choosing the correct instrument and teaching the patient the steps in taking a blood pressure reading.
✓ Supervises the patient and a family member during several trial blood pressure readings to ensure accuracy of the measurements.
✓ Suggests to the patient that the same arm and body position be used each time the blood pressure is taken.
✓ Explains that blood pressure can vary slightly with emotion, time of day, and position of the body.
✓ Explains that a slight change in readings is normal, but if a drastic change in either or both the systolic or diastolic readings occurs, the patient should contact the primary health care provider as soon as possible.

THINK CRITICALLY: PHARMACOLOGY IN PRACTICE

1. A new nurse says that she is unsure about how the adrenergic blocking drugs work. Discuss the four types of adrenergic blocking drugs and how each one works in the body.

● Test Your Knowledge

1. A patient is to receive a β-adrenergic drug for hypertension. Before the drug is administered, the most important assessment the nurse performs is _____.

   A. weighing the patient
   B. obtaining blood for laboratory tests
   C. taking a past medical history
   D. taking the blood pressure on both arms

2. When an adrenergic blocking drug is given for a life-threatening cardiac arrhythmia, which of the following activities would the nurse expect to be a part of patient care?

   A. Daily electrocardiograms
   B. Fluid restriction to 1000 mL/day
   C. Daily weights
   D. Cardiac monitoring

3. To prevent complications when administering a β-adrenergic blocking drug to an elderly patient, the nurse would be particularly alert for _____.

   A. vascular insufficiency (e.g., weak peripheral pulses and cold extremities)
   B. complaints of an occipital headache
   C. insomnia
   D. hypoglycemia

4. The patient with glaucoma will likely receive a(n) _____.

   A. α/β-adrenergic blocking drug
   B. α-adrenergic blocking drug
   C. β-adrenergic blocking drug
   D. antiadrenergic drug

● Prepare for the NCLEX

1. The primary health care provider prescribes 60 mg propranolol to be given via the GI tube. The drug is available in an oral solution with a strength of 5 mg/mL. The nurse uses 30 mL of warm water to flush before and after administering the drug. The total volume of fluid for this procedure was:

   A. 35 mL of water and drug solution
   B. 60 mL of water and drug solution
   C. 65 mL of water and drug solution
   D. 72 mL of water and drug solution

● Calculate Medication Dosages

1. A patient has just had a dose increase to 12.5 mg of carvedilol. The patient has a bottle with 3.125-mg tablets and insists on finishing the bottle before buying a different strength. The nurse tells the patient to administer_____.

To check your answers, see Appendix E.

thePoint. *For more NCLEX questions, log on to http://thepoint.lww.com to access more than 1000 questions.*

Cholinergic Drugs

LEARNING OBJECTIVES

On completion of this chapter, the student will:

1. Discuss important aspects of the parasympathetic nervous system.
2. Discuss the uses, drug actions, general adverse reactions, contraindications, precautions, and interactions of the cholinergic drugs.
3. Identify important preadministration and ongoing assessment activities the nurse should perform on the patient taking cholinergic drugs.
4. List nursing diagnoses particular to a patient taking cholinergic drugs.
5. Discuss ways to promote an optimal response to therapy, how to manage common adverse reactions, and important points to keep in mind when educating the patient about the use of cholinergic drugs.

Acetylcholine (ACh) is the substance that transmits nerve impulses across the parasympathetic branch of the autonomic nervous system. There are two types of receptors in the parasympathetic nervous branch: **muscarinic receptors** (which stimulate smooth muscle) and **nicotinic receptors** (which stimulate skeletal muscle). Stimulation of this pathway results in the opposite reactions to those triggered by the adrenergic system: blood vessels dilate, sending blood to the gastrointestinal (GI) tract; secretions and peristalsis are activated and salivary glands increase production; the heart slows and pulmonary bronchioles constrict; the smooth muscle of the bladder contracts and the pupils of the eyes constrict. Activation of these nerves is sometimes called the *rest-and-digest* response.

Conserve body energy

Cholinergic drugs mimic the activity of the parasympathetic nervous system. They also are called **parasympatho/mimetic** drugs. What makes the parasympathetic system function differently is the enzyme **acetylcholinesterase**. Acetylcholinesterase (AChE) is an enzyme that can inactivate the neurotransmitter ACh, thereby preventing the nerve synapse from continuing the nerve impulse. This interruption in neurotransmission can diminish cognitive function, which is seen in illnesses such as Alzheimer's disease. Drugs that inhibit the enzyme AChE are called *anticholinesterases* or *acetylcholinesterase inhibitors*. These drugs are discussed specifically in Chapter 28.

Actions

Cholinergic drugs that act like the neurotransmitter ACh are called *direct-acting cholinergics*. The parasympathetic branch of the autonomic nervous system partly controls the process of **micturition** (voiding of urine) by constricting the detrusor muscle and relaxing the bladder sphincter (see Table 24.1). Micturition is both a voluntary and involuntary act. Urinary retention (not caused by a mechanical obstruction, such as a stone in the bladder) results when micturition is impaired. Treatment of urinary retention with direct-acting cholinergic drugs causes contraction of the bladder smooth muscles and passage of urine.

Myasthenia gravis is a disease that involves rapid fatigue of skeletal muscles because of the lack of ACh released at the nerve endings of parasympathetic nerves. Cholinergic drugs that prolong the activity of ACh by inhibiting the release of AChE are called *indirect-acting cholinergics* or *anticholinesterase muscle stimulants*. Drugs used to treat this disorder act indirectly to inhibit the activity of AChE and promote muscle contraction.

Glaucoma is a disorder of increased pressure within the eye caused by an obstruction of the outflow of aqueous humor. Treatment of glaucoma with an indirect-acting cholinergic drug produces **miosis** (constriction of the iris). This opens the blocked channels and allows the normal passage of aqueous humor, thereby reducing intraocular pressure. Although used for many years, these drugs are rarely used today due to frequency of dosing and side effects experienced. See the Summary Drug Table: Cholinergic Drugs for a more complete listing of these drugs.

Summary Drug Table CHOLINERGIC DRUGS

Generic Name	Trade Name	Uses	Adverse Reactions	Dosage Ranges
Direct Acting Cholinergics				
bethanechol *beh-than'-eh-koll*	Duvoid, Urecholine	Acute nonobstructive urinary retention, neurogenic atony of urinary bladder with urinary retention	Abdominal discomfort, headache, diarrhea, nausea, salivation, urgency	10–50 mg orally BID to QID; 2.5–5 mg subcut TID to QID
Indirect Acting (Anticholinesterase) Muscle Stimulants				
ambenonium *am-beh-noe'-nee-um*	Mytelase	Myasthenia gravis	Increased bronchial secretions, cardiac arrhythmias, muscle weakness, urinary frequency	5–75 mg orally TID, QID
edrophonium *ed-roe-foh'-nee-yum*	Tensilon NCLEX	Diagnosis of myasthenia gravis	Increased bronchial secretions, cardiac arrhythmias, muscle weakness, urinary frequency	2–10 mg IV, look for cholinergic reaction (muscle weakness)
guanidine *goo-wan'-eh-deen*		Myasthenic syndrome (Eaton-Lambert disease)	Palpitations, numbness in lips/extremities, dry mouth, nausea, abdominal cramping	10–30 mg/kg/day, titrate until adverse reaction occurs
pyridostigmine *peer-ih-doe-stig'-meen*	Mestinon, Regonol	Myasthenia gravis *mind to grand*	Increased bronchial secretions, cardiac arrhythmias, muscle weakness	Average dose is 600 mg/day orally at spaced intervals
Topical Ophthalmics*				
carbachol, topical	Miostat	Glaucoma		
pilocarpine	Pilopine	Glaucoma		

*(see Chapter 54 for detailed information)

Uses

Major uses of the cholinergic drugs are in the treatment of the following:

• Urinary retention
• Myasthenia gravis
• Glaucoma

Adverse Reactions

Topical administration usually produces few adverse effects, but a temporary reduction of visual acuity (sharpness) and headache may occur. With the exception of those applied topically, cholinergic drugs are not selective in action. General adverse reactions include the following:

• Nausea, diarrhea, abdominal cramping
• Salivation
• Flushing of the skin
• Cardiac arrhythmias and muscle weakness

Contraindications

These drugs are contraindicated in patients with known hypersensitivity to the drugs, asthma, peptic ulcer disease, coronary artery disease, and hyperthyroidism. Bethanechol is contraindicated in those with mechanical obstruction of the GI or genitourinary tracts. Patients with secondary glaucoma, iritis, corneal abrasion, or any acute inflammatory disease of the eye should not use the ophthalmic cholinergic preparations.

Precautions

These drugs are used cautiously in patients with hypertension, epilepsy, cardiac arrhythmias, bradycardia, recent coronary occlusion, and megacolon. The safety of these drugs has not been established for use during pregnancy (category C) or lactation, or in children.

Interactions

The following interactions may occur when a cholinergic drug is administered with another agent:

Interacting Drug	Common Use	Effect of Interaction
aminoglycoside antibiotics	Anti-infective agent	Increased neuromuscular blocking effect
corticosteroids	Treatment of inflammation/respiratory	Decreased effect of the cholinergic problems

When cholinergic drugs are administered with other cholinergics, there is an increase in the effects of the drugs and greater risk for toxicity. Concurrent use of anticholinergic drugs antagonizes the effects of cholinergic drugs. Because of this property, atropine is considered an antidote for overdosage of cholinergic drugs.

NURSING PROCESS
PATIENT RECEIVING A CHOLINERGIC DRUG

ASSESSMENT

Preadministration Assessment
The preadministration assessment depends on the drug and the reason for administration.

URINARY RETENTION. If a patient receives a cholinergic drug for the treatment of urinary retention, the nurse palpates the abdomen in the pelvic area and scans the bladder to determine if urine retention is present. A rounded swelling over the pelvis usually indicates retention and a distended bladder. The patient may also complain of discomfort in the lower abdomen. In addition, the nurse takes the patient's blood pressure and pulse rate.

MYASTHENIA GRAVIS. Before the nurse gives a cholinergic drug to a patient with myasthenia gravis, the primary health care provider performs a complete neurologic assessment. The nurse assesses for signs of muscle weakness, such as drooling (i.e., the lack of ability to swallow), inability to chew and swallow, drooping of the eyelids, inability to perform repetitive movements (e.g., walking, combing hair, using eating utensils), difficulty breathing, and extreme fatigue.

Ongoing Assessment
While the patient is receiving a cholinergic drug, it is important for the nurse to monitor for drug toxicity or **cholinergic crisis.**

> **NURSING ALERT**
> Symptoms of cholinergic crisis (cholinergic drug toxicity) include severe abdominal cramping, diarrhea, excessive salivation, muscle weakness, rigidity and spasm, and clenching of the jaw. Patients exhibiting these symptoms require immediate medical treatment, and their condition must be reported immediately to the primary health care provider. In the case of overdosage, an antidote such as atropine is administered and other treatment also may be prescribed. The usual dosage of atropine is 0.4 to 0.6 mg intravenously (IV).

URINARY RETENTION. The ongoing assessment for a patient with urinary retention includes measuring and recording the fluid intake and output. The nurse must notify the primary health care provider if the patient fails to void after drug administration.

If a cholinergic drug is ordered for preventing urinary retention, the nurse measures and records the fluid intake and output. If the amount of each voiding is insufficient or the patient fails to void, the nurse palpates the bladder to determine its size, uses the bladder scanner after the patient attempts to void, and measures for urine residual. The nurse notifies the primary health care of the amount of urine the patient is unable to eliminate.

MYASTHENIA GRAVIS. Once therapy is under way, the nurse must document any increase in symptoms of the disease or adverse drug reactions before giving each dose of the drug. The nurse assesses the patient for the presence or absence of the symptoms of myasthenia gravis before each drug dose. In patients with severe myasthenia gravis, the nurse can carry out these assessments between drug doses, as well as immediately before drug administration. The nurse documents each symptom, as well as the patient's response or lack of response to drug therapy.

Assessment is important because the dosage frequently has to be increased or decreased early in therapy, depending on the patient's response. Regulation of dosage is important in keeping the symptoms of myasthenia gravis from incapacitating the patient. For many patients, the symptoms are fairly well controlled with drug therapy once the optimal drug dose is determined.

NURSING DIAGNOSIS

Drug-specific nursing diagnosis includes:

❏ **Diarrhea** related to adverse drug reaction

Nursing diagnoses related to drug administration are discussed in Chapter 4.

PLANNING

The expected outcomes of the patient depend on the reason for administration of the cholinergic drug, but may include an optimal response to therapy, meeting patient needs related to the management of adverse reactions, and an understanding therapeutic regimen.

IMPLEMENTATION

Promoting an Optimal Response to Therapy
The care of a patient receiving a cholinergic drug depends on the drug used, the reason for administration, and the patient's response to the drug.

MANAGING URINARY RETENTION. Voiding usually occurs in 5 to 15 minutes after subcutaneous drug administration and 30 to 90 minutes after oral administration. The nurse should place the call light and any other items the patient might need, such as the urinal or the bedpan, within easy reach. However, some patients are not able to reach or handle these aids easily, so the nurse must promptly answer their call light.

MANAGING MYASTHENIA GRAVIS. At the start of therapy, determining the dosage that will control symptoms may be difficult. In many cases, the dosage must be adjusted upward or downward until optimal drug effects are obtained. Patients with severe symptoms of the disease require the drug every 2 to 4 hours, even during the night. Sustained-released tablets are available that allow less frequent dosing and help the patient to have longer undisturbed periods during the night.

> **NURSING ALERT**
> Because of the need to make frequent dosage adjustments, the nurse should observe the patient closely for symptoms of drug overdosage or underdosage. Signs of drug overdosage include muscle rigidity and spasm, salivation, and clenching of the jaw. Signs of drug underdosage are signs of

the disease itself, namely, rapid fatigability of the muscles, drooping of the eyelids, and difficulty breathing. If symptoms of drug overdosage or underdosage develop, the nurse should contact the primary health care provider immediately, because a change in dosage is usually necessary.

Monitoring and Managing Patient Needs

When a cholinergic drug is given by the oral or parenteral route, adverse drug reactions may affect many systems of the body, such as the heart, respiratory and GI tracts, and the central nervous system. The nurse observes the patient closely for the appearance of adverse drug reactions, such as a change in vital signs or an increase in symptoms. The nurse documents any complaints the patient may have and notifies the primary health care provider.

DIARRHEA. When these drugs are used orally, they occasionally result in excessive salivation, abdominal cramping, flatus, and sometimes diarrhea. The patient is informed that these reactions will continue until tolerance develops, usually within a few weeks. Until tolerance develops, the nurse ensures that proper facilities, such as a bedside commode, bedpan, or bathroom, are readily available. The patient is encouraged to ambulate to assist the passing of flatus. If needed, a rectal tube may be used to assist in the passing of flatus. The nurse keeps a record of the fluid intake and output and the number, consistency, and frequency of stools if diarrhea is present. The primary health care provider is informed if diarrhea is excessive because this may be an indication of toxicity.

Educating the Patient and Family

Patients required to take a drug over a long period may incur lapses in their drug schedule. For some, it is a matter of occasionally forgetting to take a drug; for others, a lapse may be caused by other factors, such as failure to understand the importance of drug therapy, the cost of the drug, or unfamiliarity with the consequences associated with discontinuing the drug therapy.

When developing a teaching plan for the patient and family, the nurse emphasizes the importance of uninterrupted drug therapy. The nurse allows the patient and family time to ask questions. The nurse explores any problems that appear to be associated with the prescribed drug regimen and then reports them to the primary health care provider. The nurse reviews the purpose of the drug therapy with the patient and family, as well as the adverse reactions that may occur.

MYASTHENIA GRAVIS. Many patients with myasthenia gravis learn to adjust their drug dosage according to their needs, because dosage needs may vary slightly from day to day. The nurse teaches the patient and family members to recognize symptoms of overdosage and underdosage, as well as what steps the primary health care provider wishes them to take if either occurs. The dosage regimen is explained and instruction is given in how to adjust the dosage upward or downward.

The nurse gives the patient a written or printed description of the signs and symptoms of drug overdosage or underdosage. The nurse instructs the patient to keep a record of the response to drug therapy (e.g., time of day, increased or decreased muscle strength, fatigue) and to bring this to each primary health care provider or clinic visit until the symptoms are well controlled and the drug dosage is stabilized. These patients must wear or carry identification (such as a Medic Alert tag) indicating that they have myasthenia gravis.

EVALUATION

- Therapeutic effect is achieved.
- Adverse reactions are identified, reported to the primary health care provider, and managed successfully through appropriate nursing interventions.
  ☑ Patient reports adequate bowel movements.
- Patient and family demonstrate an understanding of the drug regimen.

THINK CRITICALLY: PHARMACOLOGY IN PRACTICE

1. Discuss the types of ongoing assessments made when a patient takes a cholinergic drug for urinary retention.

● Test Your Knowledge

1. A patient with glaucoma is prescribed pilocarpine eye drops. One adverse reaction that the nurse will expect with the use of this drug is _____.

   A. temporary loss of visual acuity
   B. pain in the affected eye
   C. excessive tearing of both eyes
   D. mydriasis of the eyes

2. The primary care provider allows the patient to keep pilocarpine eye drops at the bedside and to self-administer the eye drops four times daily. The nurse _____.

   A. need not check with the patient concerning the eye drops because the patient is a responsible adult
   B. must check the patient to be sure the medication is used properly and at the right time
   C. is not responsible for monitoring the patient's response to the medication
   D. does not record the administration of the drug in the patient's chart

3. A patient has received a diagnosis of myasthenia gravis and begins a regimen of ambenonium. The nursing assessment is important because the dose of the drug _____.

   A. usually must be increased every 4 hours early in therapy
   B. frequently is increased or decreased early in therapy
   C. is titrated according to the patient's blood pressure
   D. is gradually decreased as a therapeutic response is achieved

Cholinergic Drugs

● Calculate Medication Dosages

1. The dosage of pyridostigmine bromide (Mestinon) is 600 mg/day. How many tablets will the patient take if they are 60 mg each?

2. The primary care provider prescribes 2.5 mg of bethanechol subcutaneously. The drug is available in a solution of 5 mg/mL. The nurse administers _____.

To check your answers, see Appendix E.

the**Point** *For more NCLEX questions, log on to http://thepoint.lww.com to access more than 1000 questions.*

Cholinergic Blocking Drugs

LEARNING OBJECTIVES

On completion of this chapter, the student will:

1. Discuss the uses, general drug actions, general adverse reactions, contraindications, precautions, and interactions of the cholinergic blocking drugs (also called anticholinergic drugs and cholinergic blockers).
2. Discuss important preadministration and ongoing assessment activities the nurse should perform on the patient taking cholinergic blocking drugs.
3. List nursing diagnoses particular to the patient taking cholinergic blocking drugs.
4. Discuss ways to promote an optimal response to therapy, how to manage common adverse reactions, and important points to keep in mind when educating patients taking a cholinergic blocking drug.

Like adrenergic blocking drugs, the **cholinergic blocking** drugs have an effect on the autonomic nervous system. Cholinergic blocking drugs are also called **anticholinergic drugs**, *cholinergic blockers*, or **parasympatholytic** drugs.

Acetylcholine (ACh) is the primary neurotransmitter in the parasympathetic branch of the autonomic nervous system. Cholinergic blocking drugs block the action of the neurotransmitter ACh in the parasympathetic nervous system. Because parasympathetic nerves influence many areas of the body, the effects of the cholinergic blocking drugs are numerous. Examples of cholinergic blocking drugs include atropine, scopolamine, and oxybutynin (Ditropan).

Actions

Cholinergic blocking drugs inhibit the activity of ACh at the parasympathetic nerve synapse (Fig. 27.1). When the activity of ACh is inhibited, impulses traveling along the parasympathetic nerve cannot pass from the nerve ending to the effector organ or structure.

Two types of receptors are found in the parasympathetic nervous branch: muscarinic and nicotinic receptors. Cholinergic blocking drugs can specifically target one of these types of receptors. For example, antispasmodic drugs used to treat an overactive urinary bladder work by inhibiting the action of the muscarinic receptors in the parasympathetic nervous system. As a result, the detrusor muscle of the bladder does not contract, which prevents the sensations of urinary urgency. Yet, an antispasmodic drug has no effect on skeletal muscles, because it does not inhibit the nicotinic receptors in the parasympathetic nervous system.

Because of the wide distribution of parasympathetic nerves, some of these drugs that inhibit nerve impulses at both muscarinic and nicotinic receptors affect many organs and structures of the body, including the eyes, the respiratory and gastrointestinal (GI) tracts, the heart, and the bladder (Display 27.1).

However, responses to administration of a cholinergic blocking drug vary and often depend on the drug and the dose used. For example, scopolamine may occasionally cause excitement, delirium, and restlessness. This reaction is considered a **drug idiosyncrasy** (an unexpected or unusual drug effect).

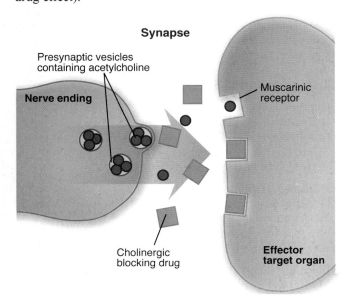

Figure 27.1 Mechanism of action of cholinergic blocking drugs.

DISPLAY 27.1 Effects of the Cholinergic Blocking Drugs

Cholinergic blocking drugs produce the following responses:

- **Central nervous system**—dreamless sleep, drowsiness; atropine may produce mild stimulation in some patients
- **Eye**—mydriasis (dilation of the pupil), cycloplegia (paralysis of accommodation or inability to focus the eye)
- **Respiratory tract**—xerostomia (drying of the secretions of the mouth); drying of the secretions of the nose, throat, bronchi; relaxation of smooth muscles of the bronchi resulting in slight bronchodilation
- **Gastrointestinal tract**—decrease in secretions of the stomach, decrease in gastric and intestinal movement (motility)
- **Cardiovascular system**—increase in pulse rate (most pronounced with atropine administration)
- **Urinary tract**—dilation of smooth muscles of the ureters and renal pelvis

Uses

The primary uses of cholinergic blocking drugs are in the treatment of the following:

- Pylorospasm and peptic ulcer
- Ureteral or biliary colic and bladder overactivity
- Vagal nerve-induced bradycardia
- Parkinsonism

In addition, the cholinergic blocking drugs are administered for the preoperative reduction of oral secretions. The Summary Drug Table: Cholinergic Blocking Drugs lists the uses of specific cholinergic blocking drugs.

Adverse Reactions

The severity of many adverse reactions is often dose dependent—that is, the larger the dose, the more intense the adverse reaction. Bodily system adverse reactions that may occur with the administration of a cholinergic blocking drug are listed in the following sections.

Gastrointestinal System Reactions

- Dry mouth, nausea, vomiting
- Difficulty in swallowing, heartburn
- Constipation

Central Nervous System Reactions

- Headache, flushing, nervousness
- Drowsiness, weakness, insomnia
- Nasal congestion, fever

Visual Reactions

- Blurred vision
- **Mydriasis**
- Photophobia
- **Cycloplegia**
- Increased ocular tension

Genitourinary System Reactions

- Urinary hesitancy and retention
- Dysuria

Cardiovascular System Reactions

- Palpitations
- Bradycardia (after low doses of atropine)
- Tachycardia (after higher doses of atropine)

Other Reactions

- Urticaria
- Decreased sweat production
- Anaphylactic shock
- Rash

Sometimes a secondary adverse reaction, such as drowsiness, is desirable. For example, when atropine is used before surgery to reduce the production of secretions in the respiratory tract, drowsiness is part of the desired response.

 LIFESPAN ALERT – Gerontology
The nurse observes the elderly patient receiving a cholinergic blocking drug at frequent intervals for excitement, agitation, mental confusion, drowsiness, urinary retention, or other adverse effects. These effects may be seen even with small doses. If any should occur, it is important to withhold the next dose of the drug and contact the primary health care provider. The nurse ensures patient safety until these adverse reactions disappear.

The nurse should observe patients receiving a cholinergic blocking drug during the hot summer months for signs of heat prostration (e.g., fever, tachycardia, flushing, warm dry skin, mental confusion) because these drugs decrease sweating.

Contraindications

Cholinergic blocking drugs are contraindicated in patients with known hypersensitivity to the drugs or glaucoma. Other patients for whom cholinergic blocking drugs are contraindicated are those with myasthenia gravis, tachyarrhythmias, myocardial infarction, and congestive heart failure (unless bradycardia is present).

Precautions

The nurse should use these drugs with caution in patients with GI infections, benign prostatic hypertrophy, urinary retention, hyperthyroidism, hepatic or renal disease, and hypertension. The nurse should use atropine with caution in patients with asthma. Cholinergic blocking drugs are classified as pregnancy category C drugs and are used only when the benefit to the woman outweighs the risk to the fetus.

This caution applies to some over-the-counter (OTC) preparations available for the relief of allergy and cold symptoms and as aids to induce sleep. Some of these products contain atropine, scopolamine, or other cholinergic blocking drugs. Although this warning is printed on the container or package, many users fail to read drug labels carefully.

Summary Drug Table CHOLINERGIC BLOCKING DRUGS

Generic Name	Trade Name	Uses	Adverse Reactions	Dosage Ranges
atropine *ah'-troe-peen*	AtroPen	Pylorospasm, reduction of bronchial and oral secretions, excessive vagal-induced bradycardia, ureteral and biliary colic	Drowsiness, blurred vision, tachycardia, dry mouth, urinary hesitancy	0.4–0.6 mg orally, IM, subcut, IV
belladonna *bel-lah-doan'-ah*		Adjunctive therapy for peptic ulcer, digestive disorders, diverticulitis, pancreatitis, diarrhea	Same as atropine	0.25–0.5 mg orally TID
dicyclomine *dye-sye'-kloe-meen*	Benty1	Functional bowel/irritable bowel syndrome	Same as atropine	80–160 mg orally QID
glycopyrrolate *glye-koe-pye'-roe-late*	Robinul	Oral: peptic ulcer Parenteral: in conjunction with anesthesia to reduce bronchial and oral secretions, to block cardiac vagal inhibitory reflexes during induction of anesthesia and intubation; protection against the peripheral muscarinic effects of cholinergic agents (e.g., neostigmine)	Blurred vision, dry mouth, altered taste perception, nausea, vomiting, dysphagia, urinary hesitancy and retention	Oral: 1–2 mg BID or TID Parenteral: peptic ulcer, 0.1–0.2 mg IM, IV, TID, QID Preanesthesia: 0.002 mg/lb IM Intraoperative: 0.1 mg IV
mepenzolate *meh-pen'-zoe-late*	Cantil	Adjunctive treatment of peptic ulcer	Same as atropine	25–50 mg orally TID or QID with meals and at bedtime
methscopolamine *meth-scoe-pol'-ah-meen*	Pamine	Adjunctive therapy for peptic ulcer	Same as atropine	2.5 mg 30 min before meals and 2.5–5 mg orally at bedtime
propantheline *proe-pan'-theh-leen*	Pro-Banthine	Adjunctive therapy for peptic ulcer	Dry mouth, constipation, hesitancy, urinary retention, blurred vision	15 mg orally 30 min before meals and at bedtime
scopolamine *scoe-pol'-ah-meen*		Preanesthetic sedation, motion sickness	Confusion, dry mouth, constipation, urinary hesitancy, urinary retention, blurred vision	0.32–0.65 mg IM, subcut, IV, diluted with sterile water for injections Transdermal: apply 1 patch 4 hr before travel q 3 days
trimethobenzamide *trye-meth-oh-ben'-zah-mide*	Tigan	Control of nausea and vomiting	Hypotension (IM use), Parkinson-like symptoms, blurred vision, drowsiness, dizziness	250 mg orally or 200 mg IM, rectal suppository TID or QID

(handwritten: no longer on market   Best for kids)

Cholinergic Blocking Urinary Antispasmodics

darifenacin *dah-ree-fen'-ah-sin*	Enablex	Overactive bladder	Dry mouth, constipation	7.5 mg orally daily
flavoxate *flah-vox'-ate*	Urispas	Urinary symptoms caused by cystitis, prostatitis, and other urinary problems	Dry mouth, drowsiness, blurred vision, headache, urinary retention	100–200 mg orally 3–4 times/day
oxybutynin *ox-see-byoo-tye'-nin*	Ditropan	Overactive bladder, neurogenic bladder	Dry mouth, nausea, headache, drowsiness, constipation, urinary retention	5 mg orally, 2–3 times/day

(table continues on page 242)

(handwritten: OTC may include AtroPen or Bentyl)

Summary Drug Table CHOLINERGIC BLOCKING DRUGS (continued)

Generic Name	Trade Name	Uses	Adverse Reactions	Dosage Ranges
solifenacin *sole-ih-fen'-ah-sin*	Vesicare	Overactive bladder	Dry mouth, constipation, blurred vision, dry eyes	5 mg orally daily
tolterodine *toll-tare'-oh-dyne*	Detrol, Detrol LA (long-acting, extended-release)	Overactive bladder	Dry mouth, constipation, headache, dizziness	2 mg orally, TID; extended–release: 4 mg daily
Ⓡ trospium *troz'-pee-um*	Sanctura	Overactive bladder	Dry mouth, constipation, headache	20 mg orally TID
Cholinergic Blocking Drugs for Parkinson's Disease				
benztropine mesylate *benz'-troe-peen*	Cogentin	Parkinson's disease, drug-induced extrapyrimidal syndrome (EPS)	Dry mouth, blurred vision, dizziness, nausea, nervousness, skin rash, urinary retention, dysuria, tachycardia, muscle weakness, disorientation, confusion	0.5–6 mg/day orally Acute dystonia: 1–2 mL IM or IV
biperiden *bye-pare'-ih-den*	Akineton	Parkinson's disease, drug-induced EPS	Same as benztropine mesylate	2 mg orally TID or QID; maximum dose 16 mg/24 hr
diphenhydramine *dye-fen-hye'-dra-meen*	Benadryl	Drug-induced EPS, allergies	Same as benztropine mesylate	25–50 mg orally TID or QID
procyclidine *pro-sye'-klih-deen*	Kemadrin	Parkinsonism symptoms, drug-induced EPS	Same as benztropine mesylate	2.5–5 mg orally TID
trihexyphenidyl *trye-hex-see-fen'-ih-dill*		Parkinsonism symptoms, drug-induced EPS	Same as benztropine mesylate	1–15 mg/day orally in divided doses
Cholinergic Blocking Drug (for acute respiratory symptom relief)				
ipratropium *ih-prah-troe'-pee-um*	Atrovent	Bronchospasm associated with chronic obstructive pulmonary disease, chronic bronchitis and emphysema, rhinorrhea	Dryness of the oropharynx, nervousness, irritation from aerosol, dizziness, headache, GI distress, dry mouth, exacerbation of symptoms, nausea, palpitations	Aerosol: two inhalations QID, not to exceed 12 inhalations; Solution: 500 mg (1 unit dose vial) TID, QID by oral nebulization Nasal spray: 2 sprays per nostril BID, TID of 0.03%, or 2 sprays per nostril TID, QID of 0.06%
tiotropium *tee-oh-troe'-pee-um*	Spiriva	Same as ipratropium	Same as ipratropium, increased stroke potential	One capsule per day using inhalation device, not for oral use

Ⓡ This drug should be administered at least 1 hour before or 2 hours after a meal.

Interactions

The following interactions may occur when a cholinergic blocking drug is administered with another agent:

Interacting Drug	Common Use	Effect of Interaction
antibiotics/antifungals	Fight infection	Decreased effectiveness of anti-infective drug
meperidine, flurazepam, phenothiazines	Preoperative sedation	Increased effect of the cholinergic blocker

Interacting Drug	Common Use	Effect of Interaction
tricyclic antidepressants	Management of depression	Increased effect of the cholinergic blocker
haloperidol	Antianxiety/antipsychotic agent	Decreased effectiveness of antipsychotic drug
digoxin	Management of cardiac problems	Increased serum levels of digoxin

NURSING PROCESS
PATIENT RECEIVING A CHOLINERGIC BLOCKING DRUG

ASSESSMENT

Preadministration Assessment
Before administering a cholinergic blocking drug to a patient for the first time, the nurse obtains a thorough health history as well as a history of the signs and symptoms of the current disorder. The focus of the initial physical assessment depends on the reason for administering the drug. In most instances, the nurse obtains the blood pressure, pulse, and respiratory rate. The nurse also may include additional assessments, such as checking the stool of the patient who has a peptic ulcer for color and signs of occult blood, determining visual acuity in the patient with glaucoma, or looking for signs of dehydration and weighing the patient if prolonged diarrhea is one of the patient's symptoms.

Ongoing Assessment
When administering a cholinergic blocking drug, the daily ongoing assessment requires that the nurse closely observe the patient. The nurse checks vital signs, observes for adverse drug reactions, and evaluates the symptoms and complaints related to the patient's diagnosis. For example, the nurse questions the patient with a peptic ulcer regarding current symptoms, then makes a comparison of these symptoms to the symptoms present before the start of therapy. The nurse reports any increase in the severity of symptoms to the primary health care provider immediately.

NURSING DIAGNOSES

Drug-specific nursing diagnoses include:

❏ **Impaired Comfort** related to **xerostomia**
❏ **Constipation** related to slowing of peristalsis in the GI tract
❏ **Risk for Injury** related to dizziness, drowsiness, mental confusion, or heat prostration
❏ **Disturbed Sensory Perception: Visual** related to adverse drug reaction
❏ **Ineffective Tissue Perfusion** related to impaired heart pumping action

Nursing diagnoses related to drug administration are discussed in Chapter 4.

PLANNING

The expected outcomes for the patient depend on the reason for administration of a cholinergic blocking drug, but may include an optimal response to therapy, meeting patient needs related to the management of adverse reactions, and an understanding of and compliance with the prescribed therapeutic regimen.

IMPLEMENTATION

Promoting an Optimal Response to Therapy

PATIENT RECEIVING A PREOPERATIVE DRUG. If a cholinergic blocking drug is administered before surgery, the nurse instructs the patient to void before the drug is given. The nurse informs the patient that his or her mouth will become extremely dry, that this is normal, and that fluid is not to be taken. The side rails of the bed are raised, and the patient is instructed to remain in bed after administration of the preoperative drug.

> **! NURSING ALERT**
> The nurse must administer the preoperative drug at the exact time prescribed, because the cholinergic blocking drug must be given time to produce the greatest effect (i.e., the drying of upper respiratory and oral secretions) before the administration of a general anesthetic. The anesthesiologist must be notified if the preoperative drug is given late.

> **LIFESPAN ALERT – Gerontology**
> Cholinergic blocking drugs are usually not included in the preoperative drugs of patients older than 60 years, because of the effects of these drugs on the eye and the central nervous system.

Monitoring and Managing Patient Needs

IMPAIRED COMFORT: XEROSTOMIA. When taking these drugs on a daily basis, mouth dryness may be severe and extremely uncomfortable in some patients. The patient may complain of a "cottonmouth" sensation, in which oral dryness feels like a mouthful of cotton. The patient may have moderate to extreme difficulty swallowing drugs and food. The patient's speech may be impeded and hard to understand because of the dry mouth.

The nurse encourages the patient to take a few sips of water before and while taking an oral drug and to sip water at intervals during meals. If allowed, hard candy slowly dissolved in the mouth and frequent sips of water during the day may help relieve persistent oral dryness. The nurse checks the oral cavity daily for soreness or ulcerations. Refer to the Patient Teaching for Improved Patient Outcomes: Combating Dry Mouth for suggestions on diminishing the discomfort.

CONSTIPATION. Constipation caused by decreased gastric motility can be a problem with cholinergic blocking drugs. The nurse urges the patient to increase fluid intake up to 2000 mL daily (if health conditions permit), eat a diet high in fiber, and obtain adequate exercise. Patients being treated for an overactive bladder may be hesitant to increase fluids because of fear of an episode of urinary incontinence. The nurse reassures the patient that increasing fluids will help minimize the adverse reactions of constipation and dry mouth, whereas the cholinergic blocking drug helps to eliminate the sensations of urinary frequency and urgency. The primary health care provider may prescribe a stool softener, if necessary, to prevent constipation.

RISK FOR INJURY. These drugs may cause drowsiness, dizziness, and blurred vision. Patients (especially older adults) may require assistance with ambulation. Blurred vision and photophobia are commonly seen with the administration of a cholinergic blocking drug. The severity of this adverse reaction is commonly dose dependent; that is, the larger the dose, the more intense the adverse reaction. The nurse monitors the patient for any disturbance in vision.

LIFESPAN ALERT – Gerontology

The nurse advises the family of an elderly patient of possible visual and mental impairments (blurred vision, confusion, agitation) that may occur during therapy with these drugs. Objects or situations that may cause falls, such as throw rugs, footstools, and wet or newly waxed floors, are removed or avoided whenever possible. The nurse instructs the family to place against the walls any items of furniture (e.g., footstools, chairs, stands) that obstruct walkways. The nurse alerts the family to the dangers of heat prostration and explains the steps to take to avoid this problem. The patient must be closely observed during the first few days of therapy, and the primary health care provider is notified if mental changes occur.

In hot weather, sweating may decrease and may be followed by heat prostration. The nurse makes sure that the patient is observed at frequent intervals for signs of heat prostration, especially if the patient is elderly or debilitated. In cases of suspected heat prostration, the next dose of the drug is withheld, and the primary health care provider contacted immediately. The older adult patient receiving a cholinergic blocking drug is also observed at frequent intervals for excitement, agitation, mental confusion, drowsiness, urinary retention, or other adverse effects. If any of these should occur, the next dose of the drug should be withheld and the primary health care provider contacted. Patient safety must be ensured until these adverse reactions subside.

DISTURBED SENSORY PERCEPTION: VISUAL. If photophobia is a problem, the patient may need to wear shaded glasses when going outside, even on cloudy days. Rooms are kept dimly lit and curtains or blinds closed to eliminate bright sunlight in the room. Those with photophobia may be more comfortable in a semidarkened room, especially on sunny days. It is a good idea to use overhead lights as little as possible.

Mydriasis (prolonged pupillary dilation) and cycloplegia (difficulty focusing resulting from paralysis of ciliary muscle), if they occur, may interfere with reading, watching television, and similar activities. If these drug effects upset the patient, the nurse discusses the problem with the primary health care provider. At times, these visual impairments will have to be tolerated because drug therapy cannot be changed or discontinued. The nurse can assist the patient to find other forms of diversional therapy, such as interaction with others or listening to the radio.

INEFFECTIVE TISSUE PERFUSION. The patient receiving atropine for third-degree heart block is placed on a cardiac monitor during and after administration of the drug. The nurse watches the monitor for a change in pulse rate or rhythm. Tachycardia, other cardiac arrhythmias, or failure of the drug to increase the heart rate must be reported to the primary health care provider immediately because other drugs or medical management may be necessary.

Educating the Patient and Family

A cholinergic blocking drug may be prescribed for a prolonged period. Some patients may discontinue drug use, especially if their original symptoms have been relieved. The nurse must make sure that the patient and family understand the prescribed drug is to be taken even though symptoms have been relieved.

When a cholinergic blocking drug is prescribed for outpatient use, the nurse informs the patient about the more common adverse reactions associated with these drugs, such as dry mouth, drowsiness, dizziness, and visual impairments. The nurse warns the patient that if drowsiness, dizziness, or blurred vision occurs, caution must be observed while driving or performing other tasks requiring alertness and clear vision.

Some of the adverse reactions associated with the cholinergic blocking drugs may be uncomfortable or distressing. The nurse encourages the patient to discuss these problems with the primary health care provider. The nurse also makes suggestions to lessen the intensity of some of these adverse reactions.

The following is a list of adverse reactions that can be included in the teaching plan, along with the measures that may lessen their intensity or allow the patient to perform tasks at times when the adverse reactions are least likely to occur.

- Photophobia—Wear sunglasses when outside, even on cloudy days. Keep rooms dimly lit, and close curtains or blinds to eliminate bright sunlight in the room; soft, indirect lighting is usually more comfortable. Schedule outdoor activities (when necessary) before the first dose of the drug is taken, such as early in the morning.
- Dry mouth—Take frequent sips of cool water during the day, before taking the drug orally, and during meals. In addition, if allowed, chew gum or dissolve hard candy in the mouth.
- Constipation—It is a good idea to drink plenty of fluids during the day, exercise if approved by the primary health care provider, and eat foods high in fiber.
- Heat prostration—Avoid going outside on hot, sunny days; use fans to cool the body if the day is extremely warm; sponge the skin with cool water if other cooling measures are not available; and wear loose-fitting clothes in warm weather.
- Drowsiness—Schedule tasks requiring alertness during times when drowsiness does not occur, such as early in the morning before the first dose of the drug is taken.

Educating the Patient Receiving a Preoperative Drug

When one of these drugs is administered before surgery, the nurse gives the patient an explanation of the preoperative drug: namely, why the drug is being given, when the drug will be given, and when the patient is going to surgery. Sufficient time is allowed for the patient to void before the preoperative drug is administered. The nurse informs the patient and family members that drowsiness and extreme dryness of the mouth and nose will occur about 20 to 30 minutes after the drug is given. The importance of remaining in bed with the side rails raised after the drug is administered is stressed.

Educating the Patient With a Peptic Ulcer

The nurse gives the patient with a peptic ulcer a full explanation of the treatment regimen, which may include drugs and a special diet. The patient is instructed to take the drug exactly as prescribed by the primary health care provider (e.g., 30 minutes before meals or between meals) to obtain the desired results. The nurse discusses the importance of diet in peptic ulcer treatment and gives a full explanation of the special diet (when ordered).

EVALUATION

- Therapeutic effect is achieved.
- Adverse reactions are identified, reported to the primary health care provider, and managed successfully through appropriate nursing interventions.
  - ☑ Mucous membranes remain moist.
  - ☑ Patient reports adequate bowel movements.
  - ☑ No evidence of injury is seen.
  - ☑ Vision remains intact.
  - ☑ Tissue perfusion is maintained.
- Patient and family demonstrate an understanding of the drug regimen.

Patient Teaching for Improved Patient Outcomes

Combating Dry Mouth

One of the most common adverse effects occurring with the use of cholinergic blocking drugs is a dry mouth. The nurse offers the following suggestions to the patient to help combat this problem:

- ✓ Perform frequent mouth care, including brushing, rinsing, and flossing.
- ✓ Keep a glass or sports bottle filled with fluid on hand at all times.
- ✓ Sip small amounts of cool water or fluids throughout the day and with meals.
- ✓ Take a few sips of water before taking any oral drugs.
- ✓ Suck on ice chips or frozen ices, such as Popsicles.
- ✓ Chew gum.
- ✓ Suck on sugar-free hard candies.
- ✓ Avoid alcohol-based mouthwashes.

THINK CRITICALLY: PHARMACOLOGY IN PRACTICE

1. A nurse assistant comes to you because she is having difficulty with Mr. Park. He is very concerned that he will be incontinent of stool in the bed. The nursing assistant is frustrated with his continual struggles to get out of bed and asks you about the purpose of preoperative drugs and why patients cannot get out of bed after receiving a preoperative drug. Describe how you would explain this to the nurse assistant.

● Test Your Knowledge

1. A patient taking solifenacin (Vesicare) for an overactive bladder complains of dry mouth. The nurse should _____.
   - **A.** consider this to be unusual and contact the primary health care provider
   - **B.** encourage the patient to take frequent sips of water
   - **C.** give the patient salt-water mouth rinses
   - **D.** ignore this reaction because it is only temporary

2. Which of the following adverse reactions would the nurse expect after the administration of atropine as part of a patient's preoperative medication regimen?
   - **A.** Enhanced action of anesthesia
   - **B.** Reduced secretions of the upper respiratory tract
   - **C.** Prolonged action of the preoperative opioid
   - **D.** Increased gastric motility

3. Because of the effect of cholinergic blocking drugs on intestinal motility, the nurse must monitor the patient taking these drugs for the development of _____.
   - **A.** esophageal ulcers
   - **B.** diarrhea
   - **C.** heartburn
   - **D.** constipation

4. Cholinergic blocking drugs are contraindicated in patients with _____.
   - **A.** gout
   - **B.** glaucoma
   - **C.** diabetes
   - **D.** bradycardia

● Calculate Medication Dosages

1. A patient is prescribed glycopyrrolate (Robinul) 0.1 mg intramuscularly (IM). The drug is available in a solution of 0.2 mg/mL. The nurse administers _____.

2. Oral trihexyphenidyl 4 mg is ordered. The drug is available as an elixir with a strength of 2 mg/5 mL. The nurse administers _____.

To check your answers, see Appendix E.

the**Point** *For more NCLEX questions, log on to* http://thepoint.lww.com *to access more than 1000 questions.*

Drugs That Affect the Neuromuscular System

Previous units in this book have examined both the central and peripheral nervous systems of our bodies and how drugs affect function both in those systems and in other selected bodily systems. The focus of unit VI is on how the nervous system connects with the muscles in our bodies to help produce movement based upon the direction given by our brains.

The musculoskeletal system comprises the bones, joints, and muscles that provide the body with movement. Although separate from the nervous system, they work together as the neuromuscular system to provide our bodies with the ability to live, work, and play. A number of degenerative diseases (Alzheimer's disease [AD], Parkinson's disease, and gout) affect both the musculoskeletal and neurologic systems.

Alzheimer's disease is a progressive deterioration of emotional, physical, and cognitive abilities. Approximately 4.8 million Americans have the disease; almost one half of Americans older than 85 years have AD. Currently, it is the ninth leading cause of death in adults older than 65 years. Typically, an individual lives on average 8 years after diagnosis; yet, some people have been known to live up to 20 years after AD is discovered. Close to $200 billion is spent annually to care for people with AD (including both direct and indirect costs). Although a cure is not known for this degenerative disease, the dementia experienced can be slowed by the use of drugs called *cholinesterase inhibitors*. Chapter 28 discusses the drugs used to enhance neurotransmission of certain substances to maintain and sometimes enhance the cognitive function of persons with dementia.

Many drugs are designed to strengthen or diminish motor messages from the brain to the muscles and other tissues. Some of these categories include antiparkinsonism, anticonvulsant (or antiseizure), and muscle relaxant drugs.

Another degenerative disorder, Parkinson's disease, affects the messages sent from the central nervous system (CNS) to the muscles of the body. The disease is caused by an imbalance of dopamine and acetylcholine in the CNS. An area of the brain, the substantia nigra, loses cells and the supply of the neurotransmitter dopamine is decreased. As a result, too much acetylcholine affects this area of the brain, which controls muscle movement; thus, causing such symptoms as trembling, rigidity, difficulty walking, and problems with balance. Parkinson's disease has no cure, but the antiparkinsonism drugs, covered in Chapter 29, are used to relieve the symptoms and assist in maintaining the patient's mobility and functioning capability as long as possible.

Neurotransmission of the brain can be overexcited by injury or disease. When this happens, seizures (or convulsions) occur. Chapter 30 discusses the drugs used to depress abnormal brain activity and lessen or prevent seizure activity. The promotion of mobility and function are the focus of Chapter 31, with discussion of drugs used as relaxants and in the treatment of bone and joint disorders.

PHARMACOLOGY IN PRACTICE

Our patient focus in this unit is Betty Peterson, an individual with anxiety. She is taking multiple drugs for different ailments. Some of her medications are given to change her neurologic or muscular functions. However, some changes occur as a result of adverse or combination reactions to the drugs she is taking. After reading the chapters in this unit, you will be asked to assess her signs and symptoms, to review her medications, and to figure out whether some of the drugs she is taking are causing her problems or whether her symptoms are the result of disease process.

Cholinesterase Inhibitors

alanine aminotransferase   dementia
Alzheimer's disease

On completion of this chapter, the student will:

1. Discuss the clinical manifestations of Alzheimer's disease.
2. List the uses, general drug actions, general adverse reactions, contraindications, precautions, and interactions associated with the administration of the cholinesterase inhibitors.
3. Discuss important preadministration and ongoing assessment activities the nurse should perform with the patient taking a cholinesterase inhibitor.
4. List nursing diagnoses particular to a patient taking a cholinesterase inhibitor.
5. Discuss ways to promote an optimal response to therapy, how to manage common adverse reactions, and important points to keep in mind when educating patients about the use of the cholinesterase inhibitors.

In **Alzheimer's disease** (AD), specific pathologic changes occur in the cortex of the brain. These changes involve the degeneration of nerves into amyloid plaques and tangled nerve bundles. AD comprises a number of symptoms that become progressively worse in three stages: early, middle, and late. Often, patients may not be diagnosed with AD until they are in the middle or late stages of the disease. Display 28.1 identifies the stages of AD and their associated clinical manifestations.

Early-stage disease is characterized by difficulties with memory, poor judgment, and withdrawal behaviors. The middle stage is typically the longest stage of the illness. As a person progresses through the middle stage, difficult behaviors appear, such as anger, wandering, and hoarding. Late-stage or the final phase of AD finds the patient becoming increasingly immobile and dysfunctional. This stage may last from a few months to several years.

One of the most debilitating symptoms of AD is dementia. **Dementia** involves a decrease in cognitive functioning. Other diseases, such as Parkinson's disease, may have a dementia component, but cholinesterase inhibitors are approved to treat mild to moderate dementia caused by AD. Drugs used to treat AD do not cure the disease, but slow the progression of dementia. Examples of the cholinesterase inhibitors include donepezil (Aricept), and rivastigmine (Exelon). Other drugs are used for symptomatic relief. For example, wandering, irritability, and aggression in people with AD are treated with antipsychotics, such as risperidone and olanzapine. Other drugs, such as antidepressants or antianxiety drugs, may be helpful in AD for symptoms of depression and anxiety; these drugs are all discussed in previous chapters.

Actions

Acetylcholine is the transmitter in the cholinergic neuropathway. Individuals with early AD experience degeneration of these cholinergic neuropathways. As a result, the patient experiences problems with memory and thinking. The cholinesterase inhibitors act to increase the level of acetylcholine in the central nervous system (CNS) by inhibiting its breakdown and slowing neural destruction. However,

DISPLAY 28.1 Clinical Manifestations of Alzheimer's Disease

Early Phase—Mild Cognitive Decline
• Increased forgetfulness
• Decreased performance in social settings
• Evidence of memory deficit when interviewed
• Mild to moderate anxiety

Early Dementia Phase—Moderately Severe Cognitive Decline
• Needs assistance for activities of daily living
• Unable to recall important aspects of current life
• Difficulty making choices (e.g., what clothes to wear, what to eat)
• Able to recall major facts (e.g., their name and family members' names)
• Needs assistance for survival

Late Dementia Phase—Severe Cognitive Decline
• Incontinent of urine
• Little verbal ability
• No basic psychomotor skills
• Needs assistance when bathing, toileting, and feeding

Adapted from *Alzheimer's disease.* Retrieved October 1, 2008, from the Family Caregiver Alliance website: www.caregiver.org/caregiver/jsp/content_node.jsp?nodeid=567.

the disease is progressive, and although these drugs alter the progress of the disease, they do not stop it. Cholinesterase inhibitors are not used in late-stage AD. A newer group of drugs, *N*-methyl-D-aspartate (NMDA) receptor antagonists, is available. Memantine (Namenda) is thought to work by decreasing the excitability of neurotransmission caused by an excess of the amino acid glutamate in the CNS.

Uses

Cholinesterase inhibitors are used to treat early and moderate stages of dementia associated with AD. Trials to see if cognitive decline can be slowed for other dementias, such as vascular or Parkinson's dementia, are being conducted.

Adverse Reactions

Generalized adverse reactions include:

• Anorexia, nausea, vomiting, diarrhea
• Dizziness and headache

Tacrine (Cognex) is particularly damaging to the liver and can result in hepatotoxicity. Patients taking tacrine should have blood drawn periodically and liver function tests performed. Family members or care providers should be instructed on adverse reactions indicating liver dysfunction, such as yellow color to skin or eyes. Additional adverse reactions are listed in the Summary Drug Table: Cholinesterase Inhibitors.

Contraindications and Precautions

Cholinesterase inhibitors are contraindicated in patients with hypersensitivity to the drugs and during pregnancy and lactation (pregnancy category B). Tacrine should not be used in patients with known liver dysfunction.

These drugs are used cautiously in patients with renal or hepatic disease, bladder obstruction, seizure disorders, sick sinus syndrome, gastrointestinal (GI) bleeding, and asthma. In individuals with a history of ulcer disease, bleeding may recur.

Interactions

The following interactions may occur when a cholinesterase inhibitor is administered with another agent:

Interacting Drug	Common Use	Effect of Interaction
anticholinergics	Decrease of bodily secretions	Decreased effectiveness of anticholinergics
nonsteroidal anti-inflammatory drugs	Pain relief	Increased risk of GI bleeding
theophylline	Breathing problems	Increased risk of theophylline toxicity

HERBAL ALERT

Ginseng has been called the "king of herbs" because of its wide use and the benefits attributed to it. In early China, the value of ginseng was as high as that of gold. Ginseng is the fourth best-selling herb in the United States, where hundreds of ginseng products (e.g., teas, chewing gum, juices) are sold. The primary use of ginseng is to improve energy and mental performance. The benefits of ginseng include improving endurance during exercise, reducing fatigue, boosting stamina and reaction times, and increasing feelings of well-being.

Adverse reactions are rare, but sleeplessness, nervousness, and diarrhea have been reported in individuals taking large amounts of the herb. The herb should not be taken in combination with stimulants, including those containing caffeine. Dosage is 200 to 500 mg daily of the standardized extract, or 1 to 4 g of powdered root a day. Ginseng is contraindicated in individuals with high blood pressure and during pregnancy.

Summary Drug Table CHOLINESTERASE INHIBITORS

Generic Name	Trade Name	Uses	Adverse Reactions	Dosage Ranges
donepezil doe-nep'-eh-zill	Aricept	Mild to moderate dementia due to AD	Headache, nausea, diarrhea, insomnia, muscle cramps	5–10 mg/day orally
galantamine gah-lan'-tah-meen	Razadyne	Mild to moderate (AD) dementia	Nausea, vomiting, diarrhea, anorexia, dizziness	16–24 mg BID orally
memantine meh-man'-teen	Namenda	Moderate to severe (AD) dementia	Dizziness, headache, confusion	5–10 mg BID orally
rivastigmine riv-ah-stig'-meen	Exelon	Mild to moderate dementia of AD and Parkinson's Disease	Nausea, vomiting, diarrhea, dyspepsia, anorexia, insomnia, fatigue, dizziness, headache	1.5–12 mg/day BID orally
® tacrine tay'-krin	Cognex	Mild to moderate (AD) dementia	Nausea, vomiting, diarrhea, dizziness, headache, elevated liver function	40–80 mg/day in 4 divided doses orally

® This drug should be administered at least 1 hour before or 2 hours after a meal.

NURSING PROCESS

PATIENT RECEIVING A CHOLINESTERASE INHIBITOR FOR MILD TO MODERATE DEMENTIA OF ALZHEIMER'S DISEASE

ASSESSMENT

Preadministration Assessment

A patient receiving a cholinesterase inhibitor may be treated in the hospital, long-term care facility, or an outpatient setting. The patient's cognitive ability and functional ability are assessed before and during therapy. Cognition can be assessed by using tools such as the Folstein Mini-Mental Status Examination. Patients are assessed on items such as orientation, calculation, recall, and language. Scoring is done by comparison with a standardized answer sheet, and the likelihood of dementia is determined. The nurse assesses the patient for agitation and impulsive behavior. Functional ability, such as performing activities of daily living and self-care, also is assessed. These assessments are used by the nurse in the ongoing monitoring of the patient's improvement (if any) after taking a cholinesterase inhibitor.

HERBAL ALERT

Ginkgo, one of the oldest herbs in the world, has many beneficial effects. It is thought to improve memory and brain function and enhance circulation to the brain, heart, limbs, and eyes. Most of the research done on ginkgo has been done on standardized extract ginkgo. The recommended dose is 40 mg standardized extract ginkgo three times daily. The effects of ginkgo may not be evident until after 4 to 24 weeks of treatment. The most common adverse reactions include mild GI discomfort, headache, and rash. Excessively large doses have been reported to cause diarrhea, nausea, vomiting, and restlessness. Ginkgo is contraindicated in patients taking monoamine oxidase inhibitors (MAOIs), because of the risk of a toxic reaction. Moreover, individuals taking anticoagulants should take ginkgo only on the advice of a primary care provider.

Before starting therapy for the hospitalized patient, the nurse obtains a complete mental health and medical history. Often, patients with AD are unable to give a reliable history of their illness. A family member or primary caregiver may be helpful in verifying or providing information needed for an accurate assessment. When taking the history, the nurse observes the patient for any behavior patterns that appear to deviate from normal. Examples of deviations include poor eye contact, failure to answer questions completely, inappropriate answers to questions, monotone speech pattern, and inappropriate laughter, sadness, or crying signifying varying stages of decline. The nurse documents the patient's cognitive ability using Display 28.1 as a guide.

Physical assessments include obtaining blood pressure measurements on both arms with the patient in a sitting position, pulse, respiratory rate, and weight. Assessing the patient's functional ability is also important.

The initial assessments of the outpatient are basically the same as those for the hospitalized patient. The nurse obtains a complete medical history and a history of the symptoms of AD from the patient (if possible), a family member, or the patient's hospital records. During the initial interview, the nurse observes the patient for what appear to be deviations from a normal behavior pattern. The nurse asks the family about unusual behaviors, such as wandering or outbursts of angry or frustrated behavior. The nurse also should assess the patient's vital signs and body weight.

Ongoing Assessment

Ongoing assessment of patients taking the cholinesterase inhibitors includes both mental and physical assessments. Cognitive and functional abilities are assessed using Display 28.1 as a guide. Initial assessments will be compared with the ongoing assessments to monitor the patient's improvement (if any) after taking the cholinesterase inhibitors.

Behavioral records should be written at periodic intervals (frequency depends on unit guidelines). An accurate description of the patient's behavior and cognitive ability aids the primary health care provider in planning therapy and thus becomes an important part of nursing management. Patients with poor response to drug therapy may require dosage changes, discontinuation of the drug therapy, or the addition of other therapies to the treatment regimen. However, response to these drugs may take several weeks. The symptoms that the patient is experiencing may improve or remain the same, or the patient may experience only a small response to therapy. It is important to remember that a treatment that slows the progression of symptoms in AD is a successful treatment.

NURSING DIAGNOSES

Drug-specific nursing diagnoses include the following:

❑ **Imbalanced Nutrition: Less Than Body Requirements** related to anorexia, nausea, or vomiting
❑ **Risk for Injury** related to dizziness, syncope, clumsiness or the disease process

Nursing diagnoses related to drug administration are discussed in Chapter 4.

PLANNING

The expected outcomes for the patient may include an optimal response to drug therapy, meeting patient needs related to the management of adverse reactions, an absence of injury, and an understanding of the therapeutic regimen.

IMPLEMENTATION

Promoting an Optimal Response to Therapy

The nurse develops a care plan to meet the patient's individual needs. If the patient is hospitalized, it is important to monitor vital signs at least daily and to

Cholinesterase Inhibitors

report any significant change in vital signs to the primary health care provider.

When administering tacrine, the nurse must monitor the patient for liver damage. This is best accomplished by monitoring levels of **alanine aminotransferase** (ALT), an enzyme found predominantly in the liver. Disease or injury to the liver causes this enzyme to be released into the bloodstream, resulting in elevated serum ALT levels. In patients taking tacrine, ALT levels should be obtained weekly from at least week 4 to week 16 after the initiation of therapy. After week 16, ALT levels are monitored every 3 months.

NURSING ALERT

The nurse immediately reports any elevated ALT level to the primary health care provider. The primary health care provider may want to continue monitoring the ALT level or discontinue use of the drug because of the danger of hepatotoxicity. However, abrupt discontinuation may cause a decline in cognitive functioning.

Within 6 weeks of the discontinuation of cholinesterase inhibitor therapy, individuals lose any benefit they have received from the drugs.

Rivastigmine (Exelon) is available in a transdermal form of the drug. The patches are changed on a daily basis and rotated to a clean, dry, and hairless area. Because the patient is experiencing dementia, the site for application should be where the patient is not able to pick at or remove the patch. The upper or lower portions of the back are recommended for the patch administration. Because the same site should not be used more than once every two weeks, the nurse makes or teaches the caregiver to make a chart of the back and indicate where patches have been applied during the last 14 days.

Monitoring and Managing Patient Needs

IMBALANCED NUTRITION: LESS THAN BODY REQUIREMENTS. When taking the cholinesterase inhibitors, patients may experience nausea and vomiting. Although this can occur with all of the cholinesterase inhibitors, patients taking rivastigmine (Exelon) appear to have more problems with nausea and severe vomiting. Nausea and vomiting should be reported to the primary health care provider who may discontinue use of the drug and then restart the drug therapy at the lowest dose possible. Restarting therapy at the lower dose helps to reduce nausea and vomiting.

Attention to the dosing of medications can decrease adverse GI reactions and promote nutrition. The cholinesterase inhibitors can be taken with or without food. Although donepezil (Aricept) is administered orally once daily at bedtime, it can also be given with a snack. When rivastigmine is administered as an oral solution, the nurse removes the oral dosing syringe provided in the protective container. The syringe provided is used to withdraw the prescribed amount. The dose may be swallowed directly from the syringe or first mixed with a small glass of water, cold fruit juice, or soda.

Weight loss and eating problems related to the inability to swallow are two major problems in the late stage of AD. These problems, coupled with anorexia and nausea associated with administration of cholinesterase inhibitors, present a challenge for the nurse or caregiver. Typically these drugs are not administered during the late stage of dementia, but there may be a period of worsening symptoms before the drugs are stopped entirely.

Mealtime should be simple and calm. The patient should be offered a well-balanced diet with foods that are easy to chew and digest. Frequent, small meals may be tolerated better than three regular meals. Offering foods of different consistency and flavor is important in case the patient can handle one form better than another. Fluid intake of six to eight glasses of water daily is encouraged to prevent dehydration.

RISK FOR INJURY. Physical decline and the adverse reactions of dizziness and syncope place the patient at risk for injury. The patient may require assistance by the nurse when ambulating. Assistive devices such as walkers or canes may reduce falls. To minimize the risk of injury, the patient's environment should be controlled and safe. Encouraging the use of side rails, keeping the bed in low position, and using night lights, as well as frequent monitoring by the nurse or caregiver, will reduce the risk of injury. The patient should wear medical identification, such as a MedicAlert bracelet.

Educating the Patient and Family

Early in the disease, the patient may be able to understand changes, yet suspicion and denial are classic symptoms of the disease; therefore, the patient may not be amenable to treatment. As cognitive abilities decrease, the nurse focuses on educating the family and primary caregiver of the patient needs. Depending on the degree of cognitive decline, the nurse discusses the drug regimen with the patient, family member, or caregiver. It is important for the nurse to evaluate accurately the patient's ability to assume responsibility for taking drugs at home. The administration of drugs to the patient with AD becomes a family responsibility when the outpatient appears to be unable to manage his or her own drug therapy.

The nurse explains any adverse reactions that may occur with a specific drug and encourages the caregiver or family members to contact the primary health care provider immediately when a serious drug reaction occurs.

The nurse includes the following points in a teaching plan for the patient or family member:

- Keep all appointments with the primary care provider or clinic, because close monitoring of therapy is essential. Dose changes may be needed to achieve the best results.
- Report any unusual changes or physical effects to the primary health care provider.

- Take the drug exactly as directed. Do not increase, decrease, or omit a dose or discontinue use of this drug unless directed to do so by the primary health care provider.
- Do not drive or perform other hazardous tasks if drowsiness occurs. As soon as the diagnosis of AD is made, patients should be evaluated for their continued ability to drive.
- Do not take any nonprescription drug unless use of a specific drug has been approved by the primary health care provider.
- Keep track of when the drug is taken. In the early stages of forgetfulness, a mark on the calendar each time the medicine is taken or a pill counter that holds the medicine for each day of the week may be used to help the patient remember to take the medication or determine whether the medication has been taken for the day.
- Notify the primary care provider if the following adverse reactions are experienced for more than a few days: nausea, diarrhea, difficulty sleeping, vomiting, or loss of appetite.
- Immediately report the occurrence of the following adverse reactions: severe vomiting, dehydration, changes in neurologic functioning, or yellowing of the skin or eyes.
- Notify the primary health care provider if the patient has a history of ulcers, feels faint, experiences severe stomach pains, vomits blood or material that resembles coffee grounds, or has bloody or black stools.
- Remember that these drugs do not cure AD but slow the mental and physical degeneration associated with the disease. The drug must be taken routinely to slow the progression.
- Remember that during tacrine therapy, the ALT level must be monitored at intervals prescribed by the primary health care provider.

EVALUATION

- Therapeutic effect is achieved and cognitive function is maintained.
- Adverse reactions are identified, reported to the primary health care provider, and managed successfully through appropriate nursing interventions.
  - ☑ Patient maintains an adequate nutritional status.
  - ☑ No injury is evident.
- Patient (if able) and family demonstrate an understanding of the drug regimen.

THINK CRITICALLY: PHARMACOLOGY IN PRACTICE

1. A female patient with AD is taking donepezil (Aricept). She attends an adult day care center during the day. She is not eating well and recently has lost 5 pounds. If you are the nurse at the center, what actions would you take, and why would you take these particular actions?

● Test Your Knowledge

1. Adverse reactions that the nurse would assess for in a patient taking rivastigmine (Exelon) include _____.
   - A. occipital headache
   - B. vomiting
   - C. hyperactivity
   - D. hypoactivity

2. When administering tacrine (Cognex) to a patient with AD, the nurse would most likely expect which laboratory tests to be prescribed?
   - A. Complete blood count
   - B. Cholesterol levels
   - C. Liver function studies
   - D. Electrolyte analysis

3. Which of the following nursing diagnoses would the nurse most likely place on the care plan of a patient with AD that is related to adverse reactions of the cholinesterase inhibitors?
   - A. Imbalanced nutrition
   - B. Confusion
   - C. Risk for suicide
   - D. Bowel incontinence

4. The nurse correctly administers donepezil (Aricept) _____.
   - A. three times daily around the clock
   - B. twice daily 1 hour before meals or 2 hours after meals
   - C. once daily in the morning
   - D. once daily at bedtime

● Prepare for the NCLEX

1. The nurse correctly disposes of the rivastigmine transdermal patch by:
   - A. placing in a tissue and discarding in trash can
   - B. flushing the patch in the patient's toilet
   - C. folding it over so the adhesive side sticks together
   - D. disposing in a sharps contaminated box in the patient room

● Calculate Medication Dosages

1. Rivastigmine (Exelon) oral solution 6 mg is prescribed. The drug is available as an oral solution of 2 mg/mL. The nurse administers _____.

2. Oral memantine (Namenda) 10 mg is prescribed for a patient with AD. On hand are 5-mg tablets. The nurse administers _____.

To check your answers, see Appendix E

the**Point** *For more NCLEX questions, log on to http://thepoint.lww.com to access more than 1000 questions.*

Antiparkinsonism Drugs

achalasia
bradykinesia
blood–brain barrier
choreiform movements

on-off phenomenon
parkinsonism
Parkinson's disease

LEARNING OBJECTIVES

On completion of this chapter, the student will:

1. Define the terms *Parkinson's disease* and *parkinsonism*.
2. Discuss the uses, general drug action, adverse drug reactions, contraindications, precautions, and interactions of the antiparkinsonism drugs.
3. Discuss important preadministration and ongoing assessment activities the nurse should perform on the patient taking antiparkinsonism drugs.
4. List nursing diagnoses particular to a patient taking antiparkinsonism drugs.
5. Discuss ways to promote an optimal response to therapy, how to manage adverse reactions, and important points to keep in mind when educating patients about the use of the antiparkinsonism drugs.

Parkinsonism is a term that refers to a group of symptoms involving motor movement. These signs are characterized by tremors, rigidity, and slow movement (**bradykinesia**). Although Parkinson-like symptoms may be seen with the use of certain drugs, head injuries, and encephalitis, **Parkinson's disease** is the most common form of parkinsonism. Because Parkinson's disease is progressive, the symptoms worsen over time. Speech becomes slurred, the face takes on a masklike and emotionless expression, and the patient may have difficulty chewing and swallowing. The patient's gait becomes unsteady and shuffled, with the upper part of the body bent forward.

Drugs used to treat the symptoms associated with parkinsonism are called *antiparkinsonism drugs*. These drugs either supplement the dopamine in the brain or block excess acetylcholine (ACh) so that better transmission of nerve impulses occurs. The Summary Drug Table: Antiparkinsonism Drugs

provides a listing of the drugs used to treat Parkinson's disease. Antiparkinsonism drugs discussed in the chapter are classified as dopaminergic agents (monoamine oxidase inhibitors [MAOIs] and dopamine receptor agonists), cholinergic blocking drugs (also known as anticholinergic drugs or cholinergic blockers), catechol-O-methyltransferase (COMT) inhibitors, and non-ergot dopamine receptor agonists.

● DOPAMINERGIC DRUGS

Dopaminergic drugs are drugs that affect the dopamine content of the brain. These drugs include levodopa, carbidopa (Lodosyn), amantadine (Symmetrel), and carbidopa/levodopa combination (Sinemet). Other drugs that work to enhance dopamine include agonists such as bromocriptine (Parlodel) or MAOIs such as selegiline (Eldepryl). (See Summary Drug Table: Antiparkinsonism Drugs).

Actions

The symptoms of parkinsonism are caused by a depletion of dopamine in the central nervous system (CNS). It is hard to supplement dopamine because of the **blood–brain barrier**. The blood–brain barrier is a meshwork of tightly packed cells in the walls of the brain's capillaries that screen out certain substances. This unique meshwork of cells in the CNS prohibits large and potentially harmful molecules from crossing into the brain. This ability to screen out certain substances has important implications for drug therapy, because some drugs can pass through the blood–brain barrier more easily than others.

Levodopa is a chemical formulation found in plants and animals that is converted into dopamine by the body. Dopamine, in the form of levodopa, crosses the blood–brain barrier only in small quantities. At one time, levodopa, used alone, caused adverse reactions because too much dopamine stayed in the peripheral nervous system. Combining levodopa with another drug (carbidopa) allows more levodopa to reach the brain, which in turn permits the drug to have a better pharmacologic effect in patients with Parkinson's disease (Fig. 29.1). Carbidopa has no effect when given alone. Therefore, the combination makes more levodopa available to the brain, and as a result, the dosage of levodopa may be reduced,

Antiparkinsonism Drugs

Summary Drug Table ANTIPARKINSONISM DRUGS

Generic Name	Trade Name	Uses	Adverse Reactions	Dosage Ranges
Dopaminergic Drugs				
amantadine *ah-man'-tah-deen*	Symmetrel	Parkinson's disease/drug-induced extra-pyramidal syndrome (EPS), prevention and treatment of infection with influenza A virus	Lightheadedness, dizziness, insomnia, confusion, nausea, constipation, dry mouth, orthostatic hypotension, depression	200–400 mg/day orally in divided doses
bromocriptine *broe-moe-krip'-teen*	Parlodel, Parlodel Snap Tabs	Parkinson's disease, female endocrine imbalances	Drowsiness, sedation, dizziness, faintness, epigastric distress, anorexia	10–40 mg/day orally
carbidopa *kar'-bih-doe-pah*	Lodosyn	Used with levodopa in the treatment of Parkinson's disease	None by its self; adverse reactions are those of levodopa	70–100 mg/day orally
carbidopa/levodopa *kar'-bih-doe-pah/lee'-voe-doe-pah*	Sinemet, Sinemet CR, Parcopa, Carbilev	Parkinson's disease	Anorexia, nausea, vomiting, abdominal pain, dysphagia, dry mouth, mental changes, headache, dizziness, increased hand tremor, choreiform or dystonic movements	Begin with 10 mg/100 mg tablet orally TID, titrated dose combination to minimize symptoms
levodopa *lee'-voe-doe-pah*		Parkinson's disease	Same as carbidopa/levodopa	0.5–1 g/day orally initially, not to exceed 8 g/day
Dopaminergic drugs - MAOIs				
rasagiline *rah-sah'-jih-leen*	Azilect	Parkinson's disease	Headache, arthralgia, depression, dyspepsia, flu syndrome	0.5–1 mg/day orally
selegiline *seh-leh'-geh-leen*	Eldepryl, Emsam, Zelapar	Agonist for levodopa/carbidopa in Parkinson's disease	Nausea, dizziness	5 mg orally at breakfast and lunch
Cholinergic Blocking Drugs (Anticholinergics)				
benztropine *benz'-troe-peen*	Cogentin	Parkinson's disease, drug-induced EPS	Dry mouth, blurred vision, dizziness, nausea, nervousness, skin rash, urinary retention, dysuria, tachycardia, muscle weakness, disorientation, confusion	0.5–6 mg/day orally Acute dystonia: 1–2 mL IM or IV
biperiden *by-pare'-ih-den*	Akineton	Parkinson's disease, drug-induced EPS	Same as benztropine	2 mg orally TID or QID; maximum dose 16 mg/24 hr
diphenhydramine *dye-fen-hye'-drah-meen*	Benadryl	Drug-induced EPS, allergies	Same as benztropine	25–50 mg orally TID or QID
procyclidine *proe-sye'-klih-deen*	Kemadrin	Parkinson's Disease, drug-induced EPS	Same as benztropine	2.5–5 mg orally TID
trihexyphenidyl *trye-hex-see-fen'-ih-dill*		Parkinson's disease, drug-induced EPS	Same as benztropine	1–15 mg/day orally in divided doses
COMT Inhibitors				
entacapone *en-tah-kap'-own*	Comtan	As adjunct to levodopa/carbidopa in Parkinson's disease	Dyskinesia, hyperkinesia, nausea, diarrhea, urine discoloration	200–1600 mg/day orally

(table continues on page 256)

involuntary twitching
paranoid, depressed
dementia, suicidal tendacies

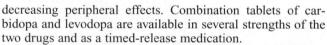

Summary Drug Table ANTIPARKINSONISM DRUGS (continued)

Generic Name	Trade Name	Uses	Adverse Reactions	Dosage Ranges
tolcapone *toll-kap'-own*	Tasmar	Parkinson's disease when refractory to levodopa/carbidopa	Orthostatic hypotension, dyskinesia, sleep disorders, dystonia, excessive dreaming, somnolence, dizziness, nausea, anorexia, muscle cramps, liver failure	100–200 mg orally TID
Dopamine Receptor Agonists, Non-Ergot				
apomorphine *ay-poe-more'-feen*	Apokyn	Parkinson's disease "off" episode	Profound hypotension, nausea, vomiting	0.2 mL as needed for "off" episode
pramipexole *pram-ih-pek'-sole*	Mirapex	Parkinson's disease	Dizziness, somnolence, insomnia, hallucinations, confusion, nausea, dyspepsia, syncope	0.125–1.5 mg orally TID
ropinirole *roe-pin'-oh-roll*	Requip	Parkinson's disease	Dizziness, somnolence, insomnia, hallucinations, confusion, nausea, dyspepsia, syncope	0.25–1 mg orally TID
Combination Drugs				
carbidopa, levodopa, entacapone	Stalevo	Parkinson's disease	See individual drugs	Titrated to individual need

decreasing peripheral effects. Combination tablets of carbidopa and levodopa are available in several strengths of the two drugs and as a timed-release medication.

Drugs that work to stimulate the dopamine receptors are called *agonists*. An example of this drug category includes bromocriptine. The action of <u>amantadine</u> is to make more of the dopamine available at the receptor site. Rasagiline (Azilect) and selegiline inhibit monoamine oxidase type B, again making more dopamine available.

Other dopamine receptor agonists are under investigation for use with Parkinson's disease and restless leg syndrome. These agents are not taken orally; instead they are manufactured as a transdermal patch to deliver the medication, which is poorly absorbed when taken by mouth.

Uses

Dopaminergic drugs are used to treat the signs and symptoms of parkinsonism and the following:

- Parkinson's disease
- Parkinson-like symptoms (extrapyramidal) as a result of injury, drug therapy, or encephalitis
- Restless leg syndrome
- Viral infections (amantadine)

Adverse Reactions

During early treatment with levodopa/carbidopa, adverse reactions are usually not a problem, because of the resolution of Parkinson-like symptoms. As the medication's effectiveness lessens, generalized adverse reactions include the following:

- Dry mouth and difficulty in swallowing
- Anorexia, nausea, and vomiting
- Abdominal pain and constipation
- Increased hand tremor
- Headache and dizziness

The most serious adverse reactions seen with levodopa include **choreiform movements** (involuntary muscular twitching of the limbs or facial muscles) and dystonic movements (muscular spasms most often affecting the tongue, jaw, eyes, and neck). Less common but still serious reactions include mental changes such as dementia, depression, psychotic episodes, paranoia, and suicidal tendencies.

Contraindications and Precautions

The dopaminergic drugs are contraindicated in patients with known hypersensitivity to the drugs. Levodopa is contraindicated in patients with narrow-angle glaucoma and those receiving MAOI antidepressants. The patient should be screened for unusual skin lesions, because levodopa can activate malignant melanoma. Levodopa is used cautiously in patients with cardiovascular or pulmonary diseases, peptic ulcer disease, renal or hepatic disease, and psychosis. Levodopa and combination antiparkinsonism drugs (e.g., carbidopa/levodopa) are classified in pregnancy category C and are used with caution during pregnancy and lactation.

The dopamine agonists, which are MAOIs, selegiline and rasagiline should not be used with the opioid meperidine (Demerol) because of antimetabolite conversion. Caution should be taken with any other opioid used with these antiparkinson drugs.

are given together, pyridoxine may be prescribed to decrease the adverse effects associated with levodopa.

• CHOLINERGIC BLOCKING DRUGS (ANTICHOLINERGICS)

Actions

ACh, a neurotransmitter, is produced in excess in Parkinson's disease. Drugs with cholinergic blocking activity block ACh in the CNS, enhancing dopamine transmission. Drugs with cholinergic blocking activity are generally less effective than levodopa in treating parkinsonism and are limited in dose by peripheral adverse reactions. Antihistamines, such as diphenhydramine (Benadryl), are used in elderly patients, because they produce fewer adverse effects.

Uses

Drugs with cholinergic blocking activity are used as adjunctive therapy in all forms of parkinsonism and in the control of drug-induced extrapyramidal disorders. Examples of drugs with cholinergic blocking activity include benztropine mesylate (Cogentin), biperiden (Akineton), diphenhydramine, procyclidine (Kemadrin), and trihexyphenidyl. See Summary Drug Table: Antiparkinsonism Drugs for specific uses of these drugs.

Adverse Reactions

Adverse reactions to drugs with cholinergic blocking activity include the following:

- Dry mouth
- Blurred vision
- Dizziness, mild nausea, and nervousness

These reactions may become less pronounced as therapy progresses. Other adverse reactions may include:

- Skin rash, urticaria (hives)
- Urinary retention, dysuria
- Tachycardia, muscle weakness
- Disorientation and confusion

If any of these reactions are severe, the drug may be discontinued for several days and restarted at a lower dosage, or a different antiparkinsonism drug may be prescribed.

 LIFESPAN ALERT – Gerontology

Individuals older than 60 years frequently develop increased sensitivity to anticholinergic drugs and require careful monitoring. Confusion and disorientation may occur. Lower doses may be required.

Contraindications and Precautions

These drugs are contraindicated in those with a hypersensitivity to the anticholinergic drugs, those with glaucoma (angle-closure glaucoma), pyloric or duodenal obstruction, peptic ulcers, prostatic hypertrophy, **achalasia** (failure of the

older

Figure 29.1 The blood–brain barrier selectively inhibits certain substances from entering the interstitial spaces of the brain and spinal fluid. It is thought that certain cells in the brain form tight junctions that prevent or slow the passage of certain substances. Levodopa passes the blood–brain barrier, whereas dopamine is unable to pass.

Interactions

The following interactions may occur when a dopaminergic drug is administered with another agent:

Interacting Drug	Common Use	Effect of Interaction
tricyclic antidepressants	Management of depression	Increased risk of hypertension and dyskinesia
antacids	Relief of gastrointestinal (GI) upset and heartburn	Increased effect of levodopa
anticonvulsants	Seizure control	Decreased effect of levodopa

Foods high in pyridoxine (vitamin B_6) or vitamin B_6 preparations reduce the effect of levodopa. However, when carbidopa is used with levodopa, pyridoxine has no effect on the action of levodopa. In fact, when levodopa and carbidopa muscles of the lower esophagus to relax, causing difficulty swallowing), myasthenia gravis, and megacolon.

These drugs are used with caution in patients with tachycardia, cardiac arrhythmias, hypertension, or hypotension, those with a tendency toward urinary retention, those with decreased liver or kidney function, and those with obstructive disease of the urinary system or GI tract. The cholinergic blocking drugs are given with caution to the older adult.

Interactions

The following interactions may occur when a cholinergic blocking drug is administered with another agent:

Interacting Drug	Common Use	Effect of Interaction
amantadine	Treatment of parkinsonism	Increased anti-cholinergic effects
digoxin	Management of cardiac disease	Increased digoxin serum levels
haloperidol	Antipsychotic agent	Increased psychotic behavior
phenothiazines	Antipsychotic agent	Increased anti-cholinergic effects

• COMT INHIBITORS

Another classification of antiparkinsonism drugs is the COMT inhibitors. Examples of the COMT inhibitors are entacapone (Comtan) and tolcapone (Tasmar).

Actions

These drugs are thought to prolong the effect of levodopa by blocking an enzyme, COMT, which eliminates dopamine. When given with levodopa, the COMT inhibitors increase the plasma concentrations and duration of action of levodopa.

Uses

The COMT inhibitors are used as adjuncts to levodopa/carbidopa in treating Parkinson's disease. Tolcapone is a potent COMT inhibitor that easily crosses the blood–brain barrier. However, the drug is associated with liver damage and liver failure. Because of the danger to the liver, tolcapone is reserved for people who are not responding to other therapies. Entacapone is a milder COMT inhibitor and is used to help manage fluctuations in the response to levodopa in individuals with Parkinson's disease.

Adverse Reactions

Adverse reactions most often associated with the administration of COMT inhibitors include the following:

• Dizziness
• Dyskinesias, hyperkinesias
• Nausea, anorexia, and diarrhea
• Orthostatic hypotension, sleep disorders, excessive dreaming
• Somnolence and muscle cramps

A serious and possibly fatal adverse reaction that can occur with the administration of tolcapone is liver failure.

Contraindications and Precautions

These drugs are contraindicated in patients with hypersensitivity to the drugs and during pregnancy and lactation (pregnancy category C). Tolcapone is contraindicated in patients with liver dysfunction. The COMT inhibitors are used with caution in patients with hypertension, hypotension, and decreased hepatic or renal function.

Interactions

The following interactions may occur when a COMT inhibitor is administered with another agent:

Interacting Drug	Common Use	Effect of Interaction
MAOI antidepressants	Management of depression	Increased risk of toxicity of both drugs
adrenergic drugs	Treatment of cardiac and blood pressure problems	Increased risk of cardiac symptoms

• DOPAMINE RECEPTOR AGONISTS

Actions

The exact mechanism of action of the non-ergot dopamine receptor agonists is not understood. It is thought that they act directly on postsynaptic dopamine receptors of nerve cells in the brain, mimicking the effects of dopamine in the brain.

Uses

Dopamine receptor agonists, such as pramipexole (Mirapex) and ropinirole (Requip), are used for the treatment of the signs and symptoms of Parkinson's disease. The drug apomorphine (Apokyn) is used for "on-off" phenomena. Antiemetic therapy must be initiated with this drug.

Adverse Reactions

The most common adverse reactions seen with pramipexole and ropinirole include the following:

• Nausea, dizziness, vomiting
• Somnolence, hallucinations, confusion, visual disturbances
• Postural hypotension, abnormal involuntary movements
• Headache

Contraindications and Precautions

Dopamine receptor agonists are contraindicated in patients with known hypersensitivity to the drugs. Dopamine receptor agonists are used with caution in patients with dyskinesia, orthostatic hypotension, hepatic or renal impairment, cardiovascular disease, and a history of hallucinations or psychosis. Both ropinirole and pramipexole are pregnancy category C drugs, and safety during pregnancy has not been established.

There is an increased risk of CNS depression when the dopamine receptor agonists are administered with other CNS depressants. When administered with levodopa, dopamine receptor agonists increase the effects of levodopa (a lower dosage of levodopa may be required). In addition, when dopamine receptor agonists are administered with levodopa, there is an increased risk of hallucinations. When administered with ciprofloxacin, there is an increased effect of the dopamine receptor agonist.

Interactions

The following interactions may occur when a dopamine receptor agonist is administered with another agent:

Interacting Drug	Common Use	Effect of Interaction
cimetidine, ranitidine	Management of GI problems	Increased dopamine agonist effectiveness
verapamil, quinidine	Management of cardiac problems	Increased dopamine agonist effectiveness
estrogen	Female hormonal supplement	Increased dopamine agonist effectiveness
phenothiazines	Antipsychotic agent	Decreased dopamine agonist effectiveness

NURSING PROCESS

PATIENT RECEIVING AN ANTIPARKINSONISM DRUG

ASSESSMENT

Preadministration Assessment

Because of memory impairment and alterations in thinking in some patients with parkinsonism, a history obtained from the patient may be unreliable. When necessary, the nurse obtains the health history from a family member. Important data to include are information regarding the symptoms of the disorder, the length of time the symptoms have been present, the ability of the patient to carry on activities of daily living, and the patient's current mental condition (e.g., impairment in memory, signs of depression, or withdrawal).

Before starting the drug therapy, the nurse performs a physical assessment of the patient to provide a baseline for future evaluations of drug therapy. It also is important to include an evaluation of the patient's neuromuscular status. Display 29.1 describes the assessments the nurse would make when evaluating the neurologic and musculoskeletal status.

Ongoing Assessment

The nurse evaluates the patient's response to drug therapy by observing the patient for various neuromuscular signs (see Display 29.1) and compares these observations with the data obtained during the initial physical assessment. For example, the patient is assessed for clinical

DISPLAY 29.1 Neuromuscular Evaluation *Know*

The neuromuscular evaluation includes observation for the following:

- Tremors of the hands or head while the patient is at rest
- Masklike facial expression
- Changes (from the normal) in walking
- Type of speech pattern (halting, monotone)
- Postural deformities
- Muscular rigidity
- Drooling, difficulty in chewing or swallowing
- Changes in thought processes
- Ability of the patient to carry out any or all of the activities of daily living (e.g., bathing, ambulating, dressing)

improvement of the symptoms of the disease, such as improvement of tremor of head or hands at rest, muscular rigidity, masklike facial expression, and ambulation stability. Although drug response may occur slowly in some patients, these observations aid the primary health care provider in adjusting the dosage to obtain the desired therapeutic results.

NURSING DIAGNOSES

Drug-specific nursing diagnoses include the following:

- ❏ **Imbalanced Nutrition: Less Than Body Requirements** related to nausea, dry mouth
- ❏ **Constipation** related to neurological changes in the bowel
- ❏ **Risk for Injury** related to dizziness, lightheadedness, orthostatic hypotension, loss of balance
- ❏ **Impaired Physical Mobility** related to alterations in balance, unsteady gait, dizziness

Nursing diagnoses related to drug administration are discussed in Chapter 4.

PLANNING

The expected outcomes for the patient may include an optimal response to drug therapy, meeting patient needs related to the management of adverse reactions, absence of injury, and an understanding of the therapeutic regimen.

IMPLEMENTATION

Promoting an Optimal Response to Therapy

Effective management of the patient with parkinsonism requires that the nurse carefully monitor the drug therapy, provide psychological support, and emphasize patient and family teaching. Optimal response to these drugs often requires titration of doses based on patient activities. To find the best response with the fewest adverse reactions, family members may be given a range of drug dosages to administer.

The antiparkinsonism drugs also may be used to treat the symptoms of parkinsonism that occur with the administration of some of the psychotherapeutic drugs. When used for this purpose, antiparkinsonism drugs may exacerbate mental symptoms and precipitate a psychotic event. The nurse must observe the patient's behavior at frequent intervals. If sudden behavioral changes are noted, the nurse withholds the next dose of the drug and immediately notifies the primary health care provider.

Monitoring and Managing Patient Needs

The nurse observes the patient daily for the development of adverse reactions. All adverse reactions are reported to the primary health care provider, because a dosage adjustment or change to a different antiparkinsonism drug may be necessary with the occurrence of more serious adverse reactions.

> **! NURSING ALERT**
>
> The nurse observes patients receiving carbidopa/ levodopa for the occurrence of choreiform and dystonic movements such as facial grimacing, protruding tongue, exaggerated chewing motions and head movements, and jerking movements of the arms and legs. If these occur, the nurse withholds the next dose of the drug and notifies the primary health care provider immediately, because it may be necessary to reduce the dosage of levodopa or discontinue use of the drug.

IMBALANCED NUTRITION: LESS THAN BODY REQUIREMENTS. Patients may experience multiple adverse reactions that can affect their dietary intake and cause them to lose weight. Some adverse reactions, although not serious, may be uncomfortable. An example of a less serious but uncomfortable adverse reaction is dryness of the mouth. The nurse can help relieve dry mouth by offering frequent sips of water, ice chips, or hard candy (if allowed). If dry mouth is so severe that there is difficulty in swallowing or speaking, or if loss of appetite and weight loss occur, the dosage of the antiparkinsonism drug may be reduced.

Some patients taking the antiparkinsonism drugs experience GI disturbances such as nausea, vomiting, or constipation. This can affect the patient's nutritional status. It is a good idea for the nurse to create a calm environment, serve small, frequent meals, and serve foods the patient prefers to help improve nutrition. The nurse also may monitor the patient's weight daily. GI disturbances are sometimes helped by taking the drug with meals. Severe nausea or vomiting may necessitate discontinuing the drug and changing to a different antiparkinsonism drug. With continued use of the drug, nausea usually decreases or resolves.

CONSTIPATION. Neurologic changes cause changes in peristalsis and dilation of the bowel, leading to chronic constipation. Also, some patients with parkinsonism may have difficulty communicating and are not able to tell the primary health care provider or nurse that bodily urges are occurring. The nurse observes the patient with parkinsonism for outward changes that may indicate the need to eliminate. For example, a sudden change in the facial expression or changes in posture may indicate abdominal pain or discomfort, which may be caused by urinary retention, paralytic ileus, or constipation. If constipation is a problem, the nurse stresses the need

for a diet high in fiber and increasing fluids in the diet. A stool softener may be needed to help prevent constipation.

> **! NURSING ALERT**
>
> A serious and potentially fatal adverse reaction to tolcapone is hepatic injury. Regular blood testing to monitor liver function is usually prescribed. The physician may order testing of serum aminotransferase levels at frequent intervals (e.g., every 2 weeks for the first year and every 8 weeks thereafter). Treatment is discontinued if the alanine aminotransferase (ALT; previously, serum glutamic pyruvic transaminase [SGPT]) exceeds the upper normal limit or signs or symptoms of liver failure develop. The patient is observed for persistent nausea, fatigue, lethargy, anorexia, jaundice, dark urine, pruritus, and right upper quadrant tenderness.

RISK FOR INJURY. Minimizing the risk for injury is an important aspect in the care of the patient with parkinsonism. The patient with visual difficulties may need assistance with ambulation. Visual difficulties (e.g., adverse reactions of blurred vision and diplopia) may be evidenced only by the patient's sudden refusal to read or watch television or by the patient bumping into objects when ambulating. The nurse carefully evaluates any sudden changes in the patient's behavior or activity and reports them to the primary health care provider. Sudden changes in behavior may indicate hallucinations, depression, or other psychotic episodes.

> **LIFESPAN ALERT – Gerontology**
>
> Hallucinations occur more often in the older adult than in the younger adult receiving antiparkinsonism drugs, especially when taking dopamine receptor agonists. The nurse should assess the older adult for signs of visual, auditory, or tactile hallucinations. The incidence of hallucinations appears to increase with age.

Adverse reactions such as dizziness, muscle weakness, and ataxia (lack of muscular coordination) may further increase difficulty with ambulatory activities. Patients with Parkinson's disease are especially prone to falls and other accidents because of the disease process and possible adverse drug reactions. The nurse assists the patient in getting out of the bed or a chair, walking, and other self-care activities. In addition, assistive devices such as a cane or walker may help with ambulation (Fig. 29.2). The nurse may suggest that the patient wear shoes with rubber soles to minimize the possibility of slipping. The room should be kept well lighted, the use of scatter or throw rugs should be avoided, and any small pieces of furniture or objects that might increase the risk of falling should be removed. The nurse carefully assesses the environment and makes necessary adjustments to ensure the patient's safety.

Patients who are prone to orthostatic hypotension as a result of the drug regimen are instructed to arise slowly from a sitting or lying position, especially after sitting or lying for a prolonged time.

Figure 29.2 The nurse provides ambulatory assistance to the patient with parkinsonian symptoms, thus promoting patient safety.

IMPAIRED PHYSICAL MOBILITY. The **on-off phenomenon** may occur in patients taking levodopa. In this condition, the patient may suddenly alternate between improved clinical status and loss of therapeutic effect. This effect is associated with long-term levodopa treatment. Low doses of the drug, reserving the drug for severe cases, or the use of a *drug holiday* may be prescribed. Should symptoms occur, the primary health care provider may order a drug holiday that includes complete withdrawal of levodopa for 5 to 14 days, followed by gradually restarting drug therapy at a lower dose. Patients on a drug holiday need to be monitored for complications.

! NURSING ALERT

Do not abruptly discontinue use of the antiparkinsonism drugs. A neuroleptic malignant-like syndrome may occur when the antiparkinsonism drugs are discontinued or the dosage of levodopa is reduced abruptly. The nurse carefully observes the patient and reports the following symptoms: muscular rigidity, elevated body temperature, and mental changes.

Educating the Patient and Family

The nurse evaluates the patient's ability to understand the therapeutic drug regimen, ability to perform self-care in the home environment, and ability to comply with the prescribed drug therapy. If any type of assistance is needed, the nurse provides a referral to the discharge planning coordinator or social worker.

If the patient requires supervision or help with daily activities and the drug regimen, the nurse encourages the family to create a home environment that is least likely to result in accidents or falls. Changes such as removing throw rugs, installing a hand rail next to the toilet, and moving obstacles that can result in tripping or falling can be made at little or no expense to the family. The nurse should include the following information in the patient and family teaching plan:

- Take this drug as prescribed. Increase, decrease, or omit a dose only as directed by the primary health care provider. If GI upset occurs, take the drug with food.
- If dizziness, drowsiness, or blurred vision occurs, avoid driving or performing other tasks that require alertness.
- Avoid the use of alcohol unless use has been approved by the primary health care provider.
- Relieve dry mouth by sucking on hard candy (unless the patient has diabetes) or frequent sips of water. Consult a dentist if dryness of the mouth interferes with wearing, inserting, or removing dentures or causes other dental problems.
- Inform patients that orthostatic hypotension may develop with or without symptoms of dizziness, nausea, fainting, and sweating. Caution the patient against rising rapidly after sitting or lying down.
- Notify the primary health care provider if any of these problems occur: severe dry mouth, inability to chew or swallow food, inability to urinate, feelings of depression, severe dizziness or drowsiness, rapid or irregular heart beat, abdominal pain, mood changes, and unusual movements of the head, eyes, tongue, neck, arms, legs, feet, mouth, or tongue.
- Keep all appointments with the primary health care provider or clinic personnel because close monitoring of therapy is necessary.
- When taking levodopa, avoid vitamin B_6 (pyridoxine), because this vitamin may interfere with the action of levodopa.
- Patients with diabetes: Levodopa may interfere with urine tests for glucose or ketones, if used. Patients who test urine should report any abnormal result to the primary care provider before adjusting the dosage of the antidiabetic medication.
- Tolcapone: Keep all appointments with the primary health care provider. Liver function tests are performed periodically and are an important part of therapy. Report any signs of liver failure, such as persistent nausea, fatigue, lethargy, anorexia, jaundice, dark urine, pruritus, and right upper quadrant tenderness.

EVALUATION

- Therapeutic effect is achieved and the symptoms of parkinsonism are controlled.
- Adverse reactions are identified, reported to the primary health care provider, and managed successfully through appropriate nursing interventions.
  - ☑ Patient maintains an adequate nutritional status.
  - ☑ Patient has adequate bowel movements.
  - ☑ No evidence of injury is seen.
  - ☑ Patient maintains adequate mobility.
- Patient and family demonstrate an understanding of the drug regimen.

THINK CRITICALLY: PHARMACOLOGY IN PRACTICE

1. A woman in the clinic waiting room comes to the front desk and says, "that lady over there is odd. She looks like she is keeping tune to a song with her hand and her head, but there is no music playing. I don't feel comfortable sitting here in the waiting area." The patient is Betty Peterson, and she was prescribed fluoxetine for depression. You assess a repetitive hand tremor, and she appears to open her mouth frequently with a dry, sticky sound. What do you think she is experiencing, and how will you document these findings for the primary health care provider? What bearing will the medications she has taken in a previous hospitalization have on drug choices (see Chapter 16)?

● Test Your Knowledge

1. The most serious adverse reactions seen with levodopa include _____.

    A. choreiform and dystonic movements
    B. depression
    C. suicidal tendencies
    D. paranoia

2. Elderly patients prescribed one of the dopamine receptor agonists are monitored closely for which of the following adverse reactions?

    A. Occipital headache
    B. Hallucinations
    C. Paralytic ileus
    D. Cardiac arrhythmias

3. When taking a cholinergic blocking drug for parkinsonism, the patient would mostly experience which of the following adverse reactions?

    A. Constipation, urinary frequency
    B. Muscle spasm, convulsions
    C. Diarrhea, hypertension
    D. Dry mouth, dizziness

4. The patient taking tolcapone for Parkinson's disease is monitored closely for _____.

    A. kidney dysfunction
    B. liver dysfunction
    C. agranulocytosis
    D. the development of an autoimmune disease

● Prepare for the NCLEX

1. The nurse reports which of the following as a diminished response to antiparkinson drug treatment rather than an adverse reaction:

    A. dry mouth and difficulty in swallowing
    B. anorexia, nausea, and vomiting
    C. abdominal pain and constipation
    D. increased hand tremor

● Calculate Medication Dosages

1. Oral levodopa 0.75 g is prescribed. The drug is available in 100-mg tablets, 250-mg tablets, and 500-mg tablets. The nurse administers _____.

2. Oral ropinirole 6 mg is prescribed. The drug is available in 2-mg tablets. The nurse administers _____.

To check your answers, see Appendix E.

the**Point** *For more NCLEX questions, log on to http://thepoint.lww.com to access more than 1000 questions.*

Anticonvulsants

anticonvulsants
convulsion
epilepsy
generalized seizures
gingival hyperplasia
motor seizures
myoclonic seizures
nystagmus

pancytopenia
partial seizures
precipitation
seizure
somatosensory seizure
status epilepticus
tonic-clonic seizure

On completion of this chapter, the student will:

1. List the different types of drugs used as anticonvulsants.
2. Discuss the general drug actions, uses, adverse reactions, contraindications, precautions, and interactions of anticonvulsants.
3. Discuss important preadministration and ongoing assessment activities the nurse should perform with the patient receiving an anticonvulsant.
4. List nursing diagnoses particular to a patient taking an anticonvulsant.
5. Discuss ways to promote an optimal response to therapy, how to manage common adverse reactions when administering the anticonvulsants, and important points to keep in mind when educating a patient about the use of anticonvulsants.

The term **convulsion** refers to a sudden, involuntary contraction of the muscles of the body, often accompanied by loss of consciousness. A **seizure** may be defined as periodic disturbances of the brain's electrical activity. The terms *convulsion* and *seizure* are often used interchangeably, having basically the same meaning. Seizure disorders are generally categorized as idiopathic, hereditary, or acquired. Idiopathic seizures have no known cause; hereditary seizure disorders are passed from parent to child in their genetic makeup; and acquired seizure disorders have a known cause; causes include high fever, electrolyte imbalances, uremia, hypoglycemia, hypoxia, brain tumors, and some drug withdrawal reactions. The primary goal is to treat the underlying pathologic process to stop the seizures. Sometimes the cause is not clear, and the seizures cannot be stopped; rather, the activity needs to be controlled.

Seizures caused by disease, such as in epilepsy, may not be easy to eliminate. **Epilepsy** may be defined as a permanent, recurrent seizure disorder. Examples of the known causes of epilepsy include brain injury at birth, head injuries, and inborn errors of metabolism. In some patients, the cause of epilepsy is never determined. Epileptic seizures are classified according to an international system. Each different type of seizure disorder is characterized by a specific pattern of events, as well as a different pattern of motor or sensory manifestation.

Partial seizures are the most common type of epileptic seizure. They arise from a localized area in the brain and cause specific symptoms. Partial seizures include simple seizures, in which consciousness is impaired and variable, and **motor seizures** with uncontrolled stiffening or jerking in one part of the body such as the finger, mouth, hand, or foot that may progress to the entire limb. Partial seizures can involve areas of the brain that interpret information; they may present as flashing lights or a change in taste or speech (**somatosensory seizure**).

Generalized seizures involve a loss of consciousness. They may or may not include convulsive movements. Manifestations of a generalized **tonic-clonic seizure** include alternate contraction (tonic phase) and relaxation (clonic phase) of muscles, a loss of consciousness, and abnormal behavior. **Myoclonic seizures** involve sudden, forceful contractions of single or multiple groups of muscles. Other classifications of epileptic seizures include localized epilepsy, generalized epilepsy, special syndromes, and unclassified.

Drugs used for managing seizure disorders are called **anticonvulsants**. Most anticonvulsants have specific uses, that is, they are of value only in treating certain types of seizure disorders. The drug categories used as anticonvulsants are the hydantoins, carboxylic acid derivatives, succinimides, oxazolidinediones, and the barbiturates and benzodiazepines. In addition, several adjunct drugs are used as anticonvulsants. All possess the ability to depress abnormal neural discharges in the central nervous system (CNS), thereby inhibiting seizure activity. The Summary Drug Table: Anticonvulsant Drugs provides a listing of the drugs used to treat seizure disorders.

Summary Drug Table ANTICONVULSANTS

Generic Name	Trade Name	Uses	Adverse Reactions	Dosage Ranges
Hydantoins				
ethotoin *eth'-ih-toe-in*	Peganone	Tonic-clonic seizures	Ataxia, CNS depression, headache, hypotension, nystagmus, mental confusion, slurred speech, dizziness, drowsiness, nausea, vomiting, gingival hyperplasia, rash	2–3 g/day orally in 4–6 divided doses
fosphenytoin *fos-fen'-ih-toe-in*	Cerebyx	Status epilepticus	Same as ethotoin	Loading dose: 15–20 mg/kg IV Maintenance dose: 4–6 mg/kg/day IV
phenytoin *fen'-ih-toe-in*	Dilantin	Tonic-clonic seizures, status epilepticus, prophylactic seizure prevention	Same as ethotoin	Oral: loading dose: 1 g divided into three doses prevention (400 mg, 300 mg, 300 mg) orally q 2 hr; Maintenance dose: started 24 hr after loading dose, 300–400 mg/day; Parenteral: 10–15 mg/kg IV
Carboxylic Acid Derivatives				
valproic acid *val-proe'-ik* (divalproex)	Depakote, Depakene	Epilepsy, migraine headache, mania	Headache, somnolence, dizziness, tremor, nausea, vomiting, diplopia	10–60 mg/kg/day orally; if dosage is more than 250 mg/day, give in divided doses
Succinimides				
ethosuximide *eth-oh-sux'-ih-mide*	Zarontin	Partial seizures	Drowsiness, ataxia, dizziness, nausea, vomiting, urinary frequency, pruritus, urticaria, gingival hyperplasia	Up to 1.5 g/day orally in divided doses; children, 250 mg/day orally
methsuximide *meth-sux'-ih-mide*	Celontin	Partial seizures	Same as ethosuximide	300–1200 mg/day orally
Oxazolidinediones				
trimethadione *trye-meth-ah-dye'-own*	Tridione	Epilepsy	Dizziness, drowsiness, nausea, vomiting, photo-sensitivity, personality changes, increased irritability, headache, fatigue	900 mg–2.4 g/day orally in equally divided doses
Benzodiazepines				
clonazepam *kloh-nay'-zeh-pam*	Klonopin	Seizure disorders, panic disorders	Drowsiness, depression, ataxia, anorexia, diarrhea, constipation, dry mouth, palpitations, visual disturbances, rash	Initial dose: do not exceed 1.5 mg/day orally in 3 divided doses; increase in increments of 0.5–1 mg q 3 day; do not exceed 20 mg/day
clorazepate *klore-az'-eh-pate*	Tranxene	Partial seizures, anxiety disorders, alcohol withdrawal	Same as clonazepam	Initial dose: 7.5 mg orally TID, maximum dose 90 mg/day
diazepam *dye-az'-eh-pam*	Valium, Diastat	Status epilepticus, seizure disorders (all forms), anxiety disorders, alcohol withdrawal	Same as clonazepam	Seizure control: 2–10 mg/day orally BID to QID; Status epilepticus: 5–10 mg IV initially, maximum dose 30 mg; Rectally: 0.2–0.5 mg/kg
lorazepam *lor-az'-eh-pam*	Ativan	Status epilepticus, preanesthetic	Same as clonazepam	Status epilepticus: 4 mg IV over 2 min

(table continues on page 265)

Summary Drug Table ANTICONVULSANTS (continued)

Generic Name	Trade Name	Uses	Adverse Reactions	Dosage Ranges
Barbiturates				
phenobarbital *fee-noe-bar'-bih-tall*	Luminal	Status epilepticus, cortical focal seizures, tonic-clonic seizures	Somnolence, agitation, confusion, ataxia, CNS depression, nervousness, nausea, vomiting, constipation, diarrhea, rash	30–200 mg/day orally BID, TID; 30–320 mg IM, IV; may repeat in 6 hr
Miscellaneous Preparations				
acetazolamide *ah-see-tah-zoll'-ah-myde*	Diamox	Epilepsy, altitude sickness	Drowsiness, dizziness, nausea, diarrhea, constipation, visual disturbances	8–30 mg/kg/day in divided doses
carbamazepine *kar-bah-maz'-eh-peen*	Tegretol, Carbatrol, Epitol, Equetro	Epilepsy, bipolar disorder, trigeminal/postherpetic neuralgia	Dizziness, nausea, drowsiness, unsteady gait, aplastic anemia and other blood cell abnormalities	Maintenance: 800–1200 mg/day orally in divided doses
felbamate *fell'-bah-mate*	Felbatol	Partial seizures in patients who fail other drug therapy first	Insomnia, headache, anxiety, acne, rash, dyspepsia, vomiting, constipation, diarrhea, upper respiratory tract infection, fatigue, rhinitis, aplastic anemia, hepatic disorders	1200–3600 mg/day orally in divided doses
gabapentin *gab-ah-pen'-tin*	Neurontin	Partial seizures (adults), postherpetic neuralgia	Somnolence, dizziness, ataxia	900–1800 mg/day orally in 3–4 divided doses
lamotrigine *lah-moe'-trih-geen*	Lamictal	Partial seizures (used with other anticonvulsants), bipolar disorder	Dizziness, insomnia, somnolence, ataxia, nausea, vomiting, diplopia, headache, Stevens-Johnson Syndrome rash	50–500 mg/day orally in 2 divided doses
levetiracetam *lee-veh-tye-rah'-seh-tam*	Keppra	Partial seizures, tonic-clonic seizures, bipolar disorder, migraine headache	Headache, dizziness, asthenia, somnolence, infection	500 mg BID orally, increasing dose every 2 weeks until reach 3,000 mg daily
magnesium *mag-nee'-ze-um*		Hypomagnesemia, seizures associated with eclampsia and acute nephritis (children)	Flushing, sweating, hypothermia, depressed reflexes, hypotension, cardiac and CNS depression	Nephritis: 20–40 mg/kg IM in a dilute solution Eclampsia: 4 g IV in dilute solution, titrate continued infusion per serum level
oxcarbazepine *ox-car-baz'-eh-peen*	Trileptal	Epilepsy	Headache, dizziness, fatigue, somnolence, ataxia, diplopia, nausea, vomiting, abdominal pain	600–1200 mg orally BID
pregabalin *preg'-ah-bal-in*	Lyrica	Partial seizures (adults), neuropathic pain, postherpetic neuralgia	Dizziness, somnolence	Seizure activity: 150 mg/day in 2–3 divided doses
primidone *prih'-mih-doan*	Mysoline	Epilepsy	Dizziness, somnolence, nausea, vomiting	Up to 500 mg orally QID
tiagabine *tye-ag'-ah-been*	Gabitril	Partial seizures	Dizziness, somnolence, asthenia, nervousness, nausea	4–56 mg/day orally
topiramate *toe-pye'-rah-mate*	Topamax	Partial/tonic-clonic seizures, migraine headache	Fatigue, concentration problems, somnolence, anorexia	Seizure activity: 200–400 mg/day orally in divided doses
zonisamide *zoe-niss'-ah-mide*	Zonegran	Partial seizures of epilepsy	Somnolence, anorexia, dizziness, headache, rash, heat stroke	100–400 mg/day orally

Anticonvulsants

Actions

Anticonvulsants depress abnormal nerve impulse discharges in the CNS. The six categories of anticonvulsants achieve this effect through different modes of action:

- Hydantoins stabilize the hyperexcitability postsynaptically in the motor cortex of the brain.
- Carboxylic acid derivatives increase levels of GABA (gamma-aminobutyric acid), which stabilizes cell membranes.
- Succinimides depress the motor cortex, creating a higher threshold before nerves react to the convulsive stimuli.
- Oxazolidinediones decrease repetitive synaptic transmissions of nerve impulses.
- Benzodiazepines and barbiturates elevate the seizure threshold by decreasing postsynaptic excitation.

Seizures are theoretically reduced in intensity and frequency of occurrence or, in some instances, are virtually eliminated. For some patients, only partial control of the seizure disorder may be obtained with anticonvulsant drug therapy.

Uses

Anticonvulsants are used prophylactically to prevent seizures after trauma or neurosurgery or in patients with tumor and in the treatment of the following:

- Seizures of all types
- Neuropathic pain
- Bipolar disorders
- Anxiety disorders

Occasionally, **status epilepticus** (an emergency characterized by continual seizure activity with no interruptions) can occur. Lorazepam (Ativan) is the drug of choice for this condition. However, because the effects of lorazepam last less than 1 hour, a longer-lasting anticonvulsant such as phenytoin (Dilantin) or phenobarbital also must be given to continue to control the seizure activity.

NURSING ALERT

Research suggests an association between the use of anticonvulsants by pregnant women with epilepsy and an increased incidence of birth defects in children born to these women. The use of anticonvulsants is not discontinued in pregnant women with a history of major seizures, because of the danger of precipitating status epilepticus. However, when seizure activity poses no serious threat to the pregnant woman, the primary health care provider may consider discontinuing use of the drug during pregnancy.

Adverse Reactions

Adverse reactions that may occur with the administration of an anticonvulsant drug include the following:

Central Nervous System Reactions

- Drowsiness, weakness, dizziness
- Headache, somnolence
- **Nystagmus** (constant, involuntary movement of the eyeball)
- Ataxia (loss of control of voluntary movements, especially gait)
- Slurred speech

Gastrointestinal System Reactions

- Nausea, vomiting
- Anorexia
- Constipation, diarrhea
- **Gingival hyperplasia** (overgrowth of gum tissue)

Other Reactions

- Skin rashes, pruritus, urticaria
- Urinary frequency
- Serious skin reactions, such as Stevens-Johnson syndrome, have been associated with the use of lamotrigine (Lamictal)
- Hematologic changes, such as **pancytopenia** (decrease in all the cellular components of the blood), leukopenia, aplastic anemia, and thrombocytopenia, have occurred with administration of selected drugs, including carbamazepine (Tegretol), felbamate (Felbatol), and trimethadione (Tridione). See the Summary Drug Table: Anticonvulsants for more information.

Contraindications

All categories of anticonvulsants are contraindicated in patients with known hypersensitivity to the drugs. Phenytoin is contraindicated in patients with sinus bradycardia, sinoatrial block, Adams-Stokes syndrome, and second- and third-degree atrioventricular (AV) block; it also is contraindicated during pregnancy and lactation (ethotoin and phenytoin are pregnancy category D drugs). Ethotoin (Peganone) is contraindicated in patients with hepatic abnormalities. The oxazolidinediones have been associated with serious adverse reactions and fetal malformations. They should be used only when other, less toxic drugs are not effective in controlling seizures. The succinimides are contraindicated in patients with bone marrow depression or hepatic or renal impairment. A higher incidence of lupus erythematosus has been found in patients taking succinimides.

Carbamazepine should not be given within 14 days of monoamine oxidase inhibitor (MAOI) antidepressants. Carbamazepine is contraindicated in patients with bone marrow depression or hepatic or renal impairment and during pregnancy (category D). Valproic acid (Depakote) is not administered to patients with renal impairment or during pregnancy (category D). Oxcarbazepine (Trileptal), a miscellaneous anticonvulsant, may exacerbate dementia.

Precautions

Anticonvulsants should be used cautiously in patients with liver or kidney disease and those with neurologic disorders. The barbiturates (e.g., phenobarbital) are used with caution in patients with pulmonary disease and in hyperactive children. The benzodiazepines are used cautiously during pregnancy (category D) and in patients with psychoses, acute narrow-angle glaucoma, and elderly or debilitated patients. Phenytoin is used cautiously in patients with hypotension, severe myocardial insufficiency, and hepatic impairment. Trimetha-

Know

dione is used with caution in patients with eye disorders (e.g., retinal or optic nerve disease).

Miscellaneous anticonvulsants are used cautiously in patients with glaucoma or increased intraocular pressure; a history of cardiac, renal or liver dysfunction; and psychiatric disorders. In addition to hepatic failure and birth defects, valproic acid is associated with an increased risk for pancreatitis.

Interactions

The following interactions may occur when an anticonvulsant is administered with another agent:

Interacting Drug	Common Use	Effect of Interaction
antibiotics/ antifungals	Fight infection	Increased effect of the anticonvulsant
tricyclic antidepressants	Manage depression	Increased effect of the anticonvulsant
salicylates	Pain relief	Increased effect of the anticonvulsant
cimetidine	Control GI upset	Increased effect of the anticonvulsant
theophylline	Treatment of respiratory problems	Decreased serum levels of the anti-convulsant
antiseizure medications	Reduce seizure activity	May increase seizure activity
protease inhibitors	Treatment of human immunodeficiency virus (HIV) infection	Increased carbamazepine levels, resulting in toxicity
oral contraceptives	Birth control	Decreased effectiveness of birth control, resulting in breakthrough bleeding or pregnancy
analgesics or alcohol	CNS depressants	Increased depressant effect
antidiabetic medications	Manage diabetes mellitus	Increased blood glucose levels

NURSING PROCESS
PATIENT RECEIVING AN ANTICONVULSANT

ASSESSMENT

Preadministration Assessment
Seizures that occur in the outpatient setting are almost always seen first by family members or friends, rather than by a member of the health care profession. The occurrence of abnormal behavior patterns or convulsive movements usually prompts the patient to visit the primary health care provider's office or a neurologic clinic. A thorough patient history is necessary to identify the type of seizure disorder. Information the nurse should

V/S ♂

DISPLAY 30.1 General Assessment of Seizure Activity

- Description of the seizures (the motor or psychic activity occurring during the seizure)
- Frequency of the seizures (approximate number per day)
- Average length of a seizure
- Description of an aura (a subjective sensation preceding a seizure), if any has occurred
- Description of the degree of impairment of consciousness
- Description of what, if anything, appears to bring on the seizure

obtain from those who have observed the seizure is listed in Display 30.1.

Additional patient information should include a family history of seizures (if any) and recent drug therapy (all drugs currently being used). Depending on the type of seizure disorder, other information may be needed, such as a history of a head or other injury or a thorough medical history.

The nurse obtains the vital signs at the time of the initial assessment to provide baseline data. The primary health care provider may order laboratory and diagnostic tests, such as an electroencephalogram, magnetic resonance imaging (MRI) scan, complete blood count, and hepatic and renal function tests, to confirm the diagnosis and identify a possible cause of the seizure disorder as well as to provide a baseline during therapy with anticonvulsants.

Ongoing Assessment
Anticonvulsants control, but do not cure, epilepsy. An accurate ongoing assessment is important for obtaining the desired effect of the anticonvulsant. The dosage of the anticonvulsant may require frequent adjustments during the initial treatment period. Dosage adjustments are based on the patient's response to therapy (e.g., the control of the seizures) as well as the occurrence of adverse reactions. Depending on the patient's response to therapy, a second anticonvulsant may be added to the therapeutic regimen, or one anticonvulsant may be changed to another. Regularly, serum plasma levels of the anticonvulsant are measured to monitor for toxicity.

The patient's seizures, along with response to drug therapy, must be observed when a hospitalized patient is receiving an anticonvulsant. The nurse must document each seizure carefully with regard to the time of occurrence, the duration, and the psychic or motor activity occurring before, during, and after the seizure. Most seizures occur without warning, and the nurse may not see the patient until after the seizure has begun or after the seizure is over.

However, any observations made during and after the seizure are important and may aid in the diagnosis of the type of seizure, as well as assist the primary health care provider in evaluating the effectiveness of drug therapy.

NURSING DIAGNOSES

Drug-specific nursing diagnoses include the following:

❑ **Risk for Injury** related to seizure disorder, drowsiness, and ataxia

Anticonvulsants

- ❏ **Risk for Impaired Skin Integrity** related to adverse reactions (rash)
- ❏ **Risk for Infection** related to immunosuppression secondary to drug therapy
- ❏ **Impaired Oral Mucous Membranes** related to gum overgrowth secondary to hydantoins
- ❏ **Disturbed Sensory Perception: Visual** related to adverse drug reactions

Nursing diagnoses related to drug administration are discussed in Chapter 4.

PLANNING

The expected outcomes for the patient depend on the type and severity of the seizure, but may include an optimal response to therapy (control of seizure), meeting patient needs related to the management of adverse reactions, and an understanding of the therapeutic regimen.

IMPLEMENTATION

Promoting an Optimal Response to Therapy

When administering an anticonvulsant, the nurse must not omit or miss a dose (except by order of the primary health care provider). An abrupt interruption in therapy by omitting a dose may result in a recurrence of the seizures.

> **! NURSING ALERT**
> Status epilepticus may result from abrupt discontinuation of the drug, even when the anticonvulsant is being administered in small daily doses.

The nurse supports continuity of anticonvulsant administration by making a notation on the care plan, as well as by informing all health care team members of the importance of the drug. If the primary health care provider discontinues the anticonvulsant therapy, the dosage is gradually withdrawn or another drug is gradually substituted.

HYDANTOINS. Phenytoin is the most commonly prescribed anticonvulsant because of its effectiveness and relatively low toxicity. However, a genetically linked inability to metabolize phenytoin has been identified. For this reason, it is important to monitor serum concentrations of the drug on a regular basis to detect signs of toxicity (slurred speech, ataxia, lethargy, dizziness, nausea, and vomiting). Phenytoin is administered orally and parenterally. When taken orally, the drug should be taken with meals to avoid GI upset. If the drug is administered parenterally, the intravenous (IV) route is preferred over the intramuscular (IM) route, because erratic absorption of phenytoin causes pain and muscle damage at the injection site.

> **LIFESPAN ALERT – Gerontology**
> The barbiturates may produce marked excitement, depression, and confusion in the elderly. In some individuals the barbiturates produce excitement, rather than depression. The nurse should monitor the older adult carefully during therapy with barbiturates and report any unusual effects to the primary health care provider.

BENZODIAZEPINES. The dosage of the benzodiazepines is highly individualized, and the nurse must increase the dosage cautiously to avoid adverse reactions, particularly in elderly and debilitated patients. IV lorazepam may bring seizures under control quickly. However, for some patients, seizure activity may resume because of the short duration of the drug effects. Drug **precipitation** can occur when diazepam (Valium) is administered IV. The nurse must not mix diazepam with other drugs. When used to control seizures, diazepam is administered by IV pushed slowly as close as possible to the IV site, allowing at least 1 minute for each 5 mg of drug.

Monitoring and Managing Patient Needs

RISK FOR INJURY. Drowsiness is a common adverse reaction to anticonvulsant drugs, especially early in therapy. Therefore, the nurse should assist the patient with all ambulatory activities until the patient is stable. The nurse helps the patient to rise from the bed slowly and sit for a few minutes before standing. Drowsiness decreases with continued use.

The nurse must use caution when giving an oral preparation because aspiration of the tablet, capsule, or liquid may occur if the patient experiences drowsiness. The nurse tests the swallowing ability of the patient by offering small sips of water before giving the drug. If the patient has difficulty swallowing, the nurse withholds the drug and notifies the primary health care provider as soon as possible. A different route of administration may be necessary. Because injury may occur when the patient has a seizure, the nurse takes precautions to prevent falls and other injuries until seizures are controlled by the drug.

> **LIFESPAN ALERT – Gerontology**
> Apnea and cardiac arrest have occurred when diazepam is administered to older adults, very ill patients, and individuals with limited pulmonary reserve. The nurse observes these patients carefully. Older or debilitated adults may require a decreased dosage of diazepam to reduce ataxia and oversedation.

RISK FOR IMPAIRED SKIN INTEGRITY. A severe and potentially fatal rash can occur in patients taking lamotrigine, and the barbiturates also can produce a hypersensitivity rash. Should a rash occur, the nurse must notify the primary health care provider immediately because the primary health care provider may discontinue the drug. The nurse carefully examines all affected areas and provides an accurate description. If pruritus is present, the nurse keeps the patient's nails short, applies an antiseptic cream (if prescribed), and tells the patient to avoid using soap until the rash subsides.

> **! NURSING ALERT**
> The nurse informs the primary health care provider immediately if a skin reaction occurs. Phenytoin is usually discontinued in such cases. If the rash is exfoliative (red rash with scaling of the skin), purpuric (small hemorrhages or bruising on the skin), or bullous (skin vesicle filled with fluid, i.e.,

blister), use of the drug is not resumed. If the rash is milder (e.g., acne/sunburn-like), therapy may be resumed after the rash completely disappears.

RISK FOR INFECTION. The nurse must also be alert for the signs of pancytopenia, such as sore throat, fever, general malaise, bleeding of the mucous membranes, epistaxis (bleeding from the nose), and easy bruising. Anticonvulsants such as carbamazepine may cause aplastic anemia and agranulocytosis. The succinimides are also particularly toxic. Routine laboratory tests, such as complete blood counts and differential counts, should be performed periodically. If bone marrow depression is evident (e.g., the patient's platelet count and white blood cell count decrease significantly), the primary health care provider is notified because the drug may be discontinued. When pancytopenia is present and blood cell counts are low, using a soft-bristled toothbrush may protect the mucous membranes from bleeding and easy bruising. The extremities also need to be protected from trauma or injury.

> **⚠ NURSING ALERT**
>
> Phenytoin can cause hematologic changes (e.g., aplastic anemia, leukopenia, and thrombocytopenia). The nurse should immediately report any signs of thrombocytopenia (bleeding gums, easy bruising, increased menstrual bleeding, tarry stools) or leukopenia (sore throat, chills, swollen glands, excessive fatigue, or shortness of breath) to the primary health care provider.

IMPAIRED ORAL MUCOUS MEMBRANE. Long-term administration of hydantoins can cause gingivitis and gingival hyperplasia (overgrowth of gum tissue). It is important to inspect periodically the mouth, teeth, and gums of patients in a hospital or long-term clinical setting who are receiving one of these drugs. Any changes in the gums or teeth are reported to the primary health care provider. Oral care needs to be given after each meal.

> **⚠ NURSING ALERT**
>
> When administering phenytoin, the nurse closely monitors the patient for the following signs of drug toxicity: slurred speech, ataxia, lethargy, dizziness, nausea, and vomiting. Phenytoin plasma levels between 10 and 20 mcg/mL give optimal anticonvulsant effect. However, many patients achieve seizure control at lower serum concentration levels. Levels greater than 20 mcg/mL are associated with toxicity. Patients with plasma levels greater than 20 mcg/mL may exhibit nystagmus, and at concentrations greater than 30 mcg/mL, ataxia and mental changes are common.

DISTURBED SENSORY PERCEPTION: VISUAL. Visual disturbances may occur with anticonvulsant therapy. The patient with a visual disturbance is assisted with ambulation and oriented carefully to the environment. The nurse ensures that the environment is safe. The patient may be especially sensitive to bright lights and may want the room light dimmed. Because photosensitivity can occur, the patient should stay out of the sun if possible and wear sunscreens and protective clothing as needed until the individual effects of the drug are known.

Educating the Patient and Family

When the patient receives a diagnosis of epilepsy, the nurse must assist the patient and the family to adjust to the diagnosis. The nurse should instruct family members in the care of the patient before, during, and after a seizure. The nurse explains the importance of restricting some activities until the seizures are controlled by drugs. Restriction of activities often depends on the age, sex, and occupation of the patient. For some patients, the restriction of activities may create problems with such activities as employment, management of the home environment, or child care. For example, the patient may be prohibited from driving while the primary health care provider attempts to control the seizure activity. The nurse should assist the patient to look for other modes of transportation to continue typical activities or employment. If a problem is recognized, a referral to a social worker, discharge planning coordinator, or public health nurse may be needed.

The nurse reviews adverse drug reactions associated with the prescribed anticonvulsant with the patient and family members. The patient and family members are instructed to contact the primary health care provider if any adverse reactions occur before the next dose of the drug is due. The patient must not stop taking the drug until the problem is discussed with the primary health care provider.

Some patients, once their seizures are under control (e.g., stop occurring or occur less frequently), may have a tendency to stop the drug abruptly or begin to omit a dose occasionally. The drug must never be abruptly discontinued or doses omitted. If the patient experiences drowsiness during initial therapy, a family member should be responsible for administering the drug. The nurse should include the following points in a patient and family teaching plan:

- Do not omit, increase, or decrease the prescribed dose.
- Anticonvulsant blood levels must be monitored at regular intervals, even if the seizures are well controlled.
- This drug should never be abruptly discontinued, except when recommended by the primary health care provider.
- Do not attempt to put anything in the mouth of a person having a seizure.
- If the primary health care provider finds it necessary to stop the drug, another drug usually is prescribed. Start taking this drug immediately (at the time the next dose of the previously used drug was due).
- Anticonvulsant drugs may cause drowsiness or dizziness. Observe caution when performing hazardous tasks. Do not drive unless the adverse reactions of drowsiness, dizziness, or blurred vision are not significant. Driving privileges will be approved or reinstated by the primary health care provider based on seizure control.
- Avoid the use of alcohol unless use has been approved by the primary health care provider.
- Carry medical identification, such as a MedicAlert tag or bracelet, indicating drug use and the type of seizure disorder.

Anticonvulsants

- Do not use any nonprescription drug unless the preparation has been approved by the primary health care provider.
- Keep a record of all seizures (date, time, length), as well as any minor problems (e.g., drowsiness, dizziness, lethargy), and take the record to each clinic or office visit.
- Contact the local branches of agencies, such as the Epilepsy Foundation of America, for information and assistance with problems, such as legal matters, insurance, driver's license, low-cost prescription services, and job training or retraining.

HYDANTOINS.

- Inform the dentist and other primary health care providers of use of this drug.
- Brush and floss the teeth after each meal and make periodic dental appointments for oral examination and care.
- Take the medication with food to reduce GI upset.
- Thoroughly shake a phenytoin suspension immediately before use.
- Do not take capsules that are discolored.
- Notify the primary health care provider if any of the following occurs: skin rash, bleeding, swollen or tender gums, yellowish discoloration of the skin or eyes, unexplained fever, sore throat, unusual bleeding or bruising, persistent headache, malaise, or pregnancy.

SUCCINIMIDES.

- If GI upset occurs, take the drug with food or milk.
- Notify the primary health care provider if any of the following occurs: skin rash, joint pain, unexplained fever, sore throat, usual bleeding or bruising, drowsiness, dizziness, blurred vision, or pregnancy.

OXAZOLIDINEDIONES.

- This drug may cause photosensitivity. Take protective measures (e.g., wear sunscreens and protective clothing) when exposed to ultraviolet light or sunlight until tolerance is determined.
- Notify the primary care provider if the following reactions occur: visual disturbances, excessive drowsiness or dizziness, sore throat, fever, skin rash, pregnancy, malaise, easy bruising, epistaxis, or bleeding tendencies.
- Avoid pregnancy while taking trimethadione; the drug has caused serious birth defects.

EVALUATION

- Therapeutic effect is achieved and convulsions are controlled.
- Adverse reactions are identified, reported to the primary health care provider, and managed successfully through appropriate nursing interventions:
  - ☑ No injury is evident.
  - ☑ Skin remains intact.
  - ☑ No evidence of infection is seen.
  - ☑ Mucous membranes are moist and intact.
  - ☑ Vision remains intact.
- Patient and family demonstrate an understanding of the drug regimen.

THINK CRITICALLY: PHARMACOLOGY IN PRACTICE

1. Ms. Chase was in a car accident last year and had a seizure on the way to the hospital. As you review her medication list and ask about her drugs, she tells you that since she has been taking phenytoin she has had no seizures. In fact, she states that she has omitted one or two doses over the last month because she is "doing so well." Explain your response to Ms. Chase's statement.

● Test Your Knowledge

1. A patient is prescribed phenytoin for a recurrent convulsive disorder. The nurse informs the patient that the most common adverse reactions are _____.

   A. related to the gastrointestinal system
   B. associated with the reproductive system
   C. associated with kidney function
   D. related to the CNS

2. When administering phenobarbital to an elderly patient, the nurse should monitor the patient for unusual effects of the drug such as _____.

   A. marked excitement
   B. excessive sweating
   C. insomnia
   D. agitation

3. When caring for a patient taking a succinimide for seizure control, the nurse monitors the patient for blood dyscrasias. Which of the following symptoms would indicate that the patient may be developing a blood dyscrasia?

   A. Constipation, blood in the stool
   B. Diarrhea, lethargy
   C. Sore throat, general malaise
   D. Hyperthermia, excitement

4. Which statement would be included when educating the patient taking trimethadione for seizures?

   A. Take this drug with milk to enhance absorption.
   B. Wear a sunscreen and protective clothing when exposed to sunlight.
   C. To minimize adverse reactions, take this drug once daily at bedtime.
   D. Visit a dentist frequently because this drug increases the risk of gum disease.

● Prepare for the NCLEX

1. Which of the following adverse reactions, if observed in a patient prescribed phenytoin, would indicate that the patient may be developing phenytoin toxicity?

A. Severe occipital headache
B. Ataxia
C. Hyperactivity
D. Somnolence

Calculate Medication Dosages

1. The nurse is preparing to administer an anticonvulsant for status epilepticus. The primary care provider prescribes lorazepam (Ativan) 4 mg IV. The drug is available in a dosage of 2 mg/mL. The nurse administers _____.

2. Zonisamide 200 mg is prescribed. The drug is available in 100-mg tablets. The nurse administers _____.

3. The primary care provider prescribes ethosuximide syrup 500 mg for a patient with absence seizures. The drug is available in a strength of 250 mg/5 mL. The nurse administers _____.

To check your answers, see Appendix E.

the**Point** *For more NCLEX questions, log on to http://thepoint.lww.com to access more than 1000 questions.*

Skeletal Muscle Relaxants and Drugs Used To Treat Bone and Joint Disorders

KEY TERMS

alopecia   osteoarthritis
gout   rheumatoid arthritis
musculoskeletal

LEARNING OBJECTIVES

On completion of this chapter, the student will:

1. List the types of drugs used to treat musculoskeletal disorders.
2. Discuss the uses, general drug actions, adverse reactions, contraindications, precautions, and interactions of the drugs used to treat musculoskeletal disorders.
3. Discuss important preadministration and ongoing assessment activities the nurse should perform on the patient taking drugs used to treat musculoskeletal disorders.
4. List nursing diagnoses particular to a patient taking a drug for the treatment of musculoskeletal disorders.
5. Discuss ways to promote an optimal response to therapy, how to manage adverse reactions, and important points to keep in mind when educating the patient about drugs used to treat musculoskeletal disorders.

A variety of drugs are used in treating **musculoskeletal** (bone and muscle) injuries and disorders. When muscles are injured, typically rest, exercise, and physical therapy are used to heal the injury. Skeletal muscle relaxants are used to assist in relaxing certain muscle groups, as strains and sprains are repaired.

Chronic disease may also affect skeletal muscles, causing limitations in function. Drugs are frequently used to maintain function due to chronic illness. Examples of the drugs discussed for musculoskeletal disorders in this chapter include bone resorption inhibitors (used to treat osteoporosis), disease-modifying antirheumatic drugs (DMARDs; used to treat **rheumatoid arthritis** [RA]), and uric acid inhibitors (used to treat **gout**). A description of these and other musculoskeletal disorders is given in Table 31.1. The drug selected is based on the musculoskeletal disorder being treated, the severity of the disorder, and the patient's positive or negative response to past therapy. For example, early cases of RA may respond well to the nonsteroidal anti-inflammatory drugs

(NSAIDs), whereas advanced RA not responding to other drug therapies may require the use of corticosteroids or immunosuppressive drugs.

Salicylates and NSAIDs are important agents used in treating arthritic conditions. For example, salicylates and NSAIDs are used for RA (a chronic disease characterized by inflammatory changes in the body's connective tissue) and **osteoarthritis** (a noninflammatory joint disease resulting in degeneration of the articular cartilage and changes in the synovial membrane), as well as for relief of pain or discomfort resulting from musculoskeletal injuries such as sprains.

• SKELETAL MUSCLE RELAXANTS

Actions

The mode of action of many skeletal muscle relaxants, such as carisoprodol (Soma), baclofen (Lioresal), and chlorzoxazone (Parafon Forte), is not clearly understood. Many of these drugs do not directly relax skeletal muscles, but their ability to relieve acute painful musculoskeletal conditions may be due to their sedative action. Cyclobenzaprine (Flexeril) appears to have an effect on muscle tone, thereby reducing muscle spasm.

The exact mode of action of diazepam (Valium), an antianxiety drug (see Chapter 20), in the relief of painful musculoskeletal conditions is unknown. The drug does have a sedative action, which may account for some of its ability to relieve muscle spasm and pain.

Uses

Skeletal muscle relaxants are used in various acute painful musculoskeletal conditions, such as muscle strains and back pain.

Adverse Reactions

Drowsiness is the most common reaction seen with the use of skeletal muscle relaxants. Additional adverse reactions are given in the Summary Drug Table: Drugs Used to Treat Musculoskeletal Disorders. Some of the adverse reactions that may occur with the administration of diazepam include drowsiness, sedation, sleepiness, lethargy, constipation or diarrhea, bradycardia or tachycardia, and rash.

(text continues on page 276)

Table 31.1 Selected Musculoskeletal Disorders

Disorder	Description
Synovitis	Inflammation of the synovial membrane of a joint resulting in pain, swelling, and inflammation. It occurs in disorders such as rheumatic fever, RA, and gout.
Arthritis	Inflammation of a joint. The term is frequently used to refer to any disease involving pain or stiffness of the musculoskeletal system.
Osteoarthritis or degenerative joint disease (DJD)	Noninflammatory DJD marked by degeneration of the articular cartilage, changes in the synovial membrane, and hypertrophy of the bone at the margins.
RA	Chronic systemic disease that produces inflammatory changes throughout the connective tissue in the body. It affects joints and other organ systems of the body. Destruction of articular cartilage occurs, affecting joint structure and mobility. RA primarily affects individuals between 20 and 40 years of age.
Gout	Form of arthritis in which uric acid accumulates in increased amounts in the blood and often is deposited in the joints. The deposit or collection of urate crystals in the joints causes the symptoms (pain, redness, swelling, joint deformity).
Osteoporosis	Loss of bone density occurring when the loss of bone substance exceeds the rate of bone formation. Bones become porous, brittle, and fragile. Compression fractures of the vertebrae are common. This disorder occurs most often in postmenopausal women, but can occur in men as well.
Hypercalcemia of malignancy	Advanced-stage malignant disease. It can occur with 10%–50% of tumors. It is associated with parathyroid hormone production and can be difficult to manage. Symptoms include lethargy, anorexia, nausea, vomiting, thirst, polydipsia, constipation, and dehydration. If untreated, it may lead to cognitive difficulties, confusion, obtundation (extreme dullness, near-coma), and coma.
Paget's disease (osteitis deformans)	Chronic bone disorder characterized by abnormal bone remodeling. The disease disrupts the growth of new bone tissue, causing the bone to thicken and become soft. This weakens the bone, which increases susceptibility to fracture or collapse of the bone (e.g., the vertebrae) even with slight trauma.

Summary Drug Table DRUGS USED TO TREAT MUSCULOSKELETAL DISORDERS

Generic Name	Trade Name	Uses	Adverse Reactions	Dosage Ranges
Skeletal Muscle Relaxants				
baclofen *bak'-loe-fen*	Lioresal	Spasticity due to multiple sclerosis, spinal cord injuries (intrathecal administration for severe spasticity)	Drowsiness, dizziness, nausea, weakness, hypotension	15–80 mg/day orally in divided doses
carisoprodol *kare-eye-soe-proe'-doll*	Soma	Relief of discomfort due to acute, painful musculoskeletal conditions	Dizziness, drowsiness, tachycardia, nausea, vomiting	350 mg orally TID or QID
chlorzoxazone *klore-zox'-ah-zone*	Parafon Forte DSC	Same as carisoprodol	GI disturbances, drowsiness, dizziness, rash	250–750 mg orally TID or QID
cyclobenzaprine *sye-kloe-ben'-zah-preen*	Flexeril, Amrix	Same as carisoprodol *more for muscle spams*	Drowsiness, dizziness, dry mouth, nausea, constipation	10–60 mg/day orally in divided doses
dantrolene *dan'-troe-leen*	Dantrium	Spasticity due to spinal cord injury, stroke, cerebral palsy, multiple sclerosis	Drowsiness, dizziness, weakness, constipation, tachycardia, malaise	Initial dose: 25 mg/day orally, then 50–400 mg/day orally in divided doses
diazepam *dye-az'-eh-pam* *antianxiety*	Valium	Relief of skeletal muscle spasm, spasticity due to cerebral palsy, epilepsy, paraplegia, anxiety	Drowsiness, sedation, sleepiness, lethargy, constipation, diarrhea, bradycardia, tachycardia, rash	2–10 mg orally BID–QID; 2–20 mg IM, IV Sustained release, 15–30 mg/day orally

(table continues on page 274)

Summary Drug Table DRUGS USED TO TREAT MUSCULOSKELETAL DISORDERS (continued)

Generic Name	Trade Name	Uses	Adverse Reactions	Dosage Ranges
metaxalone me-tax'-ah-lone	Skelaxin	Same as carisoprodol	Drowsiness, dizziness, headache, nausea, rash	800 mg orally TID or QID
methocarbamol meth-oh-kar'-bah-moll	Robaxin	Relief of discomfort due to musculoskeletal disorders	Drowsiness, dizziness, light-headedness, confusion, headache, rash, blurred vision, GI upset	1–1.5 g QID orally; limit IM, IV dose to 3 g/day
orphenadrine ore-fen'-ah-dreen	Norflex	Discomfort due to musculoskeletal disorders	Drowsiness, dizziness, light-headedness, confusion, headache, rash, blurred vision, GI upset	100 mg BID orally; 60 mg IV or IM q 12 hr
tizanidine tih-zan'-ih-deen	Zanaflex *short acting block last 4-6 hrs*	Spasticity due to spinal cord injury	Somnolence, fatigue, dizziness, dry mouth, urinary tract infections	4–8 mg orally up to TID
Bone Resorption Inhibitors: Bisphosphonates				
Ⓡ alendronate ah-len'-droe-nate	Fosamax	Treatment and prevention of postmenopausal osteoporosis; glucocorticoid-induced osteoporosis; osteoporosis in men; Paget's disease	Abdominal pain, esophageal reflux	5–70 mg orally, in daily or weekly doses
etidronate eh-tid'-roh-nate	Didronel	Hypercalcemia of malignancy, Paget's disease, prevent bone spurs after total hip replacement or spinal cord injury	Nausea, fever, fluid overload	5–20 mg/kg/day orally (treatment not to exceed 6 mo)
ibandronate ih-ban'-droe-nate	Boniva	Postmenopausal osteoporosis	Abdominal pain, nausea, diarrhea	2.5 mg/day orally, available in 150-mg tablet taken once monthly; 3 mg IV form available for dose once every 3 months
pamidronate pah-mid'-roh-nate	Aredia	Hypercalcemia of malignancy, Paget's disease	Anxiety, headache, insomnia, nausea, vomiting, diarrhea, constipation, dyspepsia, pancytopenia, fever, fatigue, bone pain	60–90 mg in a single IV dose infused over 2–24 hr
Ⓡ risedronate rih-sed'-roh-nate	Actonel	Treatment and prevention of postmenopausal osteoporosis, glucocorticoid-induced osteoporosis, osteoporosis in men, Paget's disease	Headache, abdominal pain, arthralgia, recurrent bone pain, nausea, diarrhea	5–75 mg orally, in daily or weekly doses
tiludronate tih-loo'-droe-nate	Skelid	Paget's disease	Headache, nausea, diarrhea, arthralgia, pain	400 mg/day orally for no more than 3 mo
zoledronic acid zole-eh-drone'-ik	Zometa, Reclast	Zometa: Hypercalcemia of malignancy, solid tumor bone metastases Reclast: Postmenopausal osteoporosis, Paget's disease	Hypotension, confusion, anxiety, agitation, nausea, diarrhea, constipation, fatigue	Zometa: 4 mg in a single IV dose infused over 15 min every 3–4 weeks; Reclast: 5 mg IV once per year

(table continues on page 275)

Summary Drug Table DRUGS USED TO TREAT MUSCULOSKELETAL DISORDERS (continued)

Generic Name	Trade Name	Uses	Adverse Reactions	Dosage Ranges
Disease-Modifying Antirheumatic Drugs		*RA = swelling, fluid in joints*		
adalimumab *ah-dah-lim'-mu-mab*	Humira	RA, other autoimmune disorders	Irritation at injection site, increased risk of infections	40 mg subcut every other week
anakinra *an-ah-kin'-rah*	Kineret	RA	Headache, irritation at injection site, pancytopenia	100 mg subcut daily
etanercept *ee-tah-ner'-sept*	Enbrel	RA	Headache, rhinitis, irritation at injection site, increased risk of infections	25 mg subcut twice weekly, or 50 mg subcut weekly
hydroxychloroquine *hye-drox-see-klor'-oh-kwin*	Plaquenil	RA, antimalarial	Irritability nervousness, retinal and corneal changes, anorexia, nausea, vomiting, hematologic effects	400–600 mg/day orally
infliximab *in-flick'-see-mab*	Remicade	RA in combination with methotrexate, Crohn's disease	Fever, chills, headache	3–10 mg/kg IV infusion at specified weekly intervals
leflunomide *leh-floo'-noe-mide*	Arava	RA	Hypertension, alopecia, rash, nausea, diarrhea	Initial dose: 100 mg for 3 day; Maintenance dose: 20 mg/day orally
methotrexate (MTX) *meth-oh-trex'-sate*	Rheumatrex	RA, cancer chemotherapy	Nausea, stomatitis, alopecia	7.5–20 mg orally once weekly
sulfasalazine *sul-fah-sal'-ah-zeen*	Azulfidine	RA, ulcerative colitis	Nausea, emesis, abdominal pains, crystalluria, hematuria, Stevens-Johnson syndrome, rash, headache, drowsiness, diarrhea	2–4 g/day orally in divided doses
Uric Acid Inhibitors				
allopurinol *al-oh-pyoor'-ih-noll*	Zyloprim	Management of symptoms of gout	Rash, exfoliative dermatitis, Stevens-Johnson syndrome, nausea, vomiting, diarrhea, abdominal pain, hematologic changes	100–800 mg/day orally
colchicine *koll'-chih-seen*		Relief of acute attacks of gout, prevention of gout attacks	Nausea, vomiting, diarrhea, abdominal pain, bone marrow depression	Acute attack: initial dose 0.5–1.2 mg orally or 2 mg IV, then 0.5–1.2 mg orally q 1–2 hr or 0.5 mg IV q 6 hr until attack is aborted or adverse effects occur Prophylaxis: 0.5–0.6 mg/day orally
probenecid *proe-ben'-eh-sid*		Treatment of hyperuricemia of gout and gouty arthritis; adjuvant to antibiotics	Headache, anorexia, nausea, vomiting, urinary frequency, flushing, dizziness	0.25 g orally BID for 1 wk, then 0.5 g orally BID
sulfinpyrazone *sul-fin-peer'-ah-zone*	Anturane	Treatment of gouty arthritis	Upper GI disturbances, rash	200–400 mg orally BID

main

main

Ⓡ This drug should be administered at least 1 hour before or 2 hours after a meal.

Contraindications

Skeletal muscle relaxants are contraindicated in patients with known hypersensitivity to the drugs. Baclofen is contraindicated in skeletal muscle spasms caused by rheumatic disorders. Carisoprodol is contraindicated in patients with a known hypersensitivity to meprobamate. Cyclobenzaprine is contraindicated in patients with a recent myocardial infarction, cardiac conduction disorders, and hyperthyroidism. In addition, cyclobenzaprine is contraindicated within 14 days of the administration of a monoamine oxidase inhibitor (MAOI). Oral dantrolene is contraindicated during lactation and in patients with active hepatic disease and muscle spasm caused by rheumatic disorders.

Precautions

Skeletal muscle relaxants are used with caution in patients with a history of cerebrovascular accident, cerebral palsy, parkinsonism, or seizure disorders and during pregnancy and lactation (pregnancy category C). Carisoprodol is used with caution in patients with severe liver or kidney disease and during pregnancy (category unknown) and lactation. Cyclobenzaprine is used cautiously in patients with cardiovascular disease and during pregnancy and lactation (pregnancy category B). Dantrolene, a pregnancy category C drug, is used with caution during pregnancy.

Interactions

The following interactions may occur when a skeletal muscle relaxant is administered with another agent:

Interacting Drug	Common Use	Effect of Interaction
central nervous system (CNS) depressants, such as alcohol, antihistamines, opiates, and sedatives	Promote a calming effect or provide pain relief	Increased CNS depressant effect
cyclobenzaprine		
MAOIs	Manage depression	Risk for high fever and convulsions
orphenadrine		
haloperidol	Treat psychotic behavior	Increased psychosis
tizanidine		
antihypertensives	Reduce blood pressure	Increased risk of hypotension

HEALTH SUPPLEMENT ALERT

Glucosamine and chondroitin are used, in combination or alone, to treat arthritis, particularly osteoarthritis. Chondroitin acts as the flexible connecting matrix between the protein filaments in cartilage. Chondroitin can be produced in the laboratory or can come from natural sources (e.g., shark cartilage). Some studies suggest that if chondroitin is available to the cell matrix, synthesis of tissue can occur. For this reason, it is used to treat arthritis. Although there is little information on chondroitin's long-term effects, it is generally not considered to be harmful.

Glucosamine theoretically provides a building block for regeneration of damaged cartilage. The absorption of oral glucosamine is 90% to 98%, making it widely accepted for use. Glucosamine is generally well tolerated, and no adverse reactions have been reported with its use.

• BONE RESORPTION INHIBITORS: BISPHOSPHONATES

Bisphosphonates are drugs used to treat musculoskeletal disorders such as osteoporosis and Paget's disease.

Actions

Bisphosphonates act primarily on the bone by inhibiting normal and abnormal bone resorption. This results in increased bone mineral density, reversing the progression of osteoporosis.

Uses

Bisphosphonates are used in the treatment of the following:

• Osteoporosis in postmenopausal women and men
• Hypercalcemia of malignant diseases and bony metastasis of some solid tumors
• Paget's disease of the bone

Adverse Reactions

Adverse reactions with bisphosphonates include:

• Nausea, diarrhea
• Increased or recurrent bone pain
• Headache
• Dyspepsia, acid regurgitation, dysphagia
• Abdominal pain

Contraindications and Precautions

These drugs are contraindicated in patients who are hypersensitive to the bisphosphonates. Alendronate (Fosamax) and risedronate (Actonel) are contraindicated in patients with hypocalcemia. Alendronate is a pregnancy category C drug and is contraindicated during pregnancy. These drugs are also contraindicated in patients with delayed esophageal emptying or renal impairment. Concurrent use of these drugs with hormone replacement therapy is not recommended.

These drugs are used cautiously in patients with gastrointestinal (GI) disorders or renal impairment. Although these drugs have not been studied, if a pregnant woman presents with malignancy, their use during the pregnancy may be justified if the potential benefit outweighs the potential risk to the fetus.

Interactions

The following interactions may occur when a bisphosphonate is administered with another agent:

Interacting Drug	Common Use	Effect of Interaction
calcium supplements or antacids with magnesium and aluminum	Relief of gastric upset	Decreased effectiveness of bisphosphonates
aspirin	Pain relief	Increased risk of GI bleeding
theophylline	Alleviation of breathing problems	Increased risk of theophylline toxicity

• DRUGS USED TO TREAT RHEUMATOID ARTHRITIS

RA, a chronic disorder involving the inflammation and accumulation of fluid in joints, is considered an autoimmune disease. This condition is typically treated using three classifications of drugs: NSAIDs, corticosteroids, and DMARDs. The NSAIDs and corticosteroids are discussed in Chapters 15 and 44, respectively.

• DISEASE-MODIFYING ANTIRHEUMATIC DRUGS

Actions and Uses

RA is an autoimmune disorder, in which antibodies are formed against one's own body. As a defense mechanism, white blood cells are mobilized and lodge in the joints, causing swelling, pain, and inflammation. When the immobility and pain of RA can no longer be controlled by pain relief agents and anti-inflammatory drugs, DMARDs are used. These drugs have properties to produce immunosuppression, which in turn decreases the body's autoimmune response. Therefore, in RA treatment, DMARDs are useful for their immunosuppressive ability. (DMARDs may also be used for other purposes, such as cancer therapy, in which the immunosuppression is considered an adverse reaction rather than an intended effect.)

Cytotoxic drugs, such as azathioprine (Imuran), cyclophosphamide (Cytoxan), and cyclosporine, are reserved for life-threatening problems (such as systemic vasculitis) because they are associated with a high rate of toxic adverse reactions. Gold salts and penicillamine are considered extremely toxic and used only when other drugs fail to achieve remission.

Adverse Reactions

Immunosuppressive drugs can cause the following adverse reactions:

• Nausea
• Stomatitis
• **Alopecia** (hair loss)

The adverse reactions to sulfa-based drugs include ocular changes, GI upset, and mild pancytopenia. The most common adverse reaction to the drugs given by injection is skin irritation. For more information, see the Summary Drug Table: Drugs Used to Treat Musculoskeletal Disorders.

Contraindications

All categories of DMARDs are contraindicated in patients with known hypersensitivity to the drugs. Patients with renal insufficiency, liver disease, alcohol abuse, pancytopenia, or folate deficiency should not take methotrexate. Etanercept (Enbrel), adalimumab (Humira), and infliximab (Remicade) should not be used in patients with congestive heart failure or neurologic demyelinating diseases. Anakinra (Kineret) should not be used in combination with etanercept, adalimumab, or infliximab.

Precautions

These drugs should be used with caution in patients with obesity, diabetes, and hepatitis B or C. Women should not become pregnant, and sexual partners should use barrier contraception to prevent transmission of the drug by semen.

Sulfasalazine is selected over methotrexate for patients with liver disease. Patients taking etanercept, adalimumab, or infliximab should be screened for preexisting tuberculosis because of the increase in opportunistic infections presenting after treatment.

Interactions

The following interactions may occur when a DMARD, such as methotrexate, is administered with another agent:

Interacting Drug	Common Use	Effect of Interaction
sulfa antibiotics	Fight infection	Increased risk of methotrexate toxicity
aspirin and NSAIDs	Pain relief	Increased risk of methotrexate toxicity

! NURSING ALERT
Because DMARDs are designed to produce immunosuppression, patients need to be monitored routinely for infections. Instruct patients to report any problem, no matter how minor, such as a cold or open sore—even these can become life threatening.

patient teaching

• URIC ACID INHIBITORS

Gout is a condition in which uric acid accumulates in increased amounts in the blood and often is deposited in the joints. The deposit or collection of urate crystals in the joints causes the symptoms (pain, redness, swelling, joint deformity) of gout.

Actions

Allopurinol (Zyloprim) reduces the production of uric acid, thereby decreasing serum uric acid levels and the deposit of urate crystals in joints. This probably accounts for its ability to relieve the severe pain of acute gout.

The exact mechanism of action of colchicine is unknown, but it does reduce the inflammation associated with the deposit of urate crystals in the joints. Colchicine has no effect on uric acid metabolism.

In people with gout, the serum uric acid level is usually elevated. Sulfinpyrazone (Anturane) increases the excretion of uric acid by the kidneys, which lowers serum uric acid levels and consequently retards the deposit of urate crystals in the joints. Probenecid works in the same manner and may be given alone or with colchicine as combination therapy when there are frequent, recurrent attacks of gout. Probenecid also has been used to prolong the plasma levels of penicillins and cephalosporins.

Uses

Drugs indicated for treatment of gout may be used to manage acute attacks of gout or in preventing acute attacks of gout (prophylaxis).

Adverse Reactions

Gastrointestinal System Reactions

- Nausea, vomiting, diarrhea
- Abdominal pain

Other Reactions

- Headache
- Urinary frequency

One adverse reaction associated with allopurinol is skin rash, which in some cases has been followed by serious hypersensitivity reactions, such as exfoliative dermatitis and Stevens-Johnson syndrome. Colchicine administration may result in severe nausea, vomiting, and bone marrow depression; therefore, it is used as a second line of treatment when other drugs fail.

Contraindications

The drugs used for gout are contraindicated in patients with known hypersensitivity. Sulfinpyrazone is contraindicated in patients with peptic ulcer disease and GI inflammation. Colchicine is contraindicated in patients with serious GI, renal, hepatic, or cardiac disorders and those with blood dyscrasias. Probenecid is contraindicated in patients with blood dyscrasias or uric acid kidney stones, and in children younger than 2 years.

Precautions

Uric acid inhibitors are used cautiously in patients with renal impairment and during pregnancy; these agents are either pregnancy category B or C drugs. Allopurinol is used cautiously in patients with liver impairment. Probenecid is used cautiously in patients who are hypersensitive to sulfa drugs or have peptic ulcer disease. Colchicine is used with caution in older adults.

Interactions

The following interactions may occur when a uric acid inhibitor is administered with another agent:

Interacting Drug	Common Use	Effect of Interaction
allopurinol		
ampicillin	Anti-infective agent	Increased risk of rash
theophylline	Alleviation of breathing problems	Increased risk of theophylline toxicity
aluminum-based antacids	Relief of gastric upset	Decreased effectiveness of allopurinol
probenecid		
penicillins, cephalosporins, acyclovir, rifampin, and the sulfonamides	Anti-infective agent	Increased serum level of anti-infective
barbiturates and benzodiazepines	Sedation	Increased serum level of sedative
NSAIDs	Pain relief	Increased serum level of NSAID
salicylates	Pain relief	Decreased effectiveness of probenecid
sulfinpyrazone		
oral anticoagulants	Blood thinner	Increased risk of bleeding
tolbutamide	Antidiabetic agent	Increased risk of hypoglycemia
verapamil	Management of heart problems	Increased effectiveness of verapamil

NURSING PROCESS
PATIENT RECEIVING A DRUG FOR A MUSCULOSKELETAL DISORDER

ASSESSMENT

Preadministration Assessment

The nurse obtains the patient's history—that is, a summary of the disorder, including onset, symptoms, and current treatment or therapy. In some instances, it may be necessary to question patients regarding their ability to carry out activities of daily living, including employment when applicable.

For the physical assessment, the nurse appraises the patient's physical condition and limitations. If the patient has arthritis (any type), the nurse examines the affected joints in the extremities for appearance of the skin over the joint, evidence of joint deformity, and mobility of the affected joint. Patients with osteoporosis are assessed for pain, particularly in the upper and lower back or hip. If the patient has gout, the nurse examines the affected joints and notes the appearance of the skin over the joints and any joint enlargement. Vital signs and weight are taken to provide a baseline for comparison during therapy.

The primary health care provider may order laboratory tests and bone scans to measure bone density. This is especially important for use as baseline data when a bone resorption inhibitor is prescribed for the patient.

NURSING ALERT

When bisphosphonates are administered, serum calcium levels are monitored before, during, and after therapy.

Ongoing Assessment

Periodic evaluation is an important part of therapy for musculoskeletal disorders. With some disorders, such as acute gout, the patient can be expected to respond to therapy in hours. Therefore, it is important for the nurse to inspect the joints involved every 1 to 2 hours to identify immediately a response or nonresponse to therapy. At this time, the nurse questions the patient regarding the relief of pain, as well as adverse drug reactions.

In other disorders, response is gradual and may take days, weeks, and even months of treatment. Depending on the drug administered and the disorder being treated, the evaluation of therapy may be daily or weekly. These recorded evaluations help the primary health care provider plan current and future therapy, including dosage changes, changes in the drug administered, and institution of physical therapy.

When first-line treatments are not successful, sometimes drugs that are more toxic may be prescribed. The nurse closely observes the patient for the development of adverse reactions. Should any one or more adverse reactions occur, the nurse notifies the primary health care provider before the next dose is given.

NURSING DIAGNOSES

Drug-specific nursing diagnoses include the following:

❏ **Readiness for Enhanced Fluid Balance** related to need for increased fluid intake to promote excretion of urate crystals
❏ **Impaired Comfort: Gastric Distress** related to irritation of gastric lining from medication administration
❏ **Risk for Injury** related to medication-induced drowsiness and associated risk for imbalance and falls

Nursing diagnoses related to drug administration are discussed in Chapter 4.

PLANNING

The expected outcomes for the patient depend on the reason for administration but may include an optimal response to therapy, meeting patient needs related to the management of adverse reactions, and an understanding of the therapeutic regimen.

IMPLEMENTATION

Promoting an Optimal Response to Therapy

The patient with a musculoskeletal disorder may have long-standing chronic pain, which can be just as difficult to tolerate as acute pain. Along with pain, there may be skeletal deformities, such as the joint deformities seen with advanced RA. For many musculoskeletal conditions, drug therapy is a major treatment modality. In addition to drug therapy, rest, physical therapy, and other measures may be part of treatment. Including drugs as a major part of the treatment plan may keep the disorder

under control (e.g., therapy for gout), improve the patient's ability to carry out activities of daily living, or make the pain and discomfort tolerable.

Patients with a musculoskeletal disorder often have anxiety related to the symptoms and the chronicity of the disorder. In addition to physical care, these patients often require emotional support, especially when a disorder is disabling and chronic. The nurse explains to the patient that therapy may take weeks or longer before any benefit is noted. When this is explained before therapy starts, the patient is less likely to become discouraged over slow results.

Because of the toxic nature of some drugs, they are not used as frequently as newer drugs. It is important for the nurse to be aware of the adverse toxic reactions that can occur when less frequently prescribed drugs are given. The nurse closely observes the patient taking hydroxychloroquine for adverse reactions. It is important for the nurse to be alert to reactions such as skin rash, fever, cough, or easy bruising. The nurse should be attentive to specific patient complaints such as visual changes, tinnitus, or hearing loss. The nurse immediately reports these adverse reactions. Particular attention is paid to visual changes because irreversible retinal damage may occur.

Administration of allopurinol may result in skin rash. A rash should be monitored carefully because it may precede a serious adverse reaction, such as Stevens-Johnson syndrome. The nurse immediately reports any rash to the primary health care provider.

Gold compounds and methotrexate are potentially toxic. Therefore, the nurse observes closely for development of adverse reactions, such as thrombocytopenia and leukopenia. Hematology, liver, and renal function studies are monitored every 1 to 3 months with methotrexate therapy. The primary care provider is notified of abnormal hematology, liver function, or kidney function findings. The nurse immediately brings all adverse reactions or suspected adverse reactions to the attention of the primary health care provider.

Monitoring and Managing Patient Needs

READINESS FOR ENHANCED FLUID BALANCE. When using the uric acid inhibitors, the nurse encourages liberal fluid intake and measures the intake and output. The daily urine output should be at least 2 liters. An increase in urinary output is necessary to excrete the urates (uric acid) and prevent urate acid stone formation in the genitourinary tract. The nurse provides adequate fluids and reminds the patient frequently of the importance of increasing fluid intake. If the patient fails to increase fluid intake, the nurse informs the primary health care provider. In some instances, it may be necessary to administer intravenous fluids to supplement the oral intake when the patient fails to drink about 3000 mL of fluid per day.

IMPAIRED COMFORT: GASTRIC DISTRESS. Adequate drug absorption and metabolism can depend on timing with meals. To facilitate delivery of the bone reabsorption inhibitor to the stomach and minimize adverse GI effects, the nurse instructs the patient to take the drug upon arising in the morning, with 6 to 8 oz of water while the patient is in an upright position. The patient is instructed to remain upright (avoid lying down) for at least 30 minutes after taking the drug. Etidronate is not administered within 2 hours of food, vitamin and mineral supplements, or antacids. Risedronate and etidronate are typically administered once daily.

Many bisphosphonates are becoming available in both once-a-week and once-a-month dosing forms. Although the patient has to come to the ambulatory clinic for intravenous administration; ibandronate, zoledronic acid, and pamidronate all come in parenteral form for even less frequent dosing. The nurse should check the dosage and frequency carefully to prevent drug administration errors.

The nurse administers DMARDs, uric acid inhibitors, and skeletal muscle relaxants with, or immediately after, meals to minimize gastric distress.

RISK FOR INJURY. Many of these drugs may cause drowsiness. In addition, pain or deformity may hamper mobility. These two factors place the patient at risk of injury. Therefore the nurse evaluates the patient carefully before allowing the patient to ambulate alone. If drowsiness does occur, assistance with ambulatory activities is necessary. If drowsiness is severe, the nurse notifies the primary health care provider before the next dose is due.

The patient with an arthritis disorder may experience much pain or discomfort and may require assistance with activities, such as ambulating, eating, and grooming. Patients on bed rest require position changes and skin care every 2 hours. Patients with osteoporosis may require a brace or corset when out of bed.

Educating the Patient and Family

To ensure compliance with the treatment regimen, the patient must understand the importance of the prescribed therapy and taking the drug exactly as directed to obtain the best results. To meet this goal, the nurse develops an effective plan of patient and family teaching.

The points included in a patient and family teaching plan depend on the type and severity of the patient's musculoskeletal disorder. The nurse must explain carefully that treatment for the disorder includes drug therapy, as well as other medical management, such as diet, exercise, limitations or nonlimitations of activity, and periodic physical therapy treatments. The nurse emphasizes the importance of not taking any nonprescription drugs unless their use has been approved by the primary health care provider.

The dosing schedule can be difficult for the patient to understand when the drugs are given on an outpatient basis, particularly if the person is elderly or confused and responsible for self-administering the drug.

Dosing schedules may require taking medications on alternate days (alternate-day therapy), at specific times of the day, or weekly. The patient may not see a

therapeutic response until 3 to 6 weeks of therapy and become discouraged. In some cases, a patient may stop treatment.

Some drugs used for RA require self-administered subcutaneous injections. The nurse teaches the patient and family proper injection and disposal techniques. Teaching about site rotation should be included. The patient should demonstrate proper injection technique before this becomes a self-administered procedure. Patients need to be taught how to manage the discomfort to the site of injection and to report redness, pain, and swelling to the primary health care provider.

The following points for specific drugs are included in the teaching plan:

* *Drugs used to treat osteoporosis*
  * Take these drugs with 6 to 8 oz of water first thing in the morning.
  * Do not lie down for at least 30 minutes after taking the drug and wait at least 30 minutes before taking any other food or drink.
  * Take supplemental calcium and vitamin D if dietary intake is inadequate.
* *Drugs used to treat RA*
  * When taking methotrexate, use a calendar or some other memory device to remember to take the drug on the same day each week.
  * Notify the primary health care provider immediately if any of the following occur: sore mouth or sores in the mouth, diarrhea, fever, sore throat, easy bruising, rash, itching, or nausea and vomiting.
  * Women of childbearing age should use an effective contraceptive during therapy with methotrexate and for 8 weeks after therapy.
* *Drugs used to treat gout*
  * Drink at least 10 glasses of water a day until the acute attack has subsided.
  * Take this drug with food to minimize GI upset.
  * If drowsiness occurs, avoid driving or performing other hazardous tasks.
  * Acute gout—notify the primary health care provider if pain is not relieved in a few days.
  * Notify the primary health care provider if a skin rash occurs.
* *Drugs used for muscle spasm and cramping*
  * This drug may cause drowsiness. Do not drive or perform other hazardous tasks if drowsiness occurs.
  * This drug is for short-term use. Do not use the drug for longer than 2 to 3 weeks.
  * Avoid alcohol or other CNS depressants while taking this drug.

EVALUATION

* Therapeutic drug effect is achieved, pain is decreased, and mobility is improved or maintained.
* Adverse reactions are identified, reported to the primary health care provider, and managed using appropriate nursing interventions.
  ☑ Patient improves fluid balance.

☑ GI comfort is maintained.

☑ No evidence of injury is seen.

• Patient and family demonstrate an understanding of the drug regimen.

THINK CRITICALLY: PHARMACOLOGY IN PRACTICE

1. Mary is a nurse who has returned to nursing after taking 15 years' absence to raise a family. Mary asks you what should be included in a teaching plan for a patient who has RA and who is now taking DMARDs. Discuss what information you would suggest that Mary emphasize in a teaching plan.

● Test Your Knowledge

1. When administering a skeletal muscle relaxant, the nurse observes the patient for the most common adverse reaction, which is _____.

A. drowsiness
B. GI bleeding
C. vomiting
D. constipation

2. When a patient is prescribed alendronate (Fosamax) for osteoporosis, the nurse administers the drug _____.

A. with food or milk
B. by injection
C. 30 minutes before breakfast
D. at bedtime

3. When allopurinol (Zyloprim) is used for treating gout, the nurse _____.

A. administers the drug with juice or milk
B. administers the drug after the evening meal
C. restricts fluids during evening hours
D. encourages liberal fluid intake

4. What teaching points would the nurse include when educating the patient who will begin taking risedronate?

A. The drug is administered once weekly.
B. Take a daily laxative, because the drug will likely cause constipation.
C. Take the drug with antacids to decrease gastric distress.
D. After taking the drug, remain upright for at least 30 minutes.

● Prepare for the NCLEX

1. When administering a DMARD drug subcutaneously, the nurse should:

A. use a 5 mL syringe
B. inject tissue close to the umbilicus
C. massage the area to increase blood flow to the muscles
D. rotate sites to minimize tissue irritation

● Calculate Medication Dosages

1. A patient is to receive allopurinol 300 mg orally for gout. The nurse has 100-mg tablets available. How many tablets would the nurse administer? _____

2. The physician prescribes 1.5 g methocarbamol (Robaxin) orally for a musculoskeletal disorder. Available for administration are 500-mg tablets. The nurse administers _____.

To check your answers, see Appendix E.

the**Point** *For more NCLEX questions, log on to http://thepoint.lww.com to access more than 1000 questions.*

Drugs That Affect the Respiratory System

The respiratory system consists of the upper and lower airways, the lungs, and the thoracic cavity. The respiratory system provides a mechanism for the exchange of oxygen and carbon dioxide in the lungs. Any change in the respiratory status has the potential to affect every other bodily system, because all cells need an adequate supply of oxygen for optimal functioning.

This unit focuses on drugs used to treat some of the more common disorders affecting the respiratory system. Among the most common conditions of the upper respiratory system are infections, allergic rhinitis, coughs, the common cold, and congestion. Typically, upper respiratory infections are treated with an antibiotic if bacteria are involved. When the condition is viral, then comfort measures are used to tolerate the course of the illness. These measures include (1) antihistamines to relieve allergy symptoms, (2) decongestants to reduce nasal edema, and (3) antitussives, mucolytics, and expectorants to treat accompanying cough. These drugs are discussed in Chapters 32 and 33. Many of these drugs are available as nonprescription (over-the-counter) drugs, whereas others are available only by prescription.

In Chapter 34, drugs used to treat disorders of the lower respiratory tract are discussed. These drugs include the bronchodilating drugs, which are the β_2 adrenergic agonists (which have sympathomimetic properties) and the xanthine derivatives. Along with the bronchodilating drugs, the antiasthma drugs include the corticosteroids, leukotriene modifiers, and the mast cell stabilizers.

Disorders of the lower respiratory tract include asthma (chronic inflammatory disease of the airways), emphysema (lung disorder in which the alveoli become enlarged and plugged with mucus), chronic bronchitis (chronic inflammation and possible infection of the bronchi), and chronic obstructive pulmonary disease (COPD). COPD is a slowly progressive disease of the airways characterized by a gradual loss of lung function. The symptoms of COPD range from chronic cough and sputum production to severe, disabling shortness of breath. There is no known cure for COPD; the treatment is usually supportive and designed to relieve symptoms and improve quality of life.

Asthma is a chronic inflammatory condition of the lower airway with airway constriction caused by bronchospasm and bronchoconstriction. Patients with asthma may experience periods of exacerbation alternating with periods of normal lung function. Environmental exposure to such allergens as house dust mites, tobacco smoke, pets and pet dander, mold, and cockroach wastes and physical exercise are important "triggers" for an asthma attack. Anti-inflammatory drugs play an important role in treating individuals with asthma. These drugs prevent asthma attacks by decreasing the swelling and mucus production in the airways, thereby making the airways less sensitive to asthma triggers. Drug therapy for asthma is aimed at preventing attacks and reducing swelling and mucus production in the airways.

PHARMACOLOGY IN PRACTICE

In this unit, our patient focus will be on Lillian Chase, a 36-year-old woman who had a breathing problem over the weekend and was seen in the emergency department of the local hospital. As the nurse, you are seeing her in the clinic for her first visit. After reading the chapters in this unit, you will review medications ordered by the primary care provider with the patient, establish guidelines for her self-management of asthma, and help her to create an Asthma Action Plan.

32

Antitussives, Mucolytics, and Expectorants

Upper respiratory infections are among the most common human illnesses. The drugs used to treat the discomfort associated with an upper respiratory infection include antitussives and expectorants. Many of these drugs are available as nonprescription (over-the-counter [OTC]) drugs, whereas others are available only by prescription.

The build-up of secretions in the lower respiratory system is treated with mucolytics. These agents break down the thickness of the secretions for easier removal.

• ANTITUSSIVES

Coughing is the forceful expulsion of air from the lungs. A cough may be productive or nonproductive. With a **productive cough**, secretions from the respiratory tract are expelled. A **nonproductive cough** is a dry, hacking one that produces no secretions. An **antitussive** is a drug used to relieve coughing. Many antitussive drugs are combined with another drug, such as an antihistamine or **expectorant**, and sold OTC as a nonprescription cough medicine. Other anti-

tussives, either alone or in combination with other drugs, are available by prescription only.

Actions

Most antitussives depress the cough center located in the medulla and are called centrally-acting drugs. Codeine and dextromethorphan are examples of centrally-acting antitussives. One antitussive acts peripherally by anesthetizing stretch receptors in the respiratory passages, thereby decreasing coughing. Benzonatate (Tessalon) is the peripherally-acting antitussive.

Uses

Antitussives are used to relieve a nonproductive cough. When the cough produces sputum, it should be treated by the primary health care provider, who, based on a physical examination, may or may not prescribe or recommend an antitussive.

❦ HERBAL ALERT

Eucalyptus is used as a decongestant and expectorant and is found as a component in OTC products used for the treatment of sinusitis and pharyngitis. The plant is grown throughout the world, and the leaves and oil are used to treat various respiratory conditions, such as asthma and chronic bronchitis. The lozenges are useful to soothe sore throats and as cough drops. Eucalyptus can also be used as a vapor bath for asthma or other bronchial conditions. Scientific evidence is inconclusive regarding the respiratory benefit of the herb, yet people feel a sense of well-being from its use. The herb is available in many forms, including an essential oil, fluid extract, and aqueous solution in alcohol, as well as a component of various OTC products. Eucalyptus should not be used during pregnancy and lactation and in children younger than 2 years of age. Eucalyptus may be used topically on children and adults in combination with menthol and camphor. Individuals with hypersensitivity to eucalyptus should avoid its use.

Adverse Reactions

Central Nervous System Reactions

- Lightheadedness
- Dizziness
- Drowsiness or sedation

Summary Drug Table ANTITUSSIVES, MUCOLYTIC, AND EXPECTORANT DRUGS

Generic Name	Trade Name	Uses	Adverse Reactions	Dosage Ranges
Antitussives				
Opioid Antitussives				
codeine koe'-deen		Suppression of nonproductive cough, relief of mild to moderate pain	Sedation, nausea, vomiting, dizziness, constipation, central nervous system (CNS) depression	10–20 mg orally q 4–6 hr; maximum dosage 120 mg/day
Nonopioid Antitussives				
benzonatate ben-zoe'-nah-tate	Tessalon Perles	Symptomatic relief of cough	Sedation, headache, mild dizziness, constipation, nausea, GI upset, pruritus, nasal congestion	Adults and children older than 10 yr: 100–200 mg TID (up to 600 mg/day)
dextromethorphan dex-troe-meh-thore'-fan	Benylin, DexAlone, Robitussin, Delsym, Formula 44 Cough	Symptomatic relief of cough	Drowsiness, dizziness, GI upset	Adults and children older than 12 yr: 10–30 mg q 4–8hr; sustained-release (SR) 60 mg q 12 hr orally Children 6–12 yr: 5–10 mg q 4hr or 15 mg q 6–8hr; SR 30 mg q 12 hr orally Children 2–5 yr: 2.5–7.5 mg q 4–8 hr; SR 15 mg q 12 hr orally
dextromethorphan and benzocaine ben'-zoe-cane	Cough-X, Tetra-Formula	Symptomatic relief of cough and bronchial irritation	Same as dextromethorphan HBr	Varies, depending on formulation; take as directed on package orally
diphenhydramine dye-fen-hye'-drah-meen	AllerMax, Hydramine Cough, Tusstat, Silphen Cough	Symptomatic relief of cough caused by colds, allergy, or bronchial irritation	Drowsiness, dizziness, GI upset	Adults: 25 mg q 4 hr orally, not to exceed 150 mg/day Children 6–12 yr: 12.5 mg orally q 4 hr, not to exceed 75 mg/day Children 2–5 yr: 6.25 mg q 4 hr, not to exceed 25 mg/day
Mucolytics				
acetylcysteine ah-seh-teel-sis'-tay-een	Mucomyst	Reduction of viscosity of mucus in acute and chronic bronchopulmonary diseases and diagnostic bronchial studies, acetaminophen toxicity	Stomatitis, nausea, vomiting, fever, drowsiness, bronchospasm, irritation of the trachea and bronchi	1–10 mL of 20% solution by nebulization or 2–20 mL of 10% solution q 2–6 hr PRN Acetaminophen toxicity: initially 140 mg/kg orally, then 70 mg/kg orally q 4 hr for 17 doses (total)
Expectorants				
guaifenesin (glyceryl guaiacolate) gwye-fen'-eh-sin	Hytuss, Organidin NR, Robitussin	Relief of cough associated with respiratory tract infection (sinusitis, asthma, bronchitis, pharyngitis), especially when the cough is dry and nonproductive	Nausea, vomiting, dizziness, headache, rash	Adults and children 12 yr and older: 200–400 mg orally q 4 hr Children 6–12 yr: 100–200 mg q 4 hr orally Children 2–6 yr: 50–100 mg q 4 hr
potassium iodide poe-tah'-see-um eye-oh-dyde	Pima, SSKI	Symptomatic relief of chronic pulmonary disease complicated by tenacious mucus	Iodine sensitivity or iodism (sore mouth, metallic taste, increased salivation, nausea, vomiting, epigastric pain, parotid swelling, and pain)	300–1000 mg orally after meals BID or TID, to 1.5 g orally TID

most common

 ☆

Gastrointestinal System Reactions

• Nausea
• Vomiting
• Constipation

When used as directed, nonprescription cough medicines containing two or more ingredients produce few adverse reactions. However, those that contain an antihistamine may cause drowsiness. The more common adverse reactions associated with the antitussives are listed in the Summary Drug Table: Antitussive, Mucolytic, and Expectorant Drugs.

Contraindications

Antitussives are contraindicated in patients with known hypersensitivity to the drugs. The opioid antitussives (those with codeine) are contraindicated in premature infants or during labor when delivery of a premature infant is anticipated.

Precautions

Antitussives are given with caution to patients with a persistent or chronic cough, a cough accompanied by excessive secretions, a high fever, rash, persistent headache, or nausea or vomiting.

Antitussives containing codeine are used with caution during pregnancy (category C) and labor (pregnancy category D), in patients with chronic obstructive pulmonary disease (COPD), acute asthmatic attack, preexisting respiratory disorders, acute abdominal conditions, head injury, increased intracranial pressure, convulsive disorders, hepatic or renal impairment, and prostatic hypertrophy.

Interactions

Other CNS depressants and alcohol may cause additive depressant effects when administered with antitussives containing codeine. When dextromethorphan is administered with the monoamine oxidase inhibitors antidepressants (see Chapter 22), patients may experience hypotension, fever, nausea, jerking motions to the leg, and coma.

NURSING PROCESS

PATIENT RECEIVING AN ANTITUSSIVE DRUG

ASSESSMENT

Preadministration Assessment
Ambulatory patients are most commonly prescribed an antitussive preparation. During the preadministration assessment, the nurse documents the type of cough (productive, nonproductive) and describes the color and amount of any sputum present. The patient is asked to describe actions taken or home remedies used to treat the cough independently. The nurse takes and records vital signs because some patients with a productive cough may have an infection.

A hospitalized patient may occasionally have an antitussive preparation prescribed, especially when a nonproductive cough causes discomfort or threatens to cause more serious problems, such as raising pressure in the eye (increased intraocular pressure) after eye surgery or increasing intracranial pressure in those with CNS disorders.

Ongoing Assessment
During the ongoing assessment, the nurse observes for a therapeutic effect (e.g., coughing decreases). The nurse auscultates lung sounds and takes vital signs periodically. When a patient has a cough, the nurse describes and records in the chart the type of cough (productive or nonproductive of sputum) and the frequency of coughing. The nurse also notes and records whether the cough interrupts sleep and whether it causes pain in the chest or other parts of the body.

NURSING DIAGNOSES

Drug-specific nursing diagnoses include the following:

❑ **Risk for Injury** related to drowsiness, dizziness, or sedation.
❑ **Ineffective airway clearance** related to pooling of secretions.

Nursing diagnoses related to drug administration are discussed in Chapter 4.

PLANNING

The expected outcomes for the patient depend on the reason for administration, but may include an optimal response to therapy, support of patient needs related to managing adverse reactions, and an understanding of the therapeutic regimen.

IMPLEMENTATION

Promoting an Optimal Response to Therapy
The nurse administers antitussives orally. When the nurse gives the drug as a tablet, the patient should swallow the drug whole and not chew it. For example, chewing benzonatate tablets may result in a local anesthetic effect (oropharyngeal anesthesia) with possible choking as a result.

Problems can arise from the use of a nonprescription antitussive for self-treatment of a chronic cough. Indiscriminate use of antitussives by the general public may prevent early diagnosis and treatment of serious disorders, such as lung cancer and emphysema.

> **NURSING ALERT**
> The nurse should advise the patient taking a nonprescription cough medicine that if a cough lasts more than 10 days or is accompanied by fever, chest pain, severe headache, or skin rash, the patient should consult the primary health care provider.

Monitoring and Managing Patient Needs

RISK FOR INJURY. Many of the antitussives cause drowsiness, dizziness, or sedation. These effects increase the patient's risk for falling. The nurse can minimize this risk for hospitalized patients by carefully orienting each patient to the surroundings and closely supervising the patient. A night light helps the patient to see at night. The nurse encourages the patient to ask for assistance if he or she feels dizzy or unsteady. Ingredients in antitussives may impair mental or physical abilities required to perform potentially hazardous tasks. Patients should observe caution when driving or performing tasks that require alertness, coordination, or physical dexterity. Codeine may cause orthostatic hypotension when a patient rises too quickly from a sitting or lying position. Patients should not take codeine preparations for persistent or chronic cough, such as occurs with smoking, asthma, or emphysema, or when the cough is accompanied by excessive secretions, except when under the supervision of the health care provider.

INEFFECTIVE AIRWAY CLEARANCE. One problem associated with the use of an antitussive is related to its drug action. Although not an adverse reaction, depression of the cough reflex can cause secretions to pool in the lungs. Pooling of the secretions that are normally removed by coughing may result in more serious problems, such as pneumonia and atelectasis. For this reason, using an antitussive for a productive cough is contraindicated in many situations. Patients should be encouraged to increase fluids and change position frequently to facilitate removal of secretions.

Educating the Patient and Family

The nurse instructs patients to refrain from the indiscriminate use of nonprescription antitussives, especially when coughing produces sputum. The nurse advises the patient to read the label carefully, follow the dosage recommendations, and consult the primary health care provider if the cough persists for more than 10 days or if fever or chest pain occurs. If an antitussive is prescribed for use at home, the nurse includes the following information in a teaching plan:

- Do not exceed the recommended dose.
- Avoid irritants, such as cigarette smoke, dust, or fumes, to decrease irritation to the throat.
- Drink plenty of fluids (if not contraindicated by disease process). A fluid intake of 1500 to 2000 mL is recommended.
- If taking oral capsules, do not chew or break open the capsules; swallow them whole.
- If taking a lozenge, avoid drinking fluids for 30 minutes after use to avoid losing effectiveness of the drug.
- If the cough is not relieved or becomes worse, contact the primary health care provider.
- If chills, fever, chest pain, or sputum production occurs, contact the primary health care provider as soon as possible.
- Do not use with alcohol or other CNS depressants (e.g., antidepressants, hypnotics, sedatives, tranquilizers).

EVALUATION

- Therapeutic response is achieved and coughing is relieved.
- Adverse reactions are identified, reported to the primary health care provider, and managed successfully with appropriate nursing interventions.
  - ☑ No evidence of injury is seen.
  - ☑ Patient has a clear airway.
- Patient and family demonstrate an understanding of the drug regimen.

• MUCOLYTICS AND EXPECTORANTS

thin out secretions

A **mucolytic** is a drug that breaks down thick, tenacious mucus in the lower portions of the lungs. An expectorant is a drug that thins respiratory secretions to remove them more easily from the respiratory system.

Actions

CF pt have suction Trach

A drug with mucolytic activity appears to reduce the viscosity (thickness) of respiratory secretions by direct action on the mucus. An example of a mucolytic drug is acetylcysteine (Mucomyst). One other mucolytic drug is on the market, dornase alfa (Pulmozyme). This agent is used for the treatment of cystic fibrosis.

Expectorants increase the production of respiratory secretions, which in turn appears to decrease the viscosity of the mucus. This helps to raise secretions from the respiratory passages. An example of an expectorant is guaifenesin.

Uses

The mucolytic acetylcysteine is used to treat the following:

- Acute bronchopulmonary disease (pneumonia, bronchitis, tracheobronchitis)
- Tracheostomy care
- Pulmonary complications of cystic fibrosis
- Pulmonary complications associated with surgery and during anesthesia
- Posttraumatic chest conditions
- Atelectasis due to mucus obstruction
- Acetaminophen overdosage

This drug is also used for diagnostic bronchial studies, such as bronchograms and bronchial wedge catheterizations. It is primarily given by nebulizer but also may be directly instilled into a tracheostomy to liquefy (thin) secretions.

Expectorants are used to help bring up respiratory secretions. An expectorant may also be included along with one or more additional drugs, such as an antihistamine, decongestant, or antitussive, in some prescription and nonprescription cough medicines.

Adverse Reactions

The more common adverse reactions associated with mucolytic and expectorant drugs are listed in the Summary Drug Table: Antitussive, Mucolytic, and Expectorant Drugs.

CF~Trach irritation

Contraindications

The expectorants and mucolytics are contraindicated in patients with known hypersensitivity. Mucolytics are not recommended for use by patients with asthma. The expectorant potassium iodide is contraindicated during pregnancy (category D).   COPD - may aspirate

Precautions

The expectorants are used cautiously during pregnancy and lactation (guaifenesin is a pregnancy category C drug and acetylcysteine is a pregnancy category B drug), in patients with persistent cough, severe respiratory insufficiency, or asthma, and in older adults or debilitated patients.

Interactions

No significant interactions have been reported when the expectorants are used as directed. The exception is iodine products. If used concurrently with iodine products, lithium and other antithyroid drugs may potentiate the hypothyroid effects of these drugs. When potassium-containing medications and potassium-sparing diuretics are administered with iodine products, the patient may experience hypokalemia, cardiac arrhythmias, or cardiac arrest. Thyroid function test results may also be altered by iodine.

NURSING PROCESS
PATIENT RECEIVING A MUCOLYTIC OR AN EXPECTORANT

ASSESSMENT

Preadministration Assessment
Before administering the drug, the nurse assesses the respiratory status of the patient. The nurse documents lung sounds, amount of dyspnea (if any), and consistency of sputum (if present). A description of the sputum is important as a baseline for future comparison.

Ongoing Assessment
After administering the drug, the nurse notes any increase in sputum or change in consistency. The nurse documents, on the patient's chart, a description of the sputum raised. Patients with thick, tenacious mucus may have difficulty breathing. It is important to notify the primary health care provider if the patient has difficulty breathing because of an inability to raise sputum and clear the respiratory passages.

Immediately before and after treatment with the mucolytic acetylcysteine, the nurse auscultates the lungs and records the findings of both assessments on the patient's chart. Between treatments, the nurse evaluates the patient's respiratory status and records these findings on the patient's chart. These evaluations aid the primary health care provider in determining the effectiveness of therapy. If any problem occurs during or after treatment,

or if the patient is uncooperative, the nurse discusses the problem with the primary health care provider.

When expectorants are given to those with chronic pulmonary disease, the nurse evaluates the effectiveness of drug therapy (i.e., the patient's ability to raise sputum) and records this finding in the patient's chart.

NURSING DIAGNOSES

A drug-specific nursing diagnosis may be:

❏ **Ineffective Airway Clearance** related to thick, tenacious mucus

Nursing diagnoses related to drug administration are discussed in Chapter 4.

PLANNING

The expected outcomes for the patient depend on the reason for administration, but may include an optimal response to therapy, support of patient needs related to management of adverse drug reactions, and an understanding of the therapeutic regimen.

IMPLEMENTATION

Promoting an Optimal Response to Therapy
When the mucolytic acetylcysteine is administered by nebulization, the nurse explains the treatment to the patient and demonstrates how the nebulizer will be used. The nurse informs the patient that the drug may smell odd. The nurse remains with the patient during the first few treatments, especially when the patient is elderly or exhibits anxiety. The nurse supplies the patient with tissues and places a paper bag for disposal of the tissues within the patient's reach. If acetylcysteine is ordered to be inserted into a tracheostomy, the nurse must make sure suction equipment is at the bedside to be immediately available for aspiration of secretions.

 NURSING ALERT

Acetylcysteine has a distinctive, disagreeable odor. The nurse should advise the patient that the medication may smell "like rotten eggs." Although this odor may be nauseating, the smell dissipates quickly.

Managing and Monitoring Patient Needs
INEFFECTIVE AIRWAY CLEARANCE. For the patient with thick sputum, the nurse encourages a fluid intake of up to 2000 mL per day if this amount is not contraindicated by the patient's condition or disease process. The nurse encourages the patient to take deep, diaphragmatic breaths. The amount and consistency of sputum is monitored.

Educating the Patient and Family
Acetylcysteine usually is administered in the hospital but may be prescribed for the patient being discharged and who is renting or buying respiratory therapy equipment for use at home (see Patient Teaching for Improved Patient Outcomes: Using Respiratory Equipment at Home).

Typically, the respiratory therapist gives the patient or a family member full instruction in the use and maintenance of the equipment, as well as the technique of administration of acetylcysteine. The nurse should be sure the patient or family member understands the instruction and has all questions addressed before discharge.

When an expectorant is prescribed, the nurse instructs the patient to take the drug as directed and to contact the primary health care provider if any unusual symptoms or other problems occur during use of the drug or if the drug appears to be ineffective.

EVALUATION

- Therapeutic response is achieved and secretions are thinned and easily expectorated.
- Adverse reactions are identified, reported to the primary health care provider, and managed successfully with appropriate nursing interventions.
  - ☑ Patient has a clear patent airway.
- Patient and family demonstrate an understanding of the drug regimen and use of equipment to administer the drug (mucolytic).

Patient Teaching for Improved Patient Outcomes

Using Respiratory Equipment at Home

The nurse:
- ✓ Contacts the respiratory care provider to arrange for equipment delivery to the patient's home and home services as needed.
- ✓ Assess for proper set up on sturdy surface and need for electrical power source.
- ✓ Reviews the drug therapy regimen, including the prescribed drug and solution strength, dosage, amount and type of diluent, if required, and frequency of administration.
- ✓ Demonstrates step-by-step procedure for equipment setup and drug preparation and administration.
- ✓ Evaluates return demonstration of procedure before discharge.
- ✓ Recommends sitting or high Fowler's position to maximize lung expansion and drug dispersion.
- ✓ Instructs to observe for misting as evidence of proper equipment function.
- ✓ Encourages slow, even breathing during treatment and coughing and expectorating as necessary.
- ✓ Stresses the importance of continuing treatment until the entire drug is gone. The machine should make a sputtering noise, and only a little amount of fluid will be left in the cup.
- ✓ Reviews the signs and symptoms of possible adverse reactions and impaired respiratory function, including changes in cough, color, and amount of sputum, shortness of breath, or

difficulty breathing, and stresses the need to notify the primary health care provider at once should any occur.
- ✓ Instructs to rinse equipment, following manufacturer instructions, after each use.
- ✓ Recommends storing equipment parts in safe place away from small children.
- ✓ Provides information for trouble-shooting problems such as changing filter, tightening connections, or replacing aerosol cup.
- ✓ Provides contact information for the respiratory care providers and equipment companies.

THINK CRITICALLY: PHARMACOLOGY IN PRACTICE

Mr. Peterson, Betty Peterson's husband, calls the clinic and tells you that he can't sleep due to his wife's chronic cough. He asks you to recommend the best OTC "cough medicine." What further information do you need about Mrs. Peterson's medications? Discuss the recommendations you would give to Mr. Peterson.

● Test Your Knowledge

1. Antitussives are medications that _____.
   - A. loosen respiratory secretions
   - B. depress the cough center in the brain
   - C. increase production of mucous secretion
   - D. fight microbial infections of the lungs

2. Which of these drugs is classified as an expectorant?
   - A. guaifenesin
   - B. codeine
   - C. dextromethorphan
   - D. diphenhydramine

3. Which of the following statements is appropriate for the nurse to include in discharge instructions for a patient taking an antitussive?
   - A. Increase the dosage if the drug does not relieve the cough.
   - B. Limit fluids to less than 1000 mL each day.
   - C. Expect the cough to worsen during the first few days of treatment.
   - D. Frequent sips of water may diminish coughing.

4. Which of these drugs would mostly likely be used in caring for a patient with a tracheostomy?
   - A. acetylcysteine
   - B. guaifenesin
   - C. benzonatate
   - D. dextromethorphan

● Prepare for the NCLEX

1. The nurse is to administer a mucolytic agent, which of the following nursing actions is appropriate to take to promote an effective airway?

    A. Increase fluid intake to 2000 mL per day.
    B. Limit fluids to 200 mL per day.
    C. Monitor intake and output every 8 hours.
    D. Have the patient take the mucolytic after each coughing episode

● Calculate Medication Dosages

1. A patient is prescribed 200 mg of guaifenesin syrup. The drug is available in syrup of 200 mg/5 mL. The nurse administers _____.

2. Codeine 10 mg is prescribed for a patient with a severe unproductive cough. The drug is available as an oral solution of 10 mg/5 mL. The nurse administers _____.

To check your answers, see Appendix E.

the**Point** *For more NCLEX questions, log on to http://thepoint.lww.com to access more than 1000 questions.*

Antihistamines and Decongestants

33

LEARNING OBJECTIVES

On completion of this chapter, the student will:

1. Discuss the uses, general drug action, general adverse reactions, contraindications, precautions, and interactions of the antihistamines and decongestants.
2. Discuss important preadministration and ongoing assessment activities the nurse should perform on the patient taking an antihistamine or a decongestant.
3. List nursing diagnoses particular to a patient taking an antihistamine or a decongestant.
4. Discuss ways to promote an optimal response to therapy, how to manage common patient needs (e.g., adverse reactions), and important points to keep in mind when educating a patient about the use of an antihistamine or a decongestant.

This chapter focuses on drugs used to treat some of the more common disorders affecting the upper respiratory system, particularly allergies and the congestion associated with certain respiratory disorders.

• ANTIHISTAMINES

Histamine is produced in response to an allergic reaction or tissue injury. It acts on areas such as the vascular system and smooth muscle, producing dilation of arterioles and an increased permeability of capillaries and venules. Dilation of the arterioles results in localized redness. An increase in the permeability of small blood vessels promotes an escape of fluid from these blood vessels into the surrounding tissues, which produces localized swelling. Thus, the release of histamine produces an inflammatory response. Histamine is also released from mast cells in allergic reactions or hypersensitivity reactions, such as anaphylactic shock.

There are three types of histamine cell receptors: (1) histamine type 1 (H_1) receptors contract smooth muscle and

dilate capillaries; (2) the heart rate and gastric secretions increase when H_2 receptors are activated; (3) the H_3 receptors are located throughout the nervous system.

An **antihistamine** is a drug used to block the cell receptors, thus, counteracting the effects of histamine on body organs and structures. Examples of antihistamines include diphenhydramine (Benadryl), loratadine (Claritin), fexofenadine (Allegra), and cetirizine (Zyrtec). Desloratadine(Clarinex), loratadine, and fexofenadine minimally penetrate the blood–brain barrier, which means that little of the drug is distributed in the central nervous system (CNS) so that fewer of the sedating effects are felt. Topical corticosteroid nasal sprays, such as fluticasone propionate (Flonase) or triamcinolone acetonide (Nasacort), are also used for nasal allergy symptoms. See Chapter 53 for more information on the topical corticosteroids.

Actions

Antihistamines (or H_1 receptor antagonists) block most, but not all, of the effects of histamine. They do this by competing with histamine at histamine receptor sites throughout the body, thereby preventing histamine from entering these receptor sites and producing an effect on body tissues. First-generation antihistamines bind nonselectively to central and peripheral H_1 receptors and may result in CNS stimulation or depression. CNS depression usually occurs with higher doses and allows some of these agents to be used for sedation. Other first-generation drugs may have additional effects, such as antipruritic (anti-itching) or antiemetic (antinausea) effects. Second-generation antihistamines are selective for peripheral H_1 receptors and, as a group, are less sedating. See the Summary Drug Table: Antihistamines for a listing of first- and second-generation antihistamines.

Uses

The general uses of the antihistamines include the following:

- Relief of the symptoms of seasonal and perennial allergies
- Allergic and vasomotor rhinitis
- Allergic conjunctivitis
- Mild and uncomplicated angioneurotic edema and urticaria
- Relief of allergic reactions to drugs, blood, or plasma
- Relief of coughs caused by colds or allergy
- Adjunctive therapy in anaphylactic shock
- Treatment of parkinsonism

Breaking up secretions

- Relief of nausea and vomiting
- Relief of motion sickness
- Sedation
- Adjuncts to analgesics

Each antihistamine may be used for one or more of these reasons. The more specific uses of the various antihistamine preparations are given in the Summary Drug Table: Antihistamines.

Summary Drug Table ANTIHISTAMINES

Generic Name	Trade Name	Uses	Adverse Reactions	Dosage Ranges
First-Generation Antihistamines				
brompheniramine *brome-fen-ear'-ah-meen*	LoHist 12 Hour, Bidhist, Lodrane 24, VaZol, Lodrane XR, BroveX	Temporary relief of sneezing, itchy, watery eyes, itchy nose or throat, and runny nose caused by hay fever or other respiratory allergies; VaZol also used for symptoms of the common cold; treatment of allergic reactions to blood or plasma and anaphylactic reactions	Drowsiness, sedation, dizziness, disturbed coordination, hypotension, headache, blurred vision, thickening of bronchial secretions	Adults and children 12 yr and older: 6–12 mg orally q 12 hr Sustained release: 8–12 mg orally q 12 hr Oral liquid: 4 mg QID
chlorpheniramine *klore-fen-ear'-ah-meen*	Aller-Chlor, Chlor-Trimeton Allergy 8 Hour, Chlor-Trimeton Allergy 12 Hour	Temporary relief of sneezing, itchy, watery eyes, itchy throat, and runny nose caused by hay fever, other upper respiratory allergies, and the common cold	Drowsiness, sedation, hypotension, palpitations, blurred vision, dry mouth, urinary hesitancy	Adults and children 12 yr and older: 4 mg q 4–6 hr, maximum dose 24 mg in 24 hr Extended release: 8–12 mg orally q 8–12 hr
clemastine *klem'-ah-steen*	Tavist, Dayhist-1	Allergic rhinitis, urticaria, angioedema	Drowsiness, sedation, hypotension, palpitations, blurred vision, dry mouth, urinary hesitancy	Allergic rhinitis: 1.34 mg orally BID (not to exceed 8.04 mg/day for the syrup and 2.68 mg for the tablets) Urticaria and angioedema: 2.68 mg BID orally (not to exceed 4.02 mg/day)
diphenhydramine *dye-fen-hye'-drah meen*	Benadryl, Banophen, Genahist, Tusstat, Dytan	Allergic symptoms; hypersensitivity reactions, including anaphylaxis and transfusion reactions; motion sickness; sleep aid; antitussive and antiparkinsonism effects	Drowsiness, dry mouth, anorexia, blurred vision, urinary frequency	25–50 mg orally q 4–6 hr, maximum daily dose 300 mg; 10–400 mg IM, IV
promethazine *proe-meth'-ah-zeen*	Phenergan	Antiemetic, hypersensitivity reactions, motion sickness, sedation	Excessive sedation, drowsiness, dry mouth, confusion, disorientation, dizziness, fatigue, blurred vision	Individualize dosage to smallest effective dose Allergy: 12.5–25 mg orally, 25 mg IM, IV Motion sickness: 25 mg BID Antiemetic: 12.5–25 mg orally, IM, IV Preoperative: 50 mg IM or orally the night before surgery
Second-Generation Antihistamines				
azelastine *ah-zel'-as-teen*	Astelin	Seasonal and vasomotor rhinitis	Dizziness, drowsiness, glossitis, nose bleeds	2 sprays per nostril twice daily
cetirizine *seh-teer'-ih-zeen*	Zyrtec	Seasonal or perennial rhinitis, chronic urticaria	Sedation, dry mouth, pharyngitis, somnolence, dizziness	5–10 mg/day orally; maximum dosage 20 mg/day

(table continues on page 294)

Summary Drug Table ANTIHISTAMINES (continued)

Generic Name	Trade Name	Uses	Adverse Reactions	Dosage Ranges
desloratadine *des-loe-rah'-tah-deen*	Clarinex, Clarinex RediTabs	Seasonal or perennial allergic rhinitis	Headache; fatigue; drowsiness; dry mouth, nose, and throat; flulike symptoms	Adults and children 12 yr and older: 5 mg/day orally
fexofenadine *fex-oh-fen'-ah-deen*	Allegra	Seasonal rhinitis, urticaria	Headache, nausea, drowsiness, dyspepsia, fatigue, back pain, upper respiratory infection	30–60 mg orally BID; maximum dosage 180 mg/day
levocetirizine *lee'-voe-seh-teer-ih-zeen*	Xyzal	Allergic rhinitis, urticaria	Dizziness, drowsiness	5 mg orally in evening
loratadine *lor-ah'-tah-deen*	Claritin, Claritin RediTabs, Tavist ND, Alavert	Allergic rhinitis	Dizziness, headache, tremors, insomnia, dry mouth, fatigue	10 mg/day orally

Adverse Reactions

Central Nervous System Reactions

- Drowsiness or sedation
- Disturbed coordination

Respiratory System Reactions

Anticholinergic actions of antihistamines affect the respiratory system and include the following:

- Dryness of the mouth, nose, and throat
- Thickening of bronchial secretions

Second-generation preparations (e.g., loratadine) cause less drowsiness and fewer anticholinergic effects than some of the other antihistamines. Although these drugs are sometimes used to treat allergies, a drug allergy can occur with the use of an antihistamine. Symptoms that may indicate an allergy to these drugs include skin rash, urticaria, and anaphylactic shock.

Contraindications

Although the antihistamines are classified in pregnancy category B (chlorpheniramine, cetirizine, dexchlorpheniramine, clemastine, diphenhydramine, and loratadine) and C (brompheniramine, desloratadine, fexofenadine, hydroxyzine, and promethazine), they are contraindicated during pregnancy and lactation.

The first-generation antihistamine drugs (see Summary Drug Table: Antihistamines) are contraindicated in patients with known hypersensitivity to the drugs, newborns, premature infants, and nursing mothers. These drugs are also contraindicated in individuals undergoing monoamine oxidase inhibitor antidepressant (MAOI) therapy and patients with angle-closure glaucoma, stenosing peptic ulcer, symptomatic prostatic hypertrophy, and bladder neck obstruction.

The second-generation antihistamines are contraindicated in patients with known hypersensitivity. Cetirizine is contraindicated in patients who are hypersensitive to hydroxyzine.

Precautions

The antihistamines are used cautiously in patients with bronchial asthma, cardiovascular disease, narrow-angle glaucoma, symptomatic prostatic hypertrophy, hypertension, impaired kidney function, peptic ulcer, urinary retention, pyloroduodenal obstruction, and hyperthyroidism.

Interactions

The following interactions may occur when an antihistamine is administered with another agent:

Interacting Drug	Common Use	Effect of Interaction
rifampin	Antitubercular agent	May reduce the absorption of the antihistamine (e.g., fexofenadine)
MAOIs	Antidepressant agent	Increased anticholinergic and sedative effects of the antihistamine
CNS depressants (e.g., opioid analgesics or alcohol)	Pain relief	Possible additive CNS depressant effect
β blockers	Management of cardiovascular disease	Risk for increased cardiovascular effects (e.g., with diphenhydramine)
aluminum- or magnesium-based antacids	Relief of gastrointestinal (GI) problems and upset	Decreased concentrations of drug in blood (e.g., fexofenadine)

NURSING PROCESS

PATIENT RECEIVING AN ANTIHISTAMINE

ASSESSMENT

Preadministration Assessment

The preadministration assessment of the patient receiving these drugs depends on the reason for use. Examples of assessments the nurse may perform include asking about symptoms of the involved areas (eyes, nose, and upper and lower respiratory tract) if the patient is receiving an antihistamine for the relief of allergy symptoms. Many of the medications will be used on an out-patient basis; the nurse should ask about prescription medications to minimize the potential for interactions with agents the patient is currently taking for health reasons.

 LIFESPAN ALERT – Pediatric
Promethazine (Phenergan) should not be given to children younger than 2 years due to the potential for fatal respiratory depression.

Ongoing Assessment

The nurse usually gives these drugs in the outpatient setting. If the patient is in the hospital or clinic, the nurse observes the patient for the expected effects of the antihistamine and for adverse reactions. The nurse reports adverse reactions to the primary health care provider. In some instances, drowsiness or sedation may occur. When the drug is given to relieve preoperative anxiety, these adverse reactions are expected and are allowed to occur.

If the antihistamine is given for a serious situation, such as a blood transfusion reaction or a severe drug allergy, the nurse assesses the patient at frequent intervals until the symptoms appear relieved and for about 24 hours after the incident.

NURSING DIAGNOSES

Drug-specific nursing diagnoses include the following:

❑ **Impaired Oral Mucous Membranes** related to dry mouth, nose, and throat
❑ **Risk for Injury** related drowsiness, dizziness, disturbed coordination

Nursing diagnoses related to drug administration are discussed in Chapter 4.

PLANNING

The expected outcomes for the patient depend on the reason for administration of the antihistamine, but may include an optimal response to therapy, support of patient needs related to managing adverse reactions, and an understanding of the therapeutic regimen.

IMPLEMENTATION

Promoting an Optimal Response to Therapy

Most antihistamines are given orally with food to prevent GI upset. Loratadine or other rapidly disintegrating tablets can be administered with or without water and are placed on the tongue, where the tablet dissolves almost instantly. Fexofenadine is not administered within 2 hours of an antacid. When administering antihistamines parenterally, the nurse should give the drug deep intramuscularly (IM) rather than subcutaneously (subcut) because many antihistamines irritate subcutaneous tissue.

Monitoring and Managing Patient Needs

IMPAIRED ORAL MUCOUS MEMBRANES. Dryness of the mouth, nose, and throat may occur when antihistamines are taken. The nurse offers the patient frequent sips of water or ice chips to relieve these symptoms. Sugarless gum or sugarless hard candy may also relieve these symptoms.

 LIFESPAN ALERT – Gerontology
Older adults are more likely to experience anticholinergic effects (e.g., dryness of the mouth, nose, and throat), dizziness, sedation, hypotension, and confusion from the antihistamines. The primary care provider may recommend a dosage reduction if these symptoms persist.

RISK FOR INJURY. If the patient experiences dizziness or drowsiness, it is important to provide assistance with ambulation. If drowsiness is severe or if other problems such as dizziness or a disturbance in muscle coordination occur, the patient may require assistance with ambulation and other activities. The nurse places the call light within easy reach and instructs the patient to call before attempting to get out of bed or ambulate. When the drug is taken in the home environment, the nurse cautions the patient to refrain from activities that require a clear mind or operating equipment that requires attentive detail. The nurse informs the patient that this adverse reaction may decrease with continued use of the drug.

 LIFESPAN ALERT – Gerontology
Older adults are more likely to experience injury from dizziness because with age comes an increased risk for falls. Sensorimotor deficits, such as hearing loss, visual impairments, or unsteady gait, increase the older adult's risk for injury.

Educating the Patient and Family

The nurse reviews the dosage regimen and possible adverse drug reactions with the patient. The following points are included in the patient teaching plan:

• Do not drive or perform other hazardous tasks if drowsiness occurs. This effect may diminish with continued use.
• Avoid the use of alcohol, as well as other drugs that cause sleepiness or drowsiness, while taking these drugs.
• Antihistamines may cause dryness of the mouth and throat. Frequent sips of water, sucking on hard candy, or chewing gum (preferably sugarless) may relieve this problem.
• If gastric upset occurs, take this drug with food or meals. Loratadine should be taken on an empty stomach, if possible. If the gastric upset is not relieved, discuss this with the primary health care provider.

- Do not take fexofenadine within 2 hours of taking an antacid.
- Do not crush or chew sustained-release preparations.

EVALUATION

- Therapeutic response is achieved and allergic response is lessened.
- Adverse reactions are identified, reported to the primary health care provider, and managed successfully with appropriate nursing interventions:
  - ☑ Mucous membranes are moist and intact.
  - ☑ No evidence of injury is seen.
- Patient and family demonstrate an understanding of the drug regimen.

● DECONGESTANTS

A **decongestant** is a drug that reduces swelling of the nasal passages, which, in turn, opens clogged nasal passages and enhances drainage of the sinuses. These drugs are used for the temporary relief of nasal congestion caused by the common cold, hay fever, sinusitis, and other respiratory allergies.

Actions

The nasal decongestants are sympathomimetic, in that they produce localized vasoconstriction of the small blood vessels of the nasal membranes like adrenergic-blocking drugs.

Vasoconstriction reduces swelling in the nasal passages (decongestive activity). Nasal decongestants may be applied topically, and a few are available for oral use. Examples of nasal decongestants include phenylephrine (Neo-Synephrine) and oxymetazoline (Afrin), both of which are available as nasal sprays or drops, and pseudoephedrine (Sudafed), which is taken orally. Additional nasal decongestants are listed in the Summary Drug Table: Systemic and Topical Nasal Decongestants.

Uses

Decongestants are used to treat the congestion associated with the following conditions:

- Common cold
- Hay fever
- Sinusitis
- Allergic rhinitis
- Congestion associated with rhinitis

Adverse Reactions

When used topically in prescribed doses, there are usually minimal systemic effects in most individuals. On occasion, nasal burning, stinging, and dryness may be seen. When the topical form is used frequently or if the liquid is swallowed, the same adverse reactions seen with the oral decongestants may occur. Use of oral decongestants may result in the following adverse reactions:

Summary Drug Table SYSTEMIC AND TOPICAL NASAL DECONGESTANTS

Generic Name	Trade Name	Uses	Adverse Reactions	Dosage Ranges
ephedrine *eh-fed'-rin*	Pretz-D	Nasal congestion	Nasal burning, stinging, dryness, rebound nasal congestion	2–3 drops in each nostril q 4 hr; maximum use, 3–4 day
epinephrine *ep-ih-nef'-rin*	Adrenalin Chloride	Nasal congestion	Same as ephedrine	2–3 drops or spray in each nostril q 4–6 hr
naphazoline *nah-faz'-oh-leen*	Privine	Nasal congestion	Same as ephedrine	1–2 drops or sprays in each nostril no more than q 6 hr
oxymetazoline *ox-see-meh-taz'-oh-leen*	Afrin 12 Hour, Dristan 12-Hour Nasal, Vicks Sinex	Nasal congestion	Same as ephedrine	2–3 drops or sprays q 10–12 hr
phenylephrine *fen-ill-ef'-rin*	Neo-Synephrine	Nasal congestion	Same as ephedrine	2–3 sprays of 0–25% solution q 3–4 hr
pseudoephedrine *soo-doe-eh-fed'-rin*	Sudafed	Nasal congestion	Anxiety, restlessness, anorexia, arrhythmias, nervousness, nausea, vomiting, blurred vision	60 mg orally q 4–6 hr
tetrahydrozoline *tet-trah-hye-draz'-oh-leen*	Tyzine	Nasal congestion	Same as pseu-doephedrine	2–4 drops in each nostril or 3–4 sprays in each nostril q 3 hr
xylometazoline *zye-loe-meh-taz'-oh-leen*	Otrivin, Natru-Vent	Nasal congestion	Same as ephedrine	2–3 drops or sprays in each nostril q 8–10 hr

• Tachycardia and other cardiac arrhythmias
• Nervousness, restlessness, insomnia
• Blurred vision
• Nausea and vomiting

Contraindications

The decongestants are contraindicated in patients with known hypersensitivity and in patients taking MAOI antidepressants. Sustained-released pseudoephedrine is contraindicated in children younger than 12 years.

Precautions

Decongestants are used cautiously in patients with the following:

• Thyroid disease
• Diabetes mellitus
• Cardiovascular disease
• Prostatic hypertrophy
• Coronary artery disease
• Peripheral vascular disease
• Hypertension
• Glaucoma

Safe use of the decongestants during pregnancy (category C) and lactation has not been established. Pregnant women should consult with their primary health care provider before using these drugs.

Interactions

The following interactions may occur when a decongestant is administered with another agent:

Interacting Drug	Common Use	Effect of Interaction
MAOIs	Antidepressant	Severe headache, hypertension, and possibly hypertensive crisis
β-adrenergic blocking drugs	Management of cardiovascular disease	Initial hypertension episode followed by bradycardia

NURSING PROCESS
PATIENT USING A NASAL DECONGESTANT

ASSESSMENT

Preadministration Assessment
As part of the preadministration assessment, the nurse assesses the patient's blood pressure, pulse, and level of congestion before administering a decongestant. The nurse assesses lung sounds and bronchial secretions, which are noted in the patient's record. It is important to obtain a history of the use of these products, including the name of the product used and the frequency of use.

Ongoing Assessment
Ongoing assessment usually occurs when the patient comes to an outpatient clinic for follow-up treatment with the primary health care provider. The nurse assesses the patient's blood pressure, pulse, and level of congestion. The nurse questions the patient about attaining a therapeutic effect and the presence of any adverse reactions to the drug.

NURSING DIAGNOSES

A drug-specific nursing diagnosis may be:

❏ **Ineffective Airway Clearance** related to rebound effect of nasal congestion

Nursing diagnoses related to drug administration are discussed in Chapter 4.

PLANNING

The expected outcomes for the patient depend on the reason for administration of the drug, support of patient needs related to managing adverse reactions, and an understanding of the therapeutic regimen.

IMPLEMENTATION

Promoting an Optimal Response to Therapy
Decongestants are used only occasionally in the clinical setting. Because some of these products are available without a prescription, their use may be discovered during a patient history for other medical disorders. Nonprescription nasal decongestants should not be used by those with hypertension or heart disease unless such use is approved by the primary health care provider.

> **! NURSING ALERT**
>
> Because many decongestants can be purchased over the counter, it is important for the nurse to stress to patients who have heart disease, hypertension, hyperthyroidism, benign prostatic hypertrophy, glaucoma, and diabetes that they consult with their primary health care providers before using decongestants. They should also remember to read the drug label carefully before taking a decongestant.

After administering a topical nasal decongestant, some patients may experience a mild, transient stinging sensation. This usually disappears with continued use.

> **LIFESPAN ALERT – Gerontology**
>
> Patients older than 60 years are at greater risk for experiencing adverse reactions to the decongestants. Overdosage may cause hallucinations, convulsion, and CNS depression.

Monitoring and Managing Patient Needs

INEFFECTIVE AIRWAY CLEARANCE. Overuse of the topical form of these drugs can cause "rebound" nasal congestion. This means that the congestion becomes worse with the use of the drug. Although congestion may be relieved briefly after the drug is used, it recurs within a short time, which prompts the patient to use the drug at more frequent intervals, perpetuating the rebound congestion. The patient is taught to take the drug exactly as prescribed. A simple, but uncomfortable solution to rebound congestion is to withdraw completely from the topical medication. The primary health care provider may recommend an oral decongestant. An alternative method to minimize the occurrence of rebound nasal congestion is to discontinue the drug therapy gradually by initially discontinuing the medication in one nostril, followed by withdrawal from the other nostril. The nurse may suggest saline irrigation of nasal passages in place of using a decongestant.

Educating the Patient and Family

The nurse includes the following points in the patient teaching plan:

- Use this product as directed by the primary health care provider or on the container label.
- Understand that overuse of topical nasal decongestants can make the symptoms worse, causing rebound congestion.
- Nasal burning and stinging may occur with the topical decongestants. This effect usually disappears with use. If burning or stinging becomes severe, discontinue use and discuss this problem with the primary health care provider, who may prescribe or recommend another drug.
- If using a spray, do not allow the tip of the container to touch the nasal mucosa and do not share the container with anyone.
- To administer the spray, sit upright and sniff hard for a few minutes after administration.
- To administer drops, recline on a bed and hang your head over the edge. After using the drops, remain with the head down and turn the head from side to side.
- If using inhalers, warm the inhaler in the hand before use; wipe the inhaler after each use.
- If symptoms do not improve in 7 days or are accompanied by a high fever, consult the primary health care provider before continuing use.

EVALUATION

- Therapeutic response is achieved and congestion is relieved.
- Adverse reactions are identified, reported to the primary health care provider, and managed successfully with appropriate nursing interventions:
  ☑ Patient has a clear patent airway.
- The patient and family demonstrate an understanding of the drug regimen.

THINK CRITICALLY: PHARMACOLOGY IN PRACTICE

Janna Wong, the 16-year-old gymnast with pneumonia, is experiencing nasal congestion. She has been prescribed a combination antihistamine and nasal decongestant. A number of antihistamines have anticholinergic effects. Identify nursing interactions that are important when caring for a patient who is experiencing anticholinergic effects while taking an antihistamine.

Discuss important teaching points that should be included in developing a teaching plan for Ms. Wong while taking a nasal decongestant.

● Test Your Knowledge

1. Which of the following is a common adverse reaction seen when administering an antihistamine?
   A. Sedation
   B. Blurred vision
   C. Headache
   D. Hypertension

2. Older adults are at increased risk for experiencing adverse reactions when taking the decongestants. Overdosage of the decongestants may cause _____.
   A. a hypotensive crisis
   B. migraine headaches
   C. hallucinations
   D. hypertension

3. When antihistamines are administered to patients receiving CNS depressants, the nurse monitors the patient for _____.
   A. an increase in anticholinergic effects
   B. excessive sedation
   C. seizure activity
   D. loss of hearing

4. A patient receives a prescription for phenylephrine (Neo-Synephrine). The nurse explains that overuse of this drug may _____.
   A. result in hypotensive episodes
   B. decrease sinus drainage
   C. cause rebound nasal congestion
   D. dilate capillaries in the nasal mucosa

● Prepare for the NCLEX

1. Which of the following interactions would most likely occur when diphenhydramine is administered with a β blocker drug such as propranolol (Inderal)?
   A. Increased risk for increased cardiovascular effects
   B. Increased risk for seizures
   C. Decreased risk for cardiovascular effects
   D. Decreased risk for seizures

● Calculate Medication Dosages

1. Loratadine 10 mg is prescribed. The drug is available in a syrup containing 1 mg/mL. The nurse prepares to administer _____.

2. A patient is to receive 50 mg of diphenhydramine HCl orally. The drug is available in 25-mg tablets. The nurse administers _____.

To check your answers, see Appendix E.

the**Point**. *For more NCLEX questions, log on to http://thepoint.lww.com to access more than 1000 questions.*

Bronchodilators and Antiasthma Drugs

asthma   rhinitis
dyspnea   tachypnea
leukotrienes   theophyllinization

On completion of this chapter, the student will:

1. Describe the uses, general drug action, general adverse reactions, contraindications, precautions, and interactions of the bronchodilators and antiasthma drugs.
2. Discuss important preadministration and ongoing assessment activities the nurse should perform on the patient taking bronchodilators or antiasthma drugs.
3. List nursing diagnoses particular to a patient taking a bronchodilator or an antiasthma drug.
4. Discuss ways to promote an optimal response to therapy, how to manage common adverse reactions, and important points to keep in mind when educating a patient about the use of a bronchodilator or an antiasthma drug.

The term *chronic obstructive pulmonary disease* (COPD) denotes disorders that include **asthma**, chronic bronchitis, chronic obstructive bronchitis, or emphysema, or a combination of these conditions. The patient with COPD experiences **dyspnea** (difficulty breathing) with physical exertion, has difficulty inhaling and exhaling, and may have a chronic cough. All of these disorders interfere with the exchange of gases in the lung alveoli.

More than 22 million Americans have asthma, which is a chronic inflammatory disease causing spasmodic constriction of the bronchi. It is one of the most common chronic diseases of childhood, affecting an estimated 6 million children.

During the inflammatory process, a large amount of histamine is released from the mast cells of the respiratory tract. The lung bronchi constrict, becoming hyperresponsive to the bronchoconstriction, and edema occurs. With asthma, the airways become narrow, the muscles around the airways tighten, the inner lining of the bronchi swell, and extra mucus clogs the smaller airways (Fig. 34.1). Characterized by recurrent attacks of dyspnea and wheezing, asthma also causes the patient to experience anxiety.

Patients with asthma may experience periods of exacerbation of symptoms, alternating with periods of normal respiratory function. The period of exacerbation may begin abruptly, often triggered by exercise or cold air, but usually is preceded by increasing symptoms over the previous several days:

- Cough (worse at night or early morning)
- Generalized wheezing (a whistle or squeaking sound on inspiration or expiration)
- Generalized chest tightness (may feel like someone is sitting on the chest)
- Dyspnea (shortness of breath or feeling of breathlessness)
- **Tachypnea** (rapid breathing)

These symptoms indicate that inflammation is occurring in the lungs. Stimulation of the sympathetic nervous system, the 'fight or flight' response, is the body's reaction to the inflammation.

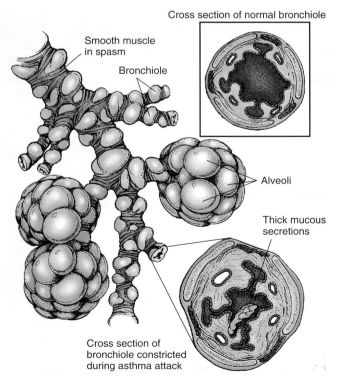

Figure 34.1 Bronchiole airflow obstruction in asthma.

Asthma medications are categorized into two major groups: (1) long-term control medications and (2) quick-relief medications used to treat acute air flow obstruction. The long-term management of asthma uses a step care approach (Display 34.1), meaning that medications and their frequency of administration are adjusted according to the severity of the patient's asthma. The most effective long-term control medications are those that reduce inflammation, with inhaled corticosteroids (ICSs) being the first-line intervention. Quick-relief medications include inhaled short-acting beta-2 (β_2) (adrenergic) agonists (SABAs) and oral steroids.

Bronchodilators are the mainstay of treatment for many chronic pulmonary disorders. SABA bronchodilators are drugs used to relieve bronchospasm associated with respiratory disorders, such as bronchial asthma, chronic bronchitis, and emphysema. These conditions are progressive disorders characterized by a decrease in the inspiratory and expiratory capacity of the lung. Examples of β_2 agonist bronchodilators include albuterol (Ventolin), epinephrine (Adrenalin), salmeterol (Serevent), and terbutaline (Brethine). Along with the bronchodilators, several types of drugs are effective in treating asthma. These include ICSs, mast cell stabilizers, leukotriene formation inhibitors, leukotriene receptor agonists, and immunomodulators.

• BRONCHODILATORS

The two major types of bronchodilators are the β_2 adrenergic agonists (or sympathomimetics) and the xanthine derivatives.

Betaz in lungs

The cholinergic blocking drug ipratropium bromide (Atrovent) is used for bronchospasm associated with COPD, chronic bronchitis, and emphysema in emergent situations. Ipratropium is featured in the Summary Drug Table: Bronchodilators. Chapter 27 provides specific information concerning the cholinergic blocking (anticholinergic) drugs.

Adrenergic Bronchodilators

When alpha (α)-adrenergic receptors (the sympathetic system) in the lungs are stimulated, bronchoconstriction results. The opposite, *bronchodilation*, occurs when β-adrenergic receptors are stimulated. Some theories propose that asthma is a lack of β-adrenergic stimulation. Many of the adrenergics used as bronchodilators have the subclassification of β_2 receptor agonists, which are either *short acting* (e.g., albuterol and terbutaline) or *long acting* (e.g., salmeterol). Additional information concerning the various adrenergic drugs is given in the Summary Drug Table: Bronchodilators.

Actions

When bronchospasm occurs, there is a decrease in the lumen (or inside diameter) of the bronchi, which decreases the amount of air taken into the lungs with each breath. A decrease in the amount of air taken into the lungs results in respiratory distress. Use of a bronchodilating drug opens the bronchi by relaxing the smooth muscles and allows more air to enter the lungs, which, in turn, completely or partially relieves respiratory distress.

rescue inhalers

Summary Drug Table BRONCHODILATORS

Generic Name	Trade Name	Uses	Adverse Reactions	Dosage Ranges
Short-Acting β_2 Agonists (SABA—Adrenergics or Sympathomimetics Used for Acute Symptom Relief)				
albuterol *al-byoo'-ter-roll*	Proventil, Ventolin	Bronchospasm, prevention of EIB	Headache, palpitations, tachycardia, tremor, dizziness, shakiness, nervousness, hyperactivity	2–4 mg TID, QID orally; 1–2 inhalations q 4–6 hr; 2 inhalations before exercise; may also be given by nebulizer
ephedrine *eh-fed'-rin*		Asthma, bronchospasm	Precordial pain, urinary hesitancy	12.5–25 mg orally q 3–4 hr PRN; 25–50 mg IM, SC, IV
epinephrine *ep-ih-nef'-rin*	Adrenalin, Epinephrine Mist, Primatene Mist	Asthma, bronchospasm	Palpitations, tremor, dizziness, drowsiness, vertigo, shakiness, nervousness, headache, nausea, vomiting, anxiety, fear, pallor	Inhalation aerosol: individualize dose; Injection: Solution 1:1000, 0.3–0.5 mL SC, IM Suspension (1:200), 0.1–0.3 mL SC only
bitolterol *bye-toll'-ter-roll*	Tornalate	Bronchospasm, Acute asthma	Same as albuterol, throat irritation	Two inhalations q 8 hr; inhalation solution, 2.5 mg over 10–15 min with continuous-flow system or 1 mg with intermittent-flow system

Short acting

A - drenergic (Beta agonist) Albuterol   fight or flight
S teroid   Pulmicort
Theophylline
Hydration IV

(table continues on page 301)

Summary Drug Table BRONCHODILATORS (continued)

Generic Name	Trade Name	Uses	Adverse Reactions	Dosage Ranges
levalbuterol *lev-al-byoo'-ter-roll*	Xopenex	Treat and prevent bronchospasm	Tachycardia, nervousness, anxiety, pain, dizziness, rhinitis, cough, cardiac arrhythmias	0.63 mg TID, q 6–8 hr by nebulization; if no response, dose may be increased to 1.25 mg TID by nebulizer
metaproterenol *met-ah-proe-ter'-eh-noll*	Alupent	Asthma, bronchospasm	Tachycardia, tremor, nervousness, shakiness, nausea, vomiting	20 mg TID orally, Aerosol 2–3 inhalations q 3–4 hr; do not exceed 12 inhalations
pirbuterol *peer-byoo'-ter-roll*	Maxair Autohaler	Asthma, bronchospasm	Tremor, dizziness, shakiness, nervousness	Two inhalations q 4–6 hr; do not exceed 12 inhalations
terbutaline *ter-byoo'-tah-leen*	Brethine	Treat and prevent bronchospasm	Palpitations, tremor, dizziness, vertigo, shakiness, nervousness, drowsiness, headache, nausea, vomiting, gastrointestinal (GI) upset	2.5–5 mg q 6 hr orally TID during waking hours; 0.25 mg SC (may repeat once if needed)

Long-Acting β₂ Agonists (LABA—Adrenergics or Sympathomimetics Used for Long-Term Management)

arformoterol *ar- for- moe'-ter-ol*	Brovana	Long-term treat and prevent bronchospasm in COPD	Nervousness, tremor, dizziness, headache, insomnia, nausea, vomiting, diarrhea, leg cramps, back pain	15 mcg inhalation BID morning and evening
formoterol *for-moh'-te-rol*	Foradil	Long-term treat and prevent bronchospasm	Palpations, tachycardia, dizziness, nervousness	One 12-mg capsule q 12 hr using inhalation device, not for oral use; EIB use 15 min before exercise
salmeterol *sal-mee'-ter-ol*	Serevent Diskus	Long-term treat and prevent bronchospasm	Tremor, headache, cough	1 inhalation BID morning and evening; inhalation powder, do not use spacer

longterm management

Xanthine Derivatives

aminophylline *am-in-off'-lin*	Truphylline (rectal suppository)	Symptomatic relief or prevention of bronchial asthma and reversible bronchospasm of chronic bronchitis and emphysema	Nausea, vomiting, restlessness, nervousness, tachycardia, tremors, headache, palpitations, hyperglycemia, electrocardiographic changes, cardiac arrhythmias *heartburn*	Individualize dosage: base adjustments on clinical responses, monitor serum aminophylline levels, maintain therapeutic range of 10–20 mcg/mL; base dosage on lean body mass
dyphylline *dye'-fi-lin*	Lufyllin	Same as aminophylline	Same as aminophylline	Up to 15 mg/kg orally q 6 hr
oxtriphylline *ox-trye'-fi-lin*	Choledyl SA	Same as aminophylline	Same as aminophylline	4.7 mg/kg orally q 8 hr; sustained-action: 1 tablet orally q 12 hr
theophylline *thee-off'-i-lin*	Theo–Dur, Theolair, Slo–bid, Uniphyl	Same as aminophylline	Same as aminophylline	Initial dosing: 16 mg/kg/day or 400 mg/day Maintenance dose: 13 mg/kg/day, not to exceed 900 mg/day

Peak > Trough

Mask O2   Magnesium Sulfate IV
Anticholinergic Atrovent

(text continues on page 302)

Summary Drug Table BRONCHODILATORS (continued)

Generic Name	Trade Name	Uses	Adverse Reactions	Dosage Ranges
Cholinergic Blocking Drug (Anticholinergics Used for Acute Symptom Relief)				
ipratropium *ih-prah-trow'-pea-um*	Atrovent	Bronchospasm associated with COPD, chronic bronchitis and emphysema, rhinorrhea	Dryness of the oropharynx, nervousness, irritation from aerosol, dizziness, headache, GI distress, dry mouth, exacerbation of symptoms, nausea, palpitations	Aerosol: two inhalations QID, not to exceed 12 inhalations; Solution: 500 mg (1 unit dose vial) TID, QID by oral nebulization Nasal spray: 2 sprays per nostril BID, TID of 0.03%, or 2 sprays per nostril TID, QID of 0.06%
tiotropium *tee-oh-tro'-pee-um*	Spiriva	Same as ipratropium	Same as ipratropium, increased stroke potential	One capsule per day using inhalation device, not for oral use

Handwritten annotations: Back door rest + digest parasympathetic / attach to cholinergic receptors / → block cholinergic release

Uses

The β₂adrenergic drugs (which mimic the sympathetic nervous system) are used in the treatment of chronic respiratory problems due to bronchoconstriction, such as:

- Bronchospasm associated with acute and chronic bronchial asthma
- Exercise-induced bronchospasm (EIB)
- Bronchitis
- Emphysema
- Bronchiectasis (chronic dilation of the bronchi and bronchioles)
- Other obstructive pulmonary diseases

Adverse Reactions

Cardiovascular System Reactions

- Tachycardia, palpitations, or cardiac arrhythmias
- Hypertension

Other Reactions

- Nervousness, anxiety
- Insomnia

When these drugs are taken by inhalation, excessive use (e.g., more than the recommended dose times) may result in paradoxical bronchospasm.

 NURSING ALERT
LABAs (e.g., salmeterol) may increase the risk of asthma-related death. ICSs should be considered first for long-term control of asthma.

Contraindications

The adrenergic bronchodilators are contraindicated in patients with known hypersensitivity to the drug, cardiac arrhythmias associated with tachycardia, organic brain damage, cerebral arteriosclerosis, and narrow-angle glaucoma. Salmeterol is contraindicated during acute bronchospasm.

Precautions

The adrenergics are used cautiously in patients with hypertension, cardiac dysfunction, hyperthyroidism, glaucoma, diabetes, prostatic hypertrophy, and a history of seizures. The adrenergic drugs are also used cautiously during pregnancy and lactation (all are in pregnancy category C, except terbutaline, which is a pregnancy category B drug).

Interactions *avoid caffine*

The following interactions may occur when an adrenergic drug is used concurrently with another agent:

Interacting Drug	Common Use	Effect of Interaction
adrenergic drugs	Treatment of hypotension and shock	Possible additive adrenergic effects
tricyclics	Treatment of depression	Possible hypotension
β adrenergic blockers	Treatment of hypertension	Inhibition of the cardiac, bronchodilating, and vasodilating effects of the adrenergic
methyldopa	Treatment of hypertension	Possible hypotension
oxytocic drugs	Uterine stimulant	Possible severe hypotension
theophylline	Treatment of asthma and COPD	Increased risk for cardiotoxicity

Xanthine Derivative Bronchodilators

Xanthine derivatives (also called *methylxanthines*) are a different class of drugs from the adrenergics and also have bronchodilating activity. Examples are theophylline (Theo-Dur) and aminophylline (Phyllocontin). Additional information concerning the xanthine derivatives is found in the Summary Drug Table: Bronchodilators.

Actions

The xanthine derivatives are drugs that stimulate the central nervous system (CNS) to promote bronchodilation. They cause direct relaxation of the smooth muscles of the bronchi.

Uses

The xanthine derivatives are used for the following:

• Symptomatic relief or prevention of bronchial asthma
• Treatment of reversible bronchospasm associated with chronic bronchitis and emphysema

Adverse Reactions

Central Nervous System Reactions

• Restlessness, irritability, headache
• Nervousness, tremors

Cardiac and Respiratory System Reactions

• Tachycardia
• Palpitations
• Electrocardiographic changes
• Increased respirations

Other Reactions

• Nausea, vomiting, fever
• Hyperglycemia, flushing, alopecia

Contraindications

The xanthine derivatives are contraindicated in those with known hypersensitivity to the drugs, peptic ulcers, seizure disorders (unless well controlled with appropriate anticonvulsant medication), and serious uncontrolled arrhythmias.

Precautions

The xanthine derivatives are used cautiously in patients with cardiac disease, hypoxemia, hypertension, congestive heart failure, and liver disease. They are also used cautiously in elderly patients and those who use alcohol habitually. Aminophylline, dyphylline, oxtriphylline, and theophylline are pregnancy category C drugs and are used cautiously during pregnancy and lactation.

Interactions

When taken with theophylline, the following agents have an effect on theophylline levels:

Interacting Drug	Common Use	Effect of Interaction
barbiturates	Sedation	
charcoal (in large amounts)	Neutralize poisoning	

Interacting Drug	Common Use	Effect of Interaction
hydantoins	Anticonvulsant	
ketoconazole	Antifungal agent	
rifampin	Antitubercular agent	
nicotine (tobacco, nicotine gum, and patches)	Effect from smoking tobacco or to aid smoking cessation	**Decreased** theophylline levels
adrenergic agents	Treatment of hypotension and shock	
isoniazid	Antitubercular agent	
loop diuretics	Treatment of hypertension	
allopurinol	Antigout agent	
β adrenergic blockers	Treatment of hypertension	
calcium channel blockers	Treatment of angina and hypertension	
cimetidine	Treatment of GI problems	
oral contraceptives	Birth control	**Increased** theophylline levels
corticosteroids	Anti-inflammatory agents	
ephedrine	Weight loss over-the-counter product	
influenza virus vaccine	Prevention of flu	
macrolide, quinolone antibiotics	Treatment of infections	
thyroid hormones	Treatment of hypothyroidism	
isoniazid	Antitubercular agent	
loop diuretics	Treatment of edema	

●ANTIASTHMA DRUGS

Long-term control medications are used daily to achieve and maintain control of persistent asthma. The most effective are those that reduce the underlying inflammation of asthma.

Inhaled Corticosteroids

ICSs are the most consistently effective long-term control medication at all steps of care for persistent asthma. ICS and LABA drugs may be combined to ease administration of the medications and produce positive outcomes in the management of asthma; these ICS/LABA combinations can be found in the Summary Drug Table: Antiasthma Drugs.

Actions

ICSs are anti-inflammatory medications that reduce airway hyperresponsiveness, reduce the number of mast cells in the airway, and block reaction to allergens. ICSs, such as

Summary Drug Table ANTIASTHMA DRUGS

Generic Name	Trade Name	Uses	Adverse Reactions	Dosage Ranges
Inhaled Corticosteroids				
beclomethasone *beh-kloe-meth'-ah-soan*	QVAR	Maintenance treatment of asthma	Oral, laryngeal, pharyngeal irritation, fungal infections, suppression of HPA function *watch for thrush*	Starting dose used with bronchodilators alone: 40–80 mcg BID; when used with ICSs: 40–160 mcg BID; maximum 320 mcg BID Children 5–12 yr: 40 mcg BID when used with bronchodilators alone or with ICSs
budesonide *byoo-dess'-oh-nyde*	Pulmicort Turbuhaler, Respules	Maintenance treatment of asthma	Same as beclomethasone	Individualized dosage by oral inhalation Adults: 200–800 mcg BID Children 6 yr and older: 200–400 mcg BID Children 12 mo to 8 yr: 0.5–1 mcg total daily dose administered once or twice daily in divided doses
flunisolide *floo-niss'-oh-lyde*	Aerospan, AeroBid, AeroBid-M	Maintenance treatment of asthma, especially those on systemic corticosteroid therapy	Same as beclomethasone	Adults: 2 inhalations BID; maximum dose, 4 inhalations BID Children 6–15 yr: 2 inhalations BID
fluticasone *floo-tik'-ah-soan*	Flovent, Flovent HFA, Flovent Diskus	Prophylactic maintenance and treatment of asthma	Same as beclomethasone	88–880 mcg BID
mometasone *moe-met'-ah-soan*	Asmanex Twisthaler	Maintenance treatment of asthma	Same as beclomethasone	One inhalation (220 mcg) QD in the evening for patients previously maintained on bronchodilators alone or ICSs; 2 inhalations (440 mcg) BID for patients previously maintained on oral corticosteroids
triamcinolone *trye-am-sin'-oh-loan*	Azmacort	Same as flunisolide	Same as beclomethasone	Adults: 2 inhalations TID, QID; maximum daily dosage 16 inhalations Children 6–12 yr: 1–2 inhalations TID, QID; maximum daily dosage, 12 inhalations
ICS/LABA Combinations				
budesonide/ formoterol *byoo-dess'-oh-nyde/ f or-moe'-ter-roll*	Symbicort	Long-term maintenance of asthma	See individual drugs	Low-medium dose (ICS) 80/4.5 mcg; medium-high dose (ICS) 160/4.5 mcg, 2 inhalations morning and evening
fluticasone/ salmeterol *floo-tik'-ah-soan/ sal-mee'-ter-roll*	Advair	Long-term maintenance of asthma, COPD	See individual drugs	2 inhalations twice daily

(text continues on page 305)

Summary Drug Table ANTIASTHMA DRUGS(continued)

Generic Name	Trade Name	Uses	Adverse Reactions	Dosage Ranges
Mast Cell Stabilizers				
cromolyn *kroe'-moe-lin* *pt vi 30min before meal* *not for attacks*	Intal, NasalCrom, Gastrocrom	Bronchial asthma, prevention of bronchospasm; prevention of EIB Nasal preparations: prevention and treatment of allergic rhinitis	Cough, wheeze, unusual taste, dizziness, headache, nausea, dry and irritated throat, rash, joint swelling and pain	Inhalation solution: 20 mg (1 ampule/vial) administered by nebulizer QID Aerosol: adults and children 5 yr and older: 2 metered sprays QID EIB: 2 metered sprays shortly (10–15 min but not more than 60 min) before exposure to the precipitating factor Nasal solution: 1 spray each nostril 3–6 times/day Oral: adults and children 13 yr and older: 2 ampules QID 30 min before meals and at bedtime Children 2–12 yr: 1 ampule QID before meals and at bedtime; do not exceed 40 mg/kg/d
nedocromil *nee-dok'-roe-mill*	Tilade	Maintenance therapy in mild to moderate bronchial asthma	Cough, nausea, pharyngitis, rhinitis, vomiting, headache, bronchospasm, unusual taste	Two inhalations QID
Leukotriene Receptor Antagonists				
montelukast *mon-teh-loo'-cast* *takes a wk! before notice* *anything*	Singulair	Prophylaxis and treatment of chronic asthma in adults and pediatric patients 12 mo of age and older, seasonal allergic rhinitis in adults and pediatric patients 2 yr of age and older	Headache, influenza-like symptoms, *cough congestion*	Adults and children older than 15 yr: 10 mg orally in the evening Children 6–14 yr: one 5-mg chewable tablet daily, in the evening Children 1–5 yr: one 4-mg chewable tablet daily, in the evening, or one 4-mg oral granule packet daily
zafirlukast *zah-fur-loo'-cast*	Accolate	Prophylaxis and treatment of chronic asthma in adults and children 5 yr or older	Same as montelukast	Adults and children older than 12 yr: 20 mg orally BID Children 5–11 yr: 10 mg orally BID
Leukotriene Formation Inhibitors				
zileuton *zye-loot'-on*	Zyflo	Prophylaxis and treatment of chronic asthma in adults and children 12 yr or older	Dyspepsia, nausea, headache	600 mg orally QID
Immunomodulators				
omalizumab *oh-mal-iz'-yoo-mab*	Xolair	Moderate to severe persistent asthma	Injection site reaction, anaphylaxis	150–375 mg SC every 2–4 wk

Bronchodilators and Antiasthma Drugs

beclomethasone (QVAR), flunisolide (AeroBid), and triamcinolone (Azmacort), are given by inhalation and decrease the inflammatory process directly in the airways. In addition, the corticosteroids increase the sensitivity of the β_2 receptors, which in turn increases the effectiveness of the β_2 receptor agonist drugs.

Uses

The ICSs are used in the management and prophylactic treatment of the inflammation associated with chronic asthma. A number of these preparations may be used intranasally for the treatment of nasal polyps and **rhinitis** (Table 34.1).

Adverse Reactions

When used to manage chronic asthma, the corticosteroids are most often given by inhalation. Adverse reactions to the corticosteroids are less likely to occur when the drugs are given by inhalation rather than taken orally. Occasionally, patients may experience reactions.

Respiratory System Reactions

- Throat irritation
- Hoarseness
- Upper respiratory tract infection
- Fungal infection of the mouth and throat

See Chapter 44 for adverse reactions after oral administration of the corticosteroids. A more complete listing of the adverse reactions associated with the ICSs is found in the Summary Drug Table: Antiasthma Drugs.

Contraindications

The ICSs are contraindicated in patients with hypersensitivity to the corticosteroids, acute bronchospasm, status asthmaticus, or other acute episodes of asthma. Beclomethasone is contraindicated for the relief of symptoms that can be controlled by a bronchodilator and other nonsteroidal medications and in the treatment of nonasthmatic bronchitis.

Table 34.1 Intranasal Steroids

Drug	Indication
beclomethasone (Beconase AQ)	Nasal polyps and rhinitis (perennial, seasonal and vasomotor)
budesonide (Rhinocort Aqua)	Rhinitis (perennial and seasonal)
flunisolide (Nasarel)	Rhinitis (perennial and seasonal)
fluticasone (Flonase, Veramyst)	Rhinitis (perennial, seasonal and vasomotor)
mometasone monohydrate (Nasonex)	Nasal polyps, rhinitis (perennial and seasonal)
triamcinolone acetonide (Nasacort AQ & HFA)	Rhinitis (perennial and seasonal)

Precautions

The ICSs are used cautiously in patients with compromised immune systems, glaucoma, kidney disease, liver disease, convulsive disorders, and diabetes. Combining ICSs with systemic corticosteroids can increase the risk of hypothalamic-pituitary-adrenal (HPA) suppression, resulting in adrenal insufficiency. These drugs are also used with caution during pregnancy (category C) and lactation (category B – budesonide).

> **NURSE ALERT**
>
> During periods of stress or a severe asthmatic attack, patients who have been withdrawn from systemic corticosteroids should be instructed to resume systemic steroids immediately and to contact the primary care provider. Patient deaths can result from adrenal insufficiency that may occur during and after transfer from systemic corticosteroids to inhaled corticosteroids.

Interactions

Ketoconazole may increase plasma levels of budesonide and fluticasone.

Mast Cell Stabilizers

Mast cell stabilizers include cromolyn (Intal) and nedocromil (Tilade).

Actions

Although their action is not fully understood, these drugs are thought to stabilize the mast cell membrane, possibly by preventing calcium ions from entering mast cells, thus preventing the release of inflammatory mediators such as histamine and **leukotrienes**.

Uses

The mast cell stabilizers are used in combination with other drugs in the treatment of asthma and allergic disorders, including allergic rhinitis (nasal solution). They are also used to prevent EIB. They are typically used in step 2 care for chronic asthma (see Display 34.1).

Adverse Reactions

Respiratory System Reactions

- Throat irritation and dryness
- Unpleasant taste sensation
- Cough or wheeze

These drugs may cause a nauseated feeling. A more complete listing of the adverse reactions associated with the mast cell stabilizers is found in the Summary Drug Table: Antiasthma Drugs.

Contraindications and Precautions

The mast cell stabilizers are contraindicated in patients with known hypersensitivity to the drugs and during attacks of

DISPLAY 34.1 Step Care Approach for Managing Asthma in Adults and Youth 12 Years and Older

Asthma Classification	Daily Medications	Rescue Drugs
Step 1: intermittent asthma	No daily medications	SABA
Step 2: mild persistent asthma	Low-dose ICS	SABA
	Alternative: cromolyn sodium or nedocromil or zafirlukast for patient aged less than 12 years or sustained-release theophylline	
Step 3: mild to moderate persistent asthma	Low-dose ICS *plus* LABA *or* medium-dose ICS	SABA
	Alternative: Low-dose ICS and zafirlukast or theophylline or zileuton	
Step 4: moderate persistent asthma	Medium-dose ICS *plus* LABA	SABA
Step 5: moderately severe persistent asthma	Daily combined use of a high-dose ICS *and* LABA, and consider immunomodulator	SABA
Step 6: severe persistent asthma	High-dose ICS *and* LABA *plus* oral corticosteroid, and consider immunomodulator	SABA

acute asthma, because they may worsen bronchospasm during the acute asthma attack.

Mast cell stabilizers are used cautiously during pregnancy (pregnancy category B) and lactation and in patients with impaired renal or hepatic function.

Interactions

No significant drug interactions have been reported.

Leukotriene Modifiers and Immunomodulators

Leukotriene receptor antagonists include montelukast (Singulair) and zafirlukast (Accolate). Zileuton (Zyflo) is classified as a leukotriene formation inhibitor. Omalizumab (Xolair) is a monoclonal antibody used in the treatment of asthma. Additional information concerning these drugs is found in the Summary Drug Table: Antiasthma Drugs.

Actions

Asthma attacks are often triggered by allergens or exercise. Inflammatory substances called *leukotrienes* are one of several substances that are released by mast cells during an asthma attack. Leukotrienes are primarily responsible for bronchoconstriction. When leukotriene production is inhibited, bronchodilation is facilitated. Zileuton (an inhibitor) acts by decreasing the formation of leukotrienes. Although the result is the same, montelukast and zafirlukast work in a manner slightly different from that of zileuton. Montelukast and zafirlukast are considered leukotriene receptor antagonists because they inhibit leukotriene receptor sites in the respiratory tract, preventing airway edema and facilitating bronchodilation. Omalizumab modulates the immune response by preventing the binding of immunoglobulin to the receptors on basophils and mast cells, thereby limiting the allergic reaction.

Uses

Leukotriene modifiers are used in the prophylaxis and treatment of chronic asthma in adults and children older than

12 years. Omalizumab is used as adjunctive therapy for patients 12 years of age who are sensitive to allergens (e.g., dust mites, cockroaches, cat or dog dander) and who require step 5 or 6 care (see Display 34.1).

Adverse Reactions

Central Nervous System Reactions

• Headache

Generalized body system reactions include flu-like symptoms. Immunomodulators may cause anaphylactic reactions, and emergency equipment should be available when administering this medication.

Contraindications and Precautions

These drugs are contraindicated in patients with known hypersensitivity, bronchospasm in acute asthma attacks, or liver disease (zileuton). They should be used cautiously in pregnancy and not at all during lactation (zafirlukast, montelukast and omalizumab are pregnancy category B drugs and zileuton is pregnancy category C).

Interactions

The following interactions may occur when a leukotriene modifier is administered with another agent:

Interacting Drug	Common Use	Effect of Interaction
aspirin	Pain relief	Increased plasma levels of zafirlukast
warfarin	Anticoagulant	Increased anticoagulant effect
theophylline	Treatment of asthma and COPD	Decreased level of zafirlukast; increased serum theophylline levels with zileuton use
erythromycin	Treatment of bacterial infection	Decreased level of zafirlukast

NURSING PROCESS

PATIENT RECEIVING A BRONCHODILATOR OR AN ANTIASTHMA DRUG

ASSESSMENT

Preadministration Assessment

Because the bronchodilators or antiasthma drugs may be given for asthma, emphysema, or chronic bronchitis, the preadministration assessment of the patient requires careful observation and documentation. Many respiratory problems are chronic conditions with acute exacerbations. Quick recognition and immediate action are essential in treating acute breathing problems. Long-term control of respiratory conditions consists of assessment and monitoring, patient education, environmental control (Display 34.2), and medication management. Patients are encouraged to establish asthma action plans for daily self-management and for acute respiratory exacerbations (Fig. 34.2).

ACUTE BREATHING DISTRESS. In situations of acute breathing distress, the nurse takes the blood pressure, pulse, and respiratory rate before therapy with a bronchodilator or antiasthma drug is initiated. Respiratory rates below 12 breaths/min or above 24 breaths/min are considered abnormal. It is important to assess the lung fields and carefully document the sounds heard before therapy is begun. The nurse notes any dyspnea, cough, wheezing, "noisy" respirations, or use of accessory muscles when breathing. If the patient is raising sputum, the nurse records a description of the sputum. The nurse notes and records the patient's general physical condition. It is important to record any signs of hypoxia, such as mental confusion, restlessness, anxiety, and cyanosis (bluish dis-

coloration of the skin and mucous membranes). In some instances, the primary heath care provider may order arterial blood gas analysis or pulmonary function tests.

The nurse questions the patient regarding possible triggers of the asthma attack causing the inability to breathe. Has the patient been around different environmental items, such as a new pet or changes in environmental temperature? Has the patient been under undo stress either physically or emotionally? Has the patient been monitoring lung function with a Peak Flow Meter, and has a change been noted?

LONG-TERM MANAGEMENT. In patients with chronic asthma, the nurse questions the patient concerning allergies, frequency of attacks, severity of attacks, factors that cause or relieve attacks, and any antiasthma drugs used currently or taken previously.

Ongoing Assessment

During an acute attack, the nurse assesses the respiratory status every 4 hours (or more often if needed) and whenever the drug is administered. The nurse notes the respiratory rate, lung sounds, and use of accessory muscles in breathing. In addition, the nurse keeps a careful record of the intake and output and reports any imbalance, which may indicate a fluid overload or excessive diuresis.

The patient monitors changes during stable chronic phases. With the asthma action plan, the primary care provider prescribes daily medications for the patient as well as quick-relief medications. The patient in turn monitors for symptoms such as wheezing and coughing, peak flow meter changes, and triggers that might be making the asthma worsen. The nurse questions the patient about changes seen on the asthma action plan. Has the patient's condition stayed within the parameters of the green zone or has the patient's status moved to the yellow or red zones (see Fig. 34.2)? It is important to monitor any patient with a history of cardiovascular problems for chest pain and changes in the electrocardiogram. The primary health care provider may order periodic pulmonary function tests, particularly for patients with emphysema or bronchitis, to help monitor respiratory status.

NURSING DIAGNOSES

Drug-specific nursing diagnoses include the following:

❑ **Anxiety** related to feelings of breathlessness
❑ **Ineffective Airway Clearance** related to bronchospasm
❑ **Impaired Oral Mucous Membranes** related to dryness or irritation
❑ **Imbalanced Nutrition: Less Than Body Requirements** related to decreased appetite caused by nausea, heartburn, or unpleasant taste

Nursing diagnoses related to drug administrations are discussed in Chapter 4.

PLANNING

The expected outcomes for the patient depend on the specific reason for administering the drug, but may

---

DISPLAY 34.2 Promoting Environmental Control for Asthma

You need to know what things bring on your asthma symptoms. Then do what you can to avoid or limit contact with these things.

- If animal dander is a problem for you, keep your pet out of the house or at least out of your bedroom, or find it a new home.
- Do not smoke or allow smoking in your home.
- If pollen is a problem for you, stay indoors with the air conditioner on, if possible, when the pollen count is high.
- To control dust mites, wash your sheets, blankets, pillows, and stuffed toys once a week in hot water. You can get special dust proof covers for your mattress and pillows.
- If cold air bothers you, wear a scarf over your mouth and nose in the winter.
- If you have symptoms when you exercise or do routine physical activities like climbing stairs, work with your doctor to find ways to be active without having asthma symptoms. Physical activity is important.
- If you are allergic to sulfites, avoid foods (like dried fruit) or beverages (like wine) that contain them.

My Asthma Plan

ENGLISH

Patient Name: _____

Medical Record #: _____

Provider's Name: _____ DOB: _____

Provider's Phone #: _____ Completed by: _____ Date: _____

Controller Medicines	How Much to Take	How Often	Other Instructions
		_____ times per day **EVERY DAY!**	❑ Gargle or rinse mouth after use
		_____ times per day **EVERY DAY!**	
		_____ times per day **EVERY DAY!**	
		_____ times per day **EVERY DAY!**	

Quick-Relief Medicines	How Much to Take	How Often	Other Instructions
❑ Albuterol (ProAir, Ventolin, Proventil) ❑ Levalbuterol (Xopenex)	❑ 2 puffs ❑ 4 puffs ❑ 1 nebulizer treatment	Take ONLY as needed (see below — starting in Yellow Zone or before excercise)	NOTE: If you need this medicine more than two days a week, call physician to consider increasing controller medications and discuss your treatment plan.

Special instructions when I am ⬤ doing well , ◯ getting worse , ⬤ having a medical alert.

GREEN ZONE

Doing well.

- No cough, wheeze, chest tightness, or shortness of breath during the day or night.
- Can do usual activities.

Peak Flow (for ages 5 and up):
is _____ or more. (80% or more of personal best)
Personal Best Peak Flow (for ages 5 and up): _____

PREVENT   asthma symptoms every day:

❑ Take my controller medicines (above) every day.

❑ Before exercise, take _____ puff(s) of _____

❑ Avoid things that make my asthma worse. (See back of form.)

YELLOW ZONE

Getting worse.

- Cough, wheeze, chest tightness, shortness of breath, or
- Waking at night due to asthma symptoms, or
- Can do some, but not all, usual activities.

Peak Flow (for ages 5 and up):
_____ to _____ (50 to 79% of personal best)

CAUTION.   Continue taking every day controller medicines, AND:

❑ Take ____ puffs or ____ one nebulizer treatment of quick relief medicine. If I am not back in the Green Zone within 20-30 minutes take ____ more puffs or nebulizer treatments. If I am not back in the Green Zone within one hour, then I should:

❑ Increase _____

❑ Add _____

❑ Call _____

❑ Continue using quick relief medicine every 4 hours as needed. Call provider if not improving in _____ days.

RED ZONE

Medical Alert

- Very short of breath, or
- Quick-relief medicines have not helped, or
- Cannot do usual activities, or
- Symptoms are same or get worse after 24 hours in Yellow Zone.

Peak Flow (for ages 5 and up):
less than _____ (50% of personal best)

MEDICAL ALERT! Get help!

❑ Take quick relief medicine: _____ puffs every _____ minutes and get help immediately.

❑ Take _____

❑ Call _____

Danger! Get help immediately! Call 911 if trouble walking or talking due to shortness of breath or if lips or fingernails are gray or blue. For child, call 911 if skin is sucked in around neck and ribs during breaths or child doesn't respond normally.

Health Care Provider: My signature provides authorization for the above written orders. I understand that all procedures will be implemented in accordance with state laws and regulations. Student may self carry asthma medications: ❑ Yes ❑ No   self administer asthma medications: ❑ Yes ❑ No (This authorization is for a maximum of one year from signature date.)

_____ _____
Healthcare Provider Signature   Date

ORIGINAL (Patient) / CANARY (School/Child Care/Work/Other Support Systems) / PINK (Chart)

Bronchodilators and Antiasthma Drugs

©2008, Public Health Institute (RAMP)

Figure 34.2 Example of asthma action plan. (Reprinted with permission from *The Asthma Action Plan*, developed by a committee facilitated by the Regional Asthma Management and Prevention (RAMP) Initiative, a program of the Public Health Institute. Source: http://www.rampasthma.org/actionplan.pdf. This publication was supported by Cooperative Agreement Number 1U58DP001016-01 from the CDC. Its contents are solely the responsibility of the authors and do not necessarily represent the official views of the CDC.)

include an optimal response to therapy, support of patient needs related to managing adverse reactions, and an understanding of the therapeutic regimen.

IMPLEMENTATION

Promoting an Optimal Response to Therapy

Nursing care of the patient receiving a bronchodilating drug or an antiasthma drug requires careful monitoring of the patient and proper administration of the various drugs. These drugs may be given orally, parenterally, or topically by inhalation or nebulization. Dosages are individualized for each patient, which allows the smallest effective dose to be given. The nurse can give oral preparations with food or milk if gastric upset occurs.

As an outpatient, the patient must understand the purposes of step care for worsening symptoms (See Display 34.1). Part of a step care program is to start the patient on the lowest number and dosage of drugs that will treat the respiratory condition. As the patient's breathing becomes distressed, doses are changed, and different medications are added at each step. As the symptoms lessen, the medications are reduced, and the patient moves down a step. The nurse provides emotional support and encouragement as the patient makes adjustments in accordance with each step.

Acute Symptom Situations. SABA bronchodilators are used to treat acute respiratory symptoms. The nurse assists the patient to administer 2 to 4 puffs of the inhaled medication. Depending upon the severity of the exacerbation, up to 3 treatments at 20-minute intervals may be administered. A nebulizer may be ordered to deliver the medication rather than an inhaler device. These treatments are given less frequently.

The nurse may administer epinephrine subcutaneously for an acute bronchospasm. Doses of drugs, such as epinephrine, are measured in tenths of a milliliter. The nurse exercises great care in reading the primary health care provider's order when preparing these drugs for administration to prevent error. Therapeutic effects occur within 5 minutes after administration and last as long as 4 hours. Anticholinergic medications or intravenous (IV) steroids may also be used when the situation is emergent.

Rapid **theophyllinization** using one of the xanthine derivatives may be required for acute respiratory symptoms. Theophyllinization is accomplished by giving the patient a higher initial dose, called a *loading dose*, to bring blood levels to a therapeutic range more quickly than waiting several days for the drug to exert a therapeutic effect. The primary health care provider may prescribe loading doses to be administered orally or IV over 12 to 24 hours. It is important for the nurse to monitor the patient closely for signs of theophylline toxicity.

NURSING ALERT

Notify the primary health care provider immediately if any of the following signs of theophylline toxicity develops: anorexia, nausea, vomiting, diarrhea, confusion, abdominal cramping, headache, restlessness, insomnia, tachycardia, arrhythmias, or seizures.

The primary health care provider may order a daily plasma theophylline level to monitor for toxicity. The therapeutic range of theophylline blood levels is 10 to 20 mcg/mL. Toxicity occurs in levels above 20 mcg/mL. In some patients, toxicity may occur with levels between 15 and 20 mcg/mL. Toxicity is more likely to occur in patients who require high doses or during prolonged therapy. The nurse reports any serum theophylline levels greater than 20 mcg/mL or any symptoms associated with toxicity.

NURSE ALERT

Theophylline dosing is determined by serum concentration. Blood samples should be taken 1 to 2 hours after administration to measure peak absorption of the drug. If a sustained-release product is being used, the lab draw should be taken 5 to 9 hours after the morning dose.

The nurse can give some of these drugs (e.g., aminophylline or theophylline) by IV infusion. When giving theophylline or aminophylline IV, the nurse monitors the patient for hypotension, cardiac arrhythmias, and tachycardia. If a bronchodilator is given IV, the nurse administers it through an infusion pump. The nurse checks the IV infusion site at frequent intervals, because these patients may be extremely restless and extravasation can occur.

LIFESPAN ALERT – Gerontology

Older adults taking the adrenergic bronchodilators are at increased risk for adverse reactions related to both the cardiovascular system (tachycardia, arrhythmias, palpitations, and hypertension) and the CNS (restlessness, agitation, insomnia).

Long-Term Control of Symptoms. Controlling respiratory mucosal inflammation is the goal of long-term medications. The step care method (See Display 34.1) is a guideline for patients and is the basis for an individualized plan made by the primary health care provider. Using the step care method, patients manage the first step without daily medications. ICSs are used in the second step of the plan. It is important to remind the patient to refrain from swallowing the medication and to rinse the mouth thoroughly after using the inhaler.

LIFESPAN ALERT – Pediatric/Gerontology

When children are taking oral corticosteroids or higher doses of the inhalant form, growth should be monitored closely. A reduction in growth may occur from corticosteroid use. The primary health care provider is kept informed of the patient's growth record. It is particularly important to monitor growth in puberty and adolescence.

For elders at risk for osteoporosis, a calcium or vitamin D supplement may be prescribed.

If the patient experiences daily distress or peak expiratory flow readings vary, medications are taken to a higher step. LABA bronchodilators are not administered more frequently than twice daily (morning and evening). LABA drugs, such as salmeterol or formoterol, do not replace the fast-acting inhalers for sudden symptoms, nor are they used to treat acute asthma symptoms. The

DISPLAY 34.3 Using a Metered-Dose Inhaler

How to Use an Inhaler

When a patient is first diagnosed with asthma and prescribed inhalation therapy, he or she may need to learn how to use the inhaler that will deliver drug therapy. The nurse may be the health care provider who supplies instructions such as these:

Metered-Dose Inhaler (MDI)

1. When using a new inhaler, or one that has not been used in several days, point the inhaler away from you and prime the inhaler 1–2 times.
2. Hold the device upright and shake it.
3. Tilt the head back slightly.
4. Exhale and open mouth.
5. Position the inhaler in one of three ways:
   • Held 1-2 inches from the mouth (this is preferred)
   • Using a spacer
   • With the inhaler between the lips
6. Start to inhale slowly and press down on the inhaler to release the medication.
7. Breathe in for 3 to 5 seconds.
8. Hold your breath for 10 seconds to allow the drug to reach deep into the lungs.
9. Repeat for the ordered number of puffs, allowing 1 minute between each puff.

Spacers are recommended for children, older adults, and anyone who has difficulty using a nebulizer alone. Spacers are indicated when using inhaled steroids.

Dry-Powder Inhaler (DPI)

1. Prepare the medication for inhalation.
2. Place the mouthpiece to the lips.
3. Inhale quickly.
4. Hold your breath for 10 seconds to allow the drug to reach deep into the lungs.
5. Capsules for inhalation (such as those used in Foradil Aerolizer or Spiriva HaniHaler) must not be swallowed.
6. Do not place your device in water.

When the patient is prescribed more than one type of inhaler, instruct the patient to use the bronchodilator first to open the air passages, and then use other prescribed medications. Percentages of drug dispersal from a MDI without a spacer (left) and with a spacer (right)

drugs may be administered by a metered-dose inhaler (Display 34.3). If a dry-powder inhaler is used for administration, the nurse teaches the patient how to use it.

! NURSE ALERT

Formoterol (Foradil Aerolizer) comes in capsule form and is administered only by oral inhalation using the Aerolizer Inhaler. Be sure to remind the patient that this capsule is not to be taken orally.

The mast cell stabilizers, such as cromolyn (Intal), may be added to the patient's existing treatment regimen (e.g., ICSs). If use of the mast cell stabilizers must be discontinued for any reason, the dosage is gradually tapered. When administered orally, cromolyn is given one half hour before meals and at bedtime. The oral form of the drug comes in an ampule. The ampule is opened and its contents poured into a glass of water. The patient or care provider stirs the mixture thoroughly. The patient must drink all of the mixture. The drug may not be mixed with any other substance (e.g., fruit juice, milk, or foods).

Leukotriene receptor antagonists, leukotriene inhibitors, and immunomodulators are drugs used for managing asthma and are never administered during an acute asthma attack. If used during an acute attack, these drugs may worsen the attack. These drugs are administered orally.

Zileuton may cause liver damage. Because of the danger of liver toxicity, the primary health care provider may order hepatic aminotransferase levels at the beginning of treatment and during therapy with zileuton. Patients are instructed to immediately report any symptoms of liver dysfunction, such as upper right quadrant pain, nausea, fatigue, lethargy, pruritus, and jaundice. Patients may be hypersensitive to monoclonal antibodies, (e.g., omalizumab), which are used to modulate the immune response. It is administered subcutaneously every 2 to 4 weeks, typically in the clinic setting, where the patient can be monitored after the injection for an anaphylactic reaction. Be sure to tell the patient a reaction may occur up to 4 days following the injection and to have emergency contact information close at hand.

Monitoring and Managing Patient Needs

ANXIETY. Patients who have difficulty breathing and are receiving a bronchodilator or antiasthma drug may experience extreme anxiety, nervousness, and restlessness, which may be caused by their breathing difficulty or by the action of the drug. In these patients, it may be difficult for the primary health care provider to determine whether the patient is having an adverse drug reaction or the problem is related to the respiratory disorder. The nurse can reassure the patient that the drug being administered will most likely relieve the respiratory distress in a short time. Patients who are extremely apprehensive are observed more frequently until their respirations are near normal. The nurse closely monitors the patient's blood pressure and pulse during therapy and reports any significant changes. The nurse speaks and acts in a calm manner, being careful not to increase the anxiety or nervousness caused by the adrenergic drug. Explaining the effects of the drug may help the patient to tolerate these uncomfortable adverse reactions.

INEFFECTIVE AIRWAY CLEARANCE. Occasionally the patient may experience an acute bronchospasm either as a result of the disease, after exposure to an allergen, or as an adverse reaction to some antiasthma drugs, such as ICSs.

! NURSING ALERT

Acute bronchospasm causes severe respiratory distress and wheezing from the forceful expiration of air and is considered a medical emergency. It is characterized by severe respiratory distress, dyspnea, forceful expiration, and wheezing. The nurse must report these symptoms to the primary health care provider immediately

During an acute bronchospasm, the nurse checks the blood pressure, pulse, respiratory rate, and response to the drug every 5 to 15 minutes until the patient's condition stabilizes, and respiratory distress is relieved.

IMPAIRED ORAL MUCOUS MEMBRANES. Inhalers, particularly the corticosteroid or mast cell aerosols, may cause throat irritation and promote infection with *Candida albicans*. The nurse instructs the patient to use strict oral hygiene, cleanse the inhaler as directed in the package directions, and use the proper technique when taking an inhalation. These interventions will decrease the incidence of candidiasis and help to soothe the throat. Occasionally an antifungal drug may be prescribed by the primary health care provider to manage the candidiasis.

IMBALANCED NUTRITION: LESS THAN BODY REQUIREMENTS. Some antiasthma drugs cause nausea. The patient with nausea should be offered frequent smaller meals rather than three large meals. Meals should be followed by good mouth care. The nurse suggests limiting fluids with meals to help with the nausea. The nurse provides a pleasant, relaxed atmosphere for meals.

The patient taking theophylline may report heartburn, because the drug relaxes the lower esophageal sphincter, allowing gastroesophageal reflux. Heartburn is minimized if the patient remains in an upright position and sleeps with the head of the bed elevated. Some antiasthma drugs may cause an unpleasant taste in the mouth. Asking the patient to take frequent sips of water, suck on sugarless candy, or chew gum helps to alleviate the problem.

Educating the Patient and Family

Due to the chronic nature of respiratory illnesses, the nurse's role is to instruct the patient and family in methods to monitor the condition, control triggers in the environment, and manage medications properly for optimal breathing.

! NURSING ALERT

Asthma Action Plans in multiple languages can be found at the Regional Asthma Management and Prevention website at http://www.rampasthma.org/index.htm. The nurse can provide the website to the patient or demonstrate how to fill out the plans during a patient teaching session. These can be printed, or the individual can fill out the information (with field version) and use to monitor daily asthma management and acute episodes.

The patient is taught to monitor breathing status and regulate medications based on the asthma action plan. The nurse helps the patient to fill in the medications prescribed to maintain optimal breathing. The patient is then instructed to monitor his or her own breathing pattern based on zones defined by specific symptoms, peak flow meter readings, and corresponding adjusted medications as defined by the primary health care provider. A commonly used method to interpret breathing status is to relate it to the three colors of a traffic light: green, yellow, and red (see Fig. 34.2).

The patient uses a peak flow meter at home to monitor breathing status and the effectiveness of the drug regimen. The nurse teaches the patient how to use the peak flow meter and when to notify the primary health care provider (see Patient Teaching for Improved Patient Outcomes: Using a Peak Flow Meter).

A majority of the medications prescribed will be delivered by inhalation. If the patient is to use an aerosol inhaler for administration of the medication, the nurse provides a thorough explanation of its use (see Display 34.3).

! NURSING ALERT

The nurse should not assume that the patient understands how to use an aerosol inhaler correctly. Many different devices are on the market; these are used with specific medications and do not all work the same. The nurse should review the written instructions as well as examine the device with the patient. Then the nurse should have the patient demonstrate the use of the inhaler to evaluate whether he or she is using the proper technique. It is important to review instructions at each follow-up visit.

The nurse also includes the following general points in the patient teaching plan:

- Take the drug regularly as prescribed by the primary health care provider, even during symptom-free times.

Long-acting medications are taken to prevent acute attacks and maintain a level of breathing–do not use to treat acute episodes of asthma.

- If symptoms become worse, increase the dose or frequency of use as directed to do so by the primary health care provider or as established in the action plan.
- Check before using nonprescription drugs or herbal preparations. Some may contain similar drugs and may cause you to increase doses unknowingly.
- Check medications weekly to be sure you can reorder prescriptions and avoid running out of medication when stores are closed. Do not chew or crush coated or sustained-release tablets.
- Because inhalers vary, the nurse carefully reviews any instruction sheets with the patient and provides information about how the unit is assembled, used, and cleaned.
- If LABAs are used for preventing EIB, the drug is administered at least 30 minutes before exercise. Additional doses are not to be given for at least 12 hours.
- For patients using adrenergic bronchodilators—These drugs may cause nervousness, insomnia, and restlessness. Contact the primary health care provider if the symptoms become severe.
- For patients using xanthine derivatives—follow your primary health care provider's instructions concerning monitoring of theophylline serum levels. Avoid foods that contain xanthine, such as colas, coffee, chocolate, and charcoal-prepared foods.
- For patients using ICSs—wear a medical alert item (e.g., bracelet) indicating the need for supplemental systemic steroids in the event of stress or severe asthmatic attack that is unresponsive to bronchodilators. Do not stop therapy abruptly.
- For patients using immunomodulators—be aware that an anaphylactic reaction can occur for up to a year after dosing. Contact the primary health care provider should you begin itching or get hives, seek emergent care if you have trouble breathing.

EVALUATION

- Therapeutic response is achieved and breathing is easier and more effective.
- Adverse reactions are identified, reported to the primary health care provider, and managed successfully with appropriate nursing interventions:
  - ☑ Anxiety is managed successfully.
  - ☑ Patient has a clear patent airway.
  - ☑ Mucous membranes are moist and intact.
  - ☑ Nutrition is adequately maintained.
- Patient and family demonstrate an understanding of the drug regimen and use of both the peak flow meter and inhalator device.

Patient Teaching for Improved Patient Outcomes

Using a Peak Flow Meter

Patients receiving bronchodilators or antiasthma drugs often need to monitor their lung function at home with a peak flow meter. Doing so provides the patient and the primary health care provider with valuable information about the status of the patient's condition and the effectiveness of therapy. Often, trends in the readings can detect changes in the patient's airway and airflow even before any signs and symptoms are experienced. This allows possible intervention before a major problem arises.

Because a variety of meters are commercially available, the nurse explains about the type of meter that will be used, how often the peak flow should be checked, and the ranges for the readings along with instructions on what to do for each range. The nurse uses the following steps to instruct the patient on the use of the peak flow meter:

- ✓ Check to make sure that the indicator is at the lowest level of the scale.
- ✓ Stand upright to allow the best inhalation possible. (Be sure to remove gum or food from your mouth.)
- ✓ Inhale as deeply as you can and then place your lips around the mouthpiece, making sure you have a tight seal.
- ✓ Exhale as forcibly and as quickly as possible in one large "huff."
- ✓ Watch the indicator rise on the scale, noting where it stops. The number below the indicator's position is your *peak flow reading*.
- ✓ Repeat the procedure two more times.
- ✓ Compare the three readings. Record the highest reading on your action plan. Do not calculate an average.
- ✓ Bring the action plan with peak flow meter readings to your follow-up visits.
- ✓ Measure the peak flow rate close to the same time each day. (Your physician may provide you with a suggested time. Some patients measure the peak flow rate twice daily between 7 and 9 AM and between 6 and 8 PM. Others measure the peak flow rate before or after taking their medication.)
- ✓ Follow the medication instructions written on your action plan next to the zone color of your reading (see Fig. 34.2).
- ✓ Clean your meter with mild soap and hot water after use.

Bronchodilators and Antiasthma Drugs

THINK CRITICALLY: PHARMACOLOGY IN PRACTICE

1. Mrs. Chase has been diagnosed with asthma by her primary care provider, and the following plan is established:
- Goal of peak flow meter should be 350.
- Azmacort 2 puffs QID, may go up to 16 inhalations if feeling breathless.
- Albuterol inhaler, 2 puffs 30 minutes before exercise, or if PEV is in yellow zone, or if feel short of breath.
- Call for medication changes if in red zone.

How will you teach her about using the peak flow meter, routine medication management, and breathless events?

Go to http://www.rampasthma.org, select Asthma Action Plan (with fields) and prepare an asthma action plan using the above parameters. Print it out and compare with classmates; did you fill it in the same way? Will you consistently teach the same information to the patient?

2. Mrs. Chase remarks that she does not want to use the inhaler because when her elderly mother used inhaled medication it smelled like rotten eggs. What medication did her mother use in the inhalation device, and how are Mrs. Chase's medications different?

Test Your Knowledge

1. Which of the following laboratory tests would the nurse expect to be ordered for a patient taking Theo-Dur?

A. Thyroid hormone levels
B. Alanine aminotransferase
C. Sodium electrolytes
D. Serum theophylline levels

2. When the SABA drugs are administered to older adults, there is an increased risk of _____.

A. GI effects
B. nephrotoxic effects
C. neurotoxic effects
D. cardiovascular effects

3. When administering aminophylline, a xanthine derivative bronchodilating drug, the nurse monitors the patient for adverse reactions, which include _____.

A. restlessness and nervousness
B. hypoglycemia and hypothyroidism
C. bradycardia and bronchospasm
D. somnolence and lethargy

4. The nurse correctly administers montelukast (Singulair) _____.

A. once daily in the evening
B. twice daily in the morning and evening
C. three times a day with meals
D. once daily in the morning

Prepare for the NCLEX

1. The following statement indicates that the patient understands the purpose of the peak flow meter.

A. "I use the peak flow meter when I am short of breath."
B. "I must wash the peak flow meter after every use."
C. "I should measure my peak flow everyday."
D. "I put the medicine in the peak flow meter."

Calculate Medication Dosages

1. A patient is prescribed 0.25 mg of terbutaline SC. The drug is available for injection in a solution of 1 mg/mL. The nurse administers _____.

2. The patient is prescribed zafirlukast 20 mg orally BID. The drug is available in 10-mg tablets. The nurse administers _____. How many milligrams of zafirlukast will the patient receive each day?

To check your answers, see Appendix E.

thePoint. *For more NCLEX questions, log on to LWW's thePoint to access more than a thousand questions.*

Drugs That Affect the Cardiovascular System

This unit discusses the cardiovascular system and the drugs used to treat disorders of the cardiovascular system. Coronary heart disease (CHD) is the single largest killer of both men and women in the United States, with nearly 2500 deaths per day. Although these numbers seem high, the death rate from CHD and stroke decreased by 36% from 1999 to 2005. Advances in diagnosis, treatment, and changes in lifestyle have much to do with this reduction; the availability of medications to treat both early and advanced disease helped to improve mortality rates. The drugs in this unit range from those used early in heart disease, such as antihyperlipidemics, to drugs used in critical care units when advanced disease is treated.

The risk of CHD increases as blood cholesterol levels increase. Elevated serum cholesterol and low-density lipoprotein (LDL) levels play a role in the development of atherosclerotic heart disease. Other risk factors, besides elevated cholesterol levels, also play a role in the development of hyperlipidemia. Uncontrollable risk factors include:

- Age (men older than 45 years and women older than 55 years)
- Gender (women after menopause, LDL cholesterol levels increase)
- Family history of early heart disease (father/brother before age 55 years and mother/sister before age 65 years)

Those factors a person can control or modify include:

- Diet (saturated fat and cholesterol in the food raises total and LDL-cholesterol levels)
- Weight (overweight can make LDL-cholesterol level go up and high-density lipoprotein [HDL] level go down)
- Physical inactivity (increased physical activity helps to lower LDL cholesterol and raise HDL cholesterol levels)

In general, the higher the LDL level and the more risk factors involved, the greater the risk for heart disease. Lowering blood cholesterol levels can arrest or reverse atherosclerosis in the vessels and can significantly decrease the incidence of heart disease. The main goal of treatment in patients with hyperlipidemia is to lower LDL concentrations to a level that will reduce the risk of heart disease. The first chapter in this unit discusses the cholesterol-lowering drugs or antihyperlipidemic drugs.

Hypertension is defined as a systolic blood pressure (SBP) greater than 140 mm Hg or a diastolic blood pressure (DBP) greater than 90 mm Hg, (or the use of an antihypertensive medication). Patients with an SBP of 120 to 139 or a DBP of 80 to 89 are considered prehypertensive and are at an increased risk for development of hypertension. Individuals at risk for hypertension require health-promoting lifestyle modifications to prevent cardiovascular disease. Hypertension, if untreated, can lead to dysfunction not only in the cardiovascular system but other systems such as the renal and respiratory systems. In individuals between the ages of 40 and 70 years, every increase of 20 mm Hg in SBP or every increase of 10 mm Hg in DBP doubles the risk of cardiovascular disease across the entire blood pressure range from 115/75 to 185/115. Treating hypertension early reduces the risk for cardiovascular disease and death and protects against hypertension-related complications, such as stroke, heart failure, and renal disease. In Chapter 36, drugs used to treat hypertension include diuretics, the β-adrenergic blocking drugs, centrally-acting antiadrenergics, peripherally-acting antiadrenergics, α/β-adrenergic blocking drugs, angiotensin-converting enzyme (ACE) inhibitors, angiotensin II receptor antagonists, calcium channel blockers, direct renin inhibitors, selective aldosterone receptor antagonists, vasodilating drugs, and drugs used for hypertensive crisis are featured.

Sharp pains in the chest, jaw, or arm may be one of the first times a person will stop and consider his or her cardiac status. Diseases of the arteries—coronary artery disease, cerebral vascular disease, and peripheral vascular disease—are caused by narrowing of the arteries and may result in pain when tissues are denied oxygen. Chapter 37 discusses the antianginal drugs: drugs whose primary purpose is to increase blood supply to an area by dilating blood vessels.

Blockage of the vessels in the form of blood clots can occur in the cardiovascular system. Chapter 38 discusses drugs used to prevent (anticoagulants or antiplatelets) and drugs used to remove (thrombolytics) blood clots from the blood vessels.

Cardiotonic drugs and miscellaneous inotropic drugs are used to treat heart failure, previously referred to as *congestive heart failure*. About 5 million Americans have heart failure. It is the most frequent cause of hospitalization for individuals older than 65 years. African Americans and obese individuals are at the highest risk for heart failure. With treatment, some patients may lead nearly normal lives, although more than 300,000 individuals with heart failure die each year. The ACE inhibitors are considered the first-choice treatment and are the cornerstones of heart failure drug therapy. These drugs are discussed in terms of their ability to reduce hypertension (see Chapter 36). The cardiotonic digoxin is discussed in Chapter 39, because it is prescribed for patients with heart failure who do not respond to the ACE inhibitors and diuretics.

The last chapter in this unit discusses the antiarrhythmic drugs used to treat cardiac arrhythmia (a conduction disorder resulting in an abnormally slow or rapid regular heart rate, or a heart that beats with an irregular pace).

Some arrhythmias do not require treatment, whereas others require immediate treatment because they are potentially fatal. Unfortunately, although these drugs are used to treat arrhythmia, they are also capable of causing or worsening an arrhythmia. The benefits of treatment must be carefully weighed by the primary health care provider against the risks of treatment with the antiarrhythmic drug.

PHARMACOLOGY IN PRACTICE

In this unit, our patient focus will be on Lillian Chase, a 36-year-old woman. Mrs. Chase has been diagnosed with asthma, yet she continues to smoke one to two packs of cigarettes daily. A year ago she presented to the emergency room with breathing difficulty, her vital signs were T = 98.7°F, P = 120, R =24, and B/P = 182/110. She was stabilized and sent to an internal medicine clinic for follow-up. At the clinic, her B/P averaged 156/98 and lab work drawn had the following values:

Cholesterol = 320
LDL = 178
HDL = 20

Mrs. Chase was diagnosed with high cholesterol and told she is at risk for heart disease. In the last year, she has attempted to follow the Dietary Approaches to Stop Hypertension (DASH) diet, but she still smokes. After reading the chapters in this unit, you will understand her disease better and help her to maintain compliance with her medications, diet, and activity habits.

Antihyperlipidemic Drugs

LEARNING OBJECTIVES

On completion of this chapter, the student will:

1. Define cholesterol, HDL, LDL, and triglyceride levels and how they contribute to the development of heart disease.
2. Define therapeutic life changes and how they affect cholesterol levels.
3. Discuss the uses, general drug actions, general adverse reactions, contraindications, precautions, and interactions of antihyperlipidemic drugs.
4. Discuss important preadministration and ongoing assessment activities the nurse should perform on the patient taking an antihyperlipidemic drug.
5. List nursing diagnoses particular to a patient taking an antihyperlipidemic drug.
6. Discuss ways to promote an optimal response to therapy, how to manage common adverse reactions, and important points to keep in mind when educating patients about the use of an antihyperlipidemic drug.

Hyperlipidemia is an increase (*hyper*) in the **lipids**, which are a group of fats or fatlike substances in the blood (*emia*). **Cholesterol** and the **triglycerides** are the two lipids in the blood. Elevation of one or both of these lipids occurs in hyperlipidemia. Serum cholesterol levels above 240 mg/dL and triglyceride levels above 150 mg/dL are associated with **atherosclerosis**. Atherosclerosis is a disorder in which lipid deposits accumulate on the lining of the blood vessels, eventually producing degenerative changes and obstructing blood flow. Atherosclerosis is considered to be a major contributor in the development of heart disease.

Triglycerides and cholesterol are insoluble in water and must be bound to a lipid-containing protein (**lipoprotein**) for transportation throughout the body. Although several lipoproteins are found in the blood, this chapter focuses on the low-density lipoproteins, the high-density lipoproteins, and cholesterol.

Lipoproteins

Low-density lipoproteins (LDL) transport cholesterol to the peripheral cells. When the cells have all the cholesterol they need, the excess cholesterol is discarded into the blood. This can result in an excess of cholesterol, which can penetrate the walls of the arteries, resulting in atherosclerotic plaque formation. Elevation of the LDL increases the risk for heart disease. **High-density lipoproteins (HDL)** take cholesterol from the peripheral cells and transport it to the liver, where it is metabolized and excreted; the higher the HDL, the lower the risk for development of atherosclerosis. Therefore, it is desirable to see an increase in the HDL (the "good" lipoprotein) level because of the protective nature of its properties against the development of atherosclerosis, and a decrease in the LDL level. A laboratory examination of blood lipids, called a *lipoprotein profile*, provides valuable information on the important cholesterol levels, such as:

- Total cholesterol
- LDL (the harmful lipoprotein)
- HDL (the protective lipoprotein)
- Triglycerides

Table 35.1 provides an analysis of cholesterol levels.

Cholesterol Levels

High-density lipoprotein cholesterol protects against heart disease, so the higher its numbers (i.e., blood level) the better. An HDL level less than 40 mg/dL is low and considered a major risk factor for heart disease. Triglyceride levels that are borderline (150–190 mg/dL) or high (above 190 mg/dL) may need treatment in some individuals.

In general, the higher the LDL level and the more risk factors involved, the greater the risk for heart disease. The main goal of treatment in patients with hyperlipidemia is to lower the LDL to a level that will reduce the risk of heart disease.

The primary health care provider may initially seek to control the cholesterol level by encouraging therapeutic life changes (TLC). This includes a cholesterol-lowering diet (the TLC diet), physical activity, quitting smoking (if applicable), and weight management. The TLC diet is a low–saturated

Level	Category
Table 35.1 Cholesterol Level Analysis	
Total Cholesterol*	
Less than 200 mg/dL	Desirable
200–239 mg/dL	Borderline
240 mg/dL and above	High
Low-Density Lipoprotein (LDL) Cholesterol*	
Less than 100 mg/dL	Optimal
100–129 mg/dL	Near optimal/above optimal
130–159 mg/dL	Borderline
160–189 mg/dL	High
190 mg/dL and above	Very high
High-Density Lipoprotein (HDL) Cholesterol*	
Less than 40 mg/dL	Low
60 mg/dL and above	High

*Cholesterol levels are measured in milligrams (mg) of cholesterol per deciliter (dL) of blood.

fat and low-cholesterol eating plan that includes less than 200 mg of dietary cholesterol per day. In addition, 30 minutes of physical activity each day is recommended for TLC. Walking at a brisk pace for 30 minutes a day 5 to 7 days a week can help raise the HDL and lower the LDL. Added benefits of a healthy diet and exercise program include a reduction of body weight. If TLC does not result in bringing blood lipids to therapeutic levels, the primary health care provider may add one of the antihyperlipidemic drugs to the treatment plan. TLC is continued along with the drug regimen.

In addition to control of the dietary intake of fat, particularly saturated fatty acids, antihyperlipidemic drug therapy is used to lower serum levels of cholesterol and triglycerides. The primary health care provider may use one drug or, in some instances, more than one antihyperlipidemic drug for those with poor response to therapy with a single drug. Three types of antihyperlipidemic drugs are currently in use, as well as miscellaneous antihyperlipidemic drugs (see Summary Drug Table: Antihyperlipidemic Drugs for a complete listing of the drugs). The various types of drugs used to treat hyperlipidemia are the following:

- HMG-CoA reductase inhibitors (statins)
- Bile acid resins
- Fibric acid derivatives
- Niacin

The target LDL level for treatment is less than 130 mg/dL. If the response to drug treatment is adequate, lipid levels are monitored every 4 months. If the response is inadequate, another drug or a combination of two drugs is used. Antihyperlipidemic drugs decrease cholesterol and triglyceride levels in several ways. Although the end result is a lower lipid blood level, each has a slightly different action.

HMG-CoA REDUCTASE INHIBITORS

Actions

The antihyperlipidemic drugs, HMG-CoA reductase inhibitors, are typically referred to as **statins**. HMG-CoA (3-hydroxy-3-methyglutaryl coenzyme A) reductase is an enzyme that is a **catalyst** (a substance that accelerates a chemical reaction without itself undergoing a change) in the manufacture of cholesterol. These drugs appear to have one of two activities, namely, inhibiting the manufacture of cholesterol or promoting the breakdown of cholesterol. Either drug activity lowers the blood levels of cholesterol, LDLs, and serum triglycerides. Examples of these drugs can be found in the Summary Drug Table: Antihyperlipidemic Drugs.

Uses

Statin drugs, along with a diet restricted in saturated fat and cholesterol, are used for the following:

- Treatment of hyperlipidemia
- Primary prevention of coronary events (in patients with hyperlipidemia without clinically evident coronary heart disease to reduce the risk of myocardial infarction and death from other cardiovascular events, including strokes, transient ischemic attacks, and cardiac revascularization procedures).
- Secondary prevention of cardiovascular events (in patients with hyperlipidemia with evident coronary heart disease to reduce the risk of coronary death, slow the progression of coronary atherosclerosis, and reduce risk of death from stroke/transient ischemic attack; and in those undergoing myocardial revascularization procedures).

Adverse Reactions

The statins are usually well tolerated. Adverse reactions, when they do occur, are often mild and transient and do not require discontinuing therapy. These reactions may include the following.

Central Nervous System Reactions

- Headache
- Dizziness
- Insomnia

Gastrointestinal System Reactions

- Flatulence, abdominal pain, cramping
- Constipation, nausea

Contraindications and Precautions

The statins are contraindicated in individuals with hypersensitivity to the drugs or serious liver disorders, and during pregnancy (category X) and lactation.

Summary Drug Table ANTIHYPERLIPIDEMIC DRUGS

Generic Name	Trade Name	Uses	Adverse Reactions	Dosage Ranges
HMG-CoA Reductase Inhibitors (Statins) statin				
atorvastatin ah-tore'-vah-stah-tin	Lipitor	Reduce risk of CHD events, hyperlipidemia, familial hypercholesterolemia	Headache, diarrhea, sinusitis	10–80 mg/day orally
fluvastatin floo-vah-stah'-tin	Lescol, Lescol XL	Atherosclerosis, hyperlipidemia, familial hypercholesterolemia	Headache, back pain, URI, flu-like syndrome	20–80 mg/day orally
lovastatin loe-vah-stah'-tin	Mevacor, Altoprev	Reduce risk of CHD events, atherosclerosis, hyperlipidemia, familial hypercholesterolemia	Headache, flatulence, infection	10–80 mg/day orally in single or divided doses Adolescents:10–40 mg/day orally
pravastatin prah-vah-stah'-tin	Pravachol	Reduce risk of CHD events, atherosclerosis, hyperlipidemia, familial hypercholesterolemia	Headache, nausea, vomiting, diarrhea, localized pain, cold symptoms	40 – 80 mg/day orally Children 8–13 yr: 20 mg/day orally Adolescents 14–18 yr: 40 mg/day orally
rosuvastatin roe-soo'-vah-stah-tin	Crestor	Hyperlipidemia	Headache	5–40 mg/day orally
simvastatin sim-vah-stah'-tin	Zocor	Reduce risk of CHD events, hyperlipidemia, familial hypercholesterolemia	Constipation	5–80 mg/day orally
Bile Acid Resins				
cholestyramine koe-less'-teer-ah-meen	Prevalite, Questran	Hyperlipidemia, relief of pruritus associated with partial biliary obstruction	Constipation (may lead to fecal impaction), exacerbation of hemorrhoids, abdominal pain, distention and cramping, nausea, increased bleeding related to vitamin K malabsorption, vitamin A and D deficiencies	4 g orally 1–6 times/day; individualize dosage based on response
colestipol koe-less'-tih-poll	Colestid	Hyperlipidemia	Same as cholestyramine	Granules: 5–30 g/day orally in divided doses Tablets: 2–16 g/day
colesevelam koe-leh-sev'-eh-lam	WelChol	Hyperlipidemia	Same as cholestyramine	3–7 tablets/day orally
Fibric Acid Derivatives (Fibrates)				
fenofibrate fen-oh-fye'-brate	TriCor, Triglide, Antara, Lipofen, Lofibra	Hyperlipidemia, hypertriglyceridemia	Abnormal liver function test results, respiratory problems, abdominal pain	Tablet: 48–145 mg/day orally
gemfibrozil jem-fye'-broe-zill	Lopid	Reduce risk of CHD events, hypertriglyceridemia	Dyspepsia, abdominal pain, diarrhea, nausea, vomiting, fatigue	1200 mg/day orally in two divided doses 30 min before morning and evening meals
Miscellaneous Preparations				
ezetimibe ee-zet'-ah-mibe	Zetia	Primary hypercholesterolemia	Diarrhea, back pain, sinusitis, dizziness, abdominal pain, arthralgia, coughing, fatigue	10 mg/day orally

(table continues on page 320)

Antihyperlipidemic Drugs

Summary Drug Table ANTIHYPERLIPIDEMIC DRUGS (continued)

Generic Name	Trade Name	Uses	Adverse Reactions	Dosage Ranges
niacin (nicotinic acid) *nye'-ah-sin*	Niaspan, Niacor	Adjunctive treatment for hyperlipidemia	Generalized flushing sensation of warmth, severe itching and tingling, nausea, vomiting, abdominal pain	Immediate-release: 1–2 g orally BID, TID Extended-release: 500–2000 mg/day orally
Combination Drugs				
amlodipine/atorvastatin Norvasc Lipitor	Caduet	Treat hypertension and hypercholesterolemia	See individual drugs	Titrate dose to no more than 10/80 mg/day combination orally
niacin/lovastatin	Advicor	Primary hypercholesterolemia	See individual drugs	Titrate dose between 500/20 mg/day combination orally, to maximum of 2000 mg of niacin
ezetimibe/simvastatin	Vytorin	Primary/familial hypercholesterolemia	See individual drugs	Titrate dose between 10/10 mg/day and 10/80 mg/day

These drugs are used cautiously in patients with a history of alcoholism, acute infection, hypotension, trauma, endocrine disorders, visual disturbances, and myopathy.

! NURSING ALERT

Studies link the drug rosuvastatin in higher doses to risks for serious muscle toxicity (myopathy/rhabdomyolysis) in certain populations. A 5-mg dose is available as a starting dose for those individuals who do not require aggressive cholesterol reductions or who have predisposing factors for myopathy. These include patients taking cyclosporine, Asian patients, and patients with severe renal insufficiency.

Interactions

The following interactions may occur when the statin drugs are administered with another agent:

Interacting Drug	Common Use	Effect of Interaction
macrolides, erythromycin, clarithromycin	Treatment of infections	Increased risk of severe myopathy or rhabdomyolysis
amiodarone	Cardiovascular problems	Increased risk of myopathy
niacin	Used to lower elevated cholesterol	Increased risk of severe myopathy or rhabdomyolysis
protease inhibitors	Treatment of human immunodeficiency virus (HIV) infection and acquired immunodeficiency syndrome (AIDS)	Elevated plasma levels of statins
verapamil	Treatment of cardiovascular problems and hypertension	Increased risk of myopathy
warfarin	Blood thinner (anticoagulant)	Increased anticoagulant effect

The statin drugs have an additive effect when used with the bile acid resins, which may provide an added benefit in treating hypercholesterolemia that does not respond to a single-drug regimen. Patients may not volunteer information regarding their use of alternative or complementary remedies. The nurse should always inquire about use of herbal products. Medical reports indicate a possible interaction with St. John's wort, used to relieve depression, causing a decrease in statin effectiveness.

• BILE ACID RESINS

Actions

Bile, which is manufactured and secreted by the liver and stored in the gallbladder, emulsifies fat and lipids as these products pass through the intestine. Once emulsified, fats and lipids are readily absorbed in the intestine. The bile acid resins bind to bile acids to form an insoluble substance that cannot be absorbed by the intestine, so it is secreted in the feces. With increased loss of bile acids, the liver uses cholesterol to manufacture more bile. This is followed by a decrease in cholesterol levels.

Uses

The bile acid resins are used to treat the following:

- Hyperlipidemia (in patients who do not have an adequate response to a diet and exercise program)
- Pruritus associated with partial biliary obstruction (cholestyramine only)

Adverse Reactions

- Constipation (may be severe and occasionally result in fecal impaction), aggravation of hemorrhoids, abdominal cramps, flatulence, nausea

- Increased bleeding tendencies related to vitamin K malabsorption, and vitamin A and D deficiencies

Contraindications and Precautions

The bile acid resins are contraindicated in patients with known hypersensitivity to the drugs. Bile acid resins are also contraindicated in those with complete biliary obstruction.

These drugs are used cautiously in patients with liver and kidney disease; they are also used cautiously during pregnancy (category C) and lactation (decreased absorption of vitamins may affect the infant).

Interactions

The following interactions may occur when the bile acid resins are administered with another agent:

Interacting Drug	Common Use	Effect of Interaction
anticoagulants	Blood thinners	Decreased effect of the anticoagulant (cholestyramine)
thyroid hormone	Treatment of hypothyroidism	Loss of efficacy of thyroid; also hypothyroidism (particularly with cholestyramine)
vitamins (A, D, E, K & folic acid)	Nutritional supplements	Reduced absorption of vitamins

When administered with the bile acid resins, a decreased serum level or decreased gastrointestinal (GI) absorption of the following drugs may occur:

- nonsteroidal anti-inflammatory drugs (NSAIDs; used to treat pain)
- penicillin G and tetracycline (used to treat infection)
- clofibrate and niacin (used to treat elevated cholesterol levels)
- digitalis glycosides (used to treat heart failure)
- furosemide and thiazide diuretics (used to treat edema)
- glipizide (used to treat diabetes)
- hydrocortisone (used to treat inflammation)
- methyldopa and propranolol (used to treat hypertension and cardiovascular problems, respectively)

Because the bile acids resins, particularly cholestyramine, can decrease the absorption of numerous drugs, the bile acid resins should be administered alone and other drugs given at least 1 hour before or 4 hours after administration of the bile acid resins.

• FIBRIC ACID DERIVATIVES

Actions

Fibric acid derivatives, also known as fibrates, are the third group of antihyperlipidemic drugs and work in a variety of ways. Clofibrate acts to stimulate the liver to increase breakdown of very-low-density lipoproteins (VLDLs) to LDLs, decreasing liver synthesis of VLDLs and inhibiting cholesterol formation. Fenofibrate acts by reducing VLDL and stimulating the catabolism of triglyceride-rich lipoproteins, resulting in a decrease in plasma triglycerides and cholesterol. Gemfibrozil increases the excretion of cholesterol in the feces and reduces the production of triglycerides by the liver, thus lowering serum lipid levels.

Uses

Although the fibric acid derivatives have antihyperlipidemic effects, their use varies depending on the drug. For example, clofibrate and gemfibrozil are used to treat individuals with very high serum triglyceride levels who are at risk for abdominal pain and pancreatitis and who do not experience a response to dietary modifications. Clofibrate is not used for the treatment of other types of hyperlipidemia and is not thought to be effective for preventing coronary heart disease. Fenofibrate is used as adjunctive treatment for reducing LDL, total cholesterol, and triglycerides in patients with hyperlipidemia.

Adverse Reactions

The adverse reactions associated with fibric acid derivatives include the following:

- Nausea, vomiting, and GI upset
- Diarrhea
- Cholelithiasis (stones in the gallbladder) or cholecystitis (inflammation of the gallbladder)

If cholelithiasis is found, the primary health care provider may discontinue the drug. See the Summary Drug Table: Antihyperlipidemic Drugs for additional adverse reactions.

Contraindications and Precautions

The fibric acid derivatives are contraindicated in patients with hypersensitivity to the drugs and in those with significant hepatic or renal dysfunction or primary biliary cirrhosis because these drugs may increase the already elevated cholesterol. The drugs are used cautiously during pregnancy (category C) and not during lactation or in patients with peptic ulcer disease or diabetes.

Interactions

The following interactions may occur when the fibric acid derivatives are administered with another agent:

Interacting Drug	Common Use	Effect of Interaction
anticoagulants	Blood thinners	Enhanced effects of the anticoagulants (particularly with gemfibrozil and fenofibrate)
cyclosporine	Immunosuppression after organ transplantation	Decreased effects of cyclosporine (particularly with gemfibrozil)
HMG-CoA reductase inhibitors (statins)	Treatment of elevated blood cholesterol levels	Increased risk of rhabdomyolysis (particularly with gemfibrozil and fenofibrate)
sulfonylureas	Treatment of diabetes	Increased hypoglycemic effects (particularly with gemfibrozil)

• MISCELLANEOUS ANTIHYPERLIPIDEMIC DRUGS

Miscellaneous antihyperlipidemic drugs include niacin and ezetimibe. Refer to the Summary Drug Table: Antihyperlipidemic Drugs for information on combinations of more than one class of antihyperlipidemic drugs in one tablet.

Actions

The mechanism by which niacin (nicotinic acid) lowers blood lipid levels is not fully understood. Ezetimibe inhibits the absorption of cholesterol in the small intestine, leading to a decrease in cholesterol in the liver.

Uses

Niacin is used as adjunctive therapy for lowering very high serum triglyceride levels in patients who are at risk for pancreatitis (inflammation of the pancreas) and whose response to dietary control is inadequate. Ezetimibe is typically used in combinations with other antihyperlipidemics in lipid lowering treatments.

Adverse Reactions

Gastrointestinal System Reactions

• Nausea, vomiting, abdominal pain
• Diarrhea

Other Reactions

• Severe, generalized flushing of the skin, sensation of warmth
• Severe itching or tingling

Contraindications, Precautions, and Interactions

Niacin is contraindicated in patients with known hypersensitivity to niacin, active peptic ulcer, hepatic dysfunction, and arterial bleeding. The drug is used cautiously in patients with renal dysfunction, high alcohol consumption, unstable angina, gout, and pregnancy (category C). Pregnant and lactating women should not use ezetimibe.

❦ HERBAL ALERT
Garlic has been used for many years throughout the world. The benefits of garlic on cardiovascular health are the best known and most extensively researched benefits of the herb. Its benefits include lowering serum cholesterol and triglyceride levels, improving the ratio of HDL to LDL cholesterol, lowering blood pressure, and helping to prevent the development of atherosclerosis. The recommended dosages of garlic are 600 to 900 mg/day of the garlic powder tablets, 10 mg of garlic oil "perles," or one moderate-sized fresh clove of garlic a day. Adverse reactions include mild stomach upset or irritation that can usually be alleviated by taking garlic supplements with food. There is an increased risk of bleeding when garlic is taken with warfarin. Although no serious reactions have occurred in pregnant women taking garlic, its use is not recommended. Garlic is excreted in breast milk and may cause colic in some infants. As with all herbal therapy, when garlic is used for therapeutic purposes, the primary health care provider should be aware of its use.

NURSING PROCESS
PATIENT RECEIVING AN ANTIHYPERLIPIDEMIC DRUG
ASSESSMENT

Preadministration Assessment
Many individuals with hyperlipidemia have no symptoms, and the disorder is not discovered until laboratory tests reveal elevated cholesterol and triglyceride levels, elevated LDL levels, and decreased HDL levels. Often, these drugs are initially prescribed on an outpatient basis, but initial administration may occur in the hospitalized patient. Serum cholesterol levels (i.e., a lipid profile) and liver functions tests (LFT) are obtained before the drugs are administered.

The nurse takes a dietary history, focusing on the types of foods normally included in the diet. Vital signs and weight are recorded. The skin and eyelids are inspected for evidence of xanthomas (flat or elevated yellowish deposits) that may be seen in the more severe forms of hyperlipidemia.

Ongoing Assessment
Patients usually take antihyperlipidemic drugs on an outpatient basis and come to the clinic or the primary health care provider's office for periodic monitoring. The primary health care provider usually prescribes frequent monitoring of blood cholesterol and triglyceride levels as a part of the ongoing assessment. Liver monitoring should occur with LFTs being drawn at 6 and 12 weeks after initiation of therapy and again at 6 month intervals. The nurse monitors these levels. Any increase in these levels is reported to the primary health care provider. If aspartate aminotransferase (AST) levels increase to three times normal, the primary health care provider may discontinue drug therapy. Because the maximum effects of these drugs are usually evident within 4 weeks, periodic lipid profiles are ordered to determine the therapeutic effect of the drug regimen. The primary health care provider may increase the dosage, add another antihyperlipidemic drug, or discontinue the drug therapy, depending on the patient's response to therapy.

⚠ NURSING ALERT
Sometimes a paradoxical elevation of blood lipid levels occurs. Should this happen, the primary health care provider is notified because he or she may prescribe a different antihyperlipidemic drug.

During the ongoing assessment, the nurse checks vital signs and assesses bowel functioning because an adverse reaction to these drugs is constipation. Constipation may become serious if not treated.

NURSING DIAGNOSES

Drug-specific nursing diagnoses include the following:

❑ **Constipation** related to antihyperlipidemic drugs
❑ **Risk for Imbalanced Nutrition: Less than Body Requirements** related to malabsorption of vitamins
❑ **Risk for Impaired Skin Integrity** related to rash and flushing
❑ **Nausea** related to antihyperlipidemic drugs
❑ **Risk for Injury** related to dizziness

Nursing diagnoses related to drug administration are discussed in depth in Chapter 4.

PLANNING

The expected outcomes of the patient depend on the specific reason for administering the drug, but may include an optimal response to therapy, support of patient needs related to the management of adverse reactions, and an understanding of the therapeutic regimen.

IMPLEMENTATION

Promoting an Optimal Response to Therapy

Because hyperlipidemia is often treated on an outpatient basis, the nurse explains the drug regimen and possible adverse reactions. If printed dietary guidelines are given to the patient, the nurse emphasizes the importance of following these recommendations. Drug therapy usually is discontinued if the antihyperlipidemic drug is not effective after 3 months of treatment.

Monitoring and Managing Patient Needs

CONSTIPATION.   Patients taking the antihyperlipidemic drugs, particularly the bile acid resins, may experience constipation. The drugs can produce or severely worsen preexisting constipation. The nurse instructs the patient to increase fluid intake, eat foods high in dietary fiber, and exercise daily to help prevent constipation. If the problem persists or becomes severe, a stool softener or laxative may be required. Some patients require decreased dosage or discontinuation of the drug therapy.

LIFESPAN ALERT – Gerontology
Older adults are particularly prone to constipation when taking the bile acid resins. The nurse should monitor older adults closely for hard, dry stools, difficulty passing stools, and any complaints of constipation. An accurate record of bowel movements must be kept.

RISK FOR IMBALANCED NUTRITION: LESS THAN BODY REQUIREMENTS.   Bile acid resins may interfere with the digestion of fats and prevent the absorption of the fat-soluble vitamins (vitamins A, D, E, and K) and folic acid. When the bile acid resins are used for long-term therapy, vitamins A and D may be given in a water-soluble form or administered parenterally.

RISK FOR IMPAIRED SKIN INTEGRITY.   Patients taking nicotinic acid may experience moderate to severe, generalized flushing of the skin, a sensation of warmth, and severe itching or tingling. Although these reactions are most often seen at higher dose levels, some patients may experience them even when small doses of nicotinic acid are administered. The sudden appearance of these reactions may frighten the patient.

! NURSING ALERT
The nurse should advise the patient taking nicotinic acid to contact their primary health care provider if the skin reactions are severe or cause extreme discomfort. Aspirin may be recommended before taking niacin preparations to reduce adverse reactions.

NAUSEA.   Some antihyperlipidemic drugs cause nausea. If nausea occurs, the drug should be taken with meals or with food. Other measures to help alleviate the nausea include providing a relaxed atmosphere for eating with no unpleasant odors or sights. The nurse can provide the patient with several small meals rather than three large meals. If nausea is severe or vomiting occurs, the primary health care provider is notified.

RISK FOR INJURY.   Injury can occur when the patient falls as the result of dizziness as an adverse reaction from the fibrates or statins. The nurse monitors the hospitalized patient carefully, placing the call light within easy reach. The patient may require assistance with ambulation until the effects of the medication are known, especially if the nurse is administering the initial doses of the antihyperlipidemic.

POTENTIAL MEDICAL COMPLICATION: VITAMIN K DEFICIENCY.   The nurse checks the patients for bruises over the body. The patient is encouraged to include foods high in vitamin K in the diet, such as asparagus, broccoli, green beans, lettuce, turnip greens, beef liver, collard greens, green tea, and spinach. If bruising is observed or if bleeding tendencies occur as the result of vitamin K deficiency, the nurse reports this to the primary health care provider. Parenteral vitamin K may be prescribed by the primary health care provider for immediate treatment, and oral vitamin K for preventing a deficiency in the future.

POTENTIAL MEDICAL COMPLICATION: RHABDOMYOLYSIS.   Antihyperlipidemic drugs, particularly the statin drugs, have been associated with skeletal muscle effects leading to rhabdomyolysis. **Rhabdomyolysis** is a rare condition in which muscle damage results in the release of muscle cell contents into the bloodstream. Rhabdomyolysis may precipitate renal dysfunction or acute renal failure. The nurse is alert for unexplained muscle pain, muscle tenderness, or weakness, especially if accompanied by malaise or fever. This reaction is more likely in Asian patients; therefore, a lower starting dose of the statin rosuvastatin is recommended. These symptoms should be reported to the primary health care provider because the drug may need to be discontinued.

Educating the Patient and Family

The nurse stresses the importance of following the diet recommended by the primary health care provider because drug therapy alone will not significantly lower cholesterol and triglyceride levels. The nurse provides a copy of the recommended diet and reviews the contents of the diet with the patient and family. The nurse should refer the patient or family member to a teaching dietitian, a dietary teaching session, internet websites, or a lecture provided by a hospital or community agency (see Patient Teaching for Improved Patient Outcomes: Using Diet and Drugs to Control High Blood Cholesterol Levels). The nurse also develops a teaching plan to include various important points for the various kinds of agents used to manage cholesterol levels.

The nurse can encourage the patient to participate in managing their ability to reduce cardiovascular risk by accessing tools on the internet. Various sites use information from the Framingham Heart Study to predict heart attack risk (See example of National Cholesterol Education Program site at http://hp2010.nhlbihin.net/atpiii/calculator.asp?usertype=pub/.). The patient uses the interactive site to enter age, gender, cholesterol and blood pressure values, and the prediction for heart attack risk in the next 10 years is calculated. Compliance will be re-enforced as the patient sees risk reduced over time.

STATINS (HMG–CoA REDUCTASE INHIBITORS). Usually, lovastatin is taken once daily, preferably with the evening meal. Fluvastatin, simvastatin, and pravastatin are taken once daily in the evening or at bedtime. The patient should not drink large quantities of grapefruit juice while taking these drugs. On the other hand:

- Advise taking rosuvastatin as a single dose once daily in the evening. If the patient is taking antacids, they should be taken at least 2 hours after the rosuvastatin.
- Inform the patient that if fluvastatin or pravastatin is prescribed with a bile acid resin, the statin should be taken 2 hours after the bile acid resin or at least 4 hours afterward.
- These drugs may cause photosensitivity; avoid exposure to the sun and wear both sunscreen and protective clothing.
- Explain that these drugs cannot be used during pregnancy (category X). Use a barrier contraceptive while taking these drugs. If the patient wishes to become pregnant while taking these drugs, the primary health care provider should be consulted before efforts at conception.
- Advise the patient to contact the primary health care provider as soon as possible if muscle pain, tenderness, or weakness occurs.

BILE ACID RESINS. The nurse advises the patient to take the drug before meals unless the primary health care provider directs otherwise. For the various forms of bile acid resins, the nurse may add teaching points such as the following:

- Cholestyramine powder: The prescribed dose must be mixed in 2 to 6 fluid ounces of water or noncarbonated beverage and shaken vigorously. The powder can also be mixed with highly fluid soups or pulpy fruits

(e.g., applesauce, crushed pineapple). The powder should not be ingested in the dry form. Other drugs are taken 1 hour before or 4 to 6 hours after cholestyramine. Cholestyramine is available combined with the artificial sweetener aspartame (Questran Light) for patients with diabetes or those who are concerned with weight gain.
- Colestipol granules: The prescribed dose must be mixed in liquids, soup, cereals, carbonated beverages, or pulpy fruits. Use approximately 90 mL of liquid and, when mixing with a liquid, slowly stir the preparation until ready to drink. The granules will not dissolve. Take the entire drug, rinse the glass with a small amount of water, and drink to ensure that all the medication is taken.
- Colestipol tablets: Tablets should be swallowed whole, one at a time, with a full glass of water or other fluid— not chewed, cut, or crushed.
- Sipping or holding the liquid preparations in the mouth can cause tooth discoloration or enamel decay.
- Constipation, nausea, abdominal pain, and distention may occur and may subside with continued therapy. The primary health care provider is notified if these effects become bothersome or if unusual bleeding or bruising occurs.

FIBRIC ACID DERIVATIVES. An important teaching point for fibric acid derivatives follows:

- Gemfibrozil: Explain that dizziness or blurred vision may occur. Observe caution when driving or performing hazardous tasks. Notify the primary health care provider if epigastric pain, diarrhea, nausea, or vomiting occurs.

MISCELLANEOUS PREPARATIONS. Teaching points to cover regarding nicotinic acid and ezetimibe include the following:

- Nicotinic acid: Advise the patient to take this drug with meals. This drug may cause mild to severe facial flushing, a sensation of warmth, severe itching, or headache. These symptoms usually subside with continued therapy, but contact the primary health care provider as soon as possible if symptoms are severe. The primary health care provider may prescribe aspirin (325 mg) to be taken about 30 minutes before nicotinic acid to decrease the flushing reaction. If dizziness occurs, avoid sudden changes in posture.
- Ezetimibe: Explain that ezetimibe should be taken at least 2 hours before or 4 hours after a bile acid sequestrant. Report unusual muscle pain, weakness or tenderness, severe diarrhea, or respiratory infections.

EVALUATION

- Therapeutic response is achieved and serum lipid levels are decreased.
- Adverse reactions are identified, reported to the primary health care provider, and managed successfully with appropriate nursing interventions:
  ☑ Patient reports adequate bowel movements.

- ☑ Patient maintains an adequate nutritional status.
- ☑ Skin remains intact.
- ☑ Nausea is controlled.
- ☑ No evidence of injury is seen.
- Patient and family demonstrate an understanding of the drug regimen.

Patient Teaching for Improved Patient Outcomes

Using Diet and Drugs to Control High Blood Cholesterol Levels

The nurse:

✓ Reviews the reasons for the drug and prescribed drug therapy, including drug name, form and method of preparation, correct dose, and frequency of administration.
✓ Emphasizes that drug therapy alone will not significantly lower blood cholesterol levels.
✓ Stresses importance of taking drug exactly as prescribed.
✓ Reinforces the importance of adhering to prescribed diet.
✓ Provides a written copy of dietary plan and reviews contents.
✓ Contacts dietitian for assistance with diet teaching.
✓ Answers questions and offers suggestions for ways to reduce dietary fat intake.
✓ Instructs in possible adverse reactions and signs and symptoms to report to primary health care provider.
✓ Reviews measures to minimize GI upset.
✓ Explains possible need for vitamin A and D therapy and high-fiber foods if patient is receiving bile acid sequestrant.
✓ Reassures that results of therapy will be monitored by periodic laboratory and diagnostic tests and follow-up with primary health care provider.

THINK CRITICALLY: PHARMACOLOGY IN PRACTICE

1. Lillian Chase is taking cholestyramine (Questran) for hyperlipidemia. The primary health care provider has prescribed therapeutic life changes for the patient. She is on a low-fat diet and walks short distances daily for exercise. Her major complaint at this visit is constipation, which is very bothersome to her. She feels depressed and has started smoking again. She tells you the medicine isn't working and wants to stop taking it. Listed below is information from her medical record today. Using the risk assessment tool at http://hp2010.nhlbihin.net/atpiii/calculator.asp?usertype=pub, calculate her 10-year heart attack risk and compare it to her risk 1 year ago. How can you use this information to help encourage Mrs. Chase to continue her medication?

    Mrs. Chase's assessment this office visit: T = 98.6°F, P = 104, R = 18, and B/P = 136/92, and lab work drawn had the following values:

    Cholesterol = 256
    HDL = 36

    What information would you give the patient concerning her constipation?

● Test Your Knowledge

1. Select the most common adverse reaction in a patient taking a bile acid resin:
    - **A.** Anorexia
    - **B.** Vomiting
    - **C.** Constipation
    - **D.** Headache

2. Lovastatin is best taken _____.
    - **A.** once daily, preferably with the evening meal
    - **B.** three times daily with meals
    - **C.** at least 1 hour before or 2 hours after meals
    - **D.** twice daily without regard to meals

3. When assessing a patient taking cholestyramine (Questran) for vitamin K deficiency, the nurse would _____.
    - **A.** check the patient for bruising
    - **B.** keep a record of the patient's intake and output
    - **C.** monitor the patient for myalgia
    - **D.** keep a dietary record of foods eaten

4. A patient taking niacin reports flushing after each dose of the niacin. Which of the following drugs would the nurse expect to be prescribed to help alleviate the flushing?
    - **A.** meperidine (Demerol)
    - **B.** aspirin
    - **C.** vitamin K
    - **D.** diphenhydramine (Benadryl)

● Prepare for the NCLEX

1. As the nurse, which of the following points is important to point out to the patient when teaching about drug and diet therapy for hyperlipidemia?
    - **A.** Fluids are taken in limited amounts when eating a low-fat diet.
    - **B.** The medication should be taken at least 1 hour before meals.
    - **C.** Medication alone will not lower cholesterol.
    - **D.** Meat is not allowed on a low-fat diet.

● Calculate Medication Dosages

1. A patient is prescribed 10-mg simvastatin orally daily for high cholesterol. The drug is available in 5-mg tablets. The nurse administers _____.

2. The primary health care provider prescribes fenofibrate for the treatment of hypertriglyceridemia. The patient is now taking 200 mg/d orally. Is this an appropriate dosage? If not, what action would you take? If the dose is appropriate, how many capsules would you administer if the drug is available in 67-mg capsules? _____

To check your answers, see Appendix E.

the**Point** *For more NCLEX questions, log on to http://thepoint.lww.com to access more than 1000 questions.*

Antihypertensive Drugs

pg 408 MS

angioedema
blood pressure
endogenous
hyperkalemia
hypertension
hypertensive emergency
hypokalemia
hyponatremia

isolated systolic
  hypertension
lumen
orthostatic hypotension
prehypertension
primary hypertension
secondary hypertension
vasodilation

On completion of this chapter, the student will:

1. Discuss the various types of hypertension and risk factors involved.
2. Identify normal and abnormal blood pressure levels for adults.
3. List the various types of drugs used to treat hypertension.
4. Discuss the general drug actions, uses, adverse reactions, contraindications, precautions, and interactions of the antihypertensive drugs.
5. Discuss important preadministration and ongoing assessment activities the nurse should perform for the patient taking an antihypertensive drug.
6. Explain why blood pressure determinations are important during therapy with an antihypertensive drug.
7. List nursing diagnoses particular to a patient taking an antihypertensive drug.
8. Discuss ways to promote an optimal response to therapy, how to manage adverse reactions, and important points to keep in mind when educating patients about the use of an antihypertensive drug.

Blood pressure is the force of the blood against the walls of the arteries. Blood pressure rises and falls throughout the day. The condition in which blood pressure stays elevated over time is known as **hypertension**. A systolic blood pressure less than 120 mm Hg and a diastolic blood pressure less than 80 mm Hg (120/80) are considered normal. **Prehypertension** is defined as a systolic pressure between 120 and 139 mm Hg or a diastolic pressure

between 80 and 89 mm Hg. Individuals with prehypertensive blood pressures are at risk for developing hypertension and should begin health-promoting lifestyle modifications. Table 36.1 identifies blood pressure classifications and management for adults.

Risks and Effects of Hypertension

Hypertension is serious, because it causes the heart to work too hard and contributes to atherosclerosis. It also increases the risk of heart disease, heart failure (HF), kidney disease, blindness, and stroke. Most cases of hypertension have no known cause. When there is no known cause of hypertension, the term **primary hypertension** is used. Primary hypertension has been linked to certain risk factors, such as diet and lifestyle. Display 36.1 identifies the risk factors associated with hypertension.

In the United States, about 72 million people have high blood pressure; this is about 1 in 3 adults. African Americans are twice as likely as whites to experience hypertension. After age 65, African-American women have the highest incidence of hypertension. Primary hypertension cannot be cured but can be controlled. Many individuals experience hypertension as they grow older, but hypertension is not a part of healthy aging. For many older individuals, the systolic pressure gives the most accurate diagnosis of hypertension. Display 36.2 discusses the importance of the systolic pressure.

Nonpharmacological Management of Hypertension

Once primary hypertension develops, management of the disorder becomes a lifetime task. When a direct cause of the hypertension can be identified, the condition is described as **secondary hypertension**. Among the known causes of secondary hypertension, kidney disease ranks first, with tumors or other abnormalities of the adrenal glands following. Most primary health care providers prescribe lifestyle changes to reduce risk factors before prescribing drugs. The primary health care provider may recommend measures such as:

- Weight loss (if the patient is overweight)
- Stress reduction (e.g., relaxation techniques, meditation, and yoga)
- Regular aerobic exercise

Table 36.1 Classification and Management of Blood Pressure for Adults

Blood Pressure Classification	Systolic Blood Pressure* (mmHg)	Diastolic Blood Pressure* (mmHg)	Lifestyle Modification	Without Compelling Indication	With Compelling Indications
Normal	<120	and <80	Encourage	n/a	n/a
Prehypertension	120–139	or 80–89	Yes	No antihypertensive drug indicated	Drug(s) for compelling indications.‡
Stage 1 hypertension	140–159	or 90–99	Yes	Thiazide-type diuretics for most.† May consider ACEI, ARB, BB, CCB, or combination.	Drug(s) for the compelling indications.‡ Other antihypertensive drugs (diuretics, ACEI, ARB, BB, CCB) as needed.
Stage 2 hypertension	≥160	or ≥100	Yes	Two-drug combination for most (usually thiazide-type diuretic and ACEI or ARB or BB or CCB).	

Drug abbreviations: ACEI, angiotensin-converting enzyme inhibitor; ARB, angiotensin receptor blocker; BB, beta blocker; CCB, calcium channel blocker.

*Treatment determined by highest BP category.

†Initial combined therapy should be used cautiously in those at risk for orthostatic hypotension.

‡Treat patients with chronic kidney disease or diabetes to BP goal of <130/80 mm Hg.

Adapted from National Heart Lung and Blood Institute (2003). *The seventh report of the Joint National Committee on Prevention, Detection, Evaluation, and Treatment of High Blood Pressure.* Bethesda, MD: National Institutes of Health. Retrieved May 7, 2009, from http://www.nhlbi.nih.gov/guidelines/hypertension/.

- Smoking cessation (if applicable)
- Moderation of alcohol consumption
- Dietary changes, such as a decrease in sodium (salt) intake

Many people with hypertension are "salt sensitive," in that any salt or sodium more than the minimum need is too much for them and leads to an increase in blood pressure. Dietitians usually recommend the Dietary Approaches to Stop Hypertension (DASH) diet. Studies indicate that blood pressure can be reduced by eating a diet low in saturated fat, total fat, and cholesterol and rich in fruits, vegetables, and low-fat dairy foods. The DASH diet includes whole grains, poultry, fish, and nuts and has reduced amounts of fats, red meats, sweets, and sugared beverages.

DISPLAY 36.1 Risk Factors in Hypertensive Patients

- Age and sex (women older than 55 years and men older than 45 years of age)
- African American race (higher rates than Asian, Caucasian or Hispanic individuals)
- Obesity
- Excessive dietary intake of salt and too little intake of potassium
- Chronic alcohol consumption
- Lack of physical activity
- Cigarette smoking
- Family history of high blood pressure and/or cardiovascular disease, diabetes, persistent stress
- Overweight in youth less than 18 years has become a risk for prehypertension in teens

Drug Therapy for Hypertension

When nonpharmacologic measures do not control high blood pressure, drug therapy usually begins, and the primary health care provider may first prescribe a diuretic (see Chapter 48) or beta (β)-adrenergic blocker (see Chapter 25), because these drugs have been highly effective (see Table 36.1 for indicators suggesting that drug therapy for hypertension should begin). However, as in many other diseases and conditions, there is no "best" single drug, drug combination, or medical regimen for hypertension treatment. After examination and evaluation of the patient, the primary health care provider selects the antihypertensive drug and therapeutic regimen that will probably be most effective. Figure 36.1 shows an algorithm for the treatment of hypertension.

DISPLAY 36.2 Importance of the Systolic Blood Pressure

Individuals with only an elevated systolic pressure have a condition known as **isolated systolic hypertension** (ISH). In ISH, systolic blood pressure is 140 mm Hg or greater with diastolic blood pressure less than 90 mm Hg. When the systolic pressure is high, blood vessels become less flexible and stiffen, leading to cardiovascular disease and kidney damage. Research indicates that treating ISH saves lives and reduces illness. The treatment is the same for ISH as for other forms of hypertension. Diastolic pressure should not be reduced lower than 70 mm Hg. Therefore, caution is advised in treating those with ISH and existing heart disease.

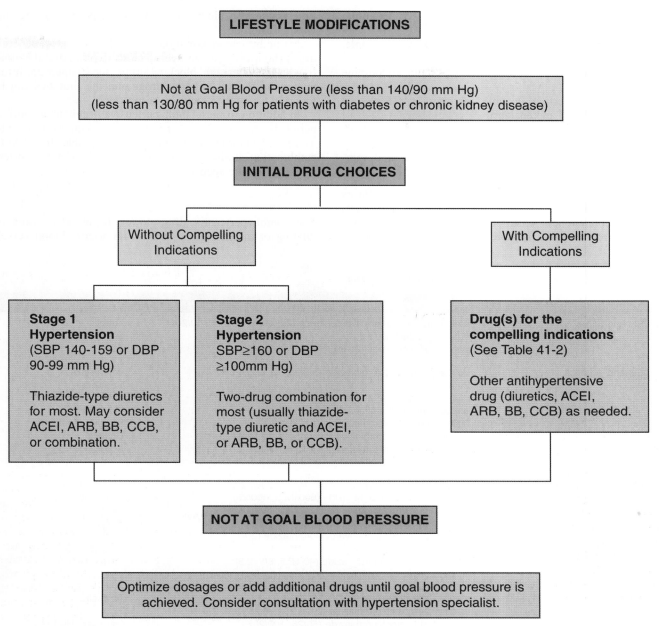

Figure 36.1 Algorithm for treatment of hypertension. Compelling Indicators include: HF, high risk for cardiovascular disease, post–myocardial infarction (MI), diabetes, stroke prevention, and chronic kidney disease. Key: DBP, diastolic blood pressure; SBP, systolic blood pressure; ACEI, angiotensin-converting enzyme inhibitor; ARB, angiotensin receptor blocker; BB, β blocker; CCB, calcium channel blocker; DBP, diastolic blood pressure; SBP, systolic blood pressure. (Adapted from National Heart Lung and Blood Institute [2003]. *The seventh report of the Joint National Committee on Prevention, Detection, Evaluation, and Treatment of High Blood Pressure.* Bethesda, MD: National Institutes of Health. Retrieved May 7, 2009, from http://www.nhlbi.nih.gov/guidelines/hypertension/.)

In some instances, it may be necessary to change to another antihypertensive drug or add a second antihypertensive drug when the patient does not experience a response to therapy. The primary health care provider also recommends that the patient continue with stress reduction, dietary modifications, and other lifestyle modifications needed for controlling hypertension. The types of drugs used for the treatment of hypertension include the following:

- Diuretics—for example, furosemide and hydrochlorothiazide
- B-adrenergic blocking drugs—for example, atenolol and propranolol

Antihypertensive Drugs

- Antiadrenergic drugs (centrally acting)—for example, clonidine and methyldopa
- Antiadrenergic drugs (peripherally acting)—for example, doxazosin and prazosin
- Calcium channel blocking drugs—for example, amlodipine and diltiazem
- Angiotensin-converting enzyme inhibitors (ACEIs)—for example, captopril and enalapril
- Angiotensin II receptor antagonists—for example, irbesartan and losartan
- Vasodilating drugs—for example, hydralazine and minoxidil

Two drug types are relatively new – direct renin inhibitors (aliskiren) and selective aldosterone receptor antagonists (SARAs; eplerenone). Aliskiren inhibits renin and subsequently prevents the angiotensin conversion process.

Eplerenone also blocks the angiotensin process by binding with aldosterone.

For additional information concerning the anti-adrenergic drugs (both centrally and peripherally acting), and the alpha (α)- and β-adrenergic blocking drugs, see Chapter 25. Information on the vasodilating drugs and the diuretics can be found in Chapters 37 and 48, respectively.

In addition to these antihypertensive drugs, many antihypertensive combinations are available, such as Capozide, Timolide, Aldoril, and Lopressor HCT (Table 36.2). Most combination antihypertensive drugs combine antihypertensive and diuretic agents.

Actions

Many antihypertensive drugs lower the blood pressure by dilating or increasing the size of the arterial blood vessels

Table 36.2 Examples of Antihypertensive Combinations

Combination Type	Fixed-Dose Combination, mg*	Trade Name
ACEIs and CCBs	amiodipine-benazepril hydrochloride (2.5/10, 5/10, 5/20, 10/20) enalapril-felodipine (5/5) trandolapril-verapamil (2/180, 1/240, 2/240, 4/240)	Lotrel Lexxel Tarka
ACEIs and diuretics	benazepril-hydrochlorothiazide (5/6.25, 10/12.5, 20/12.5, 20/25) captopril-hydrochlorothiazide (25/15, 25/25, 50/15, 50/25) enalapril-hydrochlorothiazide (5/12.5, 10/25) fosinopril-hydrochlorothiazide (10/12.5, 20/12.5) lisinopril-hydrochlorothiazide (10/12.5, 20/12.5, 20/25) moexipril-hydrochlorothiazide (7.5/12.5, 15/25) quinapril-hydrochlorothiazide (10/12.5, 20/12.5, 20/25)	Lotensin HCT Capozide Vaseretic Monopril/HCT Prinzide, Zestoretic Uniretic Accuretic
ARBs and diuretics	candesartan-hydrochlorothiazide (16/12.5, 32/12.5) eprosartan-hydrochlorothiazide (600/12.5, 600/25) irbesartan-hydrochlorothiazide (150/12.5, 300/12.5) losartan-hydrochlorothiazide (50/12.5, 100/25) olmesartan medoxomil- hydrochlorothiazide (20/12.5, 40/12.5, 40/25) telmisartan-hydrochlorothiazide (40/12.5, 80/12.5) valsartan-hydrochlorothiazide (80/12.5, 160/12.5, 160/25)	Atacand HCT Teveten-HCT Avalide Hyzaar Benicar HCT Micardis-HCT Diovan-HCT
BBs and diuretics	atenolol-chlorthalidone (50/25, 100/25) bisoprolol-hydrochlorothiazide (2.5/6.25, 5/6.25, 10/6.25) metoprolol-hydrochlorothiazide (50/25, 100/25) nadolol-bendroflumethiazide (40/5, 80/5) propranolol LA-hydrochlorothiazide (40/25, 80/25) timolol-hydrochlorothiazide (10/25)	Tenoretic Ziac Lopressor HCT Corzide Inderide LA Timolide
Centrally acting drug and diuretic	methyldopa-hydrochlorothiazide (250/15, 250/25, 500/30, 500/50) reserpine-chlorthalidone (0.125/25, 0.25/50) reserpine-chlorothiazide (0.125/250, 0.25/500) reserpine-hydrochlorothiazide (0.125/25, 0.125/50)	Aldoril Demi-Regroton, Regroton Diupres Hydropres
Diuretic and diuretic	amiloride-hydrochlorothiazide (5/50) spironolactone-hydrochlorothiazide (25/50, 50/50) triamterene-hydrochlorothiazide (37.5/25, 75/50)	Moduretic Aldactazide Dyazide, Maxzide

Drug abbreviations: BB, β-blocker; ACEI, angiotensin-converting enzyme inhibitor; ARB, angiotensin receptor blocker; CCB, calcium channel blocker.
*Some drug combinations are available in multiple fixed doses. Each drug dose is reported in milligrams.
Adapted from National Heart Lung and Blood Institute (2003). *The seventh report of the Joint National Committee on Prevention, Detection, Evaluation, and Treatment of High Blood Pressure*. Bethesda, MD: National Institutes of Health. Retrieved May 7, 2009, from http://www.nhlbi.nih.gov/guidelines/hypertension/.

(**vasodilation**). Vasodilation creates an increase in the **lumen** (the space or opening within a blood vessel) of the arterial blood vessels, which in turn increases the amount of space available for the blood to circulate. Because blood volume (the amount of blood) remains relatively constant, an increase in the space in which the blood circulates (i.e., the blood vessels) lowers the pressure of the fluid (measured as blood pressure) in the blood vessels. Although the method by which antihypertensive drugs dilate blood vessels varies, the result remains basically the same. Antihypertensive drugs that have vasodilating activity include the following:

- Adrenergic blocking drugs
- Calcium channel blocking drugs
- Vasodilating drugs

Another type of antihypertensive drug is the diuretic. The mechanism by which the diuretics reduce elevated blood pressure is unknown, but it is thought to be based, in part, on their ability to increase the excretion of sodium from the body. The actions and uses of diuretics are discussed in Chapter 48.

Action of Angiotensin-Converting Enzyme Inhibitors

The angiotensin-converting enzyme (ACE) inhibitors (ACEIs) appear to act primarily through suppression of the renin-angiotensin-aldosterone system. These drugs prevent (or inhibit) the activity of ACE, which converts angiotensin I to angiotensin II, a powerful vasoconstrictor. Both angiotensin I and ACE normally are manufactured by the body and are called **endogenous** substances. The vasoconstricting activity of angiotensin II stimulates the secretion of the endogenous hormone aldosterone by the adrenal cortex. Aldosterone promotes the retention of sodium and water, which may contribute to a rise in blood pressure. By preventing the conversion of angiotensin I to angiotensin II, this chain of events is interrupted, sodium and water are not retained, and blood pressure decreases (see Fig. 36.2).

Action of Calcium Channel Blockers

Systemic and coronary arteries are influenced by movement of calcium across cell membranes of vascular smooth muscle. The contractions of cardiac and vascular smooth muscle depend on movement of extracellular calcium ions into these walls through specific ion channels.

Calcium channel blockers act by inhibiting the movement of calcium ions across cell membranes of cardiac and arterial muscle cells. This results in less calcium available for the transmission of nerve impulses (see Fig. 36.2). As a result, these drugs relax blood vessels, increase the supply of oxygen to the heart, and reduce the heart's workload.

Action of Angiotensin II Receptor Antagonists

These drugs act to block the binding of angiotensin II at various receptor sites in the vascular smooth muscle and adrenal gland, which blocks the vasoconstrictive effect of the renin-angiotensin system and the release of aldosterone, resulting in a lowering of the blood pressure (see Fig. 36.2).

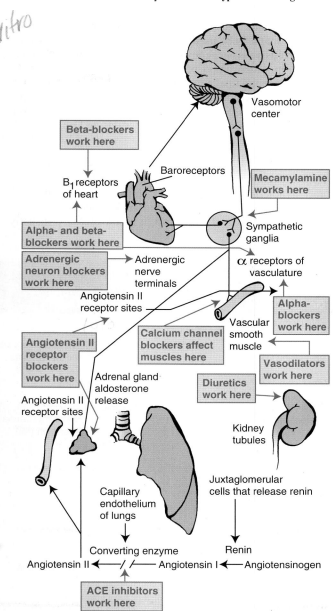

Figure 36.2 Sites of action of antihypertensive drugs.

Uses

Antihypertensive drugs are used in the treatment of hypertension. Although many antihypertensive drugs are available, not all drugs work equally well in a given patient. In some instances, the primary health care provider may find it necessary to prescribe a different antihypertensive drug when the patient does not experience a response to therapy. Some antihypertensive drugs are used only in severe cases of hypertension and when other, less potent drugs fail to lower the blood pressure. At times, two antihypertensive drugs may be given together to achieve a better response (see Fig. 36.1).

Antihypertensive Drugs

Nitroprusside (Nitropress) is an example of an intravenous (IV) drug that may be used to treat hypertensive emergencies. A **hypertensive emergency** is a case of extremely high blood pressure in which blood pressure must be lowered immediately to prevent damage to the target organs. Target organs of hypertension include the heart, kidney, and eyes (retinopathy). Additional uses of the antihypertensive drugs are given in the Summary Drug Table: Antihypertensive Drugs.

Adverse Reactions

When any antihypertensive drug is given, orthostatic (or postural) hypotension may result in some patients, especially early in therapy. **Orthostatic hypotension** occurs when the individual has a significant drop in blood pressure (usually 10 mm Hg systolic or more) when assuming an upright position. The patient can become dizzy and may fall resulting in an injury.

Central Nervous System Reactions

• Fatigue, depression, dizziness, headache, and syncope

Respiratory System Reactions

• Upper respiratory infections and cough

Gastrointestinal System Reactions

• Abdominal pain, nausea, diarrhea, constipation, gastric irritation, and anorexia

Summary Drug Table ANTIHYPERTENSIVE DRUGS

Generic Name	Trade Name	Uses	Adverse Reactions	Dosage Ranges
B-Adrenergic Blocking Drugs				
acebutolol ah-seh-byoo'-toe-loll	Sectral	Hypertension, ventricular arrhythmias	Bradycardia, dizziness, weakness, hypotension, nausea, vomiting, diarrhea, nervousness	Hypertension: 400 mg orally in 1–2 doses
atenolol ah-ten'-oh-loll	Tenormin, Tenoretic	Hypertension, angina, acute myocardial infarction (MI)	Bradycardia, dizziness, fatigue, weakness, hypotension, nausea, vomiting, diarrhea, nervousness	Hypertension/angina: 50–200 mg/day orally
betaxolol beh-tax'-oh-loll	Kerlone	Hypertension	Bradycardia, dizziness, hypotension, bronchospasm, nausea, vomiting, diarrhea, nervousness	10–20 mg/day orally, consider starting dose of 5 mg daily for elders
bisoprolol bye-soe'-proe-loll	Zebeta	Hypertension	Same as acebutolol	2.5–10 mg orally daily; maximum dose, 20 mg orally daily
carteolol kar'-tee-oh-loll		Hypertension	Same as acebutolol	2.5–10 mg/day orally
metoprolol meh-toe'-proe-loll	Lopressor, Toprol-XL	Hypertension, angina, MI, HF	Dizziness, hypotension, HF, cardiac arrhythmia, nausea, vomiting, diarrhea	Hypertension/angina: 100–450 mg/day orally; Extended release: 50–100 mg/day orally
nadolol nay-doe'-loll	Corgard	Hypertension, angina	Dizziness, hypotension nausea, vomiting, diarrhea, HF, cardiac arrhythmia	Hypertension: 40–80 mg/day orally
nebivolol neh-biv'-oh-loll	Bystolic	Hypertension	Dizziness, headache, nausea, diarrhea, tingling extremities	5–40 mg/daily
penbutolol pen-byoo'-toe-loll	Levatol	Hypertension	Bradycardia, dizziness, hypotension, nausea, vomiting, diarrhea	20 mg orally daily
pindolol pin'-doe-loll	Visken	Hypertension	Bradycardia, dizziness, hypotension, nausea, vomiting, diarrhea	5–60 mg/day orally BID

(table continues on page 333)

Summary Drug Table ANTIHYPERTENSIVE DRUGS (continued)

Generic Name	Trade Name	Uses	Adverse Reactions	Dosage Ranges
propranolol *pro-pran'-oh-loll*	Inderal	Cardiac arrhythmias, MI, angina, hypertension, migraine prophylaxis, hypertrophic subaortic stenosis, pheochromocytoma, primary tremor	Bradycardia, dizziness, hypotension, nausea, vomiting, diarrhea, bronchospasm, hyperglycemia, pulmonary edema	Hypertension: 120–240 mg/day orally in divided doses
timolol *tih'-moe-loll*	Blocadren	Hypertension, MI, migraine prophylaxis	Dizziness, hypotension, nausea, vomiting, diarrhea, pulmonary edema	Hypertension: 10–40 mg/day orally in divided doses MI: 10 mg orally BID
Antiadrenergic Drugs: Centrally Acting				
clonidine *kloe'-nih-deen*	Catapres, Catapres-TTS (transdermal)	Hypertension, Severe pain in patients with cancer ADHD	Drowsiness, dizziness, sedation, dry mouth, constipation, syncope, dreams, rash	100–600 mcg/day orally Transdermal: release rate 0.1–0.3 mg/24 hr
guanabenz *gwan'-ah-benz*		Hypertension	Dry mouth, sedation, dizziness, headache, weakness, arrhythmias	4–32 mg orally BID
guanfacine *gwan'-fah-seen*	Tenex	Hypertension	Dry mouth, somnolence, asthenia, dizziness, headache, constipation, fatigue	1–3 mg/day orally at bedtime
methyldopa or methyldopate *meth'-ill-doe-pah,* *meth'-ill-doe-pate*		Hypertension, hypertensive crisis	Bradycardia, aggravation of angina pectoris, HF, sedation, headache, rash, nausea, vomiting, nasal congestion	250 mg orally BID or TID; maintenance dose, 2 g/day; 250–500 mg q 6 hr IV
Antiadrenergic Drugs: Peripherally Acting				
doxazosin *dok-say-zoe'-sin*	Cardura	Hypertension, benign prostatic hyperplasia (BPH)	Headache, dizziness, fatigue	Hypertension: 1–8 mg orally daily; BPH: 1–16 mg orally daily
mecamylamine *mek-ah-mill'-ah-meen*	Inversine	Hypertension	Dizziness, syncope, dry mouth, nausea, constipation, urinary retention	2.5 mg orally BID
prazosin *pray-zoe'-sin*	Minipress	Hypertension	Dizziness, postural hypotension, drowsiness, headache, loss of strength, palpitation, nausea	1–20 mg orally daily in divided doses
reserpine *reh–ser'–pyne*	Serpalan	Hypertension, psychosis	Bradycardia, dizziness, nausea, vomiting, diarrhea, nasal congestion	Hypertension: 0.1–0.5 mg orally daily; psychosis: 0.1–1 mg orally daily
α/β-Adrenergic Blocking Drugs				
carvedilol *car-veh'-dih-loll*	Coreg	Hypertension, HF, left ventricular dysfunction (LVD)	Bradycardia, hypotension, cardiac insufficiency, fatigue, dizziness, diarrhea	6.25–25 mg orally BID
labetalol *lah-beh'-tah-loll*	Trandate	Hypertension	Fatigue, drowsiness, insomnia, hypotension, impotence, diarrhea	200–400 mg/day orally in divided doses IV: 20 mg over 2 min with blood pressure monitoring, may repeat

(table continues on page 334)

Summary Drug Table ANTIHYPERTENSIVE DRUGS (continued)

Generic Name	Trade Name	Uses	Adverse Reactions	Dosage Ranges
Calcium Channel Blockers				
amlodipine *am-loe'-dih-peen*	Norvasc	Hypertension, chronic stable angina, vasospastic angina (Prinzmetal's angina)	headache	Individualize dosage; 5–10 mg/day orally
diltiazem *dil-tye'-ah-zem*	Cardizem, Cardizem CD, Dilacor XR	Hypertension, chronic stable angina, atrial fibrillation/flutter, paroxysmal superventricular tachycardia	Headache, dizziness, atrioventricular block, bradycardia, edema, dyspnea, rhinitis	Extended Release Tablets/Capsules – hypertension: 120–540 mg/day
felodipine *fell-oh'-dih-peen*	Plendil	Hypertension	Headache, dizziness	2.5–10 mg/day orally
isradipine *iz-rah'-dih-peen*	DynaCirc, DynaCirc CR	Hypertension	Headache, edema	5–10 mg/day orally
nicardipine *nye-kar'-dih-peen*	Cardene, Cardene IV, Cardene SR	Hypertension, chronic stable angina	Headache	Hypertension: immediate release 20–40 mg/TID; extended release 30–60 mg/BID
nifedipine *nye-fed'-ih-peen*	Adalat, Procardia, Procardia XL	Hypertension (sustained-release only), vasospastic angina, chronic stable angina,	Headache, dizziness, weakness, edema, nausea, muscle cramps, cough, nasal congestion, wheezing	10–20 mg TID orally; may increase to 120 mg/day Sustained-release: 30–60 mg/d orally; may increase to 120 mg/day
nisoldipine *nye-sole'-dih-peen*	Sular	Hypertension	Headache, edema	20–40 mg/day orally
verapamil *ver-app'-ah-mill*	Calan, Calan SR, Isoptin, Isoptin SR, Verelan	Hypertension, chronic stable angina, vasospastic angina, chronic atrial flutter, paroxysmal superventricular tachycardia	Headache, constipation	Individualize dosage; do not exceed 480 mg/day orally in divided doses Sustained-release: 120–180 mg/day orally; maximum dose, 480 mg Extended-release: 120–180 mg/day orally, maximum dose, 480 mg/day
Angiotensin-Converting Enzyme Inhibitors Pril				
benazepril *ben-ah'-zeh-prill*	Lotensin	Hypertension	Headache, dizziness, fatigue	10–40 mg/day orally in single dose or two divided doses, maximum dose 80 mg
Ⓡ captopril *kap'-toe-prill*	Capoten	Hypertension, HF, LVD after MI, diabetic nephropathy	Rash	Hypertension: 25–100 mg/day orally in divided doses, not to exceed 450 mg/day
enalapril *eh-nal'-ah-prill*	Vasotec, Enalaprilat	Hypertension, HF, asymptomatic LVD	Headache, dizziness	Hypertension: 5–40 mg/day orally as a single dose or in two divided doses; CHF: 2.5–20 mg BID
fosinopril *foh-sin'-oh-prill*	Monopril	Hypertension, HF	Dizziness, cough	10–40 mg/day orally in a single dose or two divided doses

(table continues on page 335)

Summary Drug Table ANTIHYPERTENSIVE DRUGS (continued)

Generic Name	Trade Name	Uses	Adverse Reactions	Dosage Ranges
lisinopril *lye-sin'-oh-prill*	Prinivil, Zestril	Hypertension, HF, post-MI	Headache, dizziness, diarrhea, orthostatic hypotension, cough	Hypertension: 10–40 mg/day orally as a single dose
Ⓡ moexipril *moe-ex'-ah-prill*	Univasc	Hypertension	Dizziness, cough, bronchospasm	7.5–30 mg orally as a single dose or two divided doses
perindopril *per-in'-doh-prill*	Aceon	Hypertension	Dizziness, headache, cough, upper respiratory infection (URI) symptoms, asthenia	4–8 mg/day orally, maximum dose 16 mg
quinapril *kwin'-ah-prill*	Accupril	Hypertension, HF	Dizziness	Hypertension: 10–80 mg/day orally as a single dose or two divided doses
ramipril *rah-mih'-prill*	Altace	Hypertension, HF, decrease risk of cardiovascular disease, coronary artery disease	Dizziness, cough	Hypertension: 2.5–20 mg/day orally as a single dose or two divided doses
trandolapril *tran-dole'-ah-prill*	Mavik	Hypertension, patients post-MI with symptoms of HF and LVD	Dizziness, cough	Hypertension: 1–4 mg/day orally
Angiotensin II Receptor Antagonists				
candesartan *can-dah-sar'-tan*	Atacand	Hypertension, HF	Dizziness, URI symptoms	8–32 mg/day orally in divided doses
eprosartan *ep-roe-sar'-tan*	Teveten	Hypertension	Cough, URI, and urinary tract infection symptoms	400–800 mg/day orally in two divided doses
irbesartan *er-beh-sar'-tan*	Avapro	Hypertension, nephropathy in type 2 diabetes	Headache, URI symptoms	150–300 mg/day orally as one dose
losartan *loe-sar'-tan*	Cozaar	Hypertension, hypertension in patients with LVD, diabetic nephropathy in type 2 diabetes	Dizziness, URI symptoms	Hypertension: 25–100 mg/day orally in one or two doses
olmesartan *ol-mah-sar'-tan*	Benicar	Hypertension	Dizziness	20–40 mg/day orally
telmisartan *tell-mah-sar'-tan*	Micardis	Hypertension	Diarrhea, URI symptoms, sinusitis	40–80 mg/day orally
valsartan *val-sar'-tan*	Diovan	Hypertension, HF, post-MI	Viral infections	Hypertension: 80–320 mg/day orally
Direct Renin Inhibitors				
aliskiren *ah-liss-kye'-ren*	Tekturna	Hypertension	Diarrhea, URI symptoms	150 mg/day orally, may increase to 300 mg/day
Selective Aldosterone Receptor Antagonists				
eplerenone *eh-pler'-eh-noan*	Inspra	Hypertension, HF	Hyperkalemia	50 mg/day orally, may increase to 100 mg/day

(table continues on page 336)

Summary Drug Table ANTIHYPERTENSIVE DRUGS (continued)

Generic Name	Trade Name	Uses	Adverse Reactions	Dosage Ranges
Peripheral Vasodilators				
hydralazine *hye-drah'-lah-zeen*	Apresoline	Primary hypertension (oral) When need to lower blood pressure is urgent (parenteral)	Dizziness, palpitations, tachycardia, numb/tingling in legs, nasal congestion	10–50 mg QID orally, up to 300 mg/day; 20–40 mg IM or IV
minoxidil *mih-nok'-sih-dill*	Loniten	Severe hypertension	Dizziness, hypotension, electrocardiogram changes, tachycardia, sodium and water retention, gynecomastia, hair growth	5–100 mg/d orally; dose greater than 5 mg given in divided doses
nitroprusside *nye-troe-pruss'-syde*	Nitropress	Hypertensive crisis	Apprehension, headache, restlessness, nausea, vomiting, palpitations, diaphoresis	3 mcg/kg/min, not to exceed infusion rate of 10 mcg/min (if blood pressure is not reduced within 10 min, discontinue administration)

Ⓡ This drug should be administered at least 1 hour before or 2 hours after a meal.

Other Reactions

- Rash, pruritus, dry mouth, tachycardia, hypotension, proteinuria, and neutropenia

Additional adverse reactions that may occur when an antihypertensive drug is administered are listed in the Summary Drug Table: Antihypertensive Drugs. For the adverse reactions that may result when a diuretic is used as an antihypertensive drug, see the Summary Drug Table: Diuretics in Chapter 48.

Contraindications

Antihypertensive drugs are contraindicated in patients with known hypersensitivity to the individual drugs.

The ACEIs and angiotensin II receptor blockers are contraindicated if the patient has impaired renal function, HF, salt or volume depletion, bilateral stenosis, or angioedema. They are also contraindicated during pregnancy (category C during first trimester and category D in the second and third trimesters) or during lactation. Use of the ACEIs and the angiotensin II receptor blockers during the second and third trimesters of pregnancy is contraindicated, because use may cause fetal and neonatal injury or death.

Calcium channel blockers are contraindicated in patients who are hypersensitive to the drugs and those with sick sinus syndrome, second- or third-degree atrioventricular (AV) block (except with a functioning pacemaker), hypotension (systolic pressure less than 90 mm Hg), ventricular dysfunction, or cardiogenic shock.

HERBAL ALERT

Hawthorn, one of the most commonly used natural agents to treat various cardiovascular problems such as hypertension, angina, arrhythmias, and HF, is known for its masses of white, strong-smelling flowers. They are used, along with the fruit and leaves of the plant, in the form of capsules, fluid extract, tea, tinctures, and topical creams. Hawthorn should not be administered to individuals who are pregnant, breastfeeding, or allergic to the agent. Possible adverse reactions include hypotension, arrhythmias, sedation, nausea, and anorexia. Possible drug–hawthorn interactions include a risk of hypotension when hawthorn is used with other antihypertensive drugs, possible increased effects of inotropic drugs when inotropic drugs are administered with hawthorn, and increased risk of sedative effects when hawthorn is administered with other central nervous system (CNS) depressants. As with all substances, hawthorn should be used only under the supervision of the primary health care provider.

Precautions

Antihypertensive drugs are used cautiously in patients with renal or hepatic impairment or electrolyte imbalances, during lactation and pregnancy, and in older patients. The calcium channel blockers are used cautiously in patients with HF or renal or hepatic impairment. The calcium channel blockers are used cautiously during pregnancy (category C) and lactation. ACEIs are used cautiously in patients with sodium depletion, hypovolemia, or coronary or cerebrovascular insufficiency and in those receiving diuretic therapy or dialysis. The angiotensin II receptor agonists are used cautiously in patients with renal or hepatic dysfunction, hypovolemia, or volume or salt depletion, and in patients receiving high doses of diuretics.

Interactions

The hypotensive effects of most antihypertensive drugs are increased when administered with diuretics and other antihypertensives. Many drugs can interact with the antihypertensive drugs and decrease their effectiveness (e.g., monoamine oxidase inhibitor antidepressants, antihistamines, and sympathomimetic bronchodilators).

The following interactions may occur when the calcium channel blockers are used with another agent:

Interacting Drug	Common Use	Effect of Interaction
cimetidine or ranitidine	GI disorders	Increased effects of calcium channel blockers
theophylline	Control of asthma and chronic obstructive pulmonary disease	Increased pharmacologic and toxic effects of theophylline
digoxin	HF	Increased risk for digitalis toxicity
rifampin	Antitubercular agent	Decreased effect of calcium channel blocker

Patients may not volunteer information regarding their use of alternative or complementary remedies. The nurse should always inquire about use of herbal products. Medical reports indicate a possible interaction with St. John's wort, used to relieve depression, causing a decrease in serum levels of calcium channel blockers.

The following interactions may occur when ACEI drugs are administered with another agent:

Interacting Drug	Common Use	Effect of Interaction
nonsteroidal anti-inflammatory drugs (NSAIDs)	Relief of pain and inflammation	Reduced hypotensive effects of the ACEIs
rifampin	Antitubercular agent	Decreased pharmacologic effect of ACEIs (particularly of enalapril)
allopurinol	Antigout agent	Higher risk of hypersensitivity reaction
digoxin	Management of HF	Increased or decreased plasma digoxin levels
loop diuretics	Reduce/eliminate edema	Decreased diuretic effects

Interacting Drug	Common Use	Effect of Interaction
lithium	Management of bipolar disorder	Increased serum lithium levels, possible lithium toxicity
hypoglycemic agents and insulin	Management of diabetes	Increased risk of hypoglycemia
potassium-sparing diuretics or potassium preparations	Diuretics: reduce blood pressure and edema / Potassium preparations: control of low serum potassium levels	Elevated serum potassium level

The following interactions may occur when angiotensin II receptor antagonists are administered with other agents:

Interacting Drug	Common Use	Effect of Interaction
fluconazole	Antifungal agent	Increased antihypertensive and adverse effects (particularly with losartan)
indomethacin	Pain relief	Decreased hypotensive effect (particularly with losartan)

NURSING PROCESS
PATIENT RECEIVING AN ANTIHYPERTENSIVE DRUG

ASSESSMENT

Preadministration Assessment
Before therapy with an antihypertensive drug starts, the nurse assesses the blood pressure (Fig. 36.3) and pulse rate on both arms with the patient in standing, sitting, and lying positions. The nurse correctly identifies all pressures (e.g., the pressure readings on each arm and the three positions used to obtain the readings) and records these on the patient's chart. The nurse also obtains the patient's weight, especially if a diuretic is part of therapy or if the primary health care provider prescribes a weight-loss regimen.

Ongoing Assessment
Monitoring and recording the blood pressure is an important part of the ongoing assessment, especially early in therapy. The primary health care provider may need to adjust the dose of the drug upward or downward, try a different drug, or add another drug to the therapeutic regimen if the patient's response to drug therapy is inadequate.

Each time the blood pressure is measured, the nurse uses the same arm with the patient in the same position (e.g., standing, sitting, or lying down). In some instances, the primary health care provider may order the blood pressure taken in one or more positions, such as standing and lying down. The nurse monitors the blood pressure and pulse every 15 to 30 minutes if the patient has severe hypertension, does not have the expected response to drug therapy, or is critically ill.

❗ NURSING ALERT

The blood pressure and pulse rate must be obtained immediately before each administration of an antihypertensive drug and compared with previous readings. If the blood pressure is significantly decreased from baseline values, the nurse should not give the drug but should notify the primary health care provider. In addition, the primary health care provider must be notified if there is a significant increase in the blood pressure.

The nurse obtains daily weights during the initial period of drug therapy. Patients taking an antihypertensive drug occasionally retain sodium and water, resulting in edema and weight gain. The nurse assesses the patient's weight and examines the extremities for edema. The nurse reports a weight gain of 2 lb or more per day and any evidence of edema in the hands, fingers, feet, legs, or sacral area. The patient is also weighed at regular intervals if a weight-reduction diet is used to lower the blood pressure or if the patient is receiving a thiazide or related diuretic as part of antihypertensive therapy.

In the ambulatory setting, the nurse helps plan a schedule of regular self monitoring of weight and blood pressure. The nurse teaches the patient to record weight and blood pressure readings, and to find local resources for taking blood pressures in the community. The patient is instructed to bring these records in to the primary care provider at each appointment.

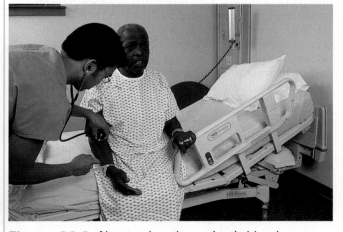

Figure 36.3 Nurse takes the patient's blood pressure before administering an antihypertensive drug.

NURSING DIAGNOSES

Drug-specific nursing diagnoses include the following:

- ❏ **Risk for Deficient Fluid Volume** related to excessive diuresis secondary to administration of a diuretic
- ❏ **Risk for Injury** related to dizziness or light-headedness secondary to postural or orthostatic hypotensive episodes
- ❏ **Risk for Ineffective Sexuality Patterns** related to impotence secondary to effects of antihypertensive drugs
- ❏ **Risk for Activity Intolerance** related to fatigue and weakness
- ❏ **Pain** (acute headache) related to antihypertensive drugs

Nursing diagnoses related to drug administration are discussed in Chapter 4.

PLANNING

The expected outcomes for the patient may include an optimal response to therapy (blood pressure maintained in an acceptable range), support of patient needs related to managing adverse reactions, and an understanding of the therapeutic regimen.

IMPLEMENTATION

Promoting an Optimal Response to Therapy

ADMINISTERING ANTIADRENERGIC DRUGS. Clonidine is available as an oral tablet (Catapres) and transdermal patch (Catapres-TTS). The nurse applies the transdermal patch to a hairless area of intact skin on the upper arm or torso; the patch is kept in place for 7 days. The adhesive overlay is applied directly over the system to ensure the patch remains in place for the required time. A different body area is selected for each application. If the patch loosens before 7 days, the edges can be reinforced with nonallergenic tape. The date the patch was placed and the date the patch is to be removed can be written on the surface of the patch with a fiber-tipped pen. (See Chapter 25 for additional information concerning the antiadrenergic drugs.)

ADMINISTERING CALCIUM CHANNEL BLOCKERS. The nurse may give these drugs without regard to meals. If gastrointestinal (GI) upset occurs, the drug may be administered with meals. Verapamil is best given with meals because of the tendency of this drug to cause gastric upset. The sustained-release capsules should not be crushed, opened, or chewed. Verapamil capsules (not sustained-release) may be opened, and the contents sprinkled in liquid or on soft foods. Diltiazem may be crushed and mixed with food or fluids for patients who have difficulty swallowing.

ADMINISTERING ACEIs. The nurse administers captopril and moexipril 1 hour before or 2 hours after meals to enhance absorption. Some patients taking an ACEI experience a dry cough that does not subside until the drug therapy is discontinued. This reaction may need to be tolerated. If the cough becomes too bothersome, the primary health care provider may discontinue use of the drug. The nurse should ensure that the patient is not pregnant before beginning therapy. These medications can cause fetal death in the second or third trimester of pregnancy. The patient should use a reliable birth control method such as barrier birth control while taking these drugs. If pregnancy is suspected, the primary health care provider is notified immediately.

The ACEIs may cause a significant drop in blood pressure after the first dose. This effect can be minimized if the primary health care provider discontinues the diuretic therapy (if the patient is taking a diuretic) or begins treatment with small doses. After the first dose of an ACEI, the nurse monitors the blood pressure every 15 to 30 minutes for at least 2 hours and afterward until the blood pressure is stable for 1 hour.

LIFESPAN ALERT – Menopause
Women experiencing the start of menopause may have irregular ovulation and periods. Some women are reluctant to use birth control as they age, because they feel they are not capable of becoming pregnant. Because the ACE inhibitors and angiotensin II receptor antagonists can cause injury and death to a developing fetus, it is important to teach the hypertensive woman who is entering menopause that pregnancy can still occur. Birth control measures should be discussed. Should a woman taking the aforementioned hypertensive medicines become pregnant, medications should be discontinued immediately.

ADMINISTERING ANGIOTENSIN II RECEPTOR ANTAGONISTS. These drugs can be administered without regard to meals. It is important to ensure that the patient is not pregnant before beginning therapy. The nurse recommends that the patient use a reliable birth control method such as barrier birth control while taking these drugs. As with the ACEIs, these medications can cause fetal death in the second or third trimester of pregnancy. If pregnancy is suspected, the primary health care provider is notified immediately.

ADMINISTERING DIRECT RENIN INHIBITORS OR SARAs. These drugs may be taken without regard to food, although absorption of aliskiren is limited when a high fat diet is taken. As with the ACEIs, direct renin inhibitors can cause fetal death in the second or third trimester of pregnancy. If pregnancy is suspected, the primary health care provider is notified immediately. Increased serum potassium, **hyperkalemia**, can occur with these medications; therefore, the nurse should teach the patient to refrain from using potassium-based salt substitutes in the preparation of foods.

NURSING ALERT
Advise patients that **angioedema** may occur at any time when taking aliskiren. If the patient experiences swelling of the face, throat, or extremities, he or she should hold the next dose of medication and call his or her primary health care provider immediately to report symptoms and instruction regarding antihypertensive treatment.

ADMINISTERING VASODILATING DRUGS. The nurse must carefully monitor the patient receiving minoxidil, because the drug increases the heart rate. The primary health care provider is notified if any of the following occur:

- Heart rate of 20 bpm or more above the normal rate
- Rapid weight gain of 5 lb or more
- Unusual swelling of the extremities, face, or abdomen
- Dyspnea, angina, severe indigestion, or fainting

ADMINISTERING DRUGS FOR HYPERTENSIVE EMERGENCIES. Nitroprusside is used to treat patients with a hypertensive emergency. When these drugs are used, hemodynamic monitoring of the patient's blood pressure and cardiovascular status is required throughout the course of therapy.

LIFESPAN ALERT – Gerontology
Older adults are particularly sensitive to the hypotensive effects of nitroprusside. To minimize hypotensive effects, the drug is initially given in lower dosages. Older adults require more frequent monitoring during the administration of nitroprusside.

Monitoring and Managing Patient Needs
The nurse observes the patient for adverse drug reactions, because their occurrence may require a change in the dose of the drug. The nurse should notify the primary health care provider if any adverse reactions occur. In some instances, the patient may have to tolerate mild adverse reactions, such as dry mouth or mild anorexia.

NURSING ALERT
If it becomes necessary to discontinue antihypertensive therapy, the nurse should never discontinue use of the drug abruptly. The primary health care provider will prescribe the parameters by which the dosage is to be discontinued. The dosage is usually gradually reduced over 2 to 4 days to avoid rebound hypertension (a rapid rise in blood pressure).

DEFICIENT FLUID VOLUME. The patient receiving a diuretic is observed for dehydration and electrolyte imbalances. A fluid volume deficit is most likely to occur if the patient fails to drink a sufficient amount of fluid. This is especially true in the elderly or confused patient. To prevent a fluid volume deficit, the nurse encourages patients to drink adequate oral fluids (up to 2000 mL/day, unless contraindicated because of a medical condition). This is especially important when a person excessively perspires or has episodes of vomiting or diarrhea.

Electrolyte imbalances that may occur during therapy with a diuretic include **hyponatremia** (low blood sodium level) and **hypokalemia** (low blood potassium level), although other imbalances may also be seen. (See Chapter 55 for the signs and symptoms of electrolyte imbalances.) When administering aliskiren or eplerenone, the nurse should monitor for hyperkalemia. The primary health care provider is notified if any signs or symptoms of an electrolyte imbalance occur.

RISK FOR INJURY. Dizziness or weakness along with orthostatic hypotension can occur with the administration of antihypertensive drugs. If orthostatic hypotension occurs, the nurse advises the patient to rise slowly from a sitting or lying position. The nurse explains that when rising from a lying position, sitting on the edge of the bed for 1 or 2 minutes often minimizes these symptoms. In addition, rising slowly from a chair and then standing for 1 to 2 minutes also minimizes the symptoms of orthostatic hypotension. When symptoms of orthostatic hypotension, dizziness, or weakness do occur, the nurse can assist the patient in getting out of bed or a chair and with ambulatory activities.

INEFFECTIVE SEXUALITY PATTERNS. Antihypertensive drugs can cause sexual dysfunction ranging from impotence to inhibition of ejaculation. The nurse must provide an open and understanding atmosphere when discussing sexuality. The nurse explains potential problems with sexual patterns that can occur with these drugs. If sexual patterns are affected negatively, suggest that the partners use other means of expressing caring, such as touching, massage, and personal closeness. The nurse allows the patient time to express feelings and concerns and encourages the patient and partner to discuss ways to satisfy intimacy needs. The nurse can suggest that the patient discuss the use of drugs for erectile dysfunction (ED) with the primary care provider. Many ED medications are safe to take with antihypertensives.

ACTIVITY INTOLERANCE. Some patients on the antihypertensive drugs have decreased exercise tolerance and feel fatigued, weak, and lethargic. In addition, patients with hypertension may have other health problems (either cardiovascular or respiratory problems) that may affect their ability to perform activities. The patient is encouraged to walk and ambulate as he or she can tolerate. Assistive devices may be used if needed. Gradually increase tolerance by increasing the daily amount of activity. Plan rest periods according to the individual's tolerance. Rest can take many forms, such as sitting in a chair, napping, watching television, or sitting with legs elevated. The nurse should inform the patient that often the fatigue diminishes after 4 to 6 weeks of therapy.

ACUTE PAIN. Patients taking the antihypertensive drugs may complain of a headache that could be an adverse reaction to the drugs, particularly antiadrenergics or the angiotensin II receptor blocking drugs. If the headache is acute, the patient may need to remain in bed with a cool cloth on the forehead, or the nurse may give the patient a back and neck rub. Relaxation techniques such as guided imagery or progressive body relaxation may prove helpful. If nursing measures are not successful, the primary health care provider is notified, because an analgesic may be required.

Educating the Patient and Family

Nurses can do much to educate others on the importance of having their blood pressure checked at periodic inter-

vals. This includes people of all ages, because hypertension is not a disease that affects only older individuals. Once hypertension is detected, patient teaching becomes an important factor in successfully returning the blood pressure to normal or near-normal levels.

To ensure lifetime compliance with the prescribed therapeutic regimen, the nurse emphasizes the importance of drug therapy, as well as other treatments recommended by the primary health care provider. The nurse describes the adverse reactions from a particular antihypertensive drug and advises the patient to contact the primary health care provider if any should occur.

The primary health care provider will want the patient or family to monitor blood pressure during therapy. The nurse teaches the technique of taking a blood pressure and pulse rate to the patient or family member, allowing sufficient time for supervised practice. If the patient or family is unable to do this, the nurse provides community resources where blood pressures are checked, such as local pharmacies or fire stations. The nurse instructs the patient to keep a record of the blood pressure and to bring this record to each visit to the primary health care provider's office or clinic. A wallet-size card can be obtained for use from the National Institutes of Health at http://www.nhlbi.nih.gov/health/public/heart/hbp/hbpwal-let.htm.

The nurse includes the following points in a teaching plan for the patient receiving an antihypertensive drug:

- Never discontinue use of this drug except on the advice of the primary health care provider. These drugs control but do not cure hypertension. Skipping doses of the drug or voluntarily discontinuing the drug may cause severe rebound hypertension.
- Avoid the use of any nonprescription drugs (some may contain drugs that can increase the blood pressure) unless approved by the primary health care provider.
- Avoid alcohol unless its use has been approved by the primary health care provider.
- This drug may produce dizziness or lightheadedness when rising suddenly from a sitting or lying position. To avoid these effects, rise slowly from a sitting or lying position (see Patient Teaching for Improved Patient Outcomes: Preventing Orthostatic Hypotension).
- If the drug causes drowsiness, avoid hazardous tasks such as driving or performing tasks that require alertness. Drowsiness may disappear with time.
- If unexplained weakness or fatigue occurs, contact the primary health care provider.
- Follow the diet restrictions recommended by the primary health care provider. Do not use salt substitutes unless a particular brand of salt substitute is approved by the primary health care provider.
- Notify the primary health care provider if the diastolic pressure suddenly increases to 130 mm Hg or higher; this may signal a hypertensive emergency.

EVALUATION

- Therapeutic response is achieved and blood pressure is controlled.
- Adverse reactions are identified, reported to the primary health care provider, and managed successfully with appropriate nursing interventions:
  - ☑ Proper fluid volume is maintained.
  - ☑ No evidence of injury is seen.
  - ☑ Patient is satisfied with sexual activity.
  - ☑ Patient engages in activity as able.
  - ☑ Patient is free of headache pain
- Patient and family demonstrate an understanding of the drug regimen.

Patient Teaching for Improved Patient Outcomes

Preventing Injury due to Orthostatic Hypotension

Many patients receiving antihypertensive therapy commonly receive more than one drug, placing them at risk for orthostatic hypotension. If it occurs, the patient may fall and be injured, so teach the following measures to follow while in the acute care facility and at home:

✓ Change your position slowly.
✓ Sit at the edge of the bed or chair for a few minutes before standing up.
✓ Stand for a few minutes before starting to walk.
✓ Ask for assistance when necessary.
✓ If you feel dizzy or lightheaded, sit or lie down immediately.
✓ Make sure to drink adequate amounts of fluid throughout the day.

THINK CRITICALLY: PHARMACOLOGY IN PRACTICE

1. Lillian Chase is feeling a lack of control due to the lifestyle changes she must make to manage both asthma and hypertension. She asks, "... what is the point of living when you can't eat the foods you love?" Mrs. Chase has been prescribed a selective aldosterone receptor antagonist for blood pressure control. Do an internet search to see what types of seasonings you can recommend that she use in cooking to enhance the flavors of foods.

2. The primary health care provider asks you to explain to a patient how to monitor blood pressure readings weekly. Access the website provided earlier and download a copy of the wallet-size card. When talking to the patient, you discover that he understands little English. Discuss how you might communicate to this patient how he should monitor weekly blood pressures.

● Test Your Knowledge

1. The nurse instructs the patient using the transdermal system Catapres TTS to _____.

   A. place the patch on the torso and keep it in place for 24 hours
   B. change placement of the patch every day after bathing
   C. place the patch on the upper arm or torso and keep it in place for 7 days
   D. avoid getting the patch wet because it might detach from the skin

2. To avoid symptoms associated with orthostatic hypotension, the nurse advises the patient to _____.

   A. sleep in a side-lying position
   B. avoid sitting for prolong periods
   C. change position slowly
   D. get up from a sitting position quickly

3. After the first dose of an ACEI, the nurse monitors _____.

   A. the patient for a hypotensive crisis
   B. the vital signs every 4 hours or more often if the patient reports being dizzy
   C. the blood pressure every hour until it is stable
   D. the blood pressure every 15 to 30 minutes for at least 2 hours

4. During the preadministration assessment of a patient prescribed an antihypertensive drug, the nurse _____.

   A. places the patient in a high Fowler's position
   B. places the patient in a supine position
   C. darkens the room to decrease stimuli
   D. takes the patient's blood pressure

● Prepare for the NCLEX

1. The nurse gives the following instruction to the patient when discontinuing use of an antihypertensive drug.

   A. monitor the blood pressure every hour for 8 hours after the drug therapy is discontinued
   B. gradually decrease the medication over a period of 2 to 4 days to avoid rebound hypertension
   C. check the blood pressure and pulse every 30 minutes after discontinuing the drug therapy

D. expect to taper the dosage of the drug over a period of 2 weeks to avoid a return of hypertension

● Calculate Medication Dosages

1. Oral nadolol 80 mg is prescribed. The drug is available in 20-mg tablets. The nurse administers _____.

2. Diltiazem 180 mg is prescribed. The drug is available in 60-mg, 90-mg, and 120-mg tablets.

Which tablet would you select? _____

How many tablets would you administer? _____

To check your answers, see Appendix E.

thePoint. *For more NCLEX questions, log on to http://thepoint.lww.com to access more than 1000 questions.*

Antianginal Drugs

angina
atherosclerosis
buccal
lumen
prophylaxis

sublingual
topical
transdermal systems
vasodilation

LEARNING OBJECTIVES

On completion of this chapter, the student will:

1. List the two types of antianginal drugs.
2. Discuss the general actions, uses, adverse reactions, contraindications, precautions, and interactions of antianginal drugs.
3. Discuss important preadministration and ongoing assessment activities the nurse should perform on the patient taking an antianginal drug.
4. List nursing diagnoses particular to a patient taking an antianginal drug.
5. Discuss ways to promote an optimal response to therapy, how to manage common adverse reactions, and important points to keep in mind when educating patients about the use of antianginal drugs.

Diseases of the arteries can cause serious problems: namely, coronary artery disease, cerebral vascular disease, and peripheral vascular disease. Drug therapy for vascular diseases may include drugs that dilate blood vessels and thereby increase blood supply to an area.

Atherosclerosis is a disease characterized by deposits of fatty plaques on the inner wall of arteries. These deposits result in a narrowing of the **lumen** (inside diameter) of the artery and a decrease in blood supply to the area served by the artery.

This chapter discusses drugs whose primary purpose is to increase blood supply to an area by dilating blood vessels around the heart. Vasodilating drugs relax the smooth muscle layer of arterial blood vessels, which results in **vasodilation**, an increase in the size of blood vessels, primarily small arteries and arterioles. Because peripheral, cerebral, or coronary artery disease usually results in decreased blood flow to an area, drugs that dilate narrowed arterial vessels permit the vessels to carry more blood, resulting in an increase in blood flow

to the affected area. Increasing the blood flow to an area may result in complete or partial relief of symptoms. Vasodilating drugs sometimes relieve the symptoms of vascular disease. In some cases, however, drug therapy provides only minimal and temporary relief. Many of the calcium channel blockers and vasodilating drugs are also used to treat hypertension. Their use as antihypertensives is discussed in Chapter 36.

• ANTIANGINAL DRUGS

Angina is a disorder characterized by atherosclerotic plaque formation in the coronary arteries, which causes decreased oxygen supply to the heart muscle and results in chest pain or pressure. Any activity that increases the workload of the heart, such as exercise or simply climbing stairs, can precipitate an angina attack. Antianginal drugs relieve chest pain or pressure by dilating coronary arteries, increasing the blood supply to the myocardium.

The antianginal drugs include the nitrates and the calcium channel blockers. Chapter 25 and its Summary Drug Table: Adrenergic Blocking Drugs discuss the adrenergic blocking drugs that also are used to treat angina and other disorders.

Actions

Nitrates and Calcium Channel Blockers

The nitrates act by relaxing the smooth muscle layer of blood vessels, increasing the lumen of the artery or arteriole, and increasing the amount of blood flowing through the vessels. An increased blood flow results in an increase in the oxygen supply to surrounding tissues.

Calcium channel blockers have several effects on the heart:

- Slowing the conduction velocity of the cardiac impulse
- Depressing myocardial contractility
- Dilating coronary arteries and arterioles, which in turn deliver more oxygen to cardiac muscle

Dilation of peripheral arteries reduces the workload of the heart. The end effect of these drugs is the same as that of the nitrates.

Uses

The antianginal drugs are used in the treatment of cardiac disease to:

- Relieve pain of acute anginal attacks
- Prevent angina attacks (**prophylaxis**)
- Treat chronic stable angina pectoris

Intravenous (IV) nitroglycerin is used to control perioperative hypertension associated with surgical procedures. Calcium channel blocking drugs are used to treat hypertension (see Chapter 36) and have additional uses. For example, verapamil affects the conduction system of the heart and is used to treat cardiac arrhythmias. See the Summary Drug Table: Antianginal Drugs for additional uses of the nitrates and calcium channel blockers.

Adverse Reactions

Adverse reactions to the calcium channel blocking drugs usually are not serious and rarely require discontinuation of the drug therapy (see Chapter 36 for specifics). Adverse reactions associated with the nitrates include the following:

- Central nervous system (CNS) reactions, such as headache (may be severe and persistent), dizziness, weakness, and restlessness
- Other body system reactions, such as hypotension, flushing (caused by dilation of small capillaries near the surface of the skin), and rash

The nitrates are available in various forms (e.g., **sublingual**, translingual spray, transdermal, and parenteral). Some adverse reactions are a result of the method of administration. For example, sublingual nitroglycerin may cause a local burning or tingling in the oral cavity. However, the patient must be aware that an absence of this effect does not indicate a decrease in the drug's potency. Contact dermatitis may occur from use of the transdermal delivery system.

In many instances, the adverse reactions associated with the nitrates lessen and often disappear with prolonged use of the drug. However, for some patients, these adverse reactions become severe, and the primary health care provider may lower the dose until symptoms subside. The dose may then be slowly increased if the lower dosage does not provide relief from the symptoms of angina. See the Summary Drug Table: Antianginal Drugs for more information.

Contraindications and Precautions

Nitrates are contraindicated in patients with known hypersensitivity to the drugs, severe anemia, closed-angle glaucoma, postural hypertension, early myocardial infarction (sublingual form), head trauma, cerebral hemorrhage (may increase intracranial hemorrhage), allergy to adhesive (transdermal system), or constrictive pericarditis. Patients taking phospho-

Summary Drug Table ANTIANGINAL DRUGS

Generic Name	Trade Name	Uses	Adverse Reactions	Dosage Ranges
Nitrates				
isosorbide *eye-soe-sor'-byde*	Isordil, Dilatate SR	Treatment and prevention of angina pectoris	Headache, hypotension, dizziness, weakness, flushing, restlessness, rash	Initial dose 5–20 mg orally; maintenance dose 10–40 mg BID, TID orally Sublingually: 2.5–5 mg; Prevention: 5–10 mg sublingually, 5 mg chewable
isosorbide mononitrate, oral *eye-soe-sor'-byde*	ISMO, Monoket	Treatment and prevention of angina pectoris	Same as isosorbide dinitrate	20 mg BID orally with the 2 doses given 7 hr apart; Extended-release tablets: 30–60 mg/day orally may be increased to 240 mg/day orally
nitroglycerin, parenteral form *nye-troe-glih'-ser-in*		Angina pectoris, heart failure, perioperative hypertension and to induce intraoperative hypotension	Same as isosorbide dinitrate	Initially 5 mcg/min by IV infusion pump; may increase to 20 mcg/min postoperative period
nitroglycerin, oral	Nitrostat (sublingual) Nitrolingual Pump Spray, NitroMist (aerosol used sublingual)	Acute relief of an attack or prophylaxis of angina pectoris	Same as isosorbide dinitrate	1 tablet under tongue or in buccal pouch at first sign of an acute anginal attack- may repeat every 5 min until relief or 3 tablets have been taken; Pump spray 1 – 2 metered doses onto or under the tongue; maximum of 3 metered doses in 15 min

(table continues on page 345)

Summary Drug Table ANTIANGINAL DRUGS (continued)

Generic Name	Trade Name	Uses	Adverse Reactions	Dosage Ranges
nitroglycerin, ointment		Prevention and treatment of angina	Same as isosorbide dinitrate	Used supplied ruled papers to give ½ – 2 inches twice daily
nitroglycerin transdermal systems	Minitran, Nitro–Dur	Prevention of angina pectoris	Same as isosorbide dinitrate	One system daily, 0.2–0.8 mg/hr
Calcium Channel Blockers				
amlodipine *am-low'-dih-peen*	Norvasc	Hypertension, chronic stable angina, vasospastic angina (Prinzmetal's angina)	Headache	Individualize dosage; 5–10 mg/day orally
diltiazem *dill-tye'-ah-zem*	Cardizem, Cardizem CD, Dilacor XR	Hypertension, chronic stable angina, atrial fibrillation/flutter, paroxysmal supraventricular tachycardia	Headache, dizziness, A-V block, bradycardia, edema, dyspnea, rhinitis	Extended Release Tablets/Capsules Angina: 120–580 mg/day Exertional angina – immediate release tablets: 30 mg/QID Heart arrhythmias – injection: 0.25 mg/kg over 2 minutes, then titrated continuous infusion
nicardipine *nye-kar'-deh-peen*	Cardene, Cardene IV, Cardene SR	Hypertension, chronic stable angina	Headache	Angina: individualize dosage; immediate-release only, 20–40 mg TID orally
nifedipine *nye-fed'-ih-peen*	Adalat, Procardia, Procardia XL	Vasospastic angina (Prinzmetal's variant angina), chronic stable angina, hypertension (sustained-release only)	Headache, dizziness, weakness, edema, nausea, muscle cramps, cough, nasal congestion, wheezing	10–20 mg TID orally; may increase to 120 mg/day Sustained-release: 30–60 mg/day orally; may increase to 120 mg/day
Nimodipine *nye-moe'-dih-peen*	Nimotop	Subarachnoid hemorrhage	Headache, hypotension, diarrhea	60 mg every 4 hours orally
Verapamil *ver-ap'-ah-mill*	Calan, Calan SR, Isoptin, Isoptin SR, Verelan	Hypertension, chronic stable angina, vasospastic angina (Prinzmetal's variant angina), chronic atrial flutter, paroxysmal supraventricular tachycardia	Headache, constipation	Individualize dosage; do not exceed 480 mg/day orally in divided doses Sustained-release: 120–180 mg/day orally; maximum dose, 480 mg Extended-release: 120–180 mg/day orally, maximum dose, 480 mg/d Parenteral: 5–10 mg IV over 2 min

diesterase inhibitors (drugs for erectile dysfunction) should not use nitrates.

Nitrates are used cautiously in patients with the following:

• Severe hepatic or renal disease
• Severe head trauma
• Hypothyroidism

These drugs are used cautiously during pregnancy and lactation (pregnancy category C).

Interactions

The following interactions may occur when the nitrates are used with another agent:

Interacting Drug	Common Use	Effect of Interaction
aspirin	Pain reliever	Increased nitrate plasma concentrations and action may occur
calcium channel blockers	Treatment of angina	Increased symptomatic orthostatic hypotension
dihydroergotamine	Migraine headache treatment	Increased risk of hypertension and decreased antianginal effect
heparin	Anticoagulant	Decreased effect of heparin
phosphodiesterase inhibitors	Erectile dysfunction (ED)	Severe hypotension and cardiovascular collapse may occur
alcohol	Relaxation and enjoyment of social situations	Severe hypotension and cardiovascular collapse may occur

NURSING PROCESS

PATIENT RECEIVING AN ANTIANGINAL DRUG

ASSESSMENT

Preadministration Assessment

Before administering an antianginal drug, the nurse obtains and records a thorough pain assessment (see Chapter 14) as well as a history of allergy to the nitrates or calcium channel blockers and of other disease processes that would contraindicate administration of the drug (Display 37.1). The nurse also assesses the physical appearance of the patient (e.g., skin color, lesions), auscultates the lungs for adventitious sounds, and obtains a baseline electrocardiogram and vital signs. Any problem with orthostatic hypotension is noted.

Ongoing Assessment

As a part of the ongoing assessment, the nurse monitors the patient for the frequency and severity of any episodes of anginal pain. With treatment, episodes of angina

---

DISPLAY 37.1 Information Regarding Anginal Pain

History
- Description of the type of pain (e.g., sharp, dull, squeezing)
- Whether the pain radiates and to where
- Events that appear to cause anginal pain (e.g., exercise, emotion)
- Events that appear to relieve the pain (e.g., resting)

Physical Assessment
- Blood pressure
- Apical and radial pulse rates
- Respiratory rate (after the patient has been at rest for about 10 minutes)
- Weight*
- Inspection of the extremities for edema*
- Auscultation of the lungs*

*These assessments may be appropriate, depending on the type of heart disease.

---

should be eliminated or decrease in frequency and severity. The nurse should report to the primary health care provider any chest pain that does not respond to three doses of nitroglycerin given every 5 minutes for 15 minutes.

The nurse takes the patient's vital signs before the drug is administered and frequently during administration of the antianginals or calcium channel blockers. If the patient's heart rate falls below 50 beats per minute or the systolic blood pressure drops below 90 mm Hg, the drug is withheld and the primary health care provider notified. A dosage adjustment may be necessary.

The nurse should assess patients receiving the calcium channel blockers for signs of heart failure: dyspnea, weight gain, peripheral edema, abnormal lung sounds (crackles/rales), and jugular vein distention. Any symptoms of heart failure are reported immediately to the primary health care provider.

The patient is monitored carefully; vital signs are taken frequently, and the patient is placed on a cardiac monitor while the drug is being titrated to a therapeutic dose. The dosage may be increased more rapidly in hospitalized patients under close supervision.

NURSING DIAGNOSES

Drug-specific nursing diagnoses include the following:

- ❏ **Risk for Injury** related to hypotension, dizziness, lightheadedness
- ❏ **Pain** related to narrowing of peripheral arteries, decreased blood supply to the extremities

Nursing diagnoses related to drug administration are discussed in Chapter 4.

PLANNING

The expected outcomes of the patient depend on the specific reason for administering the drug, but may include an optimal response to therapy, support of patient needs related to the management of adverse reactions, and an understanding of the therapeutic regimen.

IMPLEMENTATION

Promoting an Optimal Response to Therapy

NITRATES. Nitrates may be administered by the sublingual (under the tongue), **buccal** (between the cheek and gum), oral, IV, or transdermal route. If the buccal form of nitroglycerin has been prescribed, the nurse instructs the patient to place the buccal tablet between the cheek and gum or between the upper lip and gum above the incisors and allow it to dissolve. The nurse shows the patient how and where to place the tablet in the mouth. Absorption of sublingual and buccal forms depends on salivary secretion. Dry mouth decreases absorption.

Nitroglycerin may also be administered by a metered spray canister that is used to abort an acute anginal attack. The spray is directed from the canister onto or under the tongue. Each dose is metered so that when the canister top is depressed, the same dose is delivered each time. The nurse instructs the patient not to shake the canister nor inhale the spray. For some individuals, this is more convenient than placing small tablets under the tongue.

NURSING ALERT

The dose of sublingual nitroglycerin may be repeated every 5 minutes until pain is relieved or until the patient has received three doses in a 15-minute period. One to two sprays of translingual nitroglycerin may be used to relieve angina, but no more than three metered doses are recommended within a 15-minute period.

The nurse instructs the patient to call the nurse if the pain is not relieved after three doses. The primary health care provider is notified if the patient frequently has anginal pain, if the pain worsens, or if the pain is not relieved after three doses within a 15-minute period, because a change in the dosage of the drug or morphine may be ordered for pain relief.

Administering Oral Nitrates. Nitrates are also available as oral tablets that are swallowed. The nurse gives this form of nitrate to the patient whose stomach is empty, unless the primary health care provider orders otherwise. If nausea occurs after administration, the nurse notifies the primary health care provider. Taking the tablet or capsule with food may be ordered to relieve nausea. The sustained-released preparation may not be crushed or chewed.

Because of the risk of tolerance to oral nitrates developing, the primary care provider may prescribe the short-acting preparations two to three times daily, with the last dose no later than 7 PM, and the sustained-release preparations once daily or twice daily at 8 AM and 2 PM.

Administering Nitroglycerin Ointment. The dose of **topical** (ointment) nitroglycerin is measured in inches or millimeters (mm); 1 inch (25 mm) of ointment equals about 15 mg nitroglycerin. Before the drug is measured and applied and after the ambulatory patient has rested for 10 to 15 minutes, the nurse obtains the patient's blood pressure and pulse rate and compares the results with the baseline and previous vital signs. If the blood pressure is appreciably lower or the pulse rate higher than the resting baseline, the nurse contacts the primary health care provider before applying the drug. First, the nurse must remove the paper from the previous application, and cleanse the area as needed. Applicator paper is supplied with the drug; one paper is used for each application. The nurse should wear disposable plastic gloves to prevent contact with the ointment. While holding the paper, the nurse expresses the prescribed amount of ointment from the tube onto the paper. The nurse uses the applicator or dose-measured paper to gently spread a thin uniform layer over at least a $2^1/_4$ by $3^1/_2$-inch area. The ointment is usually applied to the chest or back. Application sites are rotated to prevent inflammation of the skin. Areas that may be used for appli-

cation include the chest (front and back), abdomen, and upper arms and legs. After application of the ointment, the nurse may secure the paper with non-allergenic tape.

NURSING ALERT

The nurse should not rub the nitroglycerin ointment into the patient's skin, because this will immediately deliver a large amount of the drug through the skin. Exercise care in applying topical nitroglycerin and do not allow the ointment to come in contact with the fingers or hands while measuring or applying the ointment, because the drug will be absorbed through the skin of the person applying the drug, causing a severe headache.

Administering Transdermal Nitroglycerin. For most people, nitroglycerin **transdermal systems** are more convenient and easier to use, because the drug is absorbed through the skin. A transdermal system has the drug impregnated in a pad. The primary health care provider may prescribe the pad to be applied to the skin once a day for 10 to 12 hours. Tolerance to the vascular and antianginal effects of the nitrates may develop, particularly in patients taking higher dosages, those who are prescribed longer-acting products, or those who are on more frequent dosing schedules. Patients using the transdermal nitroglycerin patches are particularly prone to tolerance, because the nitroglycerin is released at a constant rate, and steady plasma concentrations are maintained. Applying the patch in the morning and leaving it in place for 10 to 12 hours, followed by leaving the patch off for 10 to 12 hours, typically yields better results and delays tolerance to the drug.

When applying the transdermal system, the nurse inspects the skin site to be sure it is dry, free of hair, and not subject to excessive rubbing or movement. If needed, the nurse shaves the application site. The nurse applies the transdermal system at the same time each day and rotates the placement sites. Optimal sites include the chest, abdomen, and thighs. The system is not applied to distal extremities. The best time to apply the transdermal system is after daily care (bed bath, shower, tub bath), because it is important that the skin be thoroughly dry before applying the system. When removing the pad, the nurse cleanses the area as needed. To avoid errors in applying and removing the patch, the person applying the patch uses a fiber-tipped pen to write his or her name (or initials), date, and time of application on the top side of the patch. Patches should be removed before cardioversion or defibrillation to prevent patient burns.

Administering IV Nitroglycerin. The nurse administers IV nitroglycerin diluted in normal saline solution or 5% dextrose in water (D_5W) by continuous infusion using an infusion pump to ensure an accurate rate. The nurse administers the drug by using the glass IV bottles and non–polyvinyl chloride (PVC) infusions sets administration sets provided by the manufacturer. The nurse regulates the dosage according to the patient's response and the primary health care provider's instructions. Nitroglycerin solutions should not be mixed with any other drugs or blood products.

CALCIUM CHANNEL BLOCKERS. With a few exceptions, the calcium channel blockers may be taken without regard to meals. If gastrointestinal upset occurs, the drug may be taken with meals. Verapamil frequently causes gastric upset, and the nurse should routinely give tablets with meals. Verapamil tablets may be opened and sprinkled on foods or mixed in liquids. Sometimes the tablet coverings of verapamil are expelled in the stool. This causes no change in the effect of the drug and need not cause the patient concern.

For patients who have difficulty swallowing diltiazem (except Dilacor XR), tablets can be crushed and mixed with food or liquids. However, the patient should swallow the sustained-released tablets whole and not chew or divide them.

Monitoring and Managing Patient Needs

The nurse must observe carefully patients receiving these drugs for adverse reactions. Hypotension may be accompanied by paradoxical bradycardia and increased angina pectoris. Adverse reactions such as headache, flushing, and postural hypotension that are seen with the administration of the antianginal drugs often become less severe or even disappear after a period of time.

LIFESPAN ALERT – Gerontology
Quality of life has been enhanced for some patients with the advent of drugs for ED (phosphodiesterase inhibitors). When taken with nitrates, severe hypotension can occur; therefore, they are contraindicated for use together. Nurses should always assess for and discuss the use of ED drugs when a male patient is prescribed a nitrate preparation.

RISK FOR INJURY. The nurse assists patients having episodes of postural hypotension with all ambulatory activities. The nurse instructs those with episodes of postural hypotension to take the drug in a sitting or supine position and to remain in that position until symptoms disappear. The nurse monitors the blood pressure frequently in the patient with dizziness or lightheadedness. The patient may need help during ambulation if dizziness occurs.

LIFESPAN ALERT – Adolescents and Young Adults
Poppers (amyl nitrite, butyl nitrite, and isobutyl nitrite) are popular among the gay community and young people at clubs and raves. The head rush, euphoria, uncontrollable laughter or giggling, and other sensations that result from the blood pressure drop are often felt to increase sexual arousal and desire. Historically, amyl nitrite has been used to treat angina. Amyl nitrite and several other alkyl nitrites used in over-the-counter products such as air fresheners and video head cleaners may be inhaled to enhance sexual pleasure. The reduction in blood pressure can result in loss of balance and fainting, especially if people are involved in physical activity like dancing. The likelihood of accidents is increased, and people with heart conditions or high blood pressure are more at risk. Nurses should inquire about popper use when injury and low blood pressure are presenting symptoms in the urgent care or emergency department.

PAIN. The nurse must evaluate the patient's response to therapy by questioning the patient about the anginal pain. In some patients, the pain may be entirely relieved, whereas in others it may be less intense or less frequent or may occur only with prolonged exercise. The nurse records all information in the patient's chart, because this helps the primary health care provider plan future therapy as well as make dosage adjustments if required.

Educating the Patient and Family

The patient and family must have a thorough understanding of the treatment of chest pain with an antianginal drug. These drugs are used either to prevent angina from occurring or to relieve the pain of angina. The nurse explains the therapeutic regimen (dose, time of day the drug is taken, how often to take the drug, how to take or apply the drug) to the patient. The nurse adapts a teaching plan to the type of prescribed antianginal drug. The nurse should include the following general areas, as well as those points relevant to specific routes of administration of the drug, in a teaching plan:

- Avoid the use of alcohol unless use has been permitted by the primary health care provider.
- Notify the primary health care provider if the drug does not relieve pain or if pain becomes more intense despite use of this drug.
- Follow the recommendations of the primary health care provider regarding frequency of use.
- Take oral capsules or tablets (except sublingual) on an empty stomach unless the primary health care provider directs otherwise.
- Keep an adequate supply of the drug on hand for events, such as vacations, bad weather conditions, and holidays.
- Keep a record of the frequency of acute anginal attacks (date, time of the attack, drug, and dose used to relieve the acute pain), and bring this record to each primary health care provider or clinic visit.

For more teaching points related specifically to administration routes of nitrates and calcium channel blockers, see the Patient Teaching for Improved Patient Outcomes: Directions for Administering Nitrates and Calcium Channel Blockers.

EVALUATION

- Therapeutic response is achieved.
- Adverse reactions are identified, reported to the primary health care provider, and managed successfully with appropriate nursing interventions:
  ☑ No evidence of injury is seen.
  ☑ Pain is relieved.
- Patient and family demonstrate an understanding of the drug regimen.

Patient Teaching for Improved Patient Outcomes

Directions for Administering Nitrates

✓ Explain that headache is a common adverse reaction but should decrease with continued therapy. If headache persists or becomes severe, notify the primary health care provider, because a change in dosage may be needed. In patients who get headaches, the headaches may be a marker of the drug's effectiveness. Patients should not try to avoid headaches by altering the treatment schedule, because loss of headache may be associated with simultaneous loss of drug effectiveness. Aspirin or acetaminophen may be used for headache relief.

✓ Advise the patient not to change from one brand of nitrates to another without consulting the pharmacist or primary care provider. Products manufactured by different companies may not be equally effective.

Oral Nitrates

✓ Advise patients taking nitroglycerin for an acute attack of angina to sit or lie down. To relieve severe light-headedness or dizziness, lie down, elevate the extremities, move the extremities, and breathe deeply.

✓ Store capsules and tablets in their original containers, because nitroglycerin must be kept in a dark container and protected from exposure to light. Never mix this drug with any other drug in a container. Nitroglycerin will lose its potency if stored in containers made of plastic or if mixed with other drugs.

✓ Always replace the cover or cap of the container as soon as the oral drug or ointment is removed from the container or tube. Replace caps or covers tightly, because the drug deteriorates on contact with air.

✓ Seek prompt medical attention if chest pain persists, changes character, increases in severity, or is not relieved by following the recommended dosing regimen.

Sublingual or Buccal Nitrates

✓ Do not handle the tablets labeled as sublingual any more than necessary.

✓ Check the expiration date on the container of sublingual tablets. If the expiration date has passed, do not use the tablets. Instead, purchase a new supply.

✓ Do not swallow or chew sublingual or transmucosal tablets; allow them to dissolve slowly. The tablet may cause a burning or tingling in the oral cavity. Absence of this effect does not indicate a decrease in potency. Older adults are less likely to report a burning or tingling sensation on administration.

Translingual (Aerosol Spray)Nitrates

✓ Directions for use of translingual nitroglycerin are supplied with the product. Follow the instructions regarding using and cleaning the canister.

• This drug may be used prophylactically 5 to 10 minutes before engaging in activities that precipitate an anginal attack.

• Do not shake the canister before use.

✓ At the onset of an anginal attack, spray 1 to 2 metered doses onto or under the tongue. Do not exceed 3 metered doses within 15 minutes.

✓ When using the transmucosal form, insert the tablet between the lip and gum above the incisors or between the cheek and gum.

Topical Ointment or Transdermal System

✓ Instructions for application of the topical ointment or transdermal system are available with the product. Read these instructions carefully.

• Apply the topical ointment or topical transdermal system at approximately the same time each day.

• Remove the old system and inspect body to be sure no other papers or systems have been missed.

✓ Be sure the area is clean and thoroughly dry before applying the topical ointment or transdermal system, and rotate the application sites. Apply the transdermal system to the chest (front and back), abdomen, and upper or lower arms and legs. Firmly press the patch to ensure contact with the skin. If the transdermal system comes off or becomes loose, apply a new system. Apply the topical ointment to the front or the back of the chest. If applying to the back, another person should apply the ointment.

✓ When using the topical ointment form or transdermal system, cleanse old application sites with soap and warm water as soon as the ointment or transdermal system is removed.

✓ To use the topical ointment, apply a thin layer on the skin using the paper applicator (the patient or family member may need instructions regarding this technique). Avoid finger contact with the ointment.

✓ Wear disposable gloves when applying the ointment.

✓ Notify the primary health care provider if any of the following occurs: increased severity of chest pain or discomfort, irregular heartbeat, palpitations, nausea, shortness of breath, swelling of the hands or feet, or severe and prolonged episodes of light-headedness and dizziness.

✓ Make position changes slowly to minimize hypotensive effects.

✓ Because these drugs can cause dizziness or drowsiness, do not drive or engage in hazardous activities until response to the drug is known.

✓ Do not use erectile dysfunction drugs while taking nitrates.

THINK CRITICALLY: PHARMACOLOGY IN PRACTICE

1. Ms. Moore is admitted with severe chest pain and a possible myocardial infarction. After tests are done, her primary health care provider prescribes transdermal nitroglycerin for her angina. Develop a teaching plan that will show Ms. Moore how and when to apply the transdermal form of nitroglycerin.

● Test Your Knowledge

1. When administering the nitrates for angina pectoris, the nurse monitors the patient for which common adverse reaction?

A. Hyperglycemia
B. Headache
C. Fever
D. Anorexia

2. When teaching a patient about prescribed sublingual nitroglycerin, the nurse informs the patient that if pain is not relieved, the dose can be repeated in ____ minute(s).

A. 1
B. 5
C. 15
D. 30

3. When administering nitroglycerin ointment, the nurse _____.

A. rubs the ointment into the skin
B. applies the ointment every hour or until the angina is relieved
C. applies the ointment to a clean, dry area
D. rubs the ointment between his or her palms and then spreads it evenly onto the patient's chest

4. A patient taking a calcium channel blocker experiences orthostatic hypotension. The nurse instructs the patient with orthostatic hypotension to _____.

A. remain in a supine position until the effects subside
B. make position changes slowly to minimize hypotensive effects
C. increase the dosage of the calcium channel blocker
D. discontinue use of the calcium channel blocker until the hypotensive effects diminish

● Prepare for the NCLEX

1. Mr. Phillips has seen his primary health care provider for his heart condition. The provider gives you the prescription for sublingual nitrate to call into Mr. Phillip's pharmacy. Mr. Phillips hands you more prescriptions from another provider to refill. Which one should you review with the primary health care provider first:

A. cimetidine
B. ibuprofen
C. lisinopril
D. sildenafil

● Calculate Medication Dosages

1. The primary care provider prescribed verapamil hydrochloride (Calan) 120 mg TID orally. The drug is available in 40-mg tablets. The nurse administers _____.

2. The patient is prescribed isosorbide (Isordil) 40 mg orally BID. The drug form available is 20-mg tablets. The nurse administers _____.

To check your answers, see Appendix E.

the**Point** *For more NCLEX questions, log on to http://thepoint.lww.com to access more than 1000 questions.*

38

Anticoagulant and Thrombolytic Drugs

KEY TERMS

embolus
fibrolytic
hemostasis
lysis

prothrombin
thrombolytic
thrombosis
thrombus

LEARNING OBJECTIVES

On completion of this chapter, the student will:

1. Describe hemostasis and thrombosis.
2. Discuss the uses, general drug actions, adverse reactions, contraindications, precautions, and interactions of anticoagulant, antiplatelet, and thrombolytic drugs.
3. Discuss important preadministration and ongoing assessment activities the nurse should perform on the patient taking an anticoagulant, antiplatelet, or thrombolytic drug.
4. List nursing diagnoses particular to a patient taking an anticoagulant, antiplatelet, or thrombolytic drug.
5. Discuss ways to promote an optimal response to therapy, how to manage common adverse reactions, and important points to keep in mind when educating patients about the use of an anticoagulant, antiplatelet, or thrombolytic drug.

When a blood vessel is injured, a series of events occurs to form a clot and stop the bleeding. This process is called **hemostasis**. It involves a complex process also called the *coagulation cascade*. Figure 38.1 shows the blood clotting pathway and the extrinsic and intrinsic factors involved. The blood clotting or coagulation cascade is so named because as each factor is activated, it acts as a catalyst that enhances the next reaction, with the net result being a large collection of fibrin (the clot) that forms a plug in the vessel, thus stopping the bleeding. This is a normal event, taking a few minutes, that happens daily in response to tears and leaks in blood vessels throughout the body.

Thrombosis is the formation of a blood clot, or **thrombus**. A thrombus may form in any vessel (artery or vein), impeding blood flow. For example, a venous thrombus can develop as the result of venous stasis (decreased blood flow), injury to the vessel wall, or altered blood coagulation. Venous thrombosis most often occurs in the lower extremities and is associated with venous stasis. Deep vein thrombosis (DVT) occurs in the lower extremities and is the most common type of venous thrombosis.

Arterial thrombosis can occur because of atherosclerosis or arrhythmias, such as atrial fibrillation. The thrombus may begin small, but fibrin, platelets, and red blood cells attach to the thrombus, increasing its size. When a thrombus detaches itself from the wall of the vessel and is carried along through the bloodstream, it becomes an **embolus**. The embolus travels until it reaches a vessel that is too small to permit its passage. If the embolus goes to the lung and obstructs a pulmonary vessel, it is called a *pulmonary embolism* (PE). Similarly, if the embolus detaches and occludes a vessel supplying blood to the heart, it can cause a myocardial infarction (MI).

The type of drugs discussed in this chapter include drugs that prevent the formation of blood clots (anticoagulants), drugs that suppress platelet aggregation (antiplatelets), and drugs that help to eliminate the clot (thrombolytics). For more information about specific drugs, see the Drug Summary Table: Anticoagulant, Antiplatelet, Thrombolytic, and Peripheral Vasodilating Agents.

● ORAL AND PARENTERAL ANTICOAGULANTS

Anticoagulants are used to prevent the formation and extension of a thrombus. Anticoagulants have no direct effect on an existing thrombus and do not reverse any damage from the thrombus. However, once the presence of a thrombus has been established, anticoagulant therapy can prevent additional clots from forming. Although they do not thin the blood, they are commonly called *blood thinners* by patients. The anticoagulant group of drugs includes warfarin (Coumadin; a coumarin derivative), anisindione (Miradon; an indandione derivative), and fractionated and unfractionated heparin. The anticoagulant drugs are used prophylactically in patients who are at high risk for clot formation.

Warfarin is the oral anticoagulant most commonly prescribed. Although primarily given by the oral route, warfarin is also available for parenteral administration. Because it can be given orally, it is the drug of choice for patients requiring long-term therapy with an anticoagulant. Peak activity is reached 1.5 to 3 days after therapy is initiated. Anisindione is less frequently used but is an effective anticoagulant.

Heparin preparations are available as heparin sodium and the low–molecular-weight heparins (LMWHs; fractionated heparins). Heparin is not a single drug, but rather a mixture of high– and low–molecular-weight drugs. Examples of LMWH include dalteparin (Fragmin), enoxaparin (Lovenox),

EXTRINSIC

Tissue injury—Factors III, VII

INTRINSIC

Platelets Thromboplastin Precursors
Factors VIII, IX, XI, XII

Figure 38.1 Blood clotting pathway. Blood coagulation results in the formation of a stable fibrin clot. Formation of this clot involves a cascade of interactions of clotting factors, platelets, and other substances. Clotting factors exist in the blood in inactive form and must be converted to an active form before the next step in the clotting pathway can occur. Each factor is stimulated in turn until the process is complete and a fibrin clot is formed. In the intrinsic pathway, all of the components necessary for clot formation are in the circulating blood. Clot formation in the intrinsic pathway is initiated by factor XII. In the extrinsic pathway, coagulation is initiated by release of tissue thromboplastin, a factor not found in circulating blood. RBC, red blood cell; WBC, white blood cell.

Summary Drug Table ANTICOAGULANT, ANTIPLATELET, THROMBOLYTIC, AND PERIPHERAL VASODILATING AGENTS

Generic Name	Trade Name	Uses	Adverse Reactions	Dosage Ranges
Oral Anticoagulants				
anisindione *ah-nis-in-dye'-own*	Miradon	Prophylaxis/treatment of venous thrombosis	Bleeding, fatigue, dizziness, abdominal cramping	25–300 mg/day orally, individualized dose based on PT or INR
warfarin *war'-fah-rin*	Coumadin, Jantoven	Prophylaxis/treatment of venous thrombosis	Same as anisindione	2–10 mg/day orally, individualized dose based on PT or INR: IV form for injection
Parenteral Anticoagulants				
heparin *hep'-ah-rin*		Thrombosis/embolism, diagnosis and treatment of disseminated intravascular coagulation, prophylaxis of DVT, clotting prevention	Bleeding, chills, fever, urticaria, local irritation, erythema, mild pain, hematoma or bruising at the injection site (SUBCUT)	10,000–20,000 Units Subcut in divided doses q 8–12 hr; 5000–10,000 Units- q 4–6 hr intermittent IV; 5000–40,000 Units/day IV infusion
heparin sodium lock flush solution		Clearing intermittent infusion lines (heparin lock) to prevent clot formation at site	None significant	10–100 Units/mL heparin solution

(table continues on page 353)

Summary Drug Table ANTICOAGULANT, ANTIPLATELET, THROMBOLYTIC, AND PERIPHERAL VASODILATING AGENTS (continued)

Generic Name	Trade Name	Uses	Adverse Reactions	Dosage Ranges
Parenteral Anticoagulants: Low–Molecular-Weight Heparins				
dalteparin *dal-tep'-ah-rin*	Fragmin	Unstable angina/non–Q-wave MI, DVT prophylaxis	Bleeding, bruising, rash, fever, erythema and irritation at site of injection	Angina/MI: 120 Units/kg Subcut q 12 hr with concurrent oral aspirin; DVT: 2500 Units/day Subcut
enoxaparin *en-ox'-ah-par-in*	Lovenox	DVT and presurgical prophylaxis, PE treatment, unstable angina/non–Q-wave MI	Same as dalteparin	DVT prophylaxis: 30–40 mg Subcut q 12 hr; Treatment: 1 mg/kg Subcut q 12 hr
tinzaparin *ten-zah'-par-in*	Innohep	DVT treatment	Same as dalteparin	12,000–17,000 Units/day Subcut
Miscellaneous Anticoagulant Agents				
desirudin *deh-sih'-rue-din*	Iprivask	DVT prophylaxis	Bleeding (at injection site)	15 mg Subcut every 12 hr for 9 – 12 days post-operatively
fondaparinux *fon-dah-par'-ih-nux*	Arixtra	DVT prophylaxis	Bleeding (at injection site)	2.5 mg Subcut 6–8 hr following surgery, then daily for 5–9 days post-operatively
Antiplatelet Agents				
abciximab *ab-six'-ih-mab*	ReoPro	Adjunct in coronary angioplasty	Bleeding, pain	0.125 mcg/kg/min IV during procedure
anagrelide *an-ag'-greh-lyde*	Agrylin	Thrombocythemia	Heart palpitations, dizziness, headache, nausea, abdominal pain, diarrhea, edema	1 mg orally BID
cilostazol *sill-ah'-stah-zoll*	Pletal	Intermittent claudication	Heart palpitations, dizziness, diarrhea, headache, rhinitis	100 mg orally BID
clopidogrel *kloe-pid'-oh-grel*	Plavix	Recent MI, stroke, and acute coronary syndrome	Dizziness, skin rash, chest pain, constipation	Single loading dose: 300 mg; 75 mg/day orally
dipyridamole *dye-peer-id'-ah-mole*	Persantine	Post-operative thromboembolic prevention in valve replacement	Dizziness, abdominal distress	75–100 mg orally QID
eptifibatide *ep-tiff-ib'-ah-tyde*	Integrilin	Adjunct in coronary angioplasty, acute coronary syndrome	Bleeding, pain	1 mcg/kg/min IV infusion
ticlopidine *tye-kloe'-pih-deen*	Ticlid	Thrombotic stroke	Nausea, dyspepsia, diarrhea	250 mg orally BID
tirofiban *tye-roe'-fih-ban*	Aggrastat	Acute coronary syndrome	Bleeding, pain	0.4–0.1 mcg/kg/min IV infusion
Thrombolytics				
alteplase *al'-teh-plaze*	Activase, Cath-flo Activase (for IV catheter occlusions only)	Acute MI, acute ischemic stroke, PE, IV catheter clearance	Bleeding (GU, gingival, intracranial) and epistaxis, ecchymosis	Total dose of 90–100 mg IV, given as a 2- to 3-hr infusion
reteplase *ret'-ah-plaze*	Retavase	Acute MI	Bleeding (GI, GU, or at injection site), intracranial hemorrhage, anemia	Prepackaged: 2- to 10-Unit IV bolus injections

(table continues on page 354)

Anticoagulant and Thrombolytic Drugs

Summary Drug Table ANTICOAGULANT, ANTIPLATELET, THROMBOLYTIC, AND PERIPHERAL VASODILATING AGENTS (continued)

Generic Name	Trade Name	Uses	Adverse Reactions	Dosage Ranges
streptokinase *strep-toe-kye'-nase*	Streptase	Acute MI, DVT, PE, embolism	Minor bleeding (superficial and surface) and major bleeding (internal and severe)	250,000 Units IV loading dose, followed by 100,000 Units for 24–72 hr
tenecteplase *teh-nek'-tih-plaze*	TNKase	Acute MI	Bleeding (GI, GU, or at injection site), intracranial hemorrhage, anemia	Dosage based on weight, not to exceed 50 mg IV
urokinase *yoor-oh'-kye-naze*	Abbokinase	PE, lysis of coronary artery thrombi, IV catheter clearance	Minor bleeding (superficial and surface) and major bleeding (internal and severe)	PE: 4400 Units/kg IV over 10 min, followed by 4400 Units/kg/hr for 12 hr
Anticoagulant Antagonists				
phytonadione (vitamin K) *fye-toe-nah-dye'-own*	Aqua-Mephyton, Mephyton	Treatment of warfarin overdosage	Gastric upset, unusual taste, flushing, rash, urticaria, erythema, pain and/or swelling at injection site	2.5–10 mg oral, IM, may repeat orally in 12–48 hr or in 6–8 hr after parenteral dose
protamine *proe'-tah-meen*		Treatment of heparin overdose	Flushing and warm feeling, dyspnea, bradycardia, hypotension	Dose is determined by amount of heparin to be neutralized; generally, 1 mg IV neutralizes 100 Units of heparin

and tinzaparin (Innohep). LMWHs produce very stable responses when administered at recommended dosages. Because of this stability, frequent laboratory monitoring, as with heparin, is not necessary. In addition, bleeding is less likely to occur with LMWHs than with heparin.

Desirudin (Iprivask) and fondaparinux (Arixtra) are both anticoagulating drugs that inhibit portions of the coagulation cascade. They are used to prevent DVT in patients undergoing hip, knee or abdominal surgeries.

Actions

All anticoagulants interfere with the clotting mechanism of the blood. Warfarin and anisindione interfere with the manufacturing of vitamin K–dependent clotting factors by the liver. This results in the depletion of clotting factors II (**prothrombin**), VII, IX, and X. It is the depletion of prothrombin (see Fig. 38.1), a substance that is essential for the clotting of blood, that accounts for most of the action of warfarin.

By contrast, heparin inhibits the formation of fibrin clots, inhibits the conversion of fibrinogen to fibrin, and inactivates several of the factors necessary for the clotting of blood. Heparin cannot be taken orally, because it is inactivated by gastric acid in the stomach; therefore, it must be given by injection. The LMWHs act to inhibit clotting reactions by binding to antithrombin III, which inhibits the synthesis of factor X and the formation of thrombin. These drugs have no effect on clots that have already formed and aid only in preventing the formation of new blood clots.

Desirudin and fondaparinux produce strong anticoagulant effects with a different mechanism of action than heparin. Additionally, their therapeutic index is narrower than heparin and can be associated with hemorrhagic complications.

Uses

Anticoagulants are used for the following:

• Prevention (prophylaxis) and treatment of DVT
• Prevention and treatment of atrial fibrillation with embolization
• Prevention and treatment of PE
• Adjuvant treatment of MI
• Prevention of thrombus formation after valve replacement surgery

Parenteral anticoagulants are used specifically for the following:

• Prevention of postoperative DVT and PE in certain patients undergoing surgical procedures, such as major abdominal surgery
• Prevention of clotting in arterial and heart surgery, in the equipment used for extracorporeal (occurring out-side the body) circulation (e.g., in dialysis procedures), in blood transfusions, and in blood samples for laboratory purposes
• Prevention of a repeat cerebral thrombosis in some patients who have experienced a stroke
• Treatment of coronary occlusion, acute MI, and peripheral arterial embolism
• Diagnosis and treatment of disseminated intravascular coagulation (DIC), a severe hemorrhagic disorder
• Maintaining patency of intravenous (IV) catheters (very low doses of 10 to 100 units)

Adverse Reactions

The principal adverse reaction associated with anticoagulants is bleeding, which may range from very mild to severe.

Bleeding may be seen in many areas of the body, such as the skin (bruising and petechiae), bladder, bowel, stomach, uterus, and mucous membranes. Other adverse reactions are rare but may include the following:

- Nausea, vomiting, abdominal cramping, diarrhea
- Alopecia (loss of hair)
- Rash or urticaria (hives)
- Hepatitis (inflammation of the liver), jaundice (yellowish discoloration of the skin and mucous membranes), thrombocytopenia (low platelet count), and blood dyscrasias (disorders)

Additional adverse reactions include local irritation when heparin is given by the subcutaneous (subcut) route. Hypersensitivity reactions may also occur with any route of administration and include fever and chills. More serious hypersensitivity reactions include an asthma-like reaction and an anaphylactic reaction. See the Summary Drug Table: Anticoagulant, Antiplatelet, and Thrombolytic Agents for additional adverse reactions.

Contraindications

Anticoagulants are contraindicated in patients with known hypersensitivity to the drugs, active bleeding (except when caused by DIC), hemorrhagic disease, tuberculosis, leukemia, uncontrolled hypertension, gastrointestinal (GI) ulcers, recent surgery of the eye or central nervous system, aneurysms, or severe renal or hepatic disease, and during lactation. Use during pregnancy can cause fetal death (oral agents are in pregnancy category X and parenteral agents are in pregnancy category C). The LMWHs are also contraindicated in patients with a hypersensitivity to pork products.

Precautions

Anticoagulants are used cautiously in patients with fever, heart failure, diarrhea, diabetes, malignancy, hypertension, renal or hepatic disease, psychoses, or depression. Precaution is taken with patients undergoing spinal procedures (anesthesia or diagnostic) to be aware of the potential of spinal or epidural hematoma formation when parenteral anticoagulants are used. Women of childbearing age must use a reliable contraceptive to prevent pregnancy. These drugs are used with caution in all patients with a potential site for bleeding or hemorrhage.

Interactions

The following interactions may occur when an anticoagulant is administered with another agent:

Interacting Drug	Common Use	Effect of Interaction
aspirin, acetaminophen, nonsteroidal anti-inflammatory drugs (NSAIDs), and chloral hydrate	Pain relief and sedation	Increased risk for bleeding
penicillin, aminoglycosides, isoniazid, tetracyclines, and cephalosporins	Anti-infective agents	Increased risk for bleeding

Interacting Drug	Common Use	Effect of Interaction
beta blockers and loop diuretics	Treatment of cardiac problems	Increased risk for bleeding
disulfiram and cimetidine	Management of GI distress	Increased risk for bleeding
oral contraceptives, barbiturates, diuretics, and vitamin K	Birth control, sedation, treatment of cardiac problems and bleeding disorders, respectively	Decreased effectiveness of the anticoagulant

HERBAL ALERT
Warfarin, a drug with a narrow therapeutic index, has the potential to interact with many herbal remedies. For example, warfarin should not be combined with any of the following substances, because they may have additive or synergistic activity and increase the risk for bleeding: celery, chamomile, clove, dong quai, feverfew, garlic, ginger, ginkgo biloba, ginseng, green tea, onion, passion flower, red clover, St. John's wort, and turmeric. Any herbal remedy should be used with caution in patients taking warfarin.

ANTIPLATELET DRUGS

Thrombi forming in the venous system are composed primarily of fibrin and red blood cells. In contrast, it is believed that arterial thrombosis formation is due to clumping of platelet aggregates. Therefore, anticoagulant drugs prevent thrombosis in the venous system, and the antiplatelet drugs prevent thrombus formation in the arterial system. In addition to aspirin therapy, the antiplatelet drugs include adenosine diphosphate (ADP) receptor blockers and glycoprotein receptor blockers.

Actions and Uses

These drugs work by decreasing the platelets' ability to stick together (aggregate) in the blood, thus forming a clot. Aspirin works by prohibiting the aggregation of the platelets for the lifetime of the platelet. The ADP blockers alter the platelet cell membrane, preventing aggregation. Glycoprotein receptor blockers work to prevent enzyme production, again inhibiting platelet aggregation. Antiplatelet drug therapy is designed primarily to treat patients at risk for acute coronary syndrome, MI, stroke, and intermittent claudication.

Adverse Reactions

Some of the more common adverse reactions include the following:

- Heart palpitations
- Bleeding
- Dizziness and headache
- Nausea, diarrhea, constipation, dyspepsia

Contraindications and Precautions

Antiplatelet drugs are contraindicated in pregnant or lactating patients and those with known hypersensitivity to the drugs, congestive heart failure, active bleeding, or thrombotic thrombocytopenic purpura (TTP). These drugs are to be used cautiously in elderly patients, pancytopenic patients, or those with renal or hepatic impairment. If TTP is diagnosed, the antiplatelet treatment should be stopped immediately. Clopidogrel is a pregnancy category B and the others are category C, none of these drugs have been well studied in humans. Antiplatelet drugs should be discontinued 1 week before any surgical procedure.

Interactions

The following interactions may occur when an antiplatelet is administered with another agent:

Interacting Drug	Common Use	Effect of Interaction
aspirin and NSAIDs	Pain relief	Increased risk of bleeding
macrolide antibiotics	Anti-infective agents	Increased effectiveness of anti-infective
digoxin	Management of cardiac problems	Decreased digoxin serum levels
phenytoin	Control of seizure activity	Increased phenytoin serum levels

While these agents produce strong anticoagulant effects, their mechanism of action is distinct from that of heparins; thus, these agents should be used carefully using specific guidelines provided for each product. Thrombin inhibitors are effective anticoagulants; however, their therapeutic index is narrower than heparin and as such their nonoptimized use is potentially associated with hemorrhagic complications.

•THROMBOLYTIC DRUGS

Whereas the anticoagulant agents prevent thrombus formation, the **thrombolytic** class of drugs dissolves blood clots that have already formed within the walls of a blood vessel. These drugs reopen blood vessels after they become occluded. Another term used to describe the thrombolytic drugs is **fibrolytic**. Examples of the thrombolytics include alteplase recombinant (Activase), streptokinase (Streptase), and tenecteplase (TNKase).

Actions

Although the exact action of each of the thrombolytic drugs is slightly different, these drugs break down fibrin clots by converting plasminogen to plasmin. Plasmin is an enzyme that breaks down the fibrin of a blood clot. This reopens blood vessels after their occlusion and prevents tissue necrosis. Because thrombolytic drugs dissolve all clots encountered (both occlusive and those repairing vessel leaks), bleeding is a great concern when using these agents. Before these drugs are used, their potential benefits must be weighed carefully against the potential dangers of bleeding.

Uses

These drugs are used to treat the following:

- Acute MI by **lysis** (breaking up) of blood clots in the coronary arteries
- Blood clots causing pulmonary emboli and DVT
- Suspected occlusions in central venous catheters

See the Summary Drug Table: Anticoagulant, Antiplatelet, and Thrombolytic Agents for a more complete listing of the use of these drugs.

Adverse Reactions

Bleeding is the most common adverse reaction seen with the use of these drugs. Bleeding may be internal and involve areas such as the GI tract, genitourinary tract, and the brain. Bleeding may also be external (superficial) and seen at areas of broken skin, such as venipuncture sites and recent surgical wounds. Allergic reactions may also be seen.

Contraindications and Precautions

Thrombolytic drugs are contraindicated in a patient with known hypersensitivity to the drugs, active bleeding, and history of stroke, aneurysm, and recent intracranial surgery.

These drugs are used cautiously in patients who have recently undergone major surgery (within 10 days), such as coronary artery bypass grafting; who experienced stroke, trauma, vaginal or cesarean section delivery, GI bleeding, or trauma within the last 10 days; or who have hypertension, diabetic retinopathy, or any condition in which bleeding is a significant possibility; and in patients currently receiving oral anticoagulants. All of the thrombolytic drugs discussed in this chapter are classified in pregnancy category C, with the exception of urokinase, which is a pregnancy category B drug.

Interactions

When a thrombolytic is administered with medications that prevent blood clots, such as aspirin, dipyridamole, or an anticoagulant, the patient is at increased risk for bleeding.

NURSING PROCESS
PATIENT RECEIVING ANTICOAGULANT, ANTIPLATELET, OR THROMBOLYTIC DRUGS

ASSESSMENT

Preadministration Assessment
Before administering the first dose of an anticoagulant or thrombolytic, the nurse questions the patient about all drugs taken during the previous 2 to 3 weeks (if the patient was recently admitted to the hospital). If the patient took any drugs before admission, the nurse notifies the primary health care provider before the first dose is administered. Usually, the prothrombin time (PT) is

assessed and the international normalized ratio (INR) determined before therapy begins. The first dose of warfarin is not given until blood is drawn for a baseline PT/INR test. The dosage is individualized based on the results of the PT or the INR.

Before administering the first dose of heparin, the nurse obtains the patient's vital signs. The most commonly used test to monitor heparin is the activated partial thromboplastin time (aPTT). To obtain baseline data, blood is drawn for laboratory studies before giving the first dose of heparin.

If the patient has a DVT, it usually occurs in a lower extremity. The nurse examines the extremity for color and skin temperature. The nurse also checks for a pedal pulse, noting the rate and strength of the pulse. It is important to record any difference between the affected extremity and the unaffected extremity. The nurse notes areas of redness or tenderness and asks the patient to describe current symptoms. The affected extremity may appear edematous and a positive Homans' sign (pain in the calf when the foot is dorsiflexed) may be elicited. A positive Homans' sign suggests DVT.

Blood for a complete blood count is usually drawn before the administration of the thrombolytic agents. Most patients receiving a thrombolytic agent are admitted or transferred to an intensive care unit, because close monitoring is necessary for 48 hours or more after therapy. If the patient is experiencing pain because of the blood clot, the nurse does a thorough pain assessment.

Ongoing Assessment

In the ongoing assessment, a patient receiving an anticoagulant, antiplatelet, or thrombolytic drug requires close observation and careful monitoring. During the course of therapy for both oral and parenteral drugs, the nurse continually assesses the patient for any signs of bleeding and hemorrhage. Areas of assessment include the gums, nose, stools, urine, or nasogastric drainage. Level of consciousness should be assessed on a routine basis to monitor for intracranial bleeding.

Patients receiving warfarin for the first time often require daily adjustment of the dose, which is based on the daily PT/INR results. The nurse withholds the drug and notifies the primary health care provider if the PT exceeds 1.2 to 1.5 times the control value or the INR ratio exceeds 3. A daily PT/INR is performed until it stabilizes and when any other drug is added to or removed from the patient's drug regimen. After the INR has stabilized, it is monitored every 4 to 6 weeks. See Display 38.1 for more information on the laboratory tests for monitoring warfarin.

The dosage of heparin is adjusted according to daily aPTT monitoring. A therapeutic dosage is attained when the aPTT is 1.5 to 2.5 times the normal. The LMWHs have little or no effect on the aPTT values. Special monitoring of clotting times is not necessary when administering the drugs. Periodic platelet counts, hematocrit, and tests for occult blood in the stool should be performed throughout the course of heparin therapy.

DISPLAY 38.1 Understanding Prothrombin Time and International Normalized Ratio

Prothrombin time (also called pro-time or abbreviated as "PT") and the *international normalized ratio* (INR) are used to monitor the patient's response to warfarin therapy. The daily dose of the oral anticoagulant is based on the patient's daily PT/INR. The therapeutic range of the PT is 1.2 to 1.5 times the control value. Studies indicate that levels greater than 2 times the control value do not provide additional therapeutic effects in most patients and are associated with a higher incidence of bleeding.

Laboratories report results for the INR along with the patient's PT and the control value. The INR "corrects" the routine PT results from different laboratories. By measuring against a known standard, the INR gives a more consistent value. The INR is maintained between 2 and 3. Values above 5 can be dangerous, and values below 1 are ineffective.

! NURSING ALERT

Blood coagulation tests for those receiving heparin by continuous IV infusion are taken at periodic intervals (usually every 4 hours) determined by the primary health care provider. If the patient is receiving long-term heparin therapy, blood coagulation tests may be performed at less frequent intervals.

It is also important that the nurse monitor for any indication of hypersensitivity reaction. The nurse reports reactions such as chills, fever, or hives to the primary health care provider. The nurse examines the skin temperature and color in the patient with a DVT for signs of improvement. The nurse takes and records vital signs every 4 hours or more frequently, if needed. When heparin is given to prevent the formation of a thrombus, the nurse observes the patient for signs of thrombus formation every 2 to 4 hours. Because the signs and symptoms of thrombus formation vary and depend on the area or organ involved, the nurse should evaluate and report any complaint the patient may have or any change in the patient's condition to the primary health care provider.

NURSING DIAGNOSES

Drug-specific nursing diagnoses include the following:

❑ **Risk for Injury** related to excessive bleeding due to drug therapy
❑ **Individual Effective Therapeutic Regimen Management** related to inability to communicate drug use if incapacitated
❑ **Anxiety** related to fear of atypical bleeding during thrombolytic drug therapy

Nursing diagnoses related to drug administration are discussed in depth in Chapter 4.

PLANNING

The expected outcomes for the patient may include an optimal response to therapy, support of patient needs related to the management of adverse reactions, and an understanding of the postdischarge drug regimen.

IMPLEMENTATION

Promoting an Optimal Response to Therapy

ORAL ADMINISTRATION OF ANTICOAGULANTS. Before administering each dose of warfarin, the nurse checks the prothrombin flow sheet or the laboratory report to review the current PT/INR results. The nurse notifies the primary health care provider before administering the drug if these results are outside of the acceptable parameters.

To hasten the onset of the therapeutic effect, a higher dosage (loading dose) may be prescribed for 2 to 4 days, followed by a maintenance dosage adjusted according to the daily PT/INR. Otherwise, the drug takes 3 to 5 days to reach therapeutic levels. When rapid anticoagulation is required, heparin is preferred as a loading dose, followed by maintenance dose of warfarin based on the PT or INR. The dose is typically given in the evening at a specified time. This prevents errors in administration of doses too high or too low, by providing ample time to allow time for adjustments based upon lab results.

NURSING ALERT

Optimal therapeutic results are obtained when the patient's PT is 1.2 to 1.5 times the control value. In certain instances, such as in recurrent systemic embolism, a PT of 1.5 to 2 may be prescribed. Studies indicate that diet can influence the PT/INR values. A study at the Massachusetts General Hospital in Boston looked at the effect of varying dietary vitamin K intake on the INR in patients receiving anticoagulation therapy with warfarin. As vitamin K intake increased, INR became more consistent and stable. By contrast, as vitamin K intake decreased, INR became more variable and fluctuated to a greater extent. The key to vitamin K management for patients receiving warfarin is maintaining a consistent daily intake of vitamin K.

PARENTERAL ADMINISTRATION OF ANTICOAGULANTS. Heparin preparations, unlike warfarin, must be given by the parenteral route, preferably subcut or IV. The onset of anticoagulation is almost immediate after a single dose. Maximum effects occur within 10 minutes of administration. Clotting time returns to normal within 4 hours unless subsequent doses are given. Although warfarin is most often administered orally, an injectable form may be used as an alternative route for patients who are unable to receive oral drugs.

Heparin may be given by intermittent IV administration, continuous IV infusion, and the subcut route. Intramuscular (IM) administration is avoided because of the possibility of the development of local irritation, pain, or hematoma (a collection of blood in the tissue). The dosage of heparin is measured in Units and is available in various dosage strengths as Units per milliliter (e.g., 10,000 Units/mL). When selecting the strength used for administration, choose the strength closest to the prescribed dose. For example, if 5000 Units are ordered, and the available strengths are 1000, 5000, 7500, 20,000, and 40,000 Units/mL, use 1 mL of the 5000 Units/mL for administration.

NURSING ALERT

Errors have been made by misreading the numbers on the bottles of heparin. Doses of 10,000 units have been misread as 100 units; as a result, patients have been put at risk for hemorrhage when receiving these higher doses. It is important for the nurse to prepare medications without distraction to minimize risk to patients.

An infusion pump must be used for the safe administration of heparin by continuous IV infusion. The nurse checks the infusion pump every 1 to 2 hours to ensure that it is working properly. The needle site is inspected for signs of inflammation, pain, and tenderness along the pathway of the vein. If these occur, the infusion is discontinued and restarted in another vein.

When heparin or other anticoagulants are given by the subcutaneous route, administration sites are rotated and the site used is recorded on the patient's chart. The recommended sites of administration are those on the abdomen, but areas within 2 inches of the umbilicus are avoided because of the increased vascularity of that area. Other areas of administration of heparin are the buttocks, lateral thighs, and upper arms. No fluctuation in absorption has been found by using the arms and legs. Drugs for DVT prevention are available in pre-filled syringes; do not expel the air bubble. They are administered deep in subcutaneous tissue by pinching a fold of skin. The nurse inserts the needle into the tissue at a 90-degree angle so the air bubble is injected last. It is not necessary to aspirate before injecting the drug; this may activate the needle guard. Be careful not to let go of the plunger until the syringe is empty and pulled out of the skin; letting go causes the needle to withdraw into the barrel of the syringe, thus preventing injury from a needle stick following the injection. The application of firm pressure after the injection helps to prevent hematoma formation. Each time heparin is given by this route; the nurse inspects all recent injection sites for signs of inflammation (redness, swelling, tenderness) and hematoma formation.

Blood coagulation tests are usually ordered before and during heparin therapy, and the dose of heparin is adjusted to the test results. Coagulation tests are usually performed 30 minutes before the scheduled dose and from the extremity opposite the infusion site. When administering heparin by the subcutaneous route, an aPTT test is performed 4 to 6 hours after the injection. Optimal results of therapy are obtained when the aPTT is 1.5 to 2.5 times the control value. The LMWHs do not require close monitoring of blood coagulation tests.

A complete blood count, platelet count, and stool analysis for occult blood may be ordered periodically throughout therapy. Thrombocytopenia may occur during heparin or antiplatelet administration. A mild, transient thrombocytopenia may occur 2 to 3 days after heparin therapy is begun. This early development of thrombocytopenia tends to resolve itself despite continued therapy. The nurse immediately reports a platelet count of less than 100,000 mm³, because the primary health care provider may choose to discontinue the heparin therapy. Overdose of antiplatelet drugs is typically managed by withholding treatment or by infusion of platelets.

⚠ NURSING ALERT

The nurse should withhold the drug and contact the primary health care provider immediately if any of the following occurs:

The PT exceeds 1.5 times the control value.
There is evidence of bleeding.
The INR is greater than 3.

ADMINISTRATION OF THROMBOLYTICS. For optimal therapeutic effect, the thrombolytic drugs are used as soon as possible after the formation of a thrombus, preferably within 4 to 6 hours or as soon as possible after the symptoms are identified. The greatest benefit follows drug administration within 4 hours, but significant benefits occur when the agents are used within the first 24 hours. The nurse must follow the primary health care provider's orders precisely regarding dosage and time of administration. These drugs are available in powder form and must be reconstituted according to the directions in the package insert.

The nurse must assess the patient for bleeding every 15 minutes during the first 60 minutes of therapy, every 15 to 30 minutes for the next 8 hours, and at least every 4 hours until therapy is completed. Vital signs are taken at least every 4 hours for the duration of therapy.

If pain is present, the primary health care provider may order an opioid analgesic. Once the clot dissolves and blood flows freely through the obstructed blood vessel, severe pain usually decreases.

Monitoring and Managing Patient Needs

RISK FOR INJURY. Bleeding can occur any time during therapy with warfarin or the heparin preparations, even when the INR appears to be within a safe limit (e.g., 2 to 3). All nursing personnel and medical team members should be made aware of any patient receiving warfarin and the observations necessary with administration. If bleeding should occur, the primary health care provider may decrease the dose, discontinue the heparin therapy for a time, or order the administration of protamine sulfate. The nurse makes the following checks for signs of bleeding:

- If a decided drop in blood pressure or rise in the pulse rate occurs, the nurse notifies the primary health care provider, because this may indicate internal bleeding. Because hemorrhage may begin as a slight bleeding or bruising tendency, the nurse frequently observes the patient for these occurrences. Sometimes, hemorrhage occurs without warning.
- Urinal, bedpan, catheter drainage unit—Inspect the urine for a pink to red color and the stool for signs of GI bleeding (bright red to black stools). Visually check

the catheter drainage every 2 to 4 hours and when the unit is emptied. Oral anticoagulants may impart a red-orange color to alkaline urine, making hematuria difficult to detect visually. A urinalysis may be necessary to determine if blood is in the urine.
- Emesis basin, nasogastric suction units—Visually check the nasogastric suction unit every 2 to 4 hours and when the unit is emptied. Check the emesis basin each time it is emptied.
- Skin, mucous membranes—Inspect the patient's skin daily for evidence of easy bruising or bleeding. Be alert for bleeding from minor cuts and scratches, nosebleeds, or excessive bleeding after IM, Subcut, or IV injections or after a venipuncture. After oral care, check the toothbrush and gums for signs of bleeding.

⚠ NURSING ALERT

When patients using anticoagulants have spinal anesthesia or undergo spinal punctures, they are at risk for potential spinal or epidural hematoma formation, which can lead to long-term or permanent paralysis. These patients should be frequently monitored for signs and symptoms of neurologic impairment.

INDIVIDUAL EFFECTIVE THERAPEUTIC REGIMEN MANAGEMENT. The patient needs to be aware of the many food and drug interactions that can cause a higher risk for bleeding when taking anticoagulants, or make the drugs less effective. If the patient became incapacitated by accident or illness, other care providers need to know that anticoagulant or antiplatelet drugs are being taken. The nurse should instruct the patient to wear medical identification that states he or she is receiving anticoagulant or antiplatelet therapy.

The patient is instructed to notify all health care providers of the anticoagulant or antiplatelet therapy when diagnostic tests or other treatments are performed. The patient should understand why the nurse must apply prolonged pressure to needle or catheter sites after venipuncture, removal of central or peripheral IV lines, and IM and subcut injections. Laboratory personnel or those responsible for drawing blood for laboratory tests are made aware of anticoagulant therapy, because prolonged pressure on the venipuncture site is necessary. All laboratory requests should have a notation stating the patient is receiving anticoagulant therapy.

ANXIETY. Bleeding is the most common adverse reaction when thrombolytic drugs are administered. Conditions requiring thrombolytic treatment are typically of an urgent nature, and treatment occurs in special care units of the hospital such as the intensive care unit or operating room. Combined with the potential for bleeding, all this can be frightening and cause anxiety to the patient and any family members present. As the nurse monitors the patient's status, it is important to reassure the patient and communicate with family members that measures are being taken to diagnose and intervene early for any adverse reactions.

Throughout administration of the thrombolytic drug, the nurse assesses for signs of bleeding and hemorrhage. Internal bleeding may involve the GI tract, genitourinary tract, intracranial sites, or respiratory tract. Signs and symptoms of internal bleeding may include abdominal pain, coffee-ground emesis, black, tarry stools, hematuria, joint pain, and spitting or coughing up blood.

Superficial bleeding may occur at venous or arterial puncture sites or recent surgical incision sites. Again, this can be disturbing to the patient and family, and they may become anxious. Because fibrin is lysed during therapy, bleeding from recent injection sites may occur. The nurse must carefully monitor all potential bleeding sites (including catheter insertion sites, arterial and venous puncture sites, cutdown sites, and needle puncture sites). The nurse reassures the patient that bleeding will be reported to the primary health care provider and steps taken to minimize the bleeding. Minor bleeding at a puncture site can usually be controlled by applying pressure for at least 30 minutes at the site, followed by the application of a pressure dressing. The puncture site is checked frequently for evidence of further bleeding. IM injections and nonessential handling of the patient are avoided during treatment. Venipunctures are done only when absolutely necessary.

NURSING ALERT

Heparin may be given along with or after administration of a thrombolytic drug to prevent another thrombus from forming. However, administration of an anticoagulant increases the risk for bleeding. The patient must be monitored closely for internal and external bleeding.

If uncontrolled bleeding is noted or the bleeding appears to be internal, the nurse stops the drug and immediately contacts the primary health care provider, because whole blood, packed red cells, or fresh frozen plasma may be required. Vital signs are monitored every hour (or more frequently) for at least 48 hours after the drug is discontinued. The nurse contacts the primary health care provider if there is a marked change in one or more of the vital signs. Any signs of an allergic (hypersensitivity) reaction, such as difficulty breathing, wheezing, hives, skin rash, and hypotension, are reported immediately to the primary health care provider.

MANAGING ANTICOAGULANT OVERDOSAGE. *Oral Anticoagulants.* Symptoms of warfarin overdosage include blood in the stool (melena); petechiae (pinpoint-sized red hemorrhagic spots on the skin); oozing from superficial injuries, such as cuts from shaving or bleeding from the gums after brushing the teeth; or excessive menstrual bleeding. The nurse must immediately report to the primary health care provider any of these adverse reactions or evidence of bleeding.

If bleeding occurs, if the PT exceeds 1.5 times the control value, or the INR exceeds 3, the primary health care provider may either discontinue the anticoagulant therapy for a few days or order vitamin K_1 (phytonadione), an oral anticoagulant antagonist, which should be readily available when a patient is receiving warfarin. Because warfarin interferes with the synthesis of vitamin K_1–dependent clotting factors, the administration of vitamin K_1 reverses the effects of warfarin by providing the necessary ingredient to enhance clot formation and stop bleeding. However, withholding one or two doses of warfarin may quickly bring the PT to an acceptable level.

The nurse must assess the patient for additional evidence of bleeding until the PT is below 1.5 times the control value or until the bleeding episodes cease. The PT usually returns to a safe level within 6 hours of administration of vitamin K_1. Administration of whole blood or plasma may be necessary if severe bleeding occurs because of the delayed onset of action of vitamin K_1.

Parenteral Anticoagulants. In most instances, discontinuation of the drug is sufficient to correct overdosage, because the duration of action of heparin is brief. However, if hemorrhaging is severe, the primary health care provider may order protamine, the specific heparin antagonist or antidote. Protamine is also used to treat overdosage of the LMWHs. Protamine has an immediate onset of action and a duration of 2 hours. It counteracts the effects of heparin and brings blood coagulation test results to within normal limits. The drug is given slowly by the IV route over a period of 10 minutes.

If administration of this drug is necessary, the nurse monitors the patient's blood pressure and pulse rate every 15 to 30 minutes for 2 hours or more after administration of the heparin antagonist. The nurse immediately reports to the primary health care provider any sudden decrease in blood pressure or increase in the pulse rate. The nurse observes the patient for new evidence of bleeding until blood coagulation test results are within normal limits. To replace blood loss, the primary health care provider may order blood transfusions or fresh frozen plasma.

Educating the Patient and Family

In many facilities the clinical pharmacist is responsible for anticoagulant teaching. A thorough review of the dosage regimen, possible adverse drug reactions, and early signs of bleeding tendencies help the patient cooperate with the prescribed therapy. The nurse provides further explanations or validates learning on the part of the patient and family. The nurse should validate understanding of the following points in a patient and family teaching plan:

- Follow the dosage schedule prescribed by the primary health care provider, and report any signs of active bleeding immediately.
- The INR will be monitored periodically. Keep all primary health care provider and laboratory appointments, because dosage changes may be necessary during therapy.
- Do not take or stop taking other drugs except on the advice of the primary health care provider. This includes nonprescription drugs, as well as those prescribed by a primary health care provider or dentist.

- Inform the dentist or other primary health care providers of therapy of this drug before any treatment or procedure is started or drugs are prescribed.
- Take the drug at the same time each day.
- Do not change brands of anticoagulants without consulting a physician or pharmacist.
- Avoid alcohol unless use has been approved by the primary health care provider.
- Be aware of foods high in vitamin K, such as leafy green vegetables, beans, broccoli, cabbage, cauliflower, cheese, fish, and yogurt. Maintaining a healthy diet including these foods may help maintain a consistent INR value.
- Keep in mind that antiplatelet drugs can lower all blood counts, including the white cell count. Patients may be at greater risk of infection during the first 3 months of treatment.
- If evidence of bleeding occurs, such as unusual bleeding or bruising, bleeding gums, blood in the urine or stool, black stool, or diarrhea, omit the next dose of the drug and contact the primary health care provider immediately (anisindione may cause a red-orange discoloration of alkaline urine).
- Use a soft toothbrush and consult a dentist regarding routine oral hygiene, including the use of dental floss. Use an electric razor when possible to avoid small skin cuts.
- Women of childbearing age should use a reliable contraceptive to prevent pregnancy.
- Wear or carry medical identification, such as a MedicAlert bracelet, to inform medical personnel and others of therapy with this drug.

EVALUATION

- Therapeutic response is achieved and blood coagulation is controlled.
- Adverse reactions are identified, reported to the primary health care provider, and managed successfully with appropriate nursing interventions:
  - ☑ No evidence of injury is seen.
  - ☑ Patient manages the therapeutic regimen effectively.
  - ☑ Anxiety is managed successfully.
- Patient and family demonstrate an understanding of the drug regimen.

THINK CRITICALLY: PHARMACOLOGY IN PRACTICE

1. Mr. Phillip, aged 72 years, is a widower who has lived alone since his wife died 5 years ago. He has been prescribed warfarin to take at home after his dismissal from the hospital. Determine which questions concerning the home environment would be important to ask Mr. Phillip to prepare him to care for himself and prevent any complications associated with warfarin.

● Test Your Knowledge

1. The patient is receiving oral anticoagulant drug therapy. Before administering the drug, the nurse _____.
   - **A.** administers a loading dose of heparin
   - **B.** has the laboratory draw blood for a serum potassium level
   - **C.** takes the apical pulse
   - **D.** sees that blood has been drawn for a baseline PT evaluation

2. Optimal INR during therapy is _____.
   - **A.** more than 5
   - **B.** less than 1
   - **C.** between 1.8 to 2
   - **D.** between 2 and 3

3. There is an increased risk for bleeding when the patient receiving heparin is also taking _____.
   - **A.** allopurinol
   - **B.** NSAIDs
   - **C.** digoxin
   - **D.** furosemide

4. In which of the following situations would the nurse expect an dalteparin to be prescribed?
   - **A.** To prevent a DVT
   - **B.** For a patient with DIC
   - **C.** To prevent hemorrhage
   - **D.** For a patient with atrial fibrillation

● Prepare for the NCLEX

1. If bleeding is noted while a patient is receiving a thrombolytic drug, the patient may receive _____.
   - **A.** heparin
   - **B.** whole blood or fresh frozen plasma
   - **C.** a diuretic
   - **D.** protamine sulfate

● Calculate Medication Dosages

1. the patient is prescribed 5000 Units of heparin. The drug is available as a solution of 7500 Units/mL. The nurse administers _____.

2. Oral warfarin 5 mg is prescribed. On hand are 2.5-mg tablets. The nurse administers _____.

To check your answers, see Appendix E.

the**Point** *For more NCLEX questions, log on to http://thepoint.lww.com to access more than 1000 questions.*

Cardiotonics and Miscellaneous Inotropic Drugs

KEY TERMS

atrial fibrillation
cardiac output
digitalis toxicity
digitalization
heart failure
hypokalemia

left ventricular
   dysfunction
neurohormonal activity
positive inotropic activity
right ventricular
   dysfunction

LEARNING OBJECTIVES

On completion of this chapter, the student will:

1. Discuss heart failure in relationship to left ventricular failure, right ventricular failure, neurohormonal activity, and treatment options.
2. Discuss the uses, general drug action, general adverse reactions, contraindications, precautions, and interactions of the cardiotonic and inotropic drugs.
3. Discuss the use of other drugs with positive inotropic action.
4. Discuss important preadministration and ongoing assessment activities the nurse should perform on the patient taking a cardiotonic or inotropic drug.
5. List nursing diagnoses particular to a patient taking a cardiotonic or inotropic drug.
6. Identify the symptoms of digitalis toxicity.
7. Discuss ways to promote an optimal response to therapy, how to manage common adverse reactions, and important points to keep in mind when administering a cardiotonic drug.

The cardiotonics are drugs used to increase the efficiency and improve the contraction of the heart muscle, which leads to improved blood flow to all tissues of the body. These drugs have long been used to treat **heart failure** (HF), a condition in which the heart cannot pump enough blood to meet the tissue needs of the body. Although the term *congestive heart failure* is commonly used, a more accurate term is simply *heart failure*.

HF is a complex clinical syndrome that can result from any number of cardiac or metabolic disorders, such as ischemic heart disease, hypertension, or hyperthyroidism. Any condition that impairs the ability of the ventricle to

pump blood can lead to HF. In HF, the heart fails in its ability to pump enough blood to meet the needs of the body or can do so only with an elevated filling pressure. HF causes a number of neurohormonal changes as the body tries to compensate for the increased workload of the heart. Display 39.1 discusses this neurohormonal response.

The sympathetic nervous system increases the secretion of the catecholamines (the neurohormones epinephrine and norepinephrine), which results in increased heart rate and vasoconstriction. The activation of the renin-angiotensin-aldosterone (RAA) system occurs because of decreased perfusion to the kidneys. As the RAA system is activated, angiotensin II and aldosterone levels increase, which increases the blood pressure, adding to the workload of the heart. These increases in **neurohormonal activity** cause a remodeling (restructuring) of the cardiac muscle cells, leading to hypertrophy (enlargement) of the heart, increased need for oxygen, and cardiac necrosis, which worsens the HF. The tissue of the heart is changed such that there is an increase in the cellular mass of cardiac tissue, the shape of the ventricle(s) is changed, and the heart's ability to contract effectively is reduced.

HF is best described by denoting the area of initial ventricular dysfunction: left-sided (left ventricular) dysfunction or right-sided (right ventricular) dysfunction. **Left ventricular dysfunction** leads to pulmonary symptoms, such as dyspnea and moist cough with the production of frothy, pink (blood-tinged) sputum. **Right ventricular dysfunction** leads to neck vein distention, peripheral edema, weight gain, and hepatic engorgement. Because both sides of the heart work together, ultimately both sides are affected in HF. Typically the left side of the heart is affected first, followed by right ventricular involvement. The most common symptoms associated with HF include the following:

- Left ventricular dysfunction
- Shortness of breath with exercise

DISPLAY 39.1 Neurohormonal Responses Affecting Heart Failure

The body activates the neurohormonal compensatory mechanisms, which result in:

- Increased secretion of the neurohormones by the sympathetic nervous system
- Activation of the renin-angiotensin-aldosterone (RAA) system
- Remodeling of the cardiac tissue

- Dry, hacking cough or wheezing
- Orthopnea (difficulty breathing while lying flat)
- Restlessness and anxiety
- Right ventricular dysfunction
- Swollen ankles, legs, or abdomen, leading to pitting edema
- Anorexia
- Nausea
- Nocturia (the need to urinate frequently at night)
- Weakness
- Weight gain as the result of fluid retention

Other symptoms include

- Palpitations, fatigue, or pain when performing normal activities
- Tachycardia or irregular heart rate
- Dizziness or confusion

Left ventricular dysfunction, also called left ventricular systolic dysfunction, is the most common form of HF and results in decreased **cardiac output** and decreased ejection fraction (the amount of blood that the ventricle ejects per beat in relationship to the amount of blood available to eject). Typically, the ejection fraction should be greater than 60%. With left ventricular systolic dysfunction, the ejection fraction is less than 40%, and the heart is enlarged and dilated.

In the past, the cardiotonics were the mainstay in HF treatment; currently, however, they are used in the treatment of patients who continue to experience symptoms after using the angiotensin-converting enzyme (ACE) inhibitors, diuretics, and β blockers.

• CARDIOTONICS

Cardiotonic drugs are used for patients with persistent symptoms, recurrent hospitalizations, or as indicated in conjunction with ACE inhibitors, loop diuretics, and β blockers.

Digoxin (Lanoxin) is the most commonly used cardiotonic drug. Other terms used to identify the cardiotonics are cardiac glycosides or digitalis glycosides. The digitalis or cardiac glycosides are obtained from the leaves of the foxglove plant (*Digitalis purpurea* and *Digitalis lanata*).

Miscellaneous drugs with positive inotropic action, such as milrinone (Primacor), are nonglycosides used in the short-term management of HF. See the Summary Drug Table: Cardiotonics and Miscellaneous Inotropic Drugs for information concerning these drugs.

Actions

Cardiotonics, particularly digitalis drugs, increase cardiac output through **positive inotropic activity** (an increase in the force of the contraction). They slow the conduction velocity through the atrioventricular (AV) node in the heart and decrease the heart rate through a negative chronotropic effect.

Summary Drug Table CARDIOTONICS AND MISCELLANEOUS INOTROPIC DRUGS

Generic Name	Trade Name	Uses	Adverse Reactions	Dosage Ranges
Cardiotonics				
digoxin *dih-jox'-in*	Digitek, Lanoxicaps, Lanoxin	HF, atrial fibrillation	Headache, weakness, drowsiness, visual disturbances, nausea, vomiting, anorexia, arrhythmias	Loading dose*: 0.75–1.25 mg orally or 0.6–1mg IV Maintenance: 0.125–0.25 mg/day orally; Lanoxicaps: 0.1–0.3 mg/day orally
Miscellaneous Inotropic Drugs				
inamrinone *in-am'-rih-noan*		Short-term management of HF in patients with no response to digitalis, diuretics, or vasodilators	Arrhythmia, hypotension, nausea, vomiting, abdominal pain, anorexia, hepatotoxicity	IV: 0.75 mg/kg bolus, may repeat in 30 min Maintenance: 5–10 mg/kg/min IV, not to exceed 10 mg/kg/day
milrinone *mill'-rih-noan*	Primacor	Short-term management of HF	Ventricular arrhythmias, hypotension, angina/chest pain, headaches, hypokalemia	Loading dose: 50 mcg/kg IV IV: Up to 1.13 mg/kg/day
Digoxin-Specific Antidote				
digoxin immune fab	Digibind	Antidote for massive digoxin overdose	Hypokalemia, reemergence of atrial fibrillation or HF	IV: Dosage depends on serum digoxin level or estimate of the amount of digoxin ingested; average dose up to 800 mg (20 vials)

*Based on patient lean body weight of 70 kg.

Uses

The cardiotonics are used to treat the following:

• HF
• **Atrial fibrillation**

Atrial fibrillation is a cardiac arrhythmia characterized by rapid contractions and quivering of the atrial myocardium, resulting in an irregular and often rapid ventricular rate. See Chapter 40 for more information on arrhythmias and their treatment.

Adverse Reactions

Central Nervous System Reactions

• Headache
• Weakness, drowsiness
• Visual disturbances (blurring or yellow halo)

Cardiovascular and Gastrointestinal System Reactions

• Arrhythmias
• Nausea and anorexia

Because some patients are more sensitive to side effects of digoxin, dosage is calculated carefully and adjusted as the clinical condition indicates. There is a narrow margin of safety between the full therapeutic effects and the toxic effects of cardiotonic drugs. Even normal doses of a cardiotonic drug can cause toxic drug effects. Because substantial individual variations may occur, it is important to individualize the dosage. The term **digitalis toxicity** (or *digitalis intoxication*) is used to describe toxic drug effects that occur when digoxin is administered.

Contraindications and Precautions

The cardiotonics are contraindicated in the presence of digitalis toxicity and in patients with known hypersensitivity, ventricular failure, ventricular tachycardia, cardiac tamponade, restrictive cardiomyopathy, or AV block.

The cardiotonics are given cautiously to patients with electrolyte imbalance (especially **hypokalemia** [low serum potassium levels], hypocalcemia, and hypomagnesemia), thyroid disorders, severe carditis, heart block, myocardial infarction, severe pulmonary disease, acute glomerulonephritis, and impaired renal or hepatic function.

Digoxin and digoxin immune fab are classified as pregnancy category C drugs and are used cautiously during pregnancy and lactation. Exposure to digoxin in a nursing infant is typically below an infant maintenance dose, yet caution should be exercised when digoxin is taken by a nursing woman.

Interactions

When the cardiotonics are taken with food, absorption is slowed, but the amount absorbed is the same. However, if taken with high-fiber meals, absorption of the cardiotonics may be decreased. Certain drugs may increase or decrease serum digitalis levels as follows:

Interacting Drug	Common Use	Effect of Interaction
amiodarone	Cardiac problems	
benzodiazepines (alprazolam, diazepam)	Treatment of seizures and anxiety	
indomethacin	Pain relief	
itraconazole	Fungal infections	
macrolides (erythromycin, clarithromycin)	Infections	**Increased** serum digitalis levels leading to toxicity
propafenone	Cardiac problems	
quinidine	Cardiac problems	
spironolactone	Edema	
tetracyclines, macrolides	Infections	
verapamil	Cardiac problems	
oral aminoglycoside	Infections	
antacids	Gastrointestinal (GI) problems	
antineoplastics (bleomycin, carmustine, cyclophosphamide, methotrexate, and vincristine)	Anticancer agents	**Decreased** serum digitalis levels
activated charcoal	Antidote to poisoning with certain toxic substances	
cholestyramine	Agent to lower high blood cholesterol levels	
colestipol	Agent to lower high blood cholesterol levels	**Decreased** serum digitalis levels
neomycin	Agent to suppress GI bacteria before surgery	
rifampin	Antitubercular agent	

Patients may not always volunteer information regarding their use of alternative or complementary remedies. The nurse should always inquire about use of herbal products. Medical reports indicate a possible interaction with St. John's wort (used to relieve depression), causing a decrease in serum digitalis levels. The following interactions may occur with the cardiac glycosides:

Interacting Drug	Common Use	Effect of Interaction
thyroid hormones	Treatment of hypothyroidism	Decreased effectiveness of digitalis glycosides, requiring a larger dosage of digoxin
thiazide and loop diuretics	Management of edema and hypertension	Increased diuretic-induced electrolyte disturbances, predisposing the patient to digitalis-induced arrhythmias

• MISCELLANEOUS INOTROPIC DRUGS

Inamrinone and milrinone have inotropic actions and are used in the short-term management of severe HF that is not controlled by the digitalis preparations. Milrinone is used more often than inamrinone, appears to be more effective, and has fewer adverse reactions. Both drugs are given intravenously (IV), and close monitoring is required during therapy. The nurse must monitor the patient's heart rate and blood pressure continuously with administration of either drug. If hypotension occurs, the drug is discontinued or the rate of administration is reduced. Continuous cardiac monitoring is necessary. because life-threatening arrhythmias may occur. These drugs do not cure HF; rather, they control its signs and symptoms.

NURSING PROCESS
PATIENT RECEIVING A CARDIOTONIC DRUG

ASSESSMENT

Preadministration Assessment
The cardiotonics are potentially toxic drugs. Therefore, the nurse must observe the patient closely, especially during initial therapy. Before therapy is started, the physical assessment should include information that will establish a database for comparison during therapy. The physical assessment should include the following:

- Taking blood pressure, apical-radial pulse rate, respiratory rate
- Auscultating the lungs, noting any unusual sounds during inspiration and expiration
- Examining the extremities for edema
- Checking the jugular veins for distention
- Measuring weight
- Inspecting sputum raised (if any), and noting the appearance (e.g., frothy, pink-tinged, clear, yellow)
- Looking for evidence of other problems, such as cyanosis, shortness of breath on exertion (if the patient is allowed out of bed) or when lying flat, and mental changes.

The primary health care provider also may order laboratory and diagnostic tests, such as an electrocardiogram, renal and hepatic function tests, complete blood count, and serum enzyme and electrolyte levels. These tests should be reviewed before the first dose of the drug is given. Renal function is particularly important. because diminished renal function could affect the prescribed dosage of digoxin. When subsequent laboratory tests are ordered, test findings also should be reviewed when the results are recorded on the patient's record. Because digoxin interacts with many medications, the nurse must take a careful drug history. Before administering the first dose of the drug, the nurse takes the patient's vital signs and documents the apical pulse rate and rhythm.

Ongoing Assessment
Before administering each dose of a cardiotonic, the nurse takes the apical pulse rate for 60 seconds (Fig. 39.1). The nurse records the apical pulse rate in the designated area on the chart or the medication administration record. If the pulse rate is below 60 beats per minute (bpm) in adults or greater than 100 bpm, the nurse withholds the drug and notifies the primary health care provider, unless there is a written order giving different guidelines for withholding the drug.

LIFESPAN ALERT – Pediatric
The drug is withheld and the primary health care provider notified before administering the drug if the apical pulse rate in a child is below 70 bpm, or below 90 bpm in an infant.

The nurse weighs patients receiving a cardiotonic drug daily, or as ordered. Intake and output are measured, especially if the patient has edema or HF or is also receiving a diuretic. Throughout therapy, the nurse assesses the patient for peripheral edema and auscultates the lungs for rales or crackles throughout therapy. Serum electrolyte levels should be assessed periodically. Hypokalemia, hypomagnesemia, or hypercalcemia may increase the risk for toxicity. Any electrolyte imbalance is reported to the primary health care provider.

NURSING DIAGNOSES

Drug-specific nursing diagnoses include thee following:

- ❏ **Imbalanced Nutrition: Less Than Body Requirements** related to anorexia, nausea, vomiting
- ❏ **Activity Intolerance** related to weakness and drowsiness

Nursing diagnoses related to drug administration are discussed in Chapter 4.

PLANNING

The expected outcomes of the patient depend on the specific reason for administering the drug, but may

Figure 39.1 Nurse counts the apical pulse for 1 minute before administering the cardiotonic.

include an optimal response to therapy, support of patient needs related to the management of adverse reactions, and an understanding of the therapeutic regimen.

IMPLEMENTATION

Promoting an Optimal Response to Therapy

Great care must be taken when administering a cardiotonic drug. The nurse should carefully check the primary health care provider's order and the drug container. If there is any doubt about the dosage or calculation of the dosage, the nurse checks with the primary health care provider or pharmacist before giving the drug.

Dosing of digoxin is based upon individual sensitivity of the patient to the drug. The following factors are considered:

- Patient lean body weight
- Renal function as indicated by the estimated creatinine clearance
- Patient age
- Factors likely to alter the pharmacokinetics or pharmacodynamics, such as disease state or concurrent medications being taken by the patient.

DIGITALIZATION. Patients started on therapy with a cardiotonic drug are being "digitalized." **Digitalization** may be accomplished by two general methods:

- Rapid digitalization (accomplished by administering a loading dose)
- Gradual digitalization (a maintenance dose is given, allowing therapeutic drug blood levels to accumulate gradually)

Digitalization involves giving a series of doses until the drug begins to exert a full therapeutic effect. The digitalizing, or loading dose, is administered in several doses, with approximately half the total digitalization dose administered as the first dose. Additional fractions of the digitalis dose are administered at 6- to 8-hour intervals. Once a full therapeutic effect is achieved, the primary health care provider usually prescribes a maintenance dose schedule. The ranges for digitalizing (loading) and maintenance doses are given in the Summary Drug Table: Cardiotonics and Miscellaneous Inotropic Drugs. Digoxin injections are usually used for rapid digitalization; digoxin tablets or capsules are used for maintenance therapy.

During digitalization, the nurse takes the blood pressure, pulse, and respiratory rate every 2 to 4 hours or as ordered by the primary health care provider. This interval may be increased or decreased, depending on the patient's condition and the route used for drug administration.

Measurement of serum levels (digoxin) may be ordered daily during the period of digitalization and periodically during maintenance therapy. Any signs of digitalis toxicity are reported immediately to the primary health care provider (see Potential Complication: Digitalis Toxicity, later).

❗ NURSING ALERT

Plasma digoxin levels are monitored closely. Blood for plasma level measurements should be drawn immediately before the next dose or 6 to 8 hours after the last dose regardless of route. Therapeutic drug levels are between 0.8 and 2 nanograms/mL. Plasma digoxin levels greater than 2 nanograms/mL are considered toxic and are reported to the primary health care provider

Periodic electrocardiograms, serum electrolytes, hepatic and renal function tests, and other laboratory studies also may be ordered. Diuretics (see Chapter 48) may be ordered for some patients receiving a cardiotonic drug. Diuretics, along with other conditions or factors, such as GI suction, diarrhea, and old age, may produce low serum potassium levels (hypokalemia). The primary health care provider may order a potassium salt to be given orally or IV.

❗ NURSING ALERT

Hypokalemia makes the heart muscle more sensitive to digitalis, thereby increasing the possibility of developing digitalis toxicity. At frequent intervals, the nurse must observe patients with hypokalemia closely for signs of digitalis toxicity.

Patients with hypomagnesemia (low plasma magnesium levels) are at increased risk for digitalis toxicity. If low magnesium levels are detected, the primary health care provider may prescribe magnesium replacement therapy.

PARENTERAL ADMINISTRATION. The nurse may give a cardiotonic orally, IV, or intramuscularly (IM). When a cardiotonic drug is given IV, it is administered slowly (over at least 5 minutes), and the administration site is assessed for redness or infiltration. IM injection is not recommended for these drugs yet, but it may be given through this route when needed urgently and IV access is not available. When giving a cardiotonic drug IM, the nurse should give the injection deep in the muscle and follow with massage to the site. No more than 2 mL should be injected IM.

ORAL ADMINISTRATION. The nurse can administer oral preparations without regard to meals. Tablets can be crushed and mixed with food or fluids if the patient has difficulty swallowing. Do not alternate between the dosage forms (i.e., tablets and capsules). because dosages are not the same. Due to better absorption, the recommended dosage of the capsules is 80% of the dosage for tablets and elixir.

Monitoring and Managing Patient Needs

IMBALANCED NUTRITION: LESS THAN BODY REQUIREMENTS. The nurse must also closely observe the patient for other adverse drug reactions, such as anorexia, nausea, and vomiting. Some adverse drug reactions are also signs of digitalis toxicity, which can be serious. The nurse should carefully consider any patient complaint or comment, record it on the patient's chart, and bring it to the attention of the primary health care provider. If the nausea or anorexia is not a result of toxicity but an adverse reaction to the drug, the nurse may use nursing measures to help control the reactions. The nurse may offer frequent small meals, rather than three large meals. The nurse may suggest restricting fluids at meals and avoiding fluids 1 hour before and after meals to help control the nausea. Helping the patient to maintain good oral hygiene by brushing teeth or rinsing the mouth after ingesting food will also help with nausea. However, the nurse must always be aware that nausea and vomiting are symptoms of toxicity and must monitor the patient closely for other signs of digitalis toxicity.

ACTIVITY INTOLERANCE. The patient may experience weakness or drowsiness as adverse reactions associated with digoxin, which may lead to activity intolerance. The patient is encouraged to increase daily activities gradually as tolerance increases, and the nurse plans a gradual increase in activities as tolerance increases. Adequate rest periods are planned during the day. The nurse assists with activities and ambulation as necessary.

POTENTIAL MEDICAL COMPLICATION: DIGITALIS TOXICITY. The nurse observes for signs of digitalis toxicity every 2 to 4 hours during digitalization and one to two times a day when a maintenance dose is being given.

NURSING ALERT

The nurse should withhold the drug and report any of the following signs of digitalis toxicity to the primary health care provider immediately: loss of appetite (anorexia), nausea, vomiting, abdominal pain, visual disturbances (blurred, yellow, or green vision and white halos, borders around dark objects), and arrhythmias (any type). The nurse also must report immediately serum digoxin levels greater than 2.0 nanograms/mL.

Digitalis toxicity can occur even when normal doses are being administered or when the patient has been receiving a maintenance dose. Many symptoms of toxicity are similar to the symptoms of the heart conditions for which the patient is receiving the cardiotonic. This makes careful assessment of the patient by the nurse a critical aspect of care. The signs of digitalis toxicity are listed in Display 39.2. When digitalis toxicity develops, the primary health care provider may discontinue digitalis use until all signs of toxicity are gone. If severe bradycardia occurs, atropine (see Chapter 27) may be ordered. If digoxin has been given, the primary health care provider may order blood tests to determine serum drug levels.

DISPLAY 39.2 **Signs of Digitalis Toxicity**

- Gastrointestinal—anorexia (usually the first sign), nausea, vomiting, diarrhea
- Muscular—weakness, lethargy
- Central nervous system—headache, drowsiness, visual disturbances (blurred vision, disturbance in yellow green vision, halo effect around dark objects), confusion, disorientation, delirium
- Cardiac—changes in pulse rate or rhythm: electrocardiographic changes, such as bradycardia, tachycardia, premature ventricular contractions

Digoxin has a rapid onset and a short duration of action. Once the drug is withheld, the toxic effects of digoxin subside rapidly.

LIFESPAN ALERT – Gerontology

Older adults are particularly prone to digitalis toxicity. Some conditions such as dementia may have similar signs, such as confusion, as those of digitalis toxicity. All older adults must be carefully monitored for signs of digitalis toxicity.

Most often, digoxin toxicity can be treated successfully by simply withdrawing the drug. However, severe life-threatening toxicity is treated with digoxin immune fab (Digibind). Digoxin immune fab, composed of digoxin-specific antigen-binding fragments (fab), is used as an antidote in the treatment of digoxin overdosage. The dosage varies with the amount of digoxin ingested, and the drug is administered by the IV route during a 30-minute period. Most life-threatening states can be treated adequately with 800 mg of digoxin immune fab (20 vials). Few adverse reactions have been observed with the use of immune fab. However, the nurse should be alert for the possibility of worsening HF, low cardiac output, hypokalemia, or atrial fibrillation. Hypokalemia is of particular concern in patients taking digoxin immune fab, particularly because hypokalemia usually coexists with toxicity (see the Summary Drug Table: Cardiotonics and Miscellaneous Inotropic Drugs).

Educating the Patient and Family

In some instances, a cardiotonic drug may be prescribed for a prolonged period. Some patients may discontinue use of the drug, especially if they feel better and their original symptoms have been relieved. The patient and family must understand that the prescribed drug must be taken exactly as directed by the primary health care provider.

If the primary health care provider wants the patient to monitor the pulse rate daily during cardiotonic therapy, the nurse shows the patient or a family member the correct technique for taking the pulse (see Patient Teaching for Improved Patient Outcomes: Monitoring Pulse Rate).

The primary health care provider may also want the patient to omit the next dose of the drug and call him or her if the pulse rate falls below a certain level (usually 60 bpm in an adult, 70 bpm in a child, and 90 bpm in an infant). These instructions are emphasized at the time of patient teaching. The nurse includes the following points in a teaching plan for the patient taking a cardiac glycoside drug:

- Do not discontinue use of this drug without first checking with the primary health care provider (unless instructed to do otherwise). Do not miss a dose or take an extra dose.
- Take this drug at the same time each day; a compartmentalized pill container may be helpful.
- Take your pulse before taking the drug, and withhold the drug and notify the primary health care provider if your pulse rate is less than 60 bpm or greater than 100 bpm.

Cardiotonics and Miscellaneous Inotropic Drugs

- Avoid antacids and nonprescription cough, cold, allergy, antidiarrheal, and diet (weight-reducing) drugs unless their use has been approved by the primary health care provider. Some of these drugs interfere with the action of the cardiotonic drug or cause other, potentially serious problems (see Interactions, earlier).
- Contact the primary health care provider if nausea, vomiting, diarrhea, unusual fatigue, weakness, vision change (such as blurred vision, changes in colors of objects, or halos around dark objects), or mental depression occurs.
- Carry medical identification describing the disease process and your medication regimen.
- Do not substitute tablets for capsules or vice versa.
- Follow the dietary recommendations (if any) made by the primary health care provider.
- The primary health care provider will closely monitor therapy. Keep all appointments for primary health care provider visits or laboratory or diagnostic tests.

EVALUATION

- Therapeutic response is achieved, and the heart beats more efficiently.
- Adverse reactions are identified, reported to the primary health care provider, and managed successfully with appropriate nursing interventions:
  - ☑ Patient maintains an adequate nutritional status.
  - ☑ Patient carries out activities of daily living.
- Patient and family demonstrate an understanding of the drug regimen.

Patient Teaching for Improved Patient Outcomes

Monitoring Pulse Rate

Monitoring a patient's pulse rate is second nature when the patient is in an acute care facility. However, when the patient goes home with digoxin, he or she will need to monitor the pulse rate to prevent possible adverse reactions. The nurse teaches the patient or caregiver to perform the following steps:

✓ Have a watch with a second hand with you.
✓ Sit down and rest your nondominant arm on a table or chair armrest.
✓ Place the index and third fingers of your dominant hand just below the wrist bone on the thumb side of your nondominant arm.
✓ Feel lightly for a beating or pulsing sensation. This is your pulse.
✓ Count the number of beats for 30 seconds (if the pulse is regular) and multiply by 2. If the pulse is irregular, count the number of beats for 60 seconds.
✓ Record the number of beats of your pulse and keep a log of your reading.
✓ If you notice the pulse is greater than 100 bpm or less than 60 bpm, call your primary health care provider immediately.

THINK CRITICALLY: PHARMACOLOGY IN PRACTICE

1. Discuss when you would expect the primary health care provider to order digoxin immune fab. State the assessment you feel would be most important and give a rationale. Now think about the clinic patients you have learned about in this book, which ones would you suspect may be more susceptible to digoxin toxicity?

● Test Your Knowledge

1. Which of the following is commonly associated with left ventricular systolic dysfunction?
   A. Ejection fraction of 60% or more
   B. Ejection fraction below 40%
   C. Increased cardiac output
   D. Normal cardiac output

2. Which of the following serum digoxin levels in an adult would be most indicative that the patient may be experiencing digoxin toxicity?
   A. 0.5 nanograms/mL
   B. 0.8 nanograms/mL
   C. 1.0 nanograms/mL
   D. 2.0 nanograms/mL

3. In which of the following situations would the nurse withhold a dose of digoxin and notify the primary health care provider?
   A. pulse rate of 50 bpm
   B. pulse rate of 87 bpm
   C. pulse rate of 92 bpm
   D. pulse rate of 62 bpm

4. During rapid digitalization, the nurse expects the first dose to be _____.
   A. the smallest dose in case the patient is allergic to digoxin
   B. given orally, with succeeding doses given intravenously
   C. approximately half of the total digitalization dose
   D. approximately three quarters of the total digitalization dose

● Prepare for the NCLEX

1. The nurse suspects a patient is experiencing digoxin toxicity. Which of the following symptoms did the patient report to make the nurse suspicious of a toxic reaction?
   A. insatiable hunger
   B. constipation
   C. halo in vision field
   D. muscle cramping

● Calculate Medication Dosages

1. Digoxin (Lanoxin) is prescribed for a patient with HF, and digitalization is begun. The primary health care

provider prescribes digoxin (Lanoxin) 0.75 mg orally as the initial dose. Available are digoxin tablets of 0.5 and 0.25 mg. The nurse administers _____.

2. Digoxin 0.5 mg IV is prescribed. The drug is available in a solution of 0.25 mg/mL. How many milliliters will the nurse prepare?

To check your answers, see Appendix E.

the**Point** *For more NCLEX questions, log on to http://thepoint.lww.com to access more than 1000 questions.*

Antiarrhythmic Drugs

LEARNING OBJECTIVES

On completion of this chapter, the student will:

1. Describe various types of cardiac arrhythmias.
2. Discuss the uses, general drug actions, general adverse reactions, contraindications, precautions, and interactions of the antiarrhythmic drugs.
3. Discuss important preadministration and ongoing assessments the nurse should perform on a patient taking an antiarrhythmic drug.
4. List nursing diagnoses particular to a patient taking an antiarrhythmic drug.
5. Discuss ways to promote an optimal response to therapy, how to manage common adverse reactions, and important points to keep in mind when educating patients about the use of antiarrhythmic drugs.

The antiarrhythmic drugs are primarily used to treat cardiac arrhythmias. A cardiac **arrhythmia** is a disturbance or irregularity in the heart rate, rhythm, or both, which requires administration of one of the antiarrhythmic drugs. Some examples of cardiac arrhythmias are listed in Table 40.1.

An arrhythmia may occur as a result of heart disease or from a disorder that affects cardiovascular function. Conditions such as emotional stress, hypoxia, and electrolyte imbalance also may trigger an arrhythmia. An electrocardiogram (ECG) provides a record of the electrical activity of the heart. Careful interpretation of the ECG along with a thorough physical assessment are necessary to determine the cause and type of arrhythmia. The goal of antiarrhythmic drug therapy is to restore normal cardiac function and prevent life-threatening arrhythmias.

Actions

The cardiac muscle (myocardium) has attributes of both nerve and muscle and therefore has the properties of both. Some cardiac arrhythmias are caused by the generation of an abnormal number of electrical impulses (stimuli). These abnormal impulses may come from the sinoatrial (SA) node or may be generated in other areas of the myocardium. The antiarrhythmic drugs are classified according to their effects on the **action potential** of cardiac cells and their presumed mechanism of action. As understanding of the pathophysiology of cardiac arrhythmias and the drugs used to treat these arrhythmias has increased, a method of classification has been developed that includes four basic classes and several subclasses. Drugs in each group, or class, have certain similarities, yet each drug has subtle differences that make it unique.

Class I Sodium Channel Blockers

Class I antiarrhythmic drugs, such as moricizine, have a membrane-stabilizing or anesthetic effect on the cells of the

Table 40.1 Types of Arrhythmias	
Arrhythmia	**Description**
Atrial flutter	Rapid contraction of the atria (up to 300 bpm) at a rate too rapid for the ventricles to pump efficiently
Atrial fibrillation	Irregular and rapid atrial contraction, resulting in a quivering of the atria and causing an irregular and inefficient ventricular contraction
Premature ventricular	Beats originating in the contractions ventricles instead of the sinoatrial node in the atria, causing the ventricles to contract before the atria and resulting in a decrease in the amount of blood pumped to the body
Ventricular tachycardia	A rapid heart beat with a rate of more than 100 bpm, usually originating in the ventricles
Ventricular fibrillation	Rapid, disorganized contractions of the ventricles resulting in the inability of the heart to pump any blood to the body, which will result in death unless treated immediately

myocardium, making them valuable in treating cardiac arrhythmias. Class I contains the largest number of drugs of the four antiarrhythmic drug classifications. Because their actions differ slightly, the drugs are subdivided into classes IA, IB, and IC.

Class IA Drugs

In general, class IA drugs act to

• prolong the action potential
• produce moderate slowing of cardiac conduction

The drugs disopyramide (Norpace), procainamide (Procanbid), and quinidine (Quinaglute) are examples of class IA drugs. Disopyramide decreases **depolarization** of myocardial fibers during the diastolic phase of the cardiac cycle, prolongs the **refractory period**, and increases the action potential duration of normal cardiac cells (Display 40.1).

Procainamide increases the effective refractory period of the atria and, to a lesser extent, the bundle of His-Purkinje fibers. Quinidine depresses myocardial excitability or the ability of the myocardium to respond to an electrical stimulus. By depressing the myocardium and its ability to respond to some, but not all, electrical stimuli, the pulse rate decreases and the arrhythmia is corrected. Quinidine also depresses the conduction velocity and contractility. It prolongs the effective refractory period and increases conduction time. See Display 40.2 for a discussion of **polarization**, depolarization, and **repolarization**.

Class IB Drugs

Class IB drugs generally act to:

• Shorten the action potential duration
• Selectively depress cardiac conduction

Lidocaine (Xylocaine), the representative class IB drug, decreases diastolic depolarization, decreases automaticity of

DISPLAY 40.1 Understanding Action Potential and Refractory Period

Action Potential

All cells are electrically polarized, with the inside of the cell more negatively charged than the outside. The difference in the electrical charge is called the *resting membrane potential*. Nerve and muscle cells are excitable and can change the resting membrane potential in response to electrochemical stimuli. The action potential is an electrical impulse that passes from cell to cell in the myocardium, stimulating the fibers to shorten, and causing muscular contraction (systole). An action potential generated in one part of the myocardium passes almost simultaneously through all of the myocardial fibers, causing rapid contraction.

Refractory Period

Only one impulse can pass along a nerve fiber at any given time. After the passage of an impulse, there is a brief pause, or interval, before the next impulse can pass along the nerve fiber. This pause is called the *refractory period*, which is the period between the transmission of nerve impulses along a nerve fiber. Lengthening the refractory period decreases the number of impulses traveling along a nerve fiber within a given time.

ventricular cells, and raises the **threshold** of the ventricular myocardium. *Threshold* is a term applied to any stimulus of the lowest intensity that will give rise to a response in a nerve fiber. A stimulus must be of a specific intensity (strength, amplitude) to pass along a given nerve fiber (Fig. 40.1).

To illustrate further the threshold phenomenon (using round figures instead of precise electrical values), consider a certain nerve fiber as having a threshold of 10. If a stimulus rated as 9 reaches the fiber, it will not pass along the fiber, because its intensity is lower than the fiber's threshold of 10. If another stimulus reaches the fiber and is rated 14, it will pass along the fiber, because its intensity is greater than the fiber's threshold of 10. If the threshold of a fiber is raised from 10 to 15, only stimuli greater than 15 can pass along the nerve fiber.

Some cardiac arrhythmias result from many stimuli present in the myocardium. Some of these are weak or of low intensity but are still able to excite myocardial tissue. Lidocaine, by raising the threshold of myocardial fibers, reduces the number of stimuli that will pass along these fibers and therefore decreases the pulse rate and corrects the arrhythmia.

Class IC Drugs

The general action of class IC drugs includes

• Slight effect on repolarization
• Profound slowing of conduction

Flecainide (Tambocor) and propafenone (Rythmol) are examples of class IC drugs. Specifically, flecainide depresses fast sodium channels, decreases the height and rate of rise of action potentials, and slows conduction of all areas of the heart. Propafenone, which has a direct membrane-stabilizing effect on the myocardial membrane, prolongs the refractory period.

Class II β-Adrenergic Blockers

The general action of drugs in class II is to indirectly block calcium channels and block catecholamine caused dysrhythmias. Class II antiarrhythmic drugs include β-adrenergic blocking drugs, such as acebutolol (Sectral) and propranolol (Inderal). Acebutolol and propranolol act by blocking β-adrenergic receptors of the heart and kidney, reducing the influence of the sympathetic nervous system on these areas, decreasing the excitability of the heart and the release of renin (lowering heart rate and blood pressure). These drugs have membrane-stabilizing effects that contribute to their antiarrhythmic activity.

Class III Potassium Channel Blockers

The general action of class III antiarrhythmic drugs is prolongation of repolarization (phase 3). Examples are amiodarone (Cordarone) and ibutilide (Corvert). Amiodarone appears to act directly on the cardiac cell membrane, prolonging the refractory period and repolarization and increasing the ventricular fibrillation threshold. Ibutilide acts by prolonging the action potential, producing a mild slowing of the sinus rate and atrioventricular (AV) conduction.

Antiarrhythmic Drugs

DISPLAY 40.2 Polarization, Depolarization, and Repolarization

Nerve cells have positive ions on the outside and negative ions on the inside of the cell membrane when they are at rest. This is called polarization. When a stimulus passes along the nerve, the positive ions move from outside the cell into the cell, and the negative ions move from inside the cell to outside the cell. This movement of ions is called depolarization. Unless positive ions move into and negative ions move out of a nerve cell, a stimulus (or impulse) cannot pass along the nerve fiber. Once the stimulus has passed along the nerve fiber, the positive and

negative ions move back to their original place, that is, the positive ions on the outside and the negative ions on the inside of the nerve cell. This movement back to the original place is called repolarization. By decreasing the rate (or speed) of depolarization, the stimulus must literally wait for this process before it can pass along the nerve fiber. Thus, decreasing the rate (or speed) of depolarization decreases the number of impulses that can pass along a nerve fiber during a specific time period.

Polarization

When the nerve cell is polarized, positive ions (⊕) are on the outside of the cell membrane and the negative ions (⊖) are on the inside of the cell membrane.

Depolarization

In response to a stimulus, the positive ions move from the outside to the inside of the cell membrane, while the negative ions move to the outside.

Repolarization

After the stimulus has passed along the nerve fiber, the ions move back to their original place until another stimulus occurs.

Class IV Calcium Channel Blockers

In general, the class IV antiarrhythmic drugs act by

- Depressing depolarization (phase 4)
- Lengthening phase 1 and 2 of repolarization

Verapamil (Calan), a class IV antiarrhythmic drug, is also classified as a calcium channel blocker. Calcium channel blockers inhibit the movement of calcium through channels across the myocardial cell membranes and vascular smooth muscle. Cardiac and vascular smooth muscle depends on the movement of calcium ions into the muscle cells through specific ion channels. When this movement is inhibited, the coronary and peripheral arteries dilate, thereby decreasing the force of cardiac contraction. This drug also reduces heart rate by slowing conduction through the SA and AV nodes.

Additional information about the calcium channel blockers can be found in Chapter 36.

Uses

In general, the antiarrhythmic drugs are used to treat

- Premature ventricular contractions (PVCs)
- Ventricular tachycardia
- Premature atrial contractions
- Paroxysmal atrial tachycardia
- Other atrial arrhythmias, such as atrial fibrillation or flutter
- Tachycardia when rapid but short-term control of ventricular rate is desirable

Some of the antiarrhythmic drugs are used for other conditions. For example, propranolol, in addition to its use as

A stimulus must reach the threshold to cause a response in a nerve fiber. Note that stimuli **a**, **b**, and **d** do *not* reach the threshold; therefore, they do *not* cause a response in a nerve fiber. Stimuli **c**, **e**, **f**, and **g** do reach and surpass the threshold, resulting in stimulation of nerve fiber.

After receiving lidocaine hydrochloride (Xylocaine HCl), the threshold is raised to a higher level, allowing fewer stimuli to reach the threshold. This results in decreased stimulation of the nerve fiber and prevents conduction of the nerve impulses causing the arrthythmia.

Figure 40.1 Threshold phenomenon.

an antiarrhythmic, may be used for patients with myocardial infarction. This drug has reduced the risk of death and repeated myocardial infarctions in those surviving the acute phase of a myocardial infarction. See the Summary Drug Table: Antiarrhythmic Drugs for more uses.

Adverse Reactions

Adverse reactions associated with the administration of specific antiarrhythmic drugs are given in the Summary Drug Table: Antiarrhythmic Drugs. General adverse reactions common to most antiarrhythmic drugs include the following:

Central Nervous System Reactions

- Lightheadedness
- Weakness
- Somnolence

Cardiovascular System Reactions

- Hypotension
- Arrhythmias
- Bradycardia

Other Reactions

- Urinary retention
- Local inflammation

All antiarrhythmic drugs may cause new arrhythmias or worsen existing arrhythmias, even though they are administered to resolve an existing arrhythmia. This phenomenon is called the **proarrhythmic effect**. This effect ranges from an increase in frequency of PVCs to the development of more severe ventricular tachycardia, to ventricular fibrillation, and the effect may lead to death. Proarrhythmic effects may occur at any time, but they occur more often when excessive dosages are given, when the preexisting arrhythmia is life-threatening, or when the drug is given intravenously (IV).

Summary Drug Table ANTIARRHYTHMIC DRUGS

Generic Name	Trade Name	Uses	Adverse Reactions	Dosage Ranges
Class I Sodium Channel Blockers				
disopyramide *dye-soe-pee'-ah-myde*	Norpace, Norpace CR	Life-threatening ventricular arrhythmias	Dry mouth, constipation, urinary hesitancy, blurred vision, nausea, fatigue, dizziness, headache, rash, hypotension, heart failure (HF), proarrhythmic effect	Ventricular arrhythmias: dosage individualized, 400–800 mg/day orally in divided doses
flecainide *fleh-kaye'-nyde*	Tambocor	Paroxysmal atrial fibrillation/ flutter and supraventricular tachycardia	Dizziness, headache, faintness, unsteadiness, blurred vision, headache, nausea, dyspnea, HF, fatigue, palpitations, chest pain, proarrhythmic effect	Initial dose: 100 mg orally q 12 hr; maximum dosage, 390 mg/day
lidocaine *lye'-doe-kane*	Xylocaine	Ventricular arrhythmias	Lightheadedness, nervousness, bradycardia, hypotension, drowsiness, apprehension, proarrhythmic effect	50–100 mg IV bolus; 1–4 mg/min IV infusion, 20–50 mg/kg/min; 300 mg IM

(table continues on page 374)

Antiarrhythmic Drugs

Summary Drug Table ANTIARRHYTHMIC DRUGS (continued)

Generic Name	Trade Name	Uses	Adverse Reactions	Dosage Ranges
mexiletine *max-ill'-ih-teen*	Mexitil	Life-threatening ventricular arrhythmias	Palpitations, nausea, vomiting, chest pain, heartburn, dizziness, lightheadedness, rash, agranulocytosis, proarrhythmic effect	Initial dose: 200 mg orally q 8 hr; maximum dosage, 1200 mg/day orally
moricizine *mor-ih'-siz-een*	Ethmozine	Life-threatening ventricular arrhythmias	Cardiac rhythm disturbances, existing arrhythmias worsened, palpitations, dizziness, headache, nausea, anxiety, proarrhythmic effect	600–900 mg/day orally in three equally divided doses
procainamide *proe-kaye-nah'-myde*	Procanbid	Life-threatening ventricular arrhythmias	Hypotension, disturbances of cardiac rhythm, urticaria, fever, chills, nausea, vomiting, rash, confusion, dizziness, weakness, anorexia, agranulocytosis, proarrhythmic effect	Oral: 50 mg/kg/day in divided doses q 3 hr IM: 0.5–1.0 g q 4–8 hr IV: 500–600 mg over 25–30 min, then 2–6 mg/min
propafenone *proe-paff'-ah-non*	Rythmol	Atrial fibrillation, ventricular arrhythmias, paroxysmal supraventricular tachycardia	Dizziness, nausea, vomiting, constipation, unusual taste, first-degree atrioventricular block, agranulocytosis, proarrhythmic effect	Initial dose: 150 mg orally q 8 hr; may be increased to 300 mg orally q 8 hr
quinidine *kwin'-ih-deen*	Quinaglute	Premature atrial and ventricular contractions, atrial	Ringing in the ears, hearing loss, nausea, vomiting, dizziness	Administer test dose of 1 tablet orally or 200 mg IM to test for idiosyncratic reaction
quinidine sulfate quinidine polygalacturonate	Quinidex Cardioquin	Tachycardia and flutter, paroxysmal	Headache, rash, disturbed vision, hypotension, proarrhythmic effect, agranulocytosis atrial fibrillation, chronic atrial fibrillation	Oral: 200–300 mg TID, QID or 300–600 mg q 12 hr if sustained release form is used. IM: 600 mg quinidine gluconate, then 390 mg q 2 hr IV: 300 mg quinidine gluconate slow IV at 1 mL/min of diluted solution

Class II β-Adrenergic Blockers

Generic Name	Trade Name	Uses	Adverse Reactions	Dosage Ranges
acebutolol *ah-see-byoo'-toe-loll*	Sectral	Ventricular arrhythmias, hypertension	Hypotension, nausea, dizziness, bradycardia, Vomiting, diarrhea, nervousness	Arrhythmias: 400–1200 mg/day orally in divided doses
propranolol *proe-pran'-oh-loll*	Inderal	Cardiac arrhythmias, angina pectoris, hypertension, essential tremor, myocardial infarction, migraine headache, pheochromocytoma	Nausea, vomiting, bradycardia, dizziness, hypotension, hyperglycemia, diarrhea, bronchospasm, pulmonary edema	Cardiac arrhythmias: 10–30 mg orally TID or QID Life-threatening arrhythmias: 1–3 mg IV, may repeat once in 2 min Angina pectoris: 80–320 mg/day orally in 2–4 divided doses

Class III Potassium Channel Blockers

Generic Name	Trade Name	Uses	Adverse Reactions	Dosage Ranges
amiodarone *ah-mee'-oh-dah-rone*	Cordarone, Pacerone	Life-threatening ventricular arrhythmias	Malaise, fatigue, tremor, proarrhythmic effect, nausea, vomiting, constipation, ataxia, anorexia, bradycardia, photosensitivity	Loading dose: 800–1600 mg/day orally in divided doses Maintenance dose, 390 mg/day orally; up to 1000 mg/day over 24 hr IV

(table continues on page 375)

Summary Drug Table ANTIARRHYTHMIC DRUGS (continued)

Generic Name	Trade Name	Uses	Adverse Reactions	Dosage Ranges
bretylium *breh-till'-ee-um*		Prophylaxis and treatment of ventricular fibrillation	Hypotension, nausea, vomiting, vertigo, dizziness, postural hypotension, bradycardia, proarrhythmic effect	Immediate treatment: 5–10 mg/kg (diluted) IV; maintenance, rate of 1–2 mg/min by continuous IV infusion, or infuse intermittently at 5–10 mg/kg over 10–30 min q 6 hr
dofetilide *doe-feh'-tih-lyde*	Tikosyn	Conversion of atrial fibrillation/flutter to normal sinus rhythm, maintenance of normal sinus rhythm	Headache, chest pain, dizziness, respiratory tract infection, dyspnea, nausea, flu-like syndrome, insomnia, proarrhythmic effect	Dosage based on electrocardiogram response and creatinine clearance; range, 125–500 mg BID
ibutilide *eye-byoo'-tih-lyde*	Corvert	Atrial fibrillation/ flutter	Headache, nausea, hypotension or hypertension, ventricular arrhythmias, proarrhythmic effect	Adults 60 kg and more: 1 mg infused over 10 min; may repeat 10 min Adults under 60 kg: 0.1 mL/kg infused over 10 min; may repeat in 10 min
sotalol *soe'-tah-loll*	Betapace, Betapace AF	Treatment of life-threatening ventricular arrhythmias, reduction and delay of atrial fibrillation and flutter for ventricular arrhythmias (Betapace AF)	Drowsiness, difficulty sleeping, unusual tiredness or weakness, depression, decreased libido, bradycardia, HF, cold hands and feet, nausea, vomiting, nasal congestion, anxiety, life-threatening arrhythmias, proarrhythmic effect	Initially: 80 mg BID orally; may increase up to 239–320 mg/day (Betapace); up to 120 mg BID (Betapace AF)
Class IV Calcium Channel Blockers				
verapamil *ver-ap'-ah-mill*	Calan, Covera HS, Isoptin, Verelan, Verelan PM	Supraventricular tachyarrhythmias, temporary control of rapid ventricular rate in atrial flutter/fibrillation, angina, unstable angina, hypertension	Constipation, dizziness, lightheadedness, headache, asthenia, nausea, vomiting, peripheral edema, hypotension, mental depression, agranulocytosis, proarrhythmic effect	Adults: oral—initial dose 80–120 mg TID; maintenance, 320–480 mg/day Hypertension: 239 mg/day orally; sustained-release, in AM 80 mg TID; extended-release capsules, 100–300 mg orally at bedtime · Parenteral: IV use only; initial dose 5–10 mg over 2 min; may repeat 10 mg 30 min later

Contraindications

The antiarrhythmic drugs are reserved for emergency situations and are contraindicated in patients with known hypersensitivity to these drugs. They are contraindicated during pregnancy and lactation. The antiarrhythmic drug amiodarone is a pregnancy category D drug, indicating that fetal harm can occur when the agent is administered to a pregnant woman. It is used only if the potential benefits outweigh the potential hazards to the fetus. Antiarrhythmic drugs are contraindicated in patients with second- or third-degree AV block (if the patient has no artificial pacemaker), severe HF, aortic stenosis, hypotension, and cardiogenic shock. Quinidine and procainamide are contraindicated in patients with myasthenia gravis or systemic lupus.

Precautions

Antiarrhythmic drugs are used cautiously in patients with hepatic disease, electrolyte disturbances, HF (quinidine, flecainide, procainamide, and disopyramide), and renal impairment. Most antiarrhythmics are pregnancy category B or C drugs, indicating that safe use of these drugs during pregnancy or lactation, or in children, has not been established. Disopyramide is used cautiously in patients with myasthenia gravis, urinary retention, or glaucoma, and in men with prostate enlargement.

Interactions

When antiarrhythmics are used with other medications, various interactions may occur. See Table 40.2 for more information.

Table 40.2 Interactions of Class A Antiarrhythmics and Other Agents

Interacting Drug	Common Uses	Effect of Interaction
Disopyramide		
clarithromycin, erythromycin	Bacterial infections	Increased serum disopyramide levels
fluoroquinolones	Infections	Risk of life-threatening arrhythmias
quinidine	Cardiac problems	Increased serum levels of disopyramide
rifampin	Antitubercular agent	Decreased disopyramide serum levels
thioridazine, ziprasidone	Management of mental illness	Increased risk of life-threatening arrhythmias
Procainamide		
amiodarone	Cardiac problems	Increased serum procainamide level
cholinergic blocking drugs	Gastrointestinal (GI) problems	Additive antivagal effects on atrioventricular conduction
cimetidine, ranitidine	GI problems	Increased serum procainamide level
thioridazine, ziprasidone	Management of mental illness	Life-threatening cardiac arrhythmias
Quinidine		
barbiturates	Sleep aid	Possibly, decreased serum levels of quinidine
cholinergic drugs	Treatment of glaucoma	Failure to terminate paroxysmal supraventricular tachycardia
cimetidine	GI problems	Increased serum quinidine level
hydantoins	Seizure control	Decreased therapeutic effect of quinidine
nifedipine	Treatment of angina	Decreased action and serum level of quinidine
cholinergic blocking drugs	GI problems	Additive vagolytic effect
Lidocaine		
β blockers	Hypertension and angina	Increased lidocaine levels
cimetidine	GI problems	Decreased lidocaine clearance with possible toxicity
procainamide	Cardiac problems	Additive cardiodepressant action
Flecainide		
amiodarone	Cardiac problems	Increased serum flecainide levels
cimetidine	GI problems	Increased serum flecainide levels
disopyramide, verapamil	Cardiovascular problems	May increase negative inotropic properties (see Chapter 38). Avoid using either of these drugs with flecainide.
propranolol	Cardiovascular problems	Increased serum levels of propranolol and flecainide, and additive negative inotropic effects

(table continues on page 377)

Table 40.2 Interactions of Class A Antiarrhythmics and Other Agents (continued)

Interacting Drug	Common Uses	Effect of Interaction
Propafenone		
local anesthetics	Anesthesia	Concurrent use (e.g., during pacemaker implantation, surgery or dental use) may increase the risk of central nervous system (CNS) side effects
quinidine	Cardiac problems	Increased serum propafenone levels
selective serotonin reuptake inhibitors (SSRIs)	Relief of depression	Increased serum propafenone levels
anticoagulants (e.g., warfarin)	Blood thinners	Increased prothrombin time and increased plasma warfarin levels
β blockers	Cardiovascular problems	Increased effects of the β blockers
digoxin	Heart failure	Increased serum digoxin level
theophylline	Management of asthma and chronic obstructive pulmonary disease (COPD)	Increased serum theophylline level

NURSING PROCESS

PATIENT RECEIVING AN ANTIARRHYTHMIC DRUG

ASSESSMENT

Preadministration Assessment

Antiarrhythmic drugs are used to treat various types of cardiac arrhythmias. Certain initial preadministration assessments the nurse performs before starting therapy are the same for all antiarrhythmic drugs. These assessments include the following:

- Taking and recording the blood pressure, apical and radial pulses, and respiratory rate. This provides a database for comparison during therapy.
- Assessing the patient's general condition and including observations such as skin color (pale, cyanotic, flushed), orientation, level of consciousness, and the patient's general status (e.g., appears acutely ill or appears somewhat ill). All observations must be recorded to provide a means of evaluating the response to drug therapy.
- Recording any symptoms (subjective data) described by the patient.

Because all antiarrhythmic drugs may produce proarrhythmic effects, a careful preadministration assessment is essential. It is often difficult to distinguish a proarrhythmic effect from the patient's underlying rhythm disorder, so it is important that the nurse assess each patient taking an antiarrhythmic drug through the use of cardiac monitoring before therapy begins and in the ongoing assessment to determine if the patient is experiencing a therapeutic response to the drug, developing another arrhythmia, or experiencing worsening of the original arrhythmia.

The primary health care provider may also order laboratory and diagnostic tests, renal and hepatic function tests, complete blood count, and serum enzymes and electrolyte analyses. The nurse reviews these test results before the first dose of an antiarrhythmic drug is given and reports any abnormalities to the primary health care provider. The patient is usually placed on a cardiac monitor before antiarrhythmic drug therapy is initiated. In addition, the primary health care provider may order an ECG to provide baseline data for comparison during therapy.

Ongoing Assessment

During ongoing therapy with the antiarrhythmic drugs, the nurse takes the patient's blood pressure, apical and radial pulses, and respiratory rate at periodic intervals, usually every 1 to 4 hours. Specific intervals depend on the primary health care provider's order or on nursing judgment and are based on the patient's general condition. The nurse closely observes the patient for a response to drug therapy, signs of HF, the development of a new cardiac arrhythmia, or worsening of the arrhythmia being treated.

The nurse should immediately report to the primary health care provider any significant changes in the blood pressure, pulse rate or rhythm, respiratory rate or rhythm, or the patient's general condition.

NURSING ALERT

When giving an oral antiarrhythmic drug, the nurse withholds the drug and notifies the primary health care provider immediately when the pulse rate is above 120 beats per minute (bpm) or below 60 bpm. In some instances, the primary health care provider may establish additional or different guidelines for withholding the drug.

Continual cardiac monitoring assists the nurse in assessing the patient for adverse drug reactions. If the

ECG Deflections

P

R

Q S

T

Atrial depolarization

Ventricular depolarization

Ventricular repolarization

ECG Intervals

P

S–T segment

T

P–R interval

0.12–0.20 sec

Q R S

Under
0.10 sec

Q-T interval
under 0.38 sec

Figure 40.2 Normal QRS complex.

patient is acutely ill or is receiving one of the antiarrhythmics parenterally, the nurse measures and records the fluid intake and output. The primary health care provider may order subsequent laboratory tests to monitor the patient's progress for comparison with tests performed in the preadministration assessment, such as an ECG, renal and hepatic function tests, complete blood count, and serum enzyme and electrolyte analyses. The nurse reports to the primary health care provider any abnormalities or significant interval changes of the ECG, such as prolongation of the PR or QT interval or widening of the QRS complex. Prolongation of the QT interval is particularly associated with life-threatening ventricular arrhythmias (see Fig. 40.2 for a diagram of a normal QRS complex). In addition, when subsequent laboratory tests are ordered, the nurse reviews the results and reports any abnormalities to the primary health care provider.

NURSING DIAGNOSES

Drug-specific nursing diagnoses may be:

❑ **Nausea** related to antiarrhythmic drugs
❑ **Urinary Retention** related to cholinergic blocking effects of drugs
❑ **Impaired Oral Mucous Membranes** related to dry mouth
❑ **Risk for Injury** related to dizziness, light-headedness
❑ **Risk for Infection** related to agranulocytosis

Nursing diagnoses related to drug administration are discussed in Chapter 4.

PLANNING

The expected outcomes for the patient depend on the reason for administration of the antiarrhythmic drug, but may include obtaining an optimal therapeutic response to drug therapy, support of patient needs related to managing adverse reactions, and an understanding of the therapeutic regimen.

IMPLEMENTATION

Promoting an Optimal Response to Therapy

ADMINISTERING QUINIDINE. When quinidine is administered orally, the drug is not crushed or chewed. GI upset can be reduced if the drug is given with food. The nurse must monitor serum quinidine levels during administration of the drug. Normal therapeutic levels range between 2 and 7 mcg/mL.

ADMINISTERING PROCAINAMIDE. If procainamide is given IV, the nurse maintains continuous and close cardiac monitoring. Hypotension may occur with IV administration; therefore, the blood pressure must be monitored every 15 minutes while the drug is being infused. The nurse may keep the patient supine during IV administration to minimize hypotension. If hypotension should occur, the primary health care provider is notified immediately.

When the drug is given orally, the nurse instructs the patient not to chew the capsule or tablet but to swallow it whole. If GI upset occurs, the nurse can administer the drug with or immediately after meals. Sustained-released tablets should not be crushed or divided.

ADMINISTERING DISOPYRAMIDE. Oral disopyramide is administered to the patient with a full 8-oz glass of water every 6 hours, or every 12 hours if in controlled-release form. Effective and safe blood plasma levels are between 2 and 8 mcg/mL. The nurse monitors cardiac rhythm and blood pressure frequently during therapy.

ADMINISTERING LIDOCAINE. Lidocaine is most often administered IV continuously diluted in dextrose 5% in water (D_5W) at 1 to 4 mg/min (or 20–50 mcg/kg/min). The arrhythmia is usually controlled within 24 hours of continuous administration. Constant cardiac monitoring is essential when this drug is administered IV. Lidocaine is titrated to the patient's response and in accord with institutional protocols. The nurse must observe the patient closely for signs of respiratory depression, bradycardia, change in mental status, respiratory arrest, convulsions, and hypotension. The infusion is discontinued when the heart rhythm is stable or at the earliest sign of lidocaine toxicity. Blood concentration levels exceeding 6 mcg/mL are associated with significant risk of CNS and cardiovascular depression. An oropharyngeal airway and suction equipment are kept at the bedside in case convulsions occur. Life support equipment and vasopressors are also readily available in case of adverse reaction. Any sudden change in mental state should be reported to the primary health care provider immediately, because a decrease in the dosage may be necessary.

ADMINISTERING MEXILETINE. Mexiletine is administered at 8-hour intervals and with food (or an antacid) to prevent GI upset. The dosage of mexiletine must be individualized; therefore, the nurse monitors vital signs at frequent intervals during initial therapy. The nurse reports any changes in the pulse rate or rhythm to the primary health care provider. Onset of tremors indicates that the maximum dosage of mexiletine has been reached. Adverse effects related to the CNS or GI tract may occur during initial therapy and must be reported to the primary health care provider.

ADMINISTERING FLECAINIDE AND PROPAFENONE. It is advisable to hospitalize the patient during withdrawal of a previously given antiarrhythmic drug before initiating flecainide therapy, because life-threatening arrhythmias may occur. When administering flecainide, the nurse must carefully monitor the patient for cardiac arrhythmias. Therapeutic serum levels fall between 0.2 and 1 mcg/mL. Life support equipment, including a pacemaker, should be kept on standby during administration. The nurse closely observes the patient for a response to drug therapy, signs of HF, the development of a new cardiac arrhythmia, or worsening of the arrhythmia being treated.

Propafenone is administered orally every 8 hours. Any previously given antiarrhythmic drug should be discontinued before propafenone therapy is started. During the initiation of therapy, patients taking propafenone must be monitored carefully. To minimize adverse reactions, the primary health care provider may increase the dosage slowly at a minimum of 3- to 4-day intervals. Periodic

ECG monitoring is usually ordered to evaluate the effects of the drug on cardiac conduction.

ADMINISTERING PROPRANOLOL. Cardiac monitoring is recommended when propranolol is given IV, because severe bradycardia and hypotension may occur. The nurse obtains written instructions from the primary health care provider for propranolol administration. For example, the primary health care provider may want the drug to be withheld for a systolic blood pressure less than 90 mm Hg or a pulse rate less than 50 bpm. The nurse monitors the ECG frequently for cardiac arrhythmias. Patients receiving IV propranolol must have continuous cardiac monitoring. The nurse must monitor the blood pressure and pulse frequently during the dosage adjustment period and periodically throughout therapy.

ADMINISTERING BRETYLIUM. Bretylium is used in the emergency treatment of life-threatening ventricular arrhythmias. Because of its adverse reactions, bretylium is used only when the arrhythmia is unresponsive to the other antiarrhythmic drugs. Baseline data come from routine assessments made before the emergency. The nurse administers this drug IM or IV and uses continuous cardiac monitoring. The patient is placed in a supine position with suction equipment readily available in case vomiting occurs.

❗ NURSING ALERT

A transient increase in arrhythmias and hypertension may occur within 1 hour after initial therapy with bretylium is begun. The nurse should take the blood pressure and respiratory rate every 5 to 15 minutes and obtain the pulse rate from the cardiac monitor. These activities are continued until the arrhythmia is corrected.

The nurse monitors cardiac rhythm and blood pressure continuously during administration. Hypotension and postural hypotension occur in about 50% of the patients receiving bretylium. If systolic pressure is less than 75 mm Hg, the nurse should notify the primary health care provider. The patient remains supine until tolerance of postural hypotension develops. The nurse instructs the patient to change position slowly. Most individuals adjust to blood pressure changes within a few days.

To discontinue use of the drug, dosage should be reduced gradually over 3 to 5 days. After administering the drug, the nurse observes the patient closely. An oral antiarrhythmic drug may be prescribed to provide continued stability to the cardiac muscle.

ADMINISTERING VERAPAMIL. This drug is used to manage supraventricular arrhythmias and rapid ventricular rates in atrial flutter or fibrillation. Continuous cardiac monitoring is necessary during IV administration. The nurse monitors the patient's blood pressure and cardiac rhythm carefully while the drug is being titrated (dosage increased or decreased based on criteria established by the primary health care provider). The dosage may be increased more rapidly in a hospital setting. The nurse notifies the primary health care provider if bradycardia or hypotension occurs. When verapamil is administered orally, it may be given with food to minimize gastric upset.

Monitoring and Managing Patient Needs

NAUSEA. Most of the antiarrhythmic drugs cause nausea. The nurse advises the patient that eating small meals frequently may be better tolerated than three full meals daily. The nurse tells the patient to avoid lying flat for approximately 2 hours after meals. When the patient rests or reclines, the head should be at least 4 inches higher than the feet. The nurse administers the drug with meals to decrease GI effects.

URINARY RETENTION. Because of the cholinergic blocking effects of disopyramide (see Chapter 27), urinary retention may occur. The nurse monitors the urinary output closely, especially during the initial period of therapy. If the patient's intake is sufficient but the output is low, the lower abdomen is palpated for bladder distention. If urinary retention occurs, the nurse notifies the primary health care provider, because catheterization may be necessary.

IMPAIRED ORAL MUCOUS MEMBRANES. Dryness of the mouth and throat caused by the cholinergic blocking action of disopyramide may occur. The nurse provides an adequate amount of fluid and instructs the patient to take frequent sips of water to relieve this problem. The nurse instructs the patient that sucking on hard candy (preferably sugarless) will help to keep the mouth moist.

RISK FOR INJURY. Many of the antiarrhythmic drugs may cause dizziness and lightheadedness, especially during early therapy. This places the patient at risk for injury from falling. The nurse assists patients who are not on complete bed rest to ambulate until these symptoms subside.

Postural hypotension also may occur during the first few weeks of disopyramide therapy. The patient is advised to make position changes slowly. In some instances, the patient may require assistance in getting out of the bed or chair.

RISK FOR INFECTION. Some antiarrhythmic drugs, such as quinidine, procainamide, mexiletine, or verapamil, may cause agranulocytosis. The nurse reports any signs of agranulocytosis, such as fever, chills, sore throat, or unusual bleeding or bruising. A complete blood count is usually ordered every 2 to 3 weeks during the first 3 months of therapy. If decrease in the blood levels of leukocytes or platelets occurs or the hematocrit falls, the nurse reports this to the primary health care provider immediately, because the drug may be discontinued. Blood levels usually return to normal within 1 month after discontinuing the antiarrhythmic drug.

POTENTIAL MEDICAL COMPLICATION: PROARRHYTHMIC EFFECTS. Proarrhythmic effects may occur, such as ventricular tachycardia or ventricular fibrillation. It is often difficult to distinguish proarrhythmic effects from the patient's preexisting arrhythmia.

❗ NURSING ALERT

Antiarrhythmic drugs are capable of causing new arrhythmias, as well as exacerbating existing arrhythmias. The nurse must report any new arrhythmia or exacerbation of an existing arrhythmia to the primary health care provider immediately.

LIFESPAN ALERT – Gerontology

When older adults take the antiarrhythmic drugs, they are at greater risk for adverse reactions such as additional arrhythmias or aggravation of existing arrhythmias, hypotension, and HF. A dosage reduction may be indicated. Careful monitoring by the nurse is necessary for early identification and management of adverse reactions. The nurse monitors the intake and output and reports any signs of HF, such as increase in weight, decrease in urinary output, or shortness of breath.

POTENTIAL MEDICAL COMPLICATION: QUINIDINE TOXICITY. The nurse monitors the patient for the most common adverse reactions associated with quinidine (nausea, vomiting, abdominal pain, diarrhea, or anorexia). **Cinchonism** is the term used to describe quinidine toxicity. Cinchonism occurs with high blood levels of quinidine (greater than 6 mcg/mL). The nurse must report any quinidine levels greater than 6 mcg/mL and the occurrence of any of the following signs or symptoms of cinchonism: ringing in the ears (tinnitus), hearing loss, headache, nausea, dizziness, vertigo, and lightheadedness. These symptoms may be experienced after a single dose.

Educating the Patient and Family

The nurse discusses with the patient and family the adverse drug effects that may occur. To ensure compliance with the prescribed drug regimen, the nurse emphasizes the importance of taking these drugs exactly as prescribed. If necessary, the nurse may teach the patient or a family member how to take the pulse and report any changes in the pulse rate or rhythm to the primary health care provider (see Patient Teaching for Improved Patient Outcomes: Monitoring Pulse Rate in Chapter 39).

The nurse emphasizes the following points when teaching the patient and the family:

- Take the drug at the prescribed intervals. Do not omit a dose or increase or decrease the dose unless advised to do so by the primary health care provider. Do not stop taking the drug unless advised to do so by the primary health care provider.
- Do not take any nonprescription drug unless the use of a specific drug is approved by the primary health care provider.
- Avoid drinking alcoholic beverages or smoking unless these have been approved by the primary health care provider.
- Follow the directions on the drug label, such as taking the drug with food.

- Do not chew tablets or capsules; instead, swallow them whole.
- Do not attempt to drive or perform hazardous tasks if lightheadedness or dizziness occur.
- Notify the primary health care provider as soon as possible if any adverse effects occur.
- To relieve dry mouth, take frequent sips of water; allow ice chips to dissolve in the mouth, or chew (sugar-free) gum.
- Remember that the tablet matrix of sustained-release tablets of procainamide is not absorbed by the body and may be found in the stool. This is normal.
- Keep all appointments with the primary health care provider, clinic, or laboratory, because therapy will be closely monitored.
- If you have diabetes and are taking propranolol, adhere to the prescribed diet and check the blood glucose levels one to two times a day (or as recommended by the primary health care provider). Report elevated glucose levels to the primary health care provider as soon as possible, because an adjustment in the dosage of insulin or oral hypoglycemic drugs may be necessary.

EVALUATION

- Therapeutic response is achieved and the arrhythmia is controlled.
- Adverse reactions are identified, reported to the primary health care provider, and managed successfully with appropriate nursing interventions:
  ☑ Patient is free of nausea.
  ☑ Patient urinates adequately.
  ☑ Oral mucous membranes are intact and moist.
  ☑ No evidence of infection is seen.
  ☑ No evidence of injury is seen.
- Patient and family demonstrate an understanding of the drug regimen.

THINK CRITICALLY: PHARMACOLOGY IN PRACTICE

1. Mr. Phillip, aged 72 years, will be discharged in 2 hours. The primary health care provider has prescribed propranolol to treat his arrhythmia as well as his hypertension. You receive a phone call from his nephew, who is concerned about side effects his uncle may have while taking all the different medications. Unfortunately, Mr. Phillip's nephew cannot come to the hospital before discharge. Go to the Internet and do a Google search for patient teaching regarding propranolol.

   Develop a list of sites for Mr. Phillip to take home and share with his nephew.

● Test Your Knowledge

1. Which of the following adverse reactions of lidocaine (Xylocaine) should be reported immediately to the primary health care provider?
   A. Sudden change in mental status
   B. Dry mouth
   C. Occipital headache
   D. Lightheadedness

2. Which of the following drugs, when given with disopyramide (Norpace), would possibly increase the serum disopyramide levels?
   A. verapamil (Calan)
   B. propranolol (Inderal)
   C. flecainide (Tambocor)
   D. quinidine (Quinidex)

3. Common adverse reactions of the antiarrhythmic drugs include _____.
   A. lightheadedness, hypotension, and weakness
   B. headache, hypertension, and lethargy
   C. weakness, lethargy, and hyperglycemia
   D. anorexia, GI upset, and hypertension

4. Which of the following statements would the nurse include in a teaching plan for the patient taking an antiarrhythmic drug on an outpatient basis?
   A. Take the drug without regard to meals.
   B. Limit fluid intake during the evening hours.
   C. Avoid drinking alcoholic beverages unless their consumption has been approved by the primary health care provider.
   D. Eat a diet high in potassium.

● Prepare for the NCLEX

1. When administering quinidine (Quinidex), the nurse reports a blood level greater than _____.
   A. 2 mcg/mL
   B. 3 mcg/mL
   C. 4 mcg/mL
   D. 6 mcg/mL

● Calculate Medication Dosages

1. The primary health care provider prescribes verapamil 80 mg orally. The drug is available in 40-mg tablets. The nurse prepares _____.

2. Disopyramide 200 mg orally is prescribed. The pharmacy sends disopyramide (Norpace) 100-mg tablets. The nurse administers _____.

To check your answers, see Appendix E.

the**Point**. *For more NCLEX questions, log on to http://thepoint.lww.com to access more than 1000 questions.*

Antiarrhythmic Drugs

Drugs That Affect the Gastrointestinal System

The gastrointestinal (GI) system is responsible for the ingestion and exchange of body nutrients. Food and fluids are broken down in the oral cavity to begin the process of digestion in the GI system. In the stomach, foodstuffs are broken down by gastric acids and enzymes to prepare for absorption in the small intestine. Nutrients are absorbed in the small intestine. The large intestine is responsible for the reabsorption of water and the elimination of waste materials in the form of feces.

The health focus on this bodily system increases as people age. Chronic illness, such as inflammatory bowel diseases, can affect how water and nutrients are absorbed. As aging occurs, individuals experience wear and tear on their teeth and the ability to produce saliva decreases; this changes the taste of foods. Also, as the body ages, motility and absorption in the GI system slow. Drugs are used to assist in the absorption of nutrients, either by altering the gastric acids for purposes of protection or by controlling the transit of food through the system by speeding up or slowing down the process. Chapter 41 describes drugs used for protecting the structures of the upper GI system—mouth, esophagus, and stomach—from the effects of gastric acid. Drugs used to speed up or prevent emesis are also covered in this chapter.

Drugs used to slow down or facilitate transit in the lower GI system—the small and large intestines—are covered in Chapter 42. The drugs used in the treatment of chronic GI diseases are also presented in Chapter 42.

An area of concern to the nurse is the availability of nonprescription drugs for the GI system, thereby creating the potential problems of misuse and overuse of the drugs and the disguising of more serious medical problems. This issue is addressed in Chapter 42 as well.

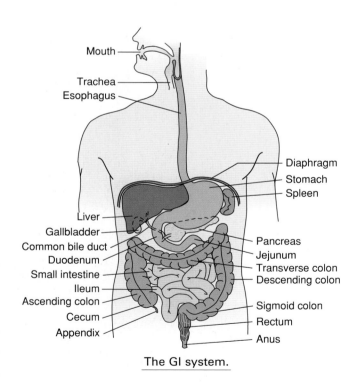

The GI system.

PHARMACOLOGY IN PRACTICE

Our patient focus in this unit is Alfredo Garcia, a 46-year-old man being seen in the clinic for an upper respiratory infection. During the intake assessment, the nurse finds that his blood pressure is high, and he complains of "heartburn." He is relatively healthy; the only medication he takes is a diuretic to maintain his blood pressure. Occasionally, he takes a pain pill for muscle aches and pains. The nurse asks him what helps relieve the heartburn, and he tells her that he thinks he might have an ulcer so he has been drinking cream and half-and-half to coat the ulcer. Mr. Garcia is attempting to use home remedies to decrease acid production in his stomach. At one time, anti-ulcer diets included the use of dairy products with the intent of coating the mucosal lining of the stomach, protecting it from acid secretion. After reading the chapters in this unit, you will learn about the current method to treat peptic ulcers in the stomach.

Drugs That Affect the Upper Gastrointestinal System

chemoreceptor trigger
  zone (CTZ)
gastric stasis
gastroesophageal reflux disease
Helicobacter pylori
hydrochloric acid (HCl)

hypersecretory
nausea
paralytic ileus
vertigo
vomiting

LEARNING OBJECTIVES

On completion of this chapter, the student will:

1. Discuss the general drug actions, uses, adverse reactions, contraindications, precautions, and interactions of drugs used to treat conditions of the upper gastrointestinal system.
2. Discuss important preadministration and ongoing assessment activities the nurse should perform with the patient receiving a drug used to treat conditions of the upper gastrointestinal system.
3. List nursing diagnoses particular to a patient receiving a drug used to treat conditions of the upper gastrointestinal system.
4. Use the nursing process when administering drugs used to treat conditions of the upper gastrointestinal system.

The gastrointestinal (GI) system is essentially a long tube in the body where ingested food and fluids are processed for absorption of nutrients. The upper GI system consists of the mouth, esophagus, and stomach. The mouth is responsible for breaking down food parts and mixing them with saliva to begin the digestion process. The tubular esophagus connects the mouth to the stomach, where food is mixed with acids and enzymes to become a solution for absorption. Some of the cells of the stomach secrete **hydrochloric acid** (HCl), a substance that aids in the initial digestive process. Problems occur when acids or stomach contents reverse direction and attempt to come back up the GI tract, which can create tissue damage and ulcers.

Drugs are presented in this chapter according to their function, whether they treat gastric acid production or prevent **vomiting**. Drugs that neutralize HCl and protect the mucosal lining are called *antacids*. Drugs that reduce the

production and release of HCl include histamine type 2 receptor (H_2) antagonists, proton pump inhibitors, and miscellaneous acid-reducing agents. The proton pump inhibitors are particularly important in the treatment of **Helicobacter pylori** infection in patients with active duodenal ulcers. *H. pylori* are believed to cause a type of chronic gastritis and some peptic and duodenal ulcers as well. GI stimulants facilitate emptying of stomach contents into the small intestine and are used both as ulcer treatments and as antiemetics. Antiemetics are used to treat and prevent **nausea** and vomiting. Some of the more common drugs are listed in the Summary Drug Table: Drugs Used in Managing Upper Gastrointestinal Disorders.

• ACID NEUTRALIZERS: ANTACIDS

Actions

Antacids ("against acids") are drugs that neutralize or reduce the acidity of stomach and duodenal contents by combining with HCl and increasing the pH of the stomach acid. Antacids do not "coat" the stomach lining, although they may increase the sphincter tone of the lower esophagus. Examples of antacids include aluminum (Amphojel), magaldrate (Riopan), and magnesium (Milk of Magnesia).

Uses

Antacids are used in the treatment of hyperacidity caused by the following:

- Heartburn, acid indigestion, or sour stomach
- **Gastroesophageal reflux disease** (GERD; a reflux or backup of gastric contents into the esophagus)
- Peptic ulcer

Antacids may be used to treat conditions that are not associated with the GI system. For example, aluminum carbonate is a phosphate-binding agent and is used in treating hyperphosphatemia (often associated with chronic renal failure) or as an adjunct to a low-phosphate diet to prevent formation of phosphate-based urinary stones. Calcium may be used in treating calcium deficiency states such as menopausal osteoporosis. Magnesium may be used for treating magnesium deficiencies or magnesium depletion from malnutrition, restricted diet, or alcoholism.

(text continues on page 338)

Summary Drug Table DRUGS USED IN MANAGING UPPER GASTROINTESTINAL DISORDERS

Generic Name	Trade Name	Uses	Adverse Reactions	Dosage Ranges
Acid Neutralizers				
aluminum carbonate *ah-loo-mih-num*	Basaljel	Symptomatic relief of peptic ulcer and stomach hyperacidity, hyperphosphatemia	Constipation, bone softening, neurotoxicity	2 tablets or capsules (10 mL of regular oral suspension) as often as q 2 hr, up to 12 times daily
aluminum hydroxide	ALternaGEL, Alu-Tab, Amphojel, Dialume	Same as aluminum carbonate	Same as aluminum carbonate	500–1500 mg (5–30 mL in oral suspension) 3–6 times daily orally between meals and bedtime
calcium carbonate *kal'-see um car'-boe nate*	Tums, Mylanta (multiple trade names)	Symptomatic relief of peptic ulcer and stomach hyperacidity, calcium deficiencies (osteoporosis)	Acid rebound *hypercalcemia*	0.5–1.5 g orally
magnesia (magnesium hydroxide) *mag-nee'-zee-ah*	Milk of Magnesia, Phillips MOM	Symptomatic relief of peptic ulcer and stomach hyperacidity, constipation	Diarrhea, <u>bone loss in patients with chronic renal failure</u>	Antacid: 622–1244 mg (5–15 mL in suspension) orally QID; Laxative: 15–60 mL orally
magnesium oxide *mag-nee'-zee-um*	Mag-Ox 400, Maox 420, Uro-Mag	Same as magnesia	Same as magnesia	140–800 mg/day orally
sodium bicarbonate *soe'-dee-um*	Bellans	Symptomatic relief of peptic ulcer and stomach hyperacidity	Electrolyte imbalance and metabolic alkalosis	0.3–2 g orally 1–4 times daily
Combined-Product Acid Neutralizer				
magaldrate (magnesium/ aluminate) *mag-al-drate*	Iosopan, Riopan	Symptomatic relief of peptic ulcer and stomach hyperacidity	Constipation, diarrhea	5–10 mL orally between meals and bedtime
Acid Reducers				
Histamine H₂ Antagonists				
cimetidine* *sye-meh'-tih-deen*	Tagamet	<u>Gastric/duodenal ulcers,</u> GERD, gastric <u>hyper-secretory conditions,</u> GI bleeding, heartburn	Headache, <u>somnolence,</u> diarrhea	800–1600 mg/day orally; 300 mg q6hr IM or IV
famotidine* *fah-moe-tih-deen*	Pepcid	Same as cimetidine	Same as cimetidine	20–40 mg orally; IV if unable to take orally
nizatidine *nih-zah'-tih-deen*	Axid	Same as cimetidine	Same as cimetidine	150–300 mg/day orally in one dose or divided doses
ranitidine* *rah-nye'-tih-deen*	Zantac	Same as cimetidine, erosive esophagitis	Same as cimetidine	150–600 mg orally in one dose or divided doses orally; 50 mg q6–8hr IM, IV (do not exceed 400 mg/day)
Proton Pump Inhibitors esomeprazole *ess-oh-meh'-prah-zoll*	Nexium	*H. pylori* Erosive esophagitis, GERD, *H. pylori* eradication, NSAID-associated gastric ulcers	Headache, nausea, diarrhea	20–40 mg/day orally

(table continues on page 387)

Summary Drug Table DRUGS USED IN MANAGING UPPER GASTROINTESTINAL DISORDERS (continued)

Generic Name	Trade Name	Uses	Adverse Reactions	Dosage Ranges
lansoprazole *lan-soe'-prah-zoll*	Prevacid	Same as esomeprazole, hypersecretory conditions, cystic fibrosis (intestinal malabsorption)	Same as esomeprazole	15–30 mg/day orally
omeprazole *oh-meh'-prah-zoll*	Prilosec, (Zegerid – combined with sodium bicarbonate)	Same as esomeprazole, hypersecretory conditions, heartburn, reduce risk of upper GI bleeding	Same as esomeprazole	20–60 mg/day orally
pantoprazole *pan-toe-prah-zoll*	Protonix	GERD, erosive esophagitis and hypersecretory conditions	Same as esomeprazole	40 mg/day orally or IV Hypersecretion: 80 mg IV q 12 hr
rabeprazole *rah-beh-prah-zoll*	Aciphex	Same as esomeprazole	Same as esomeprazole	20 mg/day orally
Miscellaneous Acid Reducers				
sucralfate *soo-kral-fate*	Carafate	Short-term duodenal ulcer treatment	Constipation	1 g/day orally in divided doses
misoprostol *mye-soe-prah'-stoll*	Cytotec	Prevention of gastric ulcers in patients taking NSAIDs	Headache, nausea, diarrhea, abdominal pain	100–200 mcg orally QID
GI Stimulants				
dexpanthenol *dex-pan'-theh-noll*	Ilopan	Immediate postoperative medication for prevention of paralytic ileus	Itching, tingling, difficulty breathing	250–500 mg IM
Ⓡ metoclopramide *meh-toe-kloe'-prah-mide*	Reglan	Diabetic gastroparesis, GERD, prevention of nausea and vomiting	Restlessness, dizziness, fatigue, extrapyramidal effects	10–15 mg orally; 10–20 mg IM, IV
Antiemetics				
Antidopaminergics chlorpromazine *klor-proe'-mah-zeen*	Thorazine	Control of nausea and vomiting, intractable hiccoughs	Drowsiness, hypotension, dry mouth, nasal congestion	Nausea and vomiting: 10–25 mg orally q 4–6 hr; 50–100 mg rectal suppository q 6–8 hr; 25–50 mg IM q 3–4 hr; Hiccoughs: 25–50 mg orally, IM, slow IV infusion
perphenazine *per-fen-ah-zeen*		Same as chlorpromazine	Same as chlorpromazine	8–16 mg/day orally in divided doses, 5–10 mg IM, IV q 6 hr
prochlorperazine *proe-klor-per'-ah-zeen*	Compazine	Control of nausea and vomiting	Same as chlorpromazine	Orally: 5–10 mg TID or QID IM, IV: 5–10 mg Rectal suppository: 25 mg BID; Sustained-release: 10–15 mg
promethazine *proe-meth'-ah-zeen*	*Phenergan*	Control of nausea and vomiting associated with anesthesia and surgery, motion sickness	Same as diphenhydramine (Benadryl)	Nausea and vomiting: 12.5–25 mg orally, IM, IV, rectally; Motion sickness: 25 mg orally 1–2 hr before travel, repeat 8–12 hr

(table continues on page 388)

Summary Drug Table DRUGS USED IN MANAGING UPPER GASTROINTESTINAL DISORDERS (continued)

Generic Name	Trade Name	Uses	Adverse Reactions	Dosage Ranges
thiethylperazine *thye-eth-ill-per-ah-zeen*	Torecan	Control of nausea and vomiting	Same as chlorpromazine	10–30 mg orally in divided doses
triflupromazine *trye-floo-proe-mah-zeen*		Control of severe nausea and vomiting	Same as chlorpromazine	5–15 mg IM q 4 hr; maximum dose, 60 mg/day; 1 mg IV, up to 3 mg/day
Cholinergic Blocking Drug				
trimethobenzamide *trye-meth-oh-ben'-zah-myde*	Tigan	Control of nausea and vomiting	Hypotension (IM use), Parkinson-like symptoms, blurred vision, drowsiness, dizziness	250 mg orally or 200 mg IM, rectal suppository TID or QID
5-HT3 Receptor Antagonists				
dolasetron[†] *doe-laz-ee-tron*	Anzemet	Prevention of chemotherapy-induced and postoperative nausea, vomiting	Headache, fatigue, fever, abdominal pain	100 mg orally or 1.8 mg/kg IV
granisetron[†] *gran-iz-ee-tron*	Kytril, Sancuso (transdermal)	Same as dolasetron	Headache, asthenia, diarrhea, constipation	1–2 mg orally or 10 mcg/kg IV; transdermal patch applied 2 days before to 5 days after chemotherapy treatment
ondansetron[†] *on-dan-see-tron*	Zofran	Same as dolasetron, bulimia, spinal analgesia–induced pruritus, levodopa-induced psychosis	Headache, fatigue, drowsiness, sedation, constipation, hypoxia	8 mg orally BID or TID; 32 mg IV
palonosetron[†] *pal-oe-noh-see-tron*	Aloxi	Same as dolasetron	Same as dolasetron	0.25–0.5 mg in a single dose
Miscellaneous Antiemetic				
aprepitant[†] *ap-re'-pih-tant*	Emend	Prevention of chemotherapy-induced and postoperative nausea, vomiting	Headache, fatigue, stomatitis, constipation	125 mg – one hour before chemotherapy and 80 mg daily for 3 days
dronabinol[†] *droe-nab-ih-nol*	Marinol	Prevention of chemotherapy-induced nausea and vomiting, appetite stimulant for patients with human immunodeficiency virus infection	Drowsiness, somnolence, euphoria, dizziness, vomiting	5 mg/m^2 1–3 hr before chemotherapy: Appetite stimulant: 2.5 mg orally BID
nabilone[†] *nab'-ih-loan*	Cesamet	Prevention of chemotherapy-induced nausea and vomiting	Drowsiness, vertigo, euphoria, dry mouth	1–2 mg BID up to 48 hours following chemotherapy dose

Ⓕ These drugs are taken at least 30 minutes before meals and at bedtime.

*These drugs are sold over the counter in smaller doses than those listed for therapeutic interventions.

[†]These drugs are administered according to specific protocols; the nurse should consult the order before administration.

Adverse Reactions

The magnesium- and sodium-containing antacids may have a laxative effect and may produce diarrhea. Aluminum- and calcium-containing products tend to produce constipation. Although the antacids have the potential for serious adverse reactions, they have a wide margin of safety, especially when used as prescribed. The less common but more serious adverse reactions include:

- Aluminum-containing antacids—constipation, intestinal impaction, anorexia, weakness, tremors, and bone pain
- Magnesium-containing antacids—severe diarrhea, dehydration, and hypermagnesemia (nausea, vomiting, hypotension, decreased respirations)
- Calcium-containing antacids—rebound hyperacidity, metabolic alkalosis, hypercalcemia, vomiting, confusion, headache, renal calculi, and neurologic impairment
- Sodium bicarbonate—systemic alkalosis and rebound hyperacidity

Contraindications and Precautions

The antacids are contraindicated in patients with severe abdominal pain of unknown cause and during lactation. Sodium-containing antacids are contraindicated in patients with cardiovascular problems, such as hypertension or congestive heart failure, and those on sodium-restricted diets. Calcium-containing antacids are contraindicated in patients with renal calculi or hypercalcemia.

Aluminum-containing antacids are used cautiously in patients with gastric outlet obstruction or those with upper GI bleeding. Magnesium- and aluminum-containing antacids are used cautiously in patients with decreased kidney function. The calcium-containing antacids are used cautiously in patients with respiratory insufficiency, renal impairment, or cardiac disease. Antacids are classified as pregnancy category C drugs and should be used with caution during pregnancy.

Interactions

The following interactions may occur when an antacid is administered with another agent:

Interacting Drug	Common Use	Effect of Interaction
digoxin, isoniazid, phenytoin, and chlorpromazine	Treatment of cardiac problems, infection, seizures, interacting drugs and nausea and vomiting, respectively	Decreased absorption of the results in a decreased effect of those drugs
tetracycline	Anti-infective agent	Decreased effectiveness of anti-infective
corticosteroids	Treatment of inflammation and respiratory problems	Decreased anti-inflammatory properties
salicylates	Pain relief	Pain reliever is excreted more rapidly in the urine
quinidine and amphetamines	Treatment of cardiac problems and central nervous system stimulant, respectively	Interacting drugs are excreted more slowly in the urine

HERBAL ALERT

Ginger, a pungent root, has been used medicinally for GI problems such as motion sickness, nausea, vomiting, and indigestion. In addition, it is recommended for the pain and inflammation of arthritis, and it may help lower cholesterol. The dosage of the dried form of ginger is 1 g (1000 mg) per day. Adverse reactions are rare, although heartburn has been reported by some individuals. Ginger should be used cautiously in patients with hypertension or gallstones and during pregnancy or lactation. As with any substance, a primary health care provider should be consulted before any ginger remedy is taken, although ginger has been consumed safely as a food by millions of individuals for centuries.

● ACID-REDUCING AGENTS

Drugs that reduce the production of HCl include histamine H_2 antagonists, proton pump inhibitors, and miscellaneous drugs such as pepsin inhibitors, prostaglandins, and cholinergic blockers.

Histamine H_2 Antagonists

Actions

These drugs inhibit the action of histamine at H_2 receptor cells of the stomach, which then reduces the secretion of gastric acid. Cholinergic blocking drugs typically block the action of histamine throughout the entire body. Histamine H_2 antagonists do not cause the effects of the cholinergic blockers, because they are selective only for the H_2 receptors in the stomach, and not the general body H_2 receptors. When ulcers are present, the decrease in acid allows the ulcerated areas to heal. Examples of histamine H_2 antagonists include cimetidine (Tagamet), famotidine (Pepcid), and ranitidine (Zantac).

Uses

These drugs are used prophylactically to treat stress-related ulcers and acute upper GI bleeding in critically ill patients. They are also used for the treatment of the following:

- Heartburn, acid indigestion, and sour stomach
- GERD
- Gastric or duodenal ulcer
- Gastric **hypersecretory** conditions (excessive gastric secretion of HCl)

Adverse Reactions

Histamine H_2 antagonist adverse reactions are usually mild and transient as well as rare (affecting less than 2% of users), and include:

- Dizziness, somnolence, headache
- Confusion, hallucinations, diarrhea, and reversible impotence *Cimetidine — Tagamet*

Contraindications and Precautions

The histamine H_2 antagonists are contraindicated in patients with a known hypersensitivity to the drugs. These drugs are used cautiously in patients with renal or hepatic impairment and in severely ill, elderly, or debilitated patients. Cimetidine is used cautiously in patients with diabetes. Histamine H_2

antagonists are pregnancy category B (cimetidine, famotidine, and ranitidine) and C (nizatidine) drugs and should be used with caution during pregnancy and lactation.

Interactions

The following interactions may occur when a histamine H_2 antagonist is administered with another agent:

Interacting Drug	Common Use	Effect of Interaction
antacids and metoclopramide	GI distress	Decreased absorption of the H_2 antagonists
carmustine	Anticancer therapy	Decreased white blood cell count
opioid analgesics	Pain relief	Increased risk of respiratory depression
oral anticoagulants	Blood thinners	Increased risk of bleeding
digoxin	Cardiac problems	May decrease serum digoxin levels

Tassimet

Proton Pump Inhibitors

Actions

Proton pump inhibitors, such as lansoprazole, omeprazole, pantoprazole, and rabeprazole, are a group of drugs with antisecretory properties. These drugs suppress gastric acid secretion by inhibition of the hydrogen-potassium adenosine triphosphatase (ATPase) enzyme system of the gastric parietal cells. The ATPase enzyme system is also called the acid (proton) pump system. The proton pump inhibitors suppress gastric acid secretion by blocking the final step in the production of gastric acid by the gastric mucosa. Examples of proton pump inhibitors include esomeprazole magnesium (Nexium) and omeprazole (Prilosec).

Uses

Proton pump inhibitors are used for treatment or symptomatic relief of various gastric disorders, including:

- Gastric and duodenal ulcers (specifically associated with *H. pylori* infections)
- GERD and erosive esophagitis
- Pathologic hypersecretory conditions

An important use of these drugs is combination therapy for the treatment of *H. pylori* infection in patients with duodenal ulcers. One treatment regimen used to treat infection with *H. pylori* is a triple-drug therapy, such as one of the proton pump inhibitors (e.g., omeprazole or lansoprazole) and two anti-infectives (e.g., amoxicillin and clarithromycin). Another triple-drug treatment regimen consists of bismuth plus two anti-infective drugs. Helidac, a triple-drug treatment regimen (bismuth, metronidazole, and tetracycline), may be given along with a histamine H_2 antagonist to treat disorders of the GI tract infected with *H. pylori*. Table 41.1 lists various drug combinations used in the treatment of *H. pylori* infection. Additional information concerning anti-infective agents is found in Chapters 6 through 10. The Summary Drug Table: Drugs Used in Managing Upper Gastrointestinal Disorders provides additional information on the proton pump inhibitor drugs used in treating H. pylori infection.

Table 41.1 Agents Used to Eradicate *H. pylori* in Patients With Duodenal Ulcers

Drug	Recommended Usage	Dosage Range
amoxicillin	In combination with lansoprazole and clarithromycin or lansoprazole alone	1 g BID for 14 days (triple therapy) or 1 g TID (double therapy)
bismuth (Bismatrol)	In combination with other products	525 mg QID
clarithromycin (Biaxin)	In combination with amoxicillin	500 mg TID
lansoprazole (Prevacid)	In combination with clarithromycin or amoxicillin	30 mg BID for 14 days (triple therapy) or 30 mg TID for 14 days (double therapy)
metronidazole (Flagyl)	In combination with other products	250 mg QID
omeprazole (Prilosec)	In combination with clarithromycin	40 mg BID for 4 wk and 20 mg/day for 15–28 days
tetracycline	In combination with other products	500 mg QID
Combination Drug Packs		
bismuth, metronidazole, tetracycline (Helidac, Pylera)	*H. pylori* eradication in patients with duodenal ulcer	Each drug provided separately in daily administration pack for QID dosing
lansoprazole, amoxicillin, clarithromycin (Prevacid)	*H. pylori* eradication in patients with duodenal ulcer	Each drug provided separately in daily administration pack for BID dosing

Adverse Reactions

The most common adverse reactions seen with the proton pump inhibitors include headache, nausea, diarrhea, and abdominal pain.

Contraindications and Precautions

Proton pump inhibitors are contraindicated in patients who are hypersensitive to any of the drugs. Proton pump inhibitors are used cautiously in older adults and in patients with hepatic impairment. Prolonged treatment may decrease the body's ability to absorb vitamin B$_{12}$, resulting in anemia. Omeprazole (pregnancy category C) and lansoprazole, rabeprazole, and pantoprazole (pregnancy category B) are contraindicated during pregnancy and lactation.

Interactions

The following interactions may occur when a proton pump inhibitor is administered with another agent:

Interacting Drug	Common Use	Effect of Interaction
sucralfate	Management of GI distress	Decreased absorption of the proton pump inhibitor
ketoconazole and ampicillin	Anti-infective agent	Decreased absorption of the anti-infective
oral anticoagulants	Blood thinners	Increased risk of bleeding
digoxin	Cardiac problems	Increased absorption of digoxin
benzodiazepines, phenytoin	Management of seizure disorders	Risk for toxic level of antiseizure drugs
clarithromycin (with omeprazole, specifically)	Anti-infective agent	Risk for an increase in plasma levels of both drugs

Miscellaneous Acid Reducers

Three other types of acid-reducing drugs that are less frequently used are the cholinergic blocking drugs (also called *anticholinergic* drugs), a pepsin inhibitor, and a prostaglandin drug. Cholinergic blocking drugs reduce gastric motility and decrease the amount of acid secreted by the stomach. These drugs have been largely replaced by histamine H$_2$ antagonists, which appear to be more effective and have fewer adverse effects. Examples of cholinergic blocking drugs used for GI disorders include propantheline (Pro-Banthine) and glycopyrrolate (Robinul). For information about specific cholinergic blocking drugs, see Chapter 27.

Sucralfate (Carafate) is known as a pepsin inhibitor or mucosal protective drug. The drug binds with protein molecules to form a viscous substance that buffers acid and protects the mucosal lining. Sucralfate is used in the short-term treatment of duodenal ulcers. The most common adverse reaction is constipation. Drug interactions of sucralfate are similar to those of the proton pump inhibitors.

A prostaglandin drug, misoprostol (Cytotec), has been used to reduce the risk of nonsteroidal anti-inflammatory drug (NSAID)–induced gastric ulcers in high-risk patients, such as older adults or the critically ill. Misoprostol both inhibits the production of gastric acid and has mucosal protective properties. Because this drug can cause abortion or birth defects, it is not recommended for use in ulcer reduction in women who are pregnant or may become pregnant, or who are lactating. Adverse reactions include headache, nausea, diarrhea, and abdominal pain. The drug effects are decreased when it is taken with antacids.

teaching topic - Dont get PG

• GASTROINTESTINAL STIMULANTS

Actions

Metoclopramide (Reglan) and dexpanthenol (Ilopan) treat delayed gastric emptying and emesis—that is, they increase the motility of the upper GI tract without increasing the production of secretions. By sensitizing tissue to the effects of acetylcholine, the tone and amplitude of gastric contractions are increased, resulting in faster emptying of gastric contents into the small intestine. Stimulation of the **chemoreceptor trigger zone** (CTZ), a group of nerve fibers located on the surface of the fourth ventricle of the brain that sends signals to the vomiting center in the medulla, is also inhibited by metoclopramide.

Uses

The GI stimulants are used in the treatment of the following:

• GERD
• **Gastric stasis** (failure to move food normally out of the stomach) in diabetic patients, in patients with nausea and vomiting associated with cancer chemotherapy, and in patients in the immediate postoperative period

Dexpanthenol may be given intravenously (IV) immediately after major abdominal surgery to reduce the risk of **paralytic ileus** (lack of peristalsis or movement of the intestines).

Adverse Reactions

Adverse reactions associated with metoclopramide are usually mild. Higher doses or prolonged administration may produce central nervous system (CNS) symptoms, such as restlessness, drowsiness, dizziness, extrapyramidal effects (tremor, involuntary movements of the limbs, muscle rigidity), facial grimacing, and depression. Dexpanthenol administration may cause itching, difficulty breathing, and urticaria.

Contraindications and Precautions

The GI stimulants are contraindicated in patients with known hypersensitivity to the drugs, GI obstruction, gastric perforation or hemorrhage, or pheochromocytoma. Patients with Parkinson's disease or a seizure disorder who are taking drugs likely to cause extrapyramidal symptoms should not take these drugs. Dexpanthenol should not be used by patients with hemophilia.

These drugs are used cautiously in patients with diabetes and cardiovascular disease. Metoclopramide is a pregnancy category B drug; dexpanthenol is a pregnancy category C drug. These drugs are secreted in breast milk and should be used with caution during pregnancy and lactation.

Interactions

The following interactions may occur when a GI stimulant is administered with another agent:

Interacting Drug	Common Use	Effect of Interaction
cholinergic blocking drugs or opioid analgesics	Management of GI distress or pain relief	Decreased effectiveness of metoclopramide
cimetidine	Management of GI distress	Decreased absorption of cimetidine
digoxin	Management of cardiac problems	Decreased absorption of digoxin
monoamine oxidase inhibitors	Management of depression	Increased risk of hypertensive episode
levodopa	Management of disease	Decreased metoclopramide and levodopa

● ANTIEMETICS

An antiemetic drug is used to treat or prevent nausea (unpleasant gastric sensation usually preceding vomiting) or vomiting (forceful expulsion of gastric contents through the mouth). The drugs discussed in this section are used to treat severe nausea and vomiting. Individuals may experience nausea due to motion sickness or a condition called **vertigo** (a sensation of spinning or a rotation-type motion). Many of the drugs used to treat motion sickness can be purchased over the counter. Table 41.2 lists examples of drugs used in the treatment of motion sickness or vertigo.

Table **41.2** **Examples of Drugs Used for Motion Sickness**	
Generic Name	**Trade Name**
buclizine	Bucladin-S
cyclizine	Marezine
dimenhydrinate	Dramamine
diphenhydramine	Benadryl
meclizine	Antivert
scopolamine	Scopace (oral), Transderm-Scop (transdermal path)

Actions

Vomiting caused by drugs, radiation, and metabolic disorders often occurs because of stimulation of the CTZ, a group of nerve fibers located on the surface of the fourth ventricle of the brain. When these nerves are stimulated by chemicals, such as drugs or toxic substances, impulses are sent to the vomiting center located in the medulla. The vomiting center may also be directly stimulated by disorders such as GI irritation, motion sickness, and vestibular neuritis (inflammation of the vestibular nerve). These drugs appear to act primarily by inhibiting the CTZ and the brain's primary neurotransmitters dopamine and acetylcholine.

A newer classification of antiemetic drugs, the 5-hydroxytryptamine type 3 (5-HT3) receptor antagonists, target serotonin receptors both at the CTZ and peripherally at the nerve endings in the stomach. This action reduces the non-GI adverse effects that are often evident when nonspecific cholinergic blocking drugs are used. Because of their localized action in the GI system, these drugs are being tested for use in irritable bowel syndrome as well.

Uses

An antiemetic is used to treat nausea and vomiting, typically by preventive administration (prophylaxis):

- Before surgery to prevent vomiting during surgery
- Immediately after surgery when the patient is recovering from anesthesia
- Before, during, and after administration of antineoplastic drugs that induce a high degree of nausea and vomiting
- During radiation therapy when the GI tract is in the treatment field

Other causes of nausea and vomiting that may be treated with an antiemetic include bacterial and viral infections and adverse drug reactions. Some antiemetics also are used for motion sickness and vertigo. Dronabinol (Marinol) is the only medically available cannabinoid (marijuana derivative) prescribed for antiemetic use. For a comprehensive listing of antiemetics, see the Summary Drug Table: Drugs Used in Managing Upper Gastrointestinal Disorders.

Adverse Reactions

The most common adverse reactions resulting from these drugs are varying degrees of drowsiness. Additional adverse reactions for each drug are listed in the Summary Drug Table: Drugs Used in Managing Upper Gastrointestinal Disorders.

Contraindications

Antiemetic drugs are contraindicated in patients with known hypersensitivity to these drugs or with severe CNS depression. The 5-HT3 receptor antagonists should not be used by patients with heart block or prolonged QT intervals. In general, these drugs are not recommended during pregnancy and lactation, or for uncomplicated vomiting in young children. Prochlorperazine is contraindicated in patients with bone marrow depression, blood dyscrasia, Parkinson's disease, or severe liver or cardiovascular disease. Thiethylperazine is a pregnancy category X drug and is contraindicated during pregnancy.

Precautions

Severe nausea and vomiting should not be treated with antiemetic drugs alone. The cause of the vomiting must be investigated. Antiemetic drugs may hamper the diagnosis of disorders such as brain tumor or injury, appendicitis, intestinal obstruction, and drug toxicity (e.g., digitalis toxicity). Delayed diagnosis of any of these disorders could have serious consequences for the patient.

Cholinergic blocking antiemetics are used cautiously in patients with glaucoma or obstructive disease of the GI or genitourinary system, those with renal or hepatic dysfunction, and in older men with possible prostatic hypertrophy. Promethazine is used cautiously in patients with hypertension, sleep apnea, or epilepsy. Trimethobenzamide is used cautiously in children with a viral illness because it is thought to increase the risk of Reye's syndrome. The 5-HT3 receptor antagonists should be used cautiously in patients with cardiac conduction problems or electrolyte imbalances.

Perphenazine, prochlorperazine, promethazine, scopolamine, chlorpromazine, and trimethobenzamide are pregnancy category C drugs. Other antiemetics are classified as pregnancy category B (except for thiethylperazine, which is classified as pregnancy category X).

Interactions

The following interactions may occur when an antiemetic is administered with another agent:

Interacting Drug	Common Use	Effect of Interaction
CNS depressants	Analgesia, sedation, or pain relief	Increased risk of sedation
antihistamines	Management of allergy and respiratory distress	Increased adverse cholinergic blocking effects
Antacids	Management of gastric distress	Decreased absorption of antiemetic
Rifampin with 5-HT3 receptor antagonist	Tuberculosis/human immunodeficiency virus infection management	Decreased effectiveness of 5-HT3 receptor antagonist
Lithium with prochlorperazine	Management of bipolar disorder	Increased risk of extrapyramidal effects

• EMETICS

An emetic is a drug that induces vomiting. This is caused by local irritation of the stomach and by stimulation of the vomiting center in the medulla. Emetics are used to empty the stomach rapidly when an individual has accidentally or intentionally ingested a poison or drug overdose. Not all poison ingestions or drug overdoses are treated with emetics.

Because more harm can occur from the vomiting of many substances, guidelines were established for the use of syrup of ipecac.*

The U.S. Food and Drug Administration approved the following warnings for the labeling of syrup of ipecac:

- Do not use in persons who are not fully conscious.
- Do not use this product unless directed by a health care professional. Do not use if turpentine, corrosives, such as alkalis (lye) or strong acids, or petroleum distillates, such as kerosene, paint thinner, cleaning fluid, or furniture polish, have been ingested.

Clinicians have expanded the contraindications for ipecac syrup to include situations in which:

- The patient is comatose or has altered mental status, and the risk of aspiration of stomach contents is high.
- The patient is having convulsions.
- The substance ingested is capable of causing altered mental status or convulsions.
- The substance ingested is a caustic or corrosive agent.
- The substance ingested is a low-viscosity petroleum distillate with the potential for pulmonary aspiration and the development of chemical pneumonitis.
- The patient has a medical condition that may be exacerbated by vomiting (e.g., severe hypertension, bradycardia, hemorrhagic diathesis).

 NURSING ALERT

Before an emetic is given, it is extremely important to know the chemicals or substances that have been ingested, the time they were ingested, and what symptoms were noted before seeking medical treatment. This information will probably be obtained from a family member or friend, but the adult patient may also contribute to the history. The primary health care provider or nurse may also contact the local poison control center to obtain information regarding treatment.

NURSING PROCESS

PATIENT RECEIVING A DRUG FOR AN UPPER GASTROINTESTINAL CONDITION

ASSESSMENT

Preadministration Assessment
The nurse questions the patient regarding the type and intensity of symptoms (e.g., pain, discomfort, nausea, vomiting) to provide a baseline for evaluating the effectiveness of drug therapy. As part of the preadministration assessment for a patient receiving a drug for nausea and vomiting, the nurse documents the number of times the patient has vomited and the approximate amount of fluid lost. Before starting therapy, the nurse takes vital signs and assesses for signs of fluid and electrolyte imbalances.

---

*Manoguerra A. S. & Cobaugh D. J. (2005). Guideline on the use of ipecac syrup in the out-of-hospital management of ingested poisons. *Clinical Toxicology, 43*(1), 1–10.

In the case of preventative administration of an antiemetic, the nurse explains the rationale for preventing an episode of nausea rather than waiting for symptoms to occur when the primary health care provider knows the drugs being given will cause this problem. The nurse questions the patient about any episodes of nausea or vomiting in anticipation of the therapy.

Ongoing Assessment

The nurse monitors the patient frequently for continued complaints of pain, sour taste, or the production of bloody or coffee-ground emesis. Suction equipment should be kept available in case a nasogastric (NG) tube must be inserted for suctioning to prevent aspiration of emesis. If vomiting is severe, the nurse observes the patient for signs and symptoms of electrolyte imbalance and monitors the blood pressure, pulse, and respiratory rate every 2 to 4 hours or as ordered by the primary health care provider. The nurse carefully measures intake and output (urine, emesis) until vomiting ceases, and the patient can take oral fluids in sufficient quantity.

The nurse documents in the patient's chart each time the patient vomits. The nurse notifies the primary health care provider if there is blood in the emesis or if vomiting suddenly becomes more severe. The nurse also may need to measure the patient's weight daily to weekly in patients with prolonged and repeated episodes of vomiting (e.g., those receiving chemotherapy for cancer). The nurse assesses the patient at frequent intervals for the effectiveness of the drug in relieving symptoms (e.g., nausea, vomiting, or vertigo) and notifies the primary health care provider if the drug fails to relieve or diminish symptoms.

NURSING DIAGNOSES

Drug-specific nursing diagnoses include the following:

❏ **Risk for Deficient Fluid Volume** related to diarrhea, nausea, and vomiting
❏ **Imbalanced Nutrition: Less Than Body Requirements** related to impaired ability to ingest and retain food and fluids, or offensive tastes and smells
❏ **Individual Effective Therapeutic Regimen Management** related to inability to take oral form of medication
❏ **Risk for Injury** related to adverse drug effects of drowsiness

Nursing diagnoses related to drug administration are discussed in Chapter 4.

PLANNING

The expected outcomes for the patient depend on the reason the upper GI drug is administered, but may include an optimal response to drug therapy, support of patient needs related to the management of adverse reactions, and an understanding of the therapeutic regimen.

IMPLEMENTATION

Promoting an Optimal Response to Therapy

ANTACIDS. The antacid may be administered hourly for the first 2 weeks when used to treat acute peptic ulcer. After the first 2 weeks, the drug is administered 1 to 2 hours after meals and at bedtime. The primary health care provider may order that the antacid be left at the patient's bedside for self-administration. The nurse ensures that an adequate supply of water and cups for measuring the dose are available.

> **❗ NURSING ALERT**
> Because of the possibility of an antacid interfering with the activity of other oral drugs, no oral drug should be administered within 1 to 2 hours of an antacid.

NON-ORAL METHODS OF DRUG ADMINISTRATION. Patients taking acid-reducing drugs may not be able to take oral medications because of preparation for an operative procedure, postoperative nausea, or physical condition. Many of these drugs come in forms for both intramuscular (IM) and IV administration. The IV route is typically preferred if the patient has an existing IV line, because these drugs are irritating, and IM injections need to be given deep into the muscular tissue to minimize harm.

> **❗ NURSING ALERT**
> When one of these drugs is given IV, the nurse monitors the rate of infusion at frequent intervals. Too rapid an infusion may induce cardiac arrhythmias.

Patients who are debilitated and require feeding from an NG tube are at risk for gastric ulcer development and may be prescribed acid-reducing drugs. The nurse always checks the medication label to see if the pill can be crushed or the capsule opened before doing so. These can be mixed with 40 mL of apple juice and injected through the NG tube. The tube is flushed with fluid afterward. Many of these drugs come in a liquid form as well as tablet or capsule. The nurse should request the liquid form when administration is in a tube to decrease the chance of a clogged NG tube due to improper flushing.

PREVENTION OF NAUSEA IN PATIENTS UNDERGOING CANCER THERAPY. Different protocols for pre-chemotherapy nausea depend on the type of cancer treatment. Some cancer (antineoplastic) drugs rarely cause nausea, and others are highly emetogenic. Granisetron (Kytril), ondansetron (Zofran), and dolasetron (Anzemet) are examples of antiemetics used when cancer chemotherapy drugs are very likely to cause nausea and vomiting. The nurse begins administering these drugs before the chemotherapy is given. The nurse may give the first dose IV during therapy, and then ask the patient to take it orally at home for a specified period. It is important for the nurse to explain to the patient that the drug prevents nausea and vomiting and to be sure to take the entire dose prescribed. Administration of antineoplastics and the preadministration of antiemetics should always be performed by a nurse trained in the administration of cancer chemotherapy.

Monitoring and Managing Patient Needs

RISK FOR DEFICIENT FLUID VOLUME. When antacids are given, the nurse keeps a record of the patient's bowel movements, because these drugs may cause constipation or diarrhea. If the patient experiences diarrhea, the nurse keeps an accurate record of fluid intake and output along with a description of the diarrhea stool. Changing to a different antacid usually alleviates the problem. Diarrhea may be controlled by combining a magnesium antacid with an antacid containing aluminum or calcium. Uncontrolled diarrhea can lead to fluid loss and dehydration.

Dehydration is a serious concern in the patient experiencing nausea and vomiting. It is important to observe the patient for signs of dehydration, which include poor skin turgor, dry mucous membranes, decrease in or absence of urinary output, concentrated urine, restlessness, irritability, increased respiratory rate, and confusion. The nurse monitors the input and output (urine and emesis) and documents findings every 8 hours. If the patient is able to take and retain small amounts of oral fluids, the nurse offers sips of water at frequent intervals. In addition, it is important to observe the patient for signs of electrolyte imbalance, particularly sodium and potassium deficit (see Chapter 55). If signs of dehydration or electrolyte imbalance are noted, the nurse contacts the primary health care provider, because parenteral administration of fluids or fluids with electrolytes may be necessary.

LIFESPAN ALERT – Chronic Care
Observations for fluid and electrolyte disturbances are particularly important in the elderly or chronically ill patients in whom severe dehydration may develop quickly. The nurse must immediately report symptoms of dehydration, such as dry mucous membranes, decreased urinary output, concentrated urine, restlessness, or confusion.

IMBALANCED NUTRITION: LESS THAN BODY REQUIREMENTS. Nausea, vomiting, vertigo, and dizziness are disagreeable sensations. The nurse provides the patient with an emesis basin and checks the basin at frequent intervals. If vomiting occurs, the nurse empties the emesis basin and measures and documents the volume in the patient's chart. The nurse may give the patient a damp washcloth and a towel to wipe the hands and face as needed. It also is a good idea to give the patient mouthwash or frequent oral rinses to remove the disagreeable taste that accompanies vomiting.

Nausea may make the patient lose his or her appetite and decrease nutritional intake. It is important to make the environment as pleasant as possible to enhance the patient's appetite. The nurse removes items with strong smells and odors. The nurse changes the patient's bedding and clothing or gown as needed, because the odor of vomit may intensify the sensations of nausea and further decrease appetite.

INDIVIDUAL EFFECTIVE THERAPEUTIC REGIMEN MANAGEMENT. When antacids are given, the nurse instructs the patient to chew the tablets thoroughly before swallowing and then drink a full glass of water or milk. If the patient expresses a dislike for the taste of the antacid or has difficulty chewing the tablet form, the nurse informs the primary health care provider. A flavored antacid may be ordered if the patient finds the taste unpleasant. A liquid form may be ordered if the patient has difficulty chewing a tablet. Liquid antacid preparations must be shaken thoroughly immediately before administration. Liquid antacids are followed by a small amount of water.

If the patient cannot retain the oral form of the drug, the nurse may give it parenterally or as a rectal suppository (if the prescribed drug is available in these forms). If only the oral form has been ordered and the patient cannot retain the drug, the nurse contacts the primary health care provider regarding an order for a parenteral or suppository form of this or another antiemetic drug.

When administering scopolamine for motion sickness, one transdermal system is applied behind the ear approximately 4 hours before the antiemetic effect is needed. Approximately 1 g of scopolamine is administered every 24 hours for 3 days. The nurse advises the individual to discard any disk that becomes detached and to replace it with a fresh disk applied behind the opposite ear. (See Patient Teaching for Improved Patient Outcomes: Applying Transdermal Scopolamine).

RISK FOR INJURY. Administration of these drugs may result in varying degrees of drowsiness. To prevent accidental falls and other injuries, the nurse assists the patient who is allowed out of bed with ambulatory activities. If extreme drowsiness is noted, the nurse instructs the patient to remain in bed and provides a call light for assistance.

LIFESPAN ALERT – Gerontology
The older adult is particularly sensitive to the effects of the histamine H_2 antagonists. The nurse must closely monitor older adults for confusion and dizziness. Dizziness increases the risk for falls in the older adult. Assistance is needed for ambulatory activities. The environment is made safe by removing throw rugs, small pieces of furniture, and the like. The nurse reports any change in orientation to the primary health care provider.

The nurse observes patients receiving high or prolonged doses of metoclopramide for adverse reactions related to the CNS (extrapyramidal effects or tardive dyskinesia). The nurse reports any sign of extrapyramidal symptoms or tardive dyskinesia to the primary health care provider before the next dose of metoclopramide is administered, because the drug therapy may be discontinued. These adverse reactions may be irreversible if therapy is continued.

Educating the Patient and Family

When a drug to treat the upper GI system is prescribed for outpatient use, the nurse includes the following information in a patient teaching plan:

• Avoid driving or performing other hazardous tasks when taking these drugs, because drowsiness may occur with use.

- Do not use an antacid indiscriminately. Check with a primary health care provider before using an antacid if other medical problems, such as a cardiac condition, exist (some laxatives contain sodium).
- Allow effervescent tablets to dissolve completely in water. Allow most of the bubbling to stop before drinking the solution.
- Adhere to the dosage schedule recommended by the primary health care provider. Do not increase the frequency of use or the dose if symptoms become worse; instead, see the primary health care provider as soon as possible.
- Because antacids impair the absorption of some drugs, do not take other drugs within 2 hours before or after taking the antacid unless use of an antacid with a drug is recommended by the primary health care provider.
- If pain or discomfort remains the same or becomes worse, if the stools turn black, or if vomitus resembles coffee grounds, contact the primary health care provider as soon as possible.
- Explain that antacids may change the color of the stool (white, white streaks); this is normal.
- Advise the patient that magnesium-containing products may produce a laxative effect and may cause diarrhea; aluminum- or calcium-containing antacids may cause constipation; magnesium-containing antacids are used to avoid bowel dysfunction.
- Taking too much antacid may cause the stomach to secrete excess stomach acid. Consult the primary health care provider or pharmacist about appropriate dose. Do not use the maximum dose for more than 2 weeks, except under the supervision of a primary health care provider.
- When taking proton pump inhibitors, swallow the tablet whole at least 1 hour before eating. Do not chew, open, or crush.
- When taking metoclopramide, immediately report any of the following signs: difficulty speaking or swallowing; masklike face; shuffling gait; rigidity; tremors; uncontrolled movements of the mouth, face, or extremities; and uncontrolled chewing or unusual movements of the tongue.
- Avoid the use of alcohol and other sedative-type drugs unless use has been approved by the primary health care provider.
- Take antiemetics for cancer chemotherapy as prescribed. Do not omit a dose. Consult the primary health care provider if you have forgotten a dose of the medication.
- When taking rectal suppositories, remove foil wrapper and immediately insert the pointed end into the rectum without using force.
- Take the drug for motion sickness about 1 hour before travel.
- Misoprostol: Because this drug may cause spontaneous abortion, advise women of childbearing age to use a reliable contraceptive. If pregnancy is suspected, discontinue use of the drug and notify the primary health

care provider. Report severe menstrual pain, bleeding, or spotting as well.

EVALUATION

- Therapeutic effect is achieved and nausea or pain is controlled.
- Adverse reactions are identified, reported to the primary health care provider, and managed successfully through appropriate nursing interventions:
  ☑ Fluid volume balance is maintained.
  ☑ Patient maintains an adequate nutritional status.
  ☑ Patient manages the therapeutic regimen effectively.
  ☑ No evidence of injury is seen.
- Patient or family demonstrates an understanding of the drug regimen.

Patient Teaching for Improved Patient Outcomes

Applying Transdermal Scopolamine

The nurse:
✓ Instructs the patient to apply the transdermal scopolamine system behind the ear.
✓ Explains that after application of the system, the hands are washed *thoroughly* with soap and water and dried. The importance of thorough handwashing to prevent any traces of the drug from coming in contact with the eyes is emphasized.
✓ Teaches that the disk will last about 3 days, at which time the patient may remove the disk and apply another disk, if needed.
✓ Instructs the patient to discard the used disk and thoroughly wash and dry the hands and previous application site.
✓ Instructs the patient to apply the new disk behind the opposite ear and again thoroughly wash and dry the hands.
✓ Emphasizes that only one disk at a time is used.
✓ Makes sure that the patient has a thorough knowledge of the adverse reactions that may occur with the use of this system: dizziness, dry mouth, and blurred vision.
✓ Stresses the importance of observing caution when driving or performing hazardous tasks.

THINK CRITICALLY: PHARMACOLOGY IN PRACTICE

1. Alfredo Garcia was found to have GERD, not a peptic ulcer. As the nurse, you would teach Mr. Garcia that using dairy products to coat the stomach lining is not helpful in reducing acid secretions. Instead, he is instructed to buy the antacid of his choice for the heartburn. As the nurse, you teach Mr. Garcia how to take the medication properly. He can't understand

why he should coat his stomach with medicine
instead of cream. Explain how antacids work.

2. He calls later because he is confused by all the
antacid preparations on the market. Considering the
fact that he is taking a diuretic for hypertension and
tends to become constipated, which products would
be the best for him, given his history?

● Test Your Knowledge

1. How would the nurse correctly administer an antacid to a
patient taking other oral medications?

   A. With the other drugs
   B. 30 minutes before or after administration of other
   drugs
   C. 2 hours before or after administration of other drugs
   D. In early morning and at bedtime

2. When a histamine H_2 antagonist drug is prescribed
for the treatment of a peptic ulcer, the nurse observes
the patient for which of the following adverse effects?

   A. Dry mouth, urinary retention
   B. Edema, tachycardia
   C. Constipation, anorexia
   D. Dizziness, somnolence

3. What is the most common adverse reaction the nurse
would expect in a patient receiving an antiemetic?

   A. Occipital headache
   B. Drowsiness
   C. Edema
   D. Nausea

4. When explaining how to use transdermal scopolamine,
the nurse tells the patient to apply the system to _____.

   A. a non-hairy region of the chest
   B. the upper back
   C. behind the ear
   D. the forearm

● Prepare for the NCLEX

1. Select the most helpful resource for the nurse assisting
the patient to determine the best antacid to purchase.

   A. Scan magazines and newspaper ads
   B. Discuss with the clinical pharmacist
   C. Search the internet for drug ads
   D. Contact the primary healthcare provider

● Calculate Medication Dosages

1. Prochlorperazine (Compazine) 10 mg orally is prescribed. Use the drug label below to prepare the correct
dosage.

   The nurse would administer _____.

Courtesy Glaxo-SmithKline.

2. The patient is to receive 400 mg cimetidine (Tagamet)
orally. Available for use is the cimetidine shown below.

   The nurse administers _____.

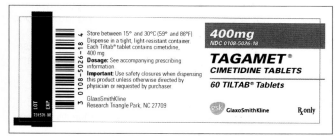

Courtesy Glaxo-SmithKline.

To check your answers, see Appendix E.

the**Point**. *For more NCLEX questions, log on to
http://thepoint.lww.com to access more than 1000 questions.*

Drugs That Affect the Lower Gastrointestinal System

KEY TERMS

antiflatulents
constipation
diarrhea
dyspepsia

inflammatory bowel
  disease
obstipation

LEARNING OBJECTIVES

On completion of this chapter, the student will:

1. Describe how inflammatory bowel disease alters function of the lower gastrointestinal system.
2. List the types of drugs prescribed or recommended for lower gastrointestinal disorders.
3. Discuss the uses, general drug actions, general adverse reactions, contraindications, precautions, and interactions associated with lower gastrointestinal drugs.
4. Discuss important preadministration and ongoing assessment activities the nurse should perform on the patient taking a lower gastrointestinal drug.
5. List nursing diagnoses particular to a patient taking a lower gastrointestinal drug.
6. Discuss ways to promote an optimal response to therapy, how to manage common adverse reactions, and important points to keep in mind when educating patients about the use of lower gastrointestinal drugs.

Figure 42.1. Disruption in bowel routine can impact the activities of daily living for the patient.

The large intestine is responsible for the absorption of water and some of the nutrients from the food and fluids we eat. The speed of transit determines what will be absorbed. Transit of contents rapidly through the bowel is called **diarrhea**. When contents move sluggishly, more water is absorbed, and the fecal material gets harder, resulting in **constipation**. Transit can be triggered by many things. Illness, such as irritable bowel syndrome or ulcerative colitis, bacterial infection, or drugs such as anti-infectives can make transit faster, resulting in diarrhea. Conditions such as Parkinson's disease can slow the bowel, causing constipation. Treatment with opioid drugs and the aftereffects of abdominal surgery can also cause constipation.

Conditions that affect the function of the lower gastrointestinal (GI) system can have a significant impact on activities of daily living; if proper absorption does not occur, people may not have the energy to engage in activities (Fig. 42.1). One such condition that affects function is **inflammatory bowel disease** (IBD). The pain and bloating of a sluggish bowel or fear of stool incontinence may prevent people from socializing, again affecting daily life. The drugs described in this chapter affect the function of the bowel. Antidiarrheals and laxatives, as well as drugs to treat IBD, are presented. Some of the more common drugs are listed in the Summary Drug Table: Drugs Used in Managing Lower Gastrointestinal Disorders.

Inflammatory Bowel Disease

According to the Crohn's and Colitis Foundation of America (2007), as many as 1.4 million Americans have IBD. The term IBD is used collectively for Crohn's disease and ulcerative colitis, diseases that cause inflammation in the intestines. The cause of these diseases is unknown, although it is thought that a virus or bacterial organism interacting with the body's immune system may be the cause. Clinical manifestations of Crohn's disease include abdominal pain and distention. As the disease progresses, other GI symptoms present, such as anorexia, diarrhea, weight loss, dehydration, and nutritional deficiencies. Ulcerative colitis has a more abrupt onset; patients experience the sudden need to defecate, resulting in severe, blood- and mucus-filled diarrhea or no stool

(text continues on page 401)

Summary Drug Table DRUGS USED IN MANAGING LOWER GASTROINTESTINAL DISORDERS

Generic Name	Trade Name	Uses	Adverse Reactions	Dosage Ranges
Drugs Used to Treat Inflammatory Bowel Disease				
Aminosalicylates				
balsalazide *bal-sal'-ah-zyde*	Colazal	Active ulcerative colitis	Headache, abdominal pain	2250 mg orally TID for 8 wk
mesalamine *meh-sal'-ah-meen*	Asacol, Pentasa, Rowasa (rectal form)	Active ulcerative colitis, proctosigmoiditis or proctitis	Headache, abdominal pain, nausea	800–1000 mg orally TID or QID Suspension enema: 4 g QD
olsalazine *ohl-sal'-ah-zeen*	Dipentum	Maintenance of remission of ulcerative colitis	Diarrhea, abdominal pain and cramping	1 g/day orally in two divided doses
sulfasalazine *sul-fah-sal'-ah-zeen*	Azulfidine	Ulcerative colitis, rheumatoid arthritis	Headache, nausea, anorexia, vomiting, gastric distress, reduced sperm count	Initial: 3–4 g/day orally in divided doses Maintenance: 2 g orally QID
Miscellaneous Drugs for Bowel Disorders				
alosetron *ah-loe'-seh-tron*	Lotronex	Second line treatment of female irritable bowel syndrome with severe diarrhea	Gastric distress, hemorrhoids, constipation	Special permission must be obtained for therapy
infliximab *in-flik'-sih-mab*	Remicade	Crohn's disease, ulcerative colitis, rheumatoid arthritis	Sore throat, cough, sinus infection, gastric distress	5 mg/kg IV every 2–8 wk
Antidiarrheals				
bismuth *biz'-muth*	Bismatrol Pepto-Bismol, Pink Bismuth	Nausea, diarrhea, abdominal cramps, *H. pylori* infection with duodenal ulcer	Same as difenoxin	2 tablets or 30 mL orally every 30 min to 1 hr, up to 8 doses in 24 hr
difenoxin with atropine *dye-fen-ok'-sin,* *ah'-troe-peen*	Motofen	Symptomatic relief of acute diarrhea	Dry skin and mucous membranes, nausea, constipation, lightheadedness	Initial dose: 2 tablets orally, then 1 tablet after each loose stool (not to exceed 8 tablets/day)
diphenoxylate with atropine *dye-fen-ok'-sih-late*	Lomotil, Lonox	Same as difenoxin	Same as difenoxin	5 mg orally QID
loperamide *loe-pare'-ah-myde*	Imodium, Kaopectate, Maalox Anti-Diarrheal Caplets	Same as difenoxin	Same as difenoxin	Initial dose 4 mg orally; then 2 mg after each loose stool (not to exceed 16 mg/day)
tincture of opium	Paregoric	Severe diarrhea	Somnolence, constipation	0.6 mL orally QID
Antiflatulents				
charcoal	CharcoCaps, Flatulex (combined with simethicone)	Intestinal gas, diarrhea, poisoning antidote	Vomiting, constipation, diarrhea, black stools	520 mg orally after meals (not to exceed 4–16 g/day)

(table continues on page 400)

Summary Drug Table DRUGS USED IN MANAGING LOWER GASTROINTESTINAL DISORDERS (continued)

Generic Name	Trade Name	Uses	Adverse Reactions	Dosage Ranges
simethicone
sye-meth'-ih-kone	Gas-X, Mylicon, Maalox Anti-Gas, Mylanta Gas	Postoperative distention, dyspepsia, irritable bowel, peptic ulcer	Bloating, constipation, diarrhea, heartburn	40–125 mg orally QID after meals and at bedtime
Laxatives				
Bulk-Producing Laxatives				
methylcellulose
meth-ill-sell'-yoo-loas	Citrucel, Unifiber	Relief of constipation, irritable bowel syndrome, severe watery diarrhea	Diarrhea, nausea, vomiting, bloating, flatulence, cramping, perianal irritation, fainting	Follow directions given on the container
psyllium
sill'-ee-um	Fiberall, Genfiber, Hydrocil, Konsyl, Metamucil, Perdiem	Same as methylcellulose	Same as methylcellulose	Powder, granules, or wafers taken as directed on package
polycarbophil
pol-ee-kar'-boe-fill	Equalactin, FiberCon, Mitrolan	Same as methylcellulose	Same as methylcellulose	1 g daily to QID or as needed (do not exceed 4 g in 24 hr)
Emollients
mineral oil	Kondremul Plain, Milkinol	Relief of constipation, and fecal impaction	Perianal discomfort and itching due to anal seepage	15–45 mL orally at bedtime
Stool Softeners/Surfactants
docusate (dioctyl; DDS)
dok'-yoo-sate	Colace, Ex-Lax Stool Softener, Modane Soft, Surfak Liquigels	Relief of constipation, prevention of straining during bowel movement	Diarrhea, nausea, vomiting, bloating, flatulence, cramping, perianal irritation, fainting	Follow directions given on the container; comes in enema form
Hyperosmotic Agents
glycerin
glih'-ser-in	Colace Suppositories, Sani-Supp, Fleet Babylax	Relief of constipation	Same as docusate sodium	Rectal suppository, use as directed
lactulose
lak'-tyoo-loas	Cephulac, Chronulac, Constilac, Duphalac	Relief of constipation, hepatic encephalopathy	Same as docusate sodium	Constipation: 15–30 mL/day orally: Hepatic encephalopathy: 30–45 mL orally QID, may give enema form
lubiprostone
loo-bih-pros'-tone	Amitiza	Chronic idiopathic constipation	Headache, nausea, diarrhea	24 mcg orally BID
Irritant or Stimulant Laxatives
cascara sagrada
kas-kar'-ah sah-grah'-dah	Aromatic Cascara	Relief of constipation	Same as docusate sodium, darkening of colon mucosa, brownish color to urine	Follow directions given on the container
sennosides
sen'-oh-sydes	Agoral, Ex-Lax, Senokot	Same as cascara	Same as cascara	Follow directions given on the container
bisacodyl
bis-ah-koe'-dill	Bisca-Evac, Dulcolax, Modane, Correctol	Same as cascara	Diarrhea, nausea, vomiting, bloating, flatulence, cramping, perianal irritation	Tablets: 10–15 mg daily orally
Rectal suppositories: 10 mg daily; comes in enema form

consume plenty of water

monitor for sodium imbalance

(table continues on page 401)

Summary Drug Table DRUGS USED IN MANAGING LOWER GASTROINTESTINAL DISORDERS (continued)

Generic Name	Trade Name	Uses	Adverse Reactions	Dosage Ranges
Saline Laxatives				
magnesium preparations *mag-nee'-zee-um*	Milk of Magnesia, Magnesium Citrate, Fleets (enema preparation)	Evacuate colon for endoscopy, relieve constipation	Same as docusate sodium	Follow directions given on the container
Bowel Evacuants				
polyethylene glycol (PEG) solution *pol-ee-eth'-ih-leen*	MiraLax	Relieve constipation	Same as sodium docusate	Follow directions given on the container
polyethylene glycol-electrolyte solution (PEG-ES) *pol-ee-eth'-ih-leen*	CoLyte, GoLYTELY, NuLytely, OCL	Evacuate colon for endoscopy, relieve constipation	Same as sodium docusate	4 L oral solution to be drunk in 3 h

at all. Pain and fatigue accompany this disorder as well. No evidence has been found to support the theory that IBD is caused by tension, anxiety, or any other psychological factor or disorder.

Drugs used to treat IBD include antibiotics, corticosteroids, biologic agents, and aminosalicylates. Aminosalicylates are described in this chapter; other drugs used in the treatment of IBD are included in their respective chapters.

• AMINOSALICYLATES

Actions and Uses

Aminosalicylates are aspirin-like compounds with anti-inflammatory action. The drugs exert a topical anti-inflammatory effect in the bowel. The exact mechanism of action of these drugs is unknown. The aminosalicylates are used to treat Crohn's disease and ulcerative colitis as well as other inflammatory diseases.

Adverse Reactions

Because these drugs are topical anti-inflammatory drugs, the most common adverse reactions happen in the GI system and include abdominal pain, nausea, and diarrhea. Other general adverse reactions include headache, dizziness, fever, and weakness.

Contraindications and Precautions

Aminosalicylates are contraindicated in patients with a known hypersensitivity to the drugs or salicylate-containing drugs. In addition, these drugs are contraindicated in patients who have hypersensitivity to sulfonamides and sulfites or intestinal obstruction, and in children younger than 2 years. Aminosalicylates are pregnancy category B drugs (except

olsalazine, which is in pregnancy category C); all are used with caution during pregnancy and lactation (safety has not been established).

Interactions

The following interactions may occur when an aminosalicylate is administered with another agent:

Interacting Drug	Common Use	Effect of Interaction
digoxin	Cardiac problems	Reduced absorption of digoxin
methotrexate	Cancer and autoimmune conditions	Increased risk of immunosuppression
oral hypoglycemic drugs	Diabetes mellitus management	Increased blood glucose level
warfarin	Blood thinner	Increased risk of bleeding

HERBAL ALERT

Chamomile has several uses in traditional herbal therapy, including as a mild sedative and for treatment of digestive upsets, menstrual cramps, and stomach ulcers. It has been used topically for skin irritation and inflammation. Chamomile is on the U.S. Food and Drug Administration (FDA) list of herbs generally recognized as safe. It is one of the most popular teas in Europe. When used as an infusion, it appears to produce an antispasmodic effect on the smooth muscle of the GI tract and to protect against the development of stomach ulcers. Although the herb is generally safe and nontoxic, the infusion is prepared from the pollen-filled flower heads and has resulted in mild symptoms of contact dermatitis to severe anaphylactic reactions in individuals hypersensitive to ragweed, asters, and chrysanthemums.

• ANTIDIARRHEALS

Actions and Uses

Antidiarrheals are used in the treatment of diarrhea. Difenoxin (Motofen) and diphenoxylate (Lomotil) are chemically related to opioid drugs; therefore, they decrease intestinal peristalsis, which often is increased when the patient has diarrhea. Because these drugs are opioid related, they may have sedative and euphoric effects, but no analgesic activity. A drug dependence potential exists; therefore, the drugs are combined with atropine (a cholinergic blocking drug), which causes dry mouth and other mild adverse effects. Abuse potential is reduced because of these unpleasant adverse effects.

Loperamide (Imodium) acts directly on the muscle wall of the bowel to slow motility, and is not related to the opioids. It therefore is also used in treating chronic diarrhea associated with IBD.

Adverse Reactions

Gastrointestinal System Reactions

• Anorexia, nausea, vomiting, constipation
• Abdominal discomfort, pain, and distention

Other System Reactions

• Dizziness, drowsiness, and headache
• Sedation and euphoria
• Rash

Contraindications and Precautions

These drugs are contraindicated in patients whose diarrhea is associated with organisms that can harm the intestinal mucosa (*Escherichia coli*, *Salmonella* and *Shigella* spp.). Patients with pseudomembranous colitis, abdominal pain of unknown origin, and obstructive jaundice also should not take antidiarrheals. Antidiarrheal drugs are contraindicated in children younger than 2 years of age.

> **❗ NURSING ALERT**
>
> If diarrhea persists for more than 2 days when over-the-counter antidiarrheal drugs are being used, the patient should discontinue use and seek treatment from the primary health care provider.

The antidiarrheal drugs are used cautiously in patients with severe hepatic impairment or IBD. Antidiarrheals are classified as pregnancy category C drugs and should be used cautiously during pregnancy and lactation. Loperamide is a pregnancy category B drug, yet is not recommended for use during pregnancy and lactation.

Interactions

The following interactions may occur when an antidiarrheal drug is administered with another agent:

Interacting Drug	Common Use	Effect of Interaction
antihistamines, opioids, sedatives, or hypnotics	Allergy treatment (antihistamines), sedation, or pain relief	Increased risk of CNS depression
antihistamines and general antidepressants	Allergy relief and depression management	Increased cholinergic blocking adverse reactions
monoamine oxidase inhibitor antidepressants	Depression management	Increased risk hypertensive crisis

MOIA MAOI

• ANTIFLATULENTS

Actions

Simethicone (Mylicon) and charcoal are used as **antiflatulents** (drugs that reduce flatus or gas in the intestinal tract). These drugs do not absorb or remove gas; rather, they act to help the body release the gas by belching or flatus. Simethicone has a defoaming action that disperses and prevents the formation of gas pockets in the intestine. Charcoal helps bind gas for expulsion.

Uses

Antiflatulents are used to relieve painful symptoms of excess gas in the digestive tract that may be caused by the following:

• Postoperative gaseous distention and air swallowing
• **Dyspepsia** (fullness or epigastric discomfort)
• Peptic ulcer
• Irritable bowel syndrome or diverticulosis

In addition to its use for the relief of intestinal gas, charcoal may be used in the prevention of nonspecific pruritus associated with kidney dialysis treatment and as an antidote in poisoning. Simethicone is in some antacid products, such as Mylanta Liquid and Di-Gel Liquid.

Adverse Reactions

No adverse reactions have been reported with the use of antiflatulents.

Contraindications and Precautions

Antiflatulents are contraindicated in patients with known hypersensitivity to any components of the drug. The pregnancy category of simethicone has not been determined; because it is not absorbed, it may be safe for use during pregnancy, although the primary health care provider should be consulted whenever any drug is to be taken. Charcoal is a pregnancy category C drug.

Interactions

There may be a decreased effectiveness of other drugs because of adsorption by charcoal, which can also adsorb other drugs in the GI tract. There are no known interactions with simethicone.

• LAXATIVES

Actions

There are various types of laxatives (see the Summary Drug Table: Drugs Used in Managing Lower Gastrointestinal Disorders). The action of each laxative is somewhat different, yet they produce the same result—relief of constipation (Display 42.1).

Uses

A laxative is most often prescribed for the short-term relief or prevention of constipation. Specific uses of laxatives include:

- Stimulant, emollient, and saline laxatives—evacuate the colon for rectal and bowel examinations
- Stool softeners or mineral oil—prevention of strain during defecation (after anorectal surgery or a myocardial infarction)
- Psyllium and polycarbophil—irritable bowel syndrome and diverticular disease
- Hyperosmotic (lactulose) agents—reduction of blood ammonia levels in hepatic encephalopathy

Adverse Reactions

Constipation may occur as an adverse drug reaction. When the patient has constipation as an adverse reaction to another drug, the primary health care provider may prescribe a stool

DISPLAY 42.1 Actions of Different Types of Laxatives

- Bulk-producing laxatives are not digested by the body and therefore add bulk and water to the contents of the intestines. The added bulk in the intestines stimulates peristalsis, moves the products of digestion through the intestine, and encourages evacuation of the stool. Examples of bulk-forming laxatives are psyllium (Metamucil) and polycarbophil (FiberCon). Sometimes these laxatives are used with severe diarrhea to add bulk to the watery bowel contents and slow transit through the bowel. *Increase water* [handwritten annotation]
- Emollient laxatives lubricate the intestinal walls and soften the stool, thereby enhancing passage of fecal material. Mineral oil is an emollient laxative.
- Stool softeners promote water retention in the fecal mass and soften the stool. One difference between emollient laxatives and stool softeners is that the emollient laxatives do not promote the retention of water in the stool. Examples of stool softeners include docusate sodium (Colace) and docusate calcium (Surfak).
- Hyperosmolar drugs dehydrate local tissues, which causes irritation and increased peristalsis, with consequent evacuation of the fecal mass. Glycerin is a hyperosmolar drug.
- Irritant or stimulant laxatives increase peristalsis by direct action on the intestine. An example of an irritant laxative is cascara sagrada and senna (Senokot).
- Saline laxatives attract or pull water into the intestine, thereby increasing pressure in the intestine, followed by an increase in peristalsis. Magnesium (Milk of Magnesia) is a saline laxative.

DISPLAY 42.2 Drugs That May Cause Constipation

- Anticholinergic (cholinergic blocking drugs)
- Antihistamines
- Phenothiazines
- Tricyclic antidepressants
- Opioids
- Non–potassium-sparing diuretics
- Iron preparations
- Barium
- Clonidine
- Antacids containing calcium or aluminum

softener or another laxative to prevent constipation during the drug therapy. Display 42.2 lists some of the drug classifications that may cause constipation.

Laxatives may cause diarrhea and a loss of water and electrolytes, abdominal pain or discomfort, nausea, vomiting, perianal irritation, fainting, bloating, flatulence, cramps, and weakness.

Prolonged use of a laxative can result in serious electrolyte imbalances, as well as the "laxative habit," that is, dependence on a laxative to have a bowel movement. Some of these products contain tartrazine (a yellow food dye), which may cause allergic-type reactions (including bronchial asthma) in susceptible individuals. Obstruction of the esophagus, stomach, small intestine, and colon has occurred when bulk-forming laxatives are administered without adequate fluid intake or in patients with intestinal stenosis.

 LIFESPAN ALERT – **Chronic Care**
The very young, the elderly, and debilitated patients are at greatest risk for aspiration of mineral oil into the lungs when it is taken orally for constipation. Aspiration of mineral oil can lead to a lipid pneumonitis.

Contraindications and Precautions

Laxatives are contraindicated in patients with known hypersensitivity and those with persistent abdominal pain, nausea, or vomiting of unknown cause or signs of acute appendicitis, fecal impaction, intestinal obstruction, or acute hepatitis. These drugs are used only as directed because excessive or prolonged use may cause physical dependence on them for normal bowel movements.

Magnesium is used cautiously in patients with any degree of renal impairment. Laxatives are used cautiously in patients with rectal bleeding, in pregnant women, and during lactation. The following laxatives are pregnancy category C drugs: cascara sagrada, docusate, glycerin, phenolphthalein, magnesium, and senna. These drugs are used during pregnancy only when the benefits clearly outweigh the risks to the fetus.

Interactions

- Mineral oil may impair the GI absorption of fat-soluble vitamins (A, D, E, and K).
- Laxatives may reduce absorption of other drugs present in the GI tract, by combining with them chemically or hastening their passage through the intestinal tract.

- When surfactants are administered with mineral oil, they may increase mineral oil absorption.
- Milk, antacids, histamine H$_2$ antagonists, and proton pump inhibitors should not be administered 1 to 2 hours before bisacodyl tablets because the enteric coating may dissolve early (before reaching the intestinal tract), resulting in gastric lining irritation or dyspepsia and decreasing the laxative effect of the drug.

[handwritten margin note: Dalcolant / Doplat]

NURSING PROCESS

PATIENT RECEIVING A DRUG FOR A LOWER GASTROINTESTINAL DISORDER

ASSESSMENT

Preadministration Assessment

During the preadministration assessment, the nurse reviews the patient's chart for the medical diagnosis and reason for administration of the prescribed drug. The nurse questions the patient regarding the type and intensity of symptoms (e.g., pain, discomfort, diarrhea, or constipation) to provide a baseline for evaluation of the effectiveness of drug therapy. The nurse listens to bowel sounds and palpates the abdomen, monitoring the patient for signs of guarding or discomfort. Loose stool may indicate diarrhea; however, hypoactive bowel sounds in severe cases of **obstipation** (liquid stool leaked around the fecal mass, presenting as loose stool) are evidence that the patient is constipated, which would indicate very different drug therapy.

Ongoing Assessment

The nurse assesses the patient receiving one of these drugs for relief of symptoms (e.g., diarrhea, pain, or constipation). The primary health care provider is notified if the drug fails to relieve symptoms. The nurse monitors vital signs daily or more frequently if the patient has severe diarrhea or another condition that may warrant more frequent observation. The nurse observes the patient for adverse drug reactions associated with the specific GI drug being administered and reports any adverse reactions to the primary health care provider before the next dose is due. The nurse evaluates the effectiveness of drug therapy by a daily comparison of symptoms with those experienced before the initiation of therapy. In some instances, frequent evaluation of the patient's response to therapy may be necessary.

NURSING DIAGNOSES

A drug-specific nursing diagnosis is the following:

❑ **Risk for Imbalance Fluid Volume** related to diarrhea

Nursing diagnoses related to drug administration are discussed in Chapter 4.

PLANNING

The expected outcomes for the patient depend on the reason for administration of the drug, but may include an optimal response to drug therapy, support of patient needs related to the management of adverse reactions, and an understanding of and compliance with the prescribed therapeutic regimen.

IMPLEMENTATION

Promoting an Optimal Response to Therapy

Ways in which the nurse can help promote an optimal response to therapy when administering lower GI drugs are listed in the following sections.

ANTIDIARRHEALS. These drugs may be ordered to be given after each loose bowel movement. The nurse inspects each bowel movement before making a decision to administer the drug.

LAXATIVES. The nurse gives bulk-producing or stool-softening laxatives with a full glass of water or juice. The administration of a bulk-producing laxative is followed by an additional full glass of water. Mineral oil preferably is given to the patient with an empty stomach in the evening. Immediately before administration, the nurse thoroughly mixes and stirs laxatives that are in powder, flake, or granule form. If the laxative has an unpleasant or salty taste, the nurse explains this to the patient. The taste of some of these preparations may be disguised by chilling, adding to juice, or pouring over cracked ice.

> **⚠ NURSING ALERT**
>
> Because activated charcoal can absorb other drugs in the GI tract, when used as an antiflatulent it should not be taken 2 hours before or 1 hour after the administration of other drugs.

Monitoring and Managing Patient Needs

RISK FOR IMBALANCED FLUID VOLUME. The nurse notifies the primary health care provider if the patient experiences an elevation in body temperature, severe abdominal pain, or abdominal rigidity or distention because this may indicate a complication of the disorder, such as infection or intestinal perforation. If diarrhea is severe, additional treatment measures, such as intravenous fluids and electrolyte replacement, may be necessary.

If diarrhea is chronic, the nurse encourages the patient to drink extra fluids. Weak tea, water, bouillon, or a commercial electrolyte preparation may be used.

The nurse closely monitors fluid intake and output. In some instances, the primary health care provider may prescribe an oral electrolyte supplement to replace electrolytes lost by frequent loose stools. Patients with fluid volume losses taking drugs that cause drowsiness or dizziness are at greater risk for injury. The patient may require assistance with ambulatory activities. For perianal irritation caused by loose stools, the nurse instructs the patient or caregiver to cleanse the area with mild soap and water after each bowel movement, dry the area with a soft cloth, and apply an emollient, such as petrolatum.

When a laxative is administered, the nurse records the bowel movement results on the patient's chart. If excessive bowel movements or severe, prolonged diarrhea occur, or if the laxative is ineffective, the nurse notifies the primary health care provider. If a laxative is ordered for constipation, the nurse encourages a liberal fluid intake and an increase in foods high in fiber to prevent a repeat of this problem.

Educating the Patient and Family

When a lower GI drug must be taken for a long time, there is a possibility that the patient may begin to skip doses or stop taking the drug. The nurse encourages patients to take the prescribed drug as directed by the primary health care provider and emphasizes the importance of not omitting doses or stopping the therapy unless advised to do so by the primary health care provider. The nurse includes the following information in a patient and family teaching plan:

ANTIDIARRHEALS.

- Do not exceed the recommended dosage.
- Observe caution when driving or performing other hazardous tasks because the drug may cause drowsiness.
- Avoid the use of alcohol or other central nervous system (CNS) depressants (e.g., tranquilizers, sleeping pills) and other nonprescription drugs unless use has been approved by the primary health care provider.
- Notify the primary health care provider if diarrhea persists or becomes more severe.

ANTIFLATULENTS.

- Take simethicone after each meal and at bedtime. Thoroughly chew tablets because complete particle dispersion enhances antiflatulent action.
- Notify the health care provider if symptoms are not relieved within several days.

LAXATIVES.

- Avoid long-term use of these products unless use of the product has been recommended by the primary health care provider. Long-term use may result in the "laxative habit," which is dependence on a laxative to have a normal bowel movement. Constipation may also occur with overuse of these drugs. Read and follow the directions on the label.
- Do not use these products in the presence of abdominal pain, nausea, or vomiting.
- Notify the primary health care provider if constipation is not relieved or if rectal bleeding or other symptoms occur.
- To avoid constipation, drink plenty of fluids, get exercise, and eat foods high in bulk or roughage.
- Cascara sagrada or senna—Pink-red, red-violet, red-brown, yellow-brown, or black discoloration of urine may occur.

EVALUATION

- Therapeutic drug effect is achieved, and bowel movements are appropriate for the patient's normal routine.

- Adverse reactions are identified, reported to the primary health care provider, and managed successfully through appropriate nursing interventions.
  - ☑ Patient maintains an adequate fluid volume.
- Patient and family demonstrate an understanding of the drug regimen.

THINK CRITICALLY: PHARMACOLOGY IN PRACTICE

1. Ms. Chase, aged 36 years, tells you that she has been using various laxatives for constipation. She states that a laxative did help, but now she is more constipated than she was before she began taking a laxative. Discuss what advice or suggestions you would give this patient.

● Test Your Knowledge

1. Which of the following is the best description of the cause of Crohn's disease?

  A. Somatic response to psychological stress
  B. Infection due to bacteria or parasites
  C. Inflammatory response in the colon
  D. Precancerous stage in the bowel

2. The patient asks how stool softeners relieve constipation. Which of the following would be the best response by the nurse? Stool softeners relieve constipation by _____.

  A. stimulating the walls of the intestine
  B. promoting the retention of sodium in the fecal mass
  C. promoting water retention in the fecal mass
  D. lubricating the intestinal walls

3. The nurse administers antidiarrheal drugs _____.

  A. after each loose bowel movement
  B. hourly until diarrhea ceases
  C. with food
  D. twice a day, in the morning and at bedtime

4. The pregnancy category for the antiflatulent drug simethicone is _____.

  A. pregnancy category A
  B. pregnancy category C
  C. pregnancy category X
  D. pregnancy category unknown

● Prepare for the NCLEX

1. When recording the administration of diphenoxylate for multiple loose stools:

  A. document the daily number of drugs given
  B. record all stools once each shift
  C. indicate all stools on the Medication Administration Record (MAR) next to the drug
  D. document each dose on the MAR

● Calculate Medication Dosages

1. A patient is to drink 4 liters of polyethylene glycol-electrolyte solution (GoLYTELY) the night before an outpatient colonoscopy. If the directions state "drink 240 mL every 10 minutes," the nurse tells the patient the solution must be completely drunk in _____ hours.

2. Balsalazide (Colazal) 2250 mg orally TID is prescribed. If the drug comes in 750-mg capsules, the nurse administers _____ capsules with each dose.

To check your answers, see Appendix E.

the**Point** *For more NCLEX questions, log onto LWW's thePoint to access more than a thousand questions.*

Drugs That Affect the Endocrine System

The endocrine system consists of a group of glands throughout the body. The work of the endocrine system is to provide hormones (chemicals that assist in function) to various organs in the body. Hormones are produced and circulated through the blood to target receptors on certain cells in specific organs to assist in function. Glands that make up the endocrine system and are discussed in this unit include the pituitary, thyroid, pancreas, adrenal glands, and sex organs.

The pituitary gland sits at the base of the brain and helps with the function of many different organs in the body. Its hormones are secreted and sent to a variety of organs to promote and regulate growth and maturation, fluid and electrolyte balance, and metabolism. These hormones and the drugs that affect them are covered in Chapter 44. The adrenal glands are crucial in the secretion of corticosteroids, which are also covered in this chapter.

Located in the lower anterior portion of the neck, the thyroid's purpose is to help control metabolism. Chapter 45 covers the function of the thyroid and its hormones as well as drugs used to supplement function of the thyroid gland.

The pancreas is part of the gastrointestinal (GI) system. This organ provides enzymes to assist in the digestion of food and provides the body with insulin to help cells use the glucose from food sources. As recently as 2008, the American Diabetes Association estimated that 7.8% (or about 23.6 million people) of the United States population has diabetes. The most up-to-date statistics can be retrieved from http://www.diabetes.org/about-diabetes.jsp. Diabetes mellitus is a chronic condition characterized by problems with the body's production or use of insulin. Chapter 43 discusses both insulin and the oral antidiabetic drugs used in treating diabetes mellitus.

Hormones play a major role in the development of the reproductive system as people go through puberty. The ovaries in the female and the testes in the male produce hormones that aid in the development of secondary sexual characteristics such as hair, voice, and musculature. Reproduction is controlled by the secretion of hormones. Chapters 46 and 47 describe the function of these hormones and the drugs used to promote optimal reproductive health. Hormones that affect the development of sexual characteristics also can alter the growth of cancer cells; these hormones are covered in Chapter 46.

PHARMACOLOGY IN PRACTICE

When Mrs. Moore, aged 85 years, was hospitalized for chest pain, it was discovered that she had not been seen by a health care provider in more than 5 years. Her chest pain was relieved her medical condition was stabilized, and she was sent home with an appointment to come to the clinic for a complete physical examination. During the clinic visit, Mrs. Moore was found to be in relatively good physical condition considering her age. Her blood chemistries showed an elevation in her blood glucose level (153 mg/dL). The HbA_{1c} reading was 9%, and she was instructed to use a blood glucometer to check her own blood daily and call the nurse after one week with the readings.

After reading the chapters in this unit, you will better understand the meaning of these laboratory values and be asked to determine both patient interventions and instruction based upon the information you learn in this unit.

43

Antidiabetic Drugs

LEARNING OBJECTIVES

On completion of this chapter, the student will:

1. Describe the two types of diabetes mellitus.
2. Discuss the types, uses, general drug actions, adverse reactions, contraindications, precautions, and interactions of the antidiabetic drugs.
3. Discuss important preadministration and ongoing assessment activities the nurse should perform with the patient taking an antidiabetic drug.
4. List nursing diagnoses particular to a patient taking an antidiabetic drug.
5. Discuss ways to promote an optimal response to therapy, how to manage common adverse reactions, and important points to keep in mind when educating patients about the use of antidiabetic drugs.

Insulin, a hormone produced by the pancreas, acts to maintain blood glucose levels within normal limits (60 to 120 mg/dL). This is accomplished by the release of small amounts of insulin into the bloodstream throughout the day in response to changes in blood glucose levels. Insulin is essential for the utilization of glucose in cellular metabolism and for the proper metabolism of protein and fat.

Diabetes mellitus is a complicated, chronic disorder characterized by either insufficient insulin production by the beta (β) cells of the pancreas or by cellular resistance to insulin. Insulin insufficiency results in elevated blood glucose levels, or **hyperglycemia**. As a result of the disease, individuals with diabetes are at greater risk for a number of disorders, including myocardial infarction, cerebrovascular accident (stroke), blindness, kidney disease, and lower limb amputations.

Insulin and oral antidiabetic drugs, along with diet and exercise, are the cornerstones of treatment for diabetes mellitus. They are used to prevent episodes of **hypoglycemia** and normalize carbohydrate metabolism.

There are two major types of diabetes mellitus:

- Type 1—formerly known as insulin-dependent diabetes mellitus or IDDM
- Type 2—formerly known as non–insulin-dependent diabetes mellitus or NIDDM

Those with type 1 diabetes mellitus produce insulin in insufficient amounts and therefore must have insulin supplementation to survive. Type 1 diabetes usually has a rapid onset, occurs before age 20 years, produces more severe symptoms than type 2 diabetes, and is more difficult to control. Major symptoms of type 1 diabetes include hyperglycemia, **polydipsia** (increased thirst), **polyphagia** (increased appetite), **polyuria** (increased urination), and weight loss. Control of type 1 diabetes is particularly difficult because of the lack of insulin production by the pancreas. Treatment requires a strict regimen that typically includes a carefully calculated diet, planned physical activity, home glucose testing several times a day, and multiple daily insulin injections.

Type 2 diabetes mellitus affects about 90% to 95% of individuals with diabetes. Those with type 2 diabetes are affected either by decreased production of insulin by the beta β cells of the pancreas or decreased sensitivity of the cells to insulin, making the cells insulin resistant. Although type 2 diabetes mellitus may occur at any age, the disorder occurs most often after age 40 years. The onset of type 2 diabetes is usually insidious. Symptoms are less severe than in type 1 diabetes mellitus, and because it tends to be more stable, type 2 diabetes is easier to control than type 1. Risk factors for type 2 diabetes include:

- Obesity
- Older age
- Family history of diabetes
- History of gestational diabetes (diabetes that develops during pregnancy but disappears when pregnancy is over)
- Impaired glucose tolerance
- Minimal or no physical activity
- Race/ethnicity (African Americans, Hispanic/Latino Americans, Native Americans, and some Asian Americans)

Obesity is thought to contribute to type 2 diabetes by placing additional stress on the pancreas, which makes it less able to respond and produce adequate insulin to meet the body's metabolic needs.

In many individuals with type 2 diabetes, the disorder can be controlled with diet, exercise, and oral antidiabetic drugs. However, about 40% of those with type 2 diabetes respond poorly to the oral antidiabetic drugs and require insulin to control the diabetes.

• INSULIN

Insulin is a hormone manufactured by the β cells of the pancreas. It is the principal hormone required for the proper use of glucose (carbohydrate) by the body. Insulin also controls the storage and utilization of amino acids and fatty acids. Insulin lowers blood glucose levels by inhibiting glucose production by the liver.

Pharmaceutical human insulin is derived from a biosynthetic process using strains of *Escherichia coli* (recombinant DNA or rDNA). Human insulin appears to cause fewer allergic reactions than does insulin obtained from animal sources. Insulin analogs, insulin lispro, and insulin aspart are newer forms of human insulin made using recombinant DNA technology and are structurally similar to human insulin.

Insulin that is biologically similar to human insulin is also available as purified extracts from beef and pork pancreas. However, these animal-source insulins are used less frequently today than in the past. They have been replaced by synthetic insulins, such as human insulin or insulin analogs.

Actions

Insulin appears to activate a process that helps glucose molecules enter the cells of striated muscle and adipose tissue. Figure 43.1 depicts normal glucose metabolism. Insulin also stimulates the synthesis of glycogen by the liver. In addition, insulin promotes protein synthesis and helps the body store fat by preventing its breakdown for energy.

Onset, Peak, and Duration of Action

Onset, peak, and duration are three clinically important properties of insulin:

- Onset—when insulin first begins to act in the body
- Peak—when the insulin is exerting maximum action
- Duration—the length of time the insulin remains in effect

To meet the needs of those with diabetes mellitus, various insulin preparations have been developed to delay the onset and prolong the duration of action of insulin. When insulin is combined with protamine (a protein), its absorption from the injection site is slowed and its duration of action is prolonged. The addition of zinc also modifies the onset and duration of action of insulin. Insulin preparations are classified as rapid acting, intermediate acting, or long acting. See the Summary Drug Table: Insulin Preparations for information concerning the onset, peak, and duration of various insulins.

Pancreas

● **Insulin**

▲ **Glucose**

Insulin receptor

Cell membrane

Figure 43.1 Normal glucose metabolism. Once insulin binds with receptors on the cell membrane, glucose can move into the cell, promoting cellular metabolism and energy production.

Know

Summary Drug Table INSULIN PREPARATIONS

Types of Insulin	Trade Name	Activity		
		Onset	Peak	Duration
Rapid-Acting Insulins				
insulin injection (regular)	Humulin R, Iletin II Regular, Novolin R, Novolin R PenFill, Novolin R Prefilled, Velosulin BR	30–60 min	2–4 hr	8–2 hr
insulin lispro (insulin analog)	Humalog, Humalog Mix 75/25	5–10 min	30 min–1.5 hr	2–5 hr	*clear*
insulin aspart (insulin analog)	NovoLog, NovoLog Mix 70/30	5–10 min	1–3 hr	3–5 hr
insulin glulisine	Apidra	10–20 min	30 min–1.5 hr	1–2.5 hr
Intermediate-Acting Insulins				
isophane insulin suspension (NPH)	Humulin N, Novolin N, Novolin N PenFill, Novolin N Prefilled, NPH Iletin II	1.5 hr	4–12 hr *6–8*	24 hr	*Cloudy*
insulin zinc suspension (Lente)	Humulin L, Lente Iletin II	1–2.5 hr	7–15 hr	24 hr
Long-Acting Insulins				
insulin glargine	Lantus	1 hr	5 hr	24 hr	*never mix*
extended insulin zinc suspension (Ultralente)	Humulin U	4–8 hr	10–30 hr	20–36 hr
insulin detemir	Levemir	In 2 hr	3–14 hr	24 hr
Mixed Insulins				
isophane insulin suspension and insulin injections (NPH)	Humulin 70/30, Novolin 70/30, Novolin 70/30 PenFill, Novolin 70/30 Prefilled	30–60 min, then 1–2 hr	2–4 hr, then 6–12 hr	6–8 hr, then 18–24 hr	*Cloudy*
isophane insulin suspension and insulin injection (Reg)	Humulin 50/50	30–60 min, then 1–2 hr	2–4 h, then 6–12 hr	6–8 h, then 18–24 hr
Inhaled Insulin				
insulin human	Exubera				*Btwn regular rapid*

Uses

Insulin is used to:

- Control type 1 diabetes
- Control type 2 diabetes when uncontrolled by diet, exercise, or weight reduction
- Treat severe **diabetic ketoacidosis** (DKA) or diabetic coma
- Treat hypokalemia in combination with glucose

Adverse Reactions

The two major adverse reactions seen with insulin administration are *hypoglycemia* (low blood glucose, or sugar, level) and *hyperglycemia* (elevated blood glucose, or sugar, level). The symptoms of hypoglycemia and hyperglycemia are listed in Table 43.1.

Hypoglycemia may occur when there is too much insulin in the bloodstream in relation to the available glucose (hyperinsulinism). Hypoglycemia may occur when:

- The patient eats too little food.
- The insulin dose is incorrectly measured and is greater than that prescribed.
- The patient has drastically increased demands (activity or illness).

Hyperglycemia may occur if there is too little insulin in the bloodstream in relation to the available glucose (hypoinsulinism). Hyperglycemia may occur when:

- The patient eats too much food.
- Too little or no insulin is given.
- The patient experiences emotional stress, infection, surgery, pregnancy, or an acute illness.

Table 43.1 Hypoglycemia Versus Hyperglycemia

Symptoms	Hypoglycemia (Insulin Reaction)	Hyperglycemia (Diabetic Coma, Ketoacidosis)
Onset	Sudden	Gradual (hours or days)
Blood glucose level	Less than 60 mg/dL	More than 200 mg/dL
Central nervous system	Fatigue, weakness, nervousness, agitation, confusion, headache, diplopia, convulsions, dizziness, unconsciousness	Drowsiness, dim vision
Respirations	Normal to rapid, shallow	Deep, rapid (air hunger)
Gastrointestinal	Hunger, nausea	Thirst, nausea, vomiting, abdominal pain, loss of appetite
Skin	Pale, moist, cool, diaphoretic	Dry, flushed, warm
Pulse	Normal or uncharacteristic	Rapid, weak
Miscellaneous	Numbness, tingling of the lips or tongue	Acetone breath, excessive urination

Another potential adverse reaction may be an allergic reaction to the animal (pig or cow) from which the insulin is obtained or to the protein or zinc added to insulin. To minimize the possibility of an allergic reaction, some health care providers prescribe human insulin or purified insulin. However, on rare occasions, some individuals become allergic to the human and purified insulins.

An individual can also become insulin resistant because antibodies develop against insulin. These patients have impaired receptor function and become so unresponsive to

DISPLAY 43.1 Drugs That Alter Insulin Effectiveness

Selected Drugs That Decrease the Effect (More Insulin May Be Required)
acetazolamide
albuterol
antipsychotics
asparaginase
calcitonin
contraceptives, oral
corticosteroids
danazol
dextrothyroxine
diazoxide
diltiazem
diuretics
dobutamine
epinephrine
estrogens
ethacrynic acid
glucagon
human immunodeficiency virus (HIV) antivirals
isoniazid
lithium
morphine sulfate
niacin
phenothiazines
phenytoin
progestogens
protease inhibitors
somatropin
terbutaline

thiazide diuretics
thyroid hormones

Drugs That Increase the Effect (Less Insulin May Be Required)
angiotensin-converting enzyme (ACE) inhibitors
alcohol
anabolic steroids
antidiabetic drugs, oral
β blocking drugs
calcium
clofibrate
clonidine
disopyramide
fluoxetine
fibrates
guanethidine
lithium
MAOIs
mebendazole
pentamidine
pentoxifylline
phenylbutazone
pyridoxine
salicylates
somatostatin analog
sulfinpyrazone
sulfonamides
tetracycline

insulin that the dose requirement may be in excess of 500 Units/day, rather than the usual 40 to 60 Units/day. High-potency insulin in a concentrated form (U500) is used for patients requiring more than 200 Units/day.

Contraindications

Specific insulin products are contraindicated in patients with hypersensitivity to any ingredient of the product (e.g., beef or pork) and when the patient is hypoglycemic.

Precautions

Insulin is used cautiously in patients with renal or hepatic impairment and during pregnancy and lactation. The insulins are grouped in pregnancy category B, except for insulin glargine and insulin aspart, which are in pregnancy category C. Insulin appears to inhibit milk production in lactating women and could interfere with breastfeeding. Lactating women may require adjustment in insulin dose and diet.

 LIFESPAN ALERT – Pregnancy

Pregnancy makes diabetes more difficult to manage. Insulin requirements usually decrease in the first trimester, increase during the second and third trimester, and decrease rapidly after delivery. The patient with diabetes or a history of gestational diabetes must be encouraged to maintain good metabolic control before conception and throughout pregnancy. Frequent monitoring is necessary.

Interactions

When certain drugs are administered with insulin, a resultant decrease or increase in hypoglycemic effect can occur. Display 43.1 identifies selected drugs that decrease and increase the hypoglycemic effect of insulin.

Patients may not volunteer information regarding their use of alternative or complementary remedies. The nurse should always inquire about use of herbal products. Although lab testing is not conclusive, medical reports indicate a possible interaction with eucalyptus products, causing decreased blood sugar.

NURSING PROCESS
PATIENT RECEIVING INSULIN

ASSESSMENT

Preadministration Assessment
If the patient has recently been diagnosed with diabetes mellitus and has not received insulin, or if the patient is known to have diabetes, the initial physical assessment before administering the first dose of insulin includes taking the blood pressure and pulse and respiratory rates and weighing the patient. The nurse makes a general assessment of the skin, mucous membranes, and extremities, with special attention given to any sores or cuts that appear to be infected or healing poorly, as well as any ulcerations or other skin or mucous membrane

changes. The nurse obtains the following information and includes it in the patient's chart:

- Dietary habits
- Family history of diabetes (if any)
- Type and duration of symptoms experienced

The nurse reviews the patient's chart for recent laboratory and diagnostic tests. If the patient has diabetes and has been receiving insulin, the nurse includes the type and dosage of insulin used, the type of diabetic diet, and the average results of glucose testing in the patient's chart. The nurse evaluates the patient's past compliance with the prescribed therapeutic regimen, such as diet, weight control, and periodic evaluation by a health care provider.

Ongoing Assessment
The number and amount of daily insulin doses, times of administration, and diet and exercise requirements require continual assessment. Dosage adjustments may be necessary when changing types of insulin, particularly when changing from the single-peak to the more pure Humulin insulins.

The nurse must assess the patient for signs and symptoms of hypoglycemia and hyperglycemia (see Table 43.1) throughout insulin therapy. The patient is particularly prone to hypoglycemic reactions at the time of peak insulin action (see the Summary Drug Table: Insulin Preparations) or when he or she has not eaten for some time or has skipped a meal. In acute care settings, frequent blood glucose monitoring is routinely done to help detect abnormalities of blood glucose. Testing usually occurs before meals and at bedtime (see the Patient Teaching for Improved Patient Outcomes: Obtaining a Blood Glucose Reading Using a Glucometer).

 NURSING ALERT

The nurse must closely observe the patient after administering any insulin, but particularly U500 insulin, because secondary hypoglycemic reactions may occur as long as 24 hours after administration.

Blood glucose levels are monitored frequently in patients with diabetes. Patients in the acute care setting are monitored closely for hyperglycemia. Insulin needs increase in times of stress or illness. The health care provider may order regular insulin as a supplement to the drug regimen to "cover" any episodes of hyperglycemia. For example, blood glucose levels are monitored every 6 hours or before meals and at bedtime, with insulin prescribed to cover any hyperglycemia detected. This coverage is sometimes referred to by the health care providers in a teaching session as a sliding scale, or insulin coverage. The nurse administers supplemental insulin based on blood glucose readings and the amount of insulin prescribed by the primary health care provider in the sliding scale. The nurse must notify the primary health care provider if the blood glucose level is greater than 400 mg/dL.

The primary health care provider may prescribe use of a sliding scale at various times, such as every 4 hours, every 6 hours, or at specified times (e.g., 7 AM, 11 AM, 4 PM, and 11 PM), depending on the patient's individual needs. Consult your institutional policy; these scales can vary.

NURSING DIAGNOSES

Drug-specific nursing diagnoses include the following:

❏ **Acute Confusion** related to hypoglycemia effects on mentation
❏ **Deficient Fluid Volume** related to fluid loss during DKA
❏ **Anxiety** related to fear of diagnosis, giving own injections, dietary restrictions, other factors (specify)

Nursing diagnoses related to drug administration are discussed in Chapter 4.

PLANNING

The expected outcomes of the patient may include an optimal response to therapy, patient needs related to the management of adverse reactions, a reduction in anxiety and fear, improved ability to cope with the diagnosis, and an understanding of and compliance with the prescribed therapeutic regimen.

IMPLEMENTATION

Nursing management of a patient with diabetes requires diligent, skillful, and comprehensive nursing care.

Promoting an Optimal Response to Therapy

There is no standard dose of insulin, as there is for most other drugs. Insulin dosage is highly individualized. Sometimes the health care provider finds that the patient achieves best control with one injection of insulin per day; sometimes the patient requires two or more injections per day. In addition, two different types of insulin may be combined, such as a rapid-acting and a long-acting preparation. The number of insulin injections, dosage, times of administration, and type of insulin are determined by the health care provider after careful evaluation of the patient's metabolic needs and response to therapy. The dosage prescribed for the patient may require changes until the dosage is found that best meets the patient's needs.

NURSING ALERT

Insulin requirements may change when the patient experiences any form of stress and with any illness, particularly illnesses resulting in nausea and vomiting.

Insulin is ordered by the generic name (e.g., insulin zinc suspension, extended) or the trade (brand) name (e.g., Humulin U; see the Summary Drug Table: Insulin Preparations). One brand of insulin must never be substituted for another unless the substitution is approved by the primary health care provider, because some patients may be sensitive to changes in brands of insulin. In addition, it is important never to substitute one type of insulin for another. For example, do not use insulin zinc suspension instead of the prescribed protamine zinc insulin.

When the nurse or patient is administering insulin, care must be taken to use the correct insulin. Names and packaging are similar and can easily be confused. The nurse carefully reads all drug labels before preparing any insulin preparation. For example, Humalog (insulin lispro) and Humulin R (regular human insulin) are easily confused because of the similar names.

Insulin cannot be administered orally, because it is a protein and readily destroyed in the GI tract. Insulin must be administered by the parenteral route, usually the subcutaneous (subcut) route. Aspiration for blood return does not need to be done when given subcutaneously. Regular insulin is the only insulin preparation given intravenously (IV). Regular insulin is given 30 to 60 minutes before a meal to achieve optimal results.

Insulin aspart is given immediately before a meal (within 5 to 10 minutes of beginning a meal). Insulin lispro is given 15 minutes before a meal or immediately after a meal. Insulin aspart and lispro make insulin administration more convenient for many patients who find taking a drug 30 to 60 minutes before meals bothersome. In addition, insulin lispro (Humalog) appears to lower the blood glucose level 1 to 2 hours after meals better than does regular human insulin, because it more closely mimics the body's natural insulin. It also lowers the risk of low blood glucose reactions from midnight to 6 AM in patients with type 1 diabetes. The longer-acting insulins are given before breakfast or at bedtime (depending on the primary health care provider's instructions). Many patients are maintained on a single dose of intermediate-acting insulin administered subcut in the morning.

Insulin glargine is given subcut once daily at bedtime. This type of insulin is used in treating adults and children with type 1 diabetes mellitus and in adults with type 2 diabetes who need long-acting insulin for the control of hyperglycemia.

Insulin is available in concentrations of U100 and U500. The nurse must read the label of the insulin bottle carefully for the name, source of insulin (e.g., human, beef, pork, beef *and* pork, purified beef), and the number of units per milliliter. The dose of insulin is measured in units. U100 insulin has 100 units in each milliliter; U500 has 500 units in each milliliter. Most people with diabetes use the U100 concentration. Patients who are resistant to insulin and require large insulin doses use the U500 concentration.

MIXING INSULINS. If the patient is to receive regular insulin and NPH (isophane insulin suspension) insulin, or regular and Lente (insulin zinc suspension) insulin, the nurse must clarify with the primary health care provider whether two separate injections are to be given or if the insulins may be mixed in the same syringe. If the two insulins are to be given in the same syringe, the short-acting insulin (regular or lispro) is drawn into the syringe first (Fig. 43.2). Even small amounts of

Figure 43.2 Drawing up two types of insulin. (**A**) After cleansing tops of both the Humulin R (regular) insulin and Humulin N (intermediate-acting insulin), with the container upright, the nurse injects air into the Humulin N insulin equal to the prescribed dosage of Humulin N. The nurse removes the needle without touching any fluid, then injects the amount of air equal to the prescribed dosage of the regular insulin and withdraws the prescribed dosage of regular insulin into the syringe. (**B**) After removing any air bubbles and determining what the total combined volume of the two insulins would measure, the nurse inverts the vial with the NPH insulin and carefully withdraws the correct volume of medication. *Note*: The nurse should have a second nurse independently check medication and dosage again before administering the insulin.

intermediate- or long-acting insulin, if mixed with the short-acting insulin, can bind with the short-acting insulin and delay its onset.

NURSING ALERT

Regular insulin is clear, whereas intermediate-and long-acting insulins are cloudy. The clear insulin should be drawn up first. When insulin lispro is mixed with a longer-acting insulin, the insulin lispro is drawn up first.

An unexpected response may be obtained when changing from mixed injections to separate injections or vice versa. If the patient had been using insulin mixtures before admission, the nurse asks whether the insulins were given separately or together.

Several types of premixed insulins are available. These insulins combine regular insulin with the longer-acting NPH insulin. The mixtures are available in ratios of 70/30 and 50/50 of NPH to regular. Although these premixed insulins are helpful for patients who have difficulty drawing up their insulin or seeing the markings on the syringe, they prohibit individualizing the dosage. For patients who have difficulty controlling their diabetes, these premixed insulins may not be effective.

NURSING ALERT

Do not mix or dilute insulin glargine with any other insulin or solution, because glucose control will be lost and the insulin will not be effective.

PREPARING INSULIN FOR ADMINISTRATION. The nurse always checks the expiration date printed on the label of the insulin bottle before withdrawing the insulin. An insulin syringe that matches the concentration of insulin to be given is always used. For example, a syringe labeled as

U100 is used only with insulin labeled U100. U500 insulin is given only by the subcut or intramuscular (IM) route, and may be administered using a tuberculin syringe if necessary.

When insulin is in a suspension (this can be seen when looking at a vial that has been untouched for about 1 hour), the nurse gently rotates the vial between the palms of the hands and tilts it gently end-to-end immediately before withdrawing the insulin. This ensures even distribution of the suspended particles. Care is taken not to shake the insulin vigorously.

The nurse carefully checks the primary health care provider's order for the type and dosage of insulin immediately before withdrawing the insulin from the vial. All air bubbles must be eliminated from the syringe barrel and hub of the needle before withdrawing the syringe from the insulin vial.

NURSING ALERT

Accuracy is of the utmost importance when measuring any insulin preparation because of the potential danger of administering an incorrect dosage. If possible, the nurse should check and consult with another nurse for accuracy of the insulin dosage by comparing the insulin container, the syringe, and the primary health care provider's order before administration.

When regular insulin and another insulin are mixed in the same syringe, the nurse must administer the insulin within 5 minutes of withdrawing the two insulins from the two vials.

ROTATING INJECTION SITES. Insulin may be injected into the arms, thighs, abdomen, or buttocks (see Patient Teaching for Improved Patient Outcomes: Rotating Insulin Injection Sites). Sites of insulin injection are rotated to pre-

Antidiabetic Drugs

vent **lipodystrophy** (atrophy of subcutaneous fat), a problem that can interfere with the absorption of insulin from the injection site. Lipodystrophy appears as a slight dimpling or pitting of the subcutaneous fat. This problem is less likely with the human insulins as compared to the animal insulin products.

Because absorption rates vary at the different sites, with the abdomen having the most rapid rate of absorption, followed by the upper arm, thigh, and buttocks, some health care providers recommend rotating the injection sites within one specific area, rather than rotating areas. For example, all available sites within the abdomen would be used before moving to the thigh.

The nurse carefully plans the injection site rotation pattern and writes this plan in the patient's chart. Before each dose of insulin is given, the nurse checks the patient's chart for the site of the previous injection and uses the next site (according to the rotation plan) for injection. After giving the injection, the nurse records the site used. Every time insulin is given, previous injection sites are inspected for inflammation, which may indicate a localized allergic reaction. The nurse notes any other inflammation or skin reactions. The nurse reports localized allergic reactions, signs of inflammation, or other skin changes to the primary health care provider as soon as possible, because a different type of insulin may be necessary.

METHODS OF ADMINISTERING INSULIN. Several methods can be used to administer insulin. The most common method is the use of a needle and syringe. Use of microfine needles has reduced the discomfort associated with an injection. Another method is the jet injection system, which uses pressure to deliver a fine stream of insulin below the skin. Another method uses a disposable needle and special syringe. The syringe has a cartridge that is prefilled with a specific type of insulin (e.g., regular human insulin, NPH insulin, or a mixture of isophane and regular insulin). The desired units are selected by turning a dial and the locking ring.

Another method of insulin delivery is the insulin pump. This system attempts to mimic the body's normal pancreatic function, uses only regular insulin, is battery powered, and requires insertion of a needle into subcutaneous tissue. The needle is changed every 1 to 3 days. The amount of insulin injected can be adjusted according to blood glucose levels, which are monitored four to eight times per day.

The insulin dosage pattern that most closely follows normal insulin production is a multiple-dose plan sometimes called *intensive insulin therapy*. In this regimen, a single dose of intermediate- or long-acting insulin is taken in the morning or at bedtime. Small doses of regular insulin are taken before meals based on the patient's blood glucose levels. This allows for greater flexibility in the patient's lifestyle, but can also be an inconvenience to the patient (e.g., the need always to carry supplies, the lack of privacy, inconvenient schedules).

Inhaled insulin delivery is designed for administration of rapid-onset and short-duration insulins. Typically the insulin is inhaled 10 minutes before mealtime. This drug may be used in addition to oral agents or insulin injection. Inhaled insulin can cause cough, dry mouth, sore throat, chest discomfort, or shortness of breath. This method is not meant to be used by those with breathing difficulties, e.g., disease or smoking.

BLOOD AND URINE TESTING. Blood glucose levels are monitored often in the patient with diabetes. The primary health care provider may order blood glucose levels to be tested before meals, after meals, and at bedtime. Less frequent monitoring may be performed if the patient's glucose levels are well controlled. The **glucometer** is a device used by the patient with diabetes or the nursing personnel to monitor blood glucose levels. Nursing or laboratory personnel are responsible for obtaining blood glucose levels during hospitalization, but the patient must be taught to monitor blood glucose levels after discharge from the acute care setting (see Patient Teaching for Improved Patient Outcomes: Obtaining a Blood Glucose Reading Using a Glucometer).

Urine testing was widely used to monitor glucose levels in the past, but this method has largely been replaced with blood glucose monitoring. Urine testing can play a role in identifying ketone excretion in patients prone to ketoacidosis. If urine testing is done, it is usually recommended that the nurse use the second voided specimen (i.e., fresh urine collected 30 minutes after the initial voiding) to check glucose or acetone levels, rather than the first specimen obtained.

The **glycosylated hemoglobin** (HbA_{1c}) test is a blood test used to monitor the patient's average blood glucose level throughout a 3- to 4-month period. When blood glucose levels are high, glucose molecules attach to hemoglobin in the red blood cell. The longer the hyperglycemia lasts, the more glucose binds to the red blood cell and the higher the glycosylated hemoglobin. This binding lasts for the life of the red blood cell (about 4 months). When the patient's diabetes is well controlled with normal or near-normal blood glucose levels, the overall HbA_{1c} level will not be greatly elevated. However, if blood glucose levels are consistently high, the HbA_{1c} level will be elevated. The test result (expressed as a percentage) refers to the average amount of glucose that has been in the blood throughout the last 4 months. Normal levels vary with the laboratory method used for analysis, but, in general, levels between 2.5% and 6% indicate good control of diabetes. Results of 10% or greater indicate poor blood glucose control for the last several months. The HbA_{1c} is useful in evaluating the success of diabetes treatment, comparing new treatment regimens with past regimens, and individualizing treatment.

Monitoring and Managing Patient Needs

ACUTE CONFUSION. Close observation of the patient with diabetes is important, especially when diabetes is newly diagnosed, the insulin dosage changes, the patient is pregnant, the patient has a medical illness or surgery, or the patient fails to adhere to the prescribed diet. Episodes of hypoglycemia are corrected as soon as the symptoms are recognized.

NURSING ALERT

The nurse should check the patient for hypoglycemia at the peak time of action of the insulin. Hypoglycemia, which can develop suddenly, may indicate a need for adjustment in the insulin dosage or other changes in treatment, such as a change in diet. Hypoglycemic reactions can occur at any time but are most likely to occur when insulin is at its peak activity.

Methods of terminating a hypoglycemic reaction include the administration of one or more of the following:

- Orange juice or other fruit juice
- Hard candy or honey
- Commercial glucose products
- **Glucagon** by the subcut, IM, or IV routes
- Glucose 10% or 50% IV

Selection of any one or more of these methods for terminating a hypoglycemic reaction, as well as other procedures to be followed, such as drawing blood for glucose levels, depends on the written order of the primary health care provider or hospital policy. The nurse should never give oral fluids or substances (such as candy) used to terminate a hypoglycemic reaction to a patient unless the swallowing and gag reflexes are present. Absence of these reflexes may result in aspiration of the oral fluid or substance into the lungs, which can result in extremely serious consequences and even death. If swallowing and gag reflexes are absent, or if the patient is unconscious, glucose or glucagon is given by the parenteral route.

Glucagon is a hormone produced by the alpha (α) cells of the pancreas; it acts to increase blood glucose by stimulating the conversion of glycogen to glucose in the liver. A return of consciousness is observed within 5 to 20 minutes after parenteral administration of glucagon. Glucagon is effective in treating hypoglycemia only if glycogen is available from the liver.

The nurse notifies the primary health care provider of any hypoglycemic reaction, the substance and amount used to terminate the reaction, blood samples drawn (if any), the length of time required for the symptoms of hypoglycemia to disappear, and the current status of the patient. After termination of a hypoglycemic reaction, the nurse closely observes the patient for additional hypoglycemic reactions. The length of time that close observation is required depends on the peak and duration of the insulin administered.

DEFICIENT FLUID VOLUME. DKA is a potentially life-threatening deficiency of insulin (hypoinsulinism), resulting in severe hyperglycemia and requiring prompt diagnosis and treatment. Because insulin is unavailable to allow glucose to enter the cell, dangerously high levels of glucose build up in the blood (hyperglycemia). The body, needing energy, begins to break down fat for energy. As fats break down, the liver produces ketones.

As more and more fat is used for energy, higher levels of ketones accumulate in the blood. This increase in ketones disrupts the acid–base balance in the body, leading to DKA. DKA is treated with fluids, correction of acidosis and hypotension, and low doses of regular insulin.

NURSING ALERT

The nurse immediately reports any of the following symptoms of hyperglycemia: elevated blood glucose levels (over 200 mg/mL), headache, increased thirst, epigastric pain, nausea, vomiting, hot, dry, flushed skin, restlessness, and diaphoresis (sweating).

ANXIETY. The patient with newly diagnosed diabetes often has many concerns regarding the diagnosis. For some, initially coping with diabetes and the methods required for controlling the disorder creates many problems. Some of the fears and concerns of these patients may include self-administering an injection, following a diet, weight control, complications associated with diabetes, and changes in eating times and habits. An effective teaching program helps relieve some of this anxiety. The patient in this situation needs time to talk about the disorder, express concerns, and ask questions.

Assisting the Patient With Impaired Adjustment, Coping, and Altered Health Maintenance

The patient with newly diagnosed diabetes may have difficulty accepting the diagnosis, and the complexity of the therapeutic regimen can seem overwhelming. Before patients can be expected to carry out treatment, they must accept that they have diabetes and deal with their feelings about having the disorder. The nurse has an important role in helping these patients gradually accept the diagnosis and begin to understand their feelings. Understanding diabetes may help patients work with health care providers and other medical personnel in managing their diabetes.

Educating the Patient and Family

Noncompliance is a problem in some patients with diabetes, making patient and family teaching vital to the proper management of diabetes. Patients may occasionally lapse in adhering to the prescribed diet, especially around holidays or other special occasions. This slip may not cause a problem if it is brief and not excessive and if the patient immediately returns to the prescribed regimen. However, some patients frequently stray from the prescribed regimen, take extra insulin to cover dietary indiscretions, fast for several days before follow-up blood glucose determinations, and engage in other dangerous behaviors. Although some patients can be convinced that failure to adhere to the prescribed therapeutic regimen is detrimental to their health, others continue to deviate from the prescribed regimen until serious complications develop. Every effort is made to stress the importance of adherence to the prescribed treatment during the initial teaching session and during follow-up office or clinic visits.

The nurse establishes a thorough teaching plan for all patients with newly diagnosed diabetes, for those who have had any change in the management of their diabetes (e.g., diet, insulin type, insulin dosage), and for those whose management has changed because of an illness or disability, such as loss of sight or disabling arthritis. The newly diagnosed patient with diabetes and the family must receive an explanation of the disease and methods of treatment as soon as the primary health care provider has revealed the diagnosis to the patient. The nurse should always individualize the teaching plan, because the needs of each patient are different.

Self-monitoring of blood glucose levels is an important component in diabetes management (see Patient Teaching for Improved Patient Outcomes: Obtaining a Blood Glucose Reading Using a Glucometer). It is the preferred method for monitoring glucose by most health care providers for all patients with diabetes, with variations only in the suggested frequency of testing. If the patient is to use a blood glucose monitoring device, the nurse reviews the method of obtaining a small sample of blood from the finger and the use of the device with the patient. Printed instructions and illustrations are supplied with the device and must be reviewed with the patient. The nurse encourages the patient to purchase the brand recommended by the primary health care provider. Time is allowed for supervised practice. The nurse includes the following information in the teaching plan for a patient with diabetes:

- Blood glucose or urine testing—the testing material recommended by the primary health care provider; a review of the instructions included with the glucometer or the materials used for urine testing; the technique of collecting the specimen; interpreting test results; number of times a day or week the blood or urine is tested (as recommended by the primary health care provider); a record of test results.
- Insulin—types; how dosage is expressed; calculating the insulin dosage; importance of using only the type, source, and brand name recommended by the primary health care provider; importance of not changing brands unless the health care provider approves; keeping a spare vial on hand; prescription for insulin purchase not required.
- Storage of insulin—insulin is kept at room temperature away from heat and direct sunlight if used within 1 month (and up to 3 months if refrigerated); vials not in use are stored in the refrigerator; prefilled insulin in glass or plastic syringes is stable for 1 week under refrigeration. Keep filled syringes in a vertical or oblique position with the needle pointing upward to avoid plugging the needle. Before injection, pull back the plunger and tip the syringe back and forth slightly to agitate and remix the insulins.
- Needle and syringe—purchase the same brand and needle size each time; parts of the syringe; reading the syringe scale. Instruction in proper disposal of used equipment and protection of others from sharp items.
- Preparation for administration—principles of aseptic technique; how to hold the syringe; how to withdraw insulin from the vial; measurement of insulin in the syringe using the syringe scale; mixing insulin in the

same syringe (when appropriate); elimination of air in the syringe and needle; what to do if the syringe or needle is contaminated.
- Administration of insulin—sites to be used; rotation of injection sites (see Patient Teaching for Improved Patient Outcomes: Rotating Insulin Injection Sites); angle of injection; administration at the time of day prescribed by the primary health care provider.
- Disposal of the needle and syringe – puncture proof containers specifically used for disposal may be obtained from pharmacies, clinics or the primary health care provider (Fig. 43.3). Patients are cautioned not to dispose in home trash, rather the filled container should be returned to where the container was purchased for disposal. Local hospitals will also take containers.
- Insulin needs may change in patients who become ill, especially with vomiting or fever, and during periods of stress or emotional disturbance. Contact the primary health care provider if these situations occur.
- Diet—importance of following the prescribed diet; calories allowed; food exchanges; planning daily menus; establishing meal schedules; selecting food from a restaurant menu; reading food labels; use of artificial sweeteners.
- Traveling—importance of carrying an extra supply of insulin and a prescription for needles and syringes; always keep medications in the original container, storage of insulin when traveling; protecting needles and syringes from theft; airports typically have disposal containers for used equipment. It is importance to discuss travel plans (especially foreign travel) with the primary health care provider.
- Hypoglycemia/hyperglycemia—signs and symptoms of hypoglycemia and hyperglycemia; food or fluid used to terminate a hypoglycemic reaction; importance of notifying the primary health care provider immediately if either reaction occurs.
- Personal hygiene—importance of good skin and foot care, personal cleanliness, frequent dental checkups, and routine eye examinations.

Figure 43.3 Puncture proof disposal containers can be obtained from hospitals, clinics and pharmacies for home use.

- Exercise—importance of following the primary health care provider's recommendations regarding physical activity.
- When to notify the primary health care provider— increase in blood glucose levels; urine positive for ketones; if pregnancy occurs; occurrence of antidiabetic or hyperglycemic episodes; occurrence of illness, infection, or diarrhea (insulin dosage may require adjustment); appearance of new problems (e.g., leg ulcers, numbness of the extremities, significant weight gain or loss).
- Identification—wear identification, such as a Medic-Alert bracelet, to inform medical personnel and others of the use of insulin to control the disease.

EVALUATION

- Therapeutic effect is achieved and normal or near-normal blood glucose levels are maintained; blood glucose levels are tested using a glucometer, and insulin is administered correctly.
- Adverse reactions are identified, reported to the health care provider, and managed successfully through appropriate nursing interventions:
  ☑ Orientation and mentation remain intact.
  ☑ Adequate fluid volume is maintained.
  ☑ Anxiety is managed successfully.
- Patient and family demonstrate an understanding of the drug regimen.

Patient Teaching for Improved Patient Outcomes

Rotating Insulin Injection Sites

If your patient must self-administer insulin at home, be sure he or she knows where to inject the insulin and how to rotate the site. Site rotation is crucial to prevent injury to the skin and fatty tissue. Review with the patient appropriate sites, including:

✓ Upper arms, outer aspect
✓ Stomach, except for a 2-inch margin around the umbilicus
✓ Back, right, and left sides just below the waist
✓ Upper thighs, both front and side
  To rotate sites, teach the patient to do the following:
✓ Note the site of the last injection
✓ Place the side of his or her thumb at the old site and measure across its width—about 1 inch
✓ Select a site on the other side of the thumb for the next injection
✓ Repeat the procedure for each subsequent injection
✓ Use the same area for a total of about 10 to 15 injections and then move to another area

Patient Teaching for Improved Patient Outcomes

Obtaining a Blood Glucose Reading Using a Glucometer

The nurse teaches the patient to:

✓ Carefully follow manufacturer's instructions, because blood glucose monitoring devices vary greatly.
✓ Read all of the manufacturer's instructions before using the glucometer.
✓ Prepare the patient's finger by cleansing with warm water to the area. (If the patient cannot prepare the area, the caregiver should wear gloves to comply with Standard Precautions, the guidelines of the Centers for Disease Control and Prevention.)
✓ Most glucometers require a small sample of capillary blood that is obtained from the fingertip using a spring-loaded lancet.
✓ Using the lancet device, perform a finger stick on the side of a finger tip where there are fewer nerve endings and more capillaries.
✓ Milk the finger to produce a large, hanging drop of blood. Using this technique to obtain a blood sample will help prevent inaccurate readings. *Note*: Do not smear the blood or try to obtain an extra drop.
✓ Drop the blood sample on a reagent test strip, wait 45 to 60 seconds, and then wipe off the excess blood with a cotton ball. *Note*: Some glucometers have eliminated the step of excess blood removal from the strip. With these devices, the reagent strip is placed in the glucometer first, allowing all of the blood to remain on the strip for the entire test. Another type of monitoring device uses a sensor cartridge instead of strips to obtain blood glucose levels. The blood is placed on the sensor, and automatic timers provide readings in a shorter time than the traditional glucometer.
✓ Place the test strip in a glucometer that automatically uses the sample to determine a numeric reading representing the current blood glucose level. *The blood glucose level reading should be between 70 and 120 mg/dL.*

• ORAL ANTIDIABETIC DRUGS AND OTHER AGENTS

Oral antidiabetic drugs are used to treat patients with type 2 diabetes that is not controlled by diet and exercise alone. These drugs are not effective for treating type 1 diabetes. A number of oral antidiabetic drugs are currently in use and can be categorized into two groups:

- Sulfonylureas
- Nonsulfonylureas

Newer agents coming on the market include those that interact or mimic the action of incretin hormones. These additional drugs are listed in the Summary Drug Table: Antidiabetic Drugs.

Uses

Oral antidiabetic drugs are of value only in the treatment of patients with type 2 diabetes mellitus whose condition cannot be controlled by diet alone. These drugs may also be used with insulin in the management of some patients with diabetes. Use of an oral antidiabetic drug with insulin may decrease the insulin dosage in some individuals. Two oral antidiabetic drugs (e.g., a sulfonylurea and metformin) may also be used together when one antidiabetic drug and diet do not control blood glucose levels in type 2 diabetes mellitus. Figure 43.4 indicates the appropriate medication regimen for type 2 diabetes.

Summary Drug Table ANTIDIABETIC DRUGS

Generic Name	Trade Name	Uses	Adverse Reactions	Dosage Ranges
Sulfonylureas				
First Generation				
acetohexamide *ah-set-oh-hek'-sah-myde*		Type 2 diabetes; adjunct to diet and exercise	Nausea, epigastric discomfort, heartburn, hypoglycemia	250 mg–1.5 g/day orally
chlorpropamide *klor-proe'-pah-myde*	Diabinese	Type 2 diabetes; adjunct to diet and exercise, diabetes insipidus	Same as acetohexamide	100–250 mg/day orally
tolazamide *toll-az'-ah-myde*		Type 2 diabetes; adjunct to diet and exercise	Same as acetohexamide	100–1000 mg/day orally
tolbutamide *toll-byoo'-tah-myde*		Type 2 diabetes; adjunct to diet and exercise	Same as acetohexamide	0.25–3 g/day orally
Second Generation glimepiride *glye-meh'-per-ryde*	Amaryl	Type 2 diabetes; adjunct to diet and exercise, may be used in conjunction with insulin	Same as acetohexamide	1–4 mg/day orally
glipizide *glip'-ih-zyde*	Glucotrol, Glucotrol XL	Type 2 diabetes; adjunct to diet and exercise	Same as acetohexamide	5–40 mg/day orally
glyburide (glibenclamide) *glye-byoo'-ryde*	DiaBeta, Micronase, Glynase	Type 2 diabetes; adjunct to diet and exercise	Same as acetohexamide	1.25–20 mg/day orally
Meglitinides nateglinide *nah-teg'-lah-nyde*	Starlix	Type 2 diabetes; in combination with metformin to improve glycemic control	Upper respiratory tract infection, back pain, flu-like symptoms	60–120 mg orally TID before meals
repaglinide *reh-pag'-lah-nyde*	Prandin	Same as nateglinide	Hypoglycemia, upper respiratory tract infection, headache	0.5–4 mg orally before meals (maximum dose, 16 mg/day)
Nonsulfonylureas				
α-Glucosidase Inhibitors acarbose *ay-kar'-bohs*	Precose	Type 2 diabetes; combination therapy with a sulfonylurea to enhance glycemic control	Flatulence, diarrhea, abdominal pain	25–100 mg orally TID
miglitol *mih'-glih-toll*	Glyset	Same as acarbose	Same as acarbose	25–100 mg orally TID

(table continues on page 421)

Summary Drug Table ANTIDIABETIC DRUGS (continued)

Generic Name	Trade Name	Uses	Adverse Reactions	Dosage Ranges
Biguanides			GI, Lactose acidosis	
metformin *met-for'-min*	Fortamet, Glucophage, Riomet	Type 2 diabetes; with a sulfonylurea or insulin to improve glycemic control	Nausea, vomiting, flatulence, diarrhea, asthenia	500–3000 mg/day orally; XR (extended-release): 500–2000 mg/day
Thiazolidinediones				
pioglitazone *pye-oh-glit'-ah-zone*	Actos	Type 2 diabetes; with sulfonylurea, metformin, or insulin to improve glycemic control	Headache, pain, myalgia, aggravated diabetes, infections, fatigue	15–30 mg/day orally
rosiglitazone *roh-zee-glit'-ah-zone*	Avandia	Type 2 diabetes; in combination with metformin to improve glycemic control	Headache, pain, diarrhea, hypoglycemia, hyperglycemia, fatigue, infections	4–8 mg/day orally
Incretin mimetic				
sitagliptin *sit-ah-glip'-tin*	Januvia *Recalled*	Type 2 diabetes	Headache, nasopharyngitis, URI	100 mg orally daily
exenatide *ex-en'-ah-tyde*	Byetta ?	Type 2 diabetes	Dizziness, headache, nausea, diarrhea	5–10 mcg subcut, within one hr of a meal
Amylinomimetics				
pramlintide *pram'-lin-tyde*	Symlin	Type 2 diabetes, Type 1 adjunct	Headache, nausea, anorexia	Type 2: 60–120 mcg subcut; Type 1: 15–60 mcg subcut
Antidiabetic Combination Drugs				
glyburide/metformin	Glucovance	Type 2 diabetes	See individual drugs	Starting dose: 1.25 mg/250 mg orally daily or BID Maximum daily dose, 20 mg/2000 mg
glipizide/metformin	Metaglip	Type 2 diabetes	See individual drugs	Individualized; maximum daily dose, 20 mg/2000 mg
rosiglitazone/metformin	Avandamet	Type 2 diabetes	See individual drugs	Individualized; maximum daily dose, 8 mg/2000 mg
pioglitazone/metformin	ActoPlus Met	Type 2 diabetes	See individual drugs	Individualized; maximum daily dose, 45 mg/2550 mg
pioglitazone/glimepiride	Duetact	Type 2 diabetes	See individual drugs	Individualized; maximum daily dose, 45 mg/8 mg
rosiglitazone/glimepiride	Avandaryl	Type 2 diabetes	See individual drugs	Individualized; maximum daily dose, 8 mg/4 mg
sitagliptin/metformin	Janumet	Type 2 diabetes	See individual drugs	Individualized; maximum daily dose, 100 mg/2000 mg
Glucose-Elevating Agents				
diazoxide *dye-az-ok'-syde*	Proglycem	Hypoglycemia due to hyperinsulinism	Sodium and fluid retention, hyperglycemia, glycosuria, tachycardia, congestive heart failure	3–8 mg/kg/day orally in two or three equal doses q 8–12 hr
glucagon *gloo-kah-gahn*	Glucagon Emergency Kit	Hypoglycemia	Nausea, vomiting, generalized allergic reactions	See instructions on the product

Antidiabetic Drugs

Figure 43.4 Pharmacologic algorithm for treating type 2 diabetes. FPG, fasting plasma glucose; HbA₁c, glycosylated hemoglobin; F/U, follow-up.

Actions

Sulfonylureas

Sulfonylureas appear to lower blood glucose by stimulating the β cells of the pancreas to release insulin. Sulfonylureas are not effective if the β cells of the pancreas cannot release a sufficient amount of insulin to meet the individual's needs. The first-generation sulfonylureas (e.g., acetohexamide, chlorpropamide (Diabinese), tolazamide, and tolbutamide) are not commonly used today because they have a long duration of action and a higher incidence of adverse reactions, and are more likely to react with other drugs. More commonly used sulfonylureas are the second- and third-generation drugs, such as glimepiride (Amaryl), glipizide (Glucotrol), and glyburide (DiaBeta, Micronase).

Like the sulfonylureas, the meglitinides act to lower blood glucose levels by stimulating the release of insulin from the pancreas. This action depends on the ability of the β cells

in the pancreas to produce some insulin. However, the action of the meglitinides is more rapid than that of the sulfonylureas and their duration of action much shorter. Because of this, they must be taken three times a day. Examples of the meglitinides include nateglinide (Starlix) and repaglinide (Prandin).

Nonsulfonylureas

The liver normally releases glucose by detecting the level of circulating insulin. When insulin levels are high, glucose is available in the blood, and the liver produces little or no glucose. When insulin levels are low, there is little circulating glucose, so the liver produces more glucose. In type 2 diabetes, the liver may not detect levels of glucose in the blood and, instead of regulating glucose production, releases glucose despite adequate blood glucose levels.

Metformin sensitizes the liver to circulating insulin levels and reduces hepatic glucose production

The a-glucosidase inhibitors, acarbose (Precose) and miglitol (Glyset), lower blood glucose levels by delaying the digestion of carbohydrates and absorption of carbohydrates in the intestine.

The thiazolidinediones, also called glitazones, decrease insulin resistance and increase insulin sensitivity by modifying several processes, resulting in decreased hepatic glucogenesis (formation of glucose from glycogen) and increased insulin-dependent muscle glucose uptake. Examples of the thiazolidinediones are rosiglitazone (Avandia) and pioglitazone (Actos).

Adverse Reactions

Sulfonylureas

Adverse reactions associated with sulfonylureas include hypoglycemia, anorexia, nausea, vomiting, epigastric discomfort, weight gain, heartburn, and various vague neurologic symptoms, such as weakness and numbness of the extremities. Often, these can be eliminated by reducing the dosage or giving the drug in divided doses. If these reactions become severe, the primary health care provider may try another oral antidiabetic drug or discontinue the use of these drugs. If the drug therapy is discontinued, it may be necessary to control the diabetes with insulin. Adverse reactions associated with the administration of the meglitinides include upper respiratory tract infection, headache, rhinitis, bronchitis, headache, back pain, and hypoglycemia.

Nonsulfonylureas

Adverse reactions associated with nonsulfonylureas include GI upset (e.g., metallic taste, abdominal bloating, nausea, cramping, flatulence, and diarrhea). These adverse reactions are self-limiting and can be reduced if the patients are started on a low dose with dosage increased slowly, and if the drug is taken with meals. Hypoglycemia rarely occurs when a nonsulfonylurea is used alone. However, patients receiving these drugs in combination with insulin or other oral hypoglycemics (e.g., sulfonylureas) are at greater risk for hypoglycemia. A reduction in the dosage of insulin or the sulfonylurea may be required to prevent episodes of hypoglycemia.

Adverse reactions associated with the administration of thiazolidinediones include upper respiratory infections, sinusitis, headache, pharyngitis, myalgia, diarrhea, and back pain.

Lactic acidosis (buildup of lactic acid in the blood) may also occur with the administration of metformin. Although lactic acidosis is a rare adverse reaction, its occurrence is serious and can be fatal. Lactic acidosis occurs mainly in patients with kidney dysfunction. Symptoms of lactic acidosis include malaise (vague feeling of bodily discomfort), abdominal pain, rapid respirations, shortness of breath, and muscular pain. In some patients, vitamin B_{12} levels are decreased. This can be reversed with vitamin B_{12} supplements or with discontinuation of the drug therapy. Because weight loss can occur, metformin is sometimes recommended for obese patients or patients with insulin-resistant diabetes.

Contraindications, Precautions, and Interactions

Sulfonylureas

Oral antidiabetic drugs are contraindicated in patients with known hypersensitivity to the drugs, DKA, severe infection, or severe endocrine disease. The first-generation sulfonylureas (chlorpropamide, tolazamide, and tolbutamide) are contraindicated in patients with coronary artery disease or liver or renal dysfunction. Other sulfonylureas are used cautiously in patients with impaired liver function because liver dysfunction can prolong the drug's effect. In addition, sulfonylureas are used cautiously in patients with renal impairment and severe cardiovascular disease. There is a risk for cross-sensitivity with sulfonylureas and sulfonamides (sulfa anti-infectives).

Many drugs may affect the action of sulfonylureas; the nurse must monitor blood glucose carefully when beginning therapy, discontinuing therapy, and any time any change is made in the drug regimen with these drugs. Sulfonylureas may have an increased hypoglycemic effect when administered with anticoagulants, chloramphenicol, clofibrate, fluconazole, histamine H_2 antagonists, methyldopa, monoamine oxidase inhibitors (MAOIs), nonsteroidal anti-inflammatory drugs (NSAIDs), salicylates, sulfonamides, and tricyclic antidepressants. The hypoglycemic effect of sulfonylureas may be decreased when the agents are administered with β blockers, calcium channel blockers, cholestyramine, corticosteroids, estrogens, hydantoins, isoniazid, oral contraceptives, phenothiazines, rifampin, thiazide diuretics, and thyroid agents.

Nonsulfonylureas

Nonsulfonylureas are contraindicated in patients with heart failure, renal disease, hypersensitivity to the individual drug, and acute or chronic metabolic acidosis, including ketoacidosis. The drug is also contraindicated in patients older than 80 years and during pregnancy (pregnancy category B, the thiazolidinediones are category C) and lactation.

Metformin use is temporarily discontinued for surgical procedures. The drug therapy is restarted when the patient's oral intake has been resumed and renal function is normal. There is a risk of acute renal failure when iodinated contrast material used for radiologic studies is administered with metformin. Metformin therapy is stopped for 48 hours before and after radiologic studies using iodinated material. There is an increased risk of lactic acidosis when metformin is administered with the glucocorticoids.

Digestive enzymes may reduce the effect of miglitol. Acarbose and miglitol are used cautiously in patients with renal impairment or preexisting GI problems, such as irritable bowel syndrome or Crohn's disease.

Thiazolidinediones are used cautiously in patients with edema, cardiovascular disease, and liver or kidney disease. These drugs may alter the effects of oral contraceptives.

HERBAL ALERT

Patients may not volunteer information regarding their use of alternative or complementary remedies. The nurse should always inquire about use of herbal products.

Although lab testing is not conclusive, medical reports indicate a possible interaction with eucalyptus products, causing decreased blood sugar.

• HORMONE MIMETIC AGENTS

These agents help control blood glucose levels by maintaining β cell function and enhancing insulin secretion, suppressing glucagon output from the liver and delaying gastric emptying, which slows carbohydrate absorption. Incretin hormones cause insulin to be made and reduce the amount of glucagon made by the liver. These hormones are released in response to increases in glucose that occur after eating.

Sitagliptin (Januvia) lowers the blood glucose level of type 2 diabetics by enhancing the secretion of the endogenous incretin hormone. Exenatide (Byetta) mimics the action of the incretin hormone. Pramlintide (Symlin) mimics the action of another secretion, amylin.

An incretin mimetic should be used cautiously in patients with chronic kidney disease or the elderly. This drug has not been studied in pregnant women, but is believed to be a category B drug from animal studies, and should be used cautiously in lactating women.

NURSING PROCESS
PATIENT RECEIVING AN ORAL ANTIDIABETIC DRUG

ASSESSMENT

Preadministration Assessment
If the patient has recently been diagnosed with diabetes mellitus and has not received an oral antidiabetic drug, or if the patient is known to have diabetes and has been taking one of these drugs, the nurse should include weight, blood pressure, pulse, and respiratory rate in the initial assessment. The nurse makes a general assessment of the skin, mucous membranes, and extremities, with special attention given to sores or cuts that appear to be healing poorly and ulcerations or other skin or mucous membrane changes. Dietary habits, a family history of diabetes (if any), and an inquiry into the type and duration of symptoms experienced are included in the history. The nurse reviews the patient's chart for recent laboratory and diagnostic tests. If the patient has diabetes and has been receiving an oral antidiabetic drug, the nurse includes the name of the drug and the dosage, the type of diabetic diet, the results of blood glucose testing, and an inquiry into adherence to the dietary and weight control regimen prescribed by the primary health care provider.

Ongoing Assessment
The most important aspect of the ongoing assessment is observation of the patient every 2 to 4 hours for symptoms of hypoglycemia (see Table 43.1), particularly during initial therapy or after a change in dosage. If both an oral antidiabetic drug and insulin are given, the nurse observes the patient more frequently for hypoglycemic episodes during the initial period of combination therapy. If the patient is receiving only an oral antidiabetic drug and a hypoglycemic reaction occurs, it is often (but not always) less intense than one seen with insulin administration.

The nurse conducts ongoing assessments, including monitoring vital signs and observing for adverse drug reactions. The primary health care provider may also order the patient be weighed daily or weekly. The nurse notifies the primary health care provider if an adverse reaction occurs or if there is a significant weight gain or loss.

As noted with the patient taking insulin, blood glucose levels are routinely monitored. When ordered by the primary health care provider, patients will need to be taught to use a glucometer for self monitoring of glucose levels (see Patient Teaching for Improved Patient Outcomes: Obtaining a Blood Glucose Reading Using a Glucometer). The best way to monitor long-term glycemic control and response to treatment is with HbA_{1c} levels measured at 3-month intervals. If the first HbA_{1c} indicates that glycemic control during the last 3 months was inadequate, the dosage may be increased for better control.

NURSING DIAGNOSES

Drug-specific nursing diagnoses include the following:

❑ **Acute Confusion** related to hypoglycemia effects on mentation
❑ **Deficient Fluid Volume** related to fluid loss during DKA
❑ **Anxiety** related to fear of diagnosis, testing own glucose levels, dietary restrictions, other factors (specify)
❑ **Ineffective Breathing Pattern** related to hyperventilation in lactic acidosis

Nursing diagnoses related to drug administration are discussed in Chapter 4.

PLANNING

The expected outcomes of the patient may include an optimal response to therapy, support of patient needs related to the management of adverse reactions, a reduction in anxiety, improved ability to cope with the diagnosis, and an understanding of and compliance with the prescribed therapeutic regimen.

IMPLEMENTATION

Promoting an Optimal Response to Therapy
There are no fixed drug dosages in antidiabetic therapy. The drug regimen is individualized on the basis of the effectiveness and tolerance of the drug(s) used and the maximum recommended dose of the drug(s). Glycemic control can often be improved when a second oral medication is added to the drug regimen. The choice of a second medication varies from patient to patient and is

prescribed by the primary health care provider. Glucovance, which includes both glyburide and metformin, is one example of the use of combination drugs for glycemic control. The combination drugs are useful for individuals needing dual therapy and those who are forgetful (only once-daily dosing is required) or mildly confused.

LIFESPAN ALERT – Chronic Care

Exposure to stress, such as infection, fever, surgery, or trauma, may cause a loss of control of blood glucose levels in patients who have been stabilized with oral antidiabetic drugs. Should this occur, the primary health care provider may discontinue use of the oral drug and administer insulin.

Oral antidiabetic drugs are given as a single daily dose or in divided doses. The following sections provide specific information for each group of oral antidiabetic drugs.

Sulfonylureas

Acetohexamide, chlorpropamide (Diabinese), tolazamide (Tolinase), and tolbutamide (Orinase) are given with food to prevent GI upset. However, because food delays absorption, the nurse gives glipizide (Glucotrol) 30 minutes before a meal. Glyburide (Micronase) is administered with breakfast or with the first main meal of the day. The primary health care provider orders the meal with which glyburide is given. Glimepiride is given once daily with breakfast or the first main meal of the day. The nurse usually gives repaglinide 15 minutes before meals but can give it immediately, or up to 30 minutes, before the meal. Nateglinide is taken up to 30 minutes before meals.

LIFESPAN ALERT – Gerontology

Older adults have an increased sensitivity to sulfonylureas and may require a dosage reduction.

After the patient has been taking sulfonylureas for a period of time, a condition called **secondary failure** may occur, in which the sulfonylurea loses its effectiveness. When the nurse notes that a normally compliant patient has a gradual increase in blood glucose levels, secondary failure may be the cause. This increase in blood glucose levels can be caused by an increase in the severity of the diabetes or a decreased response to the drug. When secondary failure occurs, the primary health care provider may prescribe another sulfonylurea or add an oral antidiabetic drug such as metformin to the drug regimen. See the Summary Drug Table: Antidiabetic Drugs for additional drugs that can be used in combination with sulfonylureas.

Nonsulfonylureas

Acarbose and miglitol are given three times as day with the first bite of the meal, because food increases absorption. Some patients begin therapy with a lower dose once daily to minimize GI effects such as abdominal discomfort, flatulence, and diarrhea. The dose is then gradually increased to three times daily. The nurse monitors the response to these drugs by periodic testing. Dosage adjustments are made at 4- to 16-week intervals based on 1-hour postprandial blood glucose levels.

The nurse instructs the patient to take metformin two or three times a day with meals. If the patient has not experienced a response in 4 weeks using the maximum dose of metformin, the primary health care provider may add an oral sulfonylurea while continuing metformin at the maximum dose. Glucophage XR (metformin, extended-release) is administered once daily with the evening meal.

The thiazolidinediones, pioglitazone and rosiglitazone, are given with or without meals. If the dose is missed at the usual meal, the drug is taken at the next meal. If the dose is missed on one day, it is not doubled the following day. If the drug is taken, the meal must not be delayed. Delay of a meal for as little as 30 minutes can cause hypoglycemia.

Monitoring and Managing Patient Needs

ACUTE CONFUSION. The nurse must immediately stop a hypoglycemic reaction. The method of stopping a hypoglycemic reaction is the same as for a hypoglycemic reaction occurring with insulin administration, with the following exception: the nurse notifies the primary health care provider as soon as possible if episodes of hypoglycemia occur, because the dosage of the oral antidiabetic drug (or insulin, when both insulin and an oral antidiabetic drug are given) may need to be changed.

NURSING ALERT

When hypoglycemia occurs in a patient taking an α-glucosidase inhibitor (e.g., acarbose or miglitol), the nurse gives the patient an oral form of glucose, such as glucose tablets or dextrose, rather than sugar (sucrose). Absorption of sugar is blocked by acarbose or miglitol.

When oral antidiabetic drugs are combined with other antidiabetic drugs (e.g., sulfonylureas) or insulin, the hypoglycemic effect may be enhanced. Elderly, debilitated, or malnourished patients are more likely to experience hypoglycemia.

LIFESPAN ALERT – Gerontology

Although older adult patients taking the oral antidiabetic drugs are particularly susceptible to hypoglycemic reactions, these reactions may be difficult to detect in the older patient. The nurse notifies the primary health care provider if blood glucose levels are elevated (consistently above 200 mg/dL) or if ketones are present in the urine.

DEFICIENT FLUID VOLUME. Capillary blood specimens are obtained and tested in the same manner as for individuals who take insulin (see Patient Teaching for Improved Patient Outcomes: Obtaining a Blood Glucose Reading Using a Glucometer). The nurse notifies the health care provider if blood glucose levels are elevated (consistently over 200 mg/dL) or if ketones are present in the urine.

ANXIETY. The patient with newly diagnosed diabetes often has many concerns about managing the disease. Some patients, when learning that management of their diabetes can be achieved by diet and an oral drug, may have a tendency to discount the seriousness of the disorder. Without creating additional anxiety, the nurse emphasizes the importance of following the prescribed treatment regimen. Then the nurse encourages the patient to talk about the disorder, express concerns, and ask questions. Allowing these patients time to talk may help them begin to cope with their diabetes.

The patient receiving an oral antidiabetic drug may also express concern about the possibility of having to take insulin in the future. The nurse encourages the patient to discuss this and other concerns with the primary health care provider.

INEFFECTIVE BREATHING PATTERN. When taking metformin, the patient is at risk for lactic acidosis. The nurse monitors the patient for symptoms of lactic acidosis, which include unexplained hyperventilation, myalgia, malaise, GI symptoms, or unusual somnolence. If the patient experiences these symptoms, the nurse should contact the primary health care provider at once. Elevated blood lactate levels exceeding 5 mmol/L are associated with lactic acidosis and should be reported immediately. Once a patient's diabetes is stabilized on metformin therapy, the adverse GI reactions that often occur at the beginning of such therapy are unlikely to be related to the drug therapy. A later occurrence of GI symptoms is more likely to be related to lactic acidosis or other serious disease.

Educating the Patient and Family

Failure to comply with the prescribed treatment regimen may be a problem with patients taking an oral antidiabetic drug because of the erroneous belief that not having to take insulin means that the disease is not serious and therefore does not require strict adherence to the recommended dietary plan. The nurse informs these patients that control of their diabetes is just as important as for patients requiring insulin and that control is achieved only when they adhere to the treatment regimen prescribed by the primary health care provider.

If the diagnosis of diabetes mellitus is new, the nurse discusses the disease and methods of control with the patient and family after the primary health care provider discloses the diagnosis to the patient. Although taking an oral antidiabetic drug is less complicated than self-administration of insulin, the patient with diabetes taking one of these drugs needs a thorough explanation of the management of the disease. The teaching plan is individualized, because the needs of each patient are different. The nurse includes the following information in a teaching plan:

- Take the drug exactly as directed on the container (e.g., with food, 30 minutes before a meal).
- To control diabetes, follow the diet and drug regimen prescribed by the primary health care provider exactly.
- An antidiabetic drug is not oral insulin and cannot be substituted for insulin.
- Never stop taking this drug or increase or decrease the dose unless told to do so by the primary health care provider.

- Take the drug at the same time or times each day.
- Eat meals at about the same time each day. Erratic meal hours or skipped meals may result in difficulty in controlling diabetes with this drug.
- Avoid alcohol, dieting, commercial weight-loss products, and strenuous exercise programs unless use or participation has been approved by the primary health care provider.
- Test blood for glucose and urine for ketones as directed by the primary health care provider. Keep a record of test results and bring this record to each visit to the primary health care provider or clinic.
- Maintain good foot and skin care and routine eye and dental examinations for the early detection of the complications that may occur.
- Exercise should be moderate; avoid strenuous exercise and erratic periods of exercise.
- Wear identification, such as a MedicAlert bracelet, to inform medical personnel and others of diabetes and the drug or drugs currently being used to treat the disease.
- Notify the primary health care provider if any of the following occur: episodes of hypoglycemia, apparent symptoms of hyperglycemia, elevated blood glucose levels, positive results of urine tests for glucose or ketone bodies, or pregnancy. Also notify the primary health care provider of any serious illness not requiring hospitalization.
- Know the symptoms of hypoglycemia and hyperglycemia and the primary health care provider's method for terminating a hypoglycemic reaction.
- Metformin—there is a risk of lactic acidosis when using this drug. Discontinue the drug therapy and notify the primary health care provider immediately if any of the following occur: respiratory distress, muscular aches, unusual somnolence, unexplained malaise, or nonspecific abdominal distress.

EVALUATION

- Therapeutic drug effect is achieved and normal or near-normal blood glucose levels are maintained.
- Hypoglycemic and other adverse reactions are identified, reported to the primary health care provider, and managed successfully through appropriate nursing interventions:
  ☑ Orientation and mentation remain intact.
  ☑ Adequate fluid volume is maintained.
  ☑ Anxiety is managed successfully.
  ☑ An adequate breathing pattern is maintained.
- Patient and family demonstrate an understanding of the drug regimen.

THINK CRITICALLY: PHARMACOLOGY IN PRACTICE

1. Ms. Moore's glycosylated hemoglobin was 9%, and she was instructed to monitor blood glucose levels at home. Her daughter was able to help, and readings indicated that she most likely has diabetes–type 2.

The primary health care provider prescribes tolbutamide (Orinase). In reviewing the medications she is taking, you see that she was prescribed the combination drug trimethoprim and sulfamethoxazole (Septra) for a bladder infection. Discuss any instructions and information you would give to Ms. Moore and her daughter in the patient education session.

● Test Your Knowledge

1. Which of the following would the nurse mostly likely choose to treat a hypoglycemic reaction?

   A. Regular insulin
   B. NPH insulin
   C. Orange juice
   D. Crackers and milk

2. Which of the following would be the correct method of administering insulin glargine?

   A. Within 10 minutes of meals
   B. Immediately before meals
   C. Any time within 30 minutes before or 30 minutes after a meal
   D. At bedtime

3. Which of the following symptoms would alert the nurse to a possible hyperglycemic reaction?

   A. Fatigue, weakness, confusion
   B. Pale skin, elevated temperature
   C. Thirst, abdominal pain, nausea
   D. Rapid, shallow respirations, headache, nervousness

4. A patient with diabetes received a glycosylated hemoglobin test result of 10%. This indicates _____.

   A. the diabetes is well controlled
   B. poor blood glucose control
   C. the need for an increase in the insulin dosage
   D. the patient is at increased risk for hypoglycemia

● Prepare for the NCLEX

1. List in order the following steps in drawing up two types of insulin.

   A. remove air bubbles from syringe, and withdraw the Humulin N insulin prescribed
   B. remove the needle from the vial without getting fluid (insulin) on the needle
   C. after cleansing both vials, inject air into the Humulin N insulin vial.
   D. inject air into the Regular insulin vial, invert and withdraw the prescribed amount.

● Calculate Medication Dosages

1. A patient is prescribed 40 units NPH insulin mixed with 5 units of regular insulin. What is the total insulin dosage? Describe how you would prepare the insulins.

2. A patient is prescribed metformin (Glucophage) 1000 mg orally BID. The drug is available in 500-mg tablets. The nurse administers _____. What is the total daily dosage of metformin?_____

3. A patient is prescribed rosiglitazone (Avandia) 8 mg orally daily. Available are 2-mg tablets. The nurse would administer ____.

To check your answers, see Appendix E.

thePoint. *For more NCLEX and review questions, log on to http://thepoint.lww.com to access more than 1000 questions.*

Pituitary and Adrenocortical Hormones

The pituitary gland lies deep within the cranial vault, connected to the brain by the infundibular stalk (a downward extension of the floor of the third ventricle) and protected by an indentation of the sphenoid bone called the *sella turcica* (Fig. 44.1). The pituitary gland, a small, gray, rounded structure, has two parts:

- Anterior pituitary (adenohypophysis)
- Posterior pituitary (neurohypophysis)

The gland secretes a number of pituitary hormones that regulate growth, metabolism, the reproductive cycle, electrolyte balance, and water retention or loss. The pituitary gland is often referred to as the "master gland" because it secretes many hormones that regulate numerous vital processes. The hormones secreted by the anterior and posterior pituitary and the organs influenced by these hormones are shown in Figure 44.2.

• POSTERIOR PITUITARY HORMONES

The posterior pituitary gland produces two hormones: vasopressin (antidiuretic hormone) and oxytocin (see Chapter 47). Posterior pituitary hormones are summarized in the Summary Drug Table: Posterior and Anterior Pituitary Hormones.

Vasopressin

Actions and Uses

Vasopressin (Pitressin Synthetic) and its derivative, desmopressin (DDAVP), regulate the reabsorption of water by the kidneys. Vasopressin is secreted by the pituitary when body fluids must be conserved. This mechanism may be activated when, for example, an individual has severe vomiting and diarrhea with little or no fluid intake. When this and similar conditions are present, the posterior pituitary releases the

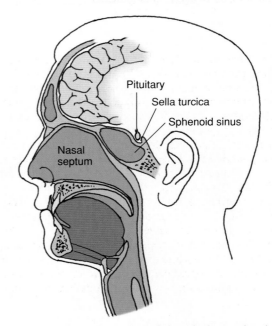

Figure 44.1 Location of the pituitary gland.

Pituitary Gland

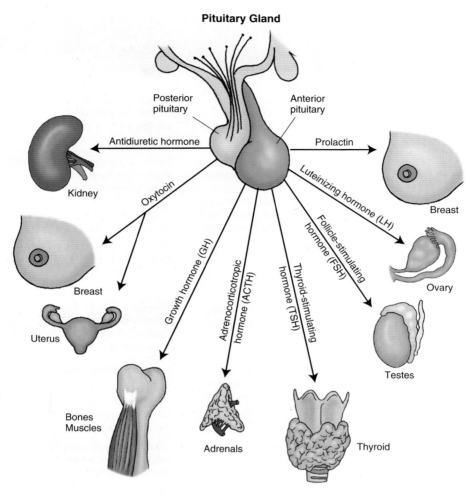

Figure 44.2 The pituitary gland and the hormones secreted by the anterior pituitary and the posterior pituitary.

hormone vasopressin, water in the kidneys is reabsorbed into the blood (i.e., conserved), and the urine becomes concentrated. Vasopressin exhibits its greatest activity on the renal tubular epithelium, where it promotes water resorption and smooth muscle contraction throughout the vascular bed. Vasopressin has some vasopressor activity.

Vasopressin and its derivative are used in treating **diabetes insipidus**, a disease resulting from the failure of the pituitary to secrete vasopressin or from surgical removal of the pituitary. Diabetes insipidus is characterized by marked increase in urination (as much as 10 L in 24 hours) and excessive thirst by inadequate secretion of vasopressin (antidiuretic hormone). Treatment with vasopressin therapy replaces the hormone in the body and restores normal urination and thirst. Vasopressin may also be used for preventing and treating postoperative abdominal distention and for dispelling gas interfering with abdominal roentgenography (x-ray studies).

Adverse Reactions

Local or systemic hypersensitivity reactions may occur in some patients receiving vasopressin, and the following may also be seen:

- Tremor, sweating, vertigo
- Nasal congestion
- Nausea, vomiting, abdominal cramps
- Water intoxication (overdosage, toxicity)

Contraindications and Precautions

Vasopressin is contraindicated in patients hypersensitive to the drug or its components. Vasopressin is used cautiously in patients with a history of seizures, migraine headaches, asthma, congestive heart failure, or vascular disease (because the substance may precipitate angina or myocardial infarction) and in those with perioperative polyuria. Vasopressin is

Pituitary and Adrenocortical Hormones

Summary Drug Table POSTERIOR AND ANTERIOR PITUITARY HORMONES

Generic Name	Trade Name	Uses	Adverse Reactions	Dosage Ranges
Posterior Pituitary Hormones				
desmopressin *des-moe-press'-in*	DDAVP, Stimate	Diabetes insipidus, hemophilia A, von Willebrand's disease, nocturnal enuresis	Headache, nausea, nasal congestion, abdominal cramps	Doses are individualized, administered orally, intranasally, or subcut
vasopressin *vay-soe-press'-in*		Diabetes insipidus, prevention and treatment of postoperative abdominal distention, to dispel gas interfering with abdominal x-ray examination	Tremor, sweating, vertigo, nausea, vomiting, abdominal cramps, headache	Diabetes insipidus: 5–10 units IM, subcut q 3–4 hr, parenteral solution may be used intranasally
Anterior Pituitary Hormones and Hormone Inhibitors				
Gonadotropins: Ovarian Stimulants				
choriogonadotropin alfa *kore-ee-oh-goe-nad'-oh-troe-pin*	Ovidrel	Ovulation induction, follicular maturation	Vasomotor flushes, breast tenderness, abdominal pain, ovarian overstimulation, nausea, vomiting	Injection following follicle stimulation drugs
gonadotropin *goe-nad'-oh-troe-pin*	Bravelle, Follistim AQ, Gonal-f, Gonal-f RFF, Luveris, Menopur, Repronex	Ovulation induction, multifollicular development, male infertility	Same as choriogonadotropin	Individualized dosing dependent on patient outcome
Gonadotropin-Releasing Hormones/Synthetics				
nafarelin *naf'-ah-rell-in*	Synarel	Endometriosis, precocious puberty	Hot flashes, decreased libido, vaginal dryness, headache, emotional lability	400 mcg/day intranasally in 2 doses
Gonadotropin-Releasing Hormone Antagonists				
cetrorelix *seh-tro'-rell-iks*	Cetrotide	Infertility	Ovarian overstimulation, nausea, vomiting	Dose individualized during cycle
ganirelix *gan-ih-rell'-iks*		Infertility	Abdominal pain, fetal death, headache	250 mcg/day subcut during cycle
Nonsteroidal Ovarian Stimulant				
clomiphene *kloe'-mih-feen*	Clomid, Milophene, Serophene	Ovulatory failure	Vasomotor flushes, breast tenderness, abdominal discomfort, ovarian enlargement, nausea, vomiting	50 mg/day orally for 5 days, may be repeated
Growth Hormone and Hormone Inhibitors				
somatropin *soe-mah-troe'-pin*	Genotropin, Humatrope, Norditropin, Nutropin, Serostim	Growth failure due to deficiency of pituitary GH in children	With injection: diarrhea, arthralgia Long term: growth problems—bone, ear, edema	Doses are individualized, administered by subcut injection weekly
octreotide *ok-tree'-oh-tyde*	Sandostatin	Reduction of GH in acromegaly and treatment of certain tumors	Nausea, diarrhea, abdominal pain, sinus bradycardia, hypoglycemia, injection site pain	50 mcg subcut or IV BID or TID
Adrenocorticotropic Hormone				
adrenocorticotropic hormone *ah-dreen-oh-core-tih-koe-troe'-pik*	ACTH	Diagnose adrenocortical function, nonsuppurative thyroiditis, hypercalcemia, multiple sclerosis	See Display 44.2	20 units IM, subcut QID

(table continues on page 431)

Summary Drug Table POSTERIOR AND ANTERIOR PITUITARY HORMONES (continued)

Generic Name	Trade Name	Uses	Adverse Reactions	Dosage Ranges
Miscellaneous Hormones and Hormone Inhibitors				
aminoglutethimide *ah-meen'-oh-gloo-tih-thye-myde*	Cytadren	Suppress adrenal function (Cushing's syndrome, metastatic breast, prostate cancers	Drowsiness, skin rash, nausea, vomiting	1–2 g/day orally
bromocriptine *broe-moe-krip'-tin*	Parlodel	Hyperprolactinemia, acromegaly, Parkinson's disease	Headache, dizziness, fatigue, nausea	5–7.5 mg/day orally
cabergoline *cah-ber'-goe-leen*		Same as bromocriptine	Same as bromocriptine	1 mg twice weekly orally
cosyntropin	Cortrosyn	Screening for adrenal insufficiency	Dizziness, nausea, vomiting	See package insert
gonadotropin, chorionic (HCG)	Pregnyl	Testicular descent induction, hypogonadism, ovulation induction	Headache, irritability, fluid retention, fatigue, gynecomastia, aggressive behavior	500–5000 units IM up to 3 times weekly depending on results

classified as a pregnancy category C drug. Desmopressin acetate (a pregnancy category B drug) is typically used when diabetes insipidus occurs during pregnancy; however, it still must be used cautiously then and during lactation.

Interactions

Interacting Drug	Common Use	Effect of Interaction
norepinephrine	Neurostimulant	Decreased antidiuretic effect
lithium	Management of psychological problems	Decreased antidiuretic effect
oral anticoagulants	Blood thinners	Decreased antidiuretic effect
carbamazepine	Anticonvulsant	Increased antidiuretic effect
chlorpropamide	Antidiabetic (diabetes mellitus) agent	Increased antidiuretic effect

NURSING PROCESS

PATIENT RECEIVING VASOPRESSIN

ASSESSMENT

Preadministration Assessment
Before administering the first dose of vasopressin for managing diabetes insipidus, the nurse takes the patient's blood pressure, pulse, and respiratory rate. The nurse weighs the patient to obtain a baseline weight for future comparison. Serum electrolyte levels and other laboratory tests may be ordered by the primary health care provider.

Before administering vasopressin to relieve abdominal distention, the nurse takes the patient's blood pressure, pulse, and respiratory rate. The nurse auscultates the abdomen and records the findings. The nurse measures and records the patient's abdominal girth.

Ongoing Assessment
During the ongoing assessment, the nurse monitors the blood pressure, pulse, and respiratory rate every 4 hours or as ordered by the primary health care provider. The patient's fluid intake and output are strictly measured. The primary health care provider is notified if there are any significant changes in these vital signs, because a dosage adjustment may be necessary.

The dosage of vasopressin or its derivatives may require periodic adjustments. After administration of the drug, the nurse observes the patient every 10 to 15 minutes for signs of an excessive dosage (e.g., blanching of the skin, abdominal cramps, and nausea). If these occur, the nurse reassures the patient that recovery from these effects will occur in a few minutes.

NURSING DIAGNOSES

Drug-specific nursing diagnoses include the following:

❑ **Deficient Fluid Volume** related to inability to replenish fluid intake secondary to diabetes insipidus
❑ **Acute Pain** related to abdominal distention

Nursing diagnoses related to drug administration are discussed in Chapter 4.

PLANNING

The expected outcomes for the patient may include an optimal response to therapy, support of patient needs related to the management of adverse reactions, and an understanding of the therapeutic regimen.

Pituitary and Adrenocortical Hormones

IMPLEMENTATION

Promoting an Optimal Response to Therapy

Vasopressin may be given intramuscularly (IM) or subcutaneously (subcut) to treat diabetes insipidus. The injection (parenteral) solution may also be administered intranasally on cotton pledgets, by nasal spray or dropper. When given parenterally, 5 to 10 Units administered two to three times daily is usually sufficient. To prevent or relieve abdominal distention, 5 Units of the drug is administered initially, which may be increased to 10 Units every 3 or 4 hours IM. When the drug is administered before abdominal roentgenography, the nurse administers two injections of 10 Units each. The first dose is given 2 hours before x-ray examination and the second dose 30 minutes before the testing. An enema may be given before the first dose.

Desmopressin may be given orally, intranasally, subcut, or intravenously (IV). The oral dose must be determined for each individual patient and adjusted according to the patient's response to therapy. A nasal spray pump may also be used. The nurse instructs the patient to hold the bottle upright with the head in a vertical position when administering the drug. Most adults require 0.2 mL daily in two divided doses to control diabetes insipidus. Patients learn to regulate their dosage based on the frequency of urination and increase of thirst. The drug may also be administered by the subcut route or direct IV injection.

Monitoring and Managing Patient Needs

The adverse reactions associated with vasopressin, such as skin blanching, abdominal cramps, and nausea, may be decreased by administering the agent with one or two glasses of water. If these adverse reactions occur, the nurse informs the patient that they are not serious and should subside within a few minutes.

! NURSING ALERT

Excessive dosage is manifested as water intoxication (fluid overload). Symptoms of water intoxication include drowsiness, listlessness, confusion, and headache (which may precede convulsions and coma). If signs of excessive dosage occur, the nurse should notify the primary health care provider before the next dose of the drug is due, because a change in the dosage, the restriction of oral or IV fluids, and the administration of a diuretic may be necessary.

Deficient Fluid Volume. The symptoms of diabetes insipidus include the voiding of a large volume of urine at frequent intervals during the day and throughout the night. Accompanying this frequent urination is the need to drink large volumes of fluid, because patients with diabetes insipidus are continually thirsty and need to be supplied with large amounts of drinking water. The nurse is careful to refill the water container at frequent intervals. This is especially important when the patient has limited ambulatory activities. Until controlled by a drug, the symptoms of frequent urination and excessive thirst may cause a great deal of anxiety. The nurse reassures the patient that with the proper drug therapy, these symptoms will most likely be reduced or eliminated.

When the patient has diabetes insipidus, the nurse measures the fluid intake and output accurately and observes the patient for signs of dehydration (dry mucous membranes, concentrated urine, poor skin turgor, flushing, dry skin, confusion). This is especially important early in treatment and until such time as the optimum dosage is determined and symptoms have diminished. If the patient's output greatly exceeds intake, the nurse notifies the primary health care provider. In some instances, the primary health care provider may order specific gravity and volume measurements of each voiding or at hourly intervals. The nurse records these results in the chart to aid the primary health care provider in adjusting the dosage to the patient's needs.

LIFESPAN ALERT – Chronic Care

If a person with diabetes insipidus is unable to take their routine medication, a fluid deficit can happen rapidly. Therefore, individuals with diabetes insipidus should wear a medical alert bracelet so emergency personnel can be aware of this need for the medication and dosing can continued if they are unable to take the drug themselves.

Acute Pain. If the patient is receiving vasopressin for abdominal distention, the nurse explains in detail the method of treating this problem and the necessity of monitoring drug effectiveness (e.g., auscultation of the abdomen for bowel sounds, insertion of a rectal tube, measurement of the abdomen). If a rectal tube is ordered after administration of vasopressin for abdominal distention, the lubricated end of the tube is inserted past the anal sphincter and taped in place. The tube is left in place for 1 hour or as prescribed by the primary health care provider. The nurse auscultates the abdomen every 15 to 30 minutes and measures abdominal girth hourly, or as ordered by the primary health care provider.

Educating the Patient and Family

If desmopressin is to be used nasally, the nurse ensures that the patient masters the technique of instillation. The nurse includes illustrated patient instructions with the drug and reviews them with the patient. The nurse should discuss the need to take the drug as directed by the primary health care provider. The patient should change the dosage (i.e., the prescribed number or frequency of sprays) only after consulting with the primary health care provider.

On occasion, a patient may need to self-administer vasopressin by the parenteral route. If so, the nurse teaches the patient or a family member how to prepare and administer the drug and measure the specific gravity of the urine.

The nurse stresses the importance of adhering to the prescribed treatment program to control symptoms. In addition to instruction in administration, the nurse includes the following in a patient and family teaching plan:

- Wear medical identification naming the disease and the drug regimen.
- Carry a sport drink bottle to be sure to have liquids available at all times.
- Monitor the amount of fluids taken each day.
- Monitor the amount and frequency of urine for each 24-hour period, reporting changes to daily patterns to your nurse.
- Carry extra doses of the drug in case you do not make it home in time for your next dose.
- Avoid the use of alcohol while taking these drugs.
- Rotate injection sites for parenteral administration.
- Contact the primary health care provider immediately if any of the following occur: a significant increase or decrease in urine output, abdominal cramps, blanching of the skin, nausea, signs of inflammation or infection at the injection sites, confusion, headache, or drowsiness.

EVALUATION

- Therapeutic effect is achieved.
- Adverse reactions are identified, reported to the primary health care provider, and managed successfully through appropriate nursing interventions:
  - ☑ Fluid volume balance is maintained.
  - ☑ Acute pain is relieved.
- Patient and family demonstrate an understanding of the drug regimen.

● ANTERIOR PITUITARY HORMONES

The hormones of the anterior pituitary include:

- Prolactin
- Luteinizing hormone (LH)
- Follicle-stimulating hormone (FSH)
- Thyroid-stimulating hormone (TSH)
- Adrenocorticotropic hormone (ACTH; corticotropin)
- Growth hormone (GH)

The anterior pituitary hormone TSH is discussed in Chapter 45. The remaining hormones can be classified into different groups. FSH and LH are called **gonadotropins** because they influence the **gonads** (the organs of reproduction). GH, also called **somatropin,** contributes to the growth of the body during childhood, especially the growth of muscles and bones. ACTH is produced by the anterior pituitary and stimulates the adrenal cortex to secrete the **corticosteroids**. Prolactin, which is also secreted by the anterior pituitary, stimulates the production of breast milk in the postpartum patient. Additional functions of prolactin are not well understood. Prolactin is the only anterior pituitary hormone that is not used medically.

Gonadotropins: Follicle-Stimulating Hormone and Luteinizing Hormone

The gonadotropins (FSH and LH) influence the secretion of sex hormones, development of secondary sex characteristics, and the reproductive cycle in both men and women.

Action and Uses

These drugs are purified preparations of the gonadotropins (FSH and LH) extracted from the urine of postmenopausal women or produced by a recombinant form of DNA. Gonadotropins are used to induce ovulation and pregnancy in anovulatory women (women whose bodies fail to produce an ovum or fail to ovulate). Menopur is also used in assisted reproductive technology (ART) programs to stimulate multiple follicles for in vitro fertilization. Besides their use in treating female infertility, some of these drugs are used in men. Human chorionic gonadotropin (HCG) is extracted from human placentas. The actions of HCG are identical to those of the pituitary LH. This drug is also used in boys to treat prepubertal **cryptorchism** (failure of the testes to descend into the scrotum) and in men to treat selected cases of hypogonadotropic hypogonadism. Follistim AQ is used to induce sperm production (spermatogenesis). For additional information on the gonadotropins, see the Summary Drug Table: Posterior and Anterior Pituitary Hormones.

Clomiphene and ganirelix are synthetic nonsteroidal compounds that bind to estrogen receptors, decreasing the amount of available estrogen receptors and causing the anterior pituitary to increase secretion of FSH and LH. These drugs are used to induce ovulation in anovulatory (nonovulating) women.

Adverse Reactions

Hormone-Associated Reactions

- Vasomotor flushes (which are like the hot flashes of menopause)
- Breast tenderness
- Abdominal discomfort, ovarian enlargement
- Hemoperitoneum (blood in the peritoneal cavity)

Generalized Reactions

- Nausea, vomiting
- Headache, irritability, restlessness, fatigue
- Edema and irritation at the injection site

LIFESPAN ALERT – Childbearing Women
Fetal effects have been demonstrated in animal studies when gonadotropins have been administered. Birth defects have been reported in human studies; therefore, gonadotropins should not be administered to women known to be pregnant.

Contraindications, Precautions, and Interactions

These drugs are contraindicated in patients who are hypersensitive to the drug or any component of the drug. The gonadotropins are contraindicated in patients with high gonadotropin levels, thyroid dysfunction, adrenal dysfunction, liver disease, abnormal bleeding, ovarian cysts, or sex hormone–dependent tumors, or those with an organic intracranial lesion (pituitary tumor). Gonadotropins are contraindicated during pregnancy (category X).

These drugs are used cautiously in patients with epilepsy, migraine headaches, asthma, or cardiac or renal dysfunction, and during lactation. There are no known clinically significant interactions with the gonadotropins.

NURSING PROCESS
PATIENT RECEIVING A GONADOTROPIN

ASSESSMENT

Preadministration Assessment
These drugs are almost always administered on an outpatient basis. Before prescribing any of these drugs, the primary health care provider takes a thorough medical history and performs a physical examination. Additional laboratory and diagnostic tests for ovarian function and tubal patency may also be performed. The nurse takes and records the patient's vital signs and weight before therapy begins. A pelvic examination may be performed by the primary health care provider to rule out ovarian enlargement, pregnancy, or uterine problems.

Ongoing Assessment
At the time of each office or clinic visit, the nurse questions the patient regarding the occurrence of adverse reactions and records the patient's vital signs and weight.

NURSING DIAGNOSES

Drug-specific nursing diagnoses include the following:

❑ **Acute Pain** related to adverse reactions (ovarian enlargement, irritation at the injection site)
❑ **Anxiety** related to inability to conceive, treatment outcome, other factors

Nursing diagnoses related to drug administration are discussed in Chapter 4.

PLANNING

The expected outcomes of the patient may include an optimal response to drug therapy, support of patient needs related to the management of adverse reactions, reduction in anxiety, and an understanding of the therapeutic regimen.

IMPLEMENTATION

Promoting an Optimal Response to Therapy
Clomiphene is an oral tablet prescribed for 5 days and is self-administered in the outpatient setting.

> **NURSING ALERT**
> If the patient complains of visual disturbances, the drug therapy is discontinued and the primary health care provider notified. An examination by an ophthalmologist is usually indicated.

The patient is observed for symptoms of ovarian stimulation (abdominal pain, distention, sudden ovarian enlargement, ascites). If symptoms occur, therapy is discontinued and the primary health care provider is notified.

Monitoring and Managing Patient Needs

ACUTE PAIN. Gonadotropin injections are given in the primary health care provider's office or clinic. These drugs are administered IM or subcut because they are destroyed in the gastrointestinal (GI) tract. The nurse should rotate sites and examine previous sites for redness and irritation. Female patients taking these drugs are usually examined by the primary health care provider every other day during treatment and at 2-week intervals to detect excessive ovarian stimulation, called **hyperstimulation syndrome** (sudden ovarian enlargement with ascites). The patient may or may not report pain. This syndrome usually develops quickly, within 3 to 4 days.

> **NURSING ALERT**
> The patient is checked for signs of excessive ovarian enlargement (abdominal distention, pain, ascites [with serious cases]). The drug is discontinued at the first sign of ovarian stimulation or enlargement. The patient is usually admitted to the hospital for supportive measures.

ANXIETY. Patients who want to become pregnant often experience a great deal of anxiety. In addition, when taking these drugs, the patient faces the possibility of multiple births. The success rate of these drugs varies and depends on many factors. The primary health care provider usually discusses the value of this, as well as other approaches, with the patient and her sexual partner. The nurse allows the patient time to talk about her problems or concerns about the proposed treatment program.

Educating the Patient and Family
Patients are instructed by the primary health care provider about the frequency of sexual intercourse. The nurse should assess whether the patient understands the directions given by the primary health care provider. When a gonadotropin is prescribed, the nurse should instruct the patient taking the hormone to keep all primary health care provider appointments and to report adverse reactions to the nurse or primary health care provider. The nurse includes the following information when a gonadotropin is prescribed:

HORMONAL OVARIAN STIMULANTS.
• Before beginning therapy, be aware of the possibility of multiple births and birth defects.
• It is a good idea to use a calendar to track the treatment schedule and ovulation.
• Report bloating, abdominal pain, flushing, breast tenderness, and pain at the injection site.

NONHORMONAL OVARIAN STIMULANTS.
• Take the drug as prescribed (5 days) and do not stop taking the drug before the course of therapy is finished unless told to do so by the primary health care provider.

- Notify the primary health care provider if bloating, stomach or pelvic pain, jaundice, blurred vision, hot flashes, breast discomfort, headache, nausea, or vomiting occurs.
- Keep in mind that if ovulation does not occur after the first course of therapy, a second or third course may be used. If therapy does not succeed after three courses, the drug is considered unsuccessful and is discontinued.

EVALUATION

- Therapeutic effect is achieved.
- Adverse reactions are identified, reported to the primary health care provider, and managed successfully through appropriate nursing interventions:
  - ☑ Patient is free of pain.
  - ☑ Anxiety is managed successfully.
- Patient demonstrates an understanding of the drug regimen.

Growth Hormone

GH, also called *somatotropic hormone*, is secreted by the anterior pituitary. This hormone regulates the growth of the individual until approximately early adulthood or the time when the person no longer gains height.

Action and Uses

GH is available as the synthetic product somatropin. Of recombinant DNA origin, somatropin is identical to human GH and produces skeletal growth in children. This drug is administered to children who have not grown because of a deficiency of pituitary GH; it must be used before closure of the child's bone epiphyses. Bone epiphyses are the ends of bones. They are separated from the main bone but joined to it by cartilage, which allows for growth or lengthening of the bone. GH is ineffective in patients with closed epiphyses, because when the epiphyses close, growth (in length) can no longer occur.

Adverse Reactions

Somatropin causes few adverse reactions when administered as directed. Antibodies to somatropin may develop in a small number of patients, resulting in a failure to experience response to therapy, namely, failure of the drug to produce growth in the child. Some patients may experience hypothyroidism or insulin resistance. Swelling, joint pain, and muscle pain may also occur.

Contraindications, Precautions, and Interactions

Somatropin is contraindicated in patients with known hypersensitivity to somatropin or sensitivity to benzyl alcohol, and those with epiphyseal closure or underlying cranial lesions (e.g., pituitary tumor). The drug is used cautiously in patients with thyroid disease or diabetes, and during pregnancy (category C) and lactation. Excessive amounts of **glucocorticoids** may decrease the response to somatropin.

NURSING PROCESS
PATIENT RECEIVING GROWTH HORMONE

ASSESSMENT

Preadministration Assessment
A thorough physical examination and laboratory and diagnostic tests are performed before a child is accepted into a GH program. Before therapy starts, the nurse takes and records the patient's vital signs, height, and weight.

Ongoing Assessment
Children may increase their growth rate from 3.5 to 4 cm/year before treatment to 8 to 10 cm/year during the first year of treatment. Each time the child visits the primary health care provider's office or clinic (usually every 3 to 6 months), the nurse measures and records the child's height and weight to evaluate the response to therapy. Bone age is monitored periodically for growth and to detect epiphyseal closure, at which time therapy must stop.

NURSING DIAGNOSES

A key nursing diagnosis for patients receiving GH therapy is:

- ❏ **Disturbed Body Image** related to changes in appearance, physical size, or failure to grow

Nursing diagnoses related to drug administration are discussed in Chapter 4.

PLANNING

The expected outcomes of the patient may include an optimal response to drug therapy, support of patient needs related to the management of adverse reactions, reduction in anxiety, and an understanding of the therapeutic regimen.

IMPLEMENTATION

Promoting an Optimal Response to Therapy
GH is administered subcutaneously. The vial containing the hormone is not shaken but swirled to mix. The solution is clear; the nurse should not administer it if it is cloudy. The weekly dosage is divided and given in three to seven doses throughout the week. The drug may (if possible) be given at bedtime to adhere most closely to the body's natural release of the hormone. Periodic testing of GH levels, glucose tolerance, and thyroid function may be done during treatment.

Monitoring and Managing Patient Needs
DISTURBED BODY IMAGE. Children requiring treatment are usually of short stature. The parents, and sometimes the children, may be concerned about the success or possible failure of treatment with GH. The child is provided with

the opportunity to share fears, concerns, or anger. The nurse acknowledges these feelings as normal and corrects any misconceptions the child or parents may have concerning treatment. Families may be surprised by the growth changes once treatment is started. Children may experience stretch marks or sizable changes in body structure and appearance. A child may become shy, reserved, or uncomfortable with his or her new body image. Time is allowed for the parents and children to ask questions not only before therapy is started but during the months of treatment.

Educating the Patient and Family

When the patient is receiving GH, the primary health care provider discusses in detail the therapeutic regimen for increasing growth (height) with the child's parents or guardians. If the drug is to be given at bedtime and not in the outpatient clinic, the nurse instructs the parents on the proper injection technique. The parents are encouraged to keep all clinic or office visits with the child. The nurse explains that the child may experience sudden growth and increase in appetite and instructs the parents to report lack of growth, symptoms of diabetes (e.g., increased hunger, increased thirst, or frequent voiding) or symptoms of hypothyroidism (e.g., fatigue, dry skin, intolerance to cold).

EVALUATION

- Therapeutic effect is achieved and the child grows in height.
- Adverse reactions are identified, reported to the primary health care provider, and managed successfully through appropriate nursing interventions:
  ☑ Positive body image is maintained.
- Patient and family demonstrate an understanding of the drug regimen.

Adrenocorticotropic Hormone (ACTH): Corticotropin

Actions and Uses

Corticotropin (ACTH) is an anterior pituitary hormone that stimulates the adrenal cortex to produce and secrete adrenocortical hormones, primarily the glucocorticoids. Corticotropin is used for diagnostic testing of adrenocortical function. This drug may also be used for managing acute exacerbations of multiple sclerosis, nonsuppurative thyroiditis, and hypercalcemia associated with cancer. It is also used as an anti-inflammatory and immunosuppressant drug when conventional glucocorticoid therapy has not been effective (Display 44.1).

Adverse Reactions

Because ACTH stimulates the release of glucocorticoids from the adrenal gland, adverse reactions seen with the administration of this hormone are similar to those seen with the glucocorticoids (Display 44.2) and affect many body systems.

Contraindications and Precautions

ACTH is contraindicated in patients with adrenocortical insufficiency or hyperfunction, allergy to pork or pork products (corticotropin is obtained from porcine pituitaries), systemic fungal infections, ocular herpes simplex, scleroderma, osteoporosis, and hypertension. Patients taking ACTH also should avoid any vaccinations with live virus.

ACTH is used cautiously in patients with diabetes, diverticulosis, renal insufficiency, myasthenia gravis, tuberculosis (may reactivate the disease), hypothyroidism, cirrhosis, nonspecific ulcerative colitis, heart failure, seizures, or febrile infections. The drug is classified as a pregnancy category C

DISPLAY 44.1 Uses of Glucocorticoids

- **Endocrine disorders:** Primary or secondary adrenal cortical insufficiency, congenital adrenal hyperplasia, nonsuppurative thyroiditis, hypercalcemia associated with cancer
- **Rheumatic disorders:** Short-term management of acute ankylosing spondylitis, acute and subacute bursitis, acute nonspecific tenosynovitis, acute gouty arthritis, psoriatic arthritis, rheumatoid arthritis, post-traumatic osteoarthritis, synovitis of osteoarthritis, epicondylitis
- **Collagen diseases:** Systemic lupus erythematosus, acute rheumatic carditis, systemic dermatomyositis
- **Dermatologic disorders:** Pemphigus, bullous dermatitis herpetiformis, severe erythema multiforme (Stevens-Johnson syndrome), exfoliative dermatitis, mycosis fungoides, severe psoriasis, severe seborrheic dermatitis, angioedema, urticaria, various skin disorders (e.g., lichen planus or keloids)
- **Allergic states:** Control of severe or incapacitating allergic conditions not controlled by other methods, bronchial asthma (including status asthmaticus), contact dermatitis, atopic dermatitis, serum sickness, drug hypersensitivity reactions

- **Ophthalmic diseases:** Severe acute and chronic allergic and inflammatory processes, keratitis, allergic corneal marginal ulcers, herpes zoster of the eye, iritis, iridocyclitis, chorioretinitis, diffuse posterior uveitis, optic neuritis, sympathetic ophthalmia, anterior segment inflammation
- **Respiratory diseases:** Seasonal allergic rhinitis, berylliosis, fulminating or disseminating pulmonary tuberculosis, aspiration pneumonia
- **Hematologic disorders:** Idiopathic or secondary thrombocytopenic purpura, hemolytic anemia, red blood cell anemia, congenital hypoplastic anemia
- **Neoplastic diseases:** Leukemia, lymphomas
- **Edematous states:** Induction of diuresis or remission of proteinuria in nephrotic syndrome
- **Gastrointestinal diseases:** During critical period of ulcerative colitis, regional enteritis, intractable sprue
- **Nervous system disorders:** Acute exacerbations of multiple sclerosis

DISPLAY 44.2 Adverse Reactions Associated With Glucocorticoids

- **Fluid and electrolyte disturbances:** Sodium and fluid retention, potassium loss, hypokalemic alkalosis, hypertension, hypocalcemia, hypotension or shocklike reactions
- **Musculoskeletal disturbances:** Muscle weakness, loss of muscle mass, tendon rupture, osteoporosis, aseptic necrosis of femoral and humeral heads, spontaneous fractures
- **Cardiovascular disturbances:** Thromboembolism or fat embolism, thrombophlebitis, necrotizing angiitis, syncopal episodes, cardiac arrhythmias, aggravation of hypertension, fatal cardiac arrhythmias with rapid, high-dose IV methylprednisolone administration, congestive heart failure in susceptible patients
- **Gastrointestinal disturbances:** Pancreatitis, abdominal distention, ulcerative esophagitis, nausea, vomiting, increased appetite and weight gain, possible peptic ulcer or bowel perforation, hemorrhage
- **Dermatologic disturbances:** Impaired wound healing, thin, fragile skin, petechiae, ecchymoses, erythema, increased sweating, suppression of skin test reactions, subcutaneous fat atrophy, purpura, striae, hirsutism, acneiform eruptions, urticaria, angioneurotic edema, perineal itch
- **Neurologic disturbances:** Convulsions, increased intracranial pressure with papilledema (usually after treatment is discontinued), vertigo, headache, neuritis or paresthesia, steroid psychosis, insomnia
- **Endocrine disturbances:** Amenorrhea, other menstrual irregularities, development of cushingoid state, suppression of growth in children, secondary adrenocortical and pituitary unresponsive (particularly in times of stress), decreased carbohydrate tolerance, manifestation of latent diabetes mellitus, increased requirements for insulin or oral hypoglycemic agents (in diabetic patients)
- **Ophthalmic disturbances:** Posterior subcapsular cataracts, increased intraocular pressure, glaucoma, exophthalmos
- **Metabolic disturbances:** Negative nitrogen balance (due to protein catabolism)
- **Other disturbances:** Anaphylactoid or hypersensitivity reactions, aggravation of existing infections, malaise, increase or decrease in sperm motility and number

drug and is used cautiously during pregnancy and lactation. ACTH also is used cautiously in children because it can inhibit skeletal growth.

Interactions

Live virus vaccines received while the patient is taking ACTH may potentiate virus replication, increase any adverse reaction to the vaccine, and decrease the patient's antibody response to the vaccine.

Interacting Drug	Common Use	Effect of Interaction
amphotericin B	Anti-infective	Increased risk of hypokalemia
diuretics	Fluid retention/cardiac problems	Increased risk of hypokalemia
insulin or oral antidiabetic	Diabetes management	Increased need for antidiabetic medication

Interacting Drug	Common Use	Effect of Interaction
barbiturates	Sedation	Decreased effect of ACTH
cholinergic blockers	Decrease of spasms or secretions; treatment of Parkinson's disease	Decreased muscle function

NURSING PROCESS
PATIENT RECEIVING CORTICOTROPIN (ACTH)

ASSESSMENT

Preadministration Assessment
Before administering ACTH, the nurse reviews the patient's chart for the diagnosis, laboratory tests, and other pertinent information. The nurse obtains the patient's weight and assesses skin integrity, lungs, and mental status. The nurse takes and records vital signs. Additional assessments depend on the patient's condition and diagnosis. The primary health care provider may order baseline diagnostic tests, such as chest or upper GI x-ray studies and serum electrolytes, urinalysis, or complete blood count.

Ongoing Assessment
The nurse monitors the patient's weight and fluid intake and output daily during therapy. The nurse observes for and reports any evidence of edema, such as weight gain, rales, increased pulse or dyspnea, or swollen extremities. The nurse monitors blood glucose levels for a rise in blood glucose concentration. In addition, the nurse checks stools for evidence of bleeding (dark or tarry in color, positive guaiac test result). Patients receiving prolonged therapy should have periodic hematologic, serum electrolyte, and serum glucose studies.

NURSING DIAGNOSES

Drug-specific nursing diagnoses include the following:

- ❏ **Risk for Infection** related to masking of signs of infection
- ❏ **Disturbed Thought Processes** related to adverse drug reactions

Nursing diagnoses related to drug administration are discussed in Chapter 4.

PLANNING

The expected outcomes of the patient may include an optimal response to therapy, support of patient needs related to the management of adverse reactions, and an understanding of the therapeutic regimen.

IMPLEMENTATION

Promoting an Optimal Response to Therapy
Nursing management depends on the patient's diagnosis and physical status and the reason for use of the drug. The nurse may need to assess vital signs every 4 hours

and observe for the adverse reactions that occur with glucocorticoid administration.

This drug may be given by the IV, subcut, or IM routes. During parenteral administration of ACTH, the nurse observes the patient for hypersensitivity reactions. Symptoms of hypersensitivity include rash, urticaria, hypotension, tachycardia, or difficulty breathing. If the drug is given IM or subcut, the nurse observes the patient for hypersensitivity reactions immediately and for about 2 hours after the drug is given. If a hypersensitivity reaction occurs, the nurse notifies the primary health care provider immediately. Long-term use increases the risk of hypersensitivity.

Monitoring and Managing Patient Needs

RISK FOR INFECTION. Corticotropin may mask signs of infection, including fungal or viral eye infections.

> **NURSING ALERT**
> The nurse instructs the patient taking ACTH to report any complaints of sore throat, cough, fever, malaise, sores that do not heal, or redness or irritation of the eyes.

There may be a decreased resistance and inability to identify the source of the infection. The nurse instructs the patient or family to observe the skin daily for localized signs of infection, especially at injection sites or IV access sites. Visitors are monitored to protect the patient against those with infectious illness.

DISTURBED THOUGHT PROCESSES. Corticotropin can also cause disturbances in the psyche. The nurse must report any evidence of behavior change, such as mental depression, insomnia, euphoria, mood swings, or nervousness. If disturbances occur, the nurse encourages communication with the staff and family members, provides a quiet, nonthreatening environment, and spends time actively listening as the patient talks. It is important to encourage verbalization of fears and concerns. Anxiety usually decreases with understanding of the therapeutic regimen. The nurse allows time for a thorough explanation of the drug regimen and answering of questions.

Educating the Patient and Family
The nurse includes the following in a teaching plan for the patient receiving ACTH:

- Report any adverse reactions.
- Avoid contact with those who have an infection, because resistance to infection may be decreased.
- Report any symptoms of infection immediately (e.g., sore throat, fever, cough, or sores that do not heal).
- Patients with diabetes—Monitor blood glucose (if self-monitoring is being done) or urine closely and notify the primary health care provider if glucose appears in the urine or the blood glucose level increases significantly. An increase in the dosage of the oral antidiabetic drug or insulin may be needed.
- Notify the primary health care provider of a marked weight gain, swelling in the extremities, muscle

weakness, persistent headache, visual disturbances, or behavior change.

EVALUATION

- Therapeutic effect is achieved.
- Adverse reactions are identified, reported to the primary health care provider, and managed using appropriate nursing interventions:
  ☑ No evidence of infection is seen.
  ☑ Orientation and mentation remain intact.
- Patient demonstrates an understanding of the drug regimen.

•ADRENOCORTICAL HORMONES

The adrenal gland lies on the superior surface of each kidney. It is a double organ composed of an outer cortex and an inner medulla. In response to ACTH secreted by the anterior pituitary, the adrenal cortex secretes several hormones (glucocorticoids, **mineralocorticoids**, and small amounts of sex hormones).

This section of the chapter discusses the hormones produced by the adrenal cortex or the adrenocortical hormones, which are the glucocorticoids and mineralocorticoids. These hormones are essential to life and influence many organs and structures of the body. The glucocorticoids and mineralocorticoids are collectively called *corticosteroids*.

Glucocorticoids

Glucocorticoids influence or regulate functions such as the immune response, glucose, fat, and protein metabolism, and the anti-inflammatory response. Table 44.1 describes the activity of glucocorticoids in the body.

Actions

Glucocorticoids enter target cells and bind to receptors, initiating many complex reactions in the body. Some of the actions are considered undesirable, depending on the indication for which these drugs are used. Examples of the glucocorticoids include cortisone, hydrocortisone, prednisone, prednisolone, and triamcinolone. The Summary Drug Table: Adrenocortical Hormones: Glucocorticoids and Mineralocorticoids provides information concerning these hormones.

Uses

Glucocorticoids are used to treat the following:

- Adrenocortical insufficiency (replacement therapy)
- Allergic reactions
- Collagen diseases (e.g., systemic lupus erythematosus)
- Dermatologic conditions
- Rheumatic disorders
- Shock
- Multiple other conditions (see Display 44.1)

Table 44.1 Activity of Glucocorticoids in the Body

Function Within the Body	Description of Bodily Activity
Anti-inflammatory	Stabilizes lysosomal membrane and prevents the release of proteolytic enzymes during the inflammatory process.
Regulation of blood pressure	Potentiates vasoconstrictor action of norepinephrine. Without glucocorticoids the vasoconstricting action is decreased, and blood pressure decreases.
Metabolism of carbohydrates and protein	Facilitates the breakdown of protein in the muscle, leading to increased plasma amino acid levels. Increases activity of enzymes necessary for glucogenesis, producing hyperglycemia, which can aggravate diabetes, precipitate latent diabetes, and cause insulin resistance.
Metabolism of fat	A complex phenomenon that promotes the use of fat for energy (a positive effect) and permits fat stores to accumulate in the body, causing buffalo hump and moon-shaped or round face (a negative effect).
Interference with the immune response	Decreases the production of lymphocytes and eosinophils in the blood by causing atrophy of the thymus gland; blocks the release of cytokines, resulting in a decreased performance of T and B monocytes in the immune response. (This action, coupled with the anti-inflammatory action, makes the corticosteroids useful in delaying organ rejection in patients with transplants.)
Protection during stress	As a protective mechanism, the corticosteroids are released during periods of stress (e.g., injury or surgery). The release of epinephrine or norepinephrine by the adrenal medulla during stress has a synergistic effect along with the corticosteroids.
Central nervous system responses	Affects mood and possibly causes neuronal or brain excitability, causing euphoria, anxiety, depression, psychosis, and an increase in motor activity in some individuals.

The anti-inflammatory activity of these hormones makes them valuable for suppressing inflammation and modifying the immune response.

Adverse Reactions

The adverse reactions that may result from the administration of the glucocorticoids are given in Display 44.2. Long- or short-term high-dose therapy may also produce many of the signs and symptoms seen with **Cushing's syndrome**, a disease caused by the overproduction of endogenous glucocorticoids. Some of the signs and symptoms of this Cushing-like (cushingoid) state include a buffalo hump (a hump on the back of the neck), moon face, oily skin and acne, osteoporosis, purple striae on the abdomen and hips, altered skin pigmentation, and weight gain. When a serious disease or disorder is treated, it is often necessary to allow these effects to occur, because therapy with these drugs is absolutely necessary.

Contraindications, Precautions, and Interactions

Glucocorticoids are contraindicated in patients with serious infections, such as tuberculosis and fungal and antibiotic-resistant infections. Glucocorticoids are administered with

caution to patients with renal or hepatic disease, hypothyroidism, ulcerative colitis, diverticulitis, peptic ulcer disease, inflammatory bowel disease, hypertension, osteoporosis, convulsive disorders, or diabetes. Glucocorticoids are classified as pregnancy category C drugs and should be used with caution during pregnancy and lactation.

Multiple drug interactions may occur with the glucocorticoids. Table 44.2 identifies selected clinically significant interactions.

Mineralocorticoids

Actions and Uses

The natural mineralocorticoids consist of aldosterone and desoxycorticosterone and play an important role in conserving sodium and increasing potassium excretion. Because of these activities, mineralocorticoids are important in controlling salt and water balance. Aldosterone is the more potent of these two hormones. Deficiencies of mineralocorticoids result in a loss of sodium and water and a retention of potassium. Fludrocortisone (Florinef) is a drug that has both glucocorticoid and mineralocorticoid activity and is the only currently available mineralocorticoid drug. Fludrocortisone is used for replacement therapy for primary and secondary adrenocortical deficiency. Even though this drug has both

Summary Drug Table ADRENOCORTICAL HORMONES: GLUCOCORTICOIDS AND MINERALOCORTICOIDS

Generic Name	Trade Name	Uses	Adverse Reactions	Dosage Ranges
Glucocorticoids				
betamethasone *bay-tah-meth'-ah-zoan*	Celestone	See Display 44.1	See Display 44.2	Individualize dosage; syrup or injectable, see package insert
budesonide *byoo-dess'-oh-nyde*	Entocort EC	Crohn's disease	See Display 44.2	9 mg QD in AM for 8 wks
cortisone *kore'-tih-zoan*		See Display 44.1	See Display 44.2	25–300 mg/day orally
dexamethasone *dex-ah-meth'-ah-zoan*	Decadron	Cerebral edema, other conditions listed in Display 44.1	See Display 44.2	Individualize dosage based on severity of condition and response
hydrocortisone (cortisol) *hye-droe-kore'-tih-zoan*	Cortef, Solu-Cortef, A-hydroCort	See Display 44.1	See Display 44.2	Individualize dosage based on severity of condition and response
methylprednisolone *meh-thill-pred-niss'-oh-loan*	Medrol, Depo-Medrol, Solu-Medrol	See Display 44.1	See Display 44.2	Individualize dosage based on severity of condition and response
prednisolone *pred-niss'-oh-loan*	Prelone	See Display 44.1	See Display 44.2	200 mg/day for 1 wk, then 80 mg every other day
prednisone *pred'-nih-zoan*		See Display 44.1	See Display 44.2	Individualize dosage: initial dose usually between 5 and 60 mg/day orally
triamcinolone *trye-am-sin'-oh-loan*	Aristospan, Kenalog	See Display 44.1	See Display 44.2	Joint and soft tissue injection: 2–80 mg
Mineralocorticoid				
fludrocortisone *floo-droe-kore'-tih-zoan*	Florinef	Partial replacement therapy for Addison's disease, salt-losing adrenogenital syndrome	See Display 44.2	0.1 mg 3 times a week to 0.2 mg/day orally

mineralocorticoid and glucocorticoid activity, it is used only for its mineralocorticoid effects.

Adverse Reactions

Adverse reactions may occur if the dosage is too high or prolonged or if withdrawal is too rapid. Administration of fludrocortisone may cause:

• Edema, hypertension, congestive heart failure, enlargement of the heart
• Increased sweating, allergic skin rash
• Hypokalemia, muscular weakness, headache, hypersensitivity reactions

Because this drug has glucocorticoid and mineralocorticoid activity and is often given with glucocorticoids, adverse reactions of glucocorticoids must be closely monitored as well (see Display 44.2).

Contraindications, Precautions, and Interactions

Fludrocortisone is contraindicated in patients with hypersensitivity to fludrocortisone and those with systemic fungal infections. Fludrocortisone is used cautiously in patients with Addison's disease or infection, and during pregnancy (category C) and lactation. Fludrocortisone decreases the effects of the barbiturates, hydantoins, and rifampin. There is a decrease in serum levels of salicylates when those agents are administered with fludrocortisone.

Table 44.2 Selected Drug Interactions of Glucocorticoids

Precipitant drug	Object drug	Description
barbiturates	corticosteroids	Decreased pharmacologic effects of the corticosteroid may be observed.
cholestyramine	hydrocortisone	Effects of hydrocortisone may be decreased.
oral contraceptives	corticosteroids	Corticosteroid concentration may be increased and clearance decreased.
estrogens	corticosteroids	Corticosteroid clearance may be decreased.
hydantoins	corticosteroids	Corticosteroid clearance may be increased, resulting in reduced therapeutic effects.
ketoconazole	corticosteroids	Corticosteroid clearance may be decreased.
rifampin	corticosteroids	Corticosteroid clearance may be increased, resulting in decreased therapeutic effects.
corticosteroids	anticholinesterases	Anticholinesterase effects may be antagonized in myasthenia gravis.
corticosteroids	oral anticoagulants	Anticoagulant dose requirements may be reduced. Corticosteroids may decrease the anticoagulant action.
corticosteroids	digitalis glycosides	Coadministration may enhance the possibility of digitalis toxicity associated with hypokalemia.
corticosteroids	isoniazid	Isoniazid serum concentrations may be decreased.
corticosteroids	potassium-depleting diuretics	Hypokalemia may occur.
corticosteroids	salicylates	Corticosteroids will reduce serum salicylate levels and may decrease their effectiveness.
corticosteroids	somatrem	Growth-promoting effect of somatrem may be inhibited.
corticosteroids	theophyllines	Alterations in the pharmacologic activity of either agent may occur.

NURSING PROCESS
PATIENT RECEIVING A GLUCOCORTICOID OR MINERALOCORTICOID

ASSESSMENT

Preadministration Assessment
Before administering a glucocorticoid or mineralocorticoid, the nurse takes and records the patient's blood pressure, pulse, and respiratory rate. Additional physical assessments depend on the reason for use and the general condition of the patient. When feasible, the nurse performs an assessment of the area of disease involvement, such as the respiratory tract or skin, and records the findings in the patient's record. These findings provide baseline data for evaluating the patient's response to drug therapy. The nurse weighs patients who are acutely ill and those with a serious systemic disease before starting therapy.

Ongoing Assessment
Ongoing assessments of the patient receiving a glucocorticoid, and the frequency of these assessments, depend largely on the disease being treated. The nurse should take and record vital signs every 4 to 8 hours. The nurse also weighs the patient daily to weekly, depending on the diagnosis and the primary health care provider's orders. The patient's response to the drug is assessed by daily evaluations. More frequent assessment may be necessary if a glucocorticoid is used for emergency situations. Because these drugs are used to treat many diseases and conditions, an evaluation of drug response is based on the patient's diagnosis and the signs and symptoms of disease.

The nurse assesses for signs of adverse effects of the mineralocorticoid or glucocorticoid, particularly signs of electrolyte imbalance, such as hypocalcemia, hypokalemia, and hypernatremia (see Chapter 55). The nurse assesses the patient's mental status for any change, especially if there is a history of depression or other psychiatric problems or if high doses of the drug are prescribed. The nurse also monitors for signs of an infection, which may be masked by glucocorticoid therapy. The blood of the patient without diabetes is checked weekly for glucose levels because glucocorticoids may aggravate latent diabetes. Those with diabetes must be checked more frequently.

When administering fludrocortisone, the nurse monitors the patient's blood pressure at frequent intervals. Hypotension may indicate insufficient dosage. The nurse weighs the patient daily and assesses for edema, particularly swelling of the feet and hands. The lungs are auscultated for adventitious sounds (e.g., rales/crackles).

NURSING DIAGNOSES

Drug-specific nursing diagnoses include the following:

❏ **Risk for Infection** related to immune suppression or impaired wound healing
❏ **Risk for Injury** related to muscle atrophy, osteoporosis, or spontaneous fractures
❏ **Acute Pain** related to epigastric distress of gastric ulcer formation
❏ **Excess Fluid Volume** related to adverse reactions (sodium and water retention)
❏ **Disturbed Body Image** related to adverse reactions (cushingoid appearance)

Nursing diagnoses related to drug administration are discussed in Chapter 4.

PLANNING

The expected outcomes of the patient include an optimal response to therapy, support of patient needs related to the management of adverse reactions, and an understanding of the therapeutic regimen.

IMPLEMENTATION

Promoting an Optimal Response to Therapy

Glucocorticoids may be administered orally, IM, subcut, IV, topically, or as an inhalant. The primary health care provider may also inject the drug into a joint (intra-articular), a lesion (intralesional), soft tissue, or bursa. The drug dosage is individualized and based on the severity of the condition and the patient's response.

> **! NURSING ALERT**
>
> The nurse must never omit a dose of a glucocorticoid. If the patient cannot take the drug orally because of nausea or vomiting, the nurse must notify the primary health care provider immediately, because the drug needs to be ordered given by the parenteral route. Patients who can receive nothing by mouth for any reason must have the glucocorticoid given by the parenteral route.

Daily oral doses are usually given before 9 AM to minimize adrenal suppression and to coincide with normal adrenal function. However, alternate-day therapy may be prescribed for patients receiving long-term therapy. Fludrocortisone is given orally and is well tolerated in the GI tract.

> **LIFESPAN ALERT – Gerontology**
>
> Corticosteroids are administered with caution in older adults, because they are more likely to have preexisting conditions, such as congestive heart failure, hypertension, osteoporosis, and arthritis, which may be worsened by use

of such agents. The nurse monitors older adults for exacerbation of existing conditions during corticosteroid therapy. In addition, lower dosages may be needed because of the effects of aging, such as decreases in muscle mass, renal function, and plasma volume.

ALTERNATE-DAY THERAPY. The alternate-day therapy approach to glucocorticoid administration is used in treating diseases and disorders requiring long-term therapy, especially arthritic disorders. This regimen involves giving twice the daily dose of the glucocorticoid every other day. The drug is given only once on the alternate day, before 9 AM. The purpose of alternate-day administration is to provide the patient requiring long-term glucocorticoid therapy with the beneficial effects of the drug while minimizing certain undesirable reactions (see Display 44.2).

Plasma levels of the endogenous adrenocortical hormones vary throughout the day and nighttime hours. They are normally higher between 2 AM and 8 AM and lower between 4 PM and midnight. When plasma levels are lower, the anterior pituitary releases ACTH, which in turn stimulates the adrenal cortex to manufacture and release glucocorticoids. When plasma levels are high, the pituitary gland does not release ACTH. The response of the pituitary to high or low plasma levels of glucocorticoids and the resulting release or nonrelease of ACTH is an example of the **feedback mechanism**, which may also be seen in other glands of the body, such as the thyroid gland.

The feedback mechanism (also called the *feedback control*) is the method by which the body maintains most hormones at relatively constant levels in the bloodstream. When the hormone concentration falls, the rate of production of that hormone increases. Likewise, when the hormone level becomes too high, the body decreases production of that hormone.

Administration of a short-acting glucocorticoid on alternate days and before 9 AM, when glucocorticoid plasma levels are still relatively high, does not affect the release of ACTH later in the day yet gives the patient the benefit of exogenous glucocorticoid therapy.

PATIENT WITH DIABETES. Patients with diabetes who are receiving a glucocorticoid may require frequent adjustment of their insulin or oral hypoglycemic drug dosage. The nurse monitors blood glucose levels several times daily or as prescribed by the primary health care provider. If the blood glucose levels increase or urine is positive for glucose or ketones, the nurse notifies the primary health care provider. Some patients may have latent (hidden) diabetes. In these cases, the corticosteroid may precipitate hyperglycemia. Therefore, all patients, those with diabetes and those without, should have blood glucose levels checked frequently.

ADRENAL INSUFFICIENCY. Administration of the glucocorticoids poses the threat of adrenal gland insufficiency (particularly if the alternate-day therapy is not prescribed). Administration of glucocorticoids several times a day and during a short time (as little as 5 to 10 days) results in shutting off the pituitary release of ACTH, because there are always high levels of glucocorticoids in the plasma (caused by the body's own glucocorticoid production plus the administration of a glucocorticoid drug). Eventually, the pituitary atrophies and ceases to release ACTH. Without ACTH, the adrenals fail to manufacture and release (endogenous) glucocorticoids. When this happens, the patient has acute **adrenal insufficiency**, which is a life-threatening situation until corrected with the administration of an exogenous glucocorticoid.

Adrenal insufficiency is a critical deficiency of mineralocorticoids and glucocorticoids; the disorder requires immediate treatment. Symptoms of adrenal insufficiency include fever, myalgia, arthralgia, malaise, anorexia, nausea, orthostatic hypotension, dizziness, fainting, dyspnea, and hypoglycemia. Death due to circulatory collapse will result unless the condition is treated promptly. Situations producing stress (e.g., trauma, surgery, severe illness) may precipitate the need for an increase in dosage of corticosteroids until the crisis or stressful situation is resolved.

! NURSING ALERT

Glucocorticoid therapy should never be discontinued suddenly. When administration of a glucocorticoid extends beyond 5 days and the drug therapy is to be discontinued, the dosage must be reduced gradually (tapered) over several days. In some instances, it may be necessary to taper the dose over 7 to 10 or more days. Abrupt discontinuation of glucocorticoid therapy usually results in acute adrenal insufficiency, which, if not recognized in time, can result in death. Tapering the dosage allows normal adrenal function to return gradually, thereby preventing adrenal insufficiency.

Monitoring and Managing Patient Needs

RISK FOR INFECTION. The nurse should report any slight rise in temperature, sore throat, or other signs of infection to the primary health care provider as soon as possible, because decreased resistance to infection may occur during glucocorticoid therapy. Nursing personnel and visitors with any type of infection or recent exposure to an infectious disease should avoid patient contact.

RISK FOR INJURY. The nurse observes patients receiving long-term glucocorticoid therapy, especially those allowed limited activity, for signs of compression fractures of the vertebrae and pathologic fractures of the long bones. If the patient reports back or bone pain, the nurse notifies the primary health care provider. Extra care is also necessary to prevent falls and other injuries when the patient is confused or is allowed out of bed. If the patient is weak, the nurse assists the patient to the bathroom or when ambulating. Edematous extremities are handled with care to prevent trauma.

ACUTE PAIN. Peptic ulcer has been associated with glucocorticoid therapy. The nurse reports to the primary health care provider any patient complaints of epigastric burning or pain, bloody or coffee-ground emesis, or the passing of tarry stools. Giving oral corticosteroids with food or a full glass of water may minimize gastric irritation.

EXCESS FLUID VOLUME. Fluid and electrolyte imbalances, particularly excess fluid volume, are common with corticosteroid therapy. The nurse checks the patient for visible edema, keeps an accurate fluid intake and output record, obtains a daily weight, and restricts sodium if indicated by the primary health care provider. Edematous extremities are elevated and the patient's position is changed frequently. The nurse informs the primary health care provider if signs of electrolyte imbalance or glucocorticoid drug effects are noted. Dietary adjustments are made for the increased potassium loss and sodium retention if necessary. Consultation with a dietitian may be indicated.

DISTURBED BODY IMAGE. A body image disturbance may occur, especially if the patient experiences cushingoid effects (e.g., buffalo hump, moon face), acne, or hirsutism. If continuation of drug therapy is necessary, the nurse thoroughly explains the cushingoid appearance reaction and emphasizes the necessity of continuing the drug regimen. The nurse assesses the patient's emotional state and helps the patient express feelings and concerns. The nurse offers positive reinforcement, when possible. The nurse instructs the patient with acne to keep the affected areas clean and use over-the-counter acne drugs and water-based cosmetics or creams.

DISTURBED THOUGHT PROCESSES. Mental and emotional changes may occur when glucocorticoids are administered. The nurse accurately documents mental changes and informs the primary health care provider of their occurrence. Patients who appear extremely depressed must be closely observed. The nurse evaluates mental status, memory, and impaired thinking (e.g., changes in orientation, impaired judgment, thoughts of hopelessness, guilt). The nurse allows time for the patient to express feeling and concerns.

Educating the Patient and Family

To prevent noncompliance, the nurse must provide the patient and family with thorough instructions and warnings about the drug regimen:

- These drugs may cause GI upset. To decrease GI effects, take the oral drug with meals or snacks.
- Take antacids between meals to help prevent peptic ulcer.

SHORT-TERM GLUCOCORTICOID THERAPY.
- Take the drug exactly as directed in the prescription container. Do not increase, decrease, or omit a dose unless advised to do so by the primary health care provider.
- Take single daily doses before 9:00 AM.
- Follow the instructions for tapering the dose, because they are extremely important.
- If the problem does not improve, contact the primary health care provider.

ALTERNATE-DAY ORAL GLUCOCORTICOID THERAPY.

- Take this drug before 9 AM once every other day. Use a calendar or some other method to identify the days of each week to take the drug.
- Do not stop taking the drug unless advised to do so by the primary health care provider.
- If the problem becomes worse, especially on the days the drug is not taken, contact the primary health care provider.

Most of the following teaching points may also apply to alternate-day therapy, especially when higher doses are used and therapy extends over many months.

LONG-TERM OR HIGH-DOSE GLUCOCORTICOID THERAPY.

- Do not omit this drug or increase or decrease the dosage except on the advice of the primary health care provider.
- Inform other primary health care providers, dentists, and all medical personnel of therapy with this drug. Wear medical identification or another form of identification to alert medical personnel of long-term therapy with a glucocorticoid.
- Do not take any nonprescription drug unless its use has been approved by the primary health care provider.
- Do not receive live virus vaccines because of the risk for a lack of antibody response. (This does not include patients receiving corticosteroids as replacement therapy.)
- Whenever possible, avoid exposure to infections. Contact the primary health care provider if minor cuts or abrasions fail to heal, persistent joint swelling or tenderness is noted, or fever, sore throat, upper respiratory infection, or other signs of infection occur.
- If the drug cannot be taken orally for any reason or if diarrhea occurs, contact the primary health care provider immediately. If you are unable to contact the primary health care provider before the next dose is due, go to the nearest hospital emergency department (preferably where the original treatment was started or where the primary health care provider is on the hospital staff), because the drug must be given by injection.
- Weigh yourself weekly. If significant weight gain or swelling of the extremities is noted, contact the primary health care provider.
- Remember that dietary recommendations made by the primary health care provider are an important part of therapy and must be followed.
- Follow the primary health care provider's recommendations regarding periodic eye examinations and laboratory tests.

INTRA-ARTICULAR OR INTRALESIONAL ADMINISTRATION.

- Do not overuse the injected joint, even if the pain is gone.
- Follow the primary health care provider's instructions concerning rest and exercise.

MINERALOCORTICOID (FLUDROCORTISONE) THERAPY.

- Take the drug as directed. Do not increase or decrease the dosage except as instructed to do so by the primary health care provider.

- Do not discontinue use of the drug abruptly.
- Inform the primary health care provider if the following adverse reactions occur: edema, muscle weakness, weight gain, anorexia, swelling of the extremities, dizziness, severe headache, or shortness of breath.
- Carry patient identification, such as a MedicAlert tag, so that drug therapy will be known to medical personnel during an emergency situation.
- Keep follow-up appointments to determine if a dosage adjustment is necessary.

EVALUATION

- Therapeutic effect is achieved.
- Adverse reactions are identified, reported to the primary health care provider, and managed successfully through appropriate nursing interventions:
  - ☑ No evidence of infection is seen.
  - ☑ No evidence of injury is seen.
  - ☑ Patient is free of pain.
  - ☑ Fluid volume balance is maintained.
  - ☑ Positive body image is maintained.
  - ☑ Orientation and mentation remain intact.
- Patient demonstrates an understanding of the drug regimen.

THINK CRITICALLY: PHARMACOLOGY IN PRACTICE

1. At the skilled nursing facility, you are implementing a policy for drug administration. Discuss the rationale for changing and assuring administering oral prednisone at 7 AM on the medication record.

● Test Your Knowledge

1. Which of the following adverse reactions would the nurse expect with the administration of clomiphene?

   A. Edema
   B. Vasomotor flushes
   C. Sedation
   D. Hypertension

2. Which of the following signs would lead the nurse to suspect a cushingoid appearance adverse reaction in a patient taking a corticosteroid?

   A. Moon face, hirsutism
   B. Kyphosis, periorbital edema
   C. Pallor of the skin, acne
   D. Exophthalmos

3. Which of the following statements, if made by the patient, would indicate a possible adverse reaction to the administration of vasopressin?

   A. "I am unable to see well at night."
   B. "My stomach is cramping."
   C. "I have a sore throat."
   D. "I am hungry all the time."

4. Adverse reactions to the administration of fludrocortisone include _____.

   A. hyperactivity and headache
   B. sedation, lethargy
   C. edema, hypertension
   D. dyspnea, confusion

● Prepare for the NCLEX

1. Which of the following assessments would be most important for the nurse to make when a child receiving GH comes to the primary health care provider's office?

   A. Blood pressure, pulse, and respiration
   B. Diet history
   C. Height and weight
   D. Measurement of abdominal girth

● Calculate Medication Dosages

1. Methylprednisolone 40 mg IM is prescribed. The drug is available in a suspension for injections in a solution of 20 mg/mL. The nurse prepares to administer _____.

2. Prednisolone 60 mg orally is prescribed. The drug is available as syrup of prednisolone 15 mg/5 mL. The nurse administers _____.

To check your answers, see Appendix E.

the**Point** *For more NCLEX questions, log on to http://thepoint.lww.com to access more than 1000 questions.*

Thyroid and Antithyroid Drugs

euthyroid
goiter
hyperthyroidism
hypothyroidism

myxedema
thyroid storm
thyrotoxicosis

On completion of this chapter, the student will:

1. Identify the hormones produced by the thyroid gland.
2. Discuss the uses, general drug actions, adverse reactions, contraindications, precautions, and interactions of thyroid and antithyroid drugs.
3. Discuss important preadministration and ongoing assessment activities the nurse should perform with the patient taking thyroid and antithyroid drugs.
4. List the signs and symptoms of iodism (too much iodine) and iodine allergy.
5. Discuss ways to promote an optimal response to therapy, how to manage adverse reactions, and important points to keep in mind when educating patients about the use of thyroid and antithyroid drugs.

The thyroid gland is located in the neck in front of the trachea. This highly vascular gland manufactures and secretes two hormones: thyroxine (T_4) and triiodothyronine (T_3). Iodine is an essential element for the manufacture of both of these hormones. The activity of the thyroid gland is regulated by thyroid-stimulating hormone, produced by the anterior pituitary gland (see Fig. 44.2 in Chapter 44). When the level of circulating thyroid hormones decreases, the anterior pituitary secretes thyroid-stimulating hormone, which then activates the cells of the thyroid to release stored thyroid hormones. This is an example of the feedback mechanism described in the nursing process section of Chapter 44.

Two diseases are related to the hormone-producing activity of the thyroid gland:

- **Hypothyroidism**—a decrease in the amount of thyroid hormones manufactured and secreted
- **Hyperthyroidism**—an increase in the amount of thyroid hormones manufactured and secreted

The symptoms of hypothyroidism and hyperthyroidism are given in Table 45.1. Thyroid hormones are used as replacement therapy when the patient is hypothyroid. By supplementing the decreased endogenous thyroid production and secretion with exogenous thyroid hormones, an attempt is made to create a **euthyroid** (normal thyroid) state.

Myxedema is a severe hypothyroidism manifested by lethargy, apathy, and memory impairment; emotional changes; slow speech and deep, coarse voice; thick, dry skin; cold intolerance; slow pulse; constipation; weight gain; and absence of menses. A severe form of hyperthyroidism, called **thyrotoxicosis** or **thyroid storm**, is characterized by high fever, extreme tachycardia, and altered mental status. Thyroid hormones are used to treat hypothyroidism and antithyroid drugs and radioactive iodine are used to treat hyperthyroidism.

•THYROID HORMONES

Thyroid hormones used in health care include both the natural and synthetic hormones. The synthetic hormones are generally preferred, because they are more uniform in potency than are the natural hormones obtained from animals. Thyroid hormones are listed in the Summary Drug Table: Thyroid and Antithyroid Drugs.

Actions

The thyroid hormones influence every organ and tissue of the body. These hormones are principally concerned with increasing the metabolic rate of tissues, which results in increases in the heart and respiratory rate, body temperature, cardiac output, oxygen consumption, and the metabolism of fats, proteins, and carbohydrates. The exact mechanisms by which the thyroid hormones exert their influence on body organs and tissues are not well understood.

Uses

Thyroid hormones are also used in the treatment or prevention of the following:

- Euthyroid **goiter** (enlargement of a normal thyroid gland)
- Thyroid nodules and multinodular goiter
- Subacute or chronic thyroiditis (Hashimoto's disease or viral thyroiditis)
- Thyroid cancer

Table 45.1 Signs and Symptoms of Thyroid Dysfunction

Bodily System or Function	Hypothyroidism	Hyperthyroidism
Metabolism	Decreased, with anorexia, intolerance to cold, low body temperature, weight gain despite anorexia	Increased, with increased appetite, intolerance to heat, elevated body temperature, weight loss despite increased appetite
Cardiovascular	Bradycardia, moderate hypotension	Tachycardia, moderate hypertension
Central nervous system	Lethargy, sleepiness	Nervousness, anxiety, insomnia, tremors, exophthalmos
Skin, skin structures	Pale, cool, dry skin; face appears puffy; coarse hair; nails thick and hard	Flushed, warm, moist skin, thinning hair, goiter
Ovarian function	Heavy menses, may be unable to conceive, loss of fetus possible	Irregular or scant menses
Testicular function	Low sperm count	

Summary Drug Table THYROID AND ANTITHYROID DRUGS

Generic Name	Trade Name	Uses	Adverse Reactions	Dosage Ranges
Thyroid Hormones				
levothyroxine (T$_4$) lee-voe-thye-rox'-een	Levothroid, Levoxyl, Synthroid, Unithroid	Hypothyroidism, thyroid-stimulating hormone suppression, thyrotoxicosis, thyroid diagnostic testing	Palpitations, tachycardia, headache, nervousness, insomnia, diarrhea, vomiting, weight loss, fatigue, sweating, flushing	100–125 mcg/day orally
liothyronine (T^3) lye'-oh-thye'-roe-neen	Cytomel, Trio stat	Same as levothyroxine	Same as levothyroxine	25–75 mcg/day orally
liotrix (T^3, T^4) lye'-oh-trix	Thyrolar	Same as levothyroxine	Same as levothyroxine	Initial: 1 Thyrolar half-grain tablet/day orally Maintenance: 1 Thyrolar, 1-grain or 2-grain tablet/day orally
thyroid, desiccated	Armour	Same as levothyroxine	Same as levothyroxine	Initial: 30 mg/day orally Maintenance: 60–120 mg/d orally
Antithyroid Preparations				
methimazole meh-thim'-ah-zoll	Tapazole	Hyperthyroidism	Numbness, headache, loss of hair, skin rash, nausea, vomiting, agranulocytosis	5–40 mg/day orally, divided doses at 8-hr intervals
propylthiouracil (PTU) proe-pill-thye-oh-yoor'-ah-sill		Same as methimazole	Same as methimazole	300–900 mg/day orally, divided doses at 8-hr intervals
Iodine Products				
sodium iodide (^{131}I) eye'-oh-dyde	Iodotope	Eradicate hyperthyroidism, selected cases of thyroid cancer	Bone marrow depression, nausea, vomiting, tachycardia, itching, rash, hives	Measured by a radioactivity calibration system before administering orally 4–10 microcuries Thyroid cancer: 50–150 mCi

Levothyroxine (Synthroid) is the drug of choice for hypothyroidism, because it is relatively inexpensive, requires once-a-day dosage, and has a more uniform potency than do other thyroid hormone replacement drugs. The hormone may be used with the antithyroid drugs to treat thyrotoxicosis. Thyroid hormones also may be used as a diagnostic measure to differentiate suspected hyperthyroidism from euthyroidism.

⚠ NURSING ALERT

All thyroid hormone replacement drugs are not equivalent. Patients should not change brands or types of thyroid hormone without first checking with their primary health care provider. The primary health care provider needs to determine the equivalent dosages when changing medication brands.

Adverse Reactions

Treatment of hypothyroidism is based on individualized doses of the hormone. During initial therapy, the most common adverse reactions are signs of overdose and hyperthyroidism as titration of the drug is being attempted (see Table 45.1). Adverse reactions other than symptoms of hyperthyroidism are rare.

Contraindications and Precautions

These drugs are contraindicated in patients with known hypersensitivity to the drug, an uncorrected adrenal cortical insufficiency, or thyrotoxicosis. These drugs should not be used as a treatment for obesity or infertility. Thyroid hormone should not be used after a recent myocardial infarction. When hypothyroidism is a cause or contributing factor to a myocardial infarction or heart disease, the physician may prescribe small doses of thyroid hormone.

These drugs are used cautiously in patients with cardiac disease and during lactation. Thyroid hormones are classified as pregnancy category A and should be continued by hypothyroid women during pregnancy.

Interactions

The following interactions may occur with thyroid hormones:

Interacting Drug	Common Use	Effect of Interaction
digoxin, beta blockers	Management of cardiac problems	Decreased effectiveness of cardiac drug
oral hypoglycemics and insulin	Treatment of diabetes	Increased risk of hypoglycemia
oral anticoagulants	Blood thinners	Prolonged bleeding
Selective serotonin reuptake inhibitors (SSRIs), antidepressants	Treatment of depression	Decreased effectiveness of thyroid drug
All other antidepressant drug categories	Treatment of depression	Increased effectiveness of thyroid drug

NURSING PROCESS
PATIENT RECEIVING A THYROID HORMONE

ASSESSMENT

Preadministration Assessment
After a patient receives a diagnosis of hypothyroidism and before therapy starts, the nurse takes vital signs and weighs the patient. A history of the patient's signs and symptoms is obtained. The nurse performs a general physical assessment to determine outward signs of hypothyroidism.

👪 LIFESPAN ALERT – Gerontology

The symptoms of hypothyroidism may be confused with symptoms associated with aging, such as depression, cold intolerance, weight gain, confusion, or unsteady gait. The presence of these symptoms should be thoroughly evaluated and documented in the preadministration assessment and periodically throughout therapy.

Ongoing Assessment
The full effects of thyroid hormone replacement therapy may not be apparent for several weeks or more, but early effects may be apparent in as little as 48 hours. During the ongoing assessment, the nurse monitors the vital signs as ordered and observes the patient for signs of hyperthyroidism, which may signal excessive drug dosage. Signs of a therapeutic response include weight loss, mild diuresis, increased appetite, an increased pulse rate, and decreased puffiness of the face, hands, and feet. The patient may also report an increased sense of well-being and increased mental activity.

NURSING DIAGNOSES

Drug-specific nursing diagnoses include the following:

❑ **Risk for Ineffective Therapeutic Regimen Management** related to discomfort of adverse reactions during titration of individualized dosing
❑ **Anxiety** related to symptoms, adverse reactions, treatment regimen, other (specify)

Nursing diagnoses related to drug administration are discussed in Chapter 4.

PLANNING

The expected outcomes of the patient may include an optimal response to therapy, support of patient needs related to the management of adverse reactions, and an understanding of the prescribed therapeutic regimen.

IMPLEMENTATION

Promoting an Optimal Response to Therapy
Thyroid hormones are administered once a day, early in the morning and preferably before breakfast. An empty stomach increases the absorption of the oral preparation. Levothyroxine (Synthroid) and liothyronine (Triostat)

also can be given intravenously and are prepared for administration immediately before use.

Monitoring and Managing Patient Needs

RISK FOR INEFFECTIVE THERAPEUTIC REGIMEN MANAGEMENT. The dosage is individualized to the needs of the patient. The nurse monitors the patient for any adverse reactions, especially during the initial stages of dosage adjustment. If the dosage is inadequate, the patient will continue to experience signs of hypothyroidism (see Table 45.1). If the dosage is excessive, the patient will exhibit signs of hyperthyroidism. It is important for the nurse to monitor reactions and document them well to provide information for correct dosing. The primary health care provider makes dose adjustments carefully based on the patient's hormone responses. At times, several upward or downward dosage adjustments must be made until the optimal therapeutic dosage is reached and the patient becomes euthyroid.

> **NURSING ALERT**
> If signs of hyperthyroidism (e.g., nervousness, anxiety, increased appetite, elevated body temperature, tachycardia, moderate hypertension or flushed, warm, moist skin) are apparent, the nurse reports them to the primary health care provider before the next dose is due, because it may be necessary to decrease the daily dosage.

ANXIETY. Some patients may exhibit anxiety related to the symptoms of their disorder, as well as concern about relief of their symptoms. The patient should be reassured that although relief may not be immediate, symptoms should begin to decrease or even disappear in a few weeks.

Thyroid hormone replacement therapy in patients with diabetes may increase the intensity of the symptoms or the diabetes. The nurse closely monitors the patient with diabetes during thyroid hormone replacement therapy for signs of hyperglycemia (see Chapter 43) and notifies the primary health care provider if this problem occurs.

The nurse carefully observes patients who have cardiovascular disease and who take the thyroid hormones. The development of chest pain or worsening of cardiovascular disease should be reported to the primary health care provider immediately, because the patient may require a reduction in the dosage of the thyroid hormone.

> **LIFESPAN ALERT – Gerontology**
> The elderly are at increased risk for adverse cardiovascular reactions when taking thyroid drugs. The initial dosage is smaller for an older adult, and increases, if they are necessary, are made in smaller increments during a period of about 8 weeks.

Educating the Patient and Family

Thyroid hormones are usually given on an outpatient basis. The nurse emphasizes the importance of taking the drug exactly as directed and not stopping the drug even though symptoms have improved. The nurse provides the following information to the patient and family when thyroid hormone replacement therapy is prescribed:

- Replacement therapy is for life, with the exception of transient hypothyroidism seen in those with thyroiditis.
- Do not increase, decrease, or skip a dose unless advised to do so by the primary health care provider.
- Take this drug in the morning, preferably before breakfast, unless advised by the primary health care provider to take it at a different time of day.
- Notify the primary health care provider if any of the following occur: headache, nervousness, palpitations, diarrhea, excessive sweating, heat intolerance, chest pain, increased pulse rate, or any unusual physical change or event.
- Normally, the dosage of this drug may require periodic adjustments. Dosage changes are based on a response to therapy and thyroid function tests.
- Therapy needs to be evaluated at periodic intervals, which may vary from every 2 weeks during the beginning of therapy to every 6 to 12 months once symptoms are controlled. Periodic thyroid function tests will be needed.
- Weigh yourself weekly and report any significant weight gain or loss to the primary health care provider.
- Do not change from one brand of this drug to another without consulting the primary health care provider.

EVALUATION

- Therapeutic effect is achieved.
- Adverse reactions are identified, reported to the primary health care provider, and managed successfully through appropriate nursing interventions:
  ☑ Patient manages the therapeutic regimen effectively.
  ☑ Anxiety is managed successfully.
- Patient and family demonstrate an understanding of the drug regimen.

• ANTITHYROID DRUGS

Antithyroid drugs or thyroid antagonists are used to treat hyperthyroidism. In addition to the antithyroid drugs, hyperthyroidism may be treated by the use of radioactive iodine (^{131}I), or by surgical removal of some or almost all of the thyroid gland (subtotal thyroidectomy).

Actions

Antithyroid drugs inhibit the manufacture of thyroid hormones. They do not affect existing thyroid hormones that are circulating in the blood or stored in the thyroid gland. For this reason, therapeutic effects of the antithyroid drugs may not be observed for 3 to 4 weeks. Antithyroid drugs are listed in the Summary Drug Table: Thyroid and Antithyroid Drugs.

Radioactive iodine is used because the thyroid has an affinity for iodine. The radioactive isotope accumulates in the cells of the thyroid gland, where destruction of thyroid cells occurs without damaging other cells throughout the body.

Not all patients respond adequately to antithyroid drugs; therefore, a thyroidectomy may be necessary. Antithyroid drugs may be administered before surgery to return the patient temporarily to an euthyroid state. When used for this reason, the vascularity of the thyroid gland is reduced typically using potassium iodide, and the tendency to bleed excessively during and immediately after surgery is decreased.

Uses

Methimazole (Tapazole) and propylthiouracil (PTU) are used for the medical management of hyperthyroidism. Potassium iodide may be given orally with methimazole or propylthiouracil to prepare for thyroid surgery. Radioactive iodine (^{131}I) may be used for treatment of hyperthyroidism and selected cases of cancer of the thyroid. The drug is given orally either as a solution or in a gelatin capsule.

Adverse Reactions

Generalized System Reactions

• Hay fever, sore throat, skin rash, fever, headache
• Nausea, vomiting, paresthesias

Severe System Reactions

• Agranulocytosis (decrease in the number of white blood cells)
• Exfoliative dermatitis, granulocytopenia, hypoprothrombinemia

Contraindications, Precautions, and Interactions

The antithyroid drugs are contraindicated in patients with hypersensitivity to the drug or any constituent of the drug. Mothers taking methimazole or propylthiouracil should not breastfeed their children. Radioactive iodine (pregnancy category X) is contraindicated during pregnancy and lactation.

Methimazole and propylthiouracil are used with extreme caution during pregnancy (category D) because they can cause hypothyroidism in the fetus. However, if an antithyroid drug is necessary during pregnancy, propylthiouracil is the preferred drug, because it does not cross the placenta. The potential for bleeding increases when these products are taken with oral anticoagulants.

NURSING PROCESS

PATIENT RECEIVING AN ANTITHYROID DRUG

ASSESSMENT

Preadministration Assessment

Before a patient starts therapy with an antithyroid drug, the nurse obtains a history of the symptoms of hyperthyroidism. It is important to include vital signs, weight, and a notation regarding the outward symptoms of the hyperthyroidism (see Table 45.1) in the physical assessment. If the patient is prescribed an iodine procedure, it is essential that the nurse take a careful allergy history,

particularly to iodine or seafood (which contains iodine).

Ongoing Assessment

During the ongoing assessment, the nurse observes the patient for adverse drug effects. During short-term therapy before surgery, adverse drug reactions are usually minimal. Long-term therapy is usually on an outpatient basis. The nurse questions the patient regarding relief of symptoms, as well as signs or symptoms indicating an adverse reaction related to a decrease in blood cells, such as fatigue, fever, sore throat, easy bruising or bleeding, fever, cough, or any other signs of infection. As the patient becomes euthyroid, signs and symptoms of hyperthyroidism become less obvious. The nurse monitors the patient for signs of thyroid storm (high fever, extreme tachycardia, and altered mental status), which can occur in patients whose hyperthyroidism is inadequately treated.

NURSING DIAGNOSES

Drug-specific nursing diagnoses include the following:

❑ **Risk for Ineffective Therapeutic Regimen Management** related to consistent dosing routine requirements
❑ **Risk for Infection** related to adverse reactions
❑ **Risk for Impaired Skin Integrity** related to adverse reactions

Nursing diagnoses related to drug administration are discussed in Chapter 4.

PLANNING

The expected outcomes of the patient may include an optimal response to therapy, support of patient needs related to the management of adverse reactions, and an understanding of the therapeutic regimen.

IMPLEMENTATION

Promoting an Optimal Response to Therapy

The patient with an enlarged thyroid gland may have difficulty swallowing the tablet. If this occurs, the nurse discusses the problem with the primary health care provider. Radioactive iodine is given by the primary health care provider, orally as a single dose. The effects of iodides are evident within 24 hours, with maximum effects attained after 10 to 15 days of continuous therapy. If the patient is hospitalized, radiation safety precautions identified by the hospital's department of nuclear medicine are followed.

Once an euthyroid state is achieved, the primary health care provider may add a thyroid hormone to the therapeutic regimen to prevent or treat hypothyroidism, which may develop slowly during long-term antithyroid drug therapy or after administration of ^{131}I.

The patient with hyperthyroidism is likely to have cardiac symptoms such as tachycardia or palpitations. Propranolol, an adrenergic blocking drug (see Chapter 25), may be prescribed by the primary health care provider as adjunctive treatment for several weeks until the therapeutic effects of the antithyroid drug are obtained.

Monitoring and Managing Patient Needs

RISK FOR INEFFECTIVE THERAPEUTIC REGIMEN MANAGEMENT. The patient with hyperthyroidism may be concerned with the results of medical treatment and with the problem of taking the drug at regular intervals around the clock (usually every 8 hours). Whereas some patients may be awake early in the morning and retire late at night, others may experience difficulty with an 8-hour dosage schedule. Another concern may be a tendency to forget the first dose early in the morning, thus causing a problem with the two following doses.

If the patient expresses a concern about the dosage schedule, the nurse may be able to offer suggestions. For example, the nurse may suggest the following 8-hour interval schedule: 7 AM, 3 PM, and 11 PM. The nurse may also suggest posting a notice on a bathroom mirror to remind the individual that the first dose is due immediately after rising. After a week or more of therapy, most patients remember to take their morning dose on time. If the first or last dose interferes with sleep, the nurse should suggest the patient discuss this with the primary health care provider.

RISK FOR INFECTION. The nurse monitors the patient throughout therapy for adverse drug reactions. The nurse monitors the patient frequently for signs of agranulocytosis. It is important that the patient be protected from individuals with infectious disease, because if agranulocytosis is present, the patient is at increased risk of contracting any infection, particularly an upper respiratory tract infection. The nurse monitors for signs of infection, particularly upper respiratory infection, in visitors and other health care personnel.

LIFESPAN ALERT – Chronic Care
Agranulocytosis is potentially the most serious adverse reaction to methimazole and propylthiouracil. The nurse instructs the patient to notify the primary health care provider if fever or sore throat are experienced in order to draw lab work and check for agranulocytosis.

RISK FOR IMPAIRED SKIN INTEGRITY. If the patient experiences a rash while taking methimazole or propylthiouracil, the nurse carefully documents the affected areas, noting size, texture, and extent of the rash, and reports the occurrence of the rash to the primary health care provider. Soothing creams or lubricants may be applied, and soap is used sparingly, if at all, until the rash subsides.

Educating the Patient and Family
The nurse reviews with the patient and family the dosage and times the drug is to be taken. The following additional teaching points are included in a teaching plan:

METHIMAZOLE AND PROPYLTHIOURACIL
- Take these drugs at regular intervals around the clock (e.g., every 8 hours) unless directed otherwise by the primary health care provider.

- Do not take these drugs in larger doses or more frequently than as directed on the prescription container.
- Notify the primary health care provider promptly if any of the following occur: sore throat, fever, cough, easy bleeding or bruising, headache, or a general feeling of malaise.
- Record weight twice a week and notify the primary health care provider if there is any sudden weight gain or loss. (Note: the primary health care provider may also want the patient to monitor pulse rate. If this is recommended, the patient needs instruction in the proper technique and a recommendation to record the pulse rate and bring the record to the primary health care provider's office or clinic.)
- Avoid the use of nonprescription drugs unless the primary health care provider has approved the use of a specific drug.

RADIOACTIVE IODINE.
- Follow the directions of the department of nuclear medicine regarding precautions to be taken. (*Note:* In some instances, the dosage is small and no special precautions may be necessary.)
- Keep in mind that tenderness and swelling of the neck, sore throat, and cough may occur in 2 to 3 days after the procedure
- Also keep in mind that thyroid hormone replacement therapy may be necessary if hypothyroidism develops.
- Schedule necessary follow-up evaluations to review the thyroid gland and the effectiveness of treatment.

EVALUATION

- Therapeutic effect is achieved.
- Adverse reactions are identified, reported to the primary health care provider, and managed successfully through appropriate nursing interventions:
  ☑ Patient manages the therapeutic regimen effectively.
  ☑ No evidence of infection is seen.
  ☑ Skin remains intact.
- Patient and family demonstrate an understanding of the drug regimen.

THINK CRITICALLY: PHARMACOLOGY IN PRACTICE

1. Betty Peterson's neighbor will receive a dose of radioactive iodine for a hyperthyroid illness. She is concerned about bringing her daughter's new baby home, thinking that her neighbor may be radioactive after the procedure. Discuss how you would present information to Betty to help deal with her fear.

● Test Your Knowledge

1. What adverse reaction is most likely to occur in the early days of therapy in a patient taking a thyroid hormone?
   A. Congestive heart failure
   B. Hyperthyroidism
   C. Hypothyroidism
   D. Euthyroidism

2. The nurse informs the patient that therapy with a thyroid hormone may not produce a therapeutic response for _____.

   A. 24 to 48 days
   B. 1 to 3 days
   C. several weeks or more
   D. 8 to 12 months

3. Which of the following symptoms best indicates that serious adverse reactions are developing in a patient receiving methimazole (Tapazole)?

   A. Fever, sore throat, bleeding from an injection site
   B. Cough, periorbital edema, constipation
   C. Constipation, anorexia, blurred vision
   D. Unsteady gait, blurred vision, insomnia

4. Which of the following statements made by a patient would indicate to the nurse that the patient is experiencing an adverse reaction to radioactive iodine?

   A. "I am sleepy most of the day."
   B. "I am unable to sleep at night."
   C. "My throat hurts when I swallow."
   D. "My body aches all over."

● Prepare for the NCLEX

1. Which of the following food allergies is of highest concern to the patient about to take radioactive iodine?

   A. Peanut or other tree nuts
   B. Seafood
   C. Wheat products
   D. Lactose intolerance

● Calculate Medication Dosages

1. Methimazole 40 mg is prescribed. The drug is available in 10-mg tablets. The nurse administers _____.

2. Levothyroxine 0.2 mg orally is prescribed. Available are 0.1-mg tablets. The nurse administers _____.

To check your answers, see Appendix E.

the**Point** *For more NCLEX questions, log on to http://thepoint.lww.com to access more than 1000 questions.*

Male and Female Hormones

46

LEARNING OBJECTIVES

On completion of this chapter, the student will:

1. Discuss the medical uses, actions, adverse reactions, contraindications, precautions, and interactions of the male and female hormones.
2. Discuss important preadministration and ongoing assessment activities the nurse should perform with the patient taking male or female hormones.
3. List nursing diagnoses particular to a patient taking male or female hormones.
4. Discuss ways to promote an optimal response to therapy, how to manage adverse reactions, and important points to keep in mind when educating the patient about the use of male or female hormones.

Male and female hormones play a vital role in the development and maintenance of secondary sex characteristics; they are necessary for human reproduction. Although hormones are naturally produced by the body, administration of a male or female hormone may be indicated in the treatment of certain disorders, such as an advanced-stage cancer, male hypogonadism, and male or female hormone deficiency. Hormones also are used as contraceptives and for treating the symptoms of menopause. Drugs to inhibit the activity of hormones are also used to treat cancers.

• MALE HORMONES

Male hormones—**testosterone** and its derivatives—are collectively called **androgens**. Androgen secretion is influenced by the anterior pituitary gland. Small amounts of male and female hormones are also produced by the adrenal cortex (see Chapter 44). The anabolic steroids are closely related to the androgen testosterone and have both androgenic and anabolic (stimulate cellular growth and repair) activity. Androgen hormone inhibitors inhibit the conversion of testosterone into a potent androgen.

Actions

Androgens

The male hormone testosterone and its derivatives actuate the reproductive potential in the adolescent boy. From puberty onward, androgens continue to aid in the development and maintenance of secondary sex characteristics: facial hair, deep voice, body hair, body fat distribution, and muscle development. Testosterone also stimulates the growth in size of the accessory sex organs (penis, testes, vas deferens, prostate) at the time of puberty. The androgens also promote tissue-building processes (**anabolism**) and reverse tissue-depleting processes (**catabolism**). Examples of androgens are fluoxymesterone, methyltestosterone (Testred), and testosterone. Additional examples of androgens are given in the Summary Drug Table: Male Hormones.

Anabolic Steroids

Anabolic steroids are synthetic drugs chemically related to the androgens. Like the androgens, they promote tissue-building processes. Given in normal doses, they have a minimal effect on the accessory sex organs and secondary sex characteristics. Examples of anabolic steroids are given in the Summary Drug Table: Male Hormones.

Androgen Hormone Inhibitor

Androgen hormone inhibitors are synthetic compound drugs that inhibit the conversion of testosterone into the potent androgen 5-alpha (a)-dihydrotestosterone (DHT). The development of the prostate gland is dependent on DHT. The lowering of serum levels of DHT reduces the effect of this hormone on the prostate gland, resulting in a decrease in the size of the gland and the symptoms associated with prostatic gland enlargement. Examples of androgen hormone inhibitors include finasteride (Proscar) and dutasteride (Avodart).

Summary Drug Table MALE HORMONES

Generic Name	Trade Name	Uses	Adverse Reactions	Dosage Ranges
Androgens				
fluoxymesterone *floo-oxi-mes'-ter-own*		Males: hypogonadism, delayed puberty Females: inoperable advanced ~~breast cancer~~	Nausea, vomiting, acne, hair thinning, headache, libido changes, anxiety, mood changes, hematopoietic and electrolyte imbalances Males: gynecomastia, testicular atrophy, erectile dysfunction Females: amenorrhea, virilization	Males: 5–20 mg/day orally; Females: 10–40 mg/day orally
methyltestosterone *meth-ill-tess-toss'-ter-own*	Testred, Virilon	Same as fluoxymesterone	Same as fluoxymesterone	Males: 10–50 mg/day orally; Females: 50–200 mg/day orally
testosterone *tess-toss'-ter-own*	Androderm, AndroGel, Testim (Transdermal) Delatestryl, Depo-Testosterone (injectable), Striant (oral, buccal)	Primary or hypogo-nadotropic hypogo-nadism, delayed puberty	Same as fluoxymesterone	Buccal: 30 mg BID Gel: apply daily Injectable: 50–400 mg every 2–4 wk; Pellet: 150–450 mg Subcut every 3–6 mo; Trans-dermal: 6 mg/day, apply patch daily
Anabolic Steroids				
nandrolone *nan'-droe-loan*		Anemia of renal insuf-ficiency, human immunodeficiency virus (HIV) wasting syndrome	Nausea, vomiting, diarrhea, acne, hair thinning, libido changes, anxiety, mood changes, edema, anemia, electrolyte imbalances Males: gynecomastia, testicular atrophy, sexual dysfunction Females: amenorrhea, virilization	50–200 mg/wk IM
oxymetholone	Anadrol-50	Anemia	Same as nandrolone decanoate	1–5 mg/kg/day orally
oxandrolone *ox-an'-droe-loan*	Oxandrin	Bone pain, weight gain, protein catabolism	Acne, hair thinning, libido changes, anxiety, mood changes, edema, electrolyte imbalances Males: gynecomastia, testicular atrophy, sexual dysfunction Females: amenorrhea, virilization	2.5–20 mg/day orally in divided doses
Androgen Hormone Inhibitors				
dutasteride	Avodart	Benign prostatic hypertrophy	Impotence, decreased libido	0.5 mg/day orally
finasteride *fin-as'-teh-ryde*	Propecia, Proscar	Male-pattern bald-ness, benign prostatic hypertrophy	Impotence, decreased libido, asthenia, dizziness, postural hypotension	1–5 mg/day orally

I: imipramine → androgen – Trt of depression → ↑ risk of paranoid behavior

Uses

Androgen therapy may be given as replacement therapy for the following:

- Testosterone deficiency
- Hypogonadism (failure of the testes to develop)
- Delayed puberty
- Development of testosterone deficiency after puberty

In the female patient, androgen therapy may be used for

- Postmenopausal, metastatic breast carcinoma
- Premenopausal, hormone-dependent metastatic breast carcinoma

The transdermal testosterone system is used as replacement therapy when **endogenous** (produced by the body) testosterone is deficient or absent.

Anabolic steroid use includes the following:

- Management of anemia of renal insufficiency
- Control of metastatic breast cancer in women
- Promotion of weight gain in those with weight loss after surgery, trauma, or infections

Androgen hormone inhibitors are used in the treatment of the following:

- Prevention of male pattern baldness
- Symptoms associated with benign prostatic hypertrophy (BPH), which includes difficulty starting the urinary stream, frequent passage of small amounts of urine, and having to urinate during the night (nocturia). Several months of therapy may be required before a significant improvement is noted and symptoms of BPH decrease.

LIFESPAN ALERT – Young Males   36

The use of anabolic steroids to promote an increase in muscle mass and strength has become a serious problem. Anabolic steroids are not intended for this use. Unfortunately, deaths in young, healthy individuals have been directly attributed to the use of these drugs. Nurses should discourage the illegal use of anabolic steroids to increase muscle mass.

Adverse Reactions

Androgens

In men, administration of an androgen may result in breast enlargement (**gynecomastia**), testicular atrophy, inhibition of testicular function, impotence, enlargement of the penis, nausea, vomiting, jaundice, headache, anxiety, male pattern baldness, acne, and depression. Fluid and electrolyte imbalances, which include sodium, water, chloride, potassium, calcium, and phosphate retention, may also occur.

In women receiving an androgen preparation for breast carcinoma, the most common adverse reactions are amenorrhea, other menstrual irregularities, and **virilization** (acquisition of male sexual characteristics by a woman). Virilization produces facial hair, a deepening of the voice, and enlargement of the clitoris. Male pattern baldness and acne may also result.

Anabolic Steroids

Virilization in the woman is the most common reaction associated with anabolic steroids, especially when higher doses are used. Acne occurs frequently in all age groups and both sexes. Nausea, vomiting, diarrhea, fluid and electrolyte imbalances (the same as for the androgens, discussed previously), testicular atrophy, jaundice, anorexia, and muscle cramps may also be seen. Blood-filled cysts of the liver and sometimes the spleen, malignant and benign liver tumors, an increased risk of atherosclerosis, and mental changes are the most serious adverse reactions that may occur during prolonged use.

Many serious adverse drug reactions are being reported in healthy individuals using anabolic steroids. There is some indication that prolonged high-dose use has resulted in psychological and possibly physical dependence, and some individuals have required treatment in drug abuse centers. Severe mental changes, such as uncontrolled rage (called "'roid rage"), severe depression, suicidal tendencies, malignant and benign liver tumors, aggressive behavior, increased risk of atherosclerosis, inability to concentrate, and personality changes are not uncommon. In addition, the incidence of the severe adverse reactions cited earlier appears to be increased in those using anabolic steroids for this purpose.

Androgen Hormone Inhibitor

Adverse reactions usually are mild and do not require discontinuing use of the drug. Adverse reactions, when they occur, are related to the sexual drive and include impotence, decreased libido, and a decreased volume of ejaculate. For more information, see Display 46.1.

Contraindications and Precautions

The male hormones and hormone inhibitors are contraindicated in patients with known hypersensitivity to the drugs,

DISPLAY 46.1 Drugs for Erectile Dysfunction

Erectile dysfunction results from a failure of the penile corpus cavernosum to become engorged with blood, preventing sexual intercourse. This condition can be a result of age-related, neurologic, or vascular changes in the tissue. A number of oral drugs are now on the market that can facilitate blood flow into the penis, resulting in an erection.

Generic Name	Trade Name	Duration of Action
sildenafil	Viagra	30 minutes to 4 hours before sexual activity
tadalafil	Cialis	Up to 36 hours before sexual activity
vardenafil	Levitra	1 hour before sexual activity

Because these drugs affect smooth muscle, patients with preexisting cardiac problems, especially those using drugs to lower blood pressure should discuss use with their primary health care provider before using the drug. Medical attention should be sought for erections sustained for more than 4 hours. Ocular problems may occur when using these drugs; again, the primary health care provider should be consulted before use.

liver disorders, or serious cardiac disease, and in men with prostate gland disorders (e.g., prostate carcinoma and prostate enlargement). These drugs are classified as pregnancy category X drugs and should not be administered during pregnancy and lactation. Anabolic steroids are contraindicated for use to enhance physical appearance or athletic performance. Anabolic steroids should be used cautiously in older men because of increased risk of prostate enlargement and prostate cancer.

14

Interactions

The following interactions may occur with the male hormones and male hormone inhibitors:

Interacting Drug	Common Use	Effect of Interaction
oral anticoagulants	Blood thinners	Increased antidiuretic effect
imipramine and androgen	Treatment of depression	Increased risk of paranoid behavior
sulfonylureas and anabolic steroids	Anti-infective	Increased risk of hypoglycemia

3
SA

> **HERBAL ALERT**
> **Saw palmetto** is used to relieve the symptoms of BPH. The herb reduces urinary frequency, increases the flow of urine, and decreases the incidence of nocturia. Saw palmetto may delay the need for prostate surgery. The dosage of the herb is:
> • 160 mg twice daily of standardized extract
> • One 585-mg capsule or tablet up to three times daily
> • 20 to 30 drops up to four times a day (tincture, 1:2 liquid extract)
>
> It is not recommended to take saw palmetto as a tea, because the active constituents are not water soluble. Improvement can be seen after 1 to 3 months of therapy. It is usually recommended that the herb be taken for 6 months, followed by evaluation by a primary health care provider.

NURSING PROCESS
PATIENT RECEIVING A MALE HORMONE

ASSESSMENT

Preadministration Assessment
Assessment of the patient receiving an androgen or anabolic steroid depends on the drug, the patient, and the reason for administration.

ANDROGENS. In most instances, androgens are administered to the man on an outpatient basis. Before and during therapy, the primary health care provider may order electrolyte studies, because use of these drugs can result in fluid and electrolyte imbalances.

When these drugs are given to the female patient with advanced breast carcinoma, the nurse evaluates the

patient's current status (physical, emotional, and nutritional) carefully and records the findings in the patient's chart. Problem areas, such as pain, any limitation of motion, and the ability to participate in the activities of daily living, are carefully evaluated and recorded in the patient's record. The nurse takes and records vital signs and weight. Baseline laboratory tests may include a complete blood count, hepatic function tests, serum electrolytes, and serum and urinary calcium levels. The nurse reviews these tests and notes any abnormalities.

ANABOLIC STEROIDS. The nurse evaluates and records the patient's physical and nutritional status before starting therapy with anabolic steroids. The nurse takes the patient's weight, blood pressure, pulse, and respiratory rate. Baseline laboratory studies may include a complete blood count, hepatic function tests, and serum electrolytes and serum lipid levels. The nurse reviews these studies and notes any abnormalities.

ANDROGEN HORMONE INHIBITOR. The nurse questions the patient at length about symptoms of BPH, such as frequency of voiding during the day and night and difficulty starting the urinary stream. The nurse records all symptoms in the patient's chart.

> **! NURSING ALERT**
> Women who are pregnant or may become pregnant should not handle crushed or broken finasteride (Propecia, Proscar) or dutasteride (Avodart) tablets or capsules. Absorption of the drug poses substantial risk for abnormal growth to a male fetus.

Ongoing Assessment
The ongoing assessment depends on the reason the drug was prescribed and the condition of the patient. Men receiving an androgen or anabolic steroid are questioned by the primary health care provider or nurse regarding the effectiveness of drug therapy.

The nurse weighs the patient with advanced breast carcinoma daily or as ordered by the primary health care provider. If the patient is on complete bed rest, the nurse may measure weight every 3 to 4 days (or as ordered) using a bed scale. The nurse notifies the primary health care provider if there is a significant (5-lb) increase or decrease in the weight. The nurse checks the lower extremities daily for signs of edema.

> **! NURSING ALERT**
> The nurse teaches the patient or caregiver to observe daily for adverse drug reactions, especially signs of fluid and electrolyte imbalance, jaundice (which may indicate hepatotoxicity), and virilization. The primary health care provider must be alerted to any signs of fluid and electrolyte imbalance or jaundice.

When hospitalized, the nurse takes vital signs every 4 to 8 hours, depending on the patient's condition, and then evaluates the patient's response to drug therapy based on original assessment findings. Possible responses include a decrease in pain, an increase in appetite, and a feeling of well-being.

Androgens given for breast cancer

LIFESPAN ALERT – Chronic Care *37*

When the androgens are administered to a patient with diabetes, blood glucose levels should be measured frequently because glucose tolerance may be altered. Adjustments may need to be made in insulin dosage, oral antidiabetic drugs, or diet. The nurse monitors the patient for signs for hypoglycemia and hyperglycemia (see Chapter 43).

When anabolic steroids are used for weight gain, the nurse weighs the patient at intervals ranging from daily to weekly. A good dietary regimen is necessary to promote weight gain. The nurse consults the dietitian if the patient eats poorly.

NURSING DIAGNOSES

Drug-specific nursing diagnoses include the following:

- ❏ **Excess Fluid Volume** related to adverse reactions (sodium and water retention)
- ❏ **Disturbed Body Image** (in the female) related to adverse reactions (virilization)

Nursing diagnoses related to drug administration are discussed in Chapter 4.

PLANNING

The expected outcomes of the patient may include an optimal response to therapy, support of patient needs related to the management of adverse reactions, and an understanding of and compliance with the prescribed therapeutic regimen.

IMPLEMENTATION

Promoting an Optimal Response to Therapy
If the androgen is to be administered as a buccal tablet, the nurse demonstrates the placement of the tablet and warns the patient not to swallow the tablet but to allow it to dissolve in the mouth. The nurse reminds the patient not to smoke or drink water until the tablet is dissolved. Oral and parenteral androgens are often taken or given by injection on an outpatient basis. When given by injection, the injection is administered deep intramuscularly (IM) into the gluteal muscle. Alternatively, a pellet dose is placed under the skin and repeated every 3 to 6 months. Oral testosterone is given with or before meals to decrease gastrointestinal (GI) upset.

Androderm is a transdermal system that is applied nightly to clean, dry skin on the abdomen, thigh, back, or upper arm. This system is not applied to the scrotum. Sites are rotated, with 7 days between applications to any specific site. The system is applied immediately after opening the pouch and removing the protective covering. If the patient has not exhibited a therapeutic response after 8 weeks of therapy, another form of testosterone replacement therapy should be considered.

Testosterone gel (AndroGel) is applied once daily (preferably in the morning) to clean, dry, intact skin of the shoulders and upper arms or abdomen. After the packet is opened, the contents are squeezed into the palm of the hand and immediately applied to the application sites. The application sites are allowed to dry before the patient gets dressed. The gel is not applied to the genitals.

Monitoring and Managing Patient Needs
The nurse observes the patient receiving an androgen or anabolic steroid for signs of adverse drug reactions.

Excess Fluid Volume. Sodium and water retention may also occur with androgen or anabolic steroid administration, causing the patient to become edematous. In addition, other electrolyte imbalances, such as hypercalcemia, may occur. The nurse monitors the patient for fluid and electrolyte disturbances.

LIFESPAN ALERT – Gerontology *14*

Older adults with cardiac problems or kidney disease are at increased risk for sodium and water retention when taking androgens or anabolic steroids.

The nurse makes a daily comparison of the patient's preadministration weight with current weights and makes sure to note the appearance of puffy eyelids and dependent swelling of the hands or feet (if the patient is ambulatory) or the sacral area (if the patient is nonambulatory) and reports any findings to the primary health care provider. The nurse monitors the daily fluid intake and output to calculate fluid balance.

Disturbed Body Image. With long-term administration of a male hormone, the female patient may experience mild to moderate masculine changes (virilization), namely, facial hair, a deepening of the voice, and enlargement of the clitoris. Male-pattern baldness, patchy hair loss, skin pigmentation, and acne may also result. Although these adverse effects are not life-threatening, they often are distressing and only add to the patient's discomfort and anxiety. These problems may be easy to identify, but they are not always easy to solve. If hair loss occurs, the nurse can suggest wearing head coverings such hats, scarves, or a wig; mild skin pigmentation may be covered with makeup, but severe and widespread pigmented areas and acne are often difficult to conceal. Each patient is different, and the emotional responses to these outward changes may range from severe depression to a positive attitude and acceptance. The nurse works with the patient as an individual, first identifying the problems, and then helping the patient, when possible, to deal with these changes.

Educating the Patient and the Family
The nurse explains the dosage regimen and possible adverse drug reactions to the patient and family and develops a teaching plan to include the following points:

Androgens.
- Notify the primary health care provider if any of the following occur: nausea, vomiting, swelling of the legs, or jaundice. Women should report any signs of virilization to the primary health care provider.
- Oral tablets—Take with food or a snack to avoid GI upset.

Male and Female Hormones

- Buccal tablets—Place the tablet between the cheek and molars and allow it to dissolve in the mouth. Do not smoke or drink water until the tablet is dissolved.
- Testosterone transdermal system—Apply according to the directions supplied with the product. Be sure the skin is clean and dry and the placement area is free of hair. Do not store outside the pouch or use damaged systems. Discard systems in household trash in a safe manner to prevent ingestion by children or pets.

ANABOLIC STEROIDS.

- Anabolic steroids may cause nausea and GI upset. Take this drug with food or meals.
- Keep all primary health care provider or clinic visits, because close monitoring of therapy is essential.
- Female patients: Notify the primary health care provider if signs of virilization occur.

ANDROGEN HORMONE INHIBITOR.

- Take this drug without regard to meals.
- Inform the primary health care provider immediately if sexual partner is or may become pregnant, because additional measures, such as discontinuing the drug or use of a condom, may be necessary.
- Women who are or may become pregnant should not handle this medication.

EVALUATION

- Therapeutic response is achieved.
- Adverse reactions are identified and reported to the primary health care provider, and managed successfully with appropriate nursing interventions:
  - ☑ Adequate fluid volume is maintained.
  - ☑ Perceptions of body changes are managed successfully.
- Patient and family demonstrate an understanding of the drug regimen.

● FEMALE HORMONES

The two endogenous (produced by the body) female hormones are **estrogen** and **progesterone**. Like the androgens, their production is under the influence of the anterior pituitary gland. The endogenous estrogens are **estradiol, estrone**, and **estriol**. The most potent of these three estrogens is estradiol. Examples of estrogens used as drugs include estropipate (Ortho-Est) and estradiol (Estrace).

There are natural and synthetic progesterones, which are collectively called **progestins**. Examples of progestins used as drugs include medroxyprogesterone (Provera) and norethindrone (Aygestin). Examples of estrogens and progestins are given in the Summary Drug Table: Female Hormones.

Actions

Estrogens

Estrogens are secreted by the ovarian follicle and in smaller amounts by the adrenal cortex. Estrogens are important in the development and maintenance of the female reproductive system and the primary and secondary sex characteristics. At puberty, they promote growth and development of the vagina, uterus, fallopian tubes, and breasts. They also affect the release of pituitary gonadotropins (see Chapter 44).

Other actions of estrogen include fluid retention, protein anabolism, thinning of the cervical mucus, and the inhibition or facilitation of ovulation. Estrogens contribute to the conservation of calcium and phosphorus, the growth of pubic and axillary hair, and pigmentation of the breast areolae and genitals. Estrogens also stimulate contraction of the fallopian tubes (which promotes movement of the ovum). They modify the physical and chemical properties of the cervical mucus, and restore the endometrium after menstruation.

Progestins

Progesterone is secreted by the corpus luteum, placenta, and (in small amounts) by the adrenal cortex. Progesterone and its derivatives (the progestins) transform the proliferative endometrium into a secretory endometrium. Progestins are necessary for the development of the placenta and inhibit the secretion of pituitary gonadotropins, which in turn prevents maturation of the ovarian follicle and ovulation. The synthetic progestins are usually preferred for medical use because of the decreased effectiveness of progesterone when administered orally.

Uses

Estrogens

Estrogen is most commonly used in combination with progesterones as a contraceptive agent or as estrogen replacement therapy (ERT) in postmenopausal women. In addition, estrogens are used in the following:

- Relief of moderate to severe vasomotor symptoms of menopause (flushing, sweating)
- Treatment of female hypogonadism
- Treatment of atrophic vaginitis
- Treatment of osteoporosis in women past menopause
- Palliative treatment of advanced prostatic carcinoma
- Selected cases of advanced breast carcinoma

The estradiol transdermal system is also used after removal of the ovaries in premenopausal women (female castration) and primary ovarian failure.

Estrogen is given IM or intravenously (IV) to treat uterine bleeding caused by hormonal imbalance. When estrogen is used to treat menopausal symptoms in a woman with an intact uterus, concurrent use of progestin is recommended to decrease the risk of endometrial cancer. After a hysterectomy, estrogen alone may be used for ERT.

Estrogens, in combination with a progestin, are also used as oral contraceptives (Table 46.1). The uses of individual estrogens are given in the Summary Drug Table: Female Hormones.

Progestins

Progestins are used in the treatment of amenorrhea, endometriosis, and functional uterine bleeding. Progestins are

Summary Drug Table FEMALE HORMONES

Generic Name	Trade Name	Uses	Adverse Reactions	Dosage Ranges
Estrogens				
estrogens, conjugated *ess'-troe-jens*	Premarin	Oral: vasomotor symptoms associated with menopause, atrophic vaginitis, osteoporosis, hypogonadism, primary ovarian failure, breast and prostate cancer palliation Parenteral: abnormal uterine bleeding from hormonal imbalance	Headache, dizziness, melasma, venous thromboembolism, nausea, vomiting, abdominal bloating and cramps, breakthrough bleeding/spotting, vaginal changes, rhinitis, changes in libido, breast enlargement and tenderness, weight changes, generalized pain	0.3–2.5 mg/day orally; IM: 25 mg/injection
estrogens, esterified	Menest	Same as conjugated estrogens	Same as conjugated estrogens	0.3–1.25 mg/day orally
estrogens, topical	EstroGel	Vaginal atrophy and vasomotor symptoms associated with menopause	Rare: minor vaginal irritation or itching	Metered dose for daily application
estrogens, vaginal	Estring, Femring; Estrace, Ogen, and Premarin Vaginal Creams	Vaginal atrophy and vasomotor symptoms associated with menopause	Rare: minor vaginal irritation or itching	See package insert; used weekly or monthly
estradiol, oral *ess-trah-dye'-ole*	Estrace, Femtrace, Gynodiol	Vasomotor symptoms associated with menopause, osteoporosis prevention, hypoestrogenism palliative therapy for breast and prostate cancer	Same as conjugated estrogens	0.5–10 mg/day orally
estradiol cypionate *ess-trah-dye'-ole 'sip-ee-oh-nate*	Depo-Estradiol	Moderate to severe vasomotor symptoms associated with menopause, female hypogonadism	Same as conjugated estrogens; pain at injection site	1–5 mg IM, every 3–4 wk
estradiol hemihydrate	Vagifem	Atrophic vaginitis	Same as conjugated estrogens	I tablet vaginally daily
estradiol transdermal system	Alora, Climara, Estraderm, Menostar, Vivelle	Same as conjugated estrogens	Same as conjugated estrogens	Variable doses, applied to skin weekly
estradiol topical emulsion	Estrasorb	Vasomotor symptoms of menopause		Two prepackaged pouches/d
estradiol valerate *ess-trah-dye'-ole val'-eh-rate*	Delestrogen	Same as estradiol cypionate	Same as conjugated estrogens; pain at injection site	10–20 mg IM monthly
estropipate *ess-troe-pye'-pate*	Ogen (cream), Ortho-Est (tablet)	Moderate to severe vasomotor symptoms associated with menopause, female hypogonadism, ovarian failure, osteoporosis	Same as conjugated estrogens	0.625–9 mg/day orally
synthetic conjugated estrogens, A	Cenestin	Moderate to severe vasomotor symptoms associated with menopause, vaginal atrophy	Same as conjugated estrogens	0.45 mg/day orally, then adjust according to symptoms

(table continues on page 460)

Male and Female Hormones

Summary Drug Table FEMALE HORMONES (continued)

Generic Name	Trade Name	Uses	Adverse Reactions	Dosage Ranges
synthetic conjugated estrogens, B	Enjuvia	Moderate to severe vasomotor symptoms associated with menopause	Same as conjugated estrogens	0.3 mg/day orally, then adjust according to symptoms
Progestins				
progesterone *pro-jess'-ter-own*	Crinone, Prometrium	Endometrial hyperplasia (oral), amenorrhea, abnormal uterine bleeding (injection), infertility (gel)	Breakthrough bleeding, spotting, change in menstrual flow, amenorrhea, breast tenderness, weight gain or loss, melasma, insomnia	Orally: 200 mg for 12 days of cycle IM: 5–10 mg/day for 6–8 days Gel: 90 mg/day
medroxy-progesterone *meh-drox'-ee-proe-jess'-ter-own*	Provera	Amenorrhea, abnormal uterine bleeding, endometrial hypoplasia	Same as progesterone	5–10 mg/day orally
norethindrone *nor-eth-in'-drone*	Aygestin	Amenorrhea, abnormal uterine bleeding, endometriosis	Same as hydroxyprogesterone caproate	2.5–10 mg/day for 5–10 day of cycle
Combination Products				
estrogens and progestins combined	Activella, Angeliq, ClimaraPro, CombiPatch, Femhrt, Prefest, Premphase, Prempro, YAZ	Treatment of moderate to severe vasomotor symptoms associated with menopause, treatment of vulval and vaginal atrophy, osteoporosis	Adverse reactions of both hormones; same as synthetic conjugated estrogens and progesterone	Oral or transdermal, variable dosing, used daily or weekly. See package insert.
Miscellaneous Drug				
raloxifene	Evista	Osteoporosis prevention and treatment	Hot flashes, flulike symptoms, arthralgia, rhinitis, increased cough	60 mg/day orally

also used as oral contraceptives, either alone or in combination with an estrogen (see the Summary Drug Table: Female Hormones; see also Table 46.1).

Contraceptive Hormones

Combination estrogens and progestins are used as oral contraceptives. There are three types of estrogen and progestin combination oral contraceptives: monophasic, biphasic, and triphasic. Monophasic oral contraceptives provide a fixed dose of estrogen and progestin throughout the cycle. The biphasic and triphasic oral contraceptives deliver hormones similar to the levels naturally produced by the body (see Table 46.1). Oral contraceptives have changed a great deal since their introduction in the 1960s. Today, lower hormone dosages provide reduced levels of hormones compared with the older formulations, while retaining the same degree of effectiveness (more than 99% when used as prescribed).

Taking contraceptive hormones provides health benefits not related to contraception, such as regulating the menstrual cycle and decreasing menstrual blood loss, the incidence of iron deficiency anemia, and dysmenorrhea. Health benefits

related to the inhibition of ovulation include a decrease in ovarian cysts and ectopic pregnancies. In addition, there is a decrease in fibrocystic breast disease, acute pelvic inflammatory disease, endometrial cancer, and ovarian cancer, improved maintenance of bone density, and a decrease in symptoms related to endometriosis in women taking contraceptive hormones. Newer combination contraceptives such as drospirenone and ethinyl estradiol combinations (YAZ) have been shown to help reduce moderate acne and maintain clear skin in women 15 years of age or older (who menstruate, want contraception, and have no response to topical antiacne medications).

Adverse Reactions: Estrogens

Administration of estrogens by any route may result in many adverse reactions, although the incidence and intensity of these reactions vary. Some of the adverse reactions seen with the administration of estrogens follow.

Central Nervous System Reactions

• Headache, migraine
• Dizziness, mental depression

Table 46.1 Oral Contraceptives	
Generic Name	**Trade Name**
Monophasic Oral Contraceptives	
50 mcg ethinyl estradiol, 1 mg norethindrone	Norinyl 1 + 50, Ortho-Novum 1/50
50 mcg ethinyl estradiol, 1 mg ethynodiol	Demulen 1/50, Zovia 1/50E
35 mcg ethinyl estradiol, 1 mg norethindrone	Norinyl 1 + 135, Ortho-Novum 1/35
35 mcg ethinyl estradiol, 0.5 mg norethindrone	Brevicon, Modicon
35 mcg ethinyl estradiol, 0.4 mg norethindrone	Ovcon-35
35 mcg ethinyl estradiol, 0.25 mg norgestimate	Ortho-Cyclen, Sprintec
35 mcg ethinyl estradiol, 1 mg ethynodiol	Demulen 1/35, Zovia 1/35E
30 mcg ethinyl estradiol, 1.5 mg norethindrone	Junel 21 1.5/30, Junel Fe, Loestrin 21 1.5/30, Loestrin Fe 1.5/30, Microgestin Fe 1.5/30
30 mcg ethinyl estradiol, 0.3 mg norgestrel	Lo/Ovral, Low-Ogestrel, Cryselle
30 mcg ethinyl estradiol, 0.15 mg desogestrel	Apri, Desogen, Ortho-Cept, Reclipsen
30 mcg ethinyl estradiol, 0.15 mg levonorgestrel	Jolessa, Levlen, Levora, Nordette, Portia, Quasense, Seasonale
30 mcg ethinyl estradiol, 3 mg drospirenone	Yasmin
20 mcg ethinyl estradiol, 3 mg drospirenone	YAZ
20 mcg ethinyl estradiol, 1 mg norethindrone	Junel 21 1/20, Junel Fe 1/20, Loestrin 21 1/20, Loestrin Fe 1/20, Microgestin Fe 1/20
20 mcg ethinyl estradiol, 0.09 mg levonorgestrel	Lybrel
20 mcg ethinyl estradiol, 0.1 mg levonorgestrel	Alesse, Aviane, Lessina, Levlite, Lutera, Sronyx
20/10 mcg ethinyl estradiol, 0.15 mg desogestrel	Kariva, Mircette
30 mcg ethinyl estradiol, 0.15 mg desogestrel	Solia
50 mcg mestranol, 1 mg norethindrone	Norinyl 1 + 50, Ortho-Novum 1/50
Biphasic Oral Contraceptives	
Phase one: 35 mcg ethinyl estradiol, 0.5 mg norethindrone Phase two: 35 mcg ethinyl estradiol, 1 mg norethindrone	Necon 10/11, Ortho-Novum 10/11
Phase one: 30 mcg ethinyl estradiol, 0.15 mg levonorgestrel	Seasonique
Phase two: 10 mcg ethinyl estradiol	
Triphasic Oral Contraceptives	
Phase one: 35 mcg ethinyl estradiol, 0.5 mg norethindrone Phase two: 35 mcg ethinyl estradiol, 1 mg norethindrone Phase three: 35 mcg ethinyl estradiol, 0.5 mg norethindrone	Aranelle, Leena, Tri-Norinyl
Phase one: 35 mcg ethinyl estradiol, 0.5 mg norethindrone Phase two: 35 mcg ethinyl estradiol, 0.75 mg norethindrone Phase three: 35 mcg ethinyl estradiol, 1 mg norethindrone	Necon7/7/7, Ortho-Novum 7/7/7
Phase one: 30 mcg ethinyl estradiol, 0.05 mg levonorgestrel Phase two: 40 mcg ethinyl estradiol, 0.075 mg levonorgestrel Phase three: 30 mcg ethinyl estradiol, 0.125 mg levonorgestrel	Triphasil, Tri-Levlen, Trivora, Enpresse

(table continues on page 462)

Male and Female Hormones

Table 46.1 Oral Contraceptives (continued)

Generic Name	Trade Name
Phase one: 35 mcg ethinyl estradiol, 0.18 mg norgestimate Phase two: 35 mcg ethinyl estradiol, 0.215 mg norgestimate Phase three: 35 mcg ethinyl estradiol, 0.25 mg norgestimate	Ortho Tri-Cyclen, Tri-Sprintec, Tri-Previfem, TriNessa
Phase one: 25 mcg ethinyl estradiol, 0.18 mg norgestimate Phase two: 25 mcg ethinyl estradiol, 0.215 mg norgestimate Phase three: 25 mcg ethinyl estradiol, 0.25 mg norgestimate	Ortho Tri-Cyclen Lo
Phase one: 1 mg norethindrone acetate, 20 mcg ethinyl estradiol Phase two: 30 mcg ethinyl estradiol, 1 mg norethindrone acetate Phase three: 35 mcg ethinyl estradiol, 1 mg norethindrone acetate	Estrostep Fe, Estrostep 21
Phase one: 25 mcg ethinyl estradiol, 0.1 mg desogestrel Phase two: 25 mcg ethinyl estradiol, 0.125 mg norgestimate Phase three: 25 mcg ethinyl estradiol, 0.15 mg norgestimate	Cesia, Cyclessa
Progestin-Only Contraceptive	
0.35 mg norethindrone	

Dermatologic Reactions

- Dermatitis, pruritus
- Chloasma (pigmentation of the skin) or melasma (discoloration of the skin), which may continue when use of the drug is discontinued

Gastrointestinal Reactions

- Nausea, vomiting
- Abdominal bloating and cramps

Genitourinary Reactions

- Breakthrough bleeding, withdrawal bleeding, spotting, change in menstrual flow
- Dysmenorrheal, premenstrual-like syndrome, amenorrhea
- Vaginal candidiasis, cervical erosion, vaginitis

Local Reactions

- Pain at injection site or sterile abscess with parenteral form of the drug
- Redness and irritation at the application site with transdermal system

Ophthalmic Reactions

- Steepening of corneal curvature
- Intolerance to contact lenses

Miscellaneous Reactions

- Edema, rhinitis, changes in libido
- Breast pain, enlargement, and tenderness
- Reduced carbohydrate tolerance
- Venous thromboembolism, pulmonary embolism

- Weight gain or loss
- Generalized and skeletal pain

Warnings associated with the administration of estrogen include an increased risk of endometrial cancer, gallbladder disease, hypertension, hepatic adenoma (a benign tumor of the liver), cardiovascular disease, and thromboembolic disease, and hypercalcemia in those with breast cancer and bone metastases.

 LIFESPAN ALERT – Menopausal Women Controversy persists over the increased risk for chronic heart disease and female cancers with the use of estrogen. Newer studies indicate that using the lower dose agents before the age of 60 may be beneficial. Alternative delivery systems are being explored to reduce the use of oral estradiol products.

Adverse Reactions: Progestins

Administration of progestins by any route may result in many adverse reactions, although the incidence and intensity of these reactions vary. Progestin administration may result in the following:

- Breakthrough bleeding, spotting, change in menstrual flow, amenorrhea
- Breast tenderness, edema, weight increase or decrease
- Acne, chloasma or melasma, insomnia, mental depression

In addition to the adverse reactions seen with progestins, the use of a levonorgestrel implant system may result in bruising after insertion, scar tissue formation at the site of insertion, and hyperpigmentation at the implant site. The use of medroxyprogesterone contraceptive injection may result in the same adverse reactions as those associated with administration of any progestin.

Adverse Reactions: Contraceptive Hormones

When estrogen–progestin combinations are used as oral contraceptives, these drugs may exhibit adverse reactions that vary depending on their estrogen or progestin content, so the adverse reactions of each must be considered. Table 46.2 identifies the symptoms of estrogen and progestin excess or deficiency. The adverse effects are minimized by adjusting the estrogen–progestin balance or dosage.

Contraindications and Precautions

Estrogen and progestin therapy is contraindicated in patients with known hypersensitivity to the drugs, breast cancer (except for metastatic disease), estrogen-dependent neoplasms, undiagnosed abnormal genital bleeding, and thromboembolic disorders. The progestins also are contraindicated in patients with cerebral hemorrhage or impaired liver function. Both the estrogens and progestins are classified as pregnancy category X drugs and are contraindicated during pregnancy.

Estrogens are used cautiously in patients with gallbladder disease, hypercalcemia (may lead to severe hypercalcemia in patients with breast cancer and bone metastasis), cardiovascular disease, and liver impairment. Cardiovascular complications are greater in women who smoke and use estrogen. Progestins are used cautiously in patients with a history of migraine headaches, epilepsy, asthma, and cardiac or renal impairment.

The warnings associated with the use of oral contraceptives are the same as those for the estrogens and progestins and include cigarette smoking, which increases the risk of cardiovascular side effects, such as venous and arterial thromboembolism, myocardial infarction, and thrombotic and hemorrhagic stroke. Also reported with oral contraceptive use are hepatic adenomas and other tumors, visual disturbances, gallbladder disease, hypertension, and fetal abnormalities.

Interactions

The following interactions may occur with female hormones:

Interacting Drug	Common Use	Effect of Interaction
Estrogens		
oral anticoagulants	Blood thinners	Decreased anticoagulant effect
tricyclic antidepressants	Treatment of depression	Increased effectiveness of antidepressant
barbiturates or rifampin	Sedation or anti-infective, respectively	Increased risk of breakthrough bleeding
hydantoins	Seizure control	Increased risk of breakthrough bleeding and pregnancy
Progestins		
anticonvulsants, barbiturates, or rifampin	Seizure control, sedation, or anti-infective, respectively	Decreased effectiveness of progestin
penicillins or tetracyclines	Anti-infective agents	Decreased effectiveness of oral contraceptives

HERBAL ALERT

Black cohosh, an herb reported to be beneficial in managing symptoms of menopause, is generally regarded as safe when used as directed. Black cohosh is a member of the buttercup family. The dosage of standardized extract is 2 tablets twice a day, or 40 drops of standardized tincture twice a day, or one 500- to 600-mg tablet or capsule three times daily. Black cohosh tea is not considered as effective as other forms. Boiling the root releases only a portion of the therapeutic constituents. The benefits of black cohosh (not to be confused with blue cohosh) include:

- Reduction in physical symptoms of menopause: hot flashes, night sweats, headaches, heart palpitations, dizziness, vaginal atrophy, and tinnitus (ringing in the ears)
- Decrease in psychological symptoms of menopause: insomnia, nervousness, irritability, and depression
- Improvement in menstrual cycle regularity by balancing the hormones and reducing uterine spasms

Adverse reactions are rare when using the recommended dosage. The most common adverse reaction is nausea. Black

Table 46.2 Estrogen and Progestin: Excess and Deficiency		
Hormone*	**Signs of Excess**	**Signs of Deficiency**
estrogen	Nausea, bloating, cervical mucorrhea (increased cervical discharge), polyposis (numerous polyps), hypertension, migraine headache, breast fullness or tenderness, edema	Early or midcycle breakthrough bleeding, increased spotting, hypomenorrhea melasma (discoloration of the skin),
progestin	Increased appetite, weight gain, tiredness, fatigue, hypomenorrhea, acne, oily scalp, hair loss, hirsutism (excessive growth of hair), depression, monilial vaginitis, breast regression	Late breakthrough bleeding, amenorrhea, hypermenorrhea.

*Hormonal balance is achieved by adjusting the estrogen/progestin dosage. Oral contraceptives have different amounts of progestin and estrogen, varying the estrogenic and progestational activity in each product

cohosh is contraindicated during pregnancy. Toxic effects include dizziness, headache, nausea, impaired vision, and vomiting. This herb is purported to be an alternative to hormone replacement therapy (HRT). In addition to its popularity as an herb for women's hormonal balance, black cohosh has been used for muscular and arthritic pain, headache, and eyestrain.

NURSING PROCESS

PATIENT RECEIVING A FEMALE HORMONE

ASSESSMENT

Preadministration Assessment

Before administering an estrogen or progestin, the nurse obtains a complete patient health history, including a menstrual history, which includes the **menarche** (age of onset of first menstruation), menstrual pattern, and any changes in the menstrual pattern (including a menopause history when applicable). In patients prescribed an estrogen (including oral contraceptives), the nurse obtains a history of thrombophlebitis or other vascular disorders, a smoking history, and a history of liver diseases. Blood pressure, pulse, and respiratory rate are taken and recorded. The primary health care provider usually performs a breast and pelvic examination and a Papanicolaou (Pap) test before starting therapy. Liver function tests may also be ordered.

If the male or female patient is being treated for a cancer, the nurse enters in the patient's record a general evaluation of the patient's physical and mental status. The primary health care provider may also order laboratory tests, such as serum electrolytes and liver function tests.

Ongoing Assessment

OUTPATIENTS. At the time of each office or clinic visit, the nurse obtains the blood pressure, pulse, respiratory rate, and weight. The nurse questions the patient regarding any adverse drug effects, as well as the result of drug therapy. For example, if the patient is receiving an estrogen for the symptoms of menopause, the nurse asks her to compare her original symptoms with the symptoms she is currently experiencing, if any. The nurse weighs the patient and reports a steady weight gain or loss. A periodic (usually annual) physical examination is performed by the primary health care provider and may include a pelvic examination, breast examination, Pap test, and laboratory tests. The patient with a prostatic or breast carcinoma usually requires more frequent evaluations of response to drug therapy.

HOSPITALIZED PATIENTS. The hospitalized patient receiving a female hormone requires careful monitoring. The nurse takes the vital signs daily or more often, depending on the patient's physical condition and the reason for drug use. The nurse observes the patient for adverse drug reactions, especially those related to the liver (the development of jaundice) or the cardiovascular system (thromboembolism). The nurse weighs the patient weekly or as ordered by the primary health care provider. The nurse reports any significant weight gain or loss to the primary health care provider.

In patients with breast or prostate cancer, the nurse observes for and evaluates signs indicating a response to therapy, including relief of pain, an increase in appetite, and a feeling of well-being. Patients with prostate cancer may respond rapidly to therapy, but patients with breast cancer usually respond slowly.

NURSING DIAGNOSES

Drug-specific nursing diagnoses include the following:

❏ **Effective Therapeutic Regimen Management** related to administration of medications routinely despite adverse reactions
❏ **Excess Fluid Volume** related to sodium and water retention
❏ **Ineffective Tissue Perfusion** related to thromboembolic effects
❏ **Imbalanced Nutrition: More or Less Than Body Requirements** related to weight gain or loss
❏ **Anxiety** related to diagnosis, use of ERT, or other factors

Nursing diagnoses related to drug administration are discussed in Chapter 4.

PLANNING

The expected outcomes of the patient may include an optimal response to therapy, support of patient needs related to the management of adverse reactions, a reduction in anxiety, and an understanding of and compliance with the prescribed therapeutic regimen.

IMPLEMENTATION

Promoting an Optimal Response to Therapy

ESTROGENS. Estrogens may be administered orally, IM, IV, transdermally, or intravaginally. Oral estrogens are administered with food or immediately after eating to reduce GI upset. Transdermal delivery has been found to be safer, especially for women with elevated triglycerides, type 2 diabetes, hypertension, migraine headaches, or those who smoke. When estrogens are given vaginally for atrophic vaginitis, the nurse gives the patient instructions on proper use.

CONTRACEPTIVE HORMONES. Monophasic oral contraceptives are administered on a 21-day regimen, with the first tablet taken on the first Sunday after the menses begin or on the day the menses begin if the menses begin on Sunday. After the 21-day regimen, the next 7 days are skipped, and then the cycle is begun again. With the biphasic oral contraceptives, the first phase is 10 days of a smaller dosage of progestin, and the second phase is a larger amount of progestin. The estrogen dosage remains constant for 21 days, followed by no estrogen for 7 days. Some regimens contain seven placebo tablets for easier management of the therapeutic regimen. With the triphasic oral contraceptives, the estrogen amount stays the same or may vary, and the progestin amount varies throughout the 21-day cycle. Progestin-only oral contraceptives are taken daily and continuously.

CONTRACEPTIVE IMPLANT SYSTEM. Levonorgestrel, a progestin, is available as an implant contraceptive system (Norplant System). Six capsules, each containing levonorgestrel, are implanted under local anesthesia in the subdermal (below the skin) tissues of the mid-portion of the upper arm. The capsules provide contraceptive protection for 5 years but may be removed at any time at the request of the patient. See Display 46.2 for more information on ways to promote an optimal response when taking the contraceptive hormones.

MEDROXYPROGESTERONE CONTRACEPTIVE INJECTION. Medroxyprogesterone (Depo-Provera), a synthetic progestin used in the treatment of abnormal uterine bleeding and secondary amenorrhea, is also used as a contraceptive. This

---

DISPLAY 46.2 Alternatives to Oral Contraceptive Hormones

Read

Patients who choose to use contraceptive hormone preparations need to be fully informed of their benefits and drawbacks. Nurses can be instrumental in educating patients about these drugs. Included here are contraceptive methods used by women in place of the traditional oral contraceptive pills.

Emergency Contraceptives (Plan B)
These preparations are used for emergency contraception after unprotected intercourse or known contraceptive failure. They prevent pregnancy; they do not work if the patient is already pregnant.

- When using high-dose levonorgestrel (Plan B), take one tablet within 72 hours after unprotected intercourse. Take the second dose of Plan B 12 hours later.
- This drug can be used any time during the menstrual cycle.
- If vomiting occurs within 1 hour after taking either dose, notify the primary health care provider.
- Emergency contraceptives are not effective in terminating an existing pregnancy.
- Emergency contraceptives should not be used as a routine form of contraception.

Etonogestrel/Ethinyl Estradiol Vaginal Ring (NuvaRing)
- The woman inserts the vaginal ring into the vagina, where it remains continuously for 3 weeks. It is removed for 1 week, during which bleeding usually occurs (usually 2 to 3 days after removal).
- Insert a new ring 1 week after the last ring was removed, on the same day of the week as it was inserted in the previous cycle. Do this even if bleeding is not finished.
- *Insertion*: Position for insertion by the woman may be standing with one leg up, squatting, or lying down. Compress the ring and insert into the vagina. (The exact position of the vaginal ring inside the vagina is not critical to its effectiveness.)
- The vaginal ring is removed after 3 weeks on the same day of the week as it was started. Removal is accomplished by hooking the index finger under the forward rim or by grasping the rim between the thumb and index finger and pulling it out. Discard the used ring in the foil pouch in a waste receptacle out of the reach of children or pets. (Do not flush the ring down the toilet.)
- Consider the menstrual cycle, timing of ovulation, and the possibility of pregnancy before beginning treatment.
- The vaginal ring may be accidentally expelled (e.g., when it was not inserted properly, during straining for defecation, while removing a tampon, or with severe constipation). If this occurs, rinse the vaginal ring with lukewarm water and reinsert promptly. (If the ring has been out of the vagina for more than 3 hours, contraceptive effectiveness may be reduced and an alternative contraceptive must be used for the next 7 days.)

- The most common adverse effects leading to discontinuation of contraceptive use involve device-related problems, such as foreign body sensations, coital problems, and device expulsion.
- Other adverse effects include vaginitis, headache, upper respiratory tract infection, leukorrhea, sinusitis, weight gain, and nausea.

Levonorgestrel Implants (Norplant System)
This is a long-term (5-year) reversible contraceptive system, and an informed consent may be required in some institutions before implementing this procedure. The patient needs to know that a surgical incision is required to insert six capsules and that removal also requires surgical intervention.

Levonorgestrel-Releasing Intrauterine System (Mirena) IUD
The capsules of the levonorgestrel-releasing intrauterine system (LRIS) are inserted during the first 7 days of the menstrual cycle or immediately after a first trimester abortion. LRIS is an intrauterine contraception device for use for not more than 5 years. Before insertion, provide the patient with the patient package insert. Also before insertion, a complete medical and social history, including that of the partner, is obtained to determine conditions that might influence the use of an intrauterine device (IUD). Several patient teaching points follow:

- Irregular menstrual bleeding, spotting, prolonged episodes of bleeding, and amenorrhea may occur. These symptoms diminish with continued use. The patient should check after each menstrual period to ensure that the thread attached to the LRIS still protrudes from the cervix. Caution her not to pull the thread.
- If pregnancy occurs with the LRIS in place, the LRIS should be removed. If the LRIS is not removed there is an increased risk of miscarriage/abortion, sepsis, premature labor, and premature delivery.
- The patient should self-monitor for flulike symptoms, fever, chills, cramping, pain, bleeding, vaginal discharge, or leakage of fluid.
- Reexamination and evaluation are done shortly after the first menses or within the first 3 months after insertion.
- Menstrual flow usually decreases after the first 3 to 6 months of LRIS use; therefore, an increase of menstrual flow may indicate expulsion of the device.
- Symptoms of partial or complete expulsion include pain and bleeding. However, the LRIS also can be expelled without any noticeable effects.

Medroxyprogesterone Contraceptive Injection (Depo-Provera)
Medroxyprogesterone is available as a long-term injectable contraceptive administered IM every 3 months. The injection is given only during the first 5 days after the onset of a normal

(box continues on page 466)

DISPLAY 46.2 **Alternatives to Oral Contraceptive Hormones** (continued)   *Read*

menstrual period, within 5 days postpartum if the woman is not breastfeeding, or at 6 weeks postpartum. Patient teaching points include the following:

- Bleeding irregularities may occur (i.e., irregular or unpredictable bleeding or spotting, or heavy continuous bleeding). Bleeding usually decreases to amenorrhea as treatment continues.
- Women tend to gain weight while using this form of contraception.
- The drug is not readministered if there is a sudden partial or complete loss of vision or if the patient experiences ptosis, diplopia, depression, or migraine.

Norelgestromin/Ethinyl Estradiol Transdermal System (Ortho Evra)
- The system is designed around a 28-day cycle, with a new patch applied each week for 3 weeks. Week 4 is patch free.
- Apply the new patch on the same day each week (note patch change day on the calendar).
- Discard used patch (only wear one patch at a time).
- Use no creams or lotions on area where patch is to be applied. Apply patch to clean, dry, intact, healthy skin on the buttock, abdomen, upper outer arm, or upper torso in a place where the

patch will not be rubbed by clothing. Patch should not be placed on the breast or on areas that are red or irritated.
- *Beginning treatment*: First day start (apply first patch on the first day of the menstrual cycle) or Sunday start (apply first patch on the first Sunday after the menstrual period begins).
- A backup contraceptive should be used for the first week of the *first* treatment cycle.
- If the patch partially or completely detaches for less than 24 hours, reapply to the same place or replace with a new patch immediately (no backup contraception needed).
- If the patch detaches for more than 24 hours, apply new patch immediately (new patch change day). Backup contraception needed for the first week (7 days) of the new cycle.
- If the patch change is forgotten, begin again immediately, making this day the new patch change day. (Backup contraception needed for the first 7 days.)
- If breakthrough bleeding continues longer than a few cycles, a cause other than the patch should be considered. Do not stop patch if bleeding occurs.
- Bleeding should occur during the patch-free week. If no bleeding occurs, consider the possibility of pregnancy.
- If pregnancy is confirmed, discontinue treatment.

---

drug is given IM every 3 months, and the initial dosage is given within the first 5 days of menstruation or within 5 days postpartum. When this drug is given IM, the solution must be shaken vigorously before use to ensure uniform suspension, and the drug is given deep IM into the gluteal or deltoid muscle.

 NURSING ALERT

If the interval is greater than 14 weeks between the IM injections of medroxyprogesterone, the nurse must be certain that the patient is not pregnant before administering the next injection.

Monitoring and Managing Patient Needs

EFFECTIVE THERAPEUTIC REGIMEN MANAGEMENT. The patient prescribed female hormones usually takes them for several months or years. Throughout that time, the patient must be monitored for adverse reactions. These drugs are self-administered at home. Patients may decide to regulate their own drug doses to alleviate adverse reactions; this can lead to ineffective dosing and more unwanted reactions such as pregnancy. Therefore, patient education is an important avenue for detecting and managing adverse reactions.

With estrogens, it is important to monitor for breakthrough bleeding. If breakthrough bleeding occurs with either estrogen or progestin, the patient notifies the primary health care provider. A dosage change may be necessary.

GI upsets such as nausea, vomiting, abdominal cramps, and bloating may also occur. Nausea usually decreases or subsides within 1 to 2 months of therapy. However, until then the discomfort may be decreased

if the drug is taken with food. If nausea is continual, frequent small meals may help. If nausea and vomiting persist, an antiemetic may be prescribed. Bloating may be alleviated with light to moderate exercise or by limiting fluid intake with meals.

The nurse carefully monitors the patient with diabetes who is taking female hormones. The primary health care provider is notified if blood glucose levels are elevated or the urine is positive for glucose or ketone bodies, because a change in the dosage of insulin or the oral hypoglycemic drug may be required. See Chapter 43 for the management of hypoglycemic and hyperglycemic episodes.

EXCESS FLUID VOLUME. Sodium and water retention may occur during female hormone therapy. In addition to reporting any swelling of the hands, ankles, or feet to the primary health care provider, the nurse weighs the hospitalized patient daily, keeps an accurate record of the intake and output, encourages ambulation (if not on bed rest), and helps the patient to eat a diet low in sodium (if prescribed by the primary health care provider).

INEFFECTIVE TISSUE PERFUSION. The nurse monitors the patient for signs of thromboembolic effects, such as pain, swelling, and tenderness in the extremities, headache, chest pain, and blurred vision. These adverse effects are reported to the primary health care provider. Patients with previous venous insufficiency, who are on bed rest for other medical reasons, or who smoke are at increased risk for thromboembolic effects. The nurse encourages the patient to elevate the lower extremities when sitting, if possible, and to exercise the lower extremities by walking.

NURSING ALERT

There is an increased risk of postoperative thromboembolic complications in women taking oral contraceptives. If possible, use of the drug is discontinued at least 4 weeks before a surgical procedure associated with thromboembolism or during prolonged immobilization.

IMBALANCED NUTRITION: MORE OR LESS THAN BODY REQUIREMENTS. Alterations in nutrition can occur, resulting in significant weight gain or loss. Weight gain occurs more frequently than weight loss. The nurse encourages a daily diet that includes adequate amounts of protein and carbohydrates and is low in fats. A variety of nutritious foods (fruits, vegetables, grains, cereals, meats, and poultry) should be included in the daily diet, with portion sizes decreased to meet individual needs. A dietitian may be consulted if necessary. An exercise program is helpful in both losing weight and maintaining weight loss.

Weight loss is often as difficult to manage as weight gain. When a patient taking the female hormones has a decrease in appetite and loses weight, the nurse encourages the individual to increase protein, carbohydrates, and calories in the diet. Small feedings with several daily snacks are usually better tolerated in those with a loss of appetite than are three larger meals. Patients are encouraged to eat foods they like. Dietary supplements may be necessary if a significant weight loss occurs. A dietitian may be consulted if necessary. Weights are usually taken on a weekly, rather than daily, basis.

ANXIETY. The woman taking female hormones may have many concerns about therapy with these drugs. Some concerns may be based on inaccurate knowledge, such as incorrect facts about certain dangers associated with female hormones. Although there are dangers associated with long-term use of female hormones, these adverse reactions occur in a small number of patients. When the patient is closely monitored by the primary health care provider, the dangers associated with long-term use are often minimized.

Some women may be anxious because of a fear of experiencing uterine cancer as the result of HRT. The nurse explains that taking progestin, which counteracts the negative effect of estrogen, can prevent estrogen-induced cancer of the uterus. Other women may fear the development of breast cancer or heart disease. Most research studies find that there is little risk for breast cancer developing and that the benefits of HRT often outweigh the risk of breast cancer. Studies questioned the effectiveness of HRT for postmenopausal women and the increased risk of cardiovascular disease. Newer studies demonstrate that lower doses orally or transdermally help reduce bone fractures in postmenopausal women.

The nurse encourages the patient to ask questions about her therapy. Information that is inaccurate is clarified before therapy is started. The nurse refers questions that cannot or should not be answered by a nurse to the primary health care provider.

The male patient with advanced prostatic carcinoma also may have concerns about taking a female hormone.

The nurse assures the patient that the dosage is carefully regulated and that feminizing effects, if they occur, are usually minimal.

Educating the Patient and Family

The instructions for starting oral contraceptive therapy vary with the product used. Each product has detailed patient instruction sheets regarding starting oral contraceptive therapy, and the nurse reviews them with the patient. The instructions for missed doses also are included in the package insert and are reviewed with the patient.

The nurse gives the patient a thorough explanation of the dosage regimen and adverse reactions that may result from the prescribed drug therapy. The nurse advises those taking oral contraceptives that skipping a dose could result in pregnancy. See Display 46.2 for more information to include in a teaching plan for a woman taking contraceptive hormones.

In most instances, the primary health care provider performs periodic examinations, such as laboratory analyses, a pelvic examination, or a Pap test. The patient is encouraged to keep all appointments for follow-up evaluation of therapy. The nurse includes several points in a teaching plan:

ESTROGENS AND PROGESTINS.

- Carefully read the patient package insert available with the drug. If there are any questions about this information, discuss them with the primary health care provider.
- If GI upset occurs, take the drug with food.
- Notify the primary health care provider if any of the following occurs: pain in the legs or groin area, sharp chest pain or sudden shortness of breath, lumps in the breast, sudden severe headache, dizziness or fainting, vision or speech disturbances, weakness or numbness in the arms, face or legs, severe abdominal pain, depression, or yellowing of the skin or eyes.
- Female patient: If pregnancy is suspected or abnormal vaginal bleeding occurs, stop taking the drug and contact the primary health care provider immediately.
- Patient with diabetes: Check the blood glucose or urine daily, or more often. Contact the primary health care provider if the blood glucose is elevated or if the urine is positive for glucose or ketones. An elevated blood glucose level or urine positive for glucose or ketones may require a change in diabetic therapy (insulin, oral hypoglycemic drug) or diet; these changes must be made by the primary health care provider.

ORAL CONTRACEPTIVES.

- A package insert is available with the drug. Read the information carefully. Begin the first dose as directed in the package insert or as directed by the primary health care provider. If there are any questions about this information, discuss them with the primary health care provider.
- To obtain a maximum effect, take this drug as prescribed and at intervals not exceeding once every

24 hours. An oral contraceptive is best taken with the evening meal or at bedtime. The effectiveness of this drug depends on following the prescribed dosage schedule. Failure to comply with the dosage schedule may result in a pregnancy.

- Use an additional method of birth control (as recommended by the primary health care provider) until after the first week in the next cycle.
- If one day's dose is missed, take the missed dose as soon as remembered or take two tablets the next day. If 2 days are missed, take two tablets for the next 2 days and continue on with the normal dosing schedule. However, another form of birth control must be used until the cycle is completed and a new cycle is begun. If 3 days in a row or more are missed, discontinue use of the drug and use another form of birth control until a new cycle can begin. Before restarting the dosage regimen, make sure a pregnancy did not result from the break in the dosage regimen.
- If there are any questions regarding what to do about a missed dose, discuss the procedure with the primary health care provider.
- Avoid smoking or excessive exposure to second-hand smoke while taking these drugs; cigarette smoking during estrogen therapy may increase the risk of cardio-vascular effects.
- Report adverse reactions such as fluid retention or edema to the extremities; weight gain; pain, swelling, or tenderness in the legs; blurred vision; chest pain; yellowed skin or eyes; dark urine; or abnormal vaginal bleeding.
- Remember that while taking these drugs, patients need periodic examinations by the primary health care provider and laboratory tests.

ESTRADIOL TRANSDERMAL SYSTEM.
- Refer to package insert for application, some systems are applied twice weekly; others are applied every 7 days.
- Apply the system immediately after opening the pouch, with the adhesive side down. Apply to clean, dry skin of the trunk, buttocks, abdomen, upper inner thigh, or upper arm. Do not apply to breasts, waistline, or a site exposed to sunlight. The area should not be oily or irritated.
- Press the system firmly in place with the palm of the hand for about 10 seconds. The application site is rotated, with at least 1-week intervals between applications to a particular site.
- Avoid areas that may be exposed to rubbing or where clothing may rub the system off or loosen the edges.
- Remove the old system before applying a new system unless the primary health care provider directs otherwise. Rotate application sites to prevent skin irritation.
- Follow the directions of the primary health care provider regarding application of the system (e.g., continuous, 3 weeks use followed by 1 week off, changed weekly, or applied twice weekly).

- If the system falls off, reapply it or apply a new system. Continue the original treatment schedule.

INTRAVAGINAL APPLICATION.
- Use the applicator correctly. Refer to the package insert for correct procedure. The applicator is marked with the correct dosage and accompanies the drug when purchased.
- Wash the applicator after each use in warm water with a mild soap and rinse well.
- Maintain a recumbent position for at least 30 minutes after instillation.
- Use a sanitary napkin or panty liner to protect clothing if necessary.
- Do not double the dosage if a dose is missed. Instead, skip the dose and resume treatment the next day (see Patient Teaching for Improved Patient Outcomes: Self-Administering Intravaginal Estrogen).
- When using the vaginal ring, press the ring into an oval and insert into the upper third of the vaginal vault.

EVALUATION

- Therapeutic effect is achieved.
- Adverse reactions are identified, reported to the primary health care provider, and managed using appropriate nursing interventions.
  - ☑ Patient manages the therapeutic regimen effectively.
  - ☑ Adequate fluid volume is maintained.
  - ☑ Tissue perfusion is maintained.
  - ☑ Patient maintains an adequate nutritional status.
  - ☑ Anxiety is managed successfully.
- Patient verbalizes the importance of complying with the prescribed therapeutic regimen.

Patient Teaching for Improved Patient Outcomes

Self-Administering Intravaginal Estrogen

The nurse:
- ✓ Explains the reason for the drug and prescribed therapy, including drug name, correct dosage, and frequency of administration.
- ✓ Describes the equipment to be used.
- ✓ Reinforces the need to empty the bladder and wash hands before administration.
- ✓ Demonstrates step-by-step procedure for filling applicator with drug and administration.
- ✓ Recommends a relaxed, supine position with knees flexed and legs spread.
- ✓ Instructs patient to insert applicator into vagina, angling it toward the tailbone and advancing it about 2 inches.
- ✓ Warns that drug may feel cold when inserted.

✓ Urges patient to remain recumbent for about 30 minutes after inserting drug.
✓ Suggests use of panty liner to prevent staining of clothes.
✓ Advises patient to wash applicator with mild soap and warm water, rinse well, and dry with paper towel after use.
✓ Cautions patient not to double dose if dose is missed but to skip dose and resume treatment the next day.
✓ Encourages daily inspection of perineal area for irritation or signs of allergic reaction.

● HORMONES FOR CANCER TREATMENT

Hormones may be used in cancer therapy especially for advanced disease. Receptors for specific hormones needed for cell growth are found on the surface of some tumor cells. By stopping the production of a hormone, blocking hormone receptors, or substituting a drug for the actual hormone, cancer cells can be killed or their growth slowed. These drugs also appear to counteract the effect of male or female hormones in hormone-dependent tumors. Hormones are not used as curative drugs in cancer treatment; rather, they have an adjuvant role because of their ability to slow or reverse tumor growth.

(handwritten notes: 13 / block production / can slow growth of cancer)

Summary Drug Table — HORMONAL THERAPY FOR CANCER

Generic Name	Trade Name	Uses	Adverse Reactions	Dosages
Adrenal Steroid Inhibitors				
aminoglutethimide *ah-meen'-oh-gloo-tih-thye-myde*	Cytadren	Metastatic breast, prostate cancers	Drowsiness, skin rash, nausea, vomiting	1–2 g/day orally
mitotane *mye'-toe-tane*	Lysodren	Adrenal cortical cancer	Leukocytosis, GI symptoms (nausea, vomiting, diarrhea, abdominal pain), fatigue, edema, hyperglycemia, dyspnea, cough, rash or itching, headaches, dizziness	2–10 g/day in divided doses
Gonadotropin-Releasing Hormone Analogs				
goserelin *goe'-seh-rell-in*	Zoladex	Prostate and breast cancer, endometriosis, endometrial thinning	Headache, emotional lability, depression, sweating, acne, breast atrophy, sexual dysfunction, vaginitis, hot flashes, pain, edema	3.6 mg monthly implant, 10.8 mg every 3 mo implant
histrelin *hiss'-trell-in*	Vantas	Prostate cancer	Hot flashes, fatigue, implant site irritation	50–60 mcg/day delivered e.g., implant changed yearly
leuprolide *loo-proe'-lyde*	Eligard, Lupron, Viadur	Prostate cancer, endometriosis, precocious puberty, uterine leiomyomata	Hot flashes, edema, bone pain, electrocardiographic changes, hypertension	1 mg/day SC, provided in monthly injection form and implant
triptorelin *trip-toe-rell'-in*	Trelstar Depot, LA	Prostate cancer	Hot flashes, skeletal pain, headache, impotence	3.75 mg IM every 28 days
Antiandrogens				
bicalutamide *bye-cal-loo'-tah-myde*	Casodex	Prostate cancer	Hot flashes, dizziness, constipation, nausea, diarrhea, nocturia, hematuria, peripheral edema, general pain, asthenia, infection	50 mg/day orally
flutamide *floo'-tah-myde*	Eulexin	Prostate cancer	Hot flashes, loss of libido, impotence, diarrhea, nausea, vomiting, gynecomastia	250 mg/orally TID

(handwritten: 12 / 15 / 15)

(table continues on page 470)

Summary Drug Table HORMONAL THERAPY FOR CANCER (continued)

Generic Name	Trade Name	Uses	Adverse Reactions	Dosages
nilutamide nah-loo'-tah-myde	Nilandron	Prostate cancer	Pain, headache, asthenia, flulike symptoms, insomnia, nausea, constipation, testicular atrophy, dyspnea	300 mg/day for 1 mo, then 150 mg/day orally
Estrogen				
estramustine	Emcyt	Prostate cancer	Breast tenderness and enlargement, nausea, diarrhea, edema	14 mg/kg/day orally in divided doses
Androgen				
testolactone tess-toe-lak'-tone	Teslac	Palliative treatment: breast cancer	Paresthesia, glossitis, anorexia, nausea, vomiting, maculopapular erythema, aches, alopecia, edema of the extremities, increase in blood pressure	250 mg orally QID
Aromatase Inhibitors				
anastrazole an-ass'-troh-zoll	Arimidex	Breast cancer	Vasodilation, mood disturbances, nausea, hot flashes, pharyngitis, asthenia, pain	1 mg/day orally
exemestane ex-ah'-mess-tane	Aromasin	Breast cancer	Same as anastrazole	25 mg/day orally
letrozole leh'-troe-zoll	Femara	Breast cancer	Same as anastrazole	2.5 mg/day orally
Progestins				
medroxyprogesterone meh-drox'-ee-proe-jess'-ter-own	Depo-Provera	Endometrial or renal cancer	Fatigue, nervousness, rash, pruritus, acne, edema	400–1000 mg/wk IM
megestrol meh-jess'-troll	Megace	Breast or endometrial cancer, appetite stimulant in HIV infection	Weight gain, nausea, vomiting, edema, breakthrough bleeding	40–320 mg/day orally in divided doses
Antiestrogens				
fulvestrant full-vess'-trant	Faslodex	Breast cancer	Nausea, vomiting, asthenia, pain, pharyngitis, headache	250 mg IM once monthly
tamoxifen tah-mox'-ih-fen	Nolvadex	Breast cancer, prophylactic therapy for women at high risk for breast cancer	Hot flashes, rashes, headaches, vaginal bleeding and discharge	20–40 mg/day orally
toremifene tore-em'-ih-feen	Fareston	Breast cancer	Hot flashes, sweating, nausea, dizziness, edema, vaginal bleeding, and discharge	60 mg/day orally

Examples of hormones used as antineoplastic drugs include the androgen testolactone (Teslac), conjugate estrogen, and the progestin megestrol (Megace). Gonadotropin-releasing hormone analogs, such as goserelin (Zoladex), appear to act by inhibiting the anterior pituitary secretion of gonadotropins, thus suppressing the release of pituitary gonadotropins. Consult the specific chapters in this book to learn the uses, cautions, adverse reactions, and nursing care associated with each category of hormone used in cancer treatment. For a listing of names, categories, and typical adverse reactions, see the Summary Drug Table: Hormonal Therapy for Cancer.

THINK CRITICALLY: PHARMACOLOGY IN PRACTICE

1. Ms. Chase calls the clinic, concerned about her mother. She has read that hormones can put a woman at risk for cancer, so she cannot understand why the primary health care provider is starting her mother on hormone therapy for her cancer. Explain how you can discuss her fears and help her to understand hormone therapy.

2. John, a friend of your brother, has started to use anabolic steroids to increase his strength and muscle mass to improve his chances of getting a football scholarship. Your brother tells you that this is acceptable, because his friend wants an education. Discuss how you would approach your brother with concerns about John's choices.

● Test Your Knowledge

1. The nurse monitors the patient taking an anabolic steroid for the more severe adverse reactions, which include _____.

   A. anorexia
   B. nausea and vomiting
   C. severe mental changes
   D. acne

2. The nurse must be aware that older men taking androgens are _____.

   A. prone to urinary problems
   B. at greater risk for hypertension
   C. at increased risk for confusion
   D. at increased risk for prostate cancer

3. When monitoring a patient taking an oral contraceptive, the nurse would observe the patient for signs of excess progestin. Which of the following reactions would indicate to the nurse that a patient has an excess of progestin?

   A. Increased appetite, hair loss
   B. Virilization, constipation
   C. Nausea, early breakthrough bleeding
   D. Deepening of the voice, lightheadedness

4. When teaching the patient taking an oral contraceptive for the first time, the nurse emphasizes the importance of taking _____.

   A. two tablets per day at the first sign of ovulation
   B. the drug at the same time each day
   C. the drug early in the morning before arising
   D. the drug each day for 20 days beginning on the first of the month

● Prepare for the NCLEX

1. A patient calls the outpatient clinic and says that she missed 1 day's dose of her "birth control pills." Which of the following statements would be most appropriate for the nurse to make to the patient?

   A. Do not take an additional tablet but resume the regular schedule today.
   B. Discontinue use of the drug and use another type of contraceptive until after your next menstrual period.
   C. Take two tablets today; then resume the regular daily schedule.
   D. Come into the office immediately for a pregnancy test.

● Calculate Medication Dosages

1. Medroxyprogesterone 650 mg IM is prescribed. The drug is available in a solution of 400 mg/mL. The nurse administers _____.

2. The physician prescribes estrone 0.5 mg IM for a postmenopausal woman with vasomotor symptoms. On hand is a vial of estrone with a solution containing 0.5 mg/mL. The nurse administers _____.

To check your answers, see Appendix E.

the**Point** *For more NCLEX questions, log on to http://thepoint.lww.com to access more than 1000 questions.*

Drugs Acting on the Uterus

ergotism   uterine atony
oxytocic   water intoxication

LEARNING OBJECTIVES

On completion of this chapter, the student will:

1. Discuss the actions, uses, adverse reactions, contraindications, precautions, and interactions of drugs acting on the uterus.
2. Discuss important preadministration and ongoing assessment activities the nurse should perform with the patient taking an oxytocic or tocolytic drug.
3. List some nursing diagnoses particular to a patient taking an oxytocic or tocolytic drug.
4. Discuss ways to promote an optimal response to therapy, how to manage adverse reactions, and important points to keep in mind when educating patients about the use of an oxytocic or tocolytic drug.

Drug therapy is beneficial for use in labor and delivery to promote the well-being of a woman and her fetus. Depending on the patient's need, drugs may be used to stimulate, intensify, or inhibit uterine contractions. The two types of drugs discussed in this chapter for their effect on the uterus are the oxytocics and the tocolytics. Drugs acting on the uterus are listed in the Summary Drug Table: Drugs Acting on the Uterus.

• OXYTOCIC DRUGS

Oxytocic drugs are used antepartum (before birth of the neonate) to induce uterine contractions similar to those of normal labor. These drugs are desirable when early vaginal delivery is in the best interest of the woman and the fetus. An oxytocic drug is one that stimulates the uterus. Included in this group of drugs are ergonovine, methylergonovine (Methergine), and oxytocin (Pitocin).

Action and Uses

Oxytocin

Oxytocin is an endogenous hormone produced by the posterior pituitary gland (see Chapter 44). This hormone has uterus-stimulating properties, acting on the smooth muscle of the uterus, especially on the pregnant uterus. As pregnancy progresses, the sensitivity of the uterus to oxytocin increases, reaching a peak immediately before the birth of the infant. This sensitivity enables oxytocic drugs to exert their full therapeutic effect on the uterus and produce the desired results. Oxytocin also has antidiuretic and vasopressor effects.

Oxytocin is administered intravenously (IV) for starting or improving labor contractions to obtain an early vaginal delivery of the fetus. An early vaginal delivery may be indicated when there are fetal or maternal problems, such as a woman with diabetes and a large fetus, Rh problems, premature rupture of the membranes, uterine inertia, and pregnancy-induced hypertension (PIH, also called eclampsia or preeclampsia). Preeclampsia is a condition of pregnancy characterized by hypertension, headache, albuminuria, and edema of the lower extremities occurring at, or near, term. The condition may progressively worsen until eclampsia (a serious condition occurring between the 20th week of pregnancy and the end of the 1st week postpartum and characterized by convulsive seizures and coma) occurs. Oxytocin may also be used in managing inevitable or incomplete abortion. Oxytocin can be given intramuscularly (IM) during the third stage of labor (period from the time the neonate is expelled until the placenta is expelled) to produce uterine contractions and control postpartum bleeding and hemorrhage. It may also be administered intranasally to stimulate the milk ejection (milk letdown) reflex.

Other Uterine Stimulants

Uterine stimulants increase the strength, duration, and frequency of uterine contractions and decrease the incidence of uterine bleeding. They are given after the delivery of the placenta and are used to prevent postpartum and postabortal hemorrhage caused by **uterine atony** (marked relaxation of

Summary Drug Table DRUGS ACTING ON THE UTERUS

Generic Name	Trade Name	Uses	Adverse Reactions	Dosage Ranges
Oxytocics				
carboprost *kar'-boe-prosst*	Hemabate	Postpartum uterine hemorrhage	Nausea, flushing	250 mcg IM may repeat in 15 –90 minutes, not to exceed 2 mg total dose
ergonovine *er-goe-noe'-veen*		Postpartum uterine atony and hemorrhage	Elevated blood pressure when spinal analgesia used	0.2 mg IM, orally q 2–4 hr
methylergonovine *meh-thill-er-goe-noe'-veen*	Methergine	Control of postpartum bleeding and hemorrhage, uterine atony	Dizziness, headache, nausea, vomiting, elevated blood pressure	0.2 mg IM, IV after delivery of the placenta; 0.2 mg orally TID, QID
misoprostol *mye-soe-prosst-ole*	Cytotec	Postpartum hemorrhage, cervical ripening	Headache, nausea, diarrhea, abdominal pain	100 mcg tablet vaginally administered
oxytocin *ox-ih-toe'-sin*	Pitocin	Antepartum: to initiate or improve uterine contractions Postpartum: control of postpartum bleeding and hemorrhage	Nausea, vomiting, pelvic hematoma, postpartum bleeding, cardiac arrhythmias, anaphylactic reactions	Induction of labor: individualize dose not to exceed 10 units/min Postpartum bleeding: IV infusion of 10–40 units in 1000 mL IV solution or 10 units IM after placenta delivery
Tocolytics				
indomethacin *in-doe-meth'-ah-sin*	Indocin	Preterm labor before 31 weeks' gestation	Headache, dizziness, nausea, vomiting, stomach upset or heartburn, prolonged vaginal bleeding	100 mg rectally, then 50 mg orally q 6 hr for a total of 8 doses
magnesium *mag-nee'-zee-um*		Preterm labor, seizure control	Fatigue, headaches, flushing, diplopia	4–6 g IV over 2 min, then infuse 1–4 g/hr
ritodrine *rih'-toe-dreen*		Preterm labor	Alterations in fetal and maternal heart rates and maternal blood pressure, palpitations, headache, nausea, vomiting	IV: 0.05–0.35 mg/min depending on patient response
terbutaline *ter-byoo'-tah-leen*	Brethine	Preterm labor	Nervousness, restlessness, tremor, headache, anxiety, hypertension, palpitations, arrhythmias, hypokalemia, pulmonary edema	Subcut: 250 mcg hourly until contractions stop Orally: 2.5 mg q 4–6 hr until delivery

the uterine muscle). These drugs include carboprost, ergonovine, methylergonovine, and misoprostol.

Adverse Reactions

Oxytocin

Administration of oxytocin may result in the following:

- Fetal bradycardia, uterine rupture, uterine hypertonicity
- Nausea, vomiting, cardiac arrhythmias, anaphylactic reactions

Because of its antidiuretic effect, serious **water intoxication** (fluid overload, fluid volume excess) may occur, partic-

ularly when the drug is administered by continuous infusion and the patient is receiving fluids by mouth. When oxytocin is used as a nasal spray, adverse reactions are rare.

Other Uterine Stimulants

Adverse reactions associated with other uterine stimulants include the following:

- Nausea, vomiting, diarrhea
- Elevated blood pressure, temporary chest pain
- Dizziness, water intoxication, headache

Allergic reactions may also occur. In some instances hypertension associated with seizure or headache may occur.

Ergotism (overdosage of ergonovine) is manifested by nausea, vomiting, abdominal pain, numbness, tingling of the extremities, and an increase in blood pressure. In severe cases, these symptoms are followed by hypotension, respiratory depression, hypothermia, gangrene of the fingers and toes, convulsions, hallucinations, and coma.

Contraindications, Precautions, and Interactions

Oxytocin is contraindicated in patients with known hypersensitivity to the drug, cephalopelvic disproportion, and unfavorable fetal position or presentation. It is also contraindicated in obstetric emergencies, situations of fetal distress when delivery is not imminent, severe toxemia (preeclampsia, eclampsia), and hypertonic uterus, as well as during pregnancy (intranasal administration) when there is total placenta previa. It is contraindicated as an agent to induce labor when vaginal delivery is contraindicated. Oxytocin is not expected to be a risk to the fetus when administered as indicated. When oxytocin is administered with vasopressors, however, severe maternal hypertension may occur.

Ergonovine and methylergonovine are not used before delivery of the placenta. They are contraindicated in those with known hypersensitivity to the drug or hypertension. These drugs are used cautiously in patients with heart disease, obliterative vascular disease, renal or hepatic disease, and during lactation. When methylergonovine is administered concurrently with vasopressors, or to patients who are heavy cigarette smokers, excessive vasoconstriction may occur.

NURSING PROCESS
PATIENT RECEIVING AN OXYTOCIC DRUG

ASSESSMENT

Preadministration Assessment
Before starting an IV infusion of oxytocin to induce labor, the nurse obtains an obstetric history (e.g., parity, gravidity, previous obstetric problems, type of labor, stillbirths, abortions, live-birth infant abnormalities) and a general health history. Immediately before starting the IV infusion of oxytocin, the nurse assesses the fetal heart rate (FHR) and the patient's blood pressure, pulse, and respiratory rate.

In addition, the nurse assesses and records the activity of the uterus (strength, duration, and frequency of contractions, if any). Monitoring uterine contractions for strength and length of the contractions can be done with an external monitor or by an internal uterine catheter with an electronic monitor. A fetal monitor is placed to assess the FHR.

The other uterine stimulants may be given orally or IM during the postpartum period to reduce the possibility of postpartum hemorrhage and to prevent relaxation of the uterus. When the patient is to receive any of these drugs after delivery, it is important to take the blood pressure, pulse, and respiratory rate before administration.

Ongoing Assessment
After injecting an oxytocic drug, the nurse monitors the patient's blood pressure, pulse, and respiratory rate at the intervals ordered by the primary health care provider.

> **NURSING ALERT**
> All patients receiving IV oxytocin must be under constant observation to identify complications. In addition, the primary health care provider should be immediately available at all times.

The nurse assesses the patient's blood pressure, pulse, and respiratory rate every 30 minutes. The FHR and uterine contractions are assessed every 15 minutes or as ordered by the primary health care provider. Three to four firm uterine contractions should occur every 10 minutes, followed by a palpable relaxation of the uterus.

> **NURSING ALERT**
> Hyperstimulation of the uterus during labor may lead to uterine tetany with marked impairment of the uteroplacental blood flow, uterine rupture, cervical rupture, amniotic fluid embolism, and trauma to the infant. Overstimulation of the uterus is dangerous to both the fetus and the mother and may occur even when the drug is administered properly in a uterus that is hypersensitive to oxytocin.

When monitoring uterine contractions, the nurse notifies the primary health care provider immediately if any of the following occurs:

- A significant change in the FHR or rhythm
- A marked change in the frequency, rate, or rhythm of uterine contractions; uterine contractions lasting more than 60 seconds; or contractions occurring more frequently than every 2 to 3 minutes, or no palpable relaxation of the uterus
- A marked increase or decrease in the patient's blood pressure or pulse or any significant change in the patient's general condition

If any of these conditions are noted, the nurse should immediately discontinue the oxytocin infusion and run the primary IV line at the rate prescribed by the primary health care provider until the primary health care provider examines the patient.

The nurse immediately reports any signs of water intoxication or fluid overload (e.g., drowsiness, confusion, headache, listlessness, and wheezing, coughing, rapid breathing) to the primary health care provider.

Oxytocin may be given IM after delivery of the placenta. After administering the drug, the nurse obtains the patient's blood pressure, pulse, and respiratory rate every 5 to 10 minutes. Then the nurse palpates the patient's uterine fundus for firmness and position. The nurse immediately reports any excess bleeding to the primary health care provider.

When administering ergonovine and methylergonovine after delivery, the nurse monitors vital signs every 4 hours and also notes the character and amount of vaginal bleeding. The patient may report abdominal cramping with the administration of these drugs. If cramping is moderately severe to severe, the nurse notifies the primary health care provider, because it may be necessary to discontinue use of the drug.

NURSING DIAGNOSES

Drug-specific nursing diagnoses include the following:

❏ **Anxiety** related to fears associated with the process of labor and delivery
❏ **Risk for Injury** (fetal) related to adverse drug effects of oxytocin on the fetus (fetal bradycardia)
❏ **Excess Fluid Volume** related to administration of IV fluids and the antidiuretic effects associated with oxytocin
❏ **Acute Pain** related to adverse reactions (abdominal cramping, nausea, headache)

Nursing diagnoses related to drug administration are discussed in Chapter 4.

PLANNING

The expected patient outcomes may include an optimal response to drug therapy (e.g., initiation of the normal labor process), adverse reactions (e.g., absence of a fluid volume excess with oxytocin administration) identified and reported to the primary health care provider, and an understanding of the treatment regimen.

IMPLEMENTATION

Promoting an Optimal Response to Therapy

OXYTOCIN. When oxytocin is prescribed, the primary health care provider orders the type and amount of IV fluid, the number of units of oxytocin added to the IV solution, and the IV infusion rate. An electronic infusion device is used to control the infusion rate. The primary health care provider establishes guidelines for administering the oxytocin solution and for increasing or decreasing the flow rate or discontinuing the administration of oxytocin. Usually, the flow rate is increased every 20 to 30 minutes, but this may vary according to the patient's response. The strength, frequency, and duration of contractions and the FHR are monitored closely.

When administering oxytocin intranasally to facilitate the letdown of milk, the nurse places the patient in an upright position, and with the squeeze bottle held upright, administers the prescribed number of sprays to one or both nostrils. The patient then waits 2 to 3 minutes before breastfeeding the infant or pumping the breasts. If the patient uses a breast pump, the nurse records the amount of milk pumped from the breasts.

The nurse notifies the primary health care provider if milk drips from the breast before or after breastfeeding or if milk drips from the opposite breast during breastfeeding, because there would be no need to continue drug therapy. The primary health care provider is notified if nasal irritation, palpitations, or uterine cramping occurs.

ERGONOVINE AND METHYLERGONOVINE. The nurse administers ergonovine and methylergonovine at the direction of the primary health care provider. Ergonovine is usually given during the third stage of labor after the placenta has been delivered. Ergonovine is primarily administered IM, but in emergencies when a quicker response is needed, the drug may be administered IV.

Methylergonovine is usually given IM at the time of the delivery of the anterior shoulder or after the delivery of the placenta. The drug is not given routinely IV because it may produce sudden hypertension and stroke. If the drug is given IV, the nurse administers the drug slowly over a period of 1 minute or more with close monitoring of the patient's blood pressure.

When ergonovine or methylergonovine is administered in the delivery room, the nurse briefly explains the purpose of the injection to the patient. If either of these drugs is given after delivery of the infant, the nurse explains the purpose of the drug, which is to improve the tone of the uterus and help the uterus to return to its (near) normal size.

Misoprostol tablets are administered vaginally to induce or augment uterine contractions. Care should be taken that hyperstimulation of the uterus causing uterine tetany does not occur.

Monitoring and Managing Patient Needs

ANXIETY. The patient receiving oxytocin to induce labor may have concern over the use of the drug to produce contractions. When given to induce or stimulate contractions, oxytocin may be given IV only. The nurse explains the purpose of the IV infusion and the expected results to the patient. Because the patient receiving oxytocin must be closely supervised, the nurse spends time with the patient and offers encouragement and reassurance to help reduce anxiety.

RISK FOR INJURY (FETAL). When oxytocin is administered, some adverse reactions must be tolerated or treated symptomatically until therapy is discontinued. For example, if the patient is nauseated, the nurse provides an emesis basin and perhaps a cool towel for the forehead. If vomiting occurs, the nurse notifies the primary health care provider.

If contractions are frequent, prolonged, or excessive, the infusion is stopped to prevent fetal anoxia or trauma to the uterus. Excessive stimulation of the uterus can cause uterine hypertonicity and possible uterine rupture. The nurse places the patient on her left side and provides supplemental oxygen. The effects of the drug diminish rapidly, because oxytocin is a short-acting drug.

EXCESS FLUID VOLUME. When oxytocin is administered IV, there is a danger of an excessive fluid volume (water intoxication), because oxytocin has an antidiuretic effect. The nurse measures the fluid intake and output. In some instances, hourly measurements of output are necessary. The nurse observes the patient for signs of fluid overload (see Chapter 55). If any of these signs or symptoms is noted, the nurse should immediately discontinue the oxytocin infusion but let the primary IV line run at the rate prescribed by the primary health care provider until the primary health care provider examines the patient.

Acute Pain. When ergonovine or methylergonovine is administered for uterine atony and hemorrhage, abdominal cramping can occur and is usually an indication of drug effectiveness. The uterus is palpated in the lower abdomen as small, firm, and round. However, the nurse should report persistent or severe cramping to the primary health care provider.

> ### ⚠ NURSING ALERT
> In some patients who are calcium deficient, the uterus may not respond to ergonovine. The nurse immediately reports a lack of response to ergonovine. Administration of calcium by IV injection usually restores response to the drug.

Although rare, ergotism or ergot poisoning can occur with the administration of excessive amounts of ergonovine or methylergonovine.

> ### ⚠ NURSING ALERT
> Symptoms of ergotism that must be reported immediately include coolness, numbness and tingling of extremities, dyspnea, nausea, confusion, tachycardia or bradycardia, chest pain, hallucinations, and convulsions. If these reactions occur, the nurse immediately reports them to the primary health care provider, because use of the drug must be discontinued.

Educating the Patient and Family
The treatment regimen is explained to the patient and family (when appropriate). The nurse answers any questions the patient may have regarding treatment and instructs the patient to report any adverse reactions. The nurse also informs the patient and family about the therapeutic response during administration of the drug, and if nasal spray is to be used, teaches the patient the proper technique.

EVALUATION

- Therapeutic effect is achieved and normal labor is initiated.
- Adverse reactions are identified, reported to the primary health care provider, and managed successfully through appropriate nursing interventions:
  - ☑ Anxiety is managed successfully.
  - ☑ No evidence of injury is seen.
  - ☑ Fluid volume balance is maintained.
  - ☑ Patient is free of pain.
- Patient demonstrates an understanding of the drug regimen.

●TOCOLYTICS

Drugs used to prevent uterine contractions are called *tocolytics*. They are useful in the management of preterm labor. These drugs decrease uterine activity and prolong the pregnancy to allow the fetus to develop more fully, thereby increasing the chance of neonatal survival. Magnesium is the most commonly used drug to decrease uterine muscle contractions, followed by the nonsteroidal anti-inflammatory drugs (NSAIDs) such as indomethacin. Ritodrine and terbutaline (Brethine) are used as second-line therapies because of the greater risks these drugs pose to the mother.

Actions and Uses

Magnesium is a calcium antagonist that works to decrease the force of uterine contractions. Typically, infusions last less than 48 hours to prevent preterm delivery until steroid prophylaxis (for fetal lung maturation) can be initiated. Magnesium is used to manage preterm labor in pregnancies of greater than 27 weeks' gestation. Magnesium administration requires hospitalization. Indomethacin is an NSAID that blocks the production of substances called *prostaglandins* (see Chapter 15), which contribute to uterine contractions.

Adverse Reactions

Adverse reactions to magnesium include the following:

- Fatigue, flushing, headache, diplopia
- Sweating, hypotension, depressed reflexes, and flaccid paralysis are other adverse reactions associated with IV administration. They are related to hypocalcemia induced by the therapy.

Adverse reactions observed with indomethacin include the following:

- Headaches, dizziness
- Nausea, vomiting, stomach upset or heartburn
- Prolonged vaginal bleeding

Contraindications, Precautions, and Interactions

Magnesium is contraindicated in patients with known hypersensitivity to the drug, heart block or myocardial damage, or eclampsia or severe preeclampsia, and within 2 hours of delivery. Magnesium is classified as a pregnancy category A drug, and indomethacin is a pregnancy category B drug. Although these drugs are given for preterm labor, they still should be given cautiously during pregnancy.

There is an increased effectiveness of central nervous system depressants (e.g., opioids, analgesics, and sedatives) when magnesium is administered. The effectiveness of neuromuscular blocking agents is enhanced as well. See Chapter 15 for drug interactions with indomethacin.

NURSING PROCESS

PATIENT RECEIVING A TOCOLYTIC AGENT

ASSESSMENT

Preadministration Assessment
Before starting an IV infusion containing a tocolytic drug, the nurse obtains the patient's vital signs. The nurse auscultates lung sounds to provide a baseline assessment. The patient has a monitoring device in place to determine uterine contractions and the FHR before and during administration.

Before magnesium is initiated, baseline blood tests (e.g., complete blood count and creatinine level) are performed. Because magnesium affects the neuromuscular system, a neurologic examination is performed as well. Mentation, cranial nerve function, and deep tendon reflexes are assessed. When indomethacin is used as the tocolytic drug, additional tests include liver function tests and amniotic fluid index (AFI).

Ongoing Assessment
During the ongoing assessment of a patient receiving a tocolytic drug, nursing activities include the following at 15- to 30-minute intervals:

- Obtaining blood pressure, pulse, and respiratory rate
- Monitoring FHR
- Checking the IV infusion rate
- Examining the area around the IV needle insertion site for signs of infiltration
- Monitoring uterine contractions (frequency, intensity, length)
- Measuring maternal intake and output

NURSING DIAGNOSES

Drug-specific nursing diagnoses include the following:

- ❏ **Anxiety** related to fears concerning preterm labor
- ❏ **Impaired Gas Exchange** related to pulmonary edema from drug therapy and IV fluids

Nursing diagnoses related to drug administration are discussed in Chapter 4.

PLANNING

The expected outcomes of the patient may include an optimal response to therapy, a reduction in anxiety, and an understanding of the treatment of preterm labor.

IMPLEMENTATION

Promoting an Optimal Response to Therapy
Nursing management for a patient receiving magnesium, ritodrine, or terbutaline is similar. For IV administration, the nurse prepares the solution according to the primary health care provider's instructions. An infusion pump is used to control the flow rate. Magnesium, ritodrine, or terbutaline may be piggybacked to the primary line, allowing the primary line to maintain patency should it become necessary temporarily to discontinue infusion of the drug. In some cases, the primary health care provider may prescribe indomethacin for administration by the rectal or oral route throughout the treatment, rather than by the IV route. Terbutaline may be given orally or by subcutaneous (subcut) injection. In any case, the nurse places a cardiac monitor on the patient and, to minimize hypotension, the nurse positions the patient in a left lateral position unless the primary health care provider orders a different position.

The primary health care provider is kept informed of the patient's response to the drug, because a dosage change may be necessary. The primary health care provider establishes guidelines for the regulation of the IV infusion rate, as well as the blood pressure and pulse ranges that require stopping the IV infusion.

Monitoring and Managing Patient Needs
During administration of the drug, the nurse monitors maternal and fetal vital signs every 15 minutes and uterine contractions frequently throughout the infusion.

ANXIETY. The patient in preterm labor may have many concerns about her pregnancy as well as the effectiveness of drug therapy. The woman is encouraged to verbalize any fears or concerns. The nurse listens to the patient's concerns and carefully and accurately answers any questions she may have concerning drug therapy. In addition, the nurse offers emotional support and encouragement while the drug is being administered. If allowed by the institution, the presence of family members may decrease anxiety in the woman experiencing preterm labor.

IMPAIRED GAS EXCHANGE. The nurse reports to the primary care provider a pulse rate of 140 bpm, persistent elevation of pulse rate, irregular pulse, or increase in respiratory rate of more than 20 respirations/min. The nurse assesses the respiratory status for symptoms of pulmonary edema (e.g., dyspnea, tachycardia, increased respiratory rate, rales, and frothy sputum). If these reactions occur, the primary health care provider is notified immediately, because use of the drug may be discontinued or the dosage may be decreased. After contractions cease, the nurse tapers the dosage to the lowest effective dose by decreasing the drug infusion rate at regular intervals prescribed by the primary health care provider. The infusion continues for at least 12 hours after uterine contractions cease. Because treatment duration is brief, mild adverse reactions must be tolerated. If adverse reactions are severe, use of the drug is discontinued or the dosage decreased.

Educating the Patient and Family
The nurse carefully explains the treatment regimen to the patient. The primary health care provider usually discusses the expected outcome of treatment with the patient and answers any questions regarding therapy. Although the patient is monitored closely during therapy,

the patient is instructed to notify the nurse immediately if any of the following occur: nausea, vomiting, palpitations, or shortness of breath. If a patient is taking ritodrine, the nurse discusses the importance of lying on the left side during IV administration.

If oral indomethacin or terbutaline is prescribed for preterm labor, the patient is instructed on use of the drug and adverse reactions to report (excessive tremor, nervousness, drowsiness, headache, nausea, dizziness, yellow coloration of skin or eyes). If contractions resume during oral therapy, the patient is instructed to notify the primary health care provider if four to six contractions per hour occur.

EVALUATION

- Therapeutic drug effect is achieved and labor is stopped.
- Adverse reactions are identified, reported to the primary health care provider, and managed successfully through appropriate nursing interventions:
  ☑ Anxiety is managed successfully.
  ☑ Gas exchange is maintained.
- Patient demonstrates an understanding of the drug regimen.

THINK CRITICALLY: PHARMACOLOGY IN PRACTICE

1. Betty Peterson's daughter has been admitted to the obstetric unit and is to receive oxytocin to induce labor. This is her daughter's first child, and Betty is extremely anxious. Analyze what information would be necessary for the family to receive from the nurse before the administration of oxytocin.

● Test Your Knowledge

1. When oxytocin is administered over a prolonged time, which of the following adverse reactions would be most likely to occur?

   A. Hyperglycemia
   B. Renal impairment
   C. Increased intracranial pressure
   D. Water intoxication

2. When the patient is receiving oxytocin, the nurse would notify the primary health care provider in which of the following conditions?

   A. Uterine contractions occur every 5 to 10 minutes
   B. Uterine contractions last more than 60 seconds or contractions occur more frequently than every 2 to 3 minutes
   C. Patient experiences pain during a uterine contraction
   D. Patient experiences increased thirst

3. Which of the following adverse reactions is most indicative of ergotism?

   A. Numbness, tingling of the extremities
   B. Headache, blurred vision
   C. Tachycardia and cardiac arrhythmias
   D. Diaphoresis, increased respirations

4. During administration of ritodrine, in what position would the nurse most probably place the patient?

   A. Supine
   B. Prone
   C. On the left side
   D. On the right side

● Prepare for the NCLEX

1. Intravenous oxytocic and tocolytic drugs should be administered as:

   A. immediate push drugs in a syringe
   B. syringe pump into a heparin lock device
   C. directly in a primarily IV line
   D. secondary or piggybacked into a primary line

● Calculate Medication Dosages

1. Terbutaline 2.5 mg is prescribed. The drug is available in 5-mg tablets. The nurse administers ____.

2. Methylergonovine 0.2 mg IM is prescribed. The drug is available as 0.2 mg/mL. The nurse administers ____.

To check your answers, see Appendix E.

the**Point** *For more NCLEX questions, log on to http://thepoint.lww.com to access more than 1000 questions.*

Drugs That Affect the Urinary System

The urinary system is responsible for the regulation and elimination body fluids. It comprises the kidneys, ureters, bladder, and urethra, as illustrated in the following figure.

The nephron is the functional unit of the kidney (see Chapter 48). Each kidney contains about one million nephrons, which filter the bloodstream to remove waste products. During this process, water and electrolytes are also selectively removed. The filtrate (i.e., the fluid removed from the blood) normally contains ions (potassium, sodium, chloride), waste products (ammonia, urea), water, and at times, other substances that are being excreted from the body, such as drugs. The filtrate then passes through the proximal tubule, the loop of Henle, and the distal tubules. At these points, selective reabsorption of amino acids, glucose, some electrolytes, and water occurs. Ions and water that are required by the body to maintain fluid and electrolyte balance are returned to the bloodstream through the minute capillaries that surround the distal and proximal tubules and the loop of Henle. Ions and water that are not needed by the body are excreted in the urine. Drugs used to control the amount and composition of the fluid excreted or reabsorbed are covered in Chapter 48.

The bladder is the storage area for urine before it is excreted from the body. The nature of the bladder and its contents make it susceptible to infection. Chapter 49 discusses drugs used specifically for treating urinary tract infections (UTIs) and the discomfort associated with those infections.

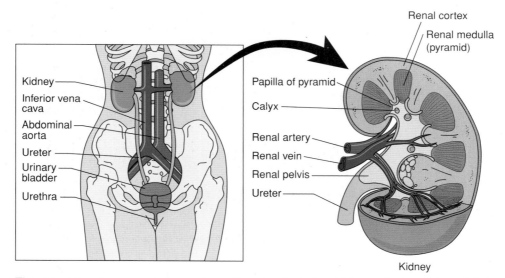

The normal urinary system, male or female, includes kidneys (enlarged at right), ureters, and bladder.

PHARMACOLOGY IN PRACTICE

Our patient focus in this unit is Mr. Phillip, a 72-year-old widower who lives alone. He was diagnosed with a UTI 8 weeks ago. Having failed to see his primary health care provider for a follow-up urine sample 2 weeks after completing the course of drug therapy, he is at the clinic to see a primary health care provider because the UTI symptoms have recurred.

After reading the chapters in this unit, you will learn about the methods to treat problems of the urinary tract system. Then you will be able to help Mr. Phillip in the treatment of his UTI.

Diuretics

anuria
diuretic
edema

gynecomastia
hyperkalemia
hypokalemia

LEARNING OBJECTIVES

On completion of this chapter, the student will:

1. List the five general types of diuretics.
2. Discuss the uses, general drug actions, adverse reactions, contraindications, precautions, and interactions of the diuretics.
3. Describe important preadministration and ongoing assessment activities the nurse should perform with the patient taking a diuretic.
4. List nursing diagnoses particular to a patient taking a diuretic.
5. Discuss ways to promote an optimal response to therapy, how to manage common adverse reactions, and important points to keep in mind when educating patients about the use of diuretics.

Many conditions or diseases, such as heart failure (HF), endocrine disturbances, and kidney and liver diseases can cause **edema** (retention of excess fluid). When the patient shows signs of excess fluid retention, the primary health care provider may order a **diuretic** to reduce the edema. A diuretic is a drug that increases the excretion of urine (i.e., water, electrolytes, and waste products) by the kidneys. There are various types of diuretic drugs, and the primary health care provider selects the one that best suits the patient's needs and effectively reduces the amount of excess fluid in body tissues. The different types of diuretic drugs are the following:

• Carbonic anhydrase inhibitors
• Loop diuretics
• Osmotic diuretics
• Potassium-sparing diuretics
• Thiazides and related diuretics

The Summary Drug Table: Diuretics lists examples of the different types of diuretic drugs. Diuretics are used in a variety of medical disorders. The primary health care provider selects the type of diuretic that will most likely be effective for treatment of a specific disorder. In some instances, hypertension may be treated with the administration of an antihypertensive drug and a diuretic. The diuretics used for this combination therapy include the loop diuretics and the thiazides and related diuretics. The specific uses of each type of diuretic drug are discussed in the following sections.

Actions

Refer to the illustration of the kidney nephron (Fig. 48.1) for a better understanding of the actions of the diuretics.

Carbonic Anhydrase Inhibitors

These drugs are sulfonamides, with nonbacteriostatic action, that inhibit the enzyme carbonic anhydrase. The carbonic anhydrase enzyme produces free hydrogen ions, which are then exchanged for sodium ions in the kidney tubules. Carbonic anhydrase inhibition results in the excretion of sodium, potassium, bicarbonate, and water. Glaucoma, a condition of increased pressure in the eye from excess aqueous humor, is treated with carbonic anhydrase inhibitors. These diuretics decrease the production of aqueous humor in the eye, which in turn decreases intraocular pressure (IOP, i.e., pressure within the eye).

Loop Diuretics

The loop diuretics furosemide (Lasix) and ethacrynic acid (Edecrin) increase the excretion of sodium and chloride by inhibiting reabsorption of these ions in the distal and proximal tubules and in the loop of Henle. These drugs act at three sites, thereby increasing their effectiveness as diuretics. Torsemide (Demadex) also increases urinary excretion of sodium, chloride, and water but acts primarily in the ascending portion of the loop of Henle. Bumetanide (Bumex) primarily increases the excretion of chloride but also has some sodium-excreting ability. This drug acts primarily on the proximal tubule of the nephron.

Osmotic Diuretics

Osmotic diuretics increase the density of the filtrate in the glomerulus. This prevents selective reabsorption of water, which allows the water to be excreted. Sodium and chloride excretion is also increased.

Summary Drug Table DIURETICS

Generic Name	Trade Name	Uses	Adverse Reactions	Dosage Ranges
Carbonic Anhydrase Inhibitors				
acetazolamide *ah-set-ah-zoll'-ah-myde*	Diamox	Open-angle glaucoma, secondary glaucoma, preoperatively to lower IOP, edema due to HF, drug-induced edema, centrencephalic epilepsy	Weakness, fatigue, anorexia, nausea, vomiting, rash, paresthesias, photosensitivity	Glaucoma: up to 1 g/day orally in divided doses; Acute glaucoma: 500 mg initially then 125–250 mg orally q 4 hr; Epilepsy: 8–30 mg kg/day in divided doses; HF and edema: 250–375 mg/day orally
methazolamide *meth-ah-zoll'-ah-myde*		Glaucoma	Same as acetazolamide	50–100 mg orally BID, TID
Loop Diuretics				
bumetanide *byoo-met'-ah-nyde*	Bumex	Edema due to HF, cirrhosis of the liver, renal disease, acute pulmonary edema	Electrolyte and hematologic imbalances, anorexia, nausea, vomiting, dizziness, rash, photosensitivity, orthostatic hypotension, glycosuria	0.5–10 mg/day orally, IV, IM
ethacrynic acid *eth-ah-krye'-nik*	Edecrin	Same as bumetanide plus ascites due to malignancy, idiopathic edema, lymphedema	Same as bumetanide plus diarrhea	50–200 mg/day orally, IV
furosemide *fur-oh-seh-myde*	Lasix	Same as bumetanide plus hypertension	Same as bumetanide	Edema: 20–80 mg/day, may go up to 600 mg/day for severe edema; Hypertension: 40 mg orally BID HF/renal failure: up to 2.5 g/day
torsemide *tor-she-myde*	Demadex	Same as bumetanide plus hypertension	Same as bumetanide plus headache	HF/renal failure: 10–20 mg/day orally, IV; Cirrhosis/hypertension: 5–10 mg/day orally, IV
Osmotic Diuretics				
glycerin (glycerol) *glíh-ser-in*		Glaucoma, before and after surgery	Headache, nausea, vomiting	1–2 g/kg orally in solution
isosorbide *eye-soe-sor-byde*		Same as glycerin	Same as glycerin	1–3 mg/kg orally, BID-QID
mannitol *man-ih-toll*	Osmitrol	To promote diuresis in acute renal failure, reduction of IOP, treatment of cerebral edema, irrigation solution in prostate surgical procedures	Edema, fluid and electrolyte imbalance, headache, blurred vision, nausea, vomiting, diarrhea, urinary retention	Diuresis: 50–200 g/24 hr IV IOP: 1.5–2 g/kg IV
urea *yoor-ee'-ah*		Reduction of IOP, reduction of intracranial pressure	Headache, nausea, vomiting, fluid and electrolyte imbalance, syncope	Up to 120 g/day IV
Potassium-Sparing Diuretics				
amiloride *ah-mill'-oh-ryde*		HF, hypertension, prevention of hypokalemia in at-risk patients, polyuria prevention with lithium use	Headache, dizziness, nausea, anorexia, diarrhea, vomiting, weakness, fatigue, rash, hypotension	5–20 mg/day orally

intracranial pressure

(table continues on page 483)

Summary Drug Table DIURETICS (continued)

Generic Name	Trade Name	Uses	Adverse Reactions	Dosage Ranges
spironolactone *speer-on-oh-lak-tone*	Aldactone	Hypertension, edema due to HF, cirrhosis, renal disease; hypokalemia, prophylaxis of hypokalemia in at-risk patients, hyperaldosteronism	Headache, diarrhea, drowsiness, lethargy, hyperkalemia, cramping, gastritis, erectile dysfunction, gynecomastia	Up to 400 mg/day orally in single dose or divided doses
triamterene *trye-am'-ter-een*	Dyrenium	Prevention of hypokalemia, edema due to HF, cirrhosis, renal disease, hyperaldosteronism	Diarrhea, nausea, vomiting, hyperkalemia, photosensitivity	Up to 300 mg/day orally in divided doses
Thiazides and Related Diuretics				
chlorothiazide *klor-oh-thye'-ah-zyde*	Diuril	Hypertension, edema due to HF, cirrhosis, corticosteroid and estrogen therapy	Orthostatic hypotension, dizziness, vertigo, light-headedness, weakness, anorexia, gastric distress, nausea, diarrhea, constipation, hematologic changes, rash, photosensitivity reactions, hyperglycemia, fluid and electrolyte imbalances, reduced libido	0.5–2 g orally or IV, QID or BID
chlorthalidone *klor-thal'-ih-doan*	Thalitone	Same as chlorothiazide	Same as chlorothiazide	Edema: 50–120 mg/day orally; Hypertension: 25–100 mg/day orally
hydrochlorothiazide *hye-droe-klor-oh-thye'-ah-zyde*	Microzide, Oretic	Same as chlorothiazide	Same as chlorothiazide	Edema: 25–200 mg/day orally; Hypertension: 12.5–50 mg/day orally
hydroflumethiazide *hye-droe-floo-meh-thye'-ah-zyde*	Saluron	Same as chlorothiazide	Same as chlorothiazide	Edema: 25–200 mg/day orally; Hypertension: 50-100 mg/day orally
indapamide *in-dap'-ah-myde*		Hypertension, edema due to HF	Same as chlorothiazide	Edema: 2.5–5 mg/day orally; Hypertension: 1.25–5 mg/day orally
metolazone *meh-toll'-ah-zoan*	Zaroxolyn	Edema in HF, cirrhosis, corticosteroids, estrogen therapy, renal dysfunction	Same as chlorothiazide	2.5–20 mg/day orally
methyclothiazide *meth-ih-kloe-thye'-ah-zyde*	Enduron	Same as chlorothiazide	Same as chlorothiazide	Edema: 2.5–10 mg/day orally; Hypertension: 2.5–5 mg/day orally

(Handwritten annotations: "lack potassium", "use is for hypokalemia", "HCTZ - can cause gout", "monitor pulse", "potassium level digoxin")

Potassium-Sparing Diuretics

Diuretics that depress the excretion of potassium are called *potassium-sparing* (or *potassium-saving*) diuretics. Potassium-sparing diuretics work in either of two ways. Triamterene (Dyrenium) and amiloride depress the reabsorption of sodium in the kidney tubules, thereby increasing sodium and water excretion. Both drugs additionally depress the excretion of potassium. Spironolactone (Aldactone) antagonizes the action of aldosterone. Aldosterone, a hormone produced by the adrenal cortex, enhances the reabsorption of sodium in the distal convoluted tubules of the kidney. When this activity of aldosterone is blocked, sodium (but not potassium) and water are excreted.

Thiazides and Related Diuretics

Thiazides and related diuretics inhibit the reabsorption of sodium and chloride ions in the ascending portion of the loop of Henle and the early distal tubule of the nephron. This action results in the excretion of sodium, chloride, and water.

Diuretics

Figure 48.1 The nephron is the functional unit of the kidney. Note the various tubules, the site of most diuretic activity. The loop of Henle is the site of action for loop diuretics. Thiazide diuretics act at the ascending portion of the loop of Henle and the distal tube of the nephron.

Uses

Diuretic drugs are used in the treatment of the following:

- Edema (fluid retention) associated with HF, corticosteroid/estrogen therapy, and cirrhosis of the liver
- Hypertension
- Renal disease (acute failure, renal insufficiency, and nephrotic syndrome)
- Cerebral edema
- Acute glaucoma and increased IOP (before and after eye surgery)

Ethacrynic acid (a loop diuretic) is also used for the short-term management of ascites caused by a malignancy, idiopathic edema, or lymphedema. When patients are at risk for potassium loss, the potassium-sparing diuretics may be used with or in place of other categories of diuretics.

Adverse Reactions

Adverse reactions associated with any category of diuretics involve various body systems.

Neuromuscular System Reactions

- Dizziness, lightheadedness, headache
- Weakness, fatigue

Cardiovascular System Reactions

- Orthostatic hypotension
- Electrolyte imbalances, glycosuria

Gastrointestinal System Reactions

- Anorexia
- Nausea, vomiting

Other System Reactions

Dermatologic reactions include rash and photosensitivity. Extremity paresthesias (numbness or tingling) or flaccid muscles may indicate **hypokalemia** (low blood potassium). **Hyperkalemia** (an increase in potassium in the blood), a serious event, may occur with the administration of potassium-sparing diuretics. Hyperkalemia is most likely to occur in patients with an inadequate fluid intake and urine output, those with diabetes or renal disease, the elderly, and those who are severely ill. In male patients taking spironolactone, **gynecomastia** (breast enlargement) may occur. This reaction appears to be related to both dosage and duration of therapy. The gynecomastia is usually reversible when therapy is discontinued, but in rare instances some breast enlargement may remain.

Additional adverse reactions of these drugs are listed in the Summary Drug Table: Diuretics. When a potassium-sparing diuretic and another diuretic are given together, the adverse reactions associated with both drugs may be evident.

Contraindications

Diuretics are contraindicated in patients with known hypersensitivity to the drugs, electrolyte imbalances, severe kidney or liver dysfunction, and **anuria** (cessation of urine production). Mannitol (an osmotic diuretic) is contraindicated in patients with active intracranial bleeding (except during craniotomy). The potassium-sparing diuretics are contraindicated in patients with hyperkalemia and are not recommended for children.

Precautions

Diuretics are used cautiously in patients with renal dysfunction. Most of the diuretics are pregnancy category C drugs (although ethacrynic acid, torsemide, isosorbide, amiloride, and triamterene are in pregnancy category B) and must be used cautiously during pregnancy and lactation. All of the thiazide diuretics are pregnancy category B drugs, with the exception of benzthiazide, hydroflumethiazide, methyclothiazide, which are pregnancy category C drugs. The safety of these drugs for use during pregnancy and lactation has not been established, so they should be used only when the drug is clearly needed and when the potential benefits to the patient outweigh the potential hazards to the fetus.

The thiazide and loop diuretics are used cautiously in patients with liver disease, diabetes, lupus erythematosus (may exacerbate or activate the disease), or diarrhea. A cross-sensitivity reaction may occur with the thiazides and sulfonamides. Some of the thiazide diuretics contain tartrazine (a yellow food dye), which may cause allergic-type reactions or bronchial asthma in individuals sensitive to tartrazine. Patients with sensitivity to sulfonamides may show allergic reactions to loop diuretics (furosemide, torsemide, or bumetanide). The potassium-sparing diuretics should be used cautiously in patients with liver disease, diabetes, or gout.

Interactions

All the diuretics may cause increased hypotension when taken with antihypertensive drugs. The interactions for specific diuretic categories are listed here.

Interacting Drug	Common Use	Effect of Interaction
Carbonic Anhydrase Inhibitors		
primidone	Treatment of seizure activity	Decreased effectiveness
Loop Diuretics		
cisplatin, aminoglycosides	Cancer treatment, anti-infective, respectively	Increased risk of ototoxicity
anticoagulants or thrombolytics	Blood thinner	Increased risk of bleeding
digitalis	Cardiac problems	Increased risk of arrhythmias
lithium	Psychotic symptoms	Increased risk of lithium toxicity
hydantoins	Treatment of seizure activity	Decreased diuretic effectiveness
nonsteroidal anti-inflammatory drugs (NSAIDs) and salicylates	Pain relief	Decreased diuretic effectiveness
Potassium-Sparing Diuretics		
angiotensin-converting enzyme inhibitors or potassium supplements	Cardiovascular problems	Increased risk of hyperkalemia
NSAIDs and salicylates; anticoagulants	Pain relief and blood thinner, respectively	Decreased diuretic effectiveness

Interacting Drug	Common Use	Effect of Interaction
Thiazides and Related Diuretics		
allopurinol	Treatment of gout	Increased risk of hypersensitivity to allopurinol
anesthetics	Surgical anesthesia	Increased anesthetic effectiveness
antineoplastic drugs	Cancer treatment	Extended leukopenia
antidiabetic drugs	Control of diabetes	Hyperglycemia

Ginger

HERBAL ALERT

Numerous **herbal diuretics** are available as over-the-counter (OTC) products. Most plant and herbal extracts available as OTC diuretics are nontoxic. However, most are either ineffective or no more effective than caffeine. The following selected herbals are reported to possess diuretic activity: celery, chicory, sassafras, juniper berries, St. John's wort, foxglove, horsetail, licorice, dandelion, digitalis purpurea, ephedra, hibiscus, parsley, and elderberry. There is very little scientific evidence to justify the use of these plants as diuretics. For example, dandelion root is a popular preparation once thought to be a strong diuretic. However, research has found dandelion root to be safe but ineffective as a diuretic. No herbal diuretic should be taken unless approved by the primary health care provider. Diuretic teas such as juniper berries and shave grass or horsetail are contraindicated. Juniper berries have been associated with renal damage, and horsetail contains severely toxic compounds. Teas with ephedrine should be avoided, especially by individuals with hypertension.

NURSING PROCESS
PATIENT RECEIVING A DIURETIC

ASSESSMENT

Preadministration Assessment
Before administering a diuretic, the nurse takes the vital signs and weighs the patient. Current laboratory test results, especially the levels of serum electrolytes, are carefully reviewed. Patients with renal dysfunction should have blood urea nitrogen (BUN) and creatinine clearance levels monitored as well. If the patient has peripheral edema, the nurse inspects the involved areas and records in the patient's chart the degree and extent of edema. If the patient is receiving a carbonic anhydrase inhibitor for increased IOP, the patient's description of pain and vital signs are obtained. The preadministration physical assessment of the patient receiving a diuretic for epilepsy includes vital signs and weight. The nurse reviews the patient's chart for a description of the seizures and their frequency.

If the patient is to receive an osmotic diuretic, the focus of the assessment is on the patient's disease or disorder and the symptoms being treated. For example, if the patient has a low urinary output and the osmotic diuretic is given to increase urinary output, the nurse reviews the intake and output ratio and symptoms the patient is experiencing. In addition, the nurse weighs the patient and takes the vital signs as part of the physical assessment before drug therapy starts.

Ongoing Assessment

During initial therapy, the nurse observes the patient for the effects of drug therapy. The type of assessment depends on such factors as the reason for the administration of the diuretic, the type of diuretic administered, the route of administration, and the condition of the patient. The nurse measures and records fluid intake and output and reports to the primary health care provider any marked decrease in the output. During ongoing therapy, the nurse weighs the patient at the same time daily, making certain that the patient is wearing the same amount or type of clothing. Depending on the specific diuretic, frequent serum electrolyte, uric acid, and liver and kidney function tests may be performed during the first few months of therapy and periodically thereafter.

NURSING DIAGNOSES

Drug-specific nursing diagnoses include the following:

❏ **Impaired Urinary Elimination** related to action of the diuretics causing increased frequency
❏ **Risk for Deficient Fluid Volume** related to excessive diuresis secondary to administration of a diuretic
❏ **Risk for Injury** related to lightheadedness, dizziness, or cardiac arrhythmias

Nursing diagnoses related to drug administration are discussed in Chapter 4.

PLANNING

The expected outcomes for the patient depend on the reason for administration of the diuretic, but may include an optimal response to drug therapy, management of patient needs related to adverse drug reactions, correction of a fluid volume deficit, absence of injury, and an understanding of the therapeutic regimen.

IMPLEMENTATION

Promoting an Optimal Response to Therapy

Diuretics are used to treat many different types of conditions. Therefore, promoting an optimal response to therapy for patients taking diuretics often depends on the specific diuretic and the patient's condition.

PATIENT WITH EDEMA. Patients with edema caused by HF or other causes are weighed daily or as ordered by the primary health care provider. A daily weight is taken to monitor fluid loss. Weight loss of about 2 lb daily is desirable to prevent dehydration and electrolyte imbalances. The nurse carefully measures and records the fluid intake and output every 8 hours. The critically ill patient

or the patient with renal disease may require more frequent measurements of urinary output. The nurse assesses the blood pressure, pulse, and respiratory rate every 4 hours or as ordered by the primary health care provider. An acutely ill patient may require more frequent monitoring of the vital signs.

The nurse examines areas of edema daily to evaluate the effectiveness of drug therapy and records the findings in the patient's chart. The nurse examines the patient's general appearance and condition daily or more often if the patient is acutely ill.

PATIENT WITH HYPERTENSION. The nurse teaches the hypertensive patient how to monitor the blood pressure and pulse rate when receiving a diuretic, or a diuretic along with an antihypertensive drug. Vital signs, including respiratory rate are more frequently monitored when the patient is critically ill or the blood pressure excessively high. *respiratory VIP*

PATIENT WITH ACUTE GLAUCOMA. If a carbonic anhydrase inhibitor is given for glaucoma, the nurse evaluates the patient's response to drug therapy (relief of eye pain) every 2 hours. If the patient is ambulatory and has reduced vision because of glaucoma, the nurse may need to assist the patient with ambulatory and self-care activities.

> **NURSING ALERT**
>
> The nurse notifies the primary health care provider immediately if eye pain increases or if it has not begun to decrease 3 to 4 hours after the first dose of diuretic. If the patient has acute closed-angle glaucoma, the nurse checks the pupil of the affected eye every 2 hours for dilation and response to light.

PATIENT WITH SEIZURE ACTIVITY. If a carbonic anhydrase inhibitor is being given for absence or nonlocalized epileptic seizures, the nurse assesses the patient at frequent intervals for the occurrence of seizures, especially early in therapy and in patients known to experience seizures at frequent intervals. If a seizure does occur, the nurse records a description of the seizure in the patient's chart, including time of onset and duration. Accurate descriptions of the pattern and number of seizures that occur each day help the primary health care provider plan future therapy and adjust drug dosages as needed.

PATIENT WITH INCREASED INTRACRANIAL PRESSURE. Mannitol is administered only by the intravenous (IV) route. The nurse inspects the solution carefully before administration, because mannitol solution may crystallize when exposed to low temperatures. If this happens, the nurse withholds the drug, returns the solution to the pharmacy, and requests another dose. The rate of administration and concentration of the drug are individualized. The nurse must monitor the urine output hourly, because the rate of administration is adjusted to maintain a urine flow of at least 30 to 50 mL/hour.

When a patient is receiving the osmotic diuretic mannitol or urea for treatment of increased intracranial pressure caused by cerebral edema, the nurse monitors the blood pressure, pulse, and respiratory rate every 30 to 60 minutes or as ordered by the primary health care provider. The nurse immediately reports to the primary health care provider any increase in blood pressure, decrease in the pulse or respiratory rate, or any changes in the neurologic status. The nurse performs neurologic assessments (e.g., vital signs, response of the pupils to light, level of consciousness, or response to a painful stimulus) at the time intervals ordered by the primary health care provider. The nurse evaluates and records the patient's response to the drug, that is, the signs and symptoms that may indicate a decrease in intracranial pressure.

PATIENT WITH RENAL COMPROMISE. When thiazide diuretics are administered, renal function should be monitored periodically. These drugs may precipitate azotemia (accumulation of nitrogenous waste in the blood). If nonprotein nitrogen (NPN) or BUN increases, the primary health care provider may consider withholding the drug or discontinuing its use. In addition, serum uric acid concentrations are monitored periodically during treatment with thiazide diuretics, because these drugs may precipitate an acute attack of gout. The patient also is monitored for any joint pain or discomfort. Because hyperglycemia may occur, insulin or oral antidiabetic drug dosages may require alterations. Serum glucose concentrations are monitored periodically.

PATIENT AT RISK FOR HYPOKALEMIA. Patients who experience cardiac arrhythmias or who are being "digitalized" (initiating digoxin therapy) may be more susceptible to significant potassium loss resulting in hypokalemia when taking diuretics. The potassium-sparing diuretics are recommended for these patients. The nurse should monitor patients taking potassium-sparing diuretics, because they are at risk for hyperkalemia. Serum potassium levels are monitored frequently, particularly during initial treatment.

The drug is discontinued and the primary health care provider is notified immediately if the patient experiences these symptoms or if the serum potassium levels exceed 5.3 mEq/mL. Treatment includes administration of IV bicarbonate (if the patient is acidotic) or oral or parenteral glucose with rapid-acting insulin. Persistent hyperkalemia may require dialysis.

NURSING ALERT

Symptoms of hyperkalemia include paresthesia (numbness, tingling, or prickling sensation), muscular weakness, fatigue, flaccid paralysis of the extremities, bradycardia, shock, and electrocardiographic abnormalities (see Display 48.1 for additional symptoms).

Monitoring and Managing Patient Needs

IMPAIRED URINARY ELIMINATION. Before the first dose of a diuretic is given, the nurse informs the patient of the drug's purpose (i.e., to rid the body of excess fluid), when diuresis may be expected to occur, and how long diuresis will last (Table 48.1). These drugs are administered early in the day to prevent any nighttime sleep disturbance caused by increased urination.

Some patients may exhibit anxiety related to the fact that it will be necessary to urinate at frequent intervals. To reduce anxiety, the nurse explains the purpose and effects of the drug. The nurse tells the patient that the

---

DISPLAY 48.1 Signs and Symptoms of Common Fluid and Electrolyte Imbalances Associated With Diuretic Therapy

Dehydration (Excessive Water Loss)
• Thirst
• Poor skin turgor
• Dry mucous membranes
• Weakness
• Dizziness
• Fever
• Low urine output

Hyponatremia (Excessive Loss of Sodium)
Note: Sodium—normal laboratory values 132–145 mEq/L

• Cold, clammy skin
• Decreased skin turgor
• Confusion
• Hypotension
• Irritability
• Tachycardia

Hypomagnesemia (Low Levels of Magnesium)
Note: Magnesium—normal laboratory values 1.5–2.5 mEq/L or 1.8–3 mg/dL

• Leg and foot cramps
• Hypertension
• Tachycardia
• Neuromuscular irritability

• Tremor
• Hyperactive deep tendon reflexes
• Confusion
• Visual or auditory hallucinations
• Paresthesias

Hypokalemia (Low Blood Potassium)
Note: Potassium—normal laboratory values 3.5–5 mEq/L

• Anorexia   *eat bananas*
• Nausea
• Vomiting
• Depression
• Confusion
• Cardiac arrhythmias
• Impaired thought processes
• Drowsiness

Hyperkalemia (High Blood Potassium)
• Irritability
• Anxiety
• Confusion
• Nausea
• Diarrhea
• Cardiac arrhythmias
• Abdominal distress

Table 48.1	Examples of Onset and Duration of Activity of Diuretics	
Drug	**Onset**	**Duration of Activity**
acetazolamide tablets	1–1.5 hr	8–12 hr
sustained-release capsules	2 hr	18–24 hr
IV	2 min	4–5 hr
amiloride	2 hr	24 hr
bumetanide oral	30–60 min	4–6 hr
IV	Within a few minutes	Less than 1 hr
ethacrynic acid oral	Within 30 min	6–8 hr
IV	Within 5 min	2 hr
furosemide oral	Within 1 hr	6–8 hr
IV	Within 5 min	2 hr
mannitol (IV)	30–60 min	6–8 hr
spironolactone	24–48 hr	48–72 hr
thiazides and related diuretics	1–2 hr	Varies*
triamterene	2–4 hr	12–16 hr
urea (IV)	30–45 min	5–6 hr

*Duration varies with drug used. Average duration is 12-24 hours. Indapamide has a duration of more than 24 hours.

need to urinate frequently will probably decrease. For some patients, the need to urinate frequently decreases after a few weeks of therapy. The nurse makes sure that the patient on bed rest has a call light and, when necessary, a bedpan or urinal within easy reach. The nurse informs the patient that the drug will be given early in the day so nighttime sleep will not be interrupted. Although the duration of activity of most diuretics is about 8 hours or less, some diuretics have a longer activity, which may result in a need to urinate during nighttime hours. This is especially true early in therapy.

RISK FOR DEFICIENT FLUID VOLUME. The most common adverse reaction associated with the administration of a diuretic is the loss of fluid and electrolytes (see Display 48.1), especially during initial therapy with the drug. In some patients, the diuretic effect is moderate, whereas in others a large volume of fluid is lost. Regardless of the amount of fluid lost, there is always the possibility of excessive electrolyte loss, which is potentially serious.

The most common imbalances are a loss of potassium and water. Other electrolytes, particularly magnesium,

sodium, and chloride, are also lost. When too much potassium is lost, hypokalemia occurs (see Patient Teaching for Improved Patient Outcomes: Preventing Potassium Imbalances). In certain patients, such as those also receiving a digitalis glycoside or those who currently have a cardiac arrhythmia, hypokalemia has the potential to create a more serious arrhythmia.

Hypokalemia is treated with potassium supplements or foods with high potassium content or by changing the diuretic to a potassium-sparing diuretic. In addition to hypokalemia, patients taking the loop diuretics are prone to magnesium deficiency (see Display 48.1). If too much water is lost, dehydration occurs, which also can be serious, especially in elderly patients.

Whether a fluid or electrolyte imbalance occurs depends on the amount of fluid and electrolytes lost and the ability of the individual to replace them. For example, if a patient receiving a diuretic eats poorly and does not drink extra fluids, an electrolyte and water imbalance is likely to occur, especially during initial therapy with the drug. However, even when a patient drinks adequate amounts of fluid and eats a balanced diet, an electrolyte imbalance may still occur and require electrolyte replacement (see Chapter 55 for additional discussion of fluid and electrolyte imbalances).

LIFESPAN ALERT – Gerontology
Older adults are particularly prone to fluid volume deficit and electrolyte imbalances while taking diuretics (see Display 48.1). The older adult is carefully monitored for hypokalemia (when taking loop or thiazide diuretics) and hyperkalemia (with potassium-sparing diuretics).

To prevent a fluid volume deficit, the nurse encourages oral fluids at frequent intervals during waking hours. A balanced diet may help prevent electrolyte imbalances. The nurse encourages patients to eat and drink all food and fluids served at mealtime. The nurse also encourages all patients, especially the elderly, to eat or drink between meals and in the evening (when allowed). The nurse monitors the fluid intake and output and notifies the primary health care provider if the patient fails to drink an adequate amount of fluid, if the urinary output is low, if the urine appears concentrated, if the patient appears dehydrated, or if signs and symptoms of an electrolyte imbalance are apparent.

NURSING ALERT
Warning signs of a fluid and electrolyte imbalance include dry mouth, thirst, weakness, lethargy, drowsiness, restlessness, muscle pains or cramps, confusion, gastrointestinal (GI) disturbances, hypotension, oliguria, tachycardia, and seizures.

The nurse must closely observe patients receiving a potassium-sparing diuretic for signs of hyperkalemia (see Display 48.1), a serious and potentially fatal electrolyte imbalance. Sometimes a potassium-sparing diuretic is prescribed along with a thiazide diuretic to keep potassium levels within normal limits. If excessive electrolyte loss occurs, the primary health care provider may reduce the dosage or withdraw the drug temporarily until the electrolyte imbalance is corrected.

RISK FOR INJURY. Patients receiving a diuretic (particularly a loop or thiazide diuretic) and a digitalis glycoside concurrently require frequent monitoring of the pulse rate and rhythm because of the possibility of cardiac arrhythmias. Any significant changes in the pulse rate and rhythm are immediately reported to the primary health care provider.

Some patients experience dizziness or lightheadedness, especially during the first few days of therapy or when a rapid diuresis has occurred. Patients who are dizzy, but who are allowed out of bed, are assisted by the nurse with ambulatory activities until these adverse drug effects disappear.

Educating the Patient and Family

The patient and the family require a full explanation of the prescribed drug therapy, including when to take the drug (diuretics taken once a day are best taken early in the morning), if the drug is to be taken with food, and the importance of following the dosage schedule printed on the container label. The nurse also explains the onset and duration of the drug's diuretic effect. The patient and family must also be made aware of the signs and symptoms of fluid and electrolyte imbalances and adverse reactions that may occur when using a diuretic.

To ensure compliance with the prescribed drug regimen, the nurse stresses the importance of diuretic therapy in treating the patient's disorder. If the patient states that taking a diuretic at a specific time will be a problem, the nurse helps the patient identify the difficulty associated with drug therapy, after which the nurse can suggest ways to overcome the barrier. The nurse includes the following points in a patient teaching plan:

- Do not stop taking the drug or omit doses, except on the advice of a primary health care provider.
- If GI upset occurs, take the drug with food or milk.
- Take the drug early in the morning (once-a-day dosage) unless directed otherwise to minimize the effects on nighttime sleep. Twice-a-day dosing should be administered early in the morning (e.g., 7 AM) and early afternoon (e.g., 2 PM) or as directed by the primary health care provider. These drugs initially cause an increase in urination, which should subside after a few weeks.
- Do not reduce fluid intake to reduce the need to urinate. Be sure to continue the fluid intake recommended by the primary health care provider.
- Avoid alcohol and nonprescription drugs unless their use has been approved by the primary health care provider. Hypertensive patients should be careful to avoid medications that increase blood pressure, such as OTC drugs for appetite suppression and cold symptoms.
- Notify the primary health care provider if any of the following occur: muscle cramps or weakness, dizziness, nausea, vomiting, diarrhea, restlessness, excessive thirst, general weakness, rapid pulse, increased heart rate or pulse, or GI distress.
- If dizziness or weakness occurs, observe caution while driving or performing hazardous tasks, rise slowly

from a sitting or lying position, and avoid standing in one place for an extended time.
- Weigh yourself weekly or as recommended by the primary health care provider. Keep a record of these weekly weights and contact the primary health care provider if weight loss exceeds 3 to 5 lb a week.
- If foods or fluids high in potassium are recommended by the primary health care provider, eat the amount recommended. Do not exceed this amount or eliminate these foods from the diet for more than 1 day, except when told to do so by the primary health care provider (see Patient Teaching for Improved Patient Outcomes: Preventing Potassium Imbalances).
- After a time, the diuretic effect of the drug may be minimal because most of the body's excess fluid has been removed. Continue therapy to prevent further accumulation of fluid.
- If taking thiazide or related diuretics, loop diuretics, potassium-sparing diuretics, carbonic anhydrase inhibitors, or triamterene, avoid exposure to sunlight or ultraviolet light (sunlamps, tanning beds), because exposure may cause exaggerated sunburn (a photosensitivity reaction). Wear sunscreen and protective clothing until tolerance is determined.
- For patients who have diabetes mellitus and who take loop or thiazide diuretics: Know that blood glucometer test results for glucose may be elevated (blood) or urine may test positive for glucose. Contact the primary health care provider if home-tested blood glucose levels increase or if urine tests positive for glucose.
- For patients who take potassium-sparing diuretics: Avoid eating foods high in potassium and avoid the use of salt substitutes containing potassium. Read food labels carefully. Do not use a salt substitute unless a particular brand has been approved by the primary health care provider. Also avoid the use of potassium supplements. Male patients who take spironolactone may experience gynecomastia. This is usually reversible when therapy is discontinued.
- For patients who take thiazide diuretics: These agents may cause gout attacks. Contact the primary health care provider if significant, sudden joint pain occurs.
- For patients who take carbonic anhydrase inhibitors: During treatment for glaucoma, contact the primary health care provider immediately if eye pain is not relieved or if it increases. When a patient with epilepsy is being treated for seizures, a family member of the patient should keep a record of all seizures witnessed and bring this to the primary health care provider at the time of the next visit. Contact the primary health care provider immediately if the number of seizures increases.

EVALUATION

- Therapeutic effect is achieved and diuresis occurs.
- Adverse reactions are identified, reported to the primary health care provider, and managed successfully through appropriate nursing interventions.

☑ Urinary elimination occurs without incident.
☑ Fluid volume problems are corrected.
☑ No injury is evident.
• Patient and family demonstrate an understanding of the drug regimen.

Patient Teaching for Improved Patient Outcomes

Preventing Potassium Imbalances

Diuretics increase the excretion of water and sodium. Some of these drugs also increase the excretion of potassium, which places the patient at risk for hypokalemia, a possibly life-threatening condition. Therefore, be sure your patient knows what foods to eat to replace the potassium lost. Patients should be taught about the following potassium-rich foods:

✓ **Meats:** Beef, chicken, pork, turkey, veal
✓ **Fish:** Flounder, haddock, halibut, salmon, sardines (canned), scallops, tuna
✓ **Fruits:** Apricots, avocado, bananas, cantaloupe, dates, dried fruit, plums, raisins, oranges and fresh orange juice, peaches, prunes, tomatoes and tomato juice (see also vegetables)
✓ **Vegetables:** Carrots, lima beans, potatoes, radishes, spinach, sweet potatoes, tomatoes
✓ **Other sources:** Coffee, gingersnaps, graham crackers, molasses, nuts, peanuts, peanut butter, tea

THINK CRITICALLY: PHARMACOLOGY IN PRACTICE

1. Mr. Park, aged 77 years, is a resident in a skilled nursing facility. His primary health care provider prescribes a thiazide diuretic for his long-standing HF. The nurse in charge advises you to evaluate Mr. Park for signs and symptoms of dehydration and hyponatremia. Discuss the assessment you would make. Identify which of these signs and symptoms might be difficult to evaluate considering the patient's age.

● Test Your Knowledge

1. When evaluating the effectiveness of acetazolamide (Diamox) given for acute glaucoma, the nurse questions the patient about _____.

   A. the amount of urine each time the patient voids
   B. the relief of eye pain
   C. the amount of fluid being taken
   D. occipital headaches

2. When administering spironolactone (Aldactone), the nurse monitors the patient closely for which of the following electrolyte imbalances?

   A. Hypernatremia
   B. Hyponatremia
   C. Hyperkalemia
   D. Hypokalemia

3. When a diuretic is being administered for HF, which of the following would be most indicative of an effective response of diuretic therapy?

   A. Output of 30 mL/hr
   B. Daily weight loss of 2 lb
   C. Increase in blood pressure
   D. Increasing edema of the lower extremities

4. Which electrolyte imbalance would the patient receiving a loop or thiazide diuretic most likely develop?

   A. Hypernatremia
   B. Hyponatremia
   C. Hyperkalemia
   D. Hypokalemia

5. Which of the following foods would the nurse most likely recommend the patient include in the daily diet to prevent hypokalemia?

   A. Green beans
   B. Apples
   C. Bananas
   D. Corn

● Prepare for the NCLEX

1. When a patient taking mannitol for increased intracranial pressure is being assessed, which of the following findings would be most important for the nurse to report?

   A. Serum potassium of 3.5 mEq/mL
   B. Urine output of 20 mL for the last 2 hours
   C. Blood pressure of 140/80 mm Hg
   D. Heart rate of 72 bpm

● Calculate Medication Dosages

1. The primary health care provider prescribes spironolactone (Aldactone) 100 mg orally. The drug is available in 50-mg tablets. The nurse administers _____.

2. Furosemide (Lasix) 20 mg oral solution is prescribed. The oral solution is available in a concentration of 40 mg/5 mL. The nurse administers _____.

To check your answers, see Appendix E.

thePoint *For more NCLEX questions, log on to http://thepoint.lww.com to access more than 1000 questions.*

Urinary Tract Anti-Infectives, Antispasmodics, and Other Urinary Drugs

LEARNING OBJECTIVES

On completion of this chapter, the student will:

1. Discuss the uses, general drug actions, adverse reactions, contraindications, precautions, and interactions of the drugs used to treat infections and symptoms associated with urinary tract infections or an overactive bladder.
2. Discuss important preadministration and ongoing assessment activities the nurse should perform with the patient taking a drug for a urinary tract infection or an overactive bladder.
3. List nursing diagnoses particular to a patient taking a drug for a urinary tract infection or an overactive bladder.
4. Discuss ways to promote an optimal response to therapy, how to manage adverse reactions, and important points to keep in mind when educating patients about the use of drugs used to treat a urinary tract infection or symptoms associated with an overactive bladder.

Urinary tract infection (UTI) is an infection caused by pathogenic microorganisms of one or more structures of the urinary tract. Because the female urethra is considerably shorter than the male urethra, women are affected by UTIs much more frequently than men. The most common structure affected is the bladder. Clinical manifestations of a UTI of the bladder (**cystitis**) include urgency, frequency, pressure, burning and pain on urination, and pain caused by spasm in the region of the bladder and the suprapubic area. With chronic UTIs, the urethra, prostate, and kidney may also be affected. Display 49.1 identifies the inflammatory disorders most frequently associated with each of these structures in the urinary system.

Overactive bladder (involuntary contractions of the detrusor or bladder muscle) is estimated to affect more than 16 million individuals in the United States. This problem sometimes results from such disorders as cystitis or prostatitis, or from abnormalities related to affected structures, such as the kidney or the urethra. Symptoms of an overactive bladder include **urinary urgency** (a strong and sudden desire to urinate), frequent urination throughout the day and night, and **urge incontinence** (involuntary urination after sudden sensation to void).

This chapter discusses drugs used to treat UTIs and drugs used to relieve the symptoms associated with an overactive bladder. When infection is present, structures of the urinary system that may be affected include the bladder (cystitis), prostate gland (**prostatitis**), the kidney (**pyelonephritis**), and the urethra. The drugs discussed in this chapter are anti-infectives. They are used in the treatment of UTIs, and they have an effect on bacteria in the urinary tract. Although administered systemically, that is, by the oral or parenteral routes, they do not achieve significant levels in the bloodstream and are of no value in treating systemic infections. They are primarily excreted by the kidneys and exert their major antibacterial effects in the urine.

Some drugs used in the treatment of UTIs, such as nitrofurantoin, do not belong to the antibiotic or sulfonamide groups of drugs. Examples of the most common drugs used in treating UTIs include amoxicillin (broad-spectrum penicillins; see Chapter 7), trimethoprim (sulfonamides; see Chapter 6), and nitrofurantoin. The anti-infective drugs known as fluoroquinolones (see Chapter 10) were initially approved for UTI treatment, but have become of greater use in systemic infection treatment. Combination drugs such as trimethoprim and sulfamethoxazole (Bactrim or Septra) are also used. The Summary Drug Table: Urinary Anti-infectives gives examples of the drugs used for UTIs.

Other drugs that treat UTIs include antispasmodic drugs, which help control the discomfort associated with irritation of the lower urinary tract mucosa caused by infection, trauma, surgery, and endoscopic procedures. Phenazopyridine (Pyridium), a urinary analgesic, is another drug used to

DISPLAY 49.1 Common Inflammatory Disorders Associated With the Urinary System

Cystitis—inflammation of the bladder
Urethritis—inflammation of the urethra
Prostatitis—inflammation of the prostate gland
Pyelonephritis—inflammation of the kidney and renal pelvis

avoiding citric

5A

Summary Drug Table URINARY TRACT ANTI-INFECTIVES

Generic Name	Trade Name	Uses	Adverse Reactions	Dosage Ranges
amoxicillin *ah-mox-ih-sill'-in*	Amoxil, Trimox, Wymox	Acute bacterial UTIs, other bacterial infections	Glossitis, stomatitis, gastritis, furry tongue, nausea, vomiting, diarrhea, rash, fever, pain at injection site, hypersensitivity reactions, hematopoietic changes	250–500 mg orally q 8 hr or 875 mg orally BID
fosfomycin *foss-foh-mye'-sin*	Monurol	Acute bacterial UTIs	Nausea, diarrhea, vaginitis, rhinitis, headache, back pain	3-g packet orally, provided in powder that must be mixed with fluid
methenamine *meth-en'-ah-meen*	Hiprex, Urex	Chronic bacterial UTIs	Nausea, vomiting, abdominal cramps, bladder irritation	1 g orally BID
℞ nalidixic *nal-ih-dix'-ic*	NegGram	Acute/chronic bacterial UTIs *c' convulsive disorders*	Abdominal pain, nausea, vomiting, anorexia, diarrhea, rash, drowsiness, dizziness, photosensitivity reactions, blurred vision, weakness, headache	1 g orally QID for 1–2 wk; may reduce to 2 g/day for prolonged therapy *discontinue*
nitrofurantoin *nye-troe-fyoor-an'-toyn*	Furadantin, Macrobid, Macrodantin	Acute bacterial UTIs	Nausea, anorexia, peripheral neuropathy, headache, bacterial superinfection	50–100 mg orally QID
trimethoprim (TMP) *trye-meth'-oh-prim*		Acute bacterial UTIs	Rash, pruritus, nausea, vomiting	200 mg/day orally
Urinary Anti-Infective Combinations				
trimethoprim and sulfamethoxazole (TMP-SMZ) *trye-meth'-oh-prim* *sul-fah-meth-ox'-ah-zoll*	Bactrim, Septra	Acute bacterial UTIs, shigellosis, and acute otitis media	Gastrointestinal (GI) disturbances, allergic skin reactions, headache, anorexia, glossitis, hypersensitivity	160 mg TMP/800 SMZ orally q 12 hr; 8–10 mg/kg/day (based on TMP) IV in 2–4 divided doses
Other Urinary Drugs (Analgesics and Antispasmodics)				
darifenacin *da-ree-fen'-ah-sin*	Enablex	Overactive bladder	Dry mouth, constipation	7.5 mg/day orally
flavoxate *fla-vox'-ate*	Urispas	Urinary symptoms caused by cystitis, prostatitis, and other urinary problems	Dry mouth, drowsiness, blurred vision, headache, urinary retention	100–200 mg orally TID or QID
oxybutynin *ox-ee-byoo-tye'-nin*	Ditropan	Overactive bladder, neurogenic bladder	Dry mouth, nausea, headache, drowsiness, constipation, urinary retention	5 mg orally BID or TID
solifenacin *soe-lih-fen'-ah-sin*	Vesicare	Overactive bladder	Dry mouth, constipation, blurred vision, dry eyes	5 mg/day orally
tolterodine *toll-tare'-oh-dyne*	Detrol, Detrol LA (long-acting, extended-release)	Overactive bladder	Dry mouth, constipation, headache, dizziness	2 mg orally TID; extended-release: 4 mg/day
℞ trospium *troz'-pee-um*	Sanctura	Overactive bladder	Dry mouth, constipation, headache	20 mg orally TID
phenazopyridine *fen-az-oh-peer'-ih-deen*	Pyridium	Relief of pain associated with irritation of the lower genitourinary tract	Headache, rash, pruritus, GI disturbances, red-orange discoloration of the urine, yellowish discoloration of the skin or sclera	200 mg orally TID

℞ Take this drug at least 1 hour before or 2 hours after meals.

relieve discomfort associated with UTI. (See Summary Drug Table: Urinary Anti-infectives for a list of drugs used to treat problems associated with the urinary system.)

Actions and Uses

Anti-Infectives

These drugs are used for UTIs that are caused by susceptible bacterial microorganisms. Many of the anti-infective drugs used for treating UTIs are chosen because of the rapid excretion rate of the drugs rather than the way they act inside the body. As a result, these anti-infectives have a high concentration in the urine and appear to act by interfering with bacterial multiplication in the urine. Nitrofurantoin (Macrodantin) may be **bacteriostatic** (slows or retards the multiplication of bacteria) or **bactericidal** (destroys bacteria), depending on the concentration of the drug in the urine. See the specific anti-infective chapters for the manner in which other anti-infective drugs work.

Antispasmodics

Antispasmodics are cholinergic blocking drugs that inhibit bladder contractions and delay the urge to void. These drugs counteract the smooth muscle spasm of the urinary tract by relaxing the detrusor and other muscles through action at the parasympathetic nerve receptors. Flavoxate (Urispas) is used to relieve symptoms of **dysuria** (painful or difficult urination), urinary urgency, **nocturia** (excessive urination during the night), suprapubic pain and frequency, and urge incontinence. The other antispasmodic drugs are also used to treat bladder instability (i.e., urgency, frequency, leakage, incontinence, and painful or difficult urination) caused by a **neurogenic bladder** (impaired bladder function caused by a nervous system abnormality, typically an injury to the spinal cord).

Phenazopyridine is a dye that exerts a topical analgesic effect on the lining of the urinary tract. It does not have anti-infective activity. Phenazopyridine is available as a separate drug but is also included in some urinary tract anti-infective combination drugs.

Adverse Reactions

Anti-Infectives

Adverse reactions are primarily GI disturbances and include the following:

- Anorexia, nausea, vomiting, and diarrhea
- Abdominal pain or stomatitis

Other generalized body system reactions include:

- Drowsiness, dizziness, headache, blurred vision, weakness, and peripheral neuropathy
- Rash, pruritus, photosensitivity reactions, and leg cramps

When these drugs are given in large doses, patients may experience burning on urination and bladder irritation; this should not be mistaken for a continued infection.

Nitrofurantoin has been known to cause acute and chronic pulmonary reactions.

Antispasmodics

Adverse reactions to these drugs are similar to those with other cholinergic blocking drugs. They include the following:

- Dry mouth, drowsiness, constipation or diarrhea, decreased production of tears, decreased sweating, GI disturbances, dim vision, and urinary hesitancy

Other generalized body system reactions include:

- Nausea and vomiting, nervousness, vertigo, headache, rash, and mental confusion (particularly in older adults)

Patients should be told that both the anti-infective and antispasmodic drugs can discolor the urine (dark orange to brown) and stain undergarments that come in contact with the urine.

Contraindications and Precautions

Anti-Infectives

Anti-infectives are contraindicated in patients with a hypersensitivity to the drugs, and during pregnancy (category C) and lactation. One exception is nitrofurantoin, which is classified as a pregnancy category B drug and is used with caution during pregnancy. Nalidixic (NegGram) is contraindicated in patients who have convulsive disorders. This drug is contraindicated in patients with a known hypersensitivity to fosfomycin. This drug should not be used during pregnancy (category B) or lactation. This drug should be used cautiously in patients taking metoclopramide (Reglan).

The anti-infectives should be used cautiously in those with renal or hepatic impairment. Patients who are allergic to tartrazine (a food dye) should not take methenamine (Hiprex). This drug is used cautiously in patients with gout, because it may cause crystals to form in the urine. Nalidixic and nitrofurantoin are used cautiously in patients with cerebral arteriosclerosis, diabetes, or a glucose-6-phosphate dehydrogenase (G6PD) deficiency.

Antispasmodics

ditropan

Antispasmodic drugs are contraindicated in those patients with known hypersensitivity to the drugs or with glaucoma. Other patients for whom antispasmodics are contraindicated are those with intestinal or gastric blockage, abdominal bleeding, myasthenia gravis, or urinary tract blockage. Phenazopyridine is contraindicated in patients with renal impairment and in undiagnosed urinary tract pain.

The nurse should use these drugs with caution in patients with GI infections, benign prostatic hypertrophy, urinary retention, hyperthyroidism, hepatic or renal disease, and hypertension. Antispasmodic drugs are classified as pregnancy category C drugs and are used only when the benefit to the woman outweighs the risk to the fetus.

Phenazopyridine is used cautiously during pregnancy (category C) and lactation. Phenazopyridine treats the symptom of pain but does not treat the cause of the disorder. No significant interactions have been reported.

Interactions

Anti-Infectives

The following interactions may occur when a specific urinary anti-infective is administered with another agent:

Interacting Drug	Common Use	Effect of Interaction
Nalidixic and Sulfamethoxazole		
oral anticoagulants	Blood thinner	Increased risk for bleeding
Nitrofurantoin		
magnesium trisilicate or magaldrate	Relieve gastric upset	Decreased absorption of anti-infective
anticholinergics	Relieve bladder spasm/ discomfort	Delay in gastric empty- ing, thereby increasing the absorption of nitrofurantoin
Fosfomycin (Monurol)		
metoclopramide (Reglan)	Relieve gastric upset	Lowers plasma concen- tration and urinary tract excretion of fosfomycin

An increased urinary pH decreases the effectiveness of methenamine. Therefore, to avoid raising the urine pH when taking methenamine, the patient should not use antacids containing sodium bicarbonate or sodium carbonate.

Antispasmodics

The following interactions may occur when an antispasmodic drug is administered with another agent:

Interacting Drug	Common Use	Effect of Interaction
antibiotics/antifungals	Fight infection	Decreased effectiveness of anti-infective drug
meperidine, flurazepam, phenothiazines	Preoperative sedation	Increased effect of the antispasmodic
tricyclic antidepressants	Management of depression	Increased effect of the antispasmodic
haloperidol (Haldol)	Antianxiety/ antipsychotic agent	Decreased effectiveness of the antipsychotic drug
digoxin	Management of cardiac problems	Increased serum levels of digoxin

HEALTH SUPPLEMENT ALERT
Cranberry juice has long been recommended for use in treating and preventing UTIs. Clinical studies have con- firmed that cranberry juice is beneficial to individuals with fre- quent UTIs. Cranberry juice inhibits bacteria from attaching to the walls of the urinary tract and prevents certain bacteria from forming dental plaque in the mouth. Cranberry juice is safe for use as a food and for urinary tract health. Cranberry juice and capsules have no contraindications, no known adverse reac- tions, and no drug interactions. The recommended dosage is 9 to 15 capsules a day (400 to 500 mg/day) or 4 to 8 ounces of juice daily.

NURSING PROCESS
PATIENT RECEIVING A URINARY TRACT ANTI-INFECTIVE OR OTHER URINARY TRACT DRUG

ASSESSMENT

Preadministration Assessment
When a UTI has been diagnosed, urine culture and sensitivity tests are performed to determine bacterial sensitivity to the drugs (antibiotics and urinary tract anti-infectives) that will control the infection. The nurse questions the patient regarding symptoms of the infec- tion before instituting therapy. The nurse records the color and appearance of the urine. The nurse takes and records the vital signs.

When miscellaneous drugs are administered, the nurse documents the symptoms the patient is experiencing to provide a baseline for future assessment. The nurse assesses for and documents pain, urinary frequency, bladder distension, and other symptoms associated with the urinary system.

Ongoing Assessment
Many UTIs are treated on an outpatient basis because hospitalization is seldom required. UTIs may affect the hospitalized patient or nursing home resident with an indwelling urethral catheter or a disorder such as a stone in the urinary tract. The primary nursing intervention to prevent UTIs in the hospitalized patient is good hand hygiene (handwashing).

When caring for a hospitalized patient with a UTI, the nurse monitors the vital signs every 4 hours or as ordered by the primary health care provider. Any signifi- cant rise in body temperature is reported to the primary health care provider, because intervention to reduce the fever or culture and sensitivity tests may need to be repeated.

The nurse monitors the patient's response to therapy daily. If after several days the symptoms of the UTI do not improve or they become worse, the nurse notifies the primary health care provider as soon as possible. Periodic urinalysis and urine culture and sensitivity tests may be ordered to monitor the effects of drug therapy.

When administering any of the other urinary drugs, such as antispasmodics, the nurse monitors the patient for a reduction in the symptoms identified in the pread- ministration assessment, such as dysuria, urinary fre- quency, urgency, and nocturia, and relief of any pain associated with irritation of the lower genitourinary tract.

NURSING DIAGNOSES

Drug-specific nursing diagnoses include the following:

❏ **Impaired Urinary Elimination** related to discomfort of urinary tract infection
❏ **Ineffective Breathing Pattern** related to adverse reaction to drug

Nursing diagnoses related to drug administration are discussed in Chapter 4.

PLANNING

The expected outcomes for the patient may include an optimal response to drug therapy, support of patient needs related to the management of adverse reactions, and an understanding of the therapeutic regimen.

IMPLEMENTATION

Promoting an Optimal Response to Therapy

To promote an optimal response to therapy, the nurse gives urinary tract anti-infectives with food to prevent GI upset. Nitrofurantoin especially should be given with food, meals, or milk, because this drug is particularly irritating to the stomach. Fosfomycin (Monurol) has special administration requirements; it comes in a 3-gram, one-dose packet that must be dissolved in 90 to 120 mL water (not hot water). The nurse administers the drug immediately after dissolving it in water. If visual disturbances occur when using nalidixic, they are noted after each dose. In many cases, they subside after a few days of therapy. The dosage of antispasmodic drugs may be reduced when the patient's symptoms improve. Phenazopyridine is administered after meals to prevent GI upset.

> ⚠ **NURSING ALERT**
>
> Phenazopyridine is not administered for more than 2 days when used in combination with an antibacterial drug to treat a UTI. When used for more than 2 days, the drug may mask the symptoms of a more serious disorder.

Monitoring and Managing Patient Needs

The nurse observes the patient for adverse drug reactions. If an adverse reaction occurs, the nurse contacts the primary health care provider before the next dose of the drug is due. However, serious drug reactions, such as a pulmonary reaction, are reported immediately.

IMPAIRED URINARY ELIMINATION. The patient is encouraged to drink at least 2000 mL of fluid daily (if condition permits) to dilute urine and decrease pain on voiding. Drinking extra fluids aids in the physical removal of bacteria from the genitourinary tract and is an important part of UTI treatment (see Patient Teaching for Improved Patient Outcomes: Preventing and Treating UTIs). The nurse offers fluids, preferably water, to the patient at hourly intervals. Cranberry or prune juice is usually given rather than orange juice or other citrus or vegetable juices. The nurse notifies the primary health care provider if the patient fails to drink extra fluids, if the

urine output is low, or if the urine appears concentrated during daytime hours. The urine of those drinking 2000 mL or more daily appears dilute and light in color.

Elderly patients often have a decreased thirst sensation and must be encouraged to increase fluid intake. This is especially true if an antispasmodic drug is also being taken. The nurse offers fluids at regular intervals to older adult patients or those who seem unable to increase their fluid intake without supervision (see Chapter 27).

When administering these drugs, the nurse monitors the fluid intake and urinary output for volume and frequency. The nurse measures and records the fluid intake and output every 8 hours, especially when the primary health care provider orders an increase in fluid intake or when a kidney infection is being treated. The primary health care provider may also order daily urinary pH levels when methenamine or nitrofurantoin is administered. These drugs work best in acid urine; failure of the urine to remain acidic may require administration of a urinary acidifier, such as ascorbic acid.

INEFFECTIVE BREATHING PATTERN. Pulmonary reactions have been reported with the use of nitrofurantoin and may occur within hours and up to 3 weeks after drug therapy is initiated. Signs and symptoms of an acute pulmonary reaction include dyspnea, chest pain, cough, fever, and chills. If these reactions occur, the nurse immediately notifies the primary health care provider and withholds the next dose of the drug until the patient is seen by a primary health care provider. In addition to the aforementioned signs and symptoms, a nonproductive cough or malaise may indicate a chronic pulmonary reaction, which may occur during prolonged therapy.

PATIENT NEEDS WHEN TAKING ANTISPASMODIC DRUGS. Common adverse reactions to cholinergic blocking drugs include dry mouth, dizziness, blurred vision, and constipation (see Chapter 27). For patients with dry mouth, the nurse suggests that the patient not only suck on hard candy, sugarless lozenges, or small pieces of ice but perform frequent mouth care. The dry mouth effect sometimes lessens with continued use of the drug. Hospitalized patients experiencing drowsiness or blurred vision may require assistance when ambulating. For patients with constipation, the nurse encourages fluids, provides a high-fiber diet, and provides times for ambulation or exercise (if the patient's condition allows). If constipation persists, the primary health care provider may prescribe a mild laxative or stool softener.

The nurse informs the patient that phenazopyridine may cause a reddish-orange discoloration of the urine that will stain clothing. In addition, the fluid that lubricates the eyes may change color, causing permanent discoloration of contact lenses. The nurse reassures the patient that this discoloration is normal and will subside when use of the drug is discontinued.

Educating the Patient and Family

The nurse stresses the importance of increasing fluid intake to at least 2000 mL/day (unless contraindicated) to help remove bacteria from the genitourinary tract (see Patient Teaching for Improving Patient Outcomes: Preventing and Treating UTIs). In many cases, symptoms are relieved after several days of drug therapy.

To ensure compliance with the prescribed drug regimen, the nurse stresses the importance of completing the full course of drug therapy even though symptoms have been relieved. A full course of therapy is necessary to ensure that all bacteria have been eliminated from the urinary tract. The nurse should include the following points in a patient and family teaching plan:

ANTI-INFECTIVES.
- Take the drug with food or meals (nitrofurantoin must be taken with food or milk). If GI upset occurs despite taking the drug with food, contact the primary health care provider.
- Take the drug at the prescribed intervals and complete the full course of therapy. Do not discontinue taking the drug even though the symptoms have disappeared, unless directed to do so by the primary health care provider.
- If drowsiness or dizziness occurs, avoid driving and performing tasks that require alertness.
- During therapy with this drug, avoid alcoholic beverages and do not take any nonprescription drug unless its use has been approved by the primary health care provider.
- Notify the primary health care provider immediately if symptoms do not improve after 3 or 4 days.
- Nitrofurantoin: Take this drug with food or milk to improve absorption. Continue therapy for at least 1 week or for 3 days after the urine shows no signs of infection. Notify the primary health care provider immediately if any of the following occur: fever, chills, cough, shortness of breath, chest pain, or difficulty breathing. Do not take the next dose of the drug until the primary health care provider has been contacted. The urine may appear brown during therapy with this drug; this is not abnormal.
- Nalidixic: Take this drug with food to prevent GI upset. Avoid prolonged exposure to sunlight or ultraviolet light (tanning beds or lamps), because an exaggerated sunburn may occur.
- Methenamine: Avoid excessive intake of citrus products, milk, and milk products.
- Fosfomycin comes in dry form as a one-dose packet to be dissolved in 90 to 120 mL water (not hot water). Drink immediately after mixing and take with food to prevent gastric upset.

ANTISPASMODIC AND OTHER DRUGS.
- For dry mouth, suck on hard candy, sugarless lozenges, or small pieces of ice and perform frequent mouth care.
- These drugs may cause drowsiness or blurred vision. Do not drive or operate dangerous machinery or participate in any activity that requires full mental alertness until you know how this medication affects you.

- If you experience constipation, drink plenty of fluids, eat a high-fiber diet, and exercise (if your condition allows). If constipation persists, the primary health care provider may prescribe a mild laxative or stool softener.
- Flavoxate: Take this drug three to four times daily as prescribed. This drug is used to treat symptoms; other drugs are given to treat the cause.
- Oxybutynin: Take this drug with or without food. Oxybutynin (Ditropan XL) contains an outer coating that may not disintegrate and sometimes may be observed in the stool. This is not a cause for concern. If using the transdermal form (patch) of the drug, be sure to apply to a clean, dry area of the hip, abdomen, or buttocks. Remove old patch and rotate sites of new application every 7 days.
- Antispasmodic drugs can cause heat prostration (fever and heat stroke caused by decreased sweating) in high temperatures. If you live in hot climates or will be exposed to high temperatures, take appropriate precautions.
- Phenazopyridine: This drug may cause a reddish-orange discoloration of the urine and tears and may stain fabrics or contact lenses. This is normal. Take the drug after meals. Do not take this drug for more than 2 days if you are also taking an antibiotic for the treatment of a UTI.

EVALUATION

- Therapeutic effect is achieved and bladder symptoms are relieved.
- Adverse reactions are identified, reported to the primary health care provider, and managed successfully through appropriate nursing interventions.
  ☑ Urinary elimination occurs without incident.
  ☑ Adequate breathing pattern is maintained.
- Patient and family demonstrate an understanding of the drug regimen.

Patient Teaching for Improved Patient Outcomes

Preventing and Treating UTIs

The nurse:
✓ Discusses UTIs and their causes, and the need for fluids and drug therapy.
✓ Reviews the drug therapy regimen, including prescribed drug, dose, and frequency of administration.
✓ Stresses the importance of continued therapy even if patient feels better after a few doses.
✓ Instructs the patient to continue therapy until all of the drug is finished or the primary care provider discontinues therapy.

✓ Explains the rationale for increasing fluid intake to at least <u>2000</u> mL/day (unless contraindicated) to aid in physical removal of bacteria.

✓ Urges patient to drink fluids every hour.

✓ Offers suggestions for fluids to drink based on patient's likes and dislikes.

✓ Demonstrates procedure for measuring intake and output using household measures.

✓ Informs patient about urine appearance when intake is increased and describes drug-induced urine color changes that can stain undergarments.

✓ Encourages continued increased fluid intake even if symptoms subside.

✓ Instructs the patient to notify primary health care provider if urine output is low, urine appears dark or concentrated during the daytime, or symptoms do not improve after 3 to 4 days.

✓ Reviews signs and symptoms of possible adverse reactions and of new infection or worsening infection, both verbally and in writing.

✓ Emphasizes the importance of follow-up visits and laboratory tests to determine the effectiveness of therapy.

THINK CRITICALLY: PHARMACOLOGY IN PRACTICE

1. Mr. Phillip, the widower, has returned to the clinic with continued UTI symptoms. The primary health care provider suspects that Mr. Phillip may not have followed instructions regarding treatment for his UTI. Analyze the situation to determine what points you would stress in a teaching plan for this patient.

● Test Your Knowledge

1. The nurse correctly administers nitrofurantoin (Macrodantin) _____.

A. with food
B. no longer than 7 days
C. without regard to food
D. no longer than 2 days

2. To avoid raising the pH when taking methenamine (Hiprex), the nurse advises the patient to _____.

A. use an antacid before taking the drug
B. take an antacid immediately after taking the drug
C. avoid antacids containing sodium bicarbonate or sodium carbonate
D. avoid the use of antacids 1 hour before or 2 hours after taking the drug

3. What instruction would be most important to give a patient prescribed fosfomycin (Monurol)?

A. Drink one to two glasses of cranberry juice daily to promote healing of the urinary tract.
B. You may take the drug without regard to meals.
C. This drug comes in a one-dose packet that must be dissolved in 90 mL or more of fluids.
D. This drug may cause mental confusion.

● Prepare for the NCLEX

1. What statement(s) would be included in a teaching plan for a patient prescribed phenazopyridine (Pyridium)?

A. There is a danger of heat prostration or heat stroke when taking phenazopyridine in a hot climate.
B. This drug may turn the urine dark brown. This is an indication of a serious condition and should be reported immediately.
C. This drug may cause photosensitivity. Take precautions when out in the sun by wearing sunscreen, a hat, and long-sleeved shirts for protection.
D. This drug may turn the urine reddish-orange. This is a normal occurrence that will disappear when use of the drug is discontinued.

● Calculate Medication Dosages

1. Amoxicillin 500 mg is prescribed. The drug is available in 250-mg tablets. The nurse administers _____.

2. Nitrofurantoin oral suspension 50 mg is prescribed. The oral suspension contains 25 mg/5 mL. The nurse administers _____.

To check your answers, see Appendix E.

the**Point** *For more NCLEX questions, log on to http://thepoint.lww.com to access more than 1000 questions.*

Drugs That Affect the Immune System

The immune system is not located in any single portion of the body. Rather, it flows through the entire body as a set of cells and fluid designed to recognize and respond to invasion. The chapters in this unit describe the drugs used to support the immune system in either recognizing invasion of an outside pathogen or by identifying the body's own cells growing out of control.

The lymphatic system plays a major role in the immune system. Cells called *T lymphocytes* (T cells) circulate in the bloodstream and lymphatics, prepared to protect the body. The various kinds of T cells include the following:

- Helper T4 cells—function in the bloodstream to identify and destroy antigens
- Helper T1 cells—increase B-lymphocyte antibody production
- Helper T2 cells—increase activity of cytotoxic (killer) T cells, which attack cells directly by altering the cell membrane and causing cell lysis (destruction)
- Suppressor T cells—suppress the immune response
- Memory T lymphocytes—recognize previous contact with antigens and activate an immune response

Immunizations, covered in Chapter 50, are individual drugs or a series of drugs given to help the body identify a pathogenic invader. In the past, communicable diseases and injuries were the primary illnesses health care providers treated. Today, some communicable diseases, such as smallpox and polio, have been almost eradicated because of the ability to immunize large populations of people at or near birth. All nurses play an important role in the continued immunization and protection of the population from easily preventable diseases.

Cancer is still a dreaded disease in our culture. At one time, a diagnosis of cancer was akin to a death sentence. With the advent of numerous drugs, known as *chemotherapy*, cancer is now viewed as a chronic illness in which people may be diagnosed and treated, then monitored for the remainder of their lives and treated again should cancer cells re-emerge. The information provided in Chapter 51 about antineoplastic drugs is meant to inform the nursing student about these medications—not to prepare students to administer them. Most hospitals and clinics require that nurses receive specialized training and standardized educational preparation before they are permitted to administer antineoplastic drugs. The Oncology Nursing Society has developed guidelines and educational tools for credentialing nurses for certification in administering chemotherapy.

The information in Chapter 51 is based on the need of all nurses to be able to assess and treat patients undergoing chemotherapy, whether they present with adverse reactions in the primary health care provider's outpatient office or hospital emergency department, or are being treated in the acute care setting for other illnesses or injuries.

Many of the treatments today are limited only by the destruction to the good cells in the body. Replacement of these cells from other people is limited by the antibodies we produce. Drugs that help to stimulate the body to make its own platelets, red and white blood cells are described in Chapter 52. With the growing ability to stimulate the body to produce its own blood cell components, many more people may live longer, improved-quality lives.

PHARMACOLOGY IN PRACTICE

Our patient focus in this unit is Betty Peterson's family. Betty's niece has been staying with her since she was laid off from her job. She received health insurance from her previous employment; without it, she has to make choices about when to go to the clinic. She cannot always find the money to pay for the visit. In this unit, you will learn about the diseases that are preventable with immunizations and the diseases that impact our immune system. After reading the chapters in this unit, you will be able to discuss the importance of various treatments and help Mrs. Peterson's family make good choices for the children at home.

Immunologic Agents

50

KEY TERMS

active immunity	humoral immunity
antibody	immune globulins
antigen	immunity
antigen–antibody response	passive immunity
attenuated antigen	toxin
booster	toxoid
cell-mediated immunity	vaccine
globulins	

LEARNING OBJECTIVES

On completion of this chapter, the student will:

1. Discuss humoral immunity and cell-mediated immunity.
2. Distinguish between and define the different types of immunity.
3. Discuss the use of vaccines, toxoids, immune globulins, and antivenins to provide immunity against disease.
4. Discuss preadministration and ongoing assessments the nurse should perform with the patient receiving an immunologic agent.
5. Identify nursing diagnoses particular to a patient receiving an immunologic agent.
6. Discuss ways to promote an optimal response, management of common adverse reactions, special considerations, and important points to keep in mind when educating a patient taking an immunologic agent.

Immunity refers to the ability of the body to identify and resist microorganisms that are potentially harmful. This ability enables the body to fight or prevent infectious disease and inhibit tissue and organ damage. The immune system is not confined to any one part of the body. Immune stem cells, formed in the bone marrow, may remain in the bone marrow until maturation, or they may migrate to different body sites for maturation. After maturation, most immune cells circulate in the body and exert specific effects. The immune system has two distinct, but overlapping, mechanisms with which to fight invading organisms:

• Cell-mediated defenses (cell-mediated immunity)
• **Antibody**-mediated defenses (**humoral immunity**)

Cell-Mediated Immunity

Cell-mediated immunity (CMI) results from the activity of many leukocyte actions, reactions, and interactions that range from simple to complex. This type of immunity depends on the actions of the T lymphocytes, which are responsible for a delayed type of immune response. The T lymphocyte becomes sensitized by its first contact with a specific **antigen**. Subsequent exposure to an antigen stimulates multiple reactions aimed at destroying or inactivating the offending antigen. T lymphocytes and macrophages (large cells that surround, engulf, and digest microorganisms and cellular debris) work together in CMI to destroy the antigen. T lymphocytes attack the antigens directly, rather than produce antibodies (as is done in humoral immunity). Cellular reactions may also occur without macrophages.

The T lymphocytes defend against viral infections, fungal infections, and some bacterial infections. If CMI is reduced, as in the case of acquired immunodeficiency syndrome (AIDS), the body is unable to protect itself against many viral, bacterial, and fungal infections.

Humoral Immunity

In humoral immunity, special lymphocytes (white blood cells), called *B lymphocytes*, produce circulating antibodies to act against a foreign substance. This type of immunity is based on the **antigen–antibody response**. An *antigen* is a substance, usually a protein, that stimulates the body to produce antibodies. An *antibody* is a globulin (protein) produced by the B lymphocytes as a defense against an antigen. Humoral immunity protects the body against bacterial and viral infections.

Specific antibodies are formed for a specific antigen—that is, chickenpox antibodies are formed when the person is exposed to the chickenpox virus (the antigen). Once manufactured, antibodies circulate in the bloodstream, sometimes only for a short time, but in other cases for the lifetime of the person. When an antigen enters the body, specific antibodies neutralize the specific invading antigen; this condition is called *immunity*. Thus, the individual with specific circulating antibodies is immune (or has immunity) to a specific antigen. Immunity is the resistance that an individual has against disease.

Cell-mediated and humoral immunity are interdependent; CMI influences the function of the B lymphocytes, and humoral immunity influences the function of the T lymphocytes.

Active and Passive Immunity

Active and passive immunity involve the use of agents that stimulate antibody formation (**active immunity**) or the injection of ready-made antibodies found in the serum of immune individuals or animals (**passive immunity**).

Active Immunity

When a person is exposed to certain infectious microorganisms (the source of antigens), the body begins to form antibodies (or build an immunity) to the invading microorganism. This is called *active immunity*. The two types of active immunity are naturally-acquired active immunity and artificially-acquired active immunity. The Summary Drug Table: Agents for Active Immunization identifies agents that produce active immunity.

Naturally-Acquired Active Immunity

Naturally-acquired active immunity occurs when the person is exposed to and experiences a disease, and the body manufactures antibodies to provide future immunity to the disease. It is called *active immunity* because the antibodies are produced by the person who had the disease (Fig. 50.1). Thus, having the disease produces immunity. Display 50.1 provides an example of naturally-acquired active immunity.

Artificially-Acquired Active Immunity

Artificially-acquired active immunity occurs when an individual is given a killed or weakened antigen, which stimulates the formation of antibodies against the antigen. The antigen does not cause the disease, but the individual still manufactures specific antibodies against the disease. When a **vaccine** containing an **attenuated** (weakened) antigen is given, the individual may experience a few minor symptoms of the disease or even a mild form of the disease, but the symptoms are almost always milder than the disease itself and usually last for a short time.

Summary Drug Table AGENTS FOR ACTIVE IMMUNIZATION

Generic Drug	Trade Name	Uses	Adverse Reactions	Dosage Ranges
Vaccines, Bacterial (Routine Immunizations)				
Hemophilus influenzae type B conjugate *hee'-mah-fill-uss in-floo-en'-zah kon'-joo-get*	ActHIB, HibTITER, PedvaxHIB	Routine immunization of children	Rare; minor local reactions such as local tenderness, pain at injection site, anorexia, fever, myalgia	0.5 mL IM, see immunization schedule
meningococcal *men-in-joe-kok'-kal*	Menomune, Menactra	Routine immunization of adolescents	Same as *H. influenzae* vaccine	0.5 mL Subcut only
pneumococcal (PCV) or (PPV) *new-moe-kok'-kal*	Pneumovax 23	Routine immunization of children, PPV is recommended for certain high-risk groups who can not take PCV	Same as *H. influenzae* vaccine	0.5 mL Subcut or IM, see immunization schedule
Vaccines, Bacterial (Special Populations)				
BCG		Prevention of pulmonary TB in negative, high-risk populations (health care workers, infants and children in high-TB areas)	Same as *H. influenzae* vaccine	0.2–0.3 mL percutaneous, repeat in 2–3 mo
pneumococcal 7-valent conjugate	Prevnar	Active immunization against *Streptococcus pneumoniae* for infants and toddlers, prevention of otitis media	Rare; minor local reactions such as local tenderness, pain at injection site, decreased appetite, irritability, drowsiness, fever	0.5 mL IM
typhoid *tye'-foyd*	Typhim Vi, Vivotif Berna	Immunization against typhoid	Same as *H. influenzae* vaccine	Oral: total of 4 capsules 1 wk before exposure Parenteral: adults and children 2 yr and older, 1 dose of 0.5 mL IM

(table continues on page 503)

Summary Drug Table AGENTS FOR ACTIVE IMMUNIZATION (continued)

Generic Drug	Trade Name	Uses	Adverse Reactions	Dosage Ranges
Vaccines, Viral (Routine Immunizations)				
measles (rubeola), mumps and rubella *mee'-zuls, roo-bee'-oh-lah, roo-bell'-ah*	MMR II (live) ProQuad (attenuated)	Routine immunization of children	Mild fever, rash, cough, rhinitis	0.5 mL Subcut
hepatitis A, inactivated *hep-ah-tye'-tuss A*	Havrix, Vaqta	Routine immunization of children	Same as measles vaccine	Administered IM; dosage varies with product; see package insert for specific dosages
hepatitis B, recombinant	Engerix-B, Recombivax HB	Routine immunization of children	Minor local reactions such as local tenderness, pain at injection site, anorexia, fever, myalgia	3–4 doses of 0.5–2 mL IM
poliovirus, inactivated (IPV) *poe'-lee-oh-vye'-russ*	IPOL	Routine immunization of children	Rare; malaise, nausea, diarrhea, fever	0.5 mL IM or Subut; see immunization schedule
varicella *var-ih-sell'-ah*	Varivax	Routine immunization of children	Minor local reactions, such as local tenderness, pain at injection site, rash, fever, cough, irritability	0.5 mL Subcut; see immunization schedule
Vaccines, Viral (Special Populations)				
human papillomavirus	Gardasil	Prevention of diseases in women caused by HPV, genital warts and certain cancers	Minor local reactions, such as local tenderness, pain at injection site	3 doses of 0.5 mL IM; initial, 2 months, 6 months
measles, live, attenuated*	Attenuvax	Selective active immunization against measles	Mild fever, rash, cough, rhinitis	0.5 mL Subcut
mumps, live*	Mumpsvax	Selective active immunization against mumps	Same as measles vaccine	0.5 mL Subcut
rubella, live*	Meruvax II	Selective active immunization against rubella	Same as measles vaccine	0.5 mL Subcut
rubella and mumps, live*	Biavax-II	Selective active immunization against rubella and mumps	Same as measles vaccine	0.5 mL Subcut
influenza *in-floo-en'-zah*	Afluria, FluMist, Fluarix, Flulaval, Fluvirin, Fluzone	Active immunization against the specific influenza virus strains contained in the formulation	Same as measles vaccine	One dose 0.5 mL IM Nasal: 1–2 doses (FluMist only)
avian influenza *ay'-vee-an in-floo-en'-zah*	H5N1	Active immunization against avian influenza in adults (18-64 years)	Headache, malaise, nausea	Two 1-mL IM doses given one month apart
rotavirus *roe'-tah-vye'-russ*	RotaTeq	Prevention of gastroenteritis caused by rotavirus serotypes contained in the vaccines	Fever, decreased appetite, abdominal cramping, irritability, decreased activity	Three 2.5-mL doses given orally

(text continues on page 504)

Immunologic Drugs

Summary Drug Table AGENTS FOR ACTIVE IMMUNIZATION (continued)

Generic Drug	Trade Name	Uses	Adverse Reactions	Dosage Ranges
rabies *ray'-beez*	Imovax Rabies Vaccine, RabAvert	Prevention of rabies in people with greater risk (e.g., veterinarians, animal handlers, forest rangers); postexposure prophylaxis: bite by an animal suspected of carrying rabies	Transient pain, erythema, swelling or itching at the injection site, headache, nausea, abdominal pain, muscle aches, dizziness	Pre-exposure prophylaxis: 1 mL IM, see package insert for dosing Postexposure: give vaccine IM after initial immune globulin injection
zoster, live	Zostavax	Prevention of shingles in elderly over 60 years of age	Transient pain, erythema, swelling or itching at the injection site	Single dose Subcut
Toxoids (Routine Immunizations)				
diphtheria and tetanus toxoids and acellular pertussis (DtaP) *dif-thair'-ee-ah, tet-ah-nuss tok'-soyds, ay-sell'-yoo-lar per-tuss'-uss*	Daptacel, Infanrix, Tripedia	Active immunization against diphtheria, tetanus, and pertussis	Headache, dizziness, rash, itching, nausea, fever	0.5 mL IM; see immunization schedule
Toxoids (Special Populations)				
diphtheria and tetanus toxoids, combined (DTTd)		Booster immunization against diphtheria and tetanus	Headache, dizziness, rash, itching, nausea, fever	0.5 mL IM, caution with site rotation; see package insert and immunization schedule
Combination Products (Viral/Bacterial Vaccine or Toxoid Together)				
hepatitis A and B combination	Twinrix	Twinrix for those over 18 y traveling to endemic areas	See individual vaccines	See package insert for specific dosing
diphtheria, tetanus toxoids, acellular pertussis, and *H. influenzae* type B	TriHIBit	See individual vaccines	See individual vaccines	See package insert for specific dosing
diphtheria, tetanus toxoids and acellular pertussis, hepatitis B [recombinant], and inactivated poliovirus	Pediarix	See individual vaccines	See individual vaccines	See package insert for specific dosing
Hemophilus influenzae type B and hepatitis B	Comvax	See individual vaccines	See individual vaccines	See package insert for specific dosing

*The trivalent measles-mumps-rubella (MMR) vaccine is the preferred immunizing agent for most children and adults.

The decision to use an attenuated, rather than a killed, virus as a vaccine to provide immunity is based on research. Many antigens, when killed, produce a poor antibody response, whereas when the antigen is merely weakened, a good antibody response occurs. Immunization against a specific disease provides artificially-acquired active immunity. Display 50.2 gives an example of artificially-acquired active immunity.

Artificially-acquired immunity against some diseases may require periodic **booster** injections to keep an adequate antibody level (or antibody titer) circulating in the blood. A booster injection is the administration of an additional dose of the vaccine to "boost" the production of antibodies to a level that will maintain the desired immunity. The booster is given months or years after the initial vaccine and may be needed because the life of some antibodies is short.

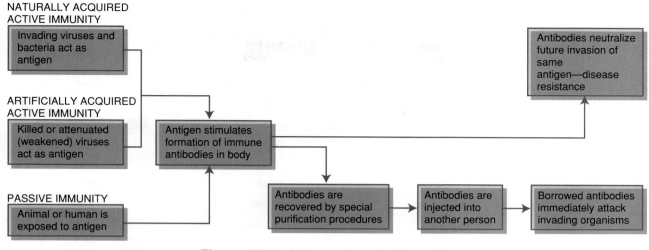

NATURALLY ACQUIRED ACTIVE IMMUNITY

Invading viruses and bacteria act as antigen

ARTIFICIALLY ACQUIRED ACTIVE IMMUNITY

Killed or attenuated (weakened) viruses act as antigen

PASSIVE IMMUNITY

Animal or human is exposed to antigen

Antigen stimulates formation of immune antibodies in body

Antibodies neutralize future invasion of same antigen—disease resistance

Antibodies are recovered by special purification procedures

Antibodies are injected into another person

Borrowed antibodies immediately attack invading organisms

Figure 50.1 Active and passive immunity.

The measles vaccine is considered an immunization. Immunization is a form of artificial active immunity and an important method of controlling some of the infectious diseases that are capable of causing serious and sometimes fatal consequences. The immunization schedule for children ages 0 to 6 years is given in Figure 50.2. The most current immunization schedules for this and other age groups and late start schedules can be obtained at http://www.cdc.gov/vaccines/. Currently, many infectious diseases may be prevented by vaccine (artificial active immunity). Examples of some of these diseases can be found in Display 50.3.

Passive Immunity

Passive immunity is obtained from the administration of ~~immune globulins~~ or antivenins. This type of immunity provides the individual with ready-made antibodies from another human or an animal (see Fig. 50.1). Passive immunity provides immediate immunity to the invading antigen, but lasts for only a short time. The Summary Drug Table: Agents for Passive Immunity identifies agents for passive immunizations. Display 50.4 provides an example of passive immunity.

DISPLAY 50.1 Example of Naturally-Acquired Active Immunity

Naturally-acquired active immunity is exemplified by an individual who is exposed to chickenpox for the first time and who has no immunity to the disease. The body immediately begins to manufacture antibodies against the chickenpox virus. However, the production of a sufficient quantity of antibodies takes time, and the individual gets the disease. At the time of exposure and while the individual still has chickenpox, the body continues to manufacture antibodies. These antibodies circulate in the individual's bloodstream for life. In the future, any exposure to the chickenpox virus results in the antibodies mobilizing to destroy the invading antigen.

DISPLAY 50.2 Example of Artificially-Acquired Active Immunity

Although chickenpox may seem like a minor illness, it can cause herpes zoster (shingles) later in life, which is a painful condition. An example of the use of an attenuated virus is the administration of the varicella virus vaccine to an individual who has not had chickenpox. The varicella (chickenpox) vaccine contains the live, attenuated varicella virus. The individual receiving the vaccine develops a mild or modified chickenpox infection, which then produces immunity against the varicella virus. The varicella vaccine protects the recipient for several years or, for some individuals, for life. An example of a killed virus used for immunization is the yearly influenza vaccine. These vaccines protect those who receive the vaccine for about 3 to 6 months.

● IMMUNOLOGIC AGENTS

Some immunologic agents capitalize on the body's natural defenses by stimulating the immune response, thereby creating protection against a specific disease within the body. Other immunologic agents supply ready-made antibodies to provide passive immunity. Examples of immunologic agents include vaccines, toxoids, and immune globulins.

Actions and Uses

Vaccines and Toxoids

Antibody-producing tissues cannot distinguish between an antigen that is capable of causing disease (a live antigen), an attenuated antigen, or a killed antigen. Because of this phenomenon, vaccines, which contain either an attenuated or a killed antigen, have been developed to create immunity to certain diseases. The live antigens are either killed or weakened during the manufacturing process. The weakened or killed antigens contained in the vaccine do not have

For those who fall behind or start late, see the catch-up schedule

(Handwritten margin note: Know for children)

Vaccine ▼ Age ▶	Birth	1 month	2 months	4 months	6 months	12 months	15 months	18 months	19–23 months	2–3 years	4–6 years
Hepatitis B[1]	HepB	HepB		see footnote 1		HepB					
Rotavirus[2]			RV	RV	RV[2]						
Diphtheria, Tetanus, Pertussis[3]			DTaP	DTaP	DTaP	see footnote 3	DTaP				DTaP
Haemophilus influenzae type b[4]			Hib	Hib	Hib[4]	Hib					
Pneumococcal[5]			PCV	PCV	PCV	PCV				PPSV	
Inactivated Poliovirus			IPV	IPV		IPV					IPV
Influenza[6]					Influenza (Yearly)						
Measles, Mumps, Rubella[7]						MMR		see footnote 7			MMR
Varicella[8]						Varicella		see footnote 8			Varicella
Hepatitis A[9]						HepA (2 doses)				HepA Series	
Meningococcal[10]										MCV	

Range of recommended ages

Certain high-risk groups

This schedule indicates the recommended ages for routine administration of currently licensed vaccines, as of December 1, 2008, for children aged 0 through 6 years. Any dose not administered at the recommended age should be administered at a subsequent visit, when indicated and feasible. Licensed combination vaccines may be used whenever any component of the combination is indicated and other components are not contraindicated and if approved by the Food and Drug Administration for that dose of the series. Providers should consult the relevant Advisory Committee on Immunization Practices statement for detailed recommendations, including high-risk conditions: http://www.cdc.gov/vaccines/pubs/acip-list.htm. Clinically significant adverse events that follow immunization should be reported to the Vaccine Adverse Event Reporting System (VAERS). Guidance about how to obtain and complete a VAERS form is available at http://www.vaers.hhs.gov or by telephone, 800-822-7967.

1. Hepatitis B vaccine (HepB). *(Minimum age: birth)*

At birth:

Administer monovalent HepB to all newborns before hospital discharge.

If mother is hepatitis B surface antigen (HBsAg)-positive, administer HepB and 0.5 mL of hepatitis B immune globulin (HBIG) within 12 hours of birth.

If mother's HBsAg status is unknown, administer HepB within 12 hours of birth. Determine mother's HBsAg status as soon as possible and, if HBsAg-positive, administer HBIG (no later than age 1 week).

After the birth dose:

The HepB series should be completed with either monovalent HepB or a combination vaccine containing HepB. The second dose should be administered at age 1 or 2 months. The final dose should be administered no earlier than age 24 weeks.

Infants born to HBsAg-positive mothers should be tested for HBsAg and antibody to HBsAg (anti-HBs) after completion of at least 3 doses of the HepB series, at age 9 through 18 months (generally at the next well-child visit).

4-month dose:

Administration of 4 doses of HepB to infants is permissible when combination vaccines containing HepB are administered after the birth dose.

2. Rotavirus vaccine (RV). *(Minimum age: 6 weeks)*

Administer the first dose at age 6 through 14 weeks (maximum age: 14 weeks 6 days). Vaccination should not be initiated for infants aged 15 weeks or older (i.e., 15 weeks 0 days or older).

Administer the final dose in the series by age 8 months 0 days.

If Rotarix® is administered at ages 2 and 4 months, a dose at 6 months is not indicated.

3. Diphtheria and tetanus toxoids and acellular pertussis vaccine (DTaP). *(Minimum age: 6 weeks)*

The fourth dose may be administered as early as age 12 months, provided at least 6 months have elapsed since the third dose.

Administer the final dose in the series at age 4 through 6 years.

4. Haemophilus influenzae type b conjugate vaccine (Hib). *(Minimum age: 6 weeks)*

If PRP-OMP (PedvaxHIB® or Comvax® [HepB-Hib]) is administered at ages 2 and 4 months, a dose at age 6 months is not indicated.

TriHiBit® (DTaP/Hib) should not be used for doses at ages 2, 4, or 6 months but can be used as the final dose in children aged 12 months or older.

5. Pneumococcal vaccine. *(Minimum age: 6 weeks for pneumococcal conjugate vaccine [PCV]; 2 years for pneumococcal polysaccharide vaccine [PPSV])*

PCV is recommended for all children aged younger than 5 years. Administer 1 dose of PCV to all healthy children aged 24 through 59 months who are not completely vaccinated for their age.

Administer PPSV to children aged 2 years or older with certain underlying medical conditions (see *MMWR* 2000;49[No. RR-9]), including a cochlear implant.

6. Influenza vaccine. *(Minimum age: 6 months for trivalent inactivated influenza vaccine [TIV]; 2 years for live, attenuated influenza vaccine [LAIV])*

Administer annually to children aged 6 months through 18 years.

For healthy nonpregnant persons (i.e., those who do not have underlying medical conditions that predispose them to influenza complications) aged 2 through 49 years, either LAIV or TIV may be used.

Children receiving TIV should receive 0.25 mL if aged 6 through 35 months or 0.5 mL if aged 3 years or older.

Administer 2 doses (separated by at least 4 weeks) to children aged younger than 9 years who are receiving influenza vaccine for the first time or who were vaccinated for the first time during the previous influenza season but only received 1 dose.

7. Measles, mumps, and rubella vaccine (MMR). *(Minimum age: 12 months)*

Administer the second dose at age 4 through 6 years. However, the second dose may be administered before age 4, provided at least 28 days have elapsed since the first dose.

8. Varicella vaccine. *(Minimum age: 12 months)*

Administer the second dose at age 4 through 6 years. However, the second dose may be administered before age 4, provided at least 3 months have elapsed since the first dose.

For children aged 12 months through 12 years the minimum interval between doses is 3 months. However, if the second dose was administered at least 28 days after the first dose, it can be accepted as valid.

9. Hepatitis A vaccine (HepA). *(Minimum age: 12 months)*

Administer to all children aged 1 year (i.e., aged 12 through 23 months). Administer 2 doses at least 6 months apart.

Children not fully vaccinated by age 2 years can be vaccinated at subsequent visits.

HepA also is recommended for children older than 1 year who live in areas where vaccination programs target older children or who are at increased risk of infection. See *MMWR* 2006;55(No. RR-7).

10. Meningococcal vaccine. *(Minimum age: 2 years for meningococcal conjugate vaccine [MCV] and for meningococcal polysaccharide vaccine [MPSV])*

Administer MCV to children aged 2 through 10 years with terminal complement component deficiency, anatomic or functional asplenia, and certain other high-risk groups. See *MMWR* 2005;54(No. RR-7).

Persons who received MPSV 3 or more years previously and who remain at increased risk for meningococcal disease should be revaccinated with MCV.

The Recommended Immunization Schedules for Persons Aged 0 Through 18 Years are approved by the Advisory Committee on Immunization Practices (www.cdc.gov/vaccines/recs/acip), the American Academy of Pediatrics (http://www.aap.org), and the American Academy of Family Physicians (http://www.aafp.org).

DEPARTMENT OF HEALTH AND HUMAN SERVICES • CENTERS FOR DISEASE CONTROL AND PREVENTION

Figure 50.2 Recommended childhood immunization schedule for persons 0 to 6 years. (From CDC [2009]. Recommendations and guidelines: 2009 child & adolescent immunization schedules for persons aged 0-6 years, 7-18 years, and "catch-up schedule." Retrieved April 27, 2009, from http://www.cdc.gov/nip/recs/child-schedule.htm#intable/.)

DISPLAY 50.3 Examples of Diseases Preventable by Vaccination

Diseases Prevented by Routine Vaccination
- *Hemophilus influenzae* type B
- Hepatitis A
- Hepatitis B
- Human papillomavirus
- Influenza
- Mumps
- Measles
- Pertussis
- Pneumococcal disease
- Poliomyelitis
- Rubella
- Tetanus
- Varicella

Diseases Preventable by Vaccination Before Travel to Endemic Areas
- Cholera
- Diphtheria
- Japanese encephalitis
- Lyme disease
- Smallpox
- Typhoid
- Yellow fever

sufficient strength to cause disease. Although it is a rare occurrence, vaccination with any vaccine may not result in a protective antibody response in all individuals given the vaccine. *tetanus, botox*

A **toxin** is a poisonous substance produced by some bacteria, such as *Clostridium tetani*, the bacterium that cause tetanus. A toxin is capable of stimulating the body to produce antitoxins, which are substances that act in the same manner as antibodies. Toxins are powerful substances, and like other antigens, they can be attenuated. A toxin that is attenuated (or weakened) but still capable of stimulating the formation of antitoxins is called a **toxoid**.

Both vaccines and toxoids are administered to stimulate the body's immune response to specific antigens or toxins. These agents must be administered before exposure to the disease-causing organism. The initiation of the immune response, in turn, produces resistance to a specific infectious disease. The immunity produced in this manner is active immunity.

Vaccines and toxoids are used for the following:

- Routine immunization of infants and children (see Fig. 50.1)
- Immunization of adults against tetanus
- Immunization of adults at high risk for certain diseases (e.g., pneumococcal and influenza vaccines)

DISPLAY 50.4 Example of Passive Immunity

An example of passive immunity is the administration of immune globulins (see Summary Drug Table: Agents for Passive Immunity) to prevent organ rejection in patients after organ transplantation surgery.

- Immunization of children or adults at risk for exposure to a particular disease (e.g., hepatitis A for those going to endemic areas or the human papilloma virus [HPV])
- Immunization of prepubertal girls or nonpregnant women of childbearing age against rubella

Immune Globulins and Antivenins

Globulins are proteins present in blood serum or plasma that contain antibodies. *Immune globulins* are solutions obtained from human or animal blood containing antibodies that have been formed by the body to specific antigens. Because they contain ready-made antibodies, they are given for passive immunity against disease. The immune globulins are administered to provide passive immunization to one or more infectious diseases. Those receiving immune globulins receive antibodies only to the diseases to which the donor blood is immune. The onset of protection is rapid but of short duration (1 to 3 months).

Antivenins are used for passive, transient protection from the toxic effects of bites by spiders (black widow and similar spiders) and snakes (rattlesnakes, copperhead and cottonmouth, and coral). The most effective response is obtained when the drug is administered within 4 hours after exposure.

Adverse Reactions

Vaccines and Toxoids

Adverse reactions from the administration of vaccines or toxoids are usually mild. Chills, fever, muscular aches and pains, rash, and lethargy may be present. Pain and tenderness at the injection site may also occur. Although rare, a hypersensitivity reaction may occur. The Summary Drug Table: Agents for Active Immunization provides a listing of the typical adverse reactions.

Immune Globulins and Antivenins

Adverse reactions to immune globulins are rare. However, local tenderness and pain at the injection site may occur. The most common adverse reactions include urticaria, angioedema, erythema, malaise, nausea, diarrhea, headache, chills, and fever. Adverse reactions, if they occur, usually last for several hours. Systemic reactions are extremely rare, with the exception of immune globulins given to prevent post-transplantation rejection. These immune globulins are made from equine (horse) or rabbit serum and can produce anaphylactic reactions. They should be administered only under the direction of a physician specializing in transplantation medicine.

The antivenins may cause various reactions, with hypersensitivity being the most severe. Some antivenins are prepared from equine serum, and if a patient is sensitive to equine serum, serious reactions or death may result. The immediate reactions usually occur within 30 minutes after administration of the antivenin. Symptoms include apprehension; flushing; itching; urticaria; edema of the face, tongue, and throat; cough; dyspnea; vomiting; cyanosis; and collapse. Other adverse reactions are included in the Summary Drug Table: Agents for Passive Immunity.

Immunologic Drugs

Summary Drug Table AGENTS FOR PASSIVE IMMUNITY

Generic Name	Trade Name	Uses	Adverse Reactions	Dosage Ranges
Immune Globulins				
botulism immune globulin (BIG-IV) *bot'-choo-lih-zum ih-mewn' glob'-yoo-lin*	BabyBIG	Treatment of infant botulism	Headache, chills, fever	Intravenous (IV) administration only; see dosing schedule
cytomegalovirus immune globulin (CMV-IGIV) *sye'-toe-meg'-ah-loe-vye-russ*	CytoGam	Prevention of CMV post-organ transplantation	Injection site: tenderness, pain, muscle stiffness Systemic: headache, chills, fever	See dosing schedule, varies weeks out from transplantation
hepatitis B immune globulin (HBIG) *hep-ah-tih'-tuss*	HepaGam B, Nabi-HB	Prevention of hepatitis B after exposure to the disease (use if not previously immunized)	Same as CMV-IGIV	0.06 mL/kg (3–5 mL) IM
immune globulin (gamma globulin; IgG)	GamaSTAN	Prevention of disease after exposure (use if not previously immunized); hepatitis A, measles (rubeola), Varicella, Rubella, immunoglobulin deficiency	Same as CMV-IGIV	See dosing schedule, varies for disease
immune globulin intravenous (IGIV)	Octogam, Gammagard, Polygam S/D	Immunodeficiency syndrome, ITP, chronic lymphocytic leukemia, bone marrow transplantation, pediatric human immunodeficiency virus infection	Headache, chills, fever	IV administration only; see dosing schedule, varies for disease
lymphocyte immune globulin* *lim'-foe-syte*	Atgam	Treatment of rejection post-organ transplantation, aplastic anemia	Chills, fever, arthralgia	After skin test dose, IV administration only; see dosing schedule, varies for disease
antithymocyte globulin*	Thymoglobulin	Treatment of acute rejection post kidney transplantation, aplastic anemia	Chills, fever, arthralgia	IV administration only; see dosing schedule
rabies immune globulin (RIG) *ray'-beez*	HyperRab, Imogam	Prevention of rabies after exposure to the disease (use if not previously immunized)	Same as CMV-IGIV	See dosing schedule
Rh immune globulin (IGIM)	BayRho-D, RhoGAM	Prevention of Rh hemolytic disease after birth	Same as CMV-IGIV	300 mcg (1 vial) IM within 72 hr of delivery
Rh immune globulin (IGIV)	WinRho SDF	Suppression of Rh isoimmunization after termination of pregnancy; ITP	Headache, chills, fever	IV administration only; see dosing schedule
Rh immune globulin microdose (IG-microdose)	BayRho-D Mini Dose, MICRho GAM	Suppression of Rh isoimmunization after termination of pregnancy before 12 weeks gestation	Same as CMV-IGIV	50 mcg (1 vial) IM

(table continues on page 509)

Summary Drug Table AGENTS FOR PASSIVE IMMUNITY (continued)

Generic Name	Trade Name	Uses	Adverse Reactions	Dosage Ranges
Respiratory syncytial virus immune globulin (RSV-IGIV) *sin-sish'-al vye'-russ*	RespiGam	Respiratory syncytial virus	Headache, chills, fever	IV administration only; see dosing schedule
tetanus immune globulin (TIG) *tet'-ah-nuss*	BayTet	Tetanus prophylaxis after injury in patients whose immunization is incomplete or uncertain	Same as CMV-IGIV	250 units IM
varicella-zoster immune globulin (VZIG) *var-ih-sell'-ah zoss'-ter*		Prevention of varicella in compromised patients after exposure to the disease (use if not previously immunized)	Same as CMV-IGIV	IM administration only; see dosing schedule
Antivenins				
crotalidae polyvalent immune Fab *kroe-tal'-ih-day pol-ee-vay'-lent*	CroFab	For treatment of mild to moderate North American rattlesnake bites	Urticaria, rash	See package insert for mixing and administration
antivenin (*Micrurus fulvius*) *an-tee-venn'-in*		Passive transient protection for toxic effects of venoms of coral snake in United States	Urticaria, rash	See package insert for mixing and administration

*Must be prescribed and administered by specialized physicians.

Contraindications and Precautions

Vaccines and Toxoids

Immunologic agents are contraindicated in patients with known hypersensitivity to the agent or any component of it. The measles, mumps, rubella, and varicella vaccines are contraindicated in patients who have had an allergic reaction to gelatin, neomycin, or a previous dose of one of the vaccines. The measles, mumps, rubella, and varicella vaccines are contraindicated during pregnancy, especially during the first trimester, because of the danger of birth defects. Women are instructed to avoid becoming pregnant at least 3 months after receiving these vaccines. Vaccines and toxoids are contraindicated during acute febrile illnesses, leukemia, lymphoma, immunosuppressive illness or drug therapy, and nonlocalized cancer. See Display 50.5 for additional information on the contraindications to immunologic agents.

Immunologic agents are used with extreme caution in individuals with a history of allergies. Sensitivity testing may be performed in individuals with a history of allergies. No adequate studies have been conducted in pregnant women, and it is not known whether these agents are excreted in breast milk. Thus, the immunologic agents (pregnancy category C) are used with caution in pregnant women and during lactation.

Immune Globulins and Antivenins

The immune globulins are contraindicated in patients with a history of allergic reactions after administration of human

DISPLAY 50.5 Contraindications to Immunization

- Moderate or severe illness, with or without fever
- Anaphylactoid reactions (e.g., hives, swelling of the mouth and throat, difficulty breathing [dyspnea], hypotension, and shock)
- Known allergy to vaccine or vaccine constituents, particularly gelatin, eggs, or neomycin
- Individuals with an immunologic deficiency should not receive a vaccine (virus is transmissible to the immunocompromised individual).
- Immunizations are postponed during the administration of steroids, radiation therapy, and antineoplastic (anticancer) drug therapy.
- Virus vaccines against measles, rubella, and mumps should not be given to pregnant women.
- Patients who experience severe systemic or neurologic reactions after a previous dose of the vaccine should not be given any additional doses.

immunoglobulin preparations and in individuals with isolated immunoglobulin A (IgA) deficiency (individuals could have an anaphylactic reaction to subsequent administration of blood products that contain IgA).

CHRONIC CARE ALERT

Human immune globulin intravenous (IGIV) products have been associated with renal impairment, acute renal failure, osmotic nephrosis, and death. Individuals with a predisposition to acute renal failure (e.g., those with preexisting renal disease), those with diabetes mellitus, individuals older than 65 years of age, or patients receiving nephrotoxic drugs should not be given human IGIV products.

The antivenins are contraindicated in patients with hypersensitivity to equine serum or any other component of the serum. The immune globulins and antivenins are administered cautiously during pregnancy and lactation (pregnancy category C) and in children.

*any chance of PG ?
don't get PG for 3 mo!*

Interactions

Vaccines and Toxoids

Vaccinations containing live organisms are not administered within 3 months of immune globulin administration, because antibodies in the globulin preparation may interfere with the immune response to the vaccination. Corticosteroids, antineoplastic drugs, and radiation therapy depress the immune system to such a degree that insufficient numbers of antibodies are produced to prevent the disease. When the salicylates are administered with the varicella vaccination, there is an increased risk of Reye's syndrome developing.

Immune Globulins and Antivenins

Antibodies in the immune globulin preparations may interfere with the immune response to live virus vaccines, particularly measles, but including others such as mumps and rubella. It is recommended that the live virus vaccines be administered 14 to 30 days before or 6 to 12 weeks after administration of immune globulins. No known interactions have been reported with antivenins.

NURSING PROCESS
PATIENT RECEIVING AN IMMUNOLOGIC AGENT

ASSESSMENT

Preadministration Assessment
Before the administration of any vaccine, the nurse obtains an allergy history. If the individual is known or thought to have allergies of any kind, the nurse tells the primary health care provider before the vaccine is given. Some vaccines contain antibodies obtained from animals, whereas other vaccines may contain proteins or preservatives to which the individual may be allergic. A highly allergic person may have an allergic reaction that could be serious and even fatal. If the patient has an allergy history, the primary health care provider may decide to perform skin tests for allergy to one or more of the components or proteins in the vaccine. The nurse also determines whether the patient has any conditions that contraindicate the administration of the agent (e.g., cancer, leukemia, lymphoma, immunosuppressive drug therapy).

Ongoing Assessment
The patient is usually not hospitalized after administration of an immunologic agent (with the exception of

transplant recipients). However, the patient may be asked to stay in the clinic or office for observation for about 30 minutes after the injection to observe for any signs of hypersensitivity (e.g., laryngeal edema, hives, pruritus, angioneurotic edema, and severe dyspnea [see Chapter 2 for additional information]). Emergency resuscitation equipment is kept available to be used in the event of a severe hypersensitivity reaction.

NURSING DIAGNOSES

Drug-specific nursing diagnoses include the following:

❑ **Acute Pain** related to adverse reactions (pain and discomfort at the injection site, muscular aches and pain)
❑ **Individual Effective Therapeutic Regimen Management** related to timing of immunization schedule

Nursing diagnoses related to drug administration are discussed in Chapter 4.

PLANNING

The expected outcomes of the patient may include an optimal response to the immunologic agent, support of patient needs related to the management of common adverse drug effects, and an understanding of and compliance with the prescribed immunization schedule.

IMPLEMENTATION

Promoting an Optimal Response to Therapy
If a vaccine is not in liquid form and must be reconstituted, the nurse must read the directions enclosed with the vaccine. It is important to follow the enclosed directions carefully. Package inserts also contain information regarding dosage, adverse reactions, method of administration, administration sites (when appropriate), and, when needed, recommended booster schedules.

LIFESPAN ALERT – Pediatric
The American Academy of Family Physicians states that children 12 to 15 months of age may receive up to seven injections during a single office visit. Many manufacturers are preparing combination products to reduce the number of injections during the vaccination process. Examples include the measle, mumps, and rubella (MMR) vaccine and the diphtheria, tetanus, pertussis, and *Hemophilus* B (TriHIBit) vaccine.

On occasion, it may be necessary to postpone the regular immunization schedule, particularly for children. This is of special concern to parents. The decision to delay immunization because of illness or for other reasons must be discussed with the primary health care provider. However, the decision to administer or delay vaccination because of febrile illness (illness causing an elevated temperature) depends on the severity of the symptoms and the specific disorder. In general, all vaccines can be administered to those with minor illness, such as a cold, and to those with a low-grade fever. However, moderate or severe febrile illness is a contraindication. In instances of moderate or severe febrile illness, vaccination is done as soon as the acute phase of the illness is over. Display 50.5 lists general contraindications to immunizations. Specific contraindications and precautions may be found in the package insert that comes with the drug.

The nurse documents the following information in the patient's chart or form provided by the institution:

- Date of vaccination
- Route and site, vaccine type, manufacturer
- Lot number and expiration date
- Name, address, and title of individual administering vaccine

Monitoring and Managing Patient Needs

Minor adverse reactions, such as fever, rashes, and aching joints, are possible with the administration of a vaccine. In most cases, these reactions subside within 48 hours.

ACUTE PAIN. General interventions, such as increasing the fluids in the diet, allowing for adequate rest, and keeping the atmosphere quiet and nonstimulating, may be beneficial. The primary health care provider may prescribe acetaminophen, every 4 hours, to control these reactions. Using the dominant arm helps aid in absorption of the injection. Also, aspiration of the syringe contents is not indicated for vaccines. If local irritation at the injection site occurs, it can be treated with warm or cool compresses, depending on the patient's preference. A lump may be palpated at the injection site after a diphtheria, pertussis, and tetanus (DPT) vaccination or other immunization. This is not abnormal and resolves itself within several days to several weeks.

INDIVIDUAL EFFECTIVE THERAPEUTIC REGIMEN MANAGEMENT. Because of the effectiveness of various types of vaccines in the prevention of disease, nurses must inform the public about the advantages of immunization. Parents are encouraged to have infants and young children receive the immunizations suggested by the primary health care provider. The nurse should provide the parents with a copy of the record of immunizations. This is especially helpful if multiple providers will be involved in the immunization schedule. Because evidence of immunization is required by schools (even at the college level), the record provided to parents by the provider is even more important. The nurse can download both information about immunizations and copies of blank record-keeping sheets from the Centers for Disease Control and Prevention (CDC) website at http://www.cdc.gov/nip/. This helps to empower the parent who cares for the child, making compliance with the routine immunization schedule likely.

 NURSING ALERT

In most cases, the risk of serious adverse reactions from an immunization is much smaller than the risk of contracting the disease for which the immunizing agent is given.

Serious viral infections of the central nervous system and fatalities have been associated with the use of vaccines. Although the number of these incidents is small, a risk factor still remains when some vaccines are given. It is also important for the parents to understand that a risk is also associated with not receiving immunization against some infectious diseases. That risk may be higher than and just as serious as the risk associated with the use of vaccines. Keep in mind that when a large segment of the population is immunized, the few not immunized are less likely to be exposed to and be infected with the disease-producing microorganism. However, when large numbers of the population are not immunized, there is a great increase in the chances of exposure to the infectious disease and a significant increase in the probability that the individual will experience the disease.

Educating the Patient and Family

When an adult or child is receiving a vaccine for immunization, the nurse explains to the patient or a family member the possible reactions that may occur, such as soreness at the injection site or fever.

The nurse advises those traveling to a foreign country to contact their primary health care provider or local health department well in advance of their departure date for information about the immunizations that will be needed. Immunizations should be given well in advance of departure, because it may take several weeks to produce adequate immunity.

The nurse encourages the parents or guardians to report any adverse reactions or serious adverse events occurring after administration of a vaccine. It may be necessary to report the event to the Vaccine Adverse Event Reporting System (VAERS) (Display 50.6).

The following list summarizes the information to be included when educating the parents of a child receiving a vaccination:

- Discuss briefly the risks of contracting vaccine-preventable diseases and the benefits of immunization.
- Instruct the parents to bring immunization records to all visits.
- Provide the date for return for the next vaccination.
- Discuss common adverse reactions (e.g., fever, soreness at the injection site) and methods to combat these reactions (e.g., acetaminophen, warm compresses).

DISPLAY 50.6 Vaccine Adverse Event Reporting System

VAERS is a national vaccine safety surveillance program cosponsored by the CDC and the U.S. Food and Drug Administration (FDA). VAERS collects and analyzes information from reports of adverse reactions after immunization. Anyone can report to VAERS. Reports are sent in by vaccine manufacturers, health care providers, and vaccine recipients and their parents or guardians. Any clinically significant adverse event that occurs after the administration of any vaccine should be reported. Individuals are encouraged to provide the information on the form even if the individual is uncertain whether the event was related to the immunization. A copy of the form can be obtained by calling 1-800-822-7967 or by submitting the information by the Internet at http://www.vaers.hhs.gov/.

Immunologic Drugs

- Instruct the parents to report any unusual or severe adverse reactions after the administration of a vaccination.

EVALUATION

- Therapeutic effect is achieved, and the disease for which immunization is given does not present itself.
- Adverse reactions are identified, reported to the primary health care provider, and managed successfully with appropriate nursing interventions:
  ☑ Acute injection pain is managed successfully.
  ☑ Patient or parents/guardians comply with the immunization schedule.
- Patient and family demonstrate an understanding of the drug regimen.

THINK CRITICALLY: PHARMACOLOGY IN PRACTICE

1. Jimmy Peterson, aged 4 months, has a slight cold with a "runny nose" when he comes for his regular well-baby checkup. His mother tells the nurse that, because Jimmy is sick, she does not think he needs his DPT injection at this time. She says that she will bring him in next month for this immunization. Looking over his records, you see that the family has no insurance at this time and has to pay out of pocket for all visits and vaccinations. Analyze the situation to determine the best response to Jimmy's mother. Discuss any assessments that you think would be important to make before giving your response.

● Test Your Knowledge

1. When discussing the possibility of adverse reactions after receiving a vaccine, the nurse tells the parents of a young child that _____.

   A. adverse reactions may be severe, and the child should be monitored closely for 24 hours
   B. adverse reactions are usually mild
   C. the child will likely experience a hypersensitivity reaction
   D. the most common adverse reaction is a severe headache

2. Which of the following statements made by the patient would alert the nurse to a possibility of an allergy to the measles vaccine? My daughter is allergic to _____.

   A. gelatin
   B. peanut butter
   C. sugar
   D. corn

3. What type of immunity does an antivenin produce?

   A. Artificially-acquired active immunity
   B. Naturally-acquired active immunity
   C. Passive immunity
   D. Cell-mediated immunity

4. What type of immunity is produced by the hepatitis B vaccine recombinant?

   A. Artificially-acquired active immunity
   B. Naturally-acquired active immunity
   C. Passive immunity
   D. Cell-mediated immunity

● Prepare for the NCLEX

1. The nurse is monitoring a patient receiving an IV infusion of RSV-IGIV globulin; which of the following symptoms may indicate an early allergic reaction?

   A. chills
   B. itching
   C. soreness at infusion site
   D. diarrhea

● Calculate Medication Dosages

1. Flulaval (influenza vaccine) is supplied in 5 mL vials. If each injection is 0.5 mL, how many vials will need to be ordered to inoculate 60 people?

To check your answers, see Appendix E.

the**Point** *For more NCLEX questions, log on to http://thepoint.lww.com to access more than 1000 questions.*

51

Antineoplastic Drugs

KEY TERMS

alopecia
anemia
anorexia
antineoplastic
bone marrow suppression
cell cycle nonspecific
cell cycle specific
chemotherapy
extravasation

leukopenia
metastasis
myelosuppression
neutropenia
oral mucositis
palliation
stomatitis
thrombocytopenia
vesicants

LEARNING OBJECTIVES

On completion of this chapter, the student will:

1. List the types of drugs used in the treatment of neoplastic diseases.
2. Discuss the uses, general drug actions, general adverse reactions, contraindications, precautions, and interactions of the antineoplastic drugs.
3. Discuss important preadministration and ongoing assessment activities the nurse should perform with the patient taking antineoplastic drugs.
4. List nursing diagnoses particular to a patient taking antineoplastic drugs.
5. Discuss ways to promote an optimal response to therapy, how to manage common adverse reactions, and important points to keep in mind when educating patients about the use of an antineoplastic drug.

Antineoplastic drugs are one of the tools used in the treatment of malignant diseases (i.e., cancer). The term **chemotherapy** is often used to refer to therapy with antineoplastic drugs. Although these drugs may not always lead to a complete cure of the cancer, they often slow the rate of tumor growth and delay **metastasis** (spreading of the cancer to other sites). These drugs can be used for cure, control, or **palliation** (comfort care, the relief of symptoms at the end of life).

● THE CELL CYCLE

All cells grow in a specific pattern of growth called the *cell cycle* (Fig. 51.1). During the cell cycle, different compo-

nents of a cell are synthesized, and the cell divides into two new cells.

Listed are the five phases of cell growth:

G_1—RNA (ribonucleic acid) and proteins are built
S—DNA (deoxyribonucleic acid) is made from the components of the G_1 phase
G_2—RNA and protein synthesis preparing for cell division
M—mitotic cell division (the cell has doubled its contents and splits into two separate cells)
G_0—the dormant or resting phase

When the cell goes into a resting phase, the cell stops performing its usual function in the body (e.g., a white blood cell might fight infection) or it prepares to start the cycle of cell division again. Some cells, such as blood cells, rapidly

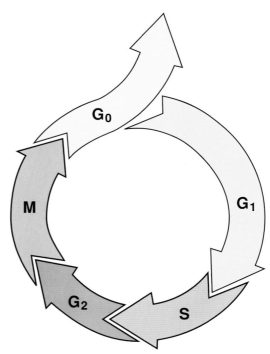

Figure 51.1 The cell cycle: **G_1**: RNA and protein synthesis; **S**: DNA synthesis; **G_2**: RNA and protein synthesis; **M**: mitotic cell division; **G_0**: cell resting phase, during which the cell either differentiates to perform its function or dies.

reproduce in a matter of hours. Other cells, such as nerve cells, complete their cell division and then go into the resting phase for years. Some cells tend to stay in the resting phase but quickly divide if the tissue is injured. Liver cells are a good example of this behavior; they do not replicate unless there is damage to the liver.

Antineoplastic drugs are designed to attack a cell during one or many of the phases of cell division. Drugs are categorized as **cell cycle specific** (meaning they target the cell in one of the phases of cell division) or as **cell cycle nonspecific** (they can target the cell at any phase of the cycle). Many subcategories of antineoplastic drugs are available to treat malignancies. The antineoplastic drugs covered in this chapter include the cell cycle nonspecific and cell cycle specific drugs. Other drugs, such as biologic and chemoprotective agents, are listed in various tables. Many hormones and antihormones are used in treating cancers associated with the sex organs (see Chapter 46), and new agents that stimulate our bodies to fight cancer are increasingly becoming available (Display 51.1).

DISPLAY 51.1 New Frontiers in Cancer Treatment: Targeted Therapies

Used in conjunction with conventional antineoplastic drugs, targeted therapies, as the term implies, are agents used to target specific malignant cell components without hurting normal cells.

Specific Targeting Agents
bortezomib (Velcade)
cetuximab (Erbitux)
dasatinib (Sprycel)
erlotinib (Tarceva)
gefitinib (Iressa)
imatinib (Gleevec)
lapatinib (Tykerb)
nilotinib (Tasigna)
sorafenib (Nexavar)
sunitinib (Sutent)
temsirolimus (Torisel)
vorinostat (Zolina)

Biologic Response Modifiers
aldesleukin (Proleukin)
BCG
denileukin diftitox (Ontak)
levamisole (Ergamisol)

Monoclonal Antibodies
alemtuzumab (Campath)
gemtuzumab ozogamicin (Mylotarg)
ibritumomab tiuxetan (Zevalin)
panitumumab (Vectibix)
rituximab (Rituxan)
trastuzumab (Herceptin)

Angiogenesis Inhibitors
bevacizumab (Avastin)
interferon-alpha (Roferon-A)
lenalidomide (Revlimid)
thalidomide (Thalomid)

The strategy of antineoplastic drug therapy is to affect cells that rapidly divide and reproduce. Malignant neoplasms or cancerous tumors usually consist of rapidly growing (abnormal) cells. Cancer cells have no biologic feedback controls to stop their growth or proliferation. Cancer cells are more sensitive to antineoplastic drugs when the cells are in the process of growing and dividing. Chemotherapy is administered at the time the cell population is dividing as part of a strategy to optimize cell death.

Because the drugs are given systemically (i.e., they circulate through the entire body), other rapidly growing cells are usually affected by these drugs. The normal cells that line the oral cavity and gastrointestinal (GI) tract, and cells of the gonads, bone marrow, hair follicles, and lymph tissue are also rapidly dividing cells. Thus, antineoplastic drugs may affect normal as well as malignant cells, causing unpleasant adverse reactions.

Chemotherapy is administered in a series of cycles to allow for recovery of normal cells and to destroy more malignant cells (Fig. 51.2). Using the cell kill theory, upon which chemotherapy is based, a drug regimen is intended to kill about 90% of the cancer cells during the first course of treatment. The second course, according to this theory, targets the remaining cancer cells and reduces those cells by another 90%. Each cycle of treatment with the antineoplastic drugs kills some, but by no means all, of the cancer cells. Theoretically, when few cells remain, the body's own immune system will be triggered and destroy what is left. By understanding the cell kill theory and the cell cycle, one can appreciate the rationale for using repeated doses of chemotherapy with different antineoplastic drugs. Various drugs that target cancer cells at various phases of the cell cycle are administered to kill as many cells as possible. Repeated courses of chemotherapy are used to kill an even greater proportion of the malignant cells until, theoretically, no cells are left.

HERBAL ALERT

Green tea and black teas come from the same plant. The difference is in the processing. Green tea is simply dried tea leaves, whereas black tea is fermented, giving it the dark color, stronger flavor, and the lowest amount of tannins and polyphenols. The beneficial effects of green tea lie in the polyphenols, or flavonoids, which have antioxidant properties. Antioxidants are thought to play a major role in preventing disease (e.g., colon cancer) and reducing the effects of aging. Green tea polyphenols are powerful antioxidants. The polyphenols are thought to act by inhibiting the reactions of free radicals in the body that are believed to play a role in aging. The benefits of green tea include an overall sense of well-being, cancer prevention, dental health, and maintenance of heart and liver health. Green tea taken as directed is safe and well tolerated. Because green tea contains caffeine, nervousness, restlessness, insomnia, and GI upset may occur. Green tea should be avoided during pregnancy because of its caffeine content. Patients with hypertension, cardiac conditions, anxiety, insomnia, diabetes, and ulcers should use green tea with caution.

Figure 51.2 The cell kill theory: rationale for repeated chemotherapy regimens.

Cell Cycle–Specific Drugs

Actions and Uses

Cell cycle–specific drugs act on the cell in one specific phase of the process of cell division, affecting both malignant and normal cells. A combination of these drugs, all acting at different phases of cell division, is typically used to treat leukemias, lymphomas, and a variety of solid tumors. The site of action of each drug depends on the drug subcategory. See the Summary Drug Table: Cell Cycle–Specific Drugs for more information.

Plant Alkaloids

Drugs that are derived from plant alkaloids include vinca alkaloids, taxanes, podophyllotoxins, and camptothecin analog drugs. The vinca alkaloids interfere with amino acid production in the S phase and formation of microtubules in the M phase. Taxanes also interfere in the M phase with microtubules. Cells are stopped during the S and G_2 phases by the podophyllotoxins and thus are unable to divide. DNA synthesis during the S phase is inhibited by camptothecin analog drugs such as topotecan (Hycamtin).

Antimetabolites

Antimetabolite drugs are substances that incorporate themselves into the cellular components during the S phase of cell division. This interferes with the synthesis of RNA and DNA, making it impossible for the cancerous cell to divide into two daughter cells. These drugs are used for many of the leukemias, lymphomas, and solid tumors as well as autoimmune diseases. Methotrexate is an example of the antimetabolite drugs.

Cell Cycle–Nonspecific Drugs

Actions and Uses

Cell cycle–nonspecific drugs interfere with the process of cell division of malignant and normal cells. Because they do not exert action specifically on one portion of the cell cycle, they are called *nonspecific* drugs. These drugs are used to cure, control, or provide palliation in the treatment of leukemias, lymphomas, and many different solid tumors, and are also used in the treatment of certain autoimmune diseases.

Summary Drug Table CELL CYCLE–SPECIFIC DRUGS

Generic Name	Trade Name	Uses	Adverse Reactions
Plant Alkaloids			
Vinca Alkaloids			
vinblastine *vin-blas'-teen*	Velban	Leukemia/lymphomas: Hodgkin's disease, other lymphomas Solid tumors: testicular, breast, Kaposi's sarcoma (KS) Nonmalignant: mycosis fungoides	Immediate: extravasation potential During therapy cycles: alopecia, anemia, leukopenia, paresthesias, nausea, vomiting, constipation Long term: fertility problems
vincristine *vin-kris'-teen*	Oncovin, Vincasar	Leukemia/lymphomas: acute leukemia, other lymphomas Solid tumors: rhabdomyosarcoma, bladder, breast, KS Nonmalignant: idiopathic thrombocytopenic purpura	Immediate: extravasation potential During therapy cycles: alopecia, anemia, leukopenia, paresthesias, nausea, vomiting, stomatitis, constipation Long term: renal, adrenal, fertility problems
vinorelbine *vin-noe'-rell-been*	Navelbine	Solid tumors: non–small cell lung cancer (NSCLC) Unlabeled use: other solid tumors, KS	Immediate: extravasation potential During therapy cycles: leukopenia, paresthesias, nausea, constipation, alopecia, radiation recall
Taxanes			
docetaxel *doe-seh-tax'-ell*	Taxotere	Solid tumors: breast, NSCLC, prostate Unlabeled use: other solid tumors	Immediate: extravasation potential During therapy cycles: nausea, peripheral neuropathy, alopecia, cutaneous changes, fever, anemia, leukopenia, vomiting, diarrhea, stomatitis, fluid retention Long term: fertility problems
paclitaxel *pak-leh-tax'-ell*	Taxol, Abraxane	Solid tumors: ovary, breast, NSCLC, KS Unlabeled use: other solid tumors	Immediate: cardiac changes, hypotension, extravasation potential During therapy cycles: nausea, vomiting, peripheral neuropathy, alopecia, fever, anemia, leukopenia, diarrhea, stomatitis Long term: fertility problems
Podophyllotoxins			
etoposide *eh-toe'-poe-syde*	Toposar, VePesid	Solid tumors: testicular, small-cell lung cancer (SCLC) Unlabeled use: other solid tumors, leukemias and lymphomas	During therapy cycles: anemia, leukopenia, thrombocytopenia, alopecia, nausea, vomiting
teniposide (VM-26) *teh-nip'-oh-syde*	Vumon	Leukemia/lymphomas: acute lymphocytic leukemia (ALL)	Immediate: extravasation potential During therapy cycles: anemia, leukopenia, thrombocytopenia, alopecia, nausea, vomiting
Camptothecin Analogs			
irinotecan *eye-rin-oh-tee'-kan*	Camptosar	Solid tumors: metastatic colon or rectal	Immediate: nausea, vomiting, diarrhea, inflammation potential (IV site) During therapy cycles: diarrhea, anemia, leukopenia, thrombocytopenia, asthenia, alopecia
topotecan *toe-poh-tee'-kan*	Hycamtin	Solid tumors: metastatic ovarian, SCLC	During therapy cycles: anemia, leukopenia, thrombocytopenia, alopecia, nausea, vomiting, diarrhea, constipation
Antimetabolites			
capecitabine *kap-eh-see'-tah-been*	Xeloda	Solid tumors: breast, colon	During therapy cycles: anemia, leukopenia, thrombocytopenia, diarrhea, hand and foot syndrome

(table continues on page 517)

Summary Drug Table CELL CYCLE–SPECIFIC DRUGS (continued)

Generic Name	Trade Name	Uses	Adverse Reactions
cladribine *kla'-drih-been*	Leustatin	Leukemia/lymphomas: hairy cell leukemia Unlabeled use: other leukemias and lymphomas	During therapy cycles: anemia, leukopenia, thrombocytopenia, fever, nausea, rash
clofarabine *kloe-far'-ah-been*	Clolar	Leukemia/lymphomas: ALL	During therapy cycles: anemia, leukopenia, thrombocytopenia, hyperuricemia
cytarabine (ara-C) *sye-tare'-ah-been*	Cytosar-U, DepoCyt	Leukemia/lymphomas: ALL, acute myelocytic leukemia (AML)	Immediate: nausea, vomiting During therapy cycles: anemia, leukopenia, thrombocytopenia
fludarabine *floo-dar'-ah-been*	Fludara	Leukemia/lymphomas: chronic lymphocytic leukemia Unlabeled use: other leukemias and lymphomas	During therapy cycles: anemia, leukopenia, thrombocytopenia
fluorouracil (5-FU) *floo-roh-yoor'-ah-sill*	Adrucil	Palliative treatment for solid tumors: breast, stomach, pancreas, colon, rectum	During therapy cycles: anemia, leukopenia, thrombocytopenia, nausea, vomiting, stomatitis, diarrhea, alopecia
gemcitabine *jem-sye'-tah-been*	Gemzar	Solid tumors: pancreatic, NSCLC	During therapy cycles: anemia, leukopenia, thrombocytopenia, fever, rash nausea, vomiting, diarrhea, proteinuria
mercaptopurine (6-MP) *mer-kap-toe-pyoor'-een*	Purinethol	Leukemia/lymphomas: ALL, AML Unlabeled use: inflammatory bowel disease	During therapy cycles: anemia, leukopenia, thrombocytopenia, hyperuricemia
methotrexate *meth-oh-trex'-ate*	Rheumatrex, Trex-all	Leukemia/lymphomas; ALL, non-Hodgkin's lymphoma Solid tumors: breast, head/neck, choriocarcinomas, osteosarcomas Nonmalignant: mycosis fungoides, severe psoriasis, rheumatoid arthritis Unlabeled use: multiple sclerosis, inflammatory bowel disease	Immediate: nausea, vomiting (high dose) During therapy cycles: anemia, leukopenia, thrombocytopenia, stomatitis, diarrhea, renal damage Long term: hepatotoxicity
nelarabine *nel-lah-rah'-been*	Arranon	Leukemia/lymphomas: T-cell acute lymphoblastic leukemia and T-cell lymphoblastic lymphoma	During therapy cycles: fatigue, neurologic toxicity
pemetrexed *pem-ah-trex'-ed*	Alimta	Solid tumors: NSCLC, malignant pleural mesothelioma	During therapy cycles: anemia, leukopenia, thrombocytopenia, skin rashes
pentostatin *pen'-toe-stat-in*	Nipent	Leukemia/lymphomas: hairy cell leukemia Unlabeled use: other leukemias and lymphomas	During therapy cycles: anemia, leukopenia, thrombocytopenia, rash, itching, nausea, vomiting, diarrhea
thioguanine *thye-oh-gwah'-neen*	Tabloid	Acute leukemias Unlabeled use: severe psoriasis, inflammatory bowel disease	During therapy cycles: anemia, leukopenia, thrombocytopenia, hyperuricemia
Miscellaneous Agents			
ixabepilone *ix'-ah-bep'-ih-loan*	Ixempra	Solid tumors: advanced breast	During therapy cycles: fatigue, peripheral neuropathy, neutropenia, alopecia, nausea, diarrhea,

Antineoplastic Drugs

Alkylating Agents

Alkylating agents make the cell a more alkaline environment, which in turn damages the cell. Malignant cells appear to be more susceptible to the effects of alkylating drugs than normal cells. A number of subcategories are included in this group of cell cycle–nonspecific drugs. Nitrogen mustard derivatives, ethyleneimines, and platinum-based drugs all break or interfere with the crosslinks in the DNA structure. The alkyl sulfonate drug busulfan interferes with DNA of granulocytes and is used primarily for leukemias. The hydrazine group interferes with multiple phases in the synthesis of RNA, DNA, and protein. Nitrosoureas are unique in that they can cross the blood–brain barrier, and therefore are used in treating brain tumors.

Antineoplastic Antibiotics

Antineoplastic antibiotics, unlike their anti-infective antibiotic relatives, do not fight infection. Rather, their action is similar to alkylating drugs. Antineoplastic antibiotics appear to interfere with DNA and RNA synthesis, thereby delaying or inhibiting cell division and blocking the reproductive ability of malignant cells. An example of an antineoplastic antibiotic is doxorubicin (Adriamycin), which is used in the treatment of many solid tumors.

Miscellaneous Antineoplastic Drugs

A number of drugs are used for their antineoplastic actions, but they do not belong to any one category. The mechanism of action of many of the drugs in this unrelated group is not entirely clear. Examples of miscellaneous antineoplastics are provided in the Summary Drug Table: Cell Cycle–Nonspecific Drugs.

Adverse Reactions

Adverse reactions to antineoplastic drugs can be viewed in three different time frames: immediate (during the actual administration), during therapy cycles, and long term (many years later, during survivorship).

Immediate adverse reactions occur as a result of administration. These include nausea and vomiting from highly emetic drugs or the potential of intravenous (IV) **extravasation** (leakage into the surrounding tissues) of irritating solutions. Antineoplastic drugs are potentially toxic, and their administration is often associated with serious adverse reactions. At times, some of these adverse effects are allowed, because the only alternative is to stop treatment of the cancer. A treatment plan is developed that will prevent, lessen, or treat most or all of the symptoms of a specific adverse reaction. An example of prevention is giving an antiemetic before administering an antineoplastic drug known to cause severe nausea and vomiting. Display 51.2 provides a list of those drugs most likely to cause nausea and vomiting.

An example of a treatment for an adverse reaction is the administration of an antiemetic and IV fluids with electrolytes when severe vomiting is anticipated. When the drugs listed in Display 51.2 are given, antiemetic protocols should always be followed to reduce adverse reactions. Some drugs,

---

DISPLAY 51.2 Emetic Potential of Antineoplastic Drugs

The following drugs have a 60% or greater chance of causing nausea and vomiting when administered to patients.

Alkylating Agents	Antibiotics
carboplatin	dactinomycin
carmustine	daunorubicin
cisplatin	doxorubicin
cyclophosphamide	mitoxantrone
dacarbazine	
ifosfamide	**Antimetabolites**
lomustine	cytarabine
mechlorethamine	methotrexate
melphalan	
procarbazine	**Plant Alkaloid**
streptozocin	irinotecan

---

such as platinum-based agents, may damage certain organs during administration. Again, prechemotherapy protocols for IV fluid administration are initiated to prevent adverse reactions.

Some of these reactions are dose dependent; that is, their occurrence is more common or their intensity is more severe when multiple doses (or cycles) are used. Because the antineoplastic drugs affect cancer cells and rapidly proliferating normal cells (i.e., cells in the bone marrow, GI tract, reproductive tract, and hair follicles), adverse reactions occur as the result of action on these cells.

Adverse reactions common to many of the antineoplastic drugs include **bone marrow suppression (anemia, leukopenia, thrombocytopenia)**, **stomatitis**, diarrhea, and hair loss. The most common reactions are leukopenia and thrombocytopenia, which may cause cycles of chemotherapy to be delayed until blood cell counts can be raised. Some drugs, especially the alkaloids, affect the nervous system. These adverse reactions can range from a peripheral tingling sensation to hand and foot syndrome (tiny capillary leaks in extremities, causing symptoms from skin color changes to numbness).

Because the drugs used to treat cancer are effective, many people are living with the disease either cured or in remission. Some of the adverse reactions to antineoplastic drugs can have long-lasting effects. These include damage to the gonads, causing fertility problems, and to other specific organ systems, leading to cardiac, pulmonary, or neurologic problems. In addition, secondary cancers like leukemia can be caused by the original cancer treatment. These problems are listed in the Summary Drug Tables. Appropriate references should be consulted when administering these drugs, because there are a variety of uses and dose ranges and, in some instances, many adverse reactions.

Contraindications and Precautions

The information discussed in this section is general, and the contraindications, precautions, and interactions for each antineoplastic drug vary. The nurse should consult appropriate sources before administering any antineoplastic drug.

(text continues on page 522)

Summary Drug Table CELL CYCLE–NONSPECIFIC DRUGS

Generic Name	Trade Name	Uses	Adverse Reactions
Alkylating Drugs			
Nitrogen Mustard Derivatives			
chlorambucil *klor-am'-byoo-sill*	Leukeran	Leukemia/lymphomas: chronic lymphocytic leukemia (CLL). lymphomas, Hodgkin's disease	During therapy cycles: anemia, leukopenia, thrombocytopenia Long term: fertility problems
cyclophosphamide *sye-kloe-foss'-fah-myde*	Cytoxan, Neosar	Leukemia/lymphomas: ALL, AML, CLL, advanced lymphomas, Hodgkin's disease Solid tumors: breast, ovary, neuroblastoma, retinoblastoma Nonmalignant: mycosis fungoides nephrotic syndrome (children), rheumatoid arthritis, systemic lupus erythematosus, multiple sclerosis	Immediate: nausea, vomiting During therapy cycles: leukopenia, hemorrhagic cystitis, thrombocytopenia Long term: fertility problems, secondary cancers
ifosfamide *eye-foss'-fah-myde*	Ifex	Leukemia/lymphomas: unlabeled use (except AML) Solid tumors: testicular Unlabeled use: lung, breast, ovary, gastric, pancreatic	Immediate: nausea, vomiting During therapy cycles: leukopenia, thrombocytopenia, hemorrhagic cystitis, alopecia, somnolence, confusion
mechlorethamine *meh-klor-eth'-ah-meen*	Mustargen	Palliative treatment for CLL, chronic myelocytic leukemia (CML), advanced lymphomas, Hodgkin's diseaseSolid tumors: lung, metastatic disease, mycosis fungoides	Immediate: nausea, vomiting, extravasation potential, lymphocytopenia During therapy cycles: anemia, leukopenia, thrombocytopenia, hyperuremia, diarrhea Long term: fertility problems, secondary cancers
melphalan *mel'-fah-lan*	Alkeran	Palliative treatment for multiple myeloma Solid tumors: ovary Unlabeled use: testicular, breast, bone marrow transplantation	Immediate: nausea, vomiting During therapy cycles: leukopenia, thrombocytopenia, diarrhea, alopecia Long term: fertility problems, secondary cancers
Ethyleneimines			
altretamine (hexamethyl melamine) *al-tret'-ah-meen*	Hexalen	Palliative treatment for solid tumors: ovary	During therapy cycles: anemia, leukopenia, thrombocytopenia, nausea, vomiting, peripheral neuropathy, dizziness
thiotepa *thye-oh-tep'-ah*	Thioplex	Solid tumors: breast, ovary, bladder	During therapy cycles: anemia, leukopenia, thrombocytopenia, alopecia Long term: fertility problems
Alkyl Sulfonate			
busulfan *byoo-sul'-fan*	Busulfex, Myleran	Palliative treatment for CML	Immediate: induce seizures During therapy cycles: anemia, leukopenia, thrombocytopenia, hyperuremia, graft-versus-host disease Long term: fertility problems
Hydrazines			
dacarbazine *dah-kar'-bah-zeen*	DTIC	Leukemia/lymphomas: Hodgkin's disease Solid tumors: melanoma Unlabeled use: pheochromocytoma, KS	Immediate: nausea, vomiting During therapy cycles: anemia, leukopenia, thrombocytopenia

(table continues on page 520)

Summary Drug Table CELL CYCLE–NONSPECIFIC DRUGS (continued)

Generic Name	Trade Name	Uses	Adverse Reactions
procarbazine *proe-kar'-bah-zeen*	Matulane	Leukemia/lymphomas: Hodgkin's disease Unlabeled use: other lymphomas, brain, small cell lung cancer, melanoma	Immediate: nausea, vomiting During therapy cycles: anemia, leukopenia, thrombocytopenia, peripheral neuropathy, alopecia
temozolomide *tem-oh-zoll'-oh-myde*	Temodar	Solid tumors: glioblastoma, astrocytoma Unlabeled use: melanoma	During therapy cycles: leukopenia, thrombocytopenia, headache, nausea, vomiting, alopecia
Nitrosoureas			
carmustine (BCNU) *car-muss'-teen*	BiCNU, Gliadel	Palliative treatment for Hodgkin's disease, multiple myeloma, various brain tumors Unlabeled use: T-cell lymphoma, melanoma	Immediate: nausea, vomiting During therapy cycles: leukopenia, thrombocytopenia Long term: pulmonary fibrosis
lomustine (CCNU) *loe-muss'-teen*	CeeNU	Leukemia/lymphomas: secondary treatment for Hodgkin's disease Solid tumors: brain	Immediate: nausea, vomiting During therapy cycles: leukopenia, thrombocytopenia, alopecia, stomatitis Long term: pulmonary fibrosis, fertility problems
streptozocin *strep'-toe-zoh-sin*	Zanosar	Solid tumors: pancreatic	Immediate: nausea, vomiting During therapy cycles: azotemia, proteinuria, stomatitis
Platinum-Based Drugs			
cisplatin *sis-plah'-tin*	Platinol-AQ	Solid tumors: ovarian, testicular, bladder	Immediate: nausea, vomiting, renal damage During therapy cycles: anemia, leukopenia, thrombocytopenia tinnitus, hyperuricemia
oxaliplatin *ox-al'-ih-plah-tin*	Eloxatin	Solid tumors: colon, rectal	During therapy cycles: leukopenia, thrombocytopenia, peripheral neuropathy
carboplatin *kar'-boe-plah-tin*	Paraplatin	Solid tumors: ovarian Unlabeled use: lung, head and neck, testicular	During therapy cycles: anemia, leukopenia, thrombocytopenia
Antibiotics			
bleomycin *blee-oh-mye'-sin*	Blenoxane	Palliative treatment for lymphomas, pleural effusion Solid tumors: testicular, various types Unlabeled use: mycosis fungoides, KS	During therapy cycles: anemia, leukopenia, thrombocytopenia, vomiting, alopecia, skin erythema, cutaneous changes Long term: pneumonitis, pulmonary fibrosis
dactinomycin *dak-tih-noe-mye'-sin*	Cosmegen	Solid tumors: various sarcomas, Wilms' tumor, gestational neoplasia, testicular	Immediate: nausea, vomiting, extravasation potential During therapy cycles: anemia, leukopenia, thrombocytopenia, alopecia, skin erythema Long term: fertility problems
daunorubicin *daw-noe-roo'-bih-sin*	DaunoXome	Leukemia/lymphomas: ALL, AML Solid tumors: KS	Immediate: nausea, vomiting, extravasation potential During therapy cycles: anemia, leukopenia, thrombocytopenia, alopecia, stomatitis, hyperuricemia, urine discoloration Long term: cardiotoxicity

(table continues on page 521)

Summary Drug Table CELL CYCLE–NONSPECIFIC DRUGS (continued)

Generic Name	Trade Name	Uses	Adverse Reactions
doxorubicin *dox-oh-roo'-bih-sin*	Adriamycin, Doxil	Leukemia/lymphomas; ALL, AML, and various lymphomas Solid tumors: Wilms' tumor, neuroblastoma, KS, various sarcomas, breast, lung, ovary, bladder, thyroid, gastric	Immediate: nausea, vomiting, extravasation potential During therapy cycles: anemia, leukopenia, thrombocytopenia, alopecia, cutaneous changes, stomatitis, hyperuricemia, urine discoloration, radiation recall, hand and foot syndrome Long term: cardiotoxicity
epirubicin *ep-pee-roo'-bih-sin*	Ellence	Solid tumors: breast Unlabeled use: advanced esophageal	Immediate: extravasation potential During therapy cycles: anemia, leukopenia, thrombocytopenia, nausea, vomiting, alopecia, stomatitis, diarrhea, urine discoloration, radiation recall Long term: cardiotoxicity, fertility problems
idarubicin *eye-dah-roo'-bih-sin*	Idamycin	Leukemia/lymphomas: AML	Immediate: extravasation potential During therapy cycles: anemia, leukopenia, thrombocytopenia, alopecia, nausea, vomiting, stomatitis, diarrhea, hyperuricemia, urine discoloration Long term: cardiotoxicity
mitomycin *mye-toe-mye'-sin*	Mutamycin	Solid tumors: stomach, pancreas	Immediate: extravasation potential During therapy cycles: anemia, leukopenia, thrombocytopenia, hyperuricemia
mitoxantrone *mye-toe-zan'-trone*	Novantrone	Leukemia/lymphomas: acute non-lymphocytic leukemia Solid tumors: advanced prostate Nonmalignant: multiple sclerosis	Immediate: nausea, vomiting, extravasation potential During therapy cycles: leukopenia, nausea, alopecia Long term: cardiotoxicity, AML
Miscellaneous Agents			
DNA Inhibitor hydroxyurea *hye-drox-ee-yoor-ee'-ah*	Hydrea, Mylocel	Solid tumors: melanoma Unlabeled use: thrombocythemia, human immunodeficiency virus infection, psoriasis	During therapy cycles: anemia, leukopenia, thrombocytopenia, radiation recall
Adrenocortical Inhibitor mitotane *mye'-toe-tane*	Lysodren	Solid tumors: adrenal cortex Unlabeled use: Cushing's disease	During therapy cycles: nausea, vomiting, diarrhea
Enzymes asparaginase *ah-spare'-ah-gih-nayce*	Elspar	Leukemia/lymphomas: ALL	During therapy cycles: anemia, leukopenia, thrombocytopenia, hyperuricemia, rash, urticaria, acute anaphylaxis
pegaspargase *peg-ah-spar'-gayce*	Oncaspar	Same as asparaginase	Same as asparaginase
Antimicrotubule Agents estramustine (estradiol/nitrogen mustard) *ess-tra-muss'-teen*	Emcyt	Palliative treatment for solid tumors e.g., prostate	Immediate: nausea, diarrhea During therapy cycles: breast tenderness, thrombophlebitis, fluid retention Long term: gynecomastia, impotence

(table continues on page 522)

Antineoplastic Drugs

Summary Drug Table CELL CYCLE–NONSPECIFIC DRUGS (continued)

Generic Name	Trade Name	Uses	Adverse Reactions
Retinoids			
tretinoin *tret'-ih-noyn*	Vesanoid	Leukemia/lymphomas: acute promyelocytic leukemia	During therapy cycles: headache, fever, weakness, fatigue, edema, retinoic acid–acute promyelocytic leukemia (RA-APL) syndrome (acute anaphylactic reaction)
bexarotene *bex-air'-oh-teen*	Targretin	Leukemia/lymphomas: cutaneous T-cell lymphoma	During therapy cycles: elevated blood lipids, rash, leukopenia, dry skin

Antineoplastic drugs are contraindicated in patients with leukopenia, thrombocytopenia, anemia, serious infections, serious renal disease, or known hypersensitivity to the drug, and during pregnancy (see Display 51.3 for pregnancy classifications of selected antineoplastic drugs) or lactation.

Antineoplastic drugs are used cautiously in patients with renal or hepatic impairment, active infection, or other debilitating illnesses, or in those who have recently completed treatment with other antineoplastic drugs or radiation therapy.

Interactions

A number of antineoplastic drugs are harmful to normal cells as well as cancer cells. Cytoprotective agents are drugs used with the antineoplastic drug to protect the normal cells or organs of the body. In this way, enough of the chemotherapeutic drug can be given to eradicate the cancer without

DISPLAY 51.3 Pregnancy Classification for Selected Antineoplastic Drugs

Pregnancy Category C

asparaginase	mitotane	streptozocin
dacarbazine	pegaspargase	

Pregnancy Category D

altretamine	doxorubicin	mitoxantrone
bleomycin	epirubicin	nelarabine
busulfan	etoposide	oxaliplatin
capecitabine	fludarabine	paclitaxel
carboplatin	fluorouracil	pemetrexed
carmustine	gemcitabine	pentostatin
chlorambucil	hydroxyurea	procarbazine
cisplatin	idarubicin	temozolomide
cladribine	ifosfamide	thioguanine
clofarabine	irinotecan	thiotepa
cyclophosphamide	ixabepilone	topotecan
cytarabine	lomustine	vinblastine
dactinomycin	mechlorethamine	vincristine
daunorubicin	melphalan	vinorelbine
docetaxel	mercaptopurine	

Pregnancy Category X

methotrexate

DISPLAY 51.4 Cytoprotective Agents

The following drugs function to protect cells or counteract adverse reactions resulting from therapeutic doses of the antineoplastic drugs.

- allopurinol, rasburicase (Elitek): Counteract the increase in uric acid and subsequent hyperuricemia resulting from the metabolic waste buildup from rapid tumor lysis (cell destruction)
- amifostine (Ethyol): Binds with metabolites of cisplatin to protect the kidneys from nephrotoxic effects, reduces xerostomia
- dexrazoxane (Zinecard): Cardioprotective agent used with doxorubicin
- leucovorin (Wellcovorin): Provides folic acid to cells after methotrexate administration
- mesna (Mesnex): Binds with metabolites of ifosfamide to protect the bladder from hemorrhagic cystitis

irreversible harm to the patient. Cytoprotective agents used with antineoplastic drugs are listed in Display 51.4.

The following table lists selected interactions of the plant alkaloids, antimetabolites, alkylating drugs, antibiotics, and miscellaneous antineoplastic drugs. Typically, additive bone marrow depressive effects occur when any category of antineoplastic drug is administered with another chemotherapy drug or radiation therapy. The nurse should consult appropriate sources for a more complete listing of interactions before any antineoplastic drug is administered.

Interacting Drug	Common Use	Effect of Interaction
Plant Alkaloids		
digoxin	Cardiac problems	Decrease serum level of digoxin
phenytoin	Seizure disorders	Increased risk of seizures
oral anticoagulants	Blood thinners	Prolonged bleeding
Antimetabolites		
digoxin	Cardiac problems	Decrease serum level of digoxin

Interacting Drug	Common Use	Effect of Interaction
phenytoin	Seizure disorders	Decreased need for antiseizure medication
Nonsteroidal anti-inflammatory drugs (NSAIDs)	Pain relief	methotrexate drugs (NSAIDs)
Alkylating Drugs		
aminoglycosides	Anti-infective agents	Increased risk of nephrotoxicity and ototoxicity
loop diuretics	Heart problems and edema	Increased risk of ototoxicity
phenytoin	Seizure disorder	Increased risk of seizure
Antineoplastic Antibiotics		
digoxin	Cardiac problems	Decrease serum level of digoxin
Miscellaneous Antineoplastic Drugs		
insulin and oral hypoglycemics	Diabetes management	Increased risk of hyperglycemia
oral anticoagulants	Blood thinners	Prolonged bleeding
antidepressants, antihistamines, opiates, or the sedatives	Depression, allergy, pain relief, or sedation, respectively	Increased risk of central nervous system depression

HERBAL ALERT

The **shiitake mushroom**, an edible variety of mushroom, is associated with general health maintenance but not with any severe adverse reactions. Mild side effects, such as skin rashes and GI upset, have been reported. Lentinan, a derivative of the shiitake mushroom, is proving to be valuable in boosting the body's immune system and may prolong the survival time of patients with cancer by supporting immunity. In Japan, lentinan is commonly used to treat cancer. Additional possible benefits of this herb include lowering cholesterol levels by increasing the rate at which cholesterol is excreted from the body. Under no circumstances should shiitake or lentinan be used for cancer or any serious illness without consulting a primary health care provider.

NURSING PROCESS

PATIENT RECEIVING AN ANTINEOPLASTIC DRUG

ASSESSMENT

Preadministration Assessment

The extent of the preadministration assessment depends on the type of cancer and the patient's general physical condition. The initial assessment of the patient scheduled for chemotherapy may include the following:

- Type and location of the neoplastic lesion
- Stage of the disease, for example, early, metastatic, or terminal
- Patient's general physical condition
- Patient's emotional response to the disease
- Anxiety or fears the patient may have regarding chemotherapy treatments
- Previous or concurrent treatments (if any), such as surgery, radiation therapy, other antineoplastic drugs
- Other current nonmalignant disease or disorder, such as congestive heart failure or peptic ulcer, that may or may not be related to the malignant disease
- Patient's knowledge or understanding of the proposed chemotherapy regimen
- Other factors, such as the patient's age, financial problems that may be associated with a long-term illness, family cooperation and interest in patient care, and the adequacy of health insurance coverage (which may be of great concern to the patient)

Immediately before administering the first dose of an antineoplastic drug, the nurse takes the patient's vital signs and obtains a current weight, because the dose of some antineoplastic drugs is based on the patient's weight in kilograms or pounds. The dosages of some antineoplastic drugs also may be based on body surface measurements and are stated as a specific amount of drug per square meter (m^2) of body surface. When an antineoplastic drug has a depressing effect on the bone marrow, laboratory tests, such as a complete blood count, are ordered to determine the effect of the previous drug dosage. Before the first dose of the drug is administered, pretreatment laboratory tests provide baseline data for future reference. The administration route of chemotherapy is routinely monitored; examples include assessment of vessel integrity for IV access or patency of venous access devices.

Some antineoplastic drugs require treatment measures before administration. An example of preadministration treatment is hydration of the patient with 1 to 2 L of IV fluid infused before administration of cisplatin (Platinol) or administration of an antiemetic before the administration of irinotecan (Camptosar). These measures are ordered by the oncology health care provider and, in some instances, may vary slightly from the manufacturer's recommendations.

Ongoing Assessment

The patient who is acutely ill with many physical problems requires different ongoing assessment activities than does one who is ambulating and able to participate in the activities of daily living. Once the patient's general condition is assessed and needs identified, the nurse develops a care plan to meet those needs. Patients receiving chemotherapy can be at different stages of their disease; therefore, nurses must individualize the nursing care of each patient based on the patient's needs, and not just on the type of drug administered.

In general, after the administration of an antineoplastic drug, the nurse bases the ongoing assessment on the following factors:

- Patient's general condition
- Patient's individual response to the drug
- Adverse reactions that may occur
- Guidelines established by the oncology health care provider or clinic
- Results of periodic laboratory tests and radiographic scans

Different types of laboratory tests may be used to monitor the patient's response to therapy. Some of these tests, such as a complete blood count, may be used to determine the response of the bone marrow to an antineoplastic drug. Other tests, such as kidney function tests, may be used to detect nephrotoxicity, an adverse reaction that sometimes occurs with the administration of some of these drugs. Abnormal laboratory test results may also require a change in the nursing care plan. For example, a significant drop in the neutrophil count may require a delay in treatment, administration of colony-stimulating factors (see Chapter 52), and patient teaching about ways to recognize and prevent infection and sepsis.

The nurse reviews the results of all laboratory tests at the time they are reported. The oncology health care provider is notified of the results before the administration of successive doses of an antineoplastic drug. If these tests indicate a severe depressant effect on the bone marrow or other test abnormalities, the primary health care provider may reduce the next drug dose or temporarily stop chemotherapy to allow the affected body systems to recover.

NURSING DIAGNOSES

The nursing diagnoses for the patient with cancer are usually extensive and are based on many factors, such as the patient's physical and emotional condition, the adverse reactions resulting from antineoplastic drug therapy, and the stage of the disease. Drug-specific nursing diagnoses include the following:

❏ **Imbalanced Nutrition: Less Than Body Requirements** related to anorexia, nausea, vomiting, and stomatitis
❏ **Fatigue** related to anemia and myelosuppression
❏ **Risk for Injury** related to thrombocytopenia and myelosuppression
❏ **Risk for Infection** related to neutropenia, leukopenia, and myelosuppression
❏ **Disturbed Body Image** related to adverse reactions of antineoplastic drugs (e.g., alopecia, weight loss)
❏ **Anxiety** related to diagnosis, necessary treatment measures, the occurrence of adverse reactions, other factors
❏ **Impaired Tissue Integrity** related to adverse reactions of the antineoplastic drugs (radiation recall and extravasation)

Nursing diagnoses related to drug administration are discussed in Chapter 4.

PLANNING

The expected outcomes of the patient may include an optimal response to therapy, support of patient needs related to the management of adverse reactions, and an understanding of the prescribed treatment modalities.

IMPLEMENTATION

Promoting an Optimal Response to Therapy

Care of the patient receiving an antineoplastic drug depends on factors such as the drug or combination of drugs given, the dosage of the drugs, the route of administration, the patient's physical response to therapy, the response of the tumor to chemotherapy, and the type and severity of adverse reactions. Some drugs may be administered by various routes, depending on the cancer being treated. For example, thiotepa may be administered by the IV route for breast cancer, intravesicular route for superficial bladder cancer, intrapleural route for malignant pleural effusions, and by the intraperitoneal route for ovarian cancer. As the methods of administration have changed, so has the location for administration. Once given as long IV infusions over days or a week in the hospital, many of the antineoplastic drugs are still given IV but as push or small-volume infusions, and they are delivered in an outpatient setting by highly skilled nurses.

GUIDELINES ESTABLISHED BY THE SETTING FOR CARE. In these settings (hospital, outpatient chemotherapy clinics, or office), policies are established to provide nursing personnel with specific guidelines for the assessment and care of patients receiving a single or combination chemotherapeutic drug regimen. During chemotherapy, the oncology health care provider may write orders for certain nursing procedures, such as measuring fluid intake and output, monitoring the vital signs at specific intervals, and increasing the fluid intake to a certain amount. Even when orders are written, the nurse should increase the frequency of certain assessments, such as monitoring vital signs, if the patient's condition changes. Some settings have written guidelines for nursing management when the patient is receiving a specific antineoplastic drug. The nurse incorporates these guidelines into the nursing care plan with nursing observations and assessments geared to the individual. The nurse adds further assessments to the nursing care plan when the patient's condition changes.

If treatment is given in a setting where guidelines are not provided, it is important for the nurse to review the drugs being given before their administration. These drugs should not be prescribed by a generalist health care provider; rather, antineoplastics should be prescribed only by a provider trained specifically in the care of oncology patients. The nurse consults appropriate references to obtain information regarding the preparation and administration of a particular drug, the average dose ranges, all the known adverse reactions, and the warnings and precautions given by the manufacturer.

PROTECTION OF THE PROVIDER. Those involved in the administration of antineoplastic drugs are at risk for many adverse reactions from accidental absorption of the drugs. Because so many of the drugs are given in the outpatient setting, personnel in clinics and offices are at high risk for exposure. It is important to follow the directions of the manufacturer regarding the type of solution to be used for preparation, dilution, or administration. The Occupational Safety and Health Administration (OSHA) guidelines state that antineoplastic drug preparation is to be performed in a biologic safety cabinet (BSC) in a designated area. This is to prevent accidental inhalation and exposure to the person preparing the drugs. In addition, nurses need to be protected during administration and cleanup from accidental ingestion, inhalation, or absorption of the drugs. Table 51.1 outlines the protective items that should be available to staff working with antineoplastic drugs.

ORAL ADMINISTRATION. A number of antineoplastic drugs are administered orally. The oral route is convenient and noninvasive. Most oral drugs are well absorbed when the GI tract is functioning normally. Antineoplastic drugs such as capecitabine (Xeloda) or temozolomide (Temodar) are given orally. Most oral drugs are administered by the patient in a home setting. The section on Educating the Patient and Family provides information to include in a teaching plan.

PARENTERAL ADMINISTRATION. Although some of these drugs are given orally, others are given by the parenteral route. Antineoplastic drugs may be administered subcutaneously (subcut), intramuscularly (IM), and IV. When giving these drugs IM, the nurse gives the injection into the large muscles using the Z-track method (see Chapter 2),

because administration can cause stinging or burning. When the subcut method of administration is used, the injection should contain no more than 1 mL, and injections are given in the usual subcut injection sites (see Chapter 2). If the injections are given frequently, the sites should be rotated and charted appropriately.

Intravenous administration may be accomplished using a vascular access device, an angiocath, or a butterfly needle. These devices have become common methods of drug delivery and, depending on the patient's individual treatment regimen, may be inserted before therapy. Selection of the device depends on the type of therapy the patient is to receive, the condition of the veins, and how long the treatment regimen is to be continued. Special directions for administration, stated by either the oncology health care provider or manufacturer, are also important. For example, cisplatin cannot be prepared or administered with needles or IV administration sets containing aluminum, because aluminum reacts with cisplatin, causing formation of a precipitate and loss of potency.

Nurses who are certified in chemotherapy drug administration administer these drugs, but any nurse may be involved in monitoring patients receiving antineoplastic drugs. Antineoplastic drugs are potentially toxic drugs that can cause a variety of effects during and after their administration. Display 51.5 summarizes important points to keep in mind when administering an antineoplastic drug.

Monitoring and Managing Patient Needs

Not all patients have the same response to a specific antineoplastic drug. For example, an antineoplastic drug may cause vomiting, but the amount of fluid and electrolytes lost through vomiting may vary from patient to

Table 51.1 Personal Protective Equipment for Safe Handling of Antineoplastic Drugs

Route of Potential Exposure	Safety Equipment
Skin	Gowns—single-use, disposable gowns with closed front and cuffs and made of impermeable or minimally permeable fabric (to the agents in use) Gloves—powder-free; made of latex, nitrile, or neoprene; labeled and tested for use with chemotherapeutic drugs
Ingestion	Safety goggles with face shield—to protect face and eyes from possible splashes
Inhalation	National Institute for Occupational Safety and Health (NIOSH)–approved respirator—when a spill must be cleaned up

Adapted from Polovich, M. (2004). Safe handling of hazardous drugs. Retrieved April 28, 2009, from http://www.guideline.gov/summary/summary.aspx?ss=15&doc_id=4152&nbr=3180/.

DISPLAY 51.5 Points to Keep in Mind About Antineoplastic Drug Administration

Great care and accuracy are important in preparing and administering these drugs. Important points to keep in mind during drug administration follow:

- Wear personal protective equipment when preparing any of these drugs for parenteral administration.
- Administer any prophylactic medications or fluids in a timely manner to prevent reactions.
- Observe the patient closely before, during, and after the administration of an antineoplastic drug.
- Observe the IV site closely to detect any signs of extravasation (leakage into the surrounding tissues). Tissue necrosis can be a serious complication. Discontinue the infusion and notify the oncology health care provider if discomfort, redness along the pathway of the vein, or infiltration occurs.
- Continually update nursing assessments, nursing diagnoses, and nursing care plans to meet the changing needs of the patient.
- Notify the oncology health care provider of all changes in the patient's general condition, the appearance of adverse reactions, and changes in laboratory test results.
- Provide the patient and family with both physical and emotional support during treatment.

patient. One patient may require additional sips of water once nausea and vomiting have subsided, whereas another may require IV fluid and electrolyte replacement. Nursing management is focused not only on what may or what did happen, but on the effects produced by a particular adverse reaction.

IMBALANCED NUTRITION: LESS THAN BODY REQUIREMENTS. Patients may not eat because they are tired or not hungry. **Anorexia** (loss of appetite resulting in the inability to eat) is a common occurrence with the antineoplastic drugs. This may be due to nausea, taste alterations, or sores in the GI system. Nausea and vomiting are common adverse reactions to some of the highly emetic antineoplastic drugs. To minimize this adverse reaction, the oncology health care provider may order an antiemetic, such as ondansetron (Zofran), to be given before treatment and continued for a few days after administration of the chemotherapy. Because this is an expensive drug, other protocols may include different (and less expensive) antiemetics. Some of these have adverse effects, such as a sedative action, which might add to the patient's lack of desire to eat. In the example of the patient who is vomiting, it is important to tract accurately all fluid intake. To prevent handling of contaminated waste, nurses should use the patient's weight to assess for fluid loss and observe the patient for signs of dehydration and electrolyte imbalances. These measurements and observations aid the oncology health care provider in determining if fluid replacement is necessary.

The nurse assesses the nutritional status of the patient before and during treatment. To stimulate appetite, the nurse provides small, frequent meals to coincide with the patient's tolerance for food. Greasy or fatty foods and unpleasant sights, smells, and tastes are avoided. Cold foods, dry foods, and salty foods may be better tolerated. It is a good idea to provide diversional activities, such as music, television, and books. Relaxation, visualization, guided imagery, hypnosis, and other nonpharmacologic measures have been helpful to some patients.

It is not uncommon for the patient to report alterations in the sense of taste during the course of chemotherapy. Some drugs give protein foods such as beef a bitter, metallic taste. Small, frequent meals (five to six meals daily) are usually better tolerated than are three large meals. Breakfast is often the best-tolerated meal of the day. The nurse stresses the importance of eating meals high in nutritive value, particularly protein (e.g., eggs, milk products, tuna, beans, peas, and lentils). Some patients prefer to have available high-protein finger foods such as cheese or peanut butter and crackers. Nutritional supplements may also be prescribed. The nurse monitors the patient's body weight weekly (or more often if necessary) and reports any weight loss. If the patient continues to lose weight, a feeding tube or total parenteral nutrition (TPN) may be used to supplement nutritional needs. Although this is not ideal, the patient who is malnourished and weak may benefit from this intervention.

Because the cells in the mouth grow rapidly, they are particularly sensitive to the effects of the antineoplastic drugs. Stomatitis (inflammation of the mouth) or **oral mucositis** (inflammation of the oral mucous membranes) may appear 5 to 7 days after chemotherapy is started and continue up to 10 days after therapy. This adverse reaction is particularly uncomfortable, because irritation of the oral mucous membranes affects the nutritional aspects of care. The patient must avoid any foods or products that are irritating to the mouth, such as alcoholic beverages, spices, alcohol-based mouthwash or toothpaste. The nurse provides soft or liquid food high in nutritive value. The oral cavity is inspected for increased irritation. The nurse reports any white patches on the tongue, throat, or gums; any burning sensation; and bleeding from the mouth or gums. Mouth care is encouraged to be performed every 4 hours, including a rinse with normal saline solution. Lemon/glycerin swabs are avoided because they tend to irritate the oral mucosa and complicate stomatitis. The oncology health care provider may order a topical viscous anesthetic, such as lidocaine viscous, to decrease discomfort.

FATIGUE, RISK FOR INJURY, AND RISK FOR INFECTION. MYELOSUPPRESSION. Many antineoplastic drugs interfere with the bone marrow's ability to make new cells. This interference is called *bone marrow suppression* or **myelosuppression** and is a potentially dangerous adverse reaction. Bone marrow suppression is manifested by abnormal laboratory test results and clinical evidence of leukopenia, thrombocytopenia, or anemia. For example, there is a decrease in the white blood cells or leukocytes (*leukopenia*), a decrease in the thrombocytes (*thrombocytopenia*), and a decrease in the red blood cells, resulting in anemia.

Anemia occurs as the result of a decreased production of red blood cells in the bone marrow and is characterized by fatigue, dizziness, shortness of breath, and palpitations. The nurse helps the patient learn to prioritize activity to conserve energy. Permission is given to the active patient to slow down and even take daytime naps. In some cases, the administration of blood transfusions may be necessary to correct the anemia.

Patients with **neutropenia** (reduction in the neutrophil type of white blood cells) have a decreased resistance to infection, and the nurse must monitor them closely for any signs of infection. Combined therapy, such as chemotherapy and radiation together, can have an additive effect on the reduction of blood cells.

NURSING ALERT

Because of the severity of leukopenia when taking temozolomide (Temodar) in conjunction with radiation to the brain, patients should be started on prophylactic therapy to prevent *Pneumocystis* pneumonia (PCP).

Patients are instructed to stay away from crowds or ill individuals while receiving myelosuppressive drugs. Sepsis, without the typical signs of infection, can affect patients because they lack neutrophils. The primary health care provider may prescribe colony-stimulating factor injections to promote the production of blood cells between the chemotherapy cycles. Low blood counts are one of the primary reasons a chemotherapy treatment may be delayed.

! **NURSING ALERT**

The nurse should report immediately any of the following signs of infection to the health care provider: temperature of 100.4°F (38°C) or higher, cough, sore throat, chills, frequent urination, or a white blood cell count of less than 2500/mm³.

Thrombocytopenia is characterized by a decrease in the platelet count (less than 100,000/mm³). The nurse monitors patients with thrombocytopenia for bleeding tendencies and takes precautions to prevent bleeding. Injections and multiple blood draws are avoided but, if necessary, the nurse applies pressure to the injection site for 3 to 5 minutes to prevent bleeding into the tissue and the formation of a hematoma. The nurse informs the patient to avoid the use of disposable razors, nail trimmers, dental floss, firm toothbrushes, or any sharp objects. The patient is taught to refrain from contact and highly physical activities at this time. The patient is monitored closely for easy bruising, skin lesions, and bleeding from any orifice (opening) of the body.

! **NURSING ALERT**

The nurse reports any of the following to the health care provider immediately: bleeding gums, easy bruising, petechiae (pinpoint hemorrhages), increased menstrual bleeding, tarry stools, bloody urine, or coffee-ground emesis.

DISTURBED BODY IMAGE. Adverse reactions seen with the administration of these drugs may range from very mild to life-threatening. Some of these reactions, such as the loss of hair (**alopecia**), may have little effect on the physical status of the patient but certainly may have a serious effect on the patient's mental health. Because nursing is concerned with the whole patient, such physically altering reactions that can have a profound effect on the patient must be considered when planning nursing management.

Some drugs cause severe hair loss, whereas others cause gradual thinning. Examples of drugs commonly associated with severe hair loss are doxorubicin and vinblastine. If hair loss is associated with the antineoplastic drug being given, the nurse informs the patient that hair loss may occur. This problem may occur 10 to 21 days after the first treatment cycle. Hair loss is usually temporary, and hair will grow again when the drug therapy is completed. The nurse forewarns the patient that hair loss may occur suddenly and in large amounts. Hair will be lost not only from the head but from the entire body. Although it is not life-threatening, alopecia can have an impact on both self-esteem and body image, serving as a reminder that the individual is undergoing treatment for cancer.

Depending on the patient, the nurse may need to assist in making plans for the purchase of a wig or cap

to disguise the hair loss until the hair grows back. The nurse should be aware that this might be as great a problem to a male patient as it is to a female patient. The patient is reminded about the importance of a head covering because of the amount of body heat that can be lost with the hair gone.

ANXIETY. The word *cancer* still evokes dread in people. Patients and family members are usually devastated by the diagnosis of cancer. Patients have to absorb much information and make quick, critical decisions about treatment. The emphasis on the safety requirements of chemotherapy administration adds to the demands and fears placed on patients. The emotional impact of the disease may be forgotten or put aside by members of the health care team as they plan and institute therapy to control the disease. Because cancer treatment happens over time, the nurse has the opportunity to offer consistent and empathetic emotional support to the patient and family members. This support can help reduce some of the fear and anxiety experienced by the patient and family during treatment.

IMPAIRED TISSUE INTEGRITY. Erythema consists of a red, warm, and sometimes painful area on the skin. Because the skin cells are rapidly growing cells, the integument is at risk for breakdown during antineoplastic drug therapy. Care should be taken by patients to avoid the sun, wear loose, protective clothing, and to watch areas of skinfolds for breakdown. Some antineoplastic drugs have the ability to sensitize skin that has previously been irradiated. The nurse makes sure to instruct the patient about this adverse reaction, because it can be both surprising and painful.

! **NURSING ALERT**

Radiation recall is a skin reaction in which an area that was previously irradiated becomes reddened when a patient is administered certain specific chemotherapy drugs. This is well differentiated from a reaction exclusive to the drugs, because of the defined outline of the previous radiation treatment field on the body.

Some antineoplastic drugs are **vesicants** (i.e., they cause tissue necrosis if they infiltrate or extravasate out of the blood vessel and into the soft tissue). If extravasation occurs, underlying tissue is damaged. The damage can be severe, causing physical deformity or loss of vascularity or tendon function. If the damage is severe, skin grafting may be necessary to preserve function. Examples of vesicant drugs are daunorubicin, doxorubicin, and vinblastine.

! **NURSING ALERT**

Patients at risk for extravasation are those unable to communicate to the nurse about the pain of extravasation, the elderly, debilitated, or confused patient, and any patient with fragile veins.

When the patient is receiving a vesicant, the nurse ensures that extravasation protocol orders are signed and that an extravasation kit is on the unit before vesicant drugs are administered. The nurse monitors the IV site continuously and checks for blood return frequently during IV push procedures (every 1 to 2 mL). If a vesicant is prescribed as an infusion, it is given through a central line only and checked every 1 to 2 hours. The nurse keeps an extravasation kit containing all materials necessary to manage an extravasation available, along with the extravasation policy and procedure guidelines.

Extravasation may occur without warning, or signs may be detected by an alert nurse. The earlier the extravasation is detected, the less likely soft tissue damage will occur.

 NURSING ALERT

Signs of extravasation include:

- Swelling (most common)
- Stinging, burning, or pain at the injection site (not always present)
- Redness
- Lack of blood return (if this is the only symptom, the IV line should be reevaluated; a lack of blood return alone is not always indicative of extravasation, and extravasation can occur even if a blood return is present)

If extravasation is suspected, the infusion is stopped immediately, antidotal procedures initiated, and the extravasation reported to the primary health care provider.

Educating the Patient and Family

The nurse explains all treatments and possible adverse effects to the patient before the initiation of therapy. The oncology health care provider usually discusses the proposed treatment and possible adverse drug reactions with the patient and family members. The nurse briefly reviews these explanations immediately before parenteral administration of a drug.

Some antineoplastic drugs are taken orally at home. The areas included in a patient and family teaching plan for this type of treatment regimen are based on the drug prescribed, the oncology health care provider's explanation of the chemotherapy regimen and instructions for taking the drug, and the needs of the individual. To prevent unintended absorption, some pills or tablets should not be handled by others when administering the drugs. Family members are taught how to take out the medication from its container without touching the drug. Some hospitals, clinics, or primary health care providers give printed instructions to the patient. The nurse reviews these instructions after the patient has read them and allows time for the patient or family member to ask questions.

In some instances, a drug to prevent nausea may be prescribed to be taken at home before administration of the antineoplastic drugs in the outpatient setting. To obtain the best possible effects, the nurse stresses to the patient that the drug must be taken at the time specified by the oncology health care provider. It is important for the patient to comply with the treatment regimen to maximize therapeutic effect. Most patients are compliant with antineoplastic therapy; however, some of the drugs have modified schedules, such as when given in conjunction with radiation therapy with certain weeks on therapy and others off therapy, and these administration schedules can become confusing. The nurse must stress the importance of maintaining the dosing schedule exactly as prescribed. A calendar indicating the doses to take and dates the drug is to be taken, with space to record each dose, is often given to the patient. The patient is instructed to bring the treatment calendar to each appointment, and he or she is questioned about any omitted or delayed doses. In general, one course of therapy is prescribed at a time to avoid inadvertent overdosing that could be life-threatening.

The nurse includes the following points in a patient and family teaching plan when oral therapy is prescribed:

- Take the drug only as directed on the prescription container. Unless otherwise indicated, take the drug on an empty stomach with water to enhance absorption. However, the patient should follow specific directions, such as "take on an empty stomach" or "take at the same time each day"; they are extremely important.
- Familiarize yourself with the brand or trade name and the generic name to avoid confusion. If you live with another person at home, ask them to help you verify the correct drug and dose of the drug before you take it.
- Never increase, decrease, or omit a dose unless advised to do so by the oncology health care provider.
- If any problems (adverse reactions) occur, no matter how minor, contact the oncology health care provider immediately.
- All recommendations given by the oncology health care provider, such as increasing the fluid intake or eating or avoiding certain foods, are important.
- Some drugs leave the body relatively unchanged; therefore, to prevent contamination men should avoid using urinals and sit to urinate for at least 48 hours following the last dose of the drug. Toilets should be 'double-flushed' with the lid down to prevent spray in the bathroom.
- The effectiveness or action of the drug could be altered if these directions are ignored. Other recommendations, such as checking the mouth for sores, rinsing the mouth thoroughly after eating or drinking, or drinking extra fluids, are given to identify or minimize some of the effects these drugs have on the body. It is important to follow these recommendations.
- Keep all appointments for chemotherapy. These drugs must be given at certain intervals to be effective.
- Do not take any nonprescription drug unless the use of a specific drug has been approved by the oncology health care provider.
- Avoid drinking alcoholic beverages unless the oncology health care provider has approved their use.

- Always inform other physicians, dentists, and medical personnel of therapy with this drug.
- Keep all appointments for the laboratory tests ordered by the oncology health care provider. If you are unable to keep a laboratory appointment, notify the oncology health care provider immediately.

EVALUATION

- Therapeutic effect is achieved.
- Adverse reactions are identified, reported to the primary health care provider, and managed successfully using nursing interventions.
  - ☑ Maintains an adequate nutritional status.
  - ☑ Patient reports fatigue is managed appropriately.
  - ☑ No evidence of injury is seen.
  - ☑ No evidence of infection is seen.
  - ☑ Perceptions of body changes are managed successfully.
  - ☑ Anxiety is managed successfully.
  - ☑ Skin remains intact.
- Patient and family demonstrate an understanding of the drug regimen.

THINK CRITICALLY: PHARMACOLOGY IN PRACTICE

1. Patients with a malignant disease need special consideration, understanding, and emotional support. On occasion, these needs are unrecognized by members of the health care profession. Suppose you recently received a diagnosis of cancer. Discuss some of the feelings you would experience at this time. Describe what you would want the nurse to do for you at this time. Discuss what you would want to know or not know. As you think about this or discuss these questions, remember that any patient may have these same emotional responses and need the same things you would expect from the nurse or other members of the medical profession.

● Test Your Knowledge

1. Which of the following findings would be most indicative to the nurse that the patient has thrombocytopenia?

- **A.** Nausea
- **B.** Blurred vision
- **C.** Headaches
- **D.** Easy bruising

2. Which of the following adverse reactions to the antineoplastic drugs is most likely to affect the patient's body image?

- **A.** Hematuria
- **B.** Alopecia
- **C.** Nausea
- **D.** Diarrhea

3. When assessing the patient for leukopenia, the nurse _____.

- **A.** checks the patient every 8 hours for hematuria
- **B.** monitors the patient for fever, sore throat, chills
- **C.** checks female patients for increased menstrual bleeding
- **D.** reports a white blood cell count of 5000/mm^3

4. Which of the following interventions would be most helpful for a patient with stomatitis?

- **A.** Mouth care should be provided at least once daily.
- **B.** Swab the mouth with lemon glycerin swabs every 4 hours.
- **C.** Provide frequent mouth care with normal saline.
- **D.** Use a hard-bristle toothbrush to cleanse the mouth and teeth of debris.

● Prepare for the NCLEX

1. Which of the following is the most common symptom of extravasation?

- **A.** Swelling around the injection site
- **B.** Redness along the vein and around the injection site
- **C.** Pain at the injection site
- **D.** Tenderness along the path of the vein

● Calculate Medication Dosages

1. Chlorambucil (Leukeran) dosage is calculated based on the patient's body weight. Mrs. Garcia weighs 142 pounds. The prescribed dosage of chlorambucil is 0.2 mg/kg of body weight per day. What is the correct daily dosage for Mrs. Garcia?

2. A patient weighing 120 pounds is to receive bleomycin (Blenoxane) 0.25 units/kg of body weight. What is the correct dosage of bleomycin?

To check your answers, see Appendix E.

the**Point**॰ *For more NCLEX questions, log on to http://thepoint.lww.com to access more than 1000 questions.*

Immunostimulant Drugs

anemia
erythrocytes RBC
erythropoiesis
folinic acid rescue
hematopoiesis
intrinsic factor
iron deficiency anemia

leucovorin rescue
leukocytes WBC
macrocytic anemia
megakaryocytes
megaloblastic anemia
thrombopoiesis

On completion of this chapter, the student will:

1. Describe the function of the different types of blood cells.
2. List the drugs used in the treatment of anemia, bleeding, and prevention of infection.
3. Discuss the actions, uses, general adverse reactions, contraindications, precautions, and interactions of the agents used to treat anemia, bleeding, and prevention of infection.
4. Discuss important preadministration and ongoing assessment activities the nurse should perform on a patient receiving an agent used to treat anemia, bleeding, and prevention of infection.
5. Identify nursing diagnoses particular to a patient receiving an agent used to treat anemia, bleeding, or prevention of infection.
6. Discuss ways to promote an optimal response to therapy and important points to keep in mind when educating patients about the use of an agent used to treat anemia, bleeding, and prevention of infection.

The hematopoietic system is comprised of fluids and particles that are known as *blood*. Blood is a complex fluid that circulates continuously through the heart and blood vessels and to the outermost cells of our body tissues. Three distinct cells circulate in the blood:

• Red blood cells (erythrocytes) that supply our cells with oxygen from the lungs to the tissues
• White blood cells (leukocytes) that protect our bodies from dangerous microorganisms   fight infection

• Platelets (megakaryocytes) that control the bleeding from microscopic to major tears in our tissues

Chronic diseases such as chronic kidney disease or medical treatments such as chemotherapy can cause a hematologic failure. When this happens, inadequate numbers of cells are produced. As a result, the body can no longer meet the demands for oxygen transportation, blood coagulation, or prevention of invasion of microorganisms. **Anemia**, bleeding, and infection can result.

The goal for treating these hematologic problems is to stimulate the body to make more of the specific blood cells. This process is called **hematopoiesis**. During this process, undifferentiated stem cells in the bone marrow are signaled to multiply and differentiate into erythrocytes, leukocytes, or megakaryocytes. Hematopoietic drugs help to enhance this process and are used to treat anemia, bleeding, and infection.

• HEMATOPOIETIC DRUGS USED IN TREATING POTENTIAL BLEEDING OR INFECTION

There are a number of different white blood cells (WBCs) that protect the body from microbial invasion and infection. The WBC known as the neutrophil is one of the major cells in the line of defense from infection. *Neutropenia* is the term for the condition that results when the neutrophil level in the blood is low. Infection is likely to occur when a patient is neutropenic. Neutrophils have an extremely short lifespan (6 to 8 hours), meaning that they rapidly grow and divide. Because of their rapid growth cycle, the neutrophil is a target of the cancer chemotherapy drugs, as well as the cancer cells themselves. Chemotherapy-induced neutropenia is a major reason that cancer treatments may be delayed or cancelled. When this happens, the patient is at a greater risk for continued growth of the cancer or illness from the treatment. Colony stimulating factors are drugs used to stimulate the growth and production of WBCs to help fight off infection.

Platelets are important to normal blood clotting. They are formed from megakaryocytes in the blood. The megakaryocyte is a large blood cell that can divide into many platelets. A low platelet count is a condition called *thrombocytopenia*. Decreased platelet production can also be caused by anemia. The interleukin drug, oprelvekin, is used when sufficient platelets are not made to meet the body's needs.

Colony Stimulating Factors

Actions and Uses

Colony stimulating factors (CSFs) are glycoproteins that act on the hematopoietic cells to stimulate proliferation, differentiation, and maturation of WBCs. CSFs are used to treat or prevent infection (by minimizing neutropenia) associated with the following:

- Chemotherapy-induced neutropenia during solid tumor cancer treatment
- Neutropenia during bone marrow transplantation (BMT)
- Production of stem cells for harvest before bone marrow transplant
- Neutropenia in those susceptible to symptomatic chronic infection

Injections of the CSF filgrastim are started at least 24 hours after the completion of a cycle of chemotherapy. The absolute neutrophil count (ANC) is monitored and therapy is continued until an ANC count of at least 10,000/mm3 is achieved. It is not recommended to use the drug for longer than 2 weeks, and treatment is discontinued at least 1 day before the next chemotherapy cycle is to begin. Special instruction is needed in cases of bone marrow transplant or stem cell harvest.

Pegfilgrastim is similar to filgrastim but is given as a single dose between chemotherapy cycles. Sargramostim is used following BMT, induction chemotherapy used with leukemia, and to stimulate stem cells for harvest.

Adverse Reactions

General System Reactions

- Bone pain
- Hypertension
- Nausea and vomiting
- Alopecia
- Hypersensitivity or allergic reactions

See the Summary Drug Table: Drugs Used in the Treatment of Anemia, Bleeding, and Infection for more information on these drugs.

Contraindications, Precautions, and Interactions

CSFs are contraindicated in patients with known hypersensitivity to the drug or any component of the drug. Filgrastim is used cautiously in patients with hypothyroid disease. The CSFs are pregnancy category C drugs, and caution is used when the patient is breast feeding. Pegfilgrastim can cause a sickle cell crisis in those with the disease. CSFs can cause hypersensitive reactions and should be treated with antihistamines, steroids, and bronchodilators to maintain their use. These drugs can stimulate cancer cell growth in cancer types that are stimulated by growth factors. An even higher increase in neutrophil count can occur when these drugs are taken with lithium, a drug used for the manic phase of mood disorders. The CSFs are currently in study phases to assess safety in children.

Oprelvekin

Actions and Uses

Oprelvekin is a drug that stimulates **thrombopoiesis**. Thrombopoiesis is the process of making platelets. The drug is used to prevent severe thrombocytopenia and reduces the need for multiple platelet transfusions. Oprelvekin is used to treat or prevent thrombocytopenia associated with chemotherapy for solid tumor cancer treatment.

Injections are started at least 6 hours after the completion of a chemotherapy cycle. Platelet counts are monitored and therapy is continued until a count of at least 50,000/mcl is achieved. It is not recommended for use for more than 21 days; treatment is discontinued at least 2 days before the next chemotherapy cycle is to begin.

Adverse Reactions

General System Reactions

- Fluid retention
- Peripheral edema
- Dyspnea
- Syncope
- Fever
- Allergic reactions

Cardiovascular System Reactions

- Tachycardia
- Palpitations
- Atrial fibrillation
- Arrhythmias resulting in stroke and pulmonary edema
- Capillary leak syndrome

See the Summary Drug Table: Drugs Used in the Treatment of Anemia, Bleeding, and Infection for more information on these drugs.

Contraindications, Precautions, and Interactions

Oprelvekin is contraindicated in patients with known hypersensitivity to the drug or any component of the drug. This drug should not be used in patients receiving chemotherapy that is extremely myelosuppressive. Oprelvekin is used cautiously in patients with renal failure, heart failure, or atrial arrhythmias. Severe hypokalemia (low potassium levels) can occur if the patient is receiving the cancer chemotherapy agent ifosfamide. It is a pregnancy category C drug and lactating patients should stop breast feeding when oprelvekin is prescribed. Safety in children has not been established.

Oprelvekin can cause anaphylactic-type reactions and should be permanently discontinued if these occur.

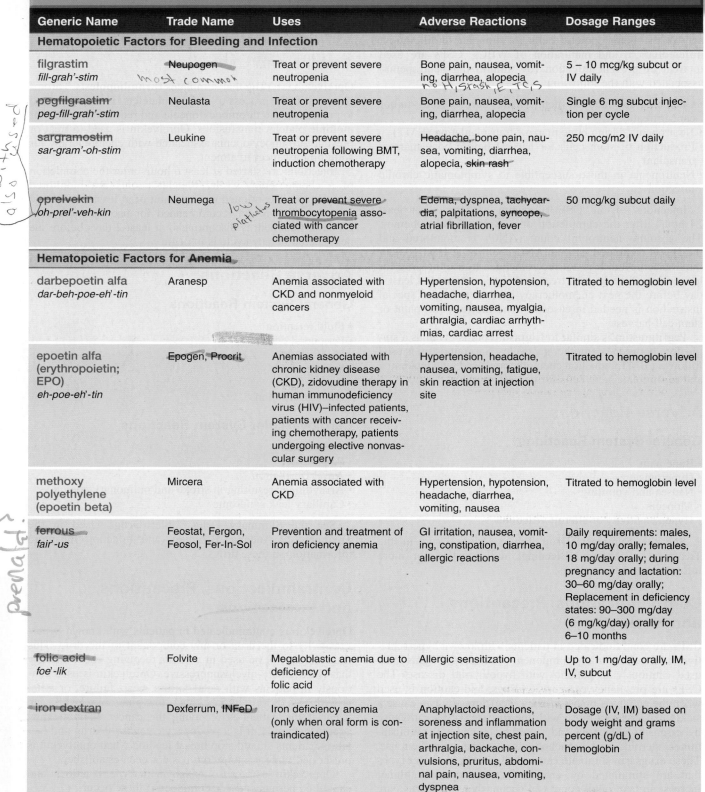

Summary Drug Table DRUGS USED IN THE TREATMENT OF ANEMIA, BLEEDING, AND INFECTION

Generic Name	Trade Name	Uses	Adverse Reactions	Dosage Ranges
Hematopoietic Factors for Bleeding and Infection				
filgrastim *fill-grah'-stim*	Neupogen *most common*	Treat or prevent severe neutropenia	Bone pain, nausea, vomiting, diarrhea, alopecia *no H, srash, E, TC, S*	5 – 10 mcg/kg subcut or IV daily
pegfilgrastim *peg-fill-grah'-stim*	Neulasta	Treat or prevent severe neutropenia	Bone pain, nausea, vomiting, diarrhea, alopecia	Single 6 mg subcut injection per cycle
sargramostim *sar-gram'-oh-stim*	Leukine	Treat or prevent severe neutropenia following BMT, induction chemotherapy	Headache, bone pain, nausea, vomiting, diarrhea, alopecia, skin rash	250 mcg/m2 IV daily
oprelvekin *oh-prel'-veh-kin*	Neumega *low platelets*	Treat or prevent severe thrombocytopenia associated with cancer chemotherapy	Edema, dyspnea, tachycardia, palpitations, syncope, atrial fibrillation, fever	50 mcg/kg subcut daily
Hematopoietic Factors for Anemia				
darbepoetin alfa *dar-beh-poe-eh'-tin*	Aranesp	Anemia associated with CKD and nonmyeloid cancers	Hypertension, hypotension, headache, diarrhea, vomiting, nausea, myalgia, arthralgia, cardiac arrhythmias, cardiac arrest	Titrated to hemoglobin level
epoetin alfa (erythropoietin; EPO) *eh-poe-eh'-tin*	Epogen, Procrit	Anemias associated with chronic kidney disease (CKD), zidovudine therapy in human immunodeficiency virus (HIV)–infected patients, patients with cancer receiving chemotherapy, patients undergoing elective nonvascular surgery	Hypertension, headache, nausea, vomiting, fatigue, skin reaction at injection site	Titrated to hemoglobin level
methoxy polyethylene (epoetin beta)	Mircera	Anemia associated with CKD	Hypertension, hypotension, headache, diarrhea, vomiting, nausea	Titrated to hemoglobin level
ferrous *fair'-us*	Feostat, Fergon, Feosol, Fer-In-Sol	Prevention and treatment of iron deficiency anemia	GI irritation, nausea, vomiting, constipation, diarrhea, allergic reactions	Daily requirements: males, 10 mg/day orally; females, 18 mg/day orally; during pregnancy and lactation: 30–60 mg/day orally; Replacement in deficiency states: 90–300 mg/day (6 mg/kg/day) orally for 6–10 months
folic acid *foe'-lik*	Folvite	Megaloblastic anemia due to deficiency of folic acid	Allergic sensitization	Up to 1 mg/day orally, IM, IV, subcut
iron dextran	Dexferrum, INFeD	Iron deficiency anemia (only when oral form is contraindicated)	Anaphylactoid reactions, soreness and inflammation at injection site, chest pain, arthralgia, backache, convulsions, pruritus, abdominal pain, nausea, vomiting, dyspnea	Dosage (IV, IM) based on body weight and grams percent (g/dL) of hemoglobin

Be familiar with used also

prenata?

(table continues on page 533)

Summary Drug Table DRUGS USED IN THE TREATMENT OF ANEMIA, BLEEDING, AND INFECTION (continued)

Generic Name	Trade Name	Uses	Adverse Reactions	Dosage Ranges
iron sucrose	Venofer	Iron deficiency anemia in kidney disease, via dialysis machine	Hypotension, cramps, leg cramps, nausea, headache, vomiting, diarrhea, dizziness	100 mg elemental iron by slow IV infusion or during dialysis session
leucovorin *loo-koe-vor'-in*	Wellcovorin	Treatment of megaloblastic anemia; leucovorin rescue after high-dose methotrexate therapy	Allergic sensitization, urticaria, anaphylaxis	See cancer therapy
sodium ferric gluconate complex	Ferrlecit	Iron deficiency	Flushing, hypotension, syncope, tachycardia, dizziness, pruritus, dyspnea, conjunctivitis, hyperkalemia	125 mg of elemental iron IV over at least 10 min
vitamin B$_{12}$ (cyanocobalamin) *sye-an-oh-koe-bal'-ah-min*		Vitamin B$_{12}$ deficiencies, GI pathology; Schilling's test	Mild diarrhea, itching, edema, anaphylaxis	Schilling's test: 100–1000 mcg/day for 2 wk, then 100–1000 mcg IM every month

● HEMATOPOIETIC DRUGS USED IN TREATING ANEMIA

Anemia is a condition caused by an insufficient amount of hemoglobin delivering oxygen to the tissues. Causes of anemia include a decrease in the number of red blood cells (RBCs), a decrease in the amount of hemoglobin in RBCs, or both. There are various types and causes of anemia. For example, anemia can result from blood loss, excessive destruction of RBCs, inadequate production of RBCs, and deficits in various nutrients, as in **iron deficiency anemia**. Once the type and cause have been identified, the primary health care provider selects a method of treatment.

The anemias discussed in this chapter include anemia in patients with chronic illness such as renal disease or caused by treatment, iron deficiency anemia, pernicious anemia, and anemia resulting from a folic acid deficiency. Table 52.1 defines these anemias.

Drugs Used in Treating Anemia Associated With Chronic Illness

Anemia may occur in patients with chronic illness as a result of disease treatment. Cancer and chronic kidney disease are two diseases that produce disease- or treatment-related anemia. Erythropoiesis-stimulating agents (ESAs) are glycoproteins that stimulate and regulate the production of erythrocytes. Chronic kidney disease reduces the kidney's ability to produce erythropoietin, which stimulates the production of RBCs. Cancer treatment reduces the bone marrow's ability to produce RBCs. Two examples of drugs used to treat anemia associated with chronic illness are epoetin alfa (Epogen) and darbepoetin alfa (Aranesp).

Table 52.1 Anemias

Type of Anemia	Description
Iron deficiency	Anemia characterized by an inadequate amount of iron in the body to produce hemoglobin
Anemia in chronic kidney disease	Anemia resulting from a reduced production of erythropoietin, a hormone secreted by the kidney that stimulates the production of RBCs
Pernicious anemia	Anemia resulting from lack of secretion by the gastric mucosa of the intrinsic factor essential to the formation of RBCs and the absorption of vitamin B$_{12}$
Folic acid deficiency	Anemia occurring because of a dietary lack of folic acid, a component necessary in the formation of RBCs

Actions and Uses

ESAs are drugs that, like natural erythropoietin, stimulate **erythropoiesis**, the process of making RBCs. ESAs are used to treat anemia associated with the following:

• Chronic kidney disease
• Chemotherapy for cancer treatment
• Zidovudine (AZT) therapy for HIV infection
• Postsurgical blood replacement in place of allogeneic transfusions

Darbepoetin alfa and methoxy polyethylene–epoetin beta are erythropoiesis-stimulating proteins used to treat anemia associated with chronic kidney disease in patients receiving dialysis, as well as in patients who are not receiving dialysis. These drugs elevate or maintain RBC levels and decrease the need for transfusions.

Adverse Reactions

Epoetin alfa (erythropoietin; EPO), darbepoetin alfa, and methoxy polyethylene are usually well tolerated when used to maintain a hemoglobin no higher than 12g/dL. The most common adverse reactions include:

- Hypertension
- Headache
- Nausea, vomiting, diarrhea
- Rashes
- Fatigue *makes symptom of fatigue worse*
- Arthralgia, and skin reaction at the injection site.

See the Summary Drug Table: Drugs Used in the Treatment of Anemia, Bleeding, and Infection for more information on these drugs.

Contraindications and Precautions

Epoetin alfa is contraindicated in patients with uncontrolled hypertension, those needing an emergency transfusion, and those with a hypersensitivity to human albumin. Darbepoetin alfa (Aranesp) is contraindicated in patients with uncontrolled hypertension or in those allergic to the drug. Polycythemia (an overload of RBCs in the circulation) can occur if the hemoglobin is not carefully monitored and the dosage is too high. This can result in increased mortality, serious cardio or thromboembolic events in any patient and possible tumor progression in cancer patients.

Epoetin alfa and darbepoetin alfa are used with caution in patients with hypertension, heart disease, congestive heart failure, or a history of seizures. Both of these drugs are pregnancy category C drugs and are used cautiously during pregnancy and lactation.

Drugs Used in Treating Iron Deficiency Anemia

When the body does not have enough iron to supply its own needs, the resulting condition is called *iron deficiency anemia*. Iron is the component in hemoglobin that picks up oxygen from the lungs and carries it to the body tissues. Iron deficiency anemia is a very common type of anemia. Approximately 50% of pregnant women and 20% of all women experience anemia. Decreased iron stores result from a decrease in RBCs; causes include heavy menstrual bleeding and poor absorption or lack of iron in the diet.

Actions and Uses

Iron preparations act by elevating the serum iron concentration, which replenishes hemoglobin and depleted iron stores. Oral iron supplements are typically used. Iron is best absorbed on an empty stomach. Supplemental iron is needed during pregnancy and lactation, because normal dietary intake rarely supplies the required amount.

Parenteral iron is used when the patient cannot take oral drugs or when the patient experiences gastrointestinal (GI) intolerance to oral iron administration. Other iron preparations, both oral and parenteral, used in treating iron deficiency anemia can be found in the Summary Drug Table: Drugs Used in the Treatment of Anemia, Bleeding, and Infection.

Adverse Reactions

Gastrointestinal Reactions

- GI irritation
- Nausea, vomiting
- Constipation, diarrhea
- Darker (black) stools

Generalized System Reactions

- Headache
- Backache
- Allergic reactions

When given parenterally, additional adverse reactions include soreness, inflammation, and sterile abscesses at the intramuscular (IM) injection site. When iron is administered by the IM route, a brownish discoloration of the skin may occur. Intravenous (IV) administration may result in phlebitis at the injection site.

Contraindications and Precautions

Iron supplements are contraindicated in patients with known hypersensitivity to the drug or any component of the drug. Iron compounds are contraindicated in patients with hemochromatosis or hemolytic anemia. Iron compounds are used cautiously in patients with hypersensitivity to aspirin, because these patients may have a hypersensitivity to the tartrazine or sulfite content of some iron compounds.

The parenteral form of iron can cause anaphylactic-type reactions and should be used only when oral supplement is contraindicated.

Interactions

The following interactions may occur when an iron preparation is administered with another agent:

Interacting Drug	Common Use	Effect of Interaction
antibiotics	Fight infection	Decreased GI absorption of the antibiotic
levothyroxine	Treatment of hypothyroidism	Decreased absorption of levothyroxine
levodopa, methyldopa	Treatment of Parkinson's disease	Decreased effect of antiparkinsonism medication
ascorbic acid (vitamin C)	Vitamin supplement	Increased absorption of iron

good interaction

Iron injection (2 track) IM - anaphalatic reaction

Drugs Used in Treating Folic Acid Deficiency Anemia

Folic acid (folate) is required for the manufacture of RBCs in the bone marrow. Folic acid is found in leafy green vegetables, fish, meat, poultry, and whole grains. A deficiency of folic acid results in **megaloblastic anemia**. Megaloblastic anemia is characterized by the presence of large, abnormal, immature erythrocytes circulating in the blood.

Actions and Uses

Folic acid is used in treating megaloblastic anemias that are caused by a deficiency of folic acid. Although neural tube defects are not related to anemia, studies indicate there is a decreased risk for embryonic neural tube defects if folic acid is taken before conception and during early pregnancy. Neural tube defects occur during early pregnancy, when the embryonic folds forming the spinal cord and brain join together. Defects of this type include anencephaly (congenital absence of brain and spinal cord), spina bifida (defect of the spinal cord), and meningocele (a saclike protrusion of the meninges in the spinal cord or skull). The U.S. Public Health Service recommends the use of folic acid for all women of childbearing age to decrease the incidence of neural tube defects. Dosages during pregnancy and lactation are as great as 0.8 mg/day.

Oral supplements are the first choice for megaloblastic anemia and folic acid deficiency treatment. If a patient is unable to take oral medications, leucovorin may be used. This drug is a derivative (an active reduced form) of folic acid. Leucovorin is more commonly used to diminish the hematologic effects of methotrexate, a drug used in treating certain types of cancer (see Chapter 51). Leucovorin "rescues" normal cells from the destruction caused by methotrexate and allows them to survive. This technique of administering leucovorin after a large dose of methotrexate is called **folinic acid rescue or leucovorin rescue**.

Adverse Reactions

Few adverse reactions are associated with the administration of folic acid. Rarely, parenteral administration may result in allergic hypersensitivity.

Contraindications and Precautions

Folic acid and leucovorin are contraindicated for treating pernicious anemia or for other anemias in which vitamin B_{12} is deficient. Folic acid is a pregnancy category A drug and is generally considered safe for use during pregnancy. Pregnant women are more likely to experience folate deficiency, because folic acid requirements increase during pregnancy. Pregnant women with a folate deficiency are at increased risk for complications of pregnancy and fetal abnormalities. The recommended dietary allowance (RDA) of folate during pregnancy is 0.4 mg/day and, during lactation, 0.26 to 0.28 mg/day. Although the potential for fetal harm appears remote, the drug should be used cautiously and only within the RDA guidelines.

Interactions

Signs of folate deficiency may occur when sulfasalazine is administered concurrently. An increase in seizure activity may occur when folic acid is administered with the hydantoins (antiseizure drugs).

Drugs Used in Treating Vitamin B_{12} Deficiency Anemia

Vitamin B_{12} is essential to growth, cell reproduction, the manufacture of myelin (which surrounds some nerve fibers), and blood cell manufacture. The **intrinsic factor**, which is produced by cells in the stomach, is necessary for the absorption of vitamin B_{12} in the intestine. A deficiency of the intrinsic factor results in abnormal formation of erythrocytes because of the body's failure to absorb vitamin B_{12}, a necessary component for blood cell formation. The resulting anemia is called **macrocytic anemia**.

Actions and Uses

Vitamin B_{12} (cyanocobalamin) is used to treat patients with a vitamin B_{12} deficiency; this condition is seen in those who have:

- A strict vegetarian (vegan) lifestyle
- Total gastrectomy or subtotal gastric resection (in which the cells producing the intrinsic factor are totally or partially removed)
- Intestinal diseases, such as ulcerative colitis or sprue
- Gastric carcinoma
- Congenital decrease in the number of gastric cells that secrete intrinsic factor

Vitamin B_{12} is also used to perform the Schilling test, which is used to diagnose pernicious anemia.

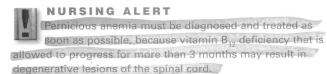

⚠ NURSING ALERT

Pernicious anemia must be diagnosed and treated as soon as possible, because vitamin B_{12} deficiency that is allowed to progress for more than 3 months may result in degenerative lesions of the spinal cord.

A deficiency of vitamin B_{12} caused by a low dietary intake is rare, because the vitamin is found in meats, milk, eggs, and cheese. The body is also able to store this vitamin. A deficiency, for any reason, will not occur for 5 to 6 years from birth. Patients should be assessed for a history of vegan diet or gastric bypass surgery.

Adverse Reactions

Mild diarrhea and itching have been reported with the administration of vitamin B_{12}. Other adverse reactions that may be seen include a marked increase in RBC production, acne, peripheral vascular thrombosis, congestive heart failure, and pulmonary edema.

Contraindications, Precautions, and Interactions

Vitamin B_{12} is contraindicated in patients who are allergic to cyanocobalamin. Vitamin B_{12} is a pregnancy category A drug if administered orally and a pregnancy category C drug if given parenterally. Vitamin B_{12} is administered cautiously during pregnancy and in patients with pulmonary disease and anemia. Alcohol, neomycin, and colchicine may decrease the absorption of oral vitamin B_{12}.

NURSING PROCESS
PATIENT RECEIVING A DRUG USED IN THE TREATMENT OF ANEMIA, BLEEDING, OR INFECTION

ASSESSMENT

Preadministration Assessment
The nurse obtains a general health history and asks about the symptoms of the anemia, bleeding, or infection. The primary health care provider may order laboratory tests to determine the type, severity, and possible cause of the anemia, bleeding, or infection. When the patient is undergoing treatment such as for cancer, the blood counts will be used to titrate the drug doses.

The nurse takes the vital signs to provide a baseline during therapy. Other physical assessments may include the patient's general appearance and, in the severely ill patient, an evaluation of the patient's ability to carry out the activities of daily living. General symptoms may include fatigue, shortness of breath, sore tongue, headache, and pallor.

If iron dextran is to be given, an allergy history is necessary, because this drug is given with caution to those with significant allergies or asthma. The patient's weight and hemoglobin level are required for calculating the dosage.

Ongoing Assessment
During the ongoing assessment, the nurse takes the vital signs daily; more frequent monitoring may be needed if the patient is moderately to acutely ill. The nurse monitors the patient for adverse reactions and reports any occurrence of adverse reactions to the primary health care provider before the next dose is due. However, the nurse immediately reports severe adverse reactions.

The nurse assesses the patient for relief of the symptoms (fatigue, shortness of breath, sore tongue, headache, pallor). Some patients may note a relief of symptoms after a few days of therapy. Periodic laboratory tests are necessary to monitor the results of therapy. The nurse monitors for signs of bleeding and infection during the first few days of therapy with the CSF since an increase in blood cells may take a few days once therapy is started.

When the patient is receiving oral iron supplements, the nurse informs the patient that the color of the stool will become darker or black. If diarrhea or constipation occurs, the nurse notifies the primary health care provider.

If parenteral iron dextran is administered, the nurse informs the patient that soreness at the injection site may occur. Injection sites are checked daily for signs of inflammation, swelling, or abscess formation.

NURSING DIAGNOSES

Drug-specific nursing diagnoses include the following:

❑ **Fatigue** related to dilutional anemia caused by fluid retention
❑ **Imbalanced Nutrition: Less Than Body Requirements** related to lack of iron, folic acid, other (specify) in the diet
❑ **Constipation** related to adverse reaction to iron therapy

Nursing diagnoses related to drug administration are discussed in Chapter 4.

PLANNING

The expected outcomes for the patient may include an optimal response to therapy, supporting the patient needs related to the management of adverse reactions, and an understanding of and compliance with the prescribed treatment regimen.

IMPLEMENTATION

Promoting an Optimal Response to Therapy

EPOETIN ALFA. When epoetin alfa is administered to a patient with hypertension, the nurse monitors the blood pressure closely. The nurse reports any rise of 20 mm Hg or more in the systolic or diastolic pressure to the primary health care provider. The hematocrit is usually measured before each dose during therapy with epoetin alfa.

The drug is given three times weekly IV or subcutaneously (subcut); if the patient is receiving dialysis, the drug is administered into the venous access line. The drug is mixed gently during preparation for administration. Shaking may denature the glycoprotein. The vial is used for only one dose; any remaining or unused portion is discarded.

> **NURSING ALERT**
> When monitoring the patient taking epoetin, the nurse reports any increase in the hematocrit of 4 points within any 2-week period, because an exacerbation of hypertension is associated with an excessive rise of hematocrit. Hematocrit is decreased by decreasing or withholding the epoetin alfa dose.

IRON. Iron supplements are preferably given between meals with water, but many people cannot tolerate this and may need to take them with food. Milk and antacids may interfere with absorption of iron and should not be taken at the same time as iron supplements. If the patient is receiving other drugs, the nurse checks with the hospital pharmacist regarding the simultaneous administration of iron salts with other drugs.

Iron dextran is given by the IM or IV route. Before iron dextran is administered, a test dose (0.5 mL iron dextran) may be administered IV at a gradual rate over a period of 30 seconds or more. A test dose is also given before administering the first dose of iron dextran IM by injecting 0.5 mL into the upper outer quadrant of the buttocks. The nurse monitors the patient for an allergic response for at least 1 hour after the test dose and before administering the remaining dose. Epinephrine is kept on standby in the event of severe anaphylactic reaction.

❗ NURSING ALERT

Parenteral administration of iron has resulted in fatal anaphylactic-type reactions. The nurse reports any of the following adverse reactions: dyspnea, urticaria, rashes, itching, and fever.

After the test dose, the prescribed dose of iron is administered IM. The drug is given into the muscle mass of the buttocks upper outer quadrant (never into an arm or other area) using the Z-track method (see Chapter 2) to prevent leakage into the subcutaneous tissue. A large-bore needle is required. If the patient is standing, have the patient place weight on the leg not receiving the injection.

VITAMIN B$_{12}$. Patients with vitamin B$_{12}$ anemia are treated with vitamin B$_{12}$ IM administered weekly. The parenteral route is used because the vitamin is ineffective orally, owing to the absence of the intrinsic factor in the stomach, which is necessary for utilization of vitamin B$_{12}$. After stabilization, maintenance (usually monthly) injections may be necessary for life. Vitamin B$_{12}$ is available in an intranasal form for those who are on maintenance therapy.

Monitoring and Managing Patient Needs

FATIGUE. When administering the CSF drugs, the patient may experience fluid retention. With the increase in fluid volume, this makes the ratio of cells to fluid in the blood less, which results in a dilutional anemia. The patient may experience fatigue due to this anemia. The nurse should explain this situation and give the patient permission to feel tired. The nurse should teach the patient and family energy-saving skills to help maintain the same level of activities of daily living.

IMBALANCED NUTRITION: LESS THAN BODY REQUIREMENTS. The nurse recommends a balanced diet with an emphasis on foods that are high in iron (e.g., lean red meats, cereals, dried beans, and leafy green vegetables), folic acid (e.g., green leafy vegetables, liver, and yeast), or vitamin B$_{12}$ (e.g., beef, pork, eggs, milk, and milk products). If the patient is a vegetarian, a dietitian may need to be consulted to provide menus with appropriate iron-rich foods.

The nurse monitors the amount of food eaten at meals. If appetite is poor or eating is inadequate to maintain normal nutrition, consultation with the dietitian may be necessary. Small portions of food may be more appealing than large or moderate portions. The nurse provides a pleasant atmosphere and allows ample time for eating. If the diet is taken poorly, the nurse

notes this on the patient's chart and discusses the problem with the primary health care provider.

CONSTIPATION. Constipation may be a problem when a patient is taking oral iron preparations. The nurse instructs the patient to increase fluid intake to 10 to 12 glasses of water daily (if the condition permits), eat a diet high in fiber, and increase activity. An active lifestyle and regular exercise (if condition permits) help to decrease the constipating effects of iron. If constipation persists, the primary health care provider may prescribe a stool softener.

Educating the Patient and Family

Read

The nurse explains the medical regimen thoroughly to the patient and family and emphasizes the importance of following the prescribed treatment regimen. The nurse includes the following points in a patient and family teaching plan:

HEMATOPOIETIC FACTORS.
- Keep all appointments with the primary health care provider. The drug is administered up to three times per week (by the subcut or IV route or through a dialysis access line). Periodic blood tests are performed to determine the effects of the drug and to determine dosage.
- Strict compliance with the antihypertensive drug regimen is important in patients with known hypertension during epoetin alfa therapy.
- The following adverse reactions may occur: dizziness, headache, fatigue, joint pain, nausea, vomiting, or diarrhea. Report any of these reactions.
- Patients might have heard about problems with the drug Leukine. The product was withdrawn temporarily, because of reports of adverse reactions including syncope (fainting). This was correlated with a change in the formulation of the drug, which included edetate disodium (EDTA). That formula has been taken off the market and Leukine is now considered safe.
- If the patient or caregiver is administering the injections at home, use puncture-resistant containers for disposal and return full containers to the proper agency for disposal.

IRON.
- Take this drug with water on an empty stomach. If GI upset occurs, take the drug with food or meals.
- Do not take antacids, tetracyclines, penicillamine, or fluoroquinolones at the same time or 2 hours before or after taking iron without first checking with the primary health care provider.
- This drug may cause a darkening of the stools, constipation, or diarrhea. If constipation or diarrhea becomes severe, contact the primary health care provider.
- Mix the liquid iron preparation with water or juice and drink through a straw to prevent staining the teeth.
- Avoid the indiscriminate use of advertised iron products. If a true iron deficiency occurs, the cause must be determined and therapy should be under the care of a health care provider.

- Have periodic blood tests during therapy to determine the therapeutic response.

FOLIC ACID.
- Avoid the use of multivitamin preparations unless it has been approved by the primary health care provider.
- Follow the diet recommended by the primary health care provider, because diet and drug are necessary to correct anemia associated with folic acid deficiency.

LEUCOVORIN.
- Megaloblastic anemia—Adhere to the diet prescribed by the primary health care provider. If the purchase of foods high in protein (which can be expensive) becomes a problem, discuss this with the primary health care provider.

VITAMIN B$_{12}$.
- Nutritional deficiency of vitamin B$_{12}$—Eat a balanced diet that includes seafood, eggs, meats, and dairy products.
- Pernicious anemia—Lifetime therapy is necessary. Eat a balanced diet that includes seafood, eggs, meats, and dairy products. Avoid contact with infections, and report any signs of infection to the primary health care provider immediately, because an increase in dosage may be necessary.
- Adhere to the treatment regimen and keep all appointments with the clinic or primary health care provider. The drug is given at periodic intervals (usually monthly for life). In some instances, parenteral or intranasal self-administration or parenteral administration by a family member is allowed (instruction in administration is necessary).

EVALUATION

- Therapeutic effect of the drug is achieved.
- Adverse reactions are identified, reported to the primary health care provider, and managed successfully with appropriate nursing interventions:
  ☑ Patient reports fatigue is manageable.
  ☑ Patient maintains an adequate nutritional status.
  ☑ Patient reports adequate bowel movements.
- Patient and family demonstrate an understanding of the drug regimen.

THINK CRITICALLY: PHARMACOLOGY IN PRACTICE

1. Mr. Phillip, aged 72 years, has chronic kidney disease. He had a friend who was on dialysis about 10 years ago and complained of being tired all the time. Mr. Phillip is concerned about his kidney disease progressing and having to start dialysis. He asks how to deal with being tired all the time. Discuss how you would answer Mr. Phillip's question.

● Test Your Knowledge

1. Which is the most common type of anemia?
   - A. Iron deficiency anemia
   - B. Folic acid anemia
   - C. Pernicious anemia
   - D. Megaloblastic anemia

2. Which of the following substances would decrease the absorption of oral iron?
   - A. antacids
   - B. levothyroxine
   - C. ascorbic acid
   - D. vitamin B$_{12}$

3. Filgrastim are contraindicated in which of the following conditions?
   - A. Hypothyroidism
   - B. Hyperthyroidism
   - C. Pernicious anemia
   - D. Pregnancy

4. When monitoring a patient taking epoetin alfa, which of the following laboratory results would be most important for the nurse to report immediately?
   - A. Any increase in hematocrit of 4 points within a 2-week period
   - B. Any increase in hematocrit of 2 points within a 2-week period
   - C. A daily change in the hematocrit of 1 point or more
   - D. A stabilization in the hematocrit in any 2-day period

● Prepare for the NCLEX

1. When teaching a patient about the use of vitamin B$_{12}$, the nurse would include which of the following statements?
   - A. Take the oral form of vitamin B$_{12}$ daily at bedtime on an empty stomach.
   - B. Take the oral form of vitamin B$_{12}$ when you begin to feel weak or experience a headache.
   - C. You will require vitamin B$_{12}$ injections monthly for life.
   - D. You will require vitamin B$_{12}$ injections every 2 weeks until remission occurs.

● Calculate Medication Dosages

1. The physician prescribes 25 mg iron dextran IM. The drug is available in a vial with 50 mg/mL. The nurse administers _____.

2. Folvite (folic acid) 1 mg subcut is prescribed. The drug is available in a vial with 5 mg/mL. The nurse administers _____.

To check your answers, see Appendix E.

thePoint. *For more NCLEX questions, log on to http://thepoint.lww.com to access more than 1000 questions.*

Drugs That Affect Other Body Systems

This unit covers a variety of drugs affecting various body systems, including topical drugs used to treat skin disorders, otic (ear) and ophthalmic (eye) preparations, and fluids and electrolytes. Chapter 53 discusses topical drugs used in the treatment of skin disorders. The skin forms a barrier between the outside environment and the structures located beneath the skin. The *epidermis* is the outermost layer of the skin. Immediately below the epidermis is the *dermis*, which contains small capillaries that supply nourishment to the dermis and epidermis, sebaceous (oil-secreting) glands, sweat glands, nerve fibers, and hair follicles. Because of the skin's proximity to the outside environment, it is subject to various types of injury and trauma, as well as to changes in the skin itself. Topical drugs discussed include anti-infectives, corticosteroids, antipsoriatics, enzymes, keratolytics, and anesthetics.

Chapter 54 discusses drugs used to treat disorders of the eye and ear. Otic drugs may be used to treat infection and inflammation of the ear or to soften and remove cerumen (wax).

Ophthalmic drugs are used for diagnostic and therapeutic purposes. As a diagnostic tool, ophthalmic drugs are used to anesthetize the eye, dilate the pupil, and stain the cornea to identify anomalies. Therapeutic purposes include the treatment of infection, allergy, and eye disorders such as glaucoma. Ophthalmic drugs discussed include an α_2-adrenergic agonist, sympathomimetics, α-adrenergic blocking drugs, β-adrenergic blocking drugs, miotics (direct acting and cholinesterase inhibitors), carbonic anhydrase inhibitors, prostaglandin agonists, mast cell stabilizers, nonsteroidal anti-inflammatory drugs, corticosteroids, cycloplegics, mydriatics, artificial tears, and various anti-infectives.

The composition of body fluids remains relatively constant despite the many demands placed on the body each day. On occasion, these demands cannot be met, and electrolytes and fluids must be given intravenously (IV) in an attempt to restore equilibrium. The solutions used in managing body fluids discussed in Chapter 55 include intravenous fluid and electrolyte replacement, blood products, and total parenteral nutrition. Electrolytes are electrically charged particles (ions) that are essential for normal cell function and are involved in various metabolic activities. The major electrolytes discussed include potassium, calcium, magnesium, sodium, and bicarbonate. Chapter 55 discusses the use of electrolytes to replace one or more electrolytes that may be lost by the body.

PHARMACOLOGY IN PRACTICE

Our patient focus in this unit is Alfredo Garcia, a 46-year-old man being seen in the clinic for an upper respiratory infection. During the intake assessment, the nurse finds that his blood pressure is high, and he complains of "heartburn." Thinking he had an ulcer, Mr. Garcia attempted to use home remedies (e.g., drinking cream) to decrease acid production. The nurse taught him about ulcer treatment, yet his heartburn persists. He continues to rely on home remedies, which are causing other problems. After reading the chapters in this unit, you will learn about some of the problems that can happen with electrolyte imbalances. Then, you will be able to help Mr. Garcia in the treatment of his heartburn.

Topical Drugs Used in the Treatment of Skin Disorders

LEARNING OBJECTIVES

On completion of this chapter, the student will:

1. List the types of drugs used in the treatment of skin disorders.
2. Discuss the general drug actions, uses, and reactions to and any contraindications, precautions, and interactions associated with drugs used in treating skin disorders.
3. Discuss important preadministration and ongoing assessment activities the nurse should perform on patients receiving a drug used to treat skin disorders.
4. List nursing diagnoses particular to a patient using a drug to treat a skin disorder.
5. Discuss ways to promote an optimal response to therapy and important points to keep in mind when educating the patient about a skin disorder.

This chapter discusses the following types of topical drugs: anti-infectives, corticosteroids, antipsoriatics, enzymes, keratolytics, and anesthetics. Each of the following sections discusses only select topical drugs. See the Summary Drug Table: Dermatologic Drugs for a more complete listing of the drugs and additional information.

•TOPICAL ANTI-INFECTIVES

Localized skin infections may require the use of a topical anti-infective. The topical anti-infectives include antibiotic, antifungal, and antiviral drugs.

Actions and Uses

Topical Antibiotic Drugs

Topical antibiotics exert a direct local effect on specific microorganisms and may be **bactericidal** (i.e., lethal to bacteria) or **bacteriostatic** (i.e., inhibit bacterial growth). Bacitracin inhibits cell wall synthesis. Bacitracin, gentamicin, and erythromycin are examples of topical antibiotics.

These drugs are used to

- Treat primary and secondary skin infections
- Prevent infection in minor cuts, wounds, scrapes, and minor burns
- Treat acne vulgaris

Topical Antifungal Drugs

Superficial mycotic infections occur on the surface of, or just below, the skin or nails. Superficial infections include **tinea pedis** (athlete's foot), **tinea cruris** (jock itch), **tinea corporis** (ringworm), **onychomycosis** (nail fungus). Antifungal drugs exert a local effect by inhibiting growth of fungi. Examples of antifungal drugs include miconazole, ketoconazole, and ciclopirox. Antifungal drugs are used for treating:

- Tinea pedis, tinea cruris, tinea corporis
- Cutaneous candidiasis
- Other superficial fungal infections of the skin

Topical Antiviral Drugs

Acyclovir and penciclovir are topical forms of antiviral drugs used to treat oral HSV. These drugs are used to inhibit viral activity during:

- Initial episodes of HSV (prodrome phase)
- Directly on lesions to speed up recovery

Docosanol is a cream sold over the counter (OTC) and speeds healing as well.

❧ HERBAL ALERT

Lemon balm is a perennial herb with heart-shaped leaves that has been used for hundreds of years. Traditionally the herb has been used for Graves' disease, as a sedative, an antispasmodic, and an antiviral agent. When used topically, lemon balm has antiviral activity against HSV. No adverse reactions have been reported when lemon balm is used topically.

Summary Drug Table DERMATOLOGIC DRUGS

Generic Name	Trade Name	Uses	Adverse Reactions	Dosage Ranges
Antibiotic Drugs				
azelaic acid *ah-zeh'-lay-ik*	Azelex, Finacea	Acne vulgaris, rosacea	Mild and transient pruritus, burning, stinging, erythema	Apply BID
bacitracin *bah-sih-tray'-sin*	Various brand names	Relief of skin infections, to help prevent infections in minor cut and burns	Rare; occasionally redness, burning, pruritus, stinging	Apply daily to TID
benzoyl peroxide *ben'-zoil per-ox'-syde*	Various brand names	Mild to moderate acne vulgaris and oily skin	Excessive drying, stinging, peeling, erythema, possible edema, allergic dermatitis	Apply daily or BID
clindamycin *clin-dah-mye'-sin*	Cleocin T, Clinda Max, Clindets, Clindagel	Acne vulgaris	Dryness, erythema, burning, itching, peeling, oily skin, diarrhea, bloody diarrhea, abdominal pain, colitis	Apply a thin film daily (Clindagel) or BID to affected area
erythromycin *ee-rith-roe-mye'-sin*	Akne-Mycin, Emgel, Erygel	Acne vulgaris	Skin irritation, tenderness, pruritus, erythema, peeling, oiliness, burning sensation	Apply to affected area BID
gentamicin *jen-tah-mye'-sin*	Various brand names	Relief of primary and secondary skin infections	Mild and transient pruritus, burning, stinging, erythema, photosensitivity	Apply TID or QID to affected area
metronidazole *meh-troe-nye'-dah-zoll*	Metro-Gel, MetroLotion, Noritate	Rosacea	Watery (tearing) eyes, redness, mild dryness, burning, skin irritation, nausea, tingling/ numbness of extremities	Apply a thin film daily or BID to affected areas
mupirocin *mew-peer'-oh-sin*	Bactroban, Bactroban Nasal	Impetigo infections caused by *Staphylococcus aureus* and *Streptococcus pyogenes* Nasal: eradication of MRSA as part of an infection control program to reduce the risk of institutional outbreaks of MRSA	Ointment: burning, stinging, pain, itching, rash, nausea, erythema, dry skin Cream: headache, rash, nausea, abdominal pain, burning at application site, dermatitis Nasal: headache, rhinitis, respiratory disorders (e.g., pharyngitis), taste perversion, burning, stinging, cough	Ointment: apply TID for 3–5 days Cream: apply TID for 10 days Nasal: divide the single-use tube between nostrils and apply BID for 5 days
retapamulin *reh'-tah-pam'-yoo-lin*	Altabax	Impetigo due to Staphylococcus or Streptococcus	Headache, pruritus	Apply a thin film daily or BID to affected areas
Antifungal Drugs				
butenafine *byoo-ten'-ah-feen*	Mentax, Lotrimin Ultra	Dermatologic infections, tinea versicolor, tinea corporis (ringworm), tinea cruris (jock itch)	Burning, stinging, itching, worsening of the condition, contact dermatis, erythema, irritation	Apply daily or BID for 2–4 wk

(table continues on page 543)

Summary Drug Table DERMATOLOGIC DRUGS (continued)

Generic Name	Trade Name	Uses	Adverse Reactions	Dosage Ranges
ciclopirox *sik-loe-peer'-ox*	Loprox, Penlac Nail Lacquer	Loprox, cream and suspension: tinea pedis (athlete's foot), tinea cruris, tinea corporis, cutaneous candidiasis Gel: interdigital tinea pedis and tinea corporis, seborrheic dermatitis of the scalp Penlac: mild to moderate onychomycosis of fingernails and toenails	Cream: pruritus at the application site, worsening of clinical signs and symptoms, burning Loprox Gel: burning sensation on application, contact dermatitis, pruritus, dry skin, acne, rash, alopecia, eye pain, facial edema Loprox shampoo: increased itching, burning, erythema, itching, rash, headache Penlac: periungual erythema, nail disorders, irritation, ingrown toenail, burning of the skin	Apply to affected areas daily or BID Shampoo: see directions Penlac: Apply daily preferably at bedtime or 8 hr before washing
clotrimazole *kloe-trim'-ah-zoll*	Cruex, Lotrimin AF, Desenex	Tinea pedis, tinea cruris, and other skin infections caused by ringworm	Burning, itching, erythema, peeling, edema, general skin irritation	Apply thin layer to affected areas BID for 2–4 wk
econazole *ee-kon'-ah-zoll*	Spectazole	Tinea pedis, tinea cruris, tinea corporis, tinea versicolor, cutaneous candidiasis	Local burning, itching, stinging, erythema, pruritic rash	Apply to affected areas daily or BID
gentian violet *jen'-shun*		External treatment of abrasions, minor cuts, surface injuries, superficial fungal infections of the skin	Local irritation or sensitivity reactions	Apply locally BID Do not bandage
ketoconazole *kee-toe-koe'-nah-zoll*	Nizoral	Cream: tinea cruris, tinea corporis, tinea versicolor Shampoo: reduction of scaling due to dandruff	Cream: Severe itching, pruritus, stinging Shampoo: increase in hair loss, abnormal hair texture, scalp pustules, mild dryness of the skin, itching, oiliness/dryness of the hair	Cream: apply daily to affected areas for 2–6 wk Shampoo: twice a week for 4 wk with at least 3 days between each shampoo
miconazole *mi-kon'-ah-zoll*	Tetterine, Micatin, Monistat-Derm, Micatin, Fungold Tincture	Tinea pedis, tinea cruris, tinea corporis, cutaneous candidiasis	Local irritation, burning, maceration, allergic contact dermatitis	Cover affected areas BID
naftifine *naf'-tih-feen*	Naftin	Topical treatment of tinea pedis, tinea cruris, tinea corporis	Burning, stinging, erythema, itching, local irritation, rash, tenderness	Apply BID for 4 wk
nystatin *nye-stat'-in*	Mycostatin, Nystex	Mycotic infections caused by *Candida albicans* and other *Candida* species	Virtually nontoxic and nonsensitizing; well tolerated by all age groups, even with prolonged administration; if irritation occurs, discontinue use	Apply BID or TID until healing is complete
oxiconazole *ox-ee-kon'-ah-zoll*	Oxistat	Tinea pedis, tinea cruris, tinea corporis	Pruritus, burning, stinging, irritation, contact dermatitis, scaling, tingling	Apply daily or BID for 1 month

(table continues on page 544)

Summary Drug Table DERMATOLOGIC DRUGS (continued)

Generic Name	Trade Name	Uses	Adverse Reactions	Dosage Ranges
suconazole *soo-kon'-ah-zoll*	Exelderm	Same as oxiconazole	Pruritus, burning, stinging, irritation	Apply daily or BID for 3–6 wk
terbinafine *ter-bin'-ah-feen*	Lamisil	Same as oxiconazole	Same as oxiconazole	Apply BID until infection clears (1–4 wk)
tolnaftate *toll-naf'-tate*	Aftate, Genaspor, Tinactin, Ting	Same as oxiconazole	Same as oxiconazole	Apply BID for 2–3 wk (4–6 wk may be needed)
Topical Antivirals				
acyclovir *ay-sye'-kloe-veer*	Zovirax	Herpes simplex virus (HSV) infections; Varicella-zoster	Ointment: Mild pain with transient burning/stinging Cream: pruritus, rash, vulvitis, edema or pain at application site	Ointment: apply to all lesions q 3 hr 6 times daily for 7 days Cream: apply 5 times daily for 4 days
Docosanol *doe-koe-nah'-zoll*	Abreva	HSV-1 and 2	Headache, skin irritation	Apply to lesions 5 times daily
imiquimod *im-ee'-kwee-mod*	Aldara	External genitalia and perianal warts	Local skin irritation, itching, excoriation, flaking	Apply externally 3 times weekly
penciclovir *pen-sye'-kloe-veer*	Denavir	HSV-1 and 2	Headache, taste perversion	Apply q 2 hr for 4 days during waking hours
vidarabine *vye-dare'-ah-been*	Ara-A, Vira-A	Keratitis, keratoconjunctivitis caused by HSV-1 and 2	Burning, itching, irritation, tearing, sensitivity to light	Ophthalmic ointment: 0.5 inch into lower conjunctival sac 2–5 times daily
Antiseptics and Germicides				
chlorhexidine *klor-hex'-eh-deen*	Bacto Shield 2, Betasept, Exidine-2 Scrub, Hibiclens	Surgical scrub, skin cleanser, preoperative skin preparation, skin wound cleanser, preoperative showering and bathing	Irritation, dermatitis, photosensitivity (rare), deafness, mild sensitivity reactions	Varies, depending on administration
hexachlorophene *hex-ah-klor'-oh-feen*	pHisoHex, Septisol	Surgical scrub and bacteriostatic skin cleanser, control of an outbreak of gram-positive infection when other procedures are unsuccessful	Dermatitis, photosensitivity, sensitivity to hexachlorophene, redness or mild scaling or dryness	Surgical wash or scrub: as indicated Bacteriostatic cleansing: wet hand with water and squeeze approx. 5 mL into palm, add water and work up lather, apply to area to be cleansed, rinse thoroughly
povidone-iodine *poe'-vih-doan*	Acu-Dyne, Aerodine, Betadine	Microbicidal against bacteria, fungi, viruses, spores, protozoa, yeasts	Dermatitis, irritation, burning, sensitivity reactions	Varies, depending on administration
sodium hypoclorite	Dakin's Solution	Antiseptic against bacteria, fungi, viruses, spores, protozoa, yeasts; deodorizing properties	Chemical reaction or burn	Varies, depending on administration
triclosan *trye'-kloe-san*	Clearasil Daily Face Wash	Skin cleanser and de-germer	None significant	Apply 5 mL on hands or face and rub thoroughly for 30 sec, rinse thoroughly, pat dry

(table continues on page 545)

Summary Drug Table DERMATOLOGIC DRUGS (continued)

Generic Name	Trade Name	Uses	Adverse Reactions	Dosage Ranges
Corticosteroids, Topical				
alclometasone *al-kloe-met'-ah-soan*	Aclovate	Treatment of various allergic/immunologic skin problems	Allergic contact dermatitis, burning, dryness, edema, irritation	Apply 1–6 times daily according to directions
amcinonide *am-sin'-oh-nyde*	Cyclocort	Same as alclometasone	Same as alclometasone	Apply 1–6 times daily according to directions
betamethasone *bay-tah-meth'-ah-soan*	Alphatrex, Betatrex, Diprolene, Diprosone, Maxivate	Same as alclometasone	Same as alclometasone	Apply 1–4 times daily according to directions
desoximetasone *dess-ox-ih-met'-ah-soan*	Topicort	Same as alclometasone	Same as alclometasone	Apply 1–4 times daily according to directions
dexamethasone *dex-ah-meth'-ah-soan*	Decadron Phosphate	Same as alclometasone	Same as alclometasone	Apply 1–4 times daily according to directions
diflorasone *dye-flor'-ah-soan*	Florone, Maxiflor	Same as alclometasone	Same as alclometasone	Apply 1–4 times daily according to directions
fluocinolone *floo-oh-sin'-oh-loan*	Fluonid, Flurosyn, Synalar	Same as alclometasone	Same as alclometasone	Apply 1–4 times daily according to directions
fluocinonide *floo-oh-sin'-oh-nyde*	Lidex	Same as alclometasone	Same as alclometasone	Apply 1–4 times daily according to directions
flurandrenolide *flor-an-dren'-oh-lyde*	Cordran	Same as alclometasone	Same as alclometasone	Apply 1–4 times daily according to directions
hydrocortisone *hye-droe-kore'-tih-soan*	Bactine, Cort-Dome, Hytone, Locoid, Pandel	Same as alclometasone	Same as alclometasone	Apply 1–4 times daily according to directions
triamcinolone *trye-am-sin'-oh-loan*	Aristocort, Flutex, Kenalog, Triacet	Same as alclometasone	Same as alclometasone	Apply 1–4 times daily according to directions
Antipsoriatic Drugs				
anthralin *an-thra'-lin*	Anthra-Derm Drithocreme, Miconal	Psoriasis	Few; transient irritation of normal skin or uninvolved skin	Apply daily
calcipotriene *cal-sip-oh-trye'-een*	Dovonex	Psoriasis	Burning, itching, skin irritation, erythema, dry skin, peeling, rash, worsening of psoriasis, dermatitis, hyperpigmentation	Apply BID
selenium sulfide *seh-leh'-nee-um*	Exsel Head and Shoulders Intensive Treatment Dandruff	Treatment of dandruff, seborrheic dermatitis of the scalp, and tinea versicolor Shampoo,	Skin irritation, greater than normal hair loss, hair discoloration, oiliness or dryness of hair Selsun Blue	Massage 5–10 mL into wet scalp and allow to remain on scalp for 2–3 min, rinse
Enzyme Preparations				
collagenase *koll-ah'-geh-nace*	Santyl	For debriding chronic dermal ulcers and severely burned areas	Well tolerated and nonirritating; transient burning sensation may occur	Apply daily according to directions

(table continues on page 546)

Summary Drug Table DERMATOLOGIC DRUGS (continued)

Generic Name	Trade Name	Uses	Adverse Reactions	Dosage Ranges
enzyme combinations	Accuzyme, Granul-Derm Granulex, Panafil	Debridement of necrotic tissue and liquefaction of slough in acute and chronic lesions such as pressure ulcers, varicose and diabetic ulcers, burns, wounds, pilonidal cyst wounds, and miscellaneous traumatic or infected wounds	Well tolerated and nonirritating; transient burning sensation may occur	Aerosol: apply BID or TID according to directions Ointment: apply daily or BID according to directions
Keratolytic Drugs				
masoprocol *mah-soe'-proe-koll*	Actinex	Actinic keratoses	Erythema, flaking, dryness, itching, edema, burning, soreness, bleeding, crusting, skin roughness	Apply BID
salicylic acid *sal-ih-sill'-ik*	Duofilm, Wart Remover, Fostex, Fung-O, Mosco, Panscol	Aids in the removal of excessive keratin in hyperkeratotic skin disorders, including warts, psoriasis, calluses, and corns	Local irritation	Apply as directed in individual product labeling
Local Anesthetics				
benzocaine *ben'-zoh-kane*	Lanacane	Topical anesthesia in local skin disorders	Rare; hypersensitivity, local burning, stinging, tenderness, sloughing	Apply to affected area
dibucaine *dih'-byoo-kane*	Nupercainal	Topical anesthesia in local skin disorders, local anesthesia of accessible mucous membranes	Same as benzocaine	Topical: apply to affected area as needed Mucous membranes: dosage varies and depends on the area to be anesthetized
lidocaine *lye'-doe-kane*	DentiPatch, ELA-Max, Lidocaine Viscous, Xylocaine	Same as dibucaine	Same as benzocaine	Topical: apply to affected area as needed Mucous membranes: dosage varies and depends on the area to be anesthetized
butamben picrate *byoo'-tam-ben*		Topical anesthesia	Rare; local burning, stinging, tenderness	Apply to affected area

Oragel

Adverse Reactions

Adverse reactions to topical anti-infectives are usually mild. Occasionally, the patient may experience a rash, itching, urticaria (hives), dermatitis, irritation, or redness, which may indicate a **hypersensitivity** (allergic) reaction to the drug. Prolonged use of topical antibiotic preparations may result in a superficial **superinfection** (an overgrowth of bacterial or fungal microorganisms not affected by the antibiotic being administered).

Contraindications, Precautions, and Interactions

These drugs are contraindicated in patients with known hypersensitivity to the drugs or any components of the drug.

The topical antibiotics are pregnancy category C drugs and are used cautiously during pregnancy and lactation. Acyclovir and penciclovir are pregnancy category B drugs and are used cautiously during pregnancy and lactation. The pregnancy categories of the antifungals are unknown except for econazole, which is in pregnancy category C, and ciclopirox, which is in pregnancy category B; both are used with caution during pregnancy and lactation. There are no significant interactions for the topical anti-infectives.

HERBAL ALERT

Aloe vera is used to prevent infection and promote healing of minor burns (e.g., sunburn) and wounds. When used externally, aloe helps to repair skin tissue and reduce inflammation. Aloe gel is naturally thick when taken from the leaf but quickly becomes watery because of the action of enzymes in the plant. Commercially available preparations have additive thickeners to make the aloe appear like the fresh gel. The agent can be applied directly from the fresh leaf by cutting the leaf in half lengthwise and gently rubbing the inner gel directly onto the skin. Commercially prepared products are applied externally as needed. Rare reports of allergy have been reported with the external use of aloe.

• TOPICAL ANTISEPTICS AND GERMICIDES

An **antiseptic** is a drug that stops, slows, or prevents the growth of microorganisms. A **germicide** is a drug that kills bacteria.

Actions

The exact mechanism of action of topical antiseptics and germicides is not well understood. These drugs affect a variety of microorganisms. Some of these drugs have a short duration of action, whereas others have a long duration of action. The action of these drugs may depend on the strength used and the time the drug is in contact with the skin or mucous membrane.

Chlorhexidine

Chlorhexidine affects a wide range of microorganisms, including gram-positive and gram-negative bacteria.

Hexachlorophene

Hexachlorophene (pHisoHex) is a bacteriostatic drug that acts against staphylococci and other gram-positive bacteria. Cumulative antibacterial action develops with repeated use.

Iodine

Iodine has anti-infective action against many bacteria, fungi, viruses, yeasts, and protozoa. Povidone–iodine (Betadine) is a combination of iodine and povidone that liberates free iodine. Povidone–iodine is often preferred over iodine solution or tincture, because it is less irritating to the skin and treated areas may be bandaged or taped.

Uses

Topical antiseptics and germicides are used for the following:

• To reduce the number of bacteria on skin surfaces
• As a surgical scrub and preoperative skin cleanser
• For washing the hands before and after caring for patients
• In the home to cleanse the skin
• On minor cuts and abrasions to prevent infection

Adverse Reactions

Topical antiseptics and germicides provoke few adverse reactions. Occasionally, an individual may be allergic to the drug, and a skin rash or itching may occur. If an allergic reaction is noted, use of the topical drug is discontinued.

Contraindications, Precautions, and Interactions

These drugs are contraindicated in patients with known hypersensitivity to the individual drug or any component of the preparation. There are no significant precautions or interactions when the drugs are used as directed.

• TOPICAL CORTICOSTEROIDS

Topical corticosteroids vary in potency, depending on the concentration (percentage) of the drug, the vehicle (lotion, cream, aerosol spray) in which the drug is suspended, and the area (open or denuded skin, unbroken skin, thickness of the skin over the treated area) to which the drug is applied. Examples of topical corticosteroids include amcinonide, betamethasone, fluocinolone, hydrocortisone, and triamcinolone.

Actions and Uses

Topical corticosteroids exert localized anti-inflammatory activity. When applied to inflamed skin, they reduce itching, redness, and swelling. These drugs are use in treating skin disorders such as:

• Psoriasis
• Dermatitis
• Rashes
• Eczema
• Insect bites
• First- and second-degree burns, including sunburn

Adverse Reactions

Localized reactions may include burning, itching, irritation, redness, dryness of the skin, allergic contact dermatitis, and secondary infection. These reactions are more likely to occur if occlusive dressings are used. Systemic reactions may also occur with hypothalamic-pituitary-adrenal axis suppression, Cushing's syndrome, hyperglycemia, and glycosuria.

Contraindications, Precautions, and Interactions

Topical corticosteroids are contraindicated in patients with known hypersensitivity to the drug or any component of the drug; as monotherapy for bacterial skin infections; for use on the face, groin, or axilla (only the high-potency corticosteroids); and for ophthalmic use (may cause steroid-induced glaucoma or cataracts). The topical corticosteroids are not used as sole therapy in widespread plaque psoriasis. The topical corticosteroids are pregnancy category C drugs and are used cautiously during pregnancy and lactation. There are no significant interactions when these drugs are administered as directed.

• TOPICAL ANTIPSORIATICS

Action and Uses

Topical **antipsoriatic** drugs are drugs used to treat psoriasis (a chronic skin disease manifested by bright red patches covered with silvery scales or plaques) by helping to remove the plaques associated with the disorder. Examples of antipsoriatics include anthralin and calcipotriene.

Adverse Reactions

These drugs may cause burning, itching, and skin irritation. Anthralin may cause skin irritation, as well as temporary discoloration of the hair and fingernails.

Contraindications, Precautions, and Interactions

Topical antipsoriatics are contraindicated in patients with known hypersensitivity to the drugs. Anthralin and calcipotriene, pregnancy category C drugs, are used cautiously during pregnancy and lactation.

• TOPICAL ENZYMES

Actions and Uses

A topical enzyme is used to help remove **necrotic** (dead) tissue from:

• Chronic dermal ulcers
• Severely burned areas

These enzymes aid in the removal of dead soft tissues by hastening the reduction of proteins into simpler substances. The process is called **proteolysis** or a **proteolytic** action. The components of certain types of wounds, namely necrotic tissues and **purulent exudates** (pus-containing fluid), prevent proper wound healing. Removal of this type of debris by application of a topical enzyme aids in healing. Examples of conditions that may respond to application of a topical enzyme include second- and third-degree burns, pressure ulcers, and ulcers caused by peripheral vascular disease. An example of a topical enzyme is collagenase.

Adverse Reactions

The application of collagenase may cause mild, transient pain and possibly numbness and dermatitis. There is a low incidence of adverse reactions to collagenase.

Contraindications, Precautions, and Interactions

Topical enzyme preparations are contraindicated in patients with known hypersensitivity to the drugs, in wounds in contact with major body cavities or where nerves are exposed, and in fungating neoplastic ulcers. These drugs are pregnancy category B drugs and are used cautiously during pregnancy and lactation. Enzymatic activity may be impaired by certain detergents and heavy metal ions, such as mercury and silver, which are used in some antiseptics. The optimal pH for collagenase is 6 to 8. Higher or lower pH conditions decrease the enzyme's activity.

• KERATOLYTICS

Actions and Uses

A **keratolytic** is a drug that removes excess growth of the epidermis (top layer of skin) in disorders such as warts. These drugs are used to remove:

• Warts
• Calluses
• Corns
• Seborrheic keratoses (benign, variously colored skin growths arising from oil glands of the skin)

Examples of keratolytics include salicylic acid and masoprocol. Some strengths of salicylic acid are available as nonprescription products for the removal of warts on the hands and feet.

Adverse Reactions

These drugs are usually well tolerated. Occasionally a transient burning sensation, rash, dry skin, scaling, or flulike syndrome may occur.

Contraindications, Precautions, and Interactions

Keratolytics are contraindicated in patients with known hypersensitivity to the drugs and for use on moles, birthmarks, or warts with hair growing from them, on genital or facial warts, on warts on mucous membranes, or on infected skin. Prolonged use of the keratolytics in infants and in patients with diabetes or impaired circulation is contraindicated. Salicylic acid may cause salicylate toxicity with prolonged use. These drugs are pregnancy category C drugs and are used cautiously during pregnancy and lactation.

• TOPICAL LOCAL ANESTHETICS

A topical anesthetic may be applied to the skin or mucous membranes.

Actions and Uses

Topical anesthetics temporarily inhibit the conduction of impulses from sensory nerve fibers. These drugs may be used to relieve itching and pain due to skin conditions, such as minor burns, fungal infections, insect bites, rashes, sunburn, and plant poisoning (e.g., poison ivy). Some are applied to mucous membranes as local anesthetics. Examples of local anesthetics include benzocaine, dibucaine, and lidocaine.

Adverse Reactions

Occasionally, local irritation, dermatitis, rash, burning, stinging, and tenderness may be noted.

Contraindications, Precautions, and Interactions

These drugs are contraindicated in those with a known hypersensitivity to any component of the preparation. Topical anesthetics are used cautiously in patients receiving class I antiarrhythmic drugs such as tocainide and mexiletine, because the toxic effects are additive and potentially synergistic. *no longer on market*

NURSING PROCESS
PATIENT RECEIVING A TOPICAL DRUG FOR A SKIN DISORDER

ASSESSMENT

Preadministration Assessment
The preadministration assessment involves a visual inspection and palpation of the involved area(s). The nurse carefully records the areas of involvement, including the size, color, and appearance. The appearance of the skin lesions, such as rough, itchy patches, cracks between the toes, and sore and reddened areas, are noted so treatment can begin with an accurate database. A specific description is important so that changes indicating worsening or improvement of the lesions can be readily identified. Terms used to describe skin lesions are found in Table 53.1. The nurse notes the presence of subjective reports, such as pain, burning or any complaint of itching. Some agencies may provide a figure on which the lesions can be drawn, indicating the shape and distribution of the involved areas.

Ongoing Assessment
At the time of each application, the nurse inspects the affected area for changes (e.g., signs of improvement or worsening of the infection) and for adverse reactions, such as redness or rash. The nurse contacts the primary health care provider, and the drug is not applied if these or other changes are noted or if the patient reports new problems, such as itching, pain, or soreness at the site. The nurse may be responsible for checking the treatment sites 1 day or more after application and

Table 53.1	Terms Used to Describe Skin Lesions
Lesion	**Description**
Macule	Flat spot on the skin
Papule	Raised spot on the skin
Nodule	Small solid swelling on the skin
Pustule	Lesion containing pus
Petechia	Pinpoint hemorrhagic areas of the skin
Erythema	Redness
Ecchymosis	Bruised area
Vesicle	Fluid-filled swelling (blister)

should inform the primary health care provider of any signs of extreme redness or infection at the application site.

LIFESPAN ALERT – Pediatric
Because infants and children have a high ratio of skin surface area to body mass, they are at greater risk than adults for systemic adverse effects when treated with topical medication.

NURSING DIAGNOSES

Drug-specific nursing diagnoses include the following:

- ❏ **Impaired Skin Integrity** related to the inflammatory process (increased sensitivity to the drug)
- ❏ **Acute Pain** related to skin condition or increased sensitivity to drug therapy
- ❏ **Risk for Infection** related to entry of pathogens into affected areas
- ❏ **Disturbed Body Image** related to changes in skin and mucous membranes

Nursing diagnoses related to drug administration are discussed in Chapter 4.

PLANNING

The expected outcomes of the patient may include an optimal response to drug therapy, support of patient needs related to management of adverse drug reactions, and an understanding of the application or the reason for use of a topical drug.

IMPLEMENTATION

Promoting an Optimal Response to Therapy
Some of the patients using these drugs will be institutionalized in acute care or long term care facilities. Drug application is carried out by a nurse in these facilities. When the patient is at home, frequently the nurse will instruct the patient or a caregiver in the methods used to apply topical drugs.

TOPICAL ANTI-INFECTIVES. Before each application, the area is cleansed with soap and warm water unless the primary health care provider orders a different method. The anti-infective is applied as prescribed (e.g., thin layer or applied liberally) and the area is either covered or left exposed as prescribed.

> **NURSING ALERT**
>
> Care must be exercised when applying anti-infectives or any topical drug near or around the eyes.

TOPICAL ANTIFUNGAL INFECTION PREPARATIONS. When these drugs are applied topically to the skin, the area is inspected at the time of each application for localized skin reactions. When these drugs are administered vaginally, the nurse questions the patient regarding any discomfort or other sensations experienced after insertion of the antifungal preparation. The nurse notes improvement or deterioration of lesions of the skin, mucous membranes, or vaginal secretions in the chart. It is important for the nurse to evaluate and chart the patient's response to therapy.

TOPICAL ANTISEPTICS AND GERMICIDES. Antiseptics and germicides are instilled or applied as directed by the primary health care provider or by the label on the product. Topical antiseptics and germicides are not a substitute for clean or aseptic techniques. Occlusive dressings are not to be used after application of these products unless a dressing is specifically ordered by the primary health care provider. Iodine permanently stains clothing and temporarily stains the skin. Care should be taken to remove or protect the patient's personal clothing when applying iodine solution or tincture.

Antiseptic and germicidal drugs kept at the patient's bedside must be clearly labeled with the name of the product, the strength, and, when applicable, the date of preparation of the solution. The nurse replaces hard-to-read or soiled, stained labels as needed. These solutions are not kept at the bedside of any patient who is confused or disoriented, because the solution may be mistaken for water or another beverage.

TOPICAL CORTICOSTEROIDS. Before drug application, the area is washed with soap and warm water unless the primary health care provider directs otherwise. Topical corticosteroids are usually ordered to be applied sparingly. The primary health care provider also may order the area of application to be covered or left exposed to the air. Some corticosteroids are applied with an occlusive dressing. The drug is applied while the skin is still moist after washing with soap and water and a dressing is applied if ordered by the primary health care provider.

> **LIFESPAN ALERT – Pediatric**
>
> Do not use tight-fitting diapers or pants on a child treated in the diaper area. These types of clothing may work like an occlusive dressing and cause more of the drug to be absorbed into the child's body, resulting in a greater risk for adverse reactions.

TOPICAL ENZYMES. Certain types of wounds may require special preparations before applying the topical enzyme. The area is cleansed or prepared and the topical enzyme is applied as directed by the primary health care provider.

TOPICAL ANTIPSORIATICS. Care is exercised so that the product is applied only to the psoriatic lesions and not to surrounding skin. The nurse instructs the patient or caregiver to bring signs of excessive irritation to the attention of the primary health care provider.

> **LIFESPAN ALERT – Gerontology**
>
> Adults older than 65 years have more skin-related adverse reactions to calcipotriene. The nurse should use calcipotriene cautiously in older adults.

TOPICAL ANESTHETICS. The anesthetic is applied as directed by the primary health care provider. Before the first application, the nurse cleanses and dries the area. For subsequent applications, all previous residue should be removed.

When a topical gel, such as lidocaine viscous, is used for oral anesthesia, the nurse instructs the patient not to eat food for 1 hour after use, because local anesthesia of the mouth or throat may impair swallowing and increase the possibility of aspiration.

Monitoring and Managing Patient Needs

Most topical drugs cause few adverse reactions and, if they occur, discontinuing use of the drug may be all that is necessary to relieve the symptoms.

IMPAIRED SKIN INTEGRITY. Dry skin increases the risk of skin breakdown from scratching. The nurse can advise the patient to keep nails short, use warm water with mild soap for cleaning the skin, and rinse and dry the skin thoroughly.

ACUTE PAIN. Occasionally, increased skin sensitivity occurs, causing greater redness, discomfort, and itching. The nurse may use cool, wet compresses for rashes or a bath to relieve the itching. Keeping the environment cool may also make the patient more comfortable.

RISK FOR INFECTION. Bath oils, creams, and lotions may be used, if necessary, as long as the primary health care provider is consulted before use. Dry, flaky skin is subject to breakdown and infection. The nurse instructs the patient or caregiver to observe the skin for signs of infection (e.g., redness, heat, pus, and elevated temperature and pulse) and immediately reports any sign of infection.

DISTURBED BODY IMAGE. Some infections such as superficial and deep fungal infections respond slowly to therapy. The lesions caused by the fungal infections may cause the patient to feel negatively about the body or a body part. In addition, many patients experience anxiety and depression over the fact that therapy must continue for a prolonged period and that results are slow to appear. Depending on the method of treatment, patients may be faced with many problems during therapy and therefore need time to talk about problems as they arise. Examples of these problems may be the cost of treatment, hospitalization (when required), the failure of treatment adequately to control the infection, and loss of income. It is important for the nurse to develop a therapeutic nurse–patient relationship that conveys an attitude of caring and fosters a sense of trust. The nurse listens to the patient's concerns and assists the patient in accepting the situation as temporary. The nurse encourages the patient to verbalize any feelings or anxiety about the effect of the disorder on body image. The nurse explains the disorder and the treatment regimen in terms the patient can understand and discusses the need at times for long-term treatment to eradicate the infection. The nurse must help the patient and the family to understand that therapy must be continued until the infection is under control. In some cases, therapy may take weeks or months.

Educating the Patient and Family

If the primary health care provider has prescribed or recommended the use of a topical drug, the nurse notes that most of the adverse effects that occur with topical drugs are a result of applying the drug improperly. Typically, if applied correctly, the drug usually is not systemically absorbed. However, sometimes patients think that if a little is good, then "more is better." Applying more than the amount necessary increases the patient's risk for systemic absorption (see Patient Teaching for Improved Patient Outcomes: Application of Topical Drugs).

GENERAL TEACHING POINTS.

- Wash the hands thoroughly before and after applying the product.
- If the enclosed directions state that the product will stain clothing, be sure clothing is moved away from the treated area. If the product stains the skin, wear disposable gloves when applying the drug.
- Follow the directions on the label or use as directed by the primary health care provider. Read any enclosed directions for use of the product carefully.
- Prepare the area to be treated as recommended by the primary health care provider or as described in the directions supplied with the product.
- Do not apply to areas other than those specified by the primary health care provider. Apply the drug as directed (e.g., thin layer or apply liberally).
- Follow the directions of the primary health care provider regarding covering the treated area or leaving it exposed to air. The effectiveness of certain drugs depends on keeping the area covered or leaving it open.
- Keep the product away from the eyes (unless use in or around the eye has been recommended or prescribed). Do not rub or put the fingers near the eyes unless the hands have been thoroughly washed and all remnants of the drug removed from the fingers. If the product is accidentally spilled, sprayed, or splashed in the eye, wash the eye immediately with copious amounts of running water. Contact the primary health care provider immediately if burning, pain, redness, discomfort, or blurred vision persists for more than a few minutes.

- The drug may cause momentary stinging or burning when applied.
- Discontinue use of the drug and contact the primary health care provider if rash, burning, itching, redness, pain, or other skin problems occur.

ANTI-INFECTIVES.

- Gentamicin may cause photosensitivity. Take measures to protect the skin from ultraviolet rays (e.g., wear protective clothing and use a sunscreen when out in the sun).
- Topical clindamycin can be absorbed in sufficient amounts to cause systemic effects. If severe diarrhea, stomach cramps, or bloody stools occur, contact the primary health care provider immediately.

ANTIFUNGALS.

- Clean the involved area and apply the ointment or cream to the skin as directed by the primary health care provider.
- Do not increase or decrease the amount used or the number of times the ointment or cream should be applied unless directed to do so by the primary health care provider.
- During treatment for a ringworm infection, keep towels and facecloths for bathing separate from those of other family members to avoid the spread of the infection. It is important to keep the affected area clean and dry.

ANTIVIRALS.

- When applying ointment, use a finger cot or glove to prevent autoinoculation of other body sites.
- This product will not prevent transmission of infection to others.
- Transient burning, itching, and rash may occur.

TOPICAL CORTICOSTEROIDS.

- Apply ointments, creams, or gels sparingly in a light film; rub in gently.
- Use only as directed. Do not use bandages, dressings, cosmetics, or other skin products over the treated area unless so directed by the primary health care provider.

ENZYME PREPARATIONS.

- If, for any reason, it becomes necessary to inactivate collagenase, this can be accomplished by washing the area with povidone–iodine.

EVALUATION

- Therapeutic drug response is achieved.
- Adverse reactions are identified, reported to the primary health care provider, and managed successfully with appropriate nursing interventions:
  - ☑ Skin remains intact.
  - ☑ Patient is free of pain.
  - ☑ No evidence of infection is seen.
  - ☑ Perceptions of body changes are managed successfully.
- Patient or family member demonstrates an understanding of the use and application of the prescribed or recommended drug.

Patient Teaching for Improved Patient Outcomes:

Application of Topical Drugs

Often patients are required to apply topical drugs in the home setting. To ensure that the patient applies the topical drug properly, the nurse includes the following points in the teaching plan:

✓ Gather all necessary supplies and wash hands before starting.

✓ Wash the area first to remove any debris and old drug.

✓ Pat the area dry with a clean cloth.

✓ Open the container (or tube) and place the lid or cap upside down on the counter or surface.

✓ Use a tongue blade, gloved finger (either with a nonsterile gloved hand or finger cot), cotton swab, or gauze pad to remove the drug, then apply it to the skin.

✓ Wipe the drug onto the affected area using long smooth strokes in the direction of hair growth.

✓ Apply a thin layer of drug to the area (more is not better).

✓ Use a new tongue blade, applicator, or clean gloved finger to remove additional drug from the container (if necessary).

✓ Apply a clean, dry dressing (if appropriate) over the area.

THINK CRITICALLY: PHARMACOLOGY IN PRACTICE

1. The medication nurse caring for Mr. Park asks you about his shingles outbreak. Her cousin has cold sores and uses an acyclovir ointment when they first appear. She understands that Mr. Park is taking acyclovir orally; she questions why he was not prescribed a topical drug to ease the pain and irritation from the shingles lesions. Discuss how you would respond to the nurse's question about Mr. Park.

● Test Your Knowledge

1. What reaction could occur with prolonged use of the topical antibiotics?

 A. Water intoxication
 B. Superficial superinfection
 C. Outbreak of eczema
 D. Cellulitis

2. Which of the following drugs has a proteolytic action?

 A. amcinonide
 B. collagenase
 C. bacitracin
 D. ciclopirox

3. A keratolytic agent would be safe to use on which of the following skin conditions?

 A. Moles
 B. Birthmarks
 C. Facial warts
 D. Calluses

4. What type of action do the corticosteroids have when used topically?

 A. Bactericidal activity
 B. Anti-inflammatory activity
 C. Antifungal activity
 D. Antiviral activity

● Prepare for the NCLEX

1. The nurse is gathering supplies to change the dressing of a patient's central line (IV). Which of the following drugs is best suited to be used as a topical antiseptic?

 A. amphotericin B
 B. benzocaine
 C. iodine
 D. povidone–iodine

● Calculate Medication Dosages

1. Dakin's solution is ordered for home irrigation of a wound. The primary health care provider orders a 3:1 solution (water:Dakin's) to be mixed with distilled water. How much water should be added to 10 mL of the Dakin's?

To check your answers, see Appendix E.

the**Point**. *For more NCLEX questions, log on to http://thepoint.lww.com to access more than 1000 questions.*

Otic and Ophthalmic Preparations

cerumen
cycloplegia
intraocular pressure
miosis
mydriasis

myopia
ophthalmic
otic
otitis media
superinfection

On completion of this chapter, the student will:

1. Discuss the general actions, uses, adverse reactions, contraindications, precautions, and interactions of otic and ophthalmic preparations.
2. Discuss important preadministration and ongoing assessment activities the nurse should perform on a patient receiving otic and ophthalmic preparations.
3. List nursing diagnoses particular to a patient taking an otic or ophthalmic preparation.
4. Discuss ways to promote an optimal response to therapy, how to administer the preparations, and important points to keep in mind when educating patients about the use of otic or ophthalmic preparations.

The eyes and ears are subject to various disorders that range from mild to serious. Because the eyes and ears are among the interpreters of our outside environment, any disease or injury that has the potential for partial or total loss of function of these organs must be treated.

• OTIC PREPARATIONS

Disorders of the ear are categorized according to the part of the ear affected: the outer, the middle, or the inner ear. The disorders most often treated with the preparations discussed in this chapter are of the outer and middle ear. **Otitis media**, by far the most common disorder of the middle ear, is fluid in the middle ear accompanied by symptoms of intense local or systemic infection. The most common causes are viruses and bacteria. Symptoms include pain in the ear, drainage of fluid from the ear canal, and hearing loss. Other symptoms that may be present if the disorder becomes systemic include fever, irritability, headache, and anorexia.

Actions

Various types of preparations are used for treating **otic** disorders. Otic preparations can be divided into three categories: antibiotics; antibiotic and steroid combinations; and miscellaneous preparations. The miscellaneous preparations usually contain one or more of the following ingredients:

- Benzocaine—a local anesthetic used to temporally relieve pain
- Phenylephrine—a vasoconstrictor decongestant
- Hydrocortisone—corticosteroid for anti-inflammatory and antipruritic effects
- Glycerin—an emollient and a solvent
- Antipyrine—an analgesic
- Acetic acid, boric acid, benzalkonium, aluminum, benzethonium—provide antifungal or antibacterial action
- Carbamide peroxide—aids in removing **cerumen** (yellowish or brownish ear wax) by softening and breaking up the wax

Examples of otic preparations are given in the Summary Drug Table: Selected Otic Preparations.

Uses

Otic preparations are instilled in the external auditory canal and may be used to:

- Relieve pain
- Treat infection and inflammation
- Aid in the removal of cerumen

When the patient has an inner ear infection, systemic antibiotic therapy is indicated.

Adverse Reactions

When otic drugs are applied topically, the amount of drug that enters the systemic circulation usually is not sufficient to produce adverse reactions. Prolonged use of otic preparations containing an antibiotic, such as ofloxacin, may result in a **superinfection** (an overgrowth of bacterial or fungal microorganisms not affected by the antibiotic being administered). Local adverse reactions that may occur include:

- Ear irritation
- Itching
- Burning

Summary Drug Table SELECTED OTIC PREPARATIONS

Generic Combinations	Trade Name	Uses	Adverse Reactions	Dosage Ranges
Corticosteroid and Antibiotic Combinations, Solutions				
1% hydrocortisone, 5 mg neomycin, 10,000 units polymyxin B	Antibiotic Ear Solution, AntibiOtic, Cortisporin Otic, Drotic, Ear-Eze, Otic-Care, OticairOtic, Otocort, Otosporin	Bacterial infections of the external auditory canal	Few; can cause ear irritation, burning, or itching; when used for prolonged periods there is a danger of a superinfection	4 gtt instilled TID or QID
0.5% hydrocortisone, 10,000 units polymyxin B	Otobiotic Otic	Same as 1% hydrocortisone solution	Same as 1% hydrocortisone solution	4 gtt instilled TID or QID
Corticosteroid and Antibiotic Combinations, Suspensions				
1% hydrocortisone, 5 mg neomycin, 10,000 units polymyxin B	AK-Spore, AntibiOtic, Antibiotic Ear Suspension, Otocort, UAD Otic, Pediotic	Same as 1% hydrocortisone solution	Same as 1% hydrocortisone solution	4 gtt instilled TID or QID
1% hydrocortisone, 4.71 mg neomycin	Coly-Mycin S Otic	Same as 1% hydrocortisone solution	Same as 1% hydrocortisone solution	4 gtt instilled TID or QID
1% hydrocortisone, 3.3 mg neomycin	Cortisporin-TC Otic	Same as 1% hydrocortisone solution	Same as 1% hydrocortisone solution	4 gtt instilled TID or QID
2 mg ciprofloxacin, 10 mg hydrocortisone/mL	Cipro HC Otic	Same as 1% hydrocortisone solution/	Same as 1% hydrocortisone solution	4 gtt instilled TID or QID
Otic Antibiotic				
ofloxacin (otic)	Floxin Otic	Otitis externa, chronic suppurative otitis media, acute otitis media	Local irritation, itching, burning, earache	Ages 1–12 yr: 5 gtt BID into affected ear for 10 day Ages 12 yr and older: 10 gtt BID into affected ear for 10–14 day
Select Miscellaneous Preparations				
1% hydrocortisone, 2% acetic acid, 3% propylene glycol, 0.015% sodium, 0.02% benzethonium chloride	Acetasol HC, VoSoL HC Otic	Relieve pain, inflammation, and irritation in the external auditory canal	Local irritation, itching, burning	Insert saturated wick into ear; leave for 24 hr, keeping moist with 3–5 gtt q 4–6 hr. Keep moist for 24 hr; remove wick and instill 5 gtt TID or QID
1% hydrocortisone, 1% pramoxine, 0.1% chloroxylenol, 3% propylene glycol and benzalkonium chloride	Cortic	Same as 1% hydrocortisone solution	Same as 1% hydrocortisone solution	Insert saturated wick into ear; leave in for 24 hr, keeping moist with 3–5 gtt q 4–6 hr; remove wick and instill 5 gtt TID or QID
1% hydrocortisone, 2% acetic acid glacial, 3% propylene glycol, 0.02% benzethonium chloride, 0.015% sodium, 0.2% citric acid	AA-HC Otic	Same as 1% hydrocortisone solution	Same as 1% hydrocortisone solution	Insert saturated wick into the ear; leave in for 24 hr, keeping moist with 3–5 gtt q 4–6 hr; remove wick and instill 5 gtt TID or QID

(table continues on page 555)

Summary Drug Table SELECTED OTIC PREPARATIONS (continued)

Generic Combinations	Trade Name	Uses	Adverse Reactions	Dosage Ranges
1.4% benzocaine, 5.4% antipyrine glycerin	Allergen Ear Drops, Auralgan Otic, Auroto Otic Ear Drops, Oto-calm Ear	Relieve ear pain	Local irritation, itching, burning	Fill ear canal with 2–4 gtt; insert saturated cotton pledget; repeat TID or QID or q 1–2 hr
20% benzocaine, 0.1% benzethoniwn chloride, 1% glycerin, PEG 300	Americaine Otic, Otocain	Relieve ear pain temporarily	Local irritation, itching, burning	Instill 4–5 gtt; insert cotton pledget; repeat q 1–2 hr
10% triethanolamine polypeptide oleate-condensate, 0.5% chlorobutanol, propylene glycol	Cerumenex Drops	Aid in the removal of ear wax	Local irritation, itching, burning	Fill ear canal, insert cotton plug, allow to remain 15–30 min, flush ear
1 mg chloroxylenol, 10 mg hydrocortisone, 10 mg/mL pramoxine	Otomar-HC	Relieve pain and irritation in the external auditory canal	Local irritation, itching, burning	Instill 5 gtt into affected ear TID or QID
2% acetic acid in aluminum acetate solution	Burow's Otic, Otic Domeboro	Relieve pain and irritation in the external auditory canal	Local irritation, itching, burning	Insert saturated wick; keep moist for 24 hr; instill 4–6 gtt q 2–3 hr

Contraindications, Precautions, and Interactions

These drugs are contraindicated in patients with a known hypersensitivity to the drugs. The otic drugs are used with caution during pregnancy and lactation. The pregnancy category of most of these drugs is unknown when they are used as otic drugs. Otic drugs available in dropper bottles may be dangerous if ingested. Therefore, the drugs are stored safely out of the reach of children and pets. Drugs to remove cerumen are not used if ear drainage, discharge, pain, or irritation is present; if the eardrum is perforated; or after ear surgery.

If an allergy is suspected, the drug is not administered. Ofloxacin is a pregnancy category C drug and should be administered in pregnancy only if the potential benefit justifies the risk to the fetus. No significant interactions have been reported with use of the otic preparations.

NURSING PROCESS
PATIENT RECEIVING AN OTIC PREPARATION

ASSESSMENT

Preadministration Assessment
Before administration of an otic preparation, the primary health care provider examines the ear and external structures surrounding the ear and prescribes the drug indicated to treat the disorder. The nurse may be responsible for examining the outer structures of the ear (i.e., the earlobe and the skin around the ear). The nurse docu-

ments a description of any drainage or impacted cerumen. Perforated eardrums may be a contraindication to some of the otic preparations. The nurse must check with the primary health care provider before administering an otic preparation to a patient with a perforated ear drum.

Ongoing Assessment
The nurse assesses the patient's response to therapy. For example, a decrease in pain or inflammation should occur. The nurse examines the outer ear and ear canal for any local redness or irritation that may indicate sensitivity to the drug.

LIFESPAN ALERT – Pediatric
When assessing the infant, the nurse looks for the infant to pull, grab, or tug at his or her ears. This may be a sign that the child's ear hurts. (However, infants do pull their ears for all kinds of reasons or for no reason at all, so if the infant seems fine otherwise, an ear infection need not be suspected). In addition, the infant may have a change in behavior, cry, be fussy or irritable, or have a fever.

NURSING DIAGNOSES

Drug-specific nursing diagnoses include the following:

❑ **Risk for Infection** (superinfection) related to prolonged use of the anti-infective otic drug
❑ **Anxiety** related to ear pain or discomfort, changes in hearing, diagnosis, or other factors

Nursing diagnoses related to drug administration are discussed in Chapter 4.

PLANNING

The expected outcomes of the patient depend on the reason for administering the drug and may include an optimal response to the drug, support of patient needs related to the management of adverse reactions, a reduction in anxiety, and an understanding of the application and use of an otic preparation.

IMPLEMENTATION

Promoting an Optimal Response to Therapy

Ear disorders may result in symptoms such as pain, a feeling of fullness in the ear, tinnitus, dizziness, or a change in hearing. Before instilling an otic solution, the nurse informs the patient that a feeling of fullness may be felt in the ear and that hearing in the treated ear may be impaired while the solution remains in the ear canal.

Before instillation of otic preparations, the nurse holds the container in the hand for a few minutes to warm it to body temperature. Cold and warm (above body temperature) preparations may cause dizziness or other sensations after being instilled into the ear.

! NURSING ALERT

Only preparations labeled as "otic" are instilled in the ear. The nurse must check the label of the preparation carefully for the name of the drug and a statement indicating that the preparation is for otic use.

Special instructions for specific ear preparations are found in the Summary Drug Table: Selected Otic Preparations. When instilling ear drops, the nurse has the patient lie on his or her side with the affected ear toward the ceiling. If the patient wishes to remain in an upright position, the head is tilted toward the untreated side with the ear toward the ceiling (Fig. 54.1). When administer-

Figure 54.1 Instilling ear drops. With the head turned toward the unaffected side, the nurse pulls the cartilaginous portion of the outer ear (pinna) up and back in the adult and instills the prescribed number of drops on the side of the auditory canal.

ing an otic drug, the ear canal should be straightened. To straighten the ear canal in the adult and children age 3 years and older, the cartilaginous portion of the outer ear is gently pulled up and back. Be particularly gentle, because some conditions make the ear canal very sensitive. Never insert the dropper or applicator tip into the ear canal.

👥 LIFESPAN ALERT – Pediatric

In children younger than 3 years of age, the ear canal is straighter and needs less manipulation. The cartilaginous portion of the outer ear is gently pulled down and back. The nurse instills the prescribed number of drops into the ear canal. If the child struggles, the nurse can gently secure the head by using the hand holding the dropper. When the child stops struggling, the nurse can administer the drops.

The patient is kept lying on the untreated side after the medication is instilled for approximately 5 minutes to facilitate the penetration of the drops into the ear canal. If medication is needed in the other ear, it is best to wait at least 5 minutes after instillation of the first ear drops before administering drops to the other ear. Once the patient is upright, the solution running out of the ear may be gently removed with gauze. A piece of cotton can be loosely inserted into the ear canal to prevent the medication from flowing out. The cotton is not inserted too deeply, because it may cause increased pressure within the ear canal.

Cerumen is a natural product of the ear and is produced by modified sweat glands in the auditory canal. Sometimes too much cerumen is produced, particularly in older adults. Drugs that loosen cerumen, such as Cerumenex, work by softening the dried ear wax inside the ear canal. Cerumenex is available by prescription and is not allowed to stay in the ear canal more than 30 minutes before irrigation. When Cerumenex is administered, the ear canal is filled with the solution and a cotton plug is inserted. The drug is allowed to remain in the ear for 15 to 30 minutes, and then the ear is flushed with warm water using a soft rubber bulb ear syringe.

👥 LIFESPAN ALERT – Gerontology

The older adult is prone to hearing loss from excess cerumen, especially the patient who is mentally impaired or debilitated. Cerumen is thicker in the elderly, making the accumulation of excess cerumen more likely. It is important for nurses in the community setting or in the nursing home to assess patients for excess cerumen.

Monitoring and Managing Patient Needs

RISK FOR INFECTION. When using the otic antibiotics there is a danger of a superinfection, or another infection on top of the original one, from prolonged use of the drug (see Chapter 7 for a discussion of superinfection). If, after administering the drops as directed for 1 week, the infection does not improve, the primary health care provider should be notified.

ANXIETY. Patients with an ear disorder or injury usually have great concern over the effect the problem will have on their hearing. The nurse reassures the patient that every effort is being made to treat the disorder and relieve the symptoms.

Educating the Patient and Family

The nurse gives the patient or a family member instructions or a demonstration of the instillation technique of an otic preparation.

LIFESPAN ALERT – Pediatric
Because some children are prone to recurrent attacks of acute **otitis media**, parents should be taught to identify signs and symptoms of otitis media and seek medical attention early when their child exhibits these symptoms. If acute or chronic otitis media is not treated, spontaneous rupture of the ear drum may occur, resulting in temporary or permanent hearing loss. The nurse needs to stress that medication should be used exactly as prescribed for the entire course of therapy.

The following information may be given to the patient when an ear ointment or solution is prescribed:

- Wash the hands thoroughly before cleansing the area around the ear (when necessary) and instilling ear drops or ointment.
- If the solution is cool or cold, warm to room temperature by holding solution in the hand for 1 to 2 minutes before administering.
- Instill the prescribed number of drops in the ear. Do not put the applicator or dropper tip in the ear or allow the tip to become contaminated from the fingers or other sources.
- Immediately after use, replace the cap or dropper and refrigerate the solution if so stated on the label.
- If the drops are in a suspension form, shake the container well for 10 seconds before using.
- Keep the head tilted or lie on the untreated side for approximately 5 minutes to allow the solution to remain in contact with the ear. Excess solution and solution running out of the ear can be wiped off with a tissue.
- Do not insert anything into the ear canal before or after applying the prescribed drug unless advised to do so by the primary health care provider. At times a soft cotton plug may be inserted into the affected ear.
- Complete a full course of treatment with the prescribed drug to achieve satisfactory results.
- Do not use nonprescription ear products during or after treatment unless such use has been approved by the primary health care provider.
- Remember that temporary changes in hearing or a feeling of fullness in the ear may occur for a short time after the drug has been instilled.
- Notify the primary health care provider if symptoms do not improve or become worse.

DRUGS USED TO REMOVE CERUMEN.

- Do not use if ear drainage, discharge, pain, or irritation occurs.
- Do not use for more than 4 days. If excessive cerumen remains, consult the primary health care provider.

- Any wax remaining after the treatment may be removed by gently flushing the ear with warm water using a soft rubber bulb ear syringe.
- If dizziness occurs, consult the primary health care provider.

EVALUATION

- Therapeutic effect is achieved.
- Adverse reactions are identified, reported to the primary health care provider, and managed successfully with appropriate nursing interventions:
  ☑ No evidence of infection is seen.
  ☑ Anxiety is managed successfully.
- Patient and family demonstrate an understanding of the drug regimen.

• OPHTHALMIC PREPARATIONS

Various types of preparations are used for treating **ophthalmic** (eye) disorders, such as glaucoma, to lower the **intraocular pressure** (IOP; the pressure within the eye); and to treat bacterial or viral infections of the eye, inflammatory conditions, and symptoms of allergy related to the eye.

Glaucoma

Glaucoma is a condition of the eye in which there is an increase in the IOP, causing progressive atrophy of the optic nerve with deterioration of vision and, if untreated, blindness. The eye's lens, iris, and cornea are continuously bathed and nourished by a fluid called *aqueous humor*. As aqueous humor is produced, excess fluid normally flows out through a complex network of tissue called *trabecular meshwork*. An angle is formed where the trabeculum and iris meet. This forms a filtration angle that maintains the normal pressure within the eye by allowing excess aqueous humor to leave the anterior chamber of the eye (Fig. 54.2).

The higher the IOP, the greater the risk of optic nerve damage, visual loss, and blindness. There are two types of

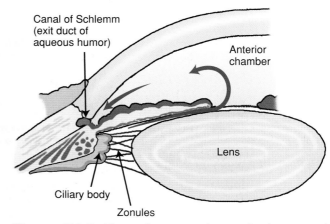

Figure 54.2 Flow of aqueous humor in the normal eye.

glaucoma: angle-closure glaucoma and open-angle, or chronic, glaucoma. In chronic or open-angle glaucoma, the angle that permits the drainage of aqueous humor appears to be normal but does not function properly. In angle-closure glaucoma, the iris blocks the trabecular meshwork and limits the flow of aqueous humor from the anterior chamber of the eye. This limitation of outflow causes an accumulation of intraocular fluid, followed by increased IOP. Some individuals have an anatomic defect that causes the angle to be more narrow than normal, but do not have any symptoms and do not develop glaucoma under normal circumstances. However, certain situations, such as medication that causes dilation of the eye, fear, or pain, may precipitate an attack. The aim of treatment in glaucoma is to lower the IOP. The Summary Drug Table: Selected Ophthalmic Preparations provides examples of the drugs used to treat both glaucoma and other ophthalmic problems.

The incidence of adverse reactions associated with the ophthalmic drugs is usually low. Because small amounts of the ophthalmic preparation may be absorbed systemically, some of the adverse effects associated with systemic administration of the particular drug may be observed. Some ophthalmic preparations produce momentary stinging or burning on instillation.

Actions and Uses

α₂-Adrenergic Drugs

Brimonidine is an alpha₂ (a₂)-adrenergic receptor agonist used to lower IOP in patients with open-angle glaucoma or ocular hypertension. This drug acts to reduce production of aqueous humor and increase the outflow of aqueous humor.

Sympathomimetic Drugs

Sympathomimetics have α- and beta (β)-adrenergic activity (see Chapter 24 for a detailed discussion of adrenergic drugs). These drugs lower the IOP by increasing the outflow of aqueous humor in the eye and are used to treat glaucoma. Apraclonidine is used to control or prevent postoperative elevations in IOP.

α-Adrenergic Blocking Drugs

Dapiprazole acts by blocking the α-adrenergic receptor in smooth muscle and produces **miosis** (constriction of the pupil) through an effect on the dilator muscle of the iris. The drug is used primarily after ophthalmic examinations to reverse the diagnostic **mydriasis** (dilation of the pupil).

(text continues on page 562)

Summary Drug Table SELECTED OPHTHALMIC PREPARATIONS

Generic Name	Trade Name	Uses	Dosage Ranges
α₂-Adrenergic Agonist			
brimonidine *brih-moe'-nih-deen*	Alphagan	Lowers IOP in patients with open-angle (chronic) glaucoma	1 gtt in affected eye(s) TID
Sympathomimetics			
apraclonidine *app-rah-kloe'-nih-deen*	Iopidine	1% Solution: control or prevention of postoperative elevations in IOP 5% Solution: short-term therapy in patients receiving maximal medical therapy who require additional IOP reduction	1% Solution: 1 gtt in operative eye 1 hr before surgery and 1 gtt immediately after surgery 5% Solution: 1–2 gtt in the affected eye(s) TID
dipivefrin *dye-pih'-veh-frin*	Propine, AKPro	Open-angle glaucoma	1 gtt into affected eye(s) q 12 hr
epinephrine *epp-ih-neff'-rin*	Epifrin, Glaucon Solution	Open-angle (chronic) glaucoma; may be used in combination with miotics, beta blockers, or carbonic anhydrase inhibitors	1–2 gtt into affected eye(s) daily or BID
α-Adrenergic Blocking Drugs			
dapiprazole *dap-ih-pray'-zoll*	Rev-Eyes	Reverse diagnostic mydriasis after ophthalmic examination	2 gtt into the conjunctiva of each eye, followed 5 min later by an additional 2 gtt
β-Adrenergic Blocking Drugs			
betaxolol *beh-tax'-oh-lahl*	Betoptic, Betoptic S	Chronic open-angle glaucoma, ocular hypertension	1–2 gtt in the affected eye(s) BID
carteolol *car'-tee-oh-lahl*	Ocupress	Same as betaxolol	1 gtt in affected eye(s) TID

(table continues on page 559)

Summary Drug Table SELECTED OPHTHALMIC PREPARATIONS (continued)

Generic Name	Trade Name	Uses	Dosage Ranges
levobetaxolol *lee'-voe-beh-tax'-oh-lahl*	Betaxon	Same as betaxolol	1 gtt in affected eye(s) BID
levobunolol *lee'-voe-byoo'-noe-lahl*	AKBeta, Betagan Liquifilm	Same as betaxolol	0.5% Solution: 1–2 gtt in affected eye(s) daily 0.25% Solution: 1–2 gtt in affected eye(s) BID
metipranolol *meh-tih-pran'-oh-lahl*	OptiPranolol	Treatment of elevated IOP in patients with ocular hypertension or open-angle glaucoma	1 gtt in affected eye(s) BID
timolol *tih'-moe-lahl*	Betimol, Timoptic, Timoptic-XE	Reduces IOP in ocular hypertension or open-angle glaucoma	1 gtt in affected eye(s) daily or BID Gel: invert the closed container and shake once before each use; administer 1 gtt/day
Miotics, Direct Acting and Cholinesterase Inhibitor			
carbachol *car'-bah-koll*	Carboptic, Isopto Carbachol	Glaucoma	1–2 gtt up to TID
pilocarpine *pye-loe-car'-peen*	Isopto Carpine, Pilopine HS	Glaucoma, preoperative and postoperative intraocular hypertension	Solution: 1–2 gtt in affected eye(s) Gel: apply a 0.5-in ribbon in the lower conjunctival sac of affected eye(s) daily at bedtime
echothiophate iodide *eck-oh-thye'-oh-fate* *eyé-oh-dyde*	Phospholine iodide	Chronic open-angle glaucoma, accommodative esotropia	Glaucoma: 2 doses/day in the morning and at bedtime or 1 dose every other day Esotropia: 1 gtt daily
Carbonic Anhydrase Inhibitors			
brinzolamide *brin-zoll'-ah-myde*	Azopt	Open-angle glaucoma, ocular hypertension	1 gtt in affected eye(s) TID
dorzolamide *dore-zoll'-ah-myde*	Trusopt	Open-angle glaucoma, ocular hypertension	1 gtt in affected eye(s) TID
Prostaglandin Agonists			
latanoprost *lah-tan'-oh-prahst*	Xalatan	First-line treatment of open-angle glaucoma, ocular hypertension	1 gtt in affected eye(s) daily in the evening
travoprost *trav'-oh-prahst*	Travatan	Reduction of increased IOP in patients with glaucoma who do not respond to or cannot take other drugs to lower IOP	1 gtt in affected eye(s) daily in the evening
bimatoprost *bih-mat'-oh-prahst*	Lumigan	Same as travoprost	1 gtt in affected eye(s) daily in the evening
unoprostone isopropyl *yoo-noh-pross'-toan*	Rescula	Same as travoprost	1 gtt in affected eye(s) BID
Combinations Used to Treat Glaucoma			
brimonidine/timolol	Combigan	Glaucoma	1 gtt in the affected eye(s) 2 times daily
dorzolamide/timolol *dore-zoll'-ah-myde*	Cosopt	Open-angle glaucoma and ocular hypertension	1 gtt into the affected eye(s) BID
Mast Cell Stabilizers			
nedocromil *neh-doe'-roe-mill*	Alocril	Allergic conjunctivitis	1–2 gtt in each eye BID

Otic and Ophthalmic Preparations

(table continues on page 560)

Summary Drug Table SELECTED OPHTHALMIC PREPARATIONS (continued)

Generic Name	Trade Name	Uses	Dosage Ranges
pemirolast peh-meer'-oh-last	Alamast	Allergic conjunctivitis	1–2 gtt in each eye QID
Nonsteroidal Anti-Inflammatory Drugs			
bromfenac brom'-fen-ak	Xibrom	Postoperative pain and inflammation after cataract surgery	1 gtt BID
diclofenac dye-kloe'-fen-ak	Voltaren	Postoperative inflammation after cataract surgery	1 gtt QID
flurbiprofen floor-bye'-proe-fen	Ocufen	Inhibition of intraoperative miosis	1 gtt q 30 min beginning 2 hr before surgery (total of 4 gtt)
ketorolac keh-tor'-oh-lak	Acular	Relief of ocular itching due to seasonal allergies, pain after corneal refractive surgery	Allergies: 1 drop QID Postoperative pain: 1 gtt in operated eye
nepafenac neh-pah'-fen-ak	Nevanac	Postoperative pain and inflammation after cataract surgery	1 gtt TID
Corticosteroids			
dexamethasone dex-ah-meth'-ah-soan	AK-Dex, Maxidex	Treatment of inflammatory conditions of the conjunctiva, eyelid, cornea, anterior segment of the eye	Solution: 1–2 gtt q hr during the day and q 2 hr at night, reduced to 1 gtt q 4 hr when response noted, then 1 gtt TID or QID Ointment: thin coating in lower conjunctival sac TID or QID
fluorometholone floo-roh-meth'-oh-loan	Flarex, Fluor-Op	Treatment of inflammatory conditions of the conjunctiva, lid, cornea, anterior segment of the eye	Suspension: 1–2 gtt BID–QID, may increase to 2 gtt q 2 hr Ointment: thin coating in lower conjunctival sac 1 to 3 times daily (up to 1 application q4hr)
loteprednol loe-teh-pred'-noll	Alrex, Lotemax	Allergic conjunctivitis	1–2 gtt QID
prednisolone pred-niss'-oh-loan	AK-Pred, Pred Forte, Pred Mild	Treatment of inflammatory conditions of the conjunctiva, lid, cornea, anterior segment of the eye	1–2 gtt/hr during the day and q 2 hr at night, reduced to 1 gtt q 4 hr, then 1 gtt TID or QID Suspensions: 1–2 gtt BID–QID
Antibiotics			
azithromycin ah-zith-roe-mye'-sin	AzaSite	Treatment of eye infections	See package insert
bacitracin bass-ih-tray'-sin	AK-Tracin	Same as azithromycin	See package insert
chloramphenicol klor-am-fen'-ih-koll	Chloromycetin	Same as azithromycin	See package insert
ciprofloxacin sih-proe-flox'-ah-sin	Ciloxan	Same as azithromycin	See package insert
erythromycin eh-rith-roe-mye'-sin	Ilotycin	Same as azithromycin	See package insert
gatifloxacin gah-tah-flox'-ah-sin	Zymar	Same as azithromycin	Days 1 and 2: instill 1 gtt in affected eye(s) q 2 hr while awake, up to 8 times daily Days 3–7: instill 1 gtt in affected eye up to QID while awake

(table continues on page 561)

Summary Drug Table SELECTED OPHTHALMIC PREPARATIONS (continued)

Generic Name	Trade Name	Uses	Dosage Ranges
gentamicin jen-tah-mye'-sin	Garamycin, Gentacidin, Gentak	Same as azithromycin	See package insert
levofloxacin lee-voe-flox'-ah-sin	Quixin	Same as azithromycin	Days 1 and 2: instill 1–2 gtt in affected eye(s) q 2 hr while awake, up to 8 times daily Days 3–7: instill 1–2 gtt in affected eye up to QID while awake
moxifloxacin mox-ah-flox'-ah-sin	Vigamox	Same as azithromycin	Adults and children at least 1 year of age: 1 drop in affected eye TID for 7 days
norfloxacin nor-flox'-ah-sin	Chibroxin	Same as azithromycin	Adults and children age 1 year and older: 1 or 2 gtt applied topically in the affected eye(s) QID for up to 7 days; dosage may be 1 or 2 gtt q 2 hr during waking hours the first day of treatment if the infection is severe
ofloxacin oh-flox'-ah-sin	Ocuflox	Same as azithromycin, corneal ulcers	Bacterial conjunctivitis: days 1 and 2: 1–2 gtt q 2–4 hr in the affected eye(s) Days 3–7: 1–2 gtt QID Bacterial corneal ulcer: Days 1 and 2: 1–2 gtt into the affected eye q 30 min while awake; awaken approximately q 4–6 hr and instill 1–2 gtt Days 3 through 7–9: instill 1–2 drops QID
polymyxin B pah-lee-mix'-in		Same as azithromycin	See package insert
tobramycin toe-brah-mye'-sin	Tobrex, Defy	Same as azithromycin	See package insert
sulfacetamide sul-fah-see'-tah-myde	Sulster, AK-Sulf, Bleph-10, Ocusulf-10	Ocular infections, trachoma	Ocular infections: 1–2 gtt q 1–4 hr Trachoma: 2 gtt q 2 hr Ointments: 0.5 in into lower conjunctival sac TID or QID
sulfisoxazole sul-fah-sox'-ah-zoll	Gantrisin	Ocular infections, trachoma	Ocular infections: 1–2 gtt q 1–4 hr Trachoma: 2 gtt q 2 hr
Silver Compound			
silver nitrate nye'-trate		Prevention of ophthalmia neonatorum	2 gtt of 1% solution in each eye
Antiviral Drugs			
ganciclovir gan-sih'-kloe-veer	Vitrasert	Cytomegalovirus (CMV) retinitis	Implant used for 5–8 months
idoxuridine eye-dox-yoor'-ih-deen	Herplex	Herpes simplex keratitis	1 gtt q hr during the day and q 2 hr at night
trifluridine tri-floor'-ih-deen	Viroptic	Keratoconjunctivitis keratitis, epithelial keratitis	Adults and children over 6 years: 1 gtt onto the corners of affected eye(s) while awake Maximum daily dose: 9 gtt until corneal ulcer has completely re-epithelialized, treat for an additional 7 day with 1 gtt q4hr for a maximum of 5 gtt/day

(table continues on page 562)

Otic and Ophthalmic Preparations

Summary Drug Table SELECTED OPHTHALMIC PREPARATIONS (continued)

Generic Name	Trade Name	Uses	Dosage Ranges
vidarabine *vye-dare'-ah-been*	Vira-A	Treatment of herpes simplex keratitis and conjunctivitis	0.5 in of ointment into lower conjunctival sac 5 times daily at 3-hr intervals
Antifungal Drug			
natamycin *nah-tah-mye'-sin*	Natacyn	Fungal infections of the eye	1 gtt q 1–2 hr
Vasoconstrictors/Mydriatics			
oxymetazoline *ox-ih-met-az'-oh-leen*	OcuClear, Visine LR	Relief of redness of eye due to minor irritation	1–2 gtt q 6 hr
phenylephrine *fen-ill-eff'-rin*	AK-Dilate 2.5%, Neo-Synephrine 10%, AK-Nephrin	0.12% for relief of redness of eye due to minor irritation; 2.5% and 10% for treatment of uveitis, glaucoma; refraction procedures, before eye surgery	0.12%: 1–2 gtt up to QID 2.5% and 10%: 1–2 gtt in the eye up to QID (may have up to 8 gtt/day)
tetrahydrozoline *tet-trah-hye-drah'-zoh-leen*	Murine Plus Eye Drops, Visine	Relief of eye redness due to minor irritation	1–2 gtt up to QID
Cycloplegics/Mydriatics			
atropine *at'-troe-peen*	Isopto-Atropine	Mydriasis/cycloplegia	1–2 gtt up to TID
homatropine hydrobromide *hoe-mah'-troe-peen*	Isopto Homatropine	Mydriasis/cycloplegia	1–2 gtt q 3–4 hr
Ocular Lubricants			
benzalkonium chloride *benz-al-koe'-nee-um*	Artificial Tears	Treatment of dry eyes	1–2 gtt TID or QID
0.25% glycerin, EDTA sodium chloride, benzalkonium chloride	Eye-Lube-A	Treatment of dry eyes	1–2 gtt TID or QID

β-Adrenergic Blocking Drugs

The β-adrenergic blocking drugs decrease the rate of production of aqueous humor and thereby lower the IOP. These drugs are used to treat glaucoma.

Miotics, Direct Acting, and Cholinesterase Inhibitors

Miotics contract the pupil of the eye (miosis), resulting in an increase in the space through which the aqueous humor flows, decreasing IOP. The miotics were, for a number of years, the drug of choice for glaucoma. These drugs have lost that first choice treatment status to the β-adrenergic blocking drugs.

Carbonic Anhydrase Inhibitors

Carbonic anhydrase is an enzyme found in many tissues of the body, including the eye. Inhibition of carbonic anhydrase

in the eye decreases aqueous humor secretion, resulting in a decrease of IOP. These drugs are used in the treatment of elevated IOP seen in open-angle glaucoma. Except for dorzolamide and brinzolamide, carbonic anhydrase inhibitors are administered systemically.

Prostaglandin Agonists

Prostaglandin agonists are used to lower IOP in patients with open-angle glaucoma and ocular hypertension in patients who do not tolerate other IOP-lowering medications or have an insufficient response to these medications. These drugs act to lower IOP by increasing the outflow of aqueous humor through the trabecular meshwork.

Mast Cell Stabilizers

Mast cell stabilizers currently approved for ophthalmic use are nedocromil and pemirolast. These drugs are used to prevent itching of the eyes caused by allergic conjunctivitis. Mast cell stabilizers inhibit the antigen-induced release of inflammatory mediators (e.g., histamine) from human mast cells.

Nonsteroidal Anti-Inflammatory Drugs

Nonsteroidal anti-inflammatory drugs (NSAIDs) inhibit prostaglandin synthesis (see Chapter 15 for a discussion of the NSAIDs), thereby exerting anti-inflammatory action. These drugs are used to treat postoperative pain and inflammation after cataract surgery, for the relief of itching of the eyes caused by seasonal allergies, and during eye surgery to prevent miosis).

Corticosteroids

These drugs possess anti-inflammatory activity and are used for inflammatory conditions, such as allergic conjunctivitis, keratitis, herpes zoster keratitis, and inflammation of the iris. Corticosteroids also may be used after injury to the cornea or after corneal transplantation to prevent rejection.

Antibiotics and Sulfonamides

Antibiotics possess antibacterial activity and are used in the treatment of eye infections. Sulfonamides possess a bacteriostatic effect against a wide range of gram-positive and gram-negative microorganisms. They are used in treating conjunctivitis, corneal ulcer, and other superficial infections of the eye. See Chapter 6 for additional information on the sulfonamides.

Silver

Silver possesses antibacterial activity against gram-positive and gram-negative microorganisms. Silver proteinate is occasionally used in the treatment of eye infections. Silver nitrate is occasionally used to prevent gonorrheal ophthalmia neonatorum (gonorrheal infection of the newborn's eyes). Ophthalmic tetracycline and erythromycin have largely replaced the use of silver nitrate in newborns.

Antiviral Drugs

Antiviral drugs interfere with viral reproduction by altering DNA synthesis. These drugs are used in the treatment of herpes simplex infections of the eye, treatment of immunocompromised patients with CMV retinitis, and for the prevention of CMV retinitis in patients undergoing transplantation.

Antifungal Drugs

Natamycin is the only ophthalmic antifungal in use. This drug possesses antifungal activity against a variety of yeast and other fungi.

Vasoconstrictors/Mydriatics

Mydriatics are drugs that dilate the pupil (mydriasis), constrict superficial blood vessels of the sclera, and decrease the formation of aqueous humor. Depending on the specific drug and strength, these drugs may be used before eye surgery in the treatment of glaucoma, for relief of minor eye irritation, and to dilate the pupil for examination of the eye.

Cycloplegic Mydriatics

Cycloplegic mydriatics cause mydriasis and **cycloplegia** (paralysis of the ciliary muscle, resulting in an inability to focus the eye). These drugs are used in the treatment of inflammatory conditions of the iris and uveal tract of the eye and for examination of the eye.

Artificial Tear Solutions

These products lubricate the eyes and are used for conditions such as dry eyes and eye irritation caused by inadequate tear production. Inactive ingredients may be found in some preparations. Examples of these inactive ingredients include preservatives, antioxidants, which prevent deterioration of the product, and drugs that slow drainage of the drug from the eye into the tear duct. Examples of the types of eye preparations are found in the Summary Drug Table: Selected Ophthalmic Preparations.

Adverse Reactions

Drugs to Treat Glaucoma

Drugs used to treat glaucoma may cause transient local reactions and systemic reactions. Although side effects are usually mild they may include:

• Locally in or near the eye—burning and stinging, headache, visual blurring, tearing, foreign body sensation, ocular allergic reactions, and ocular itching.
• Systemic effects include fatigue and drowsiness, palpations, nausea.

Corticosteroids

Local adverse reactions associated with administration of the corticosteroid ophthalmic preparations include elevated IOP with optic nerve damage, loss of visual acuity, cataract formation, delayed wound healing, secondary ocular infection, exacerbation of corneal infections, dry eyes, ptosis, blurred vision, discharge, ocular pain, foreign body sensation, and pruritus.

Antibiotics, Sulfonamides, and Silver

The antibiotic and sulfonamide ophthalmics are usually well tolerated, and few adverse reactions are seen. Local adverse reactions include occasional transient irritation, burning, itching, stinging, inflammation, and blurred vision. With prolonged or repeated use, a superinfection may occur.

Antiviral Drugs

• Administration of the antiviral ophthalmics may cause local reactions such as irritation, pain, pruritus, inflammation, edema of the eyes or eyelids, foreign body sensation, and corneal clouding.
• Systemic reactions include photophobia and allergic reactions.

Antifungal Drugs

Adverse reactions are rare. Occasional local irritation to the eye may occur.

Artificial Tear Solutions

Adverse reactions are rare, but on occasion redness or irritation may occur.

Contraindications, Precautions, and Interactions

Drugs Used to Treat Glaucoma

These drugs are contraindicated in patients with hypersensitivity to the drug or any component of the drug. Adrenergic-based drugs are contraindicated in patients taking monoamine oxidase inhibitors (MAOIs). Epinephrine is contraindicated in patients with narrow-angle glaucoma, or patients with a narrow angle but no glaucoma, and aphakia (absence of the crystalline lens of the eye). Patients wearing soft contact lenses should be cautioned, because the preservative in the drug may be absorbed by soft contact lenses and discoloration of the lenses may occur. The drug is used cautiously during pregnancy (epinephrine, category B; and apraclonidine, pregnancy category C) and lactation and in patients with cardiovascular disease, depression, cerebral or coronary insufficiency, hypertension, diabetes, hyperthyroidism, or Raynaud's phenomenon. When brimonidine is used with central nervous system (CNS) depressants, such as alcohol, barbiturates, opiates, sedatives, or anesthetics, there is a risk for an additive CNS depressant effect. Use the drugs cautiously in combination with antihypertensive drugs and cardiac glycosides, because a synergistic effect may occur.

Adrenergic blocking drugs are contraindicated in patients with bronchial asthma, obstructive pulmonary disease, sinus bradycardia, heart block, cardiac failure, or cardiogenic shock, and in patients with hypersensitivity to the drug or any components of the drug. These drugs should not be used in conditions in which pupil constriction is not desirable, such as in acute iritis (inflammation of the iris), and in the treatment of IOP in open-angle glaucoma.

These drugs are in pregnancy category C (dapiprazole is category B) and are used cautiously during pregnancy and lactation and in patients with cardiovascular disease, diabetes (may mask the symptoms of hypoglycemia), and hyperthyroidism (may mask symptoms of hyperthyroidism). The patient taking β-adrenergic blocking drugs for ophthalmic reasons may experience increased or additive effects when the drugs are administered with the oral β-adrenergic blockers. Coadministration of timolol and calcium antagonists may cause hypotension, left ventricular failure, and condition disturbances within the heart. There is a potential additive hypotensive effect when the β-adrenergic blocking ophthalmic drugs are administered with the phenothiazines.

Miotic drugs are contraindicated in patients with hypersensitivity to the drug or any component of the drug and in conditions where constriction is undesirable (e.g., iritis, uveitis, and acute inflammatory disease of the anterior chamber). The drugs are used cautiously in patients with corneal abrasion, pregnancy (category C), lactation, cardiac failure, bronchial asthma, peptic ulcer, hyperthyroidism, gastrointestinal spasm, urinary tract infection, Parkinson's disease, renal or hepatic impairment, recent myocardial infarction, hypotension, or hypertension. These drugs are also used cautiously in patients with angle-closure glaucoma, because miotics occasionally can precipitate angle-closure glaucoma by increasing the resistance to aqueous flow from posterior to anterior chamber.

Cholinesterase inhibitors are used cautiously in patients with myasthenia gravis (may cause additive adverse effects), before and after surgery, and in patients with chronic angle-closure (narrow-angle) glaucoma or those with anatomically narrow angles (may cause papillary block and increase the angle blockage). When cholinesterase inhibitors are administered with systemic anticholinesterase drugs, there is a risk for additive effects. Individuals such as farmers, warehouse workers, or gardeners working with carbamate–organophosphate insecticides or pesticides are at risk for systemic effects of cholinesterase inhibitors from absorption of the pesticide or insecticide through the respiratory tract or the skin. Individuals working with pesticides or insecticides containing carbamate–organophosphate and taking a cholinesterase inhibitor should be advised to wear respiratory masks, change clothes frequently, and wash exposed clothes thoroughly.

Drugs Used to Treat Inflammation

These drugs are contraindicated in patients with hypersensitivity to the drug or any component of the drug. The mast cell stabilizers are used cautiously in patients who wear contact lenses (preservative may be absorbed by the soft contact lenses). NSAIDs are used cautiously in patients with bleeding tendencies. When used topically, there is less risk of interactions with drugs or other substances. There is a possibility of a cross-sensitivity reaction when NSAIDs are administered to patients allergic to salicylates. Corticosteroids and antibiotics are used cautiously in patients with sulfite sensitivity, because an allergic-type reaction may result. The corticosteroid ophthalmic preparations are used cautiously in patients with infectious conditions of the eye. Prolonged use of corticosteroids may result in elevated IOP and optic nerve damage. The antibiotic and sulfonamide ophthalmics are contraindicated in patients with epithelial herpes simplex keratitis, varicella, mycobacterial infection of the eye, and fungal diseases of the eye. These drugs are pregnancy category B or C drugs and are used cautiously during pregnancy and lactation.

Artificial tears are contraindicated in patients who are allergic to any component of the solution. No precautions or interactions have been reported.

❧ HERBAL ALERT

Bilberry, also known as whortleberry, blueberry, trackleberry, and huckleberry, is a shrub with bluish flowers that appear in early spring and ripen in July and August. A beneficial use appears to be in promoting healthy eyes. Other benefits reportedly include improved visual acuity, improved night vision, prevention of free radical damage, and promotion of capillary blood flow in the eyes, hands, and feet. Bilberry extract has been used in treating nonspecific, mild diarrhea and as a mouthwash or gargle for inflammation of the mouth and throat. Bilberry fruit is a safe substance with no known adverse reactions or toxicity. There are no known contraindications to its use as directed unless the individual has an allergy to bilberry. The dosage of standard extract is 80 to 160 mg per day.

NURSING PROCESS
PATIENT RECEIVING AN OPHTHALMIC PREPARATION

ASSESSMENT

Preadministration Assessment
The primary health care provider examines the eye and external structures surrounding the eye and prescribes the drug indicated to treat the disorder. The nurse performs a baseline assessment by examining the eye for irritation, redness, and the presence of any exudate and carefully documents the findings in the patient's record. A purulent discharge is often found with infection of the eye. Pruritus (itching) is often present with allergic conditions of the eye. The nurse reviews the primary health care provider's diagnosis and comments, takes a general patient health history, and evaluates the patient's ability to carry out the activities of daily living, especially if the patient is elderly or has limited vision. The nurse also assesses the patient for any hypersensitivities to the specific medication being administered and notes any cautions to the drug as well.

Ongoing Assessment
During the ongoing assessment the nurse observes for a therapeutic drug effect and reports any increase in symptoms and the presence of any redness, irritation, or pain in the eye. Patients admitted for treatment of acute glaucoma should be assessed every 2 hours for relief of pain. Pain in the eye may indicate increased IOP.

NURSING DIAGNOSES

Drug-specific nursing diagnoses include the following:

- ❑ **Disturbed Sensory Perception: Visual** related to adverse drug effects or disease condition
- ❑ **Risk for Injury** related to adverse reactions to drug therapy (blurring of the vision)
- ❑ **Acute Pain** related to eye disorder or adverse reaction to medication
- ❑ **Anxiety** related to eye pain or discomfort, diagnosis, other factors

Nursing diagnoses related to drug administration are discussed in Chapter 4.

PLANNING

The expected outcomes of the patient depend on the reason for administration but may include an optimal response to therapy, support of patient needs related to

the management of adverse reactions, minimized anxiety, and an understanding of the application and use of an ophthalmic preparation (see the Patient Teaching for Improved Patient Outcomes: Instilling an Ophthalmic Preparation).

IMPLEMENTATION

Promoting an Optimal Response to Therapy
Before instillation, ophthalmic solutions and ointments can be warmed in the hand for a few minutes. The nurse checks the primary health care provider's order and the drug label carefully when instilling any ophthalmic preparation. The drug label must indicate that the preparation is for ophthalmic use. The nurse checks the medication to make sure the solution is clear and not discolored. Ophthalmic ointments are applied to the eyelids or dropped into the lower conjunctival sac; ophthalmic solutions are dropped into the middle of the lower conjunctival sac (Fig. 54.3). The nurse avoids touching the eye with the tip of the dropper or container to prevent contamination of the product. When eye solutions are instilled, the nurse applies gentle pressure on the inner canthus to delay drainage of the drug down the tear duct. This prevents the drug from being absorbed systemically.

The primary health care provider is consulted regarding use of this technique before the first dose is instilled, because this technique can be potentially dangerous in some eye conditions—for example, after recent eye surgery. When two eye drops are prescribed for use at the same time, the nurse waits at least 5 minutes before instilling the second drug. This helps prevent dilution of the drug and loss of some therapeutic effect from tearing.

In some instances, the patient may have been using an ophthalmic preparation for glaucoma for a long time, and the primary health care provider may allow the hos-

Figure 54.3 Instilling eye medication. While the patient looks upward, the nurse gently pulls the lower lid down and instills the correct number of drops into the lower conjunctival sac.

pitalized patient to instill his or her own eye drops. When this is stated on the patient's order sheet, the nurse can leave the drug at the patient's bedside. Even though the drug is self-administered, the nurse checks the patient at intervals to be sure that the drug is instilled at the prescribed time using the correct technique for ophthalmic instillation. Patients using the pilocarpine ocular therapeutic system must have the system replaced every 7 days. The system is inserted at bedtime because **myopia** (nearsightedness) occurs for several hours after insertion.

When a patient is scheduled for eye surgery, it is most important that the eye drops ordered by the primary health care provider are instilled at the correct time. This is especially important when the purpose of the drug is to change the size of the pupil.

> ■ **NURSING ALERT**
>
> Only preparations labeled as "ophthalmic" are instilled in the eye. The nurse must check the label of the preparation carefully for the name of the drug, the percentage of the preparation, and a statement indicating that the preparation is for ophthalmic use.

Monitoring and Managing Patient Needs

DISTURBED SENSORY PERCEPTION: VISUAL. Although adverse reactions are rare, these drugs can cause visual impairment such as blurring of vision and local irritation and burning. These reactions are most often self-limiting and resolve if the patient waits a few minutes. Visual impairment that does not clear within 30 minutes after therapy should be reported to the primary health care provider.

RISK FOR INJURY. When the ophthalmic drugs produce blurring of vision, this can result in falls and other injuries. Keeping the patient's room dimly lit at night is helpful, because night vision may be decreased. Obstacles that may hinder ambulation or result in falls, such as slippers, chairs, and tables, are placed out of the way, especially during the night. The nurse warns patients to exercise care when getting out of bed when the vision is impaired by these drugs. If needed, the nurse provides assistance with ambulation to prevent injury from falls.

ACUTE PAIN. Pain can occur with eye conditions such as glaucoma and eye infections. Patients with acute glaucoma are assessed for relief of pain. Pain in the eye may indicate increased IOP and should be reported to the primary health care provider. Pain associated with infection should decrease with administration of medication. Any increase in pain or no decrease in the symptoms after 1 to 2 days of treatment should be reported to the primary health care provider. Headache and brow ache are associated with adverse reactions of some of the ophthalmic agents and are usually self-limiting.

ANXIETY. Eye injuries and some eye infections are very painful. Other eye conditions may result in discomfort or a loss of or change in vision. The patient with an eye disorder or injury usually has great concern about the effect the problem will have on his or her vision. The

nurse reassures the patient that every effort is being made to treat the disorder.

Educating the Patient and Family

The patient or a family member will require instruction in the technique of instilling an ophthalmic preparation (see Patient Teaching for Improved Patient Outcomes: Instilling an Ophthalmic Preparation). In addition, the nurse may give the following information to the patient and family member when an eye ointment or solution is prescribed:

- Eye preparations may cause a momentary stinging or burning sensation; this is normal.
- Temporary blurring of vision may occur. Avoid activities requiring visual acuity until vision returns to normal.
- If more than one topical ophthalmic drug is being used, administer the drugs at least 5 to 10 minutes apart or as directed by the physician.
- Complete a full course of treatment with the prescribed drug to achieve satisfactory results.
- Do not rub the eyes, and keep hands away from the eyes.
- Do not use nonprescription eye products during or after treatment unless such use has been approved by the primary health care provider.
- Some of these preparations cause sensitivity (photophobia) to light; to minimize this, wear sunglasses.
- Notify the primary health care provider if symptoms do not improve or if they worsen.

DRUGS TO TREAT GLAUCOMA
- May sting on instillation, especially the first few doses.
- Do not use if solution is brown or contains a precipitate.
- Do not use while wearing soft contact lenses.
- Headache or brow ache may occur.
- Report any decrease in visual acuity. Use caution when driving at night or performing activities in poor illumination.
- If using the ocular therapeutic system, check the system before retiring at night and on arising. Follow instructions in package insert.
- If more than one ophthalmic drug is being used, administer the drugs 5 minutes apart.
- Advise patient that changes may occur to the lashes—length, thickness, pigmentation, and number—in the eye being treated.
- The color of the iris may change because of an increase in the brown pigment. This may be more noticeable in patients with blue, green, gray-brown, or other light-colored eyes. This discoloration may be permanent.

DRUGS TO TREAT INFLAMMATION
- If improvement in the condition being treated does not occur within 2 days, or pain, redness, itching, or swelling of the eye occurs, notify the primary health care provider.

EVALUATION

- Therapeutic effect is achieved.
- Adverse reactions are identified, reported to the primary health care provider, and managed successfully with appropriate nursing interventions:
  - ☑ Patient has improved visual acuity.
  - ☑ No evidence of injury is seen.
  - ☑ Patient has minimal to no pain.
  - ☑ Anxiety is reduced.
- Patient and family demonstrate an understanding of the drug regimen.

Patient Teaching for Improved Patient Outcomes

Instilling an Ophthalmic Preparation

Many eye surgeries are performed in ambulatory clinics requiring the patient to instill eye drops or ointment at home. If the patient is unable to do so, a family member or friend may have to instill the preparation. The nurse uses the following guide to evaluate whether the patient or caregiver can properly instill the eye drops or ointment.

The patient or caregiver:

- ✓ Washes hands thoroughly before beginning.
- ✓ Holds bottle (drops) or tube (ointment) in hand for a few minutes before using.
- ✓ Cleanses the area around the eye of any secretions.
- ✓ Squeezes the eye dropper bulb to release and then refill the dropper, squeezes the bottle to fill the drop chamber, or squeezes ointment to tip of the tube.
- ✓ Tilts head slightly backward and toward the eye to be treated.
- ✓ Pulls affected lower lid down.
- ✓ Positions dropper, bottle, or tube over lower conjunctival sac.
- ✓ Steadies hand by resting fingers against cheek or by resting base of hand on cheek.
- ✓ Looks up at ceiling and squeezes dropper, bottle, or tube.
- ✓ Drops ordered number of drops into the middle of lower conjunctival sac; instills prescribed amount of ointment to eyelid or lower conjunctival sac.
- ✓ Closes eye briefly and gently and releases lower lid (does not squeeze eyes shut after instilling the drug).
- ✓ Places finger on inner canthus to avoid absorption through the tear duct (when instilling drops and only if ordered).
- ✓ Repeats procedure with other eye (if ordered).
- ✓ If more than one type of ophthalmic preparation is being instilled, waits the recommended time before instilling the second drug (usually 5 minutes for drops and 10–15 minutes for ointment).
- ✓ Replaces the cap of the eye preparation immediately after instilling the eye drops or ointment. Does not touch the tip of the dropper, bottle, or tube.

THINK CRITICALLY: PHARMACOLOGY IN PRACTICE

1. Janna Wong, a 16-year-old high school student, recently switched from eyeglasses to contact lenses. She is experiencing minor eye irritation. The primary health care provider has prescribed eye drops. Janna is fidgety and tells you she just can't put those drops in her eyes. Design an age-appropriate teaching plan for this individual.

● Test Your Knowledge

1. Which of the following adverse reactions would the nurse suspect in a patient receiving prolonged treatment with an antibiotic otic drug?
   A. Congestive heart failure
   B. Superinfection
   C. Anemia
   D. Hypersensitivity reactions

2. When administering an ophthalmic solution, the drug is instilled into the ___.
   A. inner canthus
   B. upper conjunctival sac
   C. lower conjunctival sac
   D. upper canthus

3. Which of the following instructions would be included in a teaching plan for the patient prescribed an ophthalmic solution?
   A. Squeeze the eyes tightly after the solution is instilled.
   B. Immediately wipe the eye using pressure to squeeze out excess medication.
   C. After the drug is instilled, remain upright with the head bent slightly forward for about 2 minutes.
   D. A temporary stinging or burning may be felt at the time the drug is instilled.

● Prepare for the NCLEX

1. What is the rationale for warming an otic solution that has been refrigerated before instilling the drops into the patient's ear?
   A. The drug becomes thick when refrigerated, and warming liquefies the solution.
   B. It helps to prevent dizziness on instillation.
   C. A cold solution can significantly increase the patient's blood pressure.
   D. A cold solution could damage the tympanic membrane.

● Calculate Medication Dosages

1. The primary health care provider orders 0.5 mL of Burow solution for ear pain. If the dropper used delivers 0.1 mL/drop, how many drops should be instilled into the ear?

To check your answers, see Appendix E.

thePoint *For more NCLEX questions, log on to http://thepoint.lww.com to access more than 1000 questions.*

55

Fluids, Electrolytes and Parenteral Therapy

LEARNING OBJECTIVES

On completion of this chapter, the student will:

1. List the types and uses of solutions used in the parenteral management of body fluids.
2. List the types of intravenous administration of a solution or electrolyte used in the management of body fluids.
3. Describe the calculations used to establish intravenous flow rates.
4. List the types and uses of electrolytes used in the management of electrolyte imbalances.
5. Discuss the more common signs and symptoms of electrolyte imbalance.
6. Discuss preadministration and ongoing assessment activities the nurse should perform with the patient administered an electrolyte or a IV solution to manage body fluids.
7. List nursing diagnoses particular to a patient receiving an electrolyte or a solution to manage body fluids.
8. Discuss ways to promote an optimal response to therapy and important points to keep in mind when educating patients about the use of an electrolyte or a solution to manage body fluids.

Fluid makes up a major portion of our bodily tissues. When individuals become ill, they may lose excess amounts of fluid or not feel well enough to maintain the daily intake of fluid needed for basic survival. Without fluids, the body's ability to transported oxygen and nutrients to the various tissues is compromised. Individual cells or organs are not able to function and the person becomes even more ill. Various solutions are used in the management of body fluids. These solutions are used when the body cannot sustain the fluid or electrolyte balance needed for normal functioning.

Parenteral Management of Body Fluids

Parenteral administration includes the injecting of drugs or solutions directly into a vein. In the acute care or urgent care setting, solutions used to manage body fluids are usually administered intravenously (IV). Intravenous replacement solutions are used for the following:

- As a parenteral source of electrolytes, calories, or water for hydration
- To facilitate nutrition and maintain electrolyte balance when the patient can not eat
- As a method to deliver drugs when a less invasive method is not suitable due to drug pharmacokinetics or patient status

Establishing Intravenous Access

All facilities have specific policies and procedures for cleaning, access, and stabilization of IV sites. Basic steps are outlined in this section. When selecting a vein for IV access, the non-dominant arm is typically selected. The nurse inspects the limb, and a site is often selected at the most distal point. Larger, more proximal veins may be selected, depending upon the need of the IV therapy.

When a site has been selected for venipuncture, the nurse places a tourniquet above the selected vein. It is important to tighten the tourniquet so that venous blood flow is blocked but arterial blood flow is not. The vein fills (distends) and then the nurse pulls the skin taut (to anchor the vein and the skin) and inserts the needle into the vein, bevel up, and at a low angle to the skin. Blood should immediately flow into the syringe if the needle is properly inserted into the vein. The needle is then removed, and a flexible cannula remains in the vein. The cannula is secured in place, and the device is ready for drugs or fluids.

Performing a venipuncture requires practice. A suitable vein for venipuncture may be hard to find, and some veins are difficult to enter. The nurse should never repeatedly and unsuccessfully attempt a venipuncture. Depending on clinical judgment, two unsuccessful attempts on the same patient warrant having a more skilled individual attempt the procedure.

Maintaining Intravenous Access

Intermittent Intravenous Access

Fluids, electrolytes, and drugs are given by direct IV push, intermittent infusion, or continuous infusion. When the direct

Figure 55.1 Intravenous access (heparin lock) for inter-mittent infusions or direct administration of drugs.

Figure 55.2 The nurse sets the electronic intravenous device to deliver a specific amount of IV fluid.

IV method or intermittent infusion is used, the cannula that stays in the vein, an adapter and small tubing are called a **heparin** lock, and it is secured to the arm (Fig. 55.1). The device allows the nurse to give the dose directly into a vein or intermittent IV administration without having to maintain an infusion. A heparin lock also gives the patient the ability to move about more freely without cumbersome IV lines or machines to impede activities such as ambulation.

To maintain the patency of the heparin lock, a solution of dilute heparin may be ordered for injection into the heparin lock before and after the administration of a drug adminis-tered via IV route. This is called a *heparin lock flush*. The flush solution aids in preventing small clots from obstructing the cannula of the IV administration set. To prevent incom-patibility of heparin with other drugs, the heparin lock is flushed with sterile **normal saline** solution before and after any drug is given through the IV line. The primary health care provider or institutional policy dictates the use and type of heparin lock flush solution.

Continuous Infusion Access

Continuous infusion involves a continual flow of fluid into a vein for replacement purposes and continuous or frequent drug administration. When fluid replacement is indicated, the amount (or volume) of fluid to be administered is ordered over a specified time period, such as 125 mL/hour or 1000 mL over 8 hours.

Electronic infusion devices monitor the rate and flow of intravenous fluids (Fig. 55.2). The purpose of the device is to monitor the flow of the intravenous solution. An alarm is set to sound if the rate of infusion is more or less than the preset rate. These machines are classified as either infusion con-trollers or infusion pumps. The primary difference between the two is that an infusion pump adds pressure to the infusion, whereas an infusion controller does not.

When any problem is detected by the device, an alarm is activated to alert the nurse. Controllers and pumps have detectors and alarms that sound when various problems occur, such as air in the line, an occlusion, low battery, com-pletion of an infusion, or an inability to deliver the preset rate.

> **! NURSING ALERT**
>
> Use of an infusion pump or controller still requires nursing supervision and frequent monitoring of the IV infusion. It is important to monitor frequently for signs of **infiltration** (the collection of fluid into tissues), such as edema or redness at the site. Infiltration can progress rapidly, because with the increased pressure, the infusion will not slow until con-siderable edema has occurred. Careful monitoring of the pump or controller is also necessary to make sure the flow rate is cor-rect. When the patient needs fluid replacement and drugs are to be administered, a secondary line is established using the IV route. Intermittent IV infusion is given using "Y" tubing while another solution is being given on a continuous basis. When this method is used, the nurse may clamp off the IV fluid given on a continuous basis while the drug is allowed to infuse or the two solutions may infuse at the same time.

Calculating Intravenous Flow Rates

To allow the IV fluid to infuse over a specified period, the IV flow rate must be determined. Before using one of the fol-lowing methods, the drop factor must be known. Drip chambers on the various types of IV fluid administration sets vary. Some deliver 15 drops/mL and others deliver more or less than this number. This is called the *drop factor*. The drop factor (number of drops/mL) is given on the package contain-ing the drip chamber and IV tubing. Three methods for deter-mining the IV infusion rate follow. Methods 1 and 2 can be used when the known factors are the total amount of solution, the drop factor, and the number of hours over which the solu-tion is to be infused.

Method 1

Step 1. Total amount of solution ÷ number of hours = number of mL/hr

Step 2. mL/hr ÷ 60 min/hr = number of mL/min

Step 3. mL/min × drop factor = number of drops/min

Example

1000 mL of an IV solution is to infuse over a period of 8 hours. The drop factor is 15.

Step 1. 1000 mL ÷ 8 hours = 125 mL/hr
Step 2. 125 mL ÷ 60 minutes = 2.08 mL/min
Step 3. 2.08 × 15 = 31.2 or 31-32 drops/min

Method 2

Step 1. Total amount of solution ÷ number of hours = number of mL/hr
Step 2. mL/hr × drop factor ÷ 60 = number of drops/min

Example

1000 mL of an IV solution is to infuse over a period of 6 hours. The drop factor is 10.

Step 1. 1000 mL ÷ 6 hours = 166.6 mL/hr
Step 2. 166.6 × 10 ÷ 60 = 26.66 or 26 to 27) drops/min

Method 3

This method may be used when the desired amount of solution to be infused in 1 hour is known or written as a physician's order.

$$\frac{\text{drops/mL of given set (drop facter)}}{60 \times \text{(minutes in an hour)}} \times \text{total hourly volume} = \text{drops/min}$$

Example

If a set delivers 15 drops/min and 240 mL is to be infused in 1 hour:

$$\frac{15}{60} \times 240 = \frac{1}{4} \times 240 = 60 \text{ drops/min}$$

Fluid Overload

One problem commonly associated with all solutions administered by the parenteral route is fluid overload, that is, the administration of more fluid than the body is able to handle.

The term **fluid overload** (also *circulatory overload*) describes a condition when the body's fluid requirements are met, and the administration of fluid occurs at a rate that is greater than the rate at which the body can use or eliminate the fluid. Thus, the amount of fluid and the rate of administration of fluid that will cause fluid overload depend on several factors, such as the patient's cardiac status and adequacy of renal function. The signs and symptoms of fluid overload are listed in Display 55.1.

• SOLUTIONS USED IN THE MANAGEMENT OF BODY FLUIDS

The next section gives a brief overview of the following intravenous replacement solutions: electrolytes, blood products and expanders, and **total parenteral nutrition** (TPN).

Actions and Uses

One of the primary purposes of administering an intravenous solution is to provide proper electrolyte balance in the body.

DISPLAY 55.1 Signs and Symptoms of Fluid Overload

• Headache	• Rapid breathing
• Weakness	• Wheezing
• Blurred vision	• Coughing
• Behavioral changes (confusion, disorientation, delirium, drowsiness)	• Rise in blood pressure
	• Distended neck veins
• Weight gain	• Elevated central venous pressure
• Isolated muscle twitching	• Convulsions
• Hyponatremia	

• ELECTROLYTES

An *electrolyte* is an electrically charged particle essential to the normal functioning of all cells. Intracellular and extracellular fluids have specific chemical compositions of electrolytes. Major electrolytes in intracellular fluid include:

- Potassium
- Magnesium

Major electrolytes in extracellular fluid include:

- Sodium
- Calcium

Electrolytes circulate in the blood at specific levels, where they are available for use when needed by the cells. An electrolyte imbalance occurs when the concentration of an electrolyte in the blood is either too high or too low. In some instances, an electrolyte imbalance may be present without an appreciable disturbance in fluid balance. An electrolyte imbalance can profoundly affect a patient's physiologic functioning, the body's water distribution, neuromuscular activity, and acid-base balance. An electrolyte imbalance can occur from any disorder that alters electrolyte levels in the body's fluid compartments. An imbalance can also occur from vomiting, surgery, diagnostic tests, or drug administration. For example, a patient taking a diuretic is able to maintain fluid balance by an adequate oral intake of water, which replaces the water lost through diuresis. However, the patient is likely to be unable to replace the potassium that is also lost during diuresis. When the potassium concentration in the blood is too low, as may occur with the administration of a diuretic, an imbalance may occur that requires the addition of potassium. Electrolyte replacement drugs are inorganic or organic salts that increase deficient electrolyte levels that help to maintain homeostasis. Commonly used electrolyte replacement drugs are listed in the Summary Drug Table: Electrolytes.

Intracellular Electrolytes

Action and Uses

Potassium (K+)

Potassium is the major electrolyte in intracellular fluid and must be consumed daily because it cannot be stored. It is necessary for the transmission of impulses; the contraction of smooth, cardiac, and skeletal muscles; and other important physiologic processes. Potassium may be given to correct

Summary Drug Table ELECTROLYTES

Generic Name	Trade Name	Uses	Adverse Reactions	Dosage Ranges
calcium	PhosLo	Control of hyperphosphatemia in end-stage renal failure	See Display 55.2	3–4 tablets orally with each meal
calcium carbonate	Calcium-600, Apo-Cal, Caltrate, Oyster Shell Calcium Tums, Rolaids, Calcium Rich, Tums E-X	Dietary supplement for prevention or treatment of calcium deficiency for conditions such as pregnancy and lactation, chronic diarrhea, osteoporosis, osteomalacia, rickets, and latent tetany, and to reduce the symptoms of premenstrual syndrome	Rare; see Display 55.2 for signs of hypercalcemia	500–2000 mg/day orally
calcium citrate	Citracal, Citracal Liquitab	Same as calcium carbonate	Same as calcium carbonate	500–2000 mg/day orally
calcium gluconate		Hypocalcemic tetany, hyperkalemia with secondary cardiac toxicity, magnesium intoxication, exchange transfusion	Same as calcium carbonate	Adults: dosage range 1.35–70 mEq/day IV Children: 2.3 mEq/kg/day well diluted; give slowly in divided doses
calcium lactate	Cal-Lac	Same as calcium carbonate	Same as calcium carbonate	500–2000 mg/day orally
magnesium	Magonate, Mag-Ox 400, Magtrate, Mag-200, Slow-Mag	Dietary supplement, hypomagnesemia	Rare; see Display 55.2 for signs of hypermagnesemia	54–483 mg/day orally
magnesium sulfate		Mild to severe hypomagnesemia, seizures	Toxicity, weak or absent deep tendon reflexes, flaccid paralysis, drowsiness, stupor, weak pulse, arrhythmias, hypotension, circulatory collapse, respiratory paralysis	Hypomagnesemia: 2–5 g IV in 1 L of solution; 4–5 g over 3 hr Seizures: 4–5 g magnesium sulfate in 250 mL D_5 W; simultaneously give 4–5 g magnesium sulfate (undiluted) IM to each buttock for initial dose of 10–14 g; followed by 1–2 g/hr IV infusion until seizure controlled
oral electrolyte mixtures	Infalyte Oral Solution, Naturalyte, Pedialyte, Pedialyte Electrolyte, Pedialyte Freezer Pops, Rehydralyte, Resol Solution	Maintenance of water and electrolytes after corrective parenteral therapy of severe diarrhea; maintenance to replace mild to moderate fluid losses when food and liquid intake are discontinued, to restore fluid and minerals lost in diarrhea and vomiting in infants and children	Rare	Individualize dosage following the guidelines on the product labeling

Fluids, Electrolytes, and Parenteral Therapy

(text continues on page 572)

Summary Drug Table ELECTROLYTES (continued)

Generic Name	Trade Name	Uses	Adverse Reactions	Dosage Ranges
potassium replacements	Effer-K, K Norm, Kaon Cl, K-Dur, Klor-Con, K-Lyte, K-Tab, Micro-K, Slow-K	Hypokalemia	See Display 55.2; most common: nausea, vomiting, diarrhea, flatulence, abdominal discomfort, skin rash	40–100 mEq/day orally
sodium chloride	Slo-Salt	Prevention or treatment of extracellular volume depletion, dehydration, sodium depletion, aid in the prevention of heat prostration	Nausea, vomiting, diarrhea, abdominal cramps, edema, irritability, restlessness, weakness, hypertension, tachycardia, fluid accumulation, pulmonary edema, respiratory arrest (see Display 55.2)	Individualize dosage
Alkalinizing Drugs				
bicarbonate		Metabolic acidosis, cardiac arrest, systemic and urinary alkalinization	Tetany, edema, gastric distention, flatulence, belching, hypokalemia, metabolic alkalosis	Metabolic acidosis and cardiac arrest: dosage varies depending on laboratory results and patient's condition Urinary alkalinization: 4 g orally initially, followed by 1–2 g orally q 6 hr
tromethamine	Tham	Metabolic acidosis during cardiac bypass surgery or cardiac arrest	Fever, hypoglycemia, hyperkalemia, respiratory depression, hemorrhagic hepatic necrosis, venospasm, vein necrosis	9 mL/kg (not to exceed total single dose of 500 mL)
Acidifying Drug				
ammonium chloride		Metabolic alkalosis	Loss of electrolytes, especially potassium, metabolic acidosis	Varies depending on patient's tolerance and condition

hypokalemia (low blood potassium) resulting from increased potassium excretion or depletion. Examples of causes of hypokalemia are a marked loss of gastrointestinal (GI) fluids (severe vomiting, diarrhea, nasogastric suction, draining intestinal fistulas), diabetic acidosis, marked diuresis, severe malnutrition, use of a potassium-depleting diuretic, excess antidiuretic hormone, and excessive urination. Potassium as a drug is available as potassium chloride (KCl) and potassium gluconate, and is measured in milliequivalents (mEq)—for example, 40 mEq in 20 mL or 8 mEq controlled-release tablet.

Magnesium (Mg^{++})

Magnesium plays an important role in the transmission of nerve impulses. It is also important in the activity of many enzyme reactions, such as carbohydrate metabolism. Magnesium sulfate (MgSO$_4$) is used as replacement therapy in hypomagnesemia. Magnesium is also used in the prevention and control of seizures in obstetric patients with pregnancy-induced hypertension (PIH; also referred to as *eclampsia* and *preeclampsia*). It may also be added to TPN mixtures.

Adverse Reactions, Contraindications, Precautions, and Interactions

Potassium (K$^+$)

Nausea, vomiting, diarrhea, abdominal pain, and phlebitis have been seen with oral and IV administration of potassium. Adverse reactions related to hypokalemia or hyperkalemia are listed in Display 55.2.

Potassium is contraindicated in patients who are at risk for hyperkalemia, such as those with renal failure, oliguria, azotemia (the presence of nitrogen-containing compounds in the blood), anuria, severe hemolytic reactions, untreated Addison's disease, acute dehydration, heat cramps, and any form of hyperkalemia. Potassium is used cautiously in patients with renal impairment or adrenal insufficiency, heart disease, metabolic acidosis, or prolonged or severe diarrhea.

Concurrent use of potassium with angiotensin-converting enzyme (ACE) inhibitors may result in an elevated serum

lisinopirl-
spironolactine
cozaar

DISPLAY 55.2 **Signs and Symptoms of Electrolyte Imbalances**

Calcium
Normal laboratory values: 4.5–5.3 mEq/L or 9–11 mg/dL*

Hypocalcemia
Hyperactive reflexes, carpopedal spasm, perioral paresthesias, positive Trousseau's sign, positive Chvostek's sign, muscle twitching, muscle cramps, tetany (numbness, tingling, and muscular twitching usually of the extremities), laryngospasm, cardiac arrhythmias, nausea, vomiting, anxiety, confusion, emotional lability, convulsions

Hypercalcemia
Anorexia, nausea, vomiting, lethargy, bone tenderness or pain, polyuria, polydipsia, constipation, dehydration, muscle weakness and atrophy, stupor, coma, cardiac arrest

Magnesium
Normal laboratory values: 1.5–2.5 mEq/L or 1.8–3 mg/dL*

Hypomagnesemia
Leg and foot cramps, hypertension, tachycardia, neuromuscular irritability, tremor, hyperactive deep tendon reflexes, confusion, disorientation, visual or auditory hallucinations, painful paresthesias, positive Trousseau's sign, positive Chvostek's sign, convulsions

Hypermagnesemia
Lethargy, drowsiness, impaired respiration, flushing, sweating, hypotension, weak to absent deep tendon reflexes

Potassium
Normal laboratory values: 3.5–5 mEq/L*

Hypokalemia
Anorexia, nausea, vomiting, mental depression, confusion, delayed or impaired thought processes, drowsiness, abdominal distention, decreased bowel sounds, paralytic ileus, muscle weakness or fatigue, flaccid paralysis, absent or diminished deep tendon reflexes, weak, irregular pulse, paresthesias, leg cramps, electrocardiographic changes

Hyperkalemia
Irritability, anxiety, listlessness, mental confusion, nausea, diarrhea, abdominal distress, GI hyperactivity, paresthesias, weakness and heaviness of the legs, flaccid paralysis, hypotension, cardiac arrhythmias, electrocardiographic changes

Sodium
Normal laboratory values: 132–145 mEq/L*

Hyponatremia
Cold, clammy skin, decreased skin turgor, apprehension, confusion, irritability, anxiety, hypotension, postural hypotension, tachycardia, headache, tremors, convulsions, abdominal cramps, nausea, vomiting, diarrhea

Hypernatremia
Fever; hot, dry skin; dry, sticky mucous membranes; rough, dry tongue; edema, weight gain, intense thirst, excitement, restlessness, agitation, oliguria or anuria

*These laboratory values may not concur with the normal range of values in all hospitals and laboratories. The hospital policy manual or laboratory values sheet should be consulted for the normal ranges of all laboratory tests.

potassium level. Potassium-sparing diuretics and salt substitutes used with potassium can produce severe hyperkalemia. The use of digitalis with potassium increases the risk of digoxin toxicity.

Magnesium (Mg^{++})

Adverse reactions from magnesium administration are most likely related to overdose and may include flushing, sweating, hypotension, depressed reflexes, muscle weakness, respiratory failure, and circulatory collapse (see Display 55.2). Magnesium is contraindicated in patients with heart block or myocardial damage and in women with PIH during the 2 hours before delivery. Magnesium is a pregnancy category A drug, and studies indicate no increased risk of fetal abnormalities if the agent is used during pregnancy. Nevertheless, caution is used when administering magnesium during pregnancy.

Magnesium is used with caution in patients with renal function impairment. When magnesium is used with alcohol, antidepressants, antipsychotics, barbiturates, hypnotics, general anesthetics, and opioids, an increase in central nervous system depression may occur. Prolonged respiratory depression and apnea may occur when magnesium is administered with the neuromuscular blocking agents. When magnesium is used with digoxin, heart block may occur.

Extracellular Electrolytes

Action and Uses

Sodium (Na$^+$)

Sodium is a major electrolyte in extracellular fluid and is important in maintaining acid-base balance and normal heart action, and in the regulation of osmotic pressure in body cells (water balance). Sodium is administered for hyponatremia (low blood sodium). Examples of causes of hyponatremia are excessive diaphoresis, severe vomiting or diarrhea, excessive diuresis, diuretic use, wound drainage, and draining intestinal fistulas.

Sodium, as sodium chloride (NaCl), may be given IV. A solution containing 0.9% NaCl is called *normal saline*, and a solution containing 0.45% NaCl is called *half-normal saline*. Sodium also is available combined with dextrose, such as dextrose 5% and sodium chloride 0.9% (D5NS).

Calcium (Ca^{++})

Calcium is necessary for the functioning of nerves and muscles, the clotting of blood, the building of bones and teeth, and other physiologic processes. Examples of calcium salts are calcium gluconate and calcium carbonate. Calcium may be given for the treatment of hypocalcemia (low blood calcium), which may be seen in those with parathyroid disease or after accidental removal of the parathyroid glands during surgery of the thyroid gland. Calcium may also be given during cardiopulmonary resuscitation, particularly after open heart surgery, when epinephrine fails to improve weak or ineffective myocardial contractions. Calcium may be used as adjunct therapy of insect bites or stings to reduce muscle cramping, such as occurs with black widow spider bites. Calcium may also be recommended for those eating a diet low in calcium or as a dietary supplement when there is an increased need for calcium, such as during pregnancy.

Combined Electrolyte Solutions

Combined electrolyte solutions are available for oral and IV administration. The IV solutions contain various electrolytes and dextrose. The amount of electrolytes, given as milliequivalents per liter (mEq/L), also varies. The IV solutions are used to replace fluid and electrolytes that have been lost and to provide calories through their carbohydrate content. Examples of IV electrolyte solutions are dextrose 5% with 0.9% NaCl, lactated Ringer's, and Plasma-Lyte. The primary health care provider selects the type of combined electrolyte solution that will meet the patient's needs.

Oral electrolyte solutions contain a carbohydrate and various electrolytes. Examples of combined oral electrolyte solutions are Pedialyte and Rehydralyte. Oral electrolyte solutions are most often used to replace lost electrolytes and fluids in conditions such as severe vomiting or diarrhea.

Adverse Reactions, Contraindications, Precautions, and Interactions

Sodium (Na⁺)

Sodium as the salt (e.g., NaCl) has no adverse reactions except those related to overdose (see Display 55.2). In some instances, excessive oral use may produce nausea and vomiting.

Sodium is contraindicated in patients with hypernatremia or fluid retention, and when the administration of sodium or chloride could be detrimental. Sodium is used cautiously in surgical patients and those with circulatory insufficiency, hypoproteinemia, urinary tract obstruction, heart failure (HF), edema, or renal impairment. Sodium is a pregnancy category C drug and is used cautiously during pregnancy.

Calcium (Ca⁺⁺)

Irritation of the vein used for administration, tingling, a metallic or chalky taste, and "heat waves" may occur when calcium is given intravenously. Rapid IV administration (calcium gluconate) may result in bradycardia, vasodilation, decreased blood pressure, cardiac arrhythmias, and cardiac arrest. Oral administration may result in GI disturbances. Administration of calcium chloride may cause peripheral vasodilation, a temporary fall in blood pressure, and a local burning. Display 55.2 lists adverse reactions associated with hypercalcemia and hypocalcemia.

● BLOOD PRODUCTS AND EXPANDERS

Actions and Uses

Blood Plasma

Blood plasma is the liquid part of blood, containing water, sugar, electrolytes, fats, gases, proteins, bile pigment, and clotting factors. Human plasma, also called human pooled plasma, is obtained from donated blood. Although whole blood must be typed and crossmatched because it contains red blood cells carrying blood type and Rh factors, human plasma does not require this procedure. Because of this, plasma can be given in acute emergencies.

Plasma administered IV is used to increase blood volume when severe hemorrhage has occurred and it is necessary partially to restore blood volume while waiting for whole blood to be typed and crossmatched or when plasma alone has been lost, as may be seen in severe burns.

Plasma Protein Fractions

Plasma protein fractions include human plasma protein fraction 5% and normal serum albumin 5% (Albuminar-5, Buminate 5%) and 25% (Albuminar-25, Buminate 25%). Plasma protein fraction 5% is an IV solution containing 5% human plasma proteins. Serum albumin is obtained from donated whole blood and is a protein found in plasma. The albumin fraction of human blood acts to maintain plasma colloid osmotic pressure and as a carrier of intermediate metabolites in the transport and exchange of tissue products. It is critical in regulating the volume of circulating blood. When blood is lost from shock, such as in hemorrhage, there is a reduced plasma volume. When blood volume is reduced, albumin quickly restores the volume in most situations.

Plasma protein fractions are used to treat hypovolemic (low blood volume) shock that occurs as the result of burns, trauma, surgery, and infections, or in conditions where shock is not currently present but likely to occur. As with human pooled plasma, blood type and crossmatch are not needed when plasma protein fractions are given. Adverse reactions are rare when plasma protein fractions are administered, but nausea, chills, fever, urticaria, and hypotensive episodes may occasionally be seen. Plasma proteins are contraindicated in those with a history of allergic reactions to albumin, severe anemia, or cardiac failure; in the presence of normal or increased intravascular volume; and in patients on cardiopulmonary bypass. Plasma protein fractions are used cautiously in patients who are in shock or dehydrated and in those with HF or hepatic or renal failure.

Most of these solutions should not be combined with any other solutions or drugs but should be administered alone. The nurse should consult the drug insert or other appropriate sources before combining any drug with any plasma protein fraction. Solutions used in the management of body fluids are contraindicated in patients with hypersensitivity to any component of the solution. All solutions used to manage body fluids discussed in this chapter are pregnancy category C drugs and are used cautiously during pregnancy and lactation. No interactions have been reported.

Plasma Expanders

The IV solutions of plasma expanders include hetastarch (Hespan), low–molecular-weight dextran (Dextran 40), and high–molecular-weight dextran (Dextran 70, Dextran 75).

Plasma expanders are used to expand plasma volume when shock is caused by burns, hemorrhage, surgery, and other trauma or for prophylaxis of venous thrombosis and thromboembolism. When used in the treatment of shock, plasma expanders are not a substitute for whole blood or plasma, but they are of value as emergency measures until the latter substances can be used.

Administration of hetastarch, a plasma expander, may be accompanied by vomiting, a mild temperature elevation, itching, and allergic reactions. Allergic reactions are evidenced by wheezing, swelling around the eyes (periorbital edema), and urticaria. Other plasma expanders may result in mild cutaneous eruptions, generalized urticaria, hypotension, nausea, vomiting, headache, dyspnea, fever, tightness of the chest, bronchospasm, wheezing, and, rarely, anaphylactic shock.

Plasma expanders are contraindicated in patients with hypersensitivity to any component of the solution and those with severe bleeding disorders, severe cardiac failure, renal failure with oliguria, or anuria. Plasma expanders are used cautiously in patients with renal disease, HF, pulmonary edema, and severe bleeding disorders. Plasma expanders are pregnancy category C drugs and are used cautiously during pregnancy and lactation. The nurse should consult the drug insert or other appropriate sources before combining a plasma expander with another drug for IV administration.

•TOTAL PARENTERAL NUTRITION

When normal enteral feeding in not possible or is inadequate to meet an individual's nutritional needs, IV nutritional therapy or TPN is required. TPN is a method of administering nutrients to the body by an IV route. TPN uses a complex admixture of chemicals combined in a single container. The components of the TPN mixture may include proteins (amino acids), fats, glucose, electrolytes, vitamins, minerals, and sterile water. Products used to meet the IV nutritional requirements of the patient include protein substrates (amino acids), energy substrates (dextrose and fat emulsions), fluids, electrolytes, and trace minerals.

Total parenteral nutrition is used to prevent nitrogen and weight loss or to treat negative nitrogen balance (a situation in which more nitrogen is used by the body than is taken in) in the following situations:

- Oral, gastrostomy, or jejunostomy route cannot or should not be used.
- GI absorption of protein is impaired by obstruction.
- Inflammatory disease or antineoplastic therapy prevents normal GI functioning.
- Bowel rest is needed (e.g., after bowel surgery).
- Metabolic requirements for protein are significantly increased (e.g., in hypermetabolic states such as serious burns, infections, or trauma).
- Morbidity and mortality may be reduced by replacing amino acids lost from tissue breakdown (e.g., renal failure).
- Tube feeding alone cannot provide adequate nutrition.

If a patient's intake of protein nutrients is significantly less than is required by the body to meet energy expenditures, a state of negative nitrogen balance occurs. The body begins to convert protein from the muscle into carbohydrate for energy to be used by the body. This results in weight loss and muscle wasting. In these situations, traditional IV fluids do not provide sufficient calories or nitrogen to meet the body's daily requirements. TPN may be administered through a peripheral vein or a central venous catheter in a highly concentrated form to improve nutritional status, establish a positive nitrogen balance, and enhance the healing process. Peripheral TPN is used for relatively short periods (no more than 5 to 7 days) and when the central venous route is not possible or necessary. An example of a solution used in TPN is amino acids with electrolytes. These solutions may be used alone or combined with dextrose (5% or 10%) solutions.

Total parenteral nutrition through a central vein is indicated to promote protein synthesis in patients who are severely hypercatabolic or severely depleted of nutrients, or who require long-term parenteral nutrition. For example, amino acids combined with hypertonic dextrose and IV fat emulsions are infused through a central venous catheter to promote protein synthesis. Vitamins, trace minerals, and electrolytes may be added to the TPN mixture to meet the patient's individual needs. The daily dose depends on the patient's daily protein requirement and his or her metabolic state and clinical responses.

TPN is delivered with an infusion pump. The pump infuses a small amount (0.1 to 10 mL/hr) continuously to keep the vein open. Feeding schedules vary; one example is administration of the feeding continuously over a few hours, leveling off the rate for several hours, and then increasing the rate of administration for several hours to simulate a normal set of meal times.

> **NURSING ALERT**
>
> Hyperglycemia is a common metabolic complication. A too-rapid infusion of TPN may result in hyperglycemia, glycosuria, mental confusion, and loss of consciousness. Blood glucose levels may be assessed every 4 to 6 hours to monitor for hyperglycemia and guide the dosage of dextrose and insulin (if required). To minimize these complications, the primary health care provider may decrease the rate of administration, reduce the dextrose concentration, or administer insulin.

To prevent a rebound hypoglycemic reaction from the sudden withdrawal of TPN containing a concentrated dose of dextrose, the rate of administration is slowly reduced or the concentration of dextrose gradually decreased. If TPN must be abruptly withdrawn, a solution of 5% or 10% dextrose is begun to reduce gradually the amount of dextrose administered. The primary health care provider is notified if the patient exhibits symptoms of hypoglycemia, including weakness, tremors, diaphoresis, headache, hunger, and apprehension. Other complications of TPN include bacterial infection, sepsis, embolism, metabolic problems, and hemothorax or pneumothorax.

An IV fat emulsion contains soybean or safflower oil and a mixture of natural triglycerides, predominantly unsaturated fatty acids. It is used in the prevention and treatment of essential fatty acid deficiency. It also provides nonprotein calories

metabolic acidosis

for those receiving TPN when calorie requirements cannot be met by glucose. Examples of IV fat emulsion include Intralipid 10% and 20%, Liposyn II 10% and 20%, and Liposyn III 10% and 20%. Fat emulsion is used as a source of calories and essential fatty acids for patients requiring parenteral nutrition for extended periods (usually more than 5 days). No more than 60% of the patient's total caloric intake should come from fat emulsion, with carbohydrates and amino acids comprising the remaining 40% or more of caloric intake.

The most common adverse reaction associated with the administration of fat emulsion is sepsis caused by administration equipment and thrombophlebitis caused by venous irritation from concurrently administering hypertonic solutions. Less frequent adverse reactions include dyspnea, cyanosis, hyperlipidemia, hypercoagulability, nausea, vomiting, headache, flushing, increased body temperature, sweating, sleepiness, chest and back pain, slight pressure over the eyes, and dizziness. Intravenous fat emulsions are contraindicated in conditions that interfere with normal fat metabolism (e.g., acute pancreatitis) and in patients allergic to eggs. IV fat emulsions are used with caution in those with severe liver impairment, pulmonary disease, anemia, and blood coagulation disorders. These solutions are pregnancy category C drugs and are used cautiously during pregnancy and lactation.

In general, fat emulsions should not be combined with any other solutions or drugs except when combined in TPN. The nurse should consult appropriate sources before combining any drug with a fat emulsion.

• ALKALINIZING AND ACIDIFYING DRUGS

Alkalinizing and acidifying drugs are used to correct an acid-base imbalance in the blood. The acid-base imbalances are:

- Metabolic acidosis—decrease in the blood pH caused by an excess of hydrogen ions in the extracellular fluid (treated with alkalinizing drugs)
- Metabolic alkalosis—increase in the blood pH caused by an excess of bicarbonate in the extracellular fluid (treated with acidifying drugs)

Alkalinizing Drug: Bicarbonate (HCO_3^-)

Action and Uses

A low blood pH means the body is in an acidic condition, and a high blood pH indicates an alkaline condition. To raise the pH, an alkalinizing drug must be administered. Sodium bicarbonate, an alkalinizing drug, separates in the blood and the bicarbonate functions as a buffer to decrease the hydrogen ion concentration and raise the blood pH.

Bicarbonate (HCO_3^-) plays a vital role in the acid-base balance of the body. Alkalinizing drugs are used to treat metabolic acidosis and to increase blood pH. Bicarbonate may be given IV as sodium bicarbonate ($NaHCO_3$) in the treatment of metabolic acidosis, a state of imbalance that may be seen in diseases or conditions such as severe shock, diabetic acidosis, severe diarrhea, extracorporeal circulation of blood, severe renal disease, and cardiac arrest. Oral sodium bicarbonate is used as a gastric and urinary alkalinizer. It may

be used as a single drug or may be found as one of the ingredients in some antacid preparations. It is also useful in treating severe diarrhea accompanied by bicarbonate loss.

Adverse Reactions, Contraindications, Precautions, and Interactions

In some instances, excessive oral use of bicarbonate may produce nausea and vomiting. Some individuals may use sodium bicarbonate (baking soda) for the relief of GI disturbances such as pain, discomfort, symptoms of indigestion, and gas. Prolonged use of oral sodium bicarbonate or excessive doses of IV sodium bicarbonate may result in systemic alkalosis.

Bicarbonate is contraindicated in patients losing chloride by continuous GI suction or through vomiting, in patients with metabolic or respiratory alkalosis, hypocalcemia, renal failure, or severe abdominal pain of unknown cause, and in those on sodium-restricted diets.

Bicarbonate is used cautiously in patients with HF or renal impairment and those receiving glucocorticoid therapy. Bicarbonate is a pregnancy category C drug and is used cautiously during pregnancy.

Oral administration of bicarbonate may decrease the absorption of ketoconazole. Increased blood levels of quinidine, flecainide, or sympathomimetics may occur when these agents are administered with bicarbonate. There is an increased risk of crystalluria when bicarbonate is administered with the fluoroquinolones. Possible decreased effects of lithium, methotrexate, chlorpropamide, salicylates, and tetracyclines may occur when these drugs are administered with sodium bicarbonate. Sodium bicarbonate is not administered within 2 hours of enteric-coated drugs, because the protective enteric coating may disintegrate before the drug reaches the intestine.

Acidifying Drug: Ammonium Chloride

Actions and Uses

Ammonium chloride lowers the blood pH by being metabolized first into urea, then to hydrochloric acid, which is further metabolized to hydrogen ions to acidify the blood.

Adverse Reactions and Interactions

Adverse reactions to ammonium chloride include metabolic acidosis and loss of electrolytes, especially potassium. Use of ammonium chloride and spironolactone may increase systemic acidosis.

NURSING PROCESS
PATIENT RECEIVING A SOLUTION FOR MANAGEMENT OF BODY FLUIDS

ASSESSMENT

Preadministration Assessment
Before administering an IV solution, the nurse assesses the patient's general status, reviews recent laboratory test results (when appropriate), weighs the patient (when

appropriate), and takes the vital signs. Blood pressure, pulse, and respiratory rate provide a baseline, which is especially important when the patient is receiving fluids for shock or other serious disorders. The nurse assesses the patient for signs of an electrolyte imbalance (see Display 55.2). All recent laboratory and diagnostic tests appropriate to the imbalance are reviewed.

Ongoing Assessment

During the ongoing assessment, the nurse checks the needle site every 15 to 30 minutes or more frequently if the patient is restless or confused. The needle site is inspected for signs of **extravasation** (escape of fluid from a blood vessel into surrounding tissues) or infiltration (the collection of fluid into tissues). If signs of extravasation or infiltration are apparent, the nurse restarts the infusion in another vein.

When these solutions are given, the patient is in a critical condition and a central venous pressure line may be inserted to monitor the patient's response to therapy. Central venous pressure readings are taken as ordered. During administration, the nurse takes the blood pressure, pulse, and respiratory rate as ordered or at intervals determined by the patient's clinical condition. For example, a patient in shock and receiving a plasma expander may require monitoring of the blood pressure and pulse rate every 5 to 15 minutes, whereas the patient receiving dextrose 3 days after surgery may require monitoring every 30 to 60 minutes.

During therapy, the nurse periodically obtains (daily or more frequently) serum electrolyte or bicarbonate studies to monitor therapy.

POTASSIUM. Patients receiving oral potassium should have their blood pressure and pulse monitored every 4 hours, especially during early therapy. The nurse also observes the patient for signs of hyperkalemia (see Display 55.2), which would indicate that the dose of potassium is too high. Signs of hypokalemia may also occur during therapy and may indicate that the dose of potassium is too low and must be increased. If signs of hypokalemia or hyperkalemia are apparent or suspected, the nurse notifies the primary health care provider. In some instances, frequent laboratory monitoring of the serum potassium may be ordered.

The nurse inspects the IV needle site every 30 minutes for signs of extravasation. Potassium is irritating to the tissues. If extravasation occurs, the nurse discontinues the IV immediately and notifies the primary health care provider. Many facilities have protocols for treatment of the tissues to delay further tissue damage.

The acutely ill patient and the patient with severe hypokalemia require monitoring of the blood pressure and pulse rate every 15 to 30 minutes during the IV infusion. The nurse measures the intake and output every 8 hours. The infusion rate is slowed to keep the vein open, and the primary health care provider is notified if an irregular pulse is noted.

CALCIUM. Before, during, and after the administration of IV calcium, the nurse monitors the blood pressure, pulse,

and respiratory rate every 30 minutes until the patient's condition has stabilized. After administration of calcium, the nurse observes the patient for signs of hypercalcemia (see Display 55.2).

> ### NURSING ALERT
>
> Systemic overloading of calcium ions in the systemic circulation results in acute hypercalcemic syndrome. Symptoms of hypercalcemic syndrome include elevated plasma calcium, weakness, lethargy, severe nausea and vomiting, coma, and, if left untreated, death. The nurse reports any signs of hypercalcemic syndrome immediately to the primary health care provider.

To combat hypercalcemic syndrome, the primary health care provider may prescribe IV sodium chloride and a potent diuretic, such as furosemide. When used together, these two drugs markedly increase calcium renal clearance and reduce hypercalcemia.

SODIUM. When NaCl is administered by IV infusion, the nurse observes the patient during and after administration for signs of hypernatremia (see Display 55.2). The nurse checks the rate of IV infusion as ordered by the primary health care provider, usually every 15 to 30 minutes. More frequent monitoring of the infusion rate may be necessary when the patient is restless or confused. To minimize venous irritation during administration of sodium or any electrolyte solution, the nurse uses a small-bore needle placed well within the lumen of a large vein.

Patients receiving a 3% or 5% NaCl solution by IV infusion are observed closely for signs of pulmonary edema (i.e., dyspnea, cough, restlessness, bradycardia). If any one or more of these symptoms occurs, the IV infusion is slowed to keep the vein open and the primary health care provider is contacted immediately. Patients receiving NaCl by the IV route have their intake and output measured every 8 hours. The nurse observes the patient for signs of hypernatremia every 3 to 4 hours and contacts the primary health care provider if this condition is suspected.

MAGNESIUM. When magnesium is ordered to treat convulsions or severe hypomagnesemia, the patient requires constant observation. The nurse obtains the patient's blood pressure, pulse, and respiratory rate immediately before the drug is administered, as well as every 5 to 10 minutes during the time of IV infusion or place the patient on a device for continuous monitoring. The nurse continues monitoring these vital signs at frequent intervals until the patient's condition has stabilized. Because magnesium is eliminated by the kidneys, it is used with caution in patients with renal impairment. The nurse monitors the urine output to verify an output of at least 100 mL every 4 hours. Voiding less than 100 mL of urine every 4 hours is reported to the primary health care provider.

BICARBONATE. When given in the treatment of metabolic acidosis, the drug may be added to the IV fluid or given as a prepared IV sodium bicarbonate solution. Frequent laboratory monitoring of the blood pH and blood gases is usually ordered, because dosage and length of therapy depend on test results. The nurse frequently observes the patient for signs of clinical improvement and monitors the blood pressure, pulse, and respiratory rate every 15 to 30 minutes or as ordered by the primary health care provider. Extravasation of the drug requires selection of another needle site, because the drug is irritating to the tissues.

Fat Emulsions. When a fat emulsion is administered, the nurse must monitor the patient's ability to eliminate the infused fat from the circulation, because the lipidemia must clear between daily infusions. The nurse monitors for lipidemia by assessing the results of the following laboratory examinations: hemogram, blood coagulation, liver function tests, plasma lipid profile, and platelet count. The nurse reports an increase in the results of any of these laboratory examinations as abnormal.

NURSING DIAGNOSES

Drug-specific nursing diagnoses include the following:

❏ **Excess Fluid Volume** related to adverse effects resulting from too rapid intravenous infusion
❏ **Deficient Fluid Volume** related to inability to take oral fluids, abnormal fluid loss, other factors (specify cause of deficient fluid volume)
❏ **Imbalanced Nutrition: Less Than Body Requirements** related to anorexia caused by opioids
❏ **Risk for Injury** related to adverse drug effects (muscular weakness)
❏ **Disturbed Thought Processes** related to adverse drug effects
❏ **Risk for Decreased Cardiac Output** related to adverse drug effects (cardiac arrhythmias)

Nursing diagnoses related to drug administration are discussed in Chapter 4.

PLANNING

The expected outcomes of the patient depend on the specific drug, dose, route of administration, and reason for administration of an electrolyte or fluid, but may include an optimal response to therapy, supporting the patient needs related to the management of adverse reactions, and an understanding of the treatment regimen.

IMPLEMENTATION

Promoting an Optimal Response to Therapy

The extremity used for administration should be made comfortable and supported as needed by a small pillow or other device. An IV infusion pump may be ordered for the administration of these solutions. The nurse sets the alarm of the infusion pump and checks the functioning of the unit at frequent intervals.

❗ NURSING ALERT

The nurse must administer all IV solutions with great care. At no time should any IV solution be infused at a rapid rate, unless there is a specific written order to do so.

Unless otherwise directed, the IV solution should be administered at room temperature. If the solution is refrigerated, the nurse allows the solution to warm by exposing it to room temperature 30 to 45 minutes before use. The average length of time for infusion of 1000 mL of an IV solution is 4 to 8 hours. One exception is when there is a written or verbal order by the primary health care provider to give the solution at a rapid rate because of an emergency. In this instance, the order must specifically state the rate of administration as drops per minute, milliliters per minute, or the period of time over which a specific amount of fluid is to be infused (e.g., 125 mL/hr or 1000 mL in 8 hours).

In some situations, electrolytes are administered when an electrolyte imbalance may potentially occur. For example, the patient with nasogastric suction is prescribed one or more electrolytes added to an IV solution, such as 5% dextrose or a combined electrolyte solution, to be given IV to make up for the electrolytes that are lost through nasogastric suction. In other instances, electrolytes are given to replace those already lost, such as the patient admitted to the hospital with severe vomiting and diarrhea of several days' duration.

When electrolytes are administered parenterally, the dosage is expressed in milliequivalents (mEq)—for example, calcium gluconate 7 mEq IV. When administered orally, sodium bicarbonate, calcium, and magnesium dosages are expressed in milligrams (mg). Potassium liquids and effervescent tablet dosages are expressed in milliequivalents; capsule or tablet dosages may be expressed as milliequivalents or milligrams.

Electrolyte disturbances can cause varying degrees of confusion, muscular weakness, nausea, vomiting, and cardiac irregularities (see Display 55.2 for specific symptoms). Serum electrolyte blood levels have a very narrow therapeutic range. Careful monitoring is needed to determine if blood levels fall above or below normal. Normal values may vary with the laboratory, but a general range of normal values for each electrolyte is found in Display 55.2. Adverse reactions are usually controlled by maintaining blood levels of the various electrolytes within the normal range.

Administering Potassium. When given orally, potassium may cause GI distress. Therefore, it is given immediately after meals or with food and a full glass of water. Oral potassium must not be crushed or chewed. If the patient has difficulty swallowing, the nurse consults the primary health care provider regarding the use of a solution or an effervescent tablet, which fizzes and dissolves on contact with water. Potassium in the form of effervescent tablets, powder, or liquid must be thoroughly mixed with 4 to 8 oz of cold water, juice, or other beverage. Effervescent tablets must stop fizzing before the solution is sipped slowly during a period of 5 to 15 minutes. Oral liquids and soluble powders that have been mixed and dissolved in cold water or juice are also sipped slowly over a period of 5 to 15 minutes. The nurse advises patients that liquid potassium solutions have a salty taste. Some of these products are flavored to make the solution more palatable.

NURSING ALERT

Concentrated potassium solutions are for IV mixtures only and should never be used undiluted. Direct IV injection of potassium could result in sudden death. When potassium is given IV, it is always diluted in 500 to 1000 mL of an IV solution. The maximum recommended concentration of potassium is 80 mEq in 1000 mL of IV solution (although in acute emergency situations a higher concentration of potassium may be required).

ADMINISTERING MAGNESIUM. Magnesium sulfate may be ordered intramuscularly (IM), IV, or by IV infusion diluted in a specified type and amount of IV solution. When ordered to be given IM, this drug is given undiluted as a 50% solution for adults and a 20% solution for children. Magnesium sulfate is given deep IM in a large muscle mass, such as the gluteus muscle.

LIFESPAN ALERT – Gerontology

Older adults may need a reduced dosage of magnesium because of decreased renal function. The nurse should closely monitor serum magnesium levels when magnesium is administered to older adults.

The nurse observes the patient for early signs of hypermagnesemia (see Display 55.2) and contacts the primary health care provider immediately if this imbalance is suspected. Frequent plasma magnesium levels are usually ordered. The nurse notifies the primary health care provider if the magnesium level is higher or lower than the normal range.

NURSING ALERT

As plasma magnesium levels rise above 4 mEq/L, the deep tendon reflexes are first decreased and then disappear as the plasma levels reach 10 mEq/L. The knee jerk reflex is tested before each dose of magnesium sulfate. If the reflex is absent or a slow response is obtained, the nurse withholds the dosage and notifies the primary health care provider. IV calcium is kept available to reverse the respiratory depression and heart block that may occur with magnesium overdose.

TOTAL PARENTERAL NUTRITION. A microscopic filter is attached to the IV line when TPN solutions are administered. The filter prevents microscopic aggregates (particles that may form in the IV bag) from entering the bloodstream, where they could cause massive emboli.

LIPID SOLUTIONS. Fat solutions (emulsions) should be handled with care to decrease the risk of separation or "breaking out of the oil." Separation can be identified by yellowish streaking or the accumulation of yellowish droplets in the emulsion. Fat solutions are administered to adults at a rate no greater than 1 to 2 mL/min.

NURSING ALERT

During the first 30 minutes of infusion of a fat solution, the nurse carefully observes the patient for difficulty in breathing, headache, flushing, nausea, vomiting, or signs of a hypersensitivity reaction. If any of these reactions occur, the nurse discontinues the infusion and immediately notifies the primary health care provider.

ADMINISTERING BICARBONATE. The nurse gives oral sodium bicarbonate tablets with a full glass of water; the powdered form is dissolved in a full glass of water. If oral sodium bicarbonate is used to alkalinize the urine, the nurse checks the urine pH two or three times a day or as ordered by the primary health care provider. If the urine remains acidic, the nurse notifies the primary health care provider, because an increase in the dose of the drug may be necessary. IV sodium bicarbonate is given in emergency situations, such as metabolic acidosis or certain types of drug overdose, when alkalinization of the urine is necessary to hasten drug elimination.

Monitoring and Managing Patient Needs

When electrolyte solutions are administered, adverse reactions are most often related to overdose. Correcting the imbalance by decreasing the dosage or discontinuing the solution usually works, and the adverse reactions subside quickly. Frequent serum electrolyte levels are used to monitor blood levels.

EXCESS FLUID VOLUME. The nurse monitors patients receiving IV solutions at frequent intervals for signs of fluid overload. If signs of fluid overload (see Display 55.1) are observed, the nurse slows the IV infusion rate and immediately notifies the primary health care provider.

LIFESPAN ALERT – Gerontology

Older adults are at increased risk for fluid overload because of the increased incidence of cardiac disease and decreased renal function that may accompany old age. Careful monitoring for signs and symptoms of fluid overload is extremely important when administering fluids to older adults.

DEFICIENT FLUID VOLUME AND IMBALANCED NUTRITION: LESS THAN BODY REQUIREMENTS. Often, the solutions used in the management of body fluids are given to correct a fluid volume deficit and to supply carbohydrates (nutrition). The nurse reviews the patient's chart for a full understanding of the rationale for administration of the specific solution.

When appropriate, nursing measures that may be instituted to correct a fluid volume and carbohydrate deficit may be included in a plan of care. Examples of these measures include offering oral fluids at frequent intervals and encouraging the patient to take small amounts of nourishment between meals and to eat as much as possible at mealtime.

Electrolyte imbalances may cause nausea, vomiting, and other GI disturbances. If GI disturbances occur from oral administration, taking the drug with meals may decrease the nausea. Offering smaller, more frequent meals may help to stabilize nutritional status. Correcting the electrolyte imbalance usually solves the problem of nausea and vomiting.

RISK FOR INJURY. The patient is at increased risk of falling because of weakness or muscular cramping. Frequent observation and quickly answering the call light helps to maintain the patient's safety. If weakness or muscular cramping occurs, the nurse assists the patient when ambulating to prevent falls or other injury.

DISTURBED THOUGHT PROCESSES. The patient with an electrolyte imbalance may be confused or disoriented. The nurse approaches the patient in a calm and nurturing manner. The nurse gently reorients the individual and explains any procedures carefully before performing any procedures with the patient. The nurse reassures the patient that these symptoms are part of the imbalance but can recede as the imbalance improves (if applicable).

RISK FOR DECREASED CARDIAC OUTPUT. Some electrolytes may cause cardiac irregularities. The nurse checks the pulse rate at regular intervals, usually every 4 hours or more often if an irregularity in the heart rate is observed. Depending on the patient's condition, cardiac monitoring may be indicated when administering the electrolytes (particularly when administering potassium or calcium). For example, if potassium is administered to a patient with cardiac disease, a cardiac monitor is needed to monitor the heart rate and rhythm continuously during therapy.

> **NURSING ALERT**
>
> Mild (5.5 to 6.5 mEq/L) to moderate (6.5 to 8 mEq/L) potassium blood level increases may be asymptomatic and manifested only by increased serum potassium concentrations and characteristic electrocardiographic changes, such as disappearance of P waves or spreading (widening) of the QRS complex.

Educating the Patient and Family
The nurse gives the patient or family a brief explanation of the reason for and the method of administration of an IV solution. Sometimes, when alarms go off, patients and families may feel the staff is too busy to respond and tamper with or adjust the rate of flow of IV administration sets. The nurse emphasizes the importance of calling for the nurse if there appears to be a problem with the IV site or the IV administration set or the equipment.

To ensure accurate compliance with the prescribed drug regimen, the nurse carefully explains the dose and time intervals to the patient or a family member. Because overdose (which can be serious) may occur if the patient does not adhere to the prescribed dosage and schedule, it is most important that the patient completely understands how much and when to take the drug. The nurse stresses the importance of adhering to the prescribed dosage schedule during patient teaching.

The primary health care provider may order periodic laboratory and diagnostic tests for some patients receiving oral electrolytes. The nurse encourages the patient to keep all appointments for these tests, as well as primary health care provider or clinic visits. Persons with a history of using sodium bicarbonate (baking soda) as an antacid are warned that overuse can result in alkalosis and could disguise a more serious problem.

EVALUATION

- Therapeutic response is achieved; fluid and electrolyte imbalances are corrected.
- Adverse reactions are identified, reported to the primary health care provider, and managed successfully with appropriate nursing interventions:
  - ☑ Patient maintains an adequate fluid volume.
  - ☑ Patient maintains an adequate nutritional status.
  - ☑ No evidence of injury is seen.
  - ☑ Orientation and mentation remain intact.
  - ☑ Cardiac output is maintained.
- Patient and family demonstrate an understanding of the drug regimen.

THINK CRITICALLY: PHARMACOLOGY IN PRACTICE

1. Mr. Garcia's weight is up during the nurse's intake assessment. Looking at his legs, you note + 2 pitting edema bilaterally. He tells you that he has not deviated from the sodium-restricted diet that he was given. Mr. Garcia cannot figure out why he has gained weight. He states that, with his heartburn, he knows he has been eating less. He also mentions that the soda bicarbonate he uses does little to relieve the heartburn. Describe how you would teach him about the side effects he is experiencing from the sodium bicarbonate.

● Test Your Knowledge

1. Which of the following is a symptom of fluid overload?
   - **A.** Tinnitus
   - **B.** Hypotension
   - **C.** Decreased body temperature
   - **D.** Behavioral changes

2. Which of the following symptoms would indicate hypocalcemia?
   - **A.** Tetany
   - **B.** Constipation
   - **C.** Muscle weakness
   - **D.** Hypertension

3. Which of the following potassium plasma concentration laboratory results would the nurse report immediately to the physician?
   - **A.** 3.5 mEq/L
   - **B.** 4.0 mEq/L
   - **C.** 4.5 mEq/L
   - **D.** 5.5 mEq/mL

4. Which of the following symptoms would most likely indicate hypernatremia?
   - **A.** Fever, increased thirst
   - **B.** Cold, clammy skin
   - **C.** Decreased skin turgor
   - **D.** Hypotension

5. Which of the following is a common metabolic complication of TPN?

    A. Hypomagnesemia
    B. Hypermagnesemia
    C. Hypoglycemia
    D. Hyperglycemia

● Prepare for the NCLEX

1. When monitoring a patient with an IV line, the nurse observes that the area around the needle insertion site is swollen and red. The first action of the nurse is to _____.

    A. check the patient's blood pressure and pulse
    B. check further for possible extravasation
    C. ask the patient if the IV site has been accidentally injured
    D. immediately notify the primary health care provider

● Calculate Medication Dosages

1. The patient is to receive 1000 mL of 5% dextrose and water during a period of 10 hours. Calculate how many milliliters should be infused each hour.

2. The patient is prescribed potassium 40 mEq orally. The drug is available from the pharmacy in a solution of 20 mEq/15mL. The nurse administers _____.

To check your answers, see Appendix E.

the**Point** *For more NCLEX questions, log on to http://thepoint.lww.com to access more than 1000 questions.*

Glossary

A

acetylcholine: neurotransmitter that transmits impulses across the parasympathetic branch of the autonomic nervous system

acetylcholinesterase: enzyme that can inactivate the neurotransmitter acetylcholine

achalasia: failure to relax; usually referring to the smooth muscle fibers of the gastrointestinal tract, especially failure of the lower esophagus to relax, causing difficulty swallowing and a feeling of fullness in the sternal region

action potential: electrical impulse that passes from cell to cell in the myocardium of the heart and stimulates the fibers to shorten, causing heart muscle to contract

active immunity: type of immunity that occurs when the person is exposed to a disease and develops the disease, and the body makes antibodies to provide future protection against the disease

acute pain: pain with duration of fewer than 6 months

additive drug reaction: the combined effect of two drugs equals the sum of the effects of each drug given alone

adjuvant: see *adjunctive treatment*

adjunctive treatment: therapy used in addition to the primary treatment

adrenal insufficiency: deficiency in corticosteroids

adrenergic: pertaining to the sympathetic branch of the nervous system, which controls heart rate, breathing rate, and ability to divert blood to the skeletal muscles

adrenergic blocking: drug that blocks the neurotransmission of the sympathetic nervous system

adverse reaction: undesirable drug effect

affective domain: in regard to patient teaching, the patient's or caregiver's attitudes, feelings, beliefs, and opinions

aggregation: clumping of blood elements

agonist: drug that binds with a receptor to produce a therapeutic response

agonist-antagonist: drug with both agonist and antagonist properties

agonist (partial): agent that binds to a receptor but produces a limited response

agranulocytosis: decrease or lack of granulocytes (a type of white blood cell)

akathisia: extreme restlessness and increased motor activity

allergic reaction: immediate hypersensitive reaction by the immune system, it presents as itching, hives, swelling, difficulty breathing; see *hypersensitivity*; see also *anaphylactic shock*

alopecia: abnormal loss of hair; baldness

alpha-adrenergic blocking: drugs use to block neurotransmission in the sympathetic nervous system

alpha/beta-adrenergic blocking: drugs that block both alpha- and beta-adrenergic receptors

Alzheimer's disease: progressive disorder that affects cognition, emotion, and movement

anabolism: tissue-building process

analeptics: drugs that stimulate respiratory center of the brain

analgesic: drug that relieves pain

analysis: using data to determine patient need or nursing diagnosis

anaphylactic shock (also called *anaphylactic* reaction or *anaphylactoid reaction*): sudden, severe hypersensitivity reaction with symptoms that progress rapidly and may result in death if not treated

anaphylactoid reactions: unusual or exaggerated allergic reactions; see *anaphylactic shock*

androgen: male hormone, testosterone and its derivatives

anemia: decrease in the number of red blood cells and hemoglobin value below normal

anesthesia: loss of feeling or sensation

anesthesiologist: physician with special training in administering anesthesia

anesthetist: nurse with special training who administers anesthesia; also called *nurse anesthetist*

angina (angina pectoris): acute pain in the chest resulting from decreased blood supply to the heart muscle

angioedema: localized wheals or swellings in subcutaneous tissues or mucous membranes, which may be due to an allergic response; also called *angioneurotic edema*

anhedonia: finding no pleasure in activities

anorexia: loss of appetite

anorexiants: drugs used to suppress the appetite

antagonist: drugs that join with a receptor to prevent the action of an agonist

antiadrenergic drugs: see *adrenergic blocking drugs*; also called *sympatholytic drugs*

antibacterial: active against bacteria

antibody: molecule with the ability to bind to a specific antigen; responsible for the immune response

anticholinergic action: blockage of parasympathetic nervous system

anticholinergics: see *cholinergic blocking drugs*; also called *cholinergic blockers* or *parasympatholytic drugs*

anticonvulsants: drugs used to manage seizure disorders

antiflatulents: drugs that work against flatus (gas)

antigen: substance that is capable of inducing a specific immune response

antigen–antibody response: antibodies formed in response to exposure to a specific antigen

antihistamine: drug used to counteract the effects of histamine on body organs and structures

antineoplastic: drug used to treat neoplasia (cancer)

antipyretic: fever-reducing agent

antipsoriatic: drug used to treat psoriasis

antiseptic: agent that stops, slows, or prevents the growth of microorganisms

antitussive: drug used to relieve coughing

anuria: cessation of urine production

anxiety: feelings of apprehension, worry, or uneasiness

anxiolytics: drugs used to treat anxiety

aplastic anemia: blood disorder caused by damage to the bone marrow resulting in a marked reduction in the number of red blood cells and some white blood cells

arrhythmia: abnormal heart rate or rhythm; also called *dysrhythmia*

assessment: collection of subjective and objective data

asthma: respiratory disorder characterized by bronchospasm and difficulty in breathing, especially exhaling

ataxia: unsteady gait; muscular incoordination

atherosclerosis: disease characterized by deposits of fatty plaques on the inner walls of arteries

atrial fibrillation: quivering of the atria of the heart

attention deficit hyperactivity disorder (ADHD): disorder characterized by inattention, hyperactivity, and impulsivity

attenuate: weaken

autonomic nervous system: division of the peripheral nervous system concerned with functions essential to the life of the organism and not consciously controlled (e.g., blood pressure, heart rate, gastrointestinal activity)

B

bacterial resistance: phenomenon by which a bacteria-produced substance inactivates or destroys an antibiotic drug

bactericidal: drug or agent that destroys or kills bacteria

bacteriostatic: drug or agent that slows or retards the multiplication of bacteria

beta-adrenergic blocking drugs: drugs that decrease stimulation of the sympathetic nervous system on certain tissues in order to decrease heart rate and cardiac workload and dilate blood vessels; also called *beta blockers*

beta-lactam ring: portion of the penicillin drug molecule

biotransformation: process by which the body changes a drug to a more or less active form that can be excreted

bipolar disorder: mental health disorder characterized by severe mood swings from extreme hyperactivity to depression

blood–brain barrier: ability of the nervous system to prohibit large and potentially harmful molecules from crossing from the blood into the brain

blood dyscrasias: abnormality of blood cell structure

blood pressure: force of blood against artery walls

bone marrow suppression: decreased production of all blood cells; also called *myelosuppression*

booster: immunogen injected after a specified interval; often after the primary immunization to stimulate and sustain the immune response

bowel preparation: treatment protocol to cleanse the bowel of bacteria before surgery or other procedures

brachial plexus: network of spinal nerves affecting the arm, forearm, and hand

brachial plexus block: see *conduction block*

bradycardia: slow heart rate, usually below 60 beats per minute

bradykinesia: slow movement

broad spectrum: description of an antibiotic that affects a large number of different strains of bacteria

buccal: space in the mouth between the gum and the cheek in either the upper or lower jaw

C

cachectic: malnourished, in poor health, physically wasted

candidiasis: infection of the skin or mucous membrane with the yeast *Candida albicans*

cardiac arrhythmia: abnormal rhythm of the heart

cardiac output: volume of blood discharged from the left or right ventricle per minute

catabolism: tissue-depleting process

catalyst: substance that accelerates a chemical reaction without itself undergoing a change

cell cycle nonspecific: pertaining to a drug used in cancer treatment, effective in any phase of cell division

cell cycle specific: pertaining to a drug used in cancer treatment, affecting a specific phase of cell division

cell-mediated immunity: immune reaction caused by white blood cells

cerumen: ear wax

chemoreceptor trigger zone (CTZ): group of nerve fibers located on the surface of the fourth ventricle of the brain that, when stimulated, results in vomiting

chemotherapy: drug therapy with a chemical, often used when referring to treatment with an antineoplastic drug

cholesterol: fat-like substance produced mostly in the liver of animals

cholinergic blocking: affect the parasympathetic branch of the autonomic nervous system; also called *anticholinergics*

cholinergic crisis: cholinergic drug toxicity

choreiform movements: involuntary muscular twitching of the limbs or facial muscles

chronic pain: pain that lasts more than 6 months

cinchonism: quinidine toxicity or poisoning

circumoral: encircling the mouth

cognitive domain: intellectual activities such as thought, recall, decision making, and drawing conclusions

conduction block: type of regional anesthesia produced by injection of a local anesthetic drug into or near a nerve trunk examples include: epidural, transsacral (caudal) and brachial

constipation: hardened fecal material that is difficult to pass

controlled release: see *extended release*

controlled substances: drugs that have the potential for abuse and dependency, both physical and psychological

convulsion: paroxysm (occurring suddenly) of involuntary muscular contractions and relaxations

corticosteroids: glucocorticoid and mineralocorticoid hormones

coughing: forceful expulsion of air from the lungs

cross-allergenicity: allergy to drugs in the same or related groups

cross-sensitivity: see *cross-allergenicity*

cryptorchism: failure of the testes to descend into the scrotum

crystalluria: formation of crystals in the urine

culture and sensitivity test: culture of bacteria to determine to which antibiotic the microorganism is sensitive

cumulative drug effect: when the body is unable to metabolize and excrete one dose of a drug before the next is given

Cushing's syndrome: disease caused by the overproduction of endogenous glucocorticoids

cyclooxygenase: enzyme responsible for prostaglandin synthesis

cyclooxygenase-1 (COX-1): enzyme that helps to maintain the stomach lining

cyclooxygenase-2 (COX-2): enzyme that triggers pain and inflammation

cycloplegia: paralysis of the ciliary muscle, resulting in an inability to focus the eye

cytomegalovirus (CMV): any of a group of herpes viruses infecting humans, monkeys, or rodents; the human CMV is found in the salivary glands and causes cytomegalic inclusion disease

cystinuria: presence of cystine, an amino acid, in urine

cystitis: inflammation of the bladder

D

decongestant: drug that reduces swelling of the nasal passages, which promotes drainage of the nasal sinuses

delusion: false belief that cannot be changed with reason

dementia: decrease in cognitive function

denominator: part of a fraction (the number under the line)

depolarization: movement of ions in a nerve cell from inside to outside and vice versa

depression: feeling sad, unhappy, down in the dumps, hopeless

diabetes insipidus: disease caused by failure of the pituitary gland to secrete vasopressin or by surgical removal of the pituitary

diabetes mellitus: disease caused by insufficient insulin production

diabetic ketoacidosis: life-threatening deficiency of insulin resulting in severe hyperglycemia and excessively high levels of ketones in the blood

diarrhea: loose, watery stool

digitalis toxicity: toxic drug effects from administration of digoxin

digitalization: administration of digitalis at intervals to produce and maintain a therapeutic blood level

dimensional analysis: method of calculating drug dosages based on fractions

directly observed therapy (DOT): drug dose taken in front of the administrator

disulfiram-like: pertaining to a reaction, usually to alcohol, characterized by flushing, throbbing head, vomiting, sweating, chills, and hypotension

diuretic: drug that produces urine excretion

dosage strength: amount of drug in the given form, such as tablet or capsule

drug error: any event or activity that can cause a patient to receive the wrong dose, the wrong drug, a drug by the wrong route, or a drug given at the wrong time

drug idiosyncrasy: any unusual or abnormal response that differs from the response normally expected to a specific drug and dosage

drug tolerance: decreased response to a drug, requiring an increase in dosage to achieve the desired effect

dyspepsia: fullness or epigastric discomfort

dysphoric: characterized by extreme or exaggerated sadness, anxiety, or unhappiness

dyspnea: feelings of shortness of breath, labored or difficult breathing

dystonia: prolonged muscle contractions that may cause twisting and repetitive movements of abnormal posture

dysuria: painful or difficult urination

E

edema: accumulation of excess water in the body

electrolyte: electrically charged substance essential to the normal functioning of all cells

embolus: thrombus that detaches from a blood vessel wall and travels through the bloodstream

endogenous: pertaining to something that normally occurs or is produced within the organism

enteric coating: special coating on drug that prevents absorption until drug reaches the small bowel

epidural: outside or above the dura mater

epidural block: see *conduction block*

epilepsy: chronic, recurring seizure disorder

ergotism: overdose of an ergot drug

erythrocytes: red blood cells; one of several formed elements in the blood

erythropoiesis: process of making red blood cells

Escherichia coli (E. coli): nonpathogenic colon bacillus; may cause infection outside the colon

essential hypertension: see primary hypertension

estradiol: endogenous estrogen

estriol: endogenous estrogen

estrogens: female hormones

estrone: endogenous estrogen

euthyroid: normal thyroid function

evaluation: decision-making process determining the effectiveness of nursing actions or interventions

expected outcomes: expected behavior and physical and mental state of the patient after a therapeutic intervention

expectorant: drug that aids in raising thick, tenacious mucus from the respiratory tract

extended release: formulation in which drug is released over time

extrapulmonary: occurring outside of the lungs in the respiratory system

extrapyramidal syndrome: group of adverse reactions involving the extrapyramidal portion of the nervous system causing abnormal muscle movements, especially akathisia and dystonia

extravasation: escape of fluid from a blood vessel into surrounding tissue

F

feedback mechanism: method to control output

fibrolytic: drug that dissolves clots already formed within blood vessel walls

first-dose effect: marked adverse reaction with the first dose

first-pass effect: action by which an oral drug is absorbed and carried directly to the liver, where it is inactivated by enzymes before it enters the general bloodstream

flattened affect: absence of emotion

fluid overload: condition in which the body's fluid requirements are met and the administration of fluid occurs at a rate that is greater than the rate at which the body can use or eliminate the fluid; also called *circulatory overload*

folinic acid rescue: *in chemotherapy,* the technique of administering leucovorin after a large dose of methotrexate, thereby allowing normal cells to survive; also called *leucovorin rescue*

fungicidal: deadly to fungi

fungistatic: pertaining to agents that retard growth of fungi

fungus: single-cell, colorless plant that lacks chlorophyll, such as yeast or mold

G

gastric stasis: failure of the body to remove stomach contents normally

gastroesophageal reflux disease (GERD): reflux or backup of gastric contents into the esophagus

general anesthesia: sensation-free state of entire body

generalized seizure: loss of consciousness during seizure

germicide: an agent that kills bacteria

gingival hyperplasia: overgrowth of gum tissue

glaucoma: group of diseases of the eye characterized by increased intraocular pressure; results in changes within the eye, visual field defects, and eventually blindness (if left untreated)

globulins: plasma proteins that are insoluble in water

glossitis: inflammation of the tongue

glucagon: hormone secreted by the alpha cells of the pancreas that increases the concentration of glucose in the blood

glucocorticoid: hormone produced by adrenal gland

glucometer: device to monitor blood glucose level

glycosylated hemoglobin: blood test that monitors average blood glucose level over a 3- to 4-month period

goiter: enlargement of the thyroid gland causing a swelling in the front part of the neck, usually caused by a lack of iodine in the diet

gonadotropin: hormone that stimulates the sex glands (gonads)

gonads: glands responsible for sexual activity and characteristics

gout: uric acid accumulation in joints

gram: mass metric measure equivalent to one thousandth of a kilogram

growth hormone: *see somatropin*

gynecomastia: male breast enlargement

H

HAART: highly active antiretroviral therapy; multiple drugs used together for treatment of HIV infection

half-life: time required for the body to eliminate 50% of a drug

hallucination: false sensation or perception of reality

heart failure: condition in which the heart cannot pump enough blood to meet the tissue needs of the body

Helicobacter pylori: stomach bacterium that causes peptic ulcer; also know as ***H. pylori***

helminthiasis: invasion by helminths (worms)

hematopoiesis: undifferentiated stem cells are stimulated to become specific blood cells

hematuria: blood in the urine

hemostasis: complex process by which fibrin forms and blood clots

heparin lock: equipment consisting of an adapter and tubing introduced into a vein to maintain access to circulation

hepatic coma: coma induced by liver disease

herb: plant used as medicine or food seasoning

herbal medicine: type of complementary/alternative therapy that uses plants or herbs to treat various disorders; also called *herbalism*

high-density lipoproteins (HDL): macromolecules that carry cholesterol from the body cells to the liver to be excreted

highly active antiretroviral therapy: see *HAART*

histamine: substance found in various parts of the body (i.e., liver, lungs, intestines, skin) and produced from the amino acid histidine in response to injury to trigger the inflammatory response

HMG-CoA reductase inhibitors: drugs that inhibit the manufacture or promote breakdown of cholesterol, and are referred to as *statin* drugs.

humoral immunity: antibody-mediated immune response of the body

hydrochloric acid (HCl): stomach acid that aids in digestion

hyperglycemia: high blood glucose (sugar) level

hyperinsulinism: elevated levels of insulin in the body

hyperkalemia: increase in potassium levels in the blood

hyperlipidemia: increase in the lipids in the blood

hypersecretory: characterized by excessive secretion of a substance

hypersensitivity: undesirable reaction produced by a normal immune system

hyperstimulation syndrome: sudden ovarian enlargement caused by overstimulation

hypertension: high blood pressure which stays elevated over time

hypertensive emergency: extremely high blood pressure that must be lowered immediately to prevent damage to target organs (i.e., heart, kidneys, eyes)

hyperthyroidism: overactive thyroid function

hypnotic: drug that induces sleep

hypoglycemia: low blood glucose (sugar) level

hypokalemia: low blood potassium level

hyponatremia: low blood sodium level

hypotension: abnormally low blood pressure

hypotension, orthostatic: decrease in blood pressure occurring after standing in one place for an extended period

hypotension, postural: decrease in blood pressure after a sudden change in body position

hypothyroidism: underactive thyroid function

I

idiopathic hypertension: see primary hypertension

immune globulin: solution obtained from human or animal blood containing antibodies that have been formed by the body to specific antigens; administered to provide passive immunity to one or more infectious diseases

immunity: resistance to infection

immunocompromised: immune system incapable of fighting infection

implementation: carrying out of a plan of action

independent nursing actions: actions that do not require a physician's orders

infiltration: collection of fluid into tissue

inflammatory bowel disease: inflammation of the bowel (e.g., Crohn's disease and ulcerative colitis)

inhalation: drug administration route in which the patient inhales the drug orally or nasally

initial assessment: gathering of baseline data

insulin: hormone secreted by the pancreas; necessary for the metabolism of carbohydrates and fats (conversion of glucose to glycogen to regulate blood glucose level)

intermittent claudication: group of symptoms characterized by pain in the calf muscle of one or both legs, caused by walking and relieved by rest

intradermal: pertaining to the dermis area within the upper layers of the skin

intramuscular (IM): area within a muscle

intraocular pressure: pressure within the eye

intravenous (IV): area within a vein

intrinsic factor: substance produced by the cells in the stomach and necessary for the absorption of vitamin B_{12}

iron deficiency anemia: condition resulting when the body does not have enough iron to meet its need for iron

isolated systolic hypertension: systolic blood pressure over 140 mm Hg with diastolic blood pressure under 90 mm Hg

J

jaundice: yellow discoloration of the skin due to liver disease

K

keratolytic: agent that removes excessive growth of the epidermis (top layer of skin)

L

learning: acquisition of new knowledge or skills; outcome of learning is change in behavior, thinking, or both

left ventricular dysfunction: condition in which fluids back up previous to the left ventricle of the heart and is characterized by shortness of breath and moist cough in heart failure

leprosy: chronic, communicable disease caused by *Mycobacterium leprae*; also called *Hansen's disease*

leucovorin rescue: see *folinic acid rescue*

leukocytes: white blood cells

leukopenia: decrease in the number of leukocytes (white blood cells)

leukotriene: inflammatory substance which is released by mast cells during an asthma attack

lipids: group of fats or fatlike substances

lipodystrophy: atrophy of subcutaneous fat

lipoprotein: macromolecule consisting of lipid (fat) and protein; how fats are transported in the blood

liter: metric measure of volume, roughly equivalent to a quart in household measure

local anesthesia: provision of a pain-free state in a specific body area

low-density lipoproteins (LDL): macromolecules that carry cholesterol from the liver to the body cells

lumen: inner diameter of a tube; the space or opening within an artery

lysis: dissolution or destruction of cells

M

macrocytic anemia: anemia resulting from abnormal formation (enlargement) of erythrocytes

malaise: discomfort, uneasiness

manual redundancy system: process of medication prescription and delivery in which each person checks the drug dosage for accuracy.

megakaryocytes: precursor cell to the platelets

megaloblastic anemia: anemia characterized by large, abnormal, immature erythrocytes circulating in the blood; results from folic acid deficiency

menarche: age of onset of first menstruation

metabolite: inactive form of the original drug

metastasis: spread of cancer outside the original organ or tissue

meter: metric measure of distance

methicillin-resistant *Staphylococcus aureus* (MRSA): bacterium that is resistant to methicillin

metric system: system of measurement based on units of 10

micturition: voiding of urine

mineralocorticoids: hormones produced by the adrenal gland

miosis: constriction of the pupil

motivation: desire for action or recognition of need

motor seizure: uncontrolled muscle stiffening

mucolytic: drug that loosens and thins respiratory secretions (lowers the viscosity of the secretions)

muscarinic receptors: neurologic receptors that stimulate smooth muscle

musculoskeletal: pertaining to the bones and muscles

myasthenia gravis: condition characterized by weakness and fatigability of the muscles

Mycobacterium leprae: bacterium that causes leprosy (Hansen's disease)

Mycobacterium tuberculosis: bacterium that causes tuberculosis (TB)

mycotic infection: infection caused by fungi

mydriasis: dilation of the pupil

myelosuppression: see bone marrow suppression

myoclonic seizure: sudden, forceful muscular contraction

myopia: nearsightedness

myxedema: condition caused by hypothyroidism or deficiency of thyroxine and characterized by swelling of the face, periorbital tissues, hands, and feet

N

narcolepsy: chronic disorder that results in recurrent attacks of drowsiness and sleep during daytime

narrow spectrum: describes an antibiotic that affects only one or a few strains of bacteria

nausea: unpleasant and uncomfortable feeling in the stomach, sometimes followed by vomiting

necrotic: pertaining to death of tissue (n. *necrosis*)

nephrotoxicity: damage to the kidneys by a toxic substance

neurogenic bladder: altered bladder function caused by abnormality in nervous system

neurohormonal activity: *in heart failure*, increased secretions of epinephrine and norepinephrine, resulting in arteriolar vasoconstriction, tachycardia, and myocardial contractility resulting in a worsening of heart failure and reduced ability of the heart to contract effectively

neurohormones: secreted rather than transmitted neurosubstances

neuroleptanalgesia: altered state of consciousness or sensation

neuroleptic malignant syndrome: rare reaction to antipsychotic drug; includes extrapyramidal syndrome, hypothermia, and autonomic disturbances

neuromuscular blockade: acute muscle paralysis and apnea

neurotoxicity: damage to the nervous system by a toxic substance

neurotransmitter: chemical substances released at the nerve ending that facilitate the transmission of nerve impulses

neutropenia: abnormally small number of neutrophils (type of white blood cell)

nicotinic receptors: neurologic receptors that stimulate skeletal muscles

nocturia: excessive urination at night

nonprescription drugs: drugs that are designated by the U.S. Food and Drug Administration (FDA) to be safe (if taken as directed) and obtainable without a prescription, also called *over-the-counter* (OTC) drugs; may be purchased in various settings, such as a pharmacy, drugstore, or supermarket

nonproductive cough: dry, hacking cough that produces no secretions

normal flora: nonpathogenic microorganisms in the body

normal saline: solution of 0.9% sodium chloride and water, which is the proportion of salt and water normally circulating in body fluid

numerator: part of a fraction (the numeral above the line)

nurse anesthetist: see *anesthetist*

nursing diagnosis: description of a patient problem

nursing process: framework for nursing action, consisting of a series of problem-solving steps, which helps members of the health care team provide effective and consistent patient care

nystagmus: involuntary and constant movement of the eyeball

O

objective data: information obtained through a physical assessment or physical examination

obstipation: watery stool leakage around a hard fecal impaction

ongoing assessment: continuing assessment activities that proceed from the initial nursing assessment

on-off phenomenon: fluctuation in levodopa therapy where inconsistent absorption causes alternating improved status and loss of therapeutic effect

onychomycosis: finger or toenail fungal infection

ophthalmic: pertaining to the eye

opioid: drug having opiate properties but not necessarily derived from opium; used to relieve moderate to severe pain

opioid naive: no previous use or infrequent use of opioid medications

opportunistic infection: infection resulting from microorganisms commonly found in the environment that normally do not cause an infection unless there is an impaired immune system

optic neuritis: inflammation of the optic nerve

oral mucositis: inflammation of the oral mucous membranes

orthostatic hypotension: see *hypotension, orthostatic*

osteoarthritis: noninflammatory degeneration of joints and cartilage

otic: pertaining to the ear

otitis media: infection of the middle ear

ototoxic: see *ototoxicity*

ototoxicity: damage to the organs of hearing by a toxic substance

overactive bladder: condition characterized by involuntary contraction of bladder muscles

over-the-counter (OTC): pertaining to drugs or other substances sold without a prescription; see *nonprescription*

oxytocic: agent that stimulates contractions of the uterus, resulting in labor

P

pain: unpleasant sensory or emotional perception

palliation: therapy designed to treat symptoms, not to produce a cure

pancytopenia: reduction in all cellular elements of the blood

paradoxical: contradiction, when a drug increases the problem rather than diminishing the symptoms

paralytic ileus: paralysis of the bowel resulting in lack of movement of bowel contents

parasite: organism living in or on another organism (host) without contributing to the survival or well-being of the host

parasympathetic: pertaining to the part of the autonomic nervous system concerned with conserving body energy (i.e., slowing the heart rate, digesting food, and eliminating waste)

parasympatholytic: blocking the parasympathetic nervous system

parasympathomimetic drugs: mimic the activity of the parasympathetic nervous system; also called *cholinergic drugs*

parenteral: administration of a substance, such as a drug, by any route other than through the gastrointestinal system (e.g., oral or rectal route)

parkinsonism: referring to a cluster of symptoms associated with Parkinson's disease (i.e., fine tremors, slowing of voluntary movements, muscular weakness)

Parkinson's disease: degenerative disorder caused by an imbalance of dopamine and acetylcholine in the central nervous system

partial agonist: agent that binds to a receptor but produces a limited response

partial seizure: localized seizure in the brain

passive immunity: type of immunity occurring from the administration of ready-made antibodies from another individual or animal

pathogen: disease producing microorganism

patient-controlled analgesia: drug pump and delivery system that allows patients to administer their own analgesic medication intravenously within a preset protocol

penicillinase: enzyme produced by bacteria that deactivates penicillin

perioperative: pertaining to the preoperative, intraoperative, or postoperative period

peripheral: pertaining to the outward surface; away from the center

peripheral nervous system: all nerves outside of brain and spinal cord

peripheral neuropathy: numbness and tingling of the extremities

pharmaceutic: pertaining to the phase during which a drug dissolves in the body

pharmacodynamics: study of the drug mechanisms that produce biochemical or physiologic changes in the body

pharmacogenetics: study of how people's responses are variable to medications due to individual genetic variation.

pharmacokinetics: study of body mechanisms (or activity) after a drug is administered; these mechanisms include absorption, distribution, metabolism, and excretion

pharmacology: study of drugs and their action on living organisms

phenylketonuria: genetic disorder in which the body lacks the enzyme necessary to metabolize phenylalanine; without treatment, the disorder results in mental retardation

pheochromocytoma: tumor of the adrenal medulla characterized by hypersecretion of epinephrine and norepinephrine

phlebitis: inflammation of a vein

photophobia: aversion to or intolerance of light

photosensitivity: exaggerated sunburn reaction when the skin is exposed to sunlight or ultraviolet light

physical dependence: habitual use of a drug, where negative physical withdrawal symptoms result from abrupt discontinuation

planning: design of steps to carry out nursing actions

polarization: status of a nerve cell at rest, with positive ions on the outside of the cell membrane and negative ions on the inside

polydipsia: excessive thirst

polyphagia: eating large amounts of food

polypharmacy: taking a large number of different drugs (may be prescribed or over-the-counter drugs)

polyuria: increased urination

positive inotropic activity: increase in the force of cardiac contraction

postural hypotension: see *hypotension, postural*

preanesthetic: pertaining to status before administration of an anesthetic agent

precipitation: condensation of a solid from a solution during a chemical reaction

prehypertension: systolic blood pressure between 120 and 139 mm Hg or diastolic pressure between 80 and 89 mm Hg

prescription drugs: drugs the federal government has designated as potentially harmful unless their use is supervised by a licensed health care provider, such as a nurse practitioner, physician, or dentist

priapism: painful, persistent penile erection

primary hypertension: hypertension that has no known cause, also known as essential or idiopathic hypertension

proarrhythmic effect: creation of new arrhythmia or worsening of existing arrhythmia, resulting from administration of an antiarrhythmic drug

productive cough: cough by which secretions from the respiratory tract are expelled

progesterone: female hormone produced by the corpus luteum that works in the uterus (along with estrogen) to prepare the uterus for possible conception

progestins: natural and synthetic progesterones

prophylactic: see *prophylaxis*

prophylaxis: prevention

prostaglandins: fatty acid derivative found in almost every tissue and fluid of the body that affects the uterus and other smooth muscles; also thought to increase the sensitivity of peripheral pain receptors to painful stimuli

prostatitis: inflammation of the prostate gland

proteinuria: protein in the urine

proteolysis: enzymatic action that helps remove dead soft tissues by reducing proteins to simpler substances

proteolytic: pertaining to proteolysis (see *proteolysis*)

prothrombin: substance that is essential for the clotting of blood; clotting factor II

pruritus: itching

pseudomembranous colitis: severe, life-threatening form of diarrhea

psychological dependence: compulsion or craving to use a substance to obtain a pleasurable experience

psychomotor domain: area of education concerned with teaching and learning physical skills and tasks

pyelonephritis: inflammation of the kidney nephron

Q

quiescent: having no symptoms

R

receptor: *in pharmacology*, a reactive site on the surface of a cell; when a drug binds to and interacts with the receptor, a pharmacologic response occurs

red-man syndrome: severe adverse drug reaction characterized by a sudden and profound fall in blood pressure, fever, chills, paresthesias, and erythema (redness) of the neck and back

red-neck syndrome: see *red-man syndrome*

refractory period: quiet period between the transmission of nerve impulses along a nerve fiber

regional anesthesia: injection of a local anesthetic around nerves to block sensation

repolarization: return of positive and negative ions to their original place on the nerve cell after an impulse has passed along the nerve fiber (see *polarization*)

retrovirus: virus that uses RNA as its primary component instead of DNA

Reye's syndrome: acute and potentially fatal disease of childhood; associated with a previous viral infection

rhabdomyolysis: condition in which muscle damage results in the release of muscle cell contents into the bloodstream.

rheumatoid arthritis: inflammatory changes in connective tissue

rhinitis: inflammation of the mucous membranes of the nose

right ventricular dysfunction: condition in which fluid backs up previous to the right ventricle of the heart and is characterized by peripheral edema and venous congestion in heart failure

S

salicylism: adverse reaction to a salicylate characterized by dizziness, impaired hearing, nausea, vomiting, flushing, sweating, rapid, deep breathing, tachycardia, diarrhea, mental confusion, lassitude, drowsiness, respiratory depression, and possibly coma

secondary failure: *in diabetes mellitus*, loss of the effectiveness of sulfonylurea, an oral antidiabetic drug

secondary hypertension: hypertension with a known cause, such as kidney disease

sedative: drug producing a relaxing, calming effect

seizure: periodic disturbance in electrical activity in brain

shock: inadequate blood flow to the bodily tissues

solvent: fluid in which a solid dissolves

somatotropic hormone: growth hormone (see *somatotropin*)

somatosensory: change in sensation due to a seizure

somatropin: hormone produced by the anterior pituitary gland that contributes to the growth of muscles and bones; also called *growth hormone*

spinal anesthesia: type of regional anesthesia produced by injection of a local anesthetic drug into the subarachnoid space of the spinal cord

Standard Precautions: recommendation that gloves and/or other protective gear be worn when touching any blood or body fluids, mucous membranes, or any broken skin area; also see *Universal Precautions*

Statin drugs: see *HMG-CoA reductase inhibitors*

status epilepticus: emergency situation characterized by continual seizure activity

Stevens-Johnson syndrome: fever, cough, muscular aches and pains, headache, and lesions of the skin, mucous membranes, and eyes; the lesions appear as red wheals or blisters, often starting on the face, in the mouth, or on the lips, neck, and extremities

stomatitis: inflammation of a cavity opening such as the oral cavity

subcutaneous (subcut): under the skin or dermis layer in the fatty tissue layer.

subjective data: information supplied by the patient or family

sublingual: under the tongue

superinfection: overgrowth of bacterial or fungal microorganisms not affected by the antibiotic being administered

sustained release: see *extended release*

sympathetic: pertaining to the sympathetic nervous system

sympathetic nervous system: part of the autonomic nervous system concerned with mobilizing involuntary body systems

sympatholytic: blocking the sympathetic nervous system

sympathomimetic: drugs acting like the sympathetic nervous system, see *adrenergic*

synergism: action that occurs when two substances (drugs) interact to produce an effect that is greater than the sum of their separate actions

T

tachycardia: heart rate above 100 beats/minute

tachypnea: rapid breathing

tardive dyskinesia: rhythmic, involuntary movements of the tongue, face, mouth, jaw, and sometimes the extremities

teaching: interactive process that promotes learning

teratogen: drug or substance that causes abnormal development of the fetus, leading to deformities

testosterone: primary male sex hormone; acts to stimulate development of the male reproductive organs and secondary sex characteristics

theophyllinization: delivery of a high enough dose of theophylline to bring blood levels to a therapeutic range more quickly than over several days

threshold: term applied to any stimulus of the lowest intensity that will give rise to a response in a nerve fiber

thrombocytopenia: decreased number of platelets in the blood

thrombolytic: drug that helps to eliminate blood clots

thrombophlebitis: inflammation of a vein with clot formation

thrombopoiesis: formation of platelets (thrombocytes)

thrombosis: formation of a blood clot

thrombus: blood clot (pl. *thrombi*)

thrush: candidiasis (candidal infection) of the mouth

thyroid storm: see *thyrotoxicosis*

thyrotoxicosis: severe hyperthyroidism characterized by high fever, extreme tachycardia, and altered mental status (also called *thyroid storm*)

tinea corporis: superficial fungal infection, commonly called *ringworm*

tinea cruris: superficial fungal infection of the groin region, commonly called *jock itch*

tinea pedis: superficial fungal infection of the foot, commonly called *athlete's foot*

tinnitus: ringing in the ears

tolerance: increasingly larger dosages of a drug are required to obtain the desired effect

tonic-clonic seizure: generalized seizure activity consisting of alternating contraction (tonic) and relaxation of muscles (clonic)

topical: pertaining to a substance applied directly to the skin by patch, ointment, gel, or other formulation

total parenteral nutrition (TPN): complex admixture of nutrients combined in a single container and administered to the body by an IV route.

toxic: poisonous or harmful

toxic epidermal necrolysis (TEN): toxic skin reaction with sloughing of skin and mucous membranes

toxin: poisonous substance

toxoid: attenuated toxin that is capable of stimulating the formation of antitoxins

transdermal: through the skin

transdermal system: drug delivery system by which the drug is applied to and absorbed through the skin

transient ischemic attack (TIA): temporary interference with blood supply to the brain causing symptoms related to the portion of the brain affected (i.e., temporary blindness, aphasia, dizziness, numbness, difficulty swallowing, or paresthesias); may last a few moments to several hours, after which no residual neurologic damage is evident

transsacral block: anesthesia of caudal region of spinal cord and canal; see *conduction block*

triglycerides: types of lipids that circulate in the blood

tuberculosis: infection caused by *Mycobacterium tuberculosis*

U

unit dose: system of drug delivery by which a drug order is filled and medication dispensed to fill each medication order(s) for a 24-hour period; each drug dose (unit) is dispensed in a package labeled with the drug name and dosage

Universal Precautions: guidelines set forth by the Centers for Disease Control and Prevention (CDC) to control the spread of disease

unlabeled use: use of a drug to treat a condition which is not officially approved by the U.S. Food and Drug Administration (FDA)

urge incontinence: involuntary passage of urine

urinary tract infection (UTI): infection by pathogenic microorganisms of one or more structures of the urinary tract

urinary urgency: immediate sensation of need to void

urticaria: hives; itchy wheals on the skin resulting from contact with or ingestion of an allergenic substance or food

uterine atony: marked relaxation of the uterine muscle

V

vaccine: substance containing either weakened or killed antigens developed for the purpose of creating resistance to disease

vancomycin-resistant enterococci (VRE): bacteria resistant to the drug vancomycin

vasodilation: increase in the diameter of the blood vessels that, when widespread, results in a drop in blood pressure

vasopressors: drugs that raise the blood pressure

venous: pertaining to the veins

vertigo: feeling of a spinning or rotational motion; dizziness

vesicant: caustic drug substance

virilization: acquisition of male sexual characteristics by a woman

volatile liquids: anesthetic agents that are flammable

vomiting: spasmodic ejection of stomach contents through the mouth

W

water intoxication: fluid overload in the body when electrolytes are imbalanced

water soluble: dissolves in water

X-Y-Z

xerostomia: drying of oral secretions

Z-track technique: method of intramuscular drug injection preventing leakage onto subcutaneous or skin tissues, used when a drug is highly irritating to subcutaneous tissues or has the ability permanently to stain the skin

Drug Categories: Controlled Substances and FDA Pregnancy Risk

Schedules of Controlled Substances

Schedule I (C-I)
- High abuse potential
- Lack of accepted safety, not approved for medical use in the United States
- Examples: heroin, marijuana, ecstasy, peyote

Schedule II (C-II)
- Potential for high abuse with severe physical or psychological dependence
- Approved for medical use in the United States (and all categories below)
- Examples: opioids such as meperidine, methadone, morphine, oxycodone; amphetamines; and cocaine

Schedule III (C-III)
- Less abuse potential than schedule II drugs
- Potential for moderate physical or psychological dependence
- Examples: anabolic steroids, ketamine, hydrocodone/codeine compounded with an nonsteroidal anti-inflammatory drug

Schedule IV (C-IV)
- Less abuse potential than schedule III drugs
- Limited dependence potential
- Examples: some sedatives and anxiety agents, non-opioid analgesics, "diet drugs"

Schedule V (C-V)*
- Limited abuse potential
- Examples: small amounts of opioid (codeine) used as antitussives or antidiarrheals, pregabalin (Lyrica)

*Under federal law, limited quantities of certain schedule V drugs may be purchased without a prescription directly from a pharmacist if allowed under state law. The purchaser must be at least 18 years of age and must furnish identification. All such transactions must be recorded by the dispensing pharmacist.

FDA Pregnancy Risk Categories

Pregnancy Category A
- Adequate, well-controlled studies in pregnant women have not shown an increased risk of fetal abnormalities to the fetus in any trimester of pregnancy.

Pregnancy Category B
- Animal studies have revealed no evidence of harm to the fetus; however, there are no adequate and well-controlled studies in pregnant women.

OR
- Animal studies have shown an adverse effect, but adequate and well-controlled studies in pregnant women have failed to demonstrate a risk to the fetus in any trimester.

Pregnancy Category C
- Animal studies have shown an adverse effect and there are no adequate and well-controlled studies in pregnant women.

OR
- No animal studies have been conducted and there are no adequate and well-controlled studies in pregnant women.

Pregnancy Category D
- Adequate well-controlled or observational studies in pregnant women have demonstrated a risk to the fetus.
- However, potential benefits may outweigh the risk to the fetus. If needed in a life-threatening situation or a serious disease, the drug may be acceptable if safer drugs cannot be used or are ineffective.

Pregnancy Category X
- Adequate well-controlled or observational studies in animals or pregnant women have demonstrated positive evidence of fetal abnormalities or risks.
- The use of the product is contraindicated in women who are or may become pregnant.

  Regardless of the pregnancy category or the presumed safety of the drug, no drug should be administered during pregnancy unless it is clearly needed and the potential benefits outweigh potential harm to the fetus.

Institute for Safe Medication Practices

FDA and ISMP Lists of
Look-Alike Drug Name Sets With Recommended Tall Man Letters

The sets of look-alike drug names in the Tables below have been modified using "tall man" letters to help draw attention to the dissimilarities in their names. Several studies have shown that highlighting sections of drug names using tall man (mixed case) letters can help distinguish similar drug names,[1] making them less prone to mix-ups.[2-3] ISMP, FDA, The Joint Commission, and other safety-conscious organizations have promoted the use of tall man letters as one means of reducing confusion between similar drug names.

Table 1 provides a list of FDA-approved established drug name sets with recommended tall man letters, which were first identified during the FDA Name Differentiation Project (www.fda.gov/CDER/Drug/MedErrors/nameDiff.htm).

Table 2 provides a list of additional drug name sets with recommendations from ISMP regarding the use and placement of tall man letters. This is not an official list approved by FDA. It is intended for voluntary use by healthcare practitioners and drug information vendors. Any product label changes by manufacturers require FDA approval.

One of the difficulties with the use of tall man letters is the lack of scientific evidence regarding which name pairs would most benefit from this error-reduction strategy as well as which letters to present in uppercase. Until further evidence is available, ISMP suggests that the tall man lettering scheme provided in these Tables be followed to promote consistency.

Table 2. ISMP List of Additional Drug Names with Tall Man Letters

ALPRAZolam – LORazepam	metroNIDAZOLE – metFORMIN
amLODIPine – aMILoride	morphine – HYDROmorphone
azaCITIDine – azaTHIOprine	NexIUM* – NexAVAR*
ceFAZolin – cefTRIAXone	niMODipine – NIFEdipine
CeleBREX* – CeleXA*	NovoLOG* – NovoLIN*
chlorproMAZINE – chlordiazePOXIDE	OXcarbazepine – carBAMazepine
CISplatin – CARBOplatin	oxyCODONE – OxyCONTIN*
clonazePAM – cloNIDine	PARoxetine – FLUoxetine
clonazePAM – LORazepam	PENTobarbital – PHENobarbital
cloNIDine – KlonoPIN*	PriLOSEC* – PROzac*
DACTINomycin – DAPTOmycin	QUEtiapine – OLANZapine
ePHEDrine – EPINEPHrine	quiNINE – quiNIDine
fentaNYL – SUFentanil	riTUXimab inFLIXimab
FLUoxetine – DULoxetine	SandIMMUNE* – SandoSTATIN*
guanFACINE – guaiFENesin	SEROquel* – SINEquan*
HumaLOG* – HumuLIN*	Solu-MEDROL* – Solu-CORTEF*
HYDROcodone – oxyCODONE	SUMAtriptan – sitaGLIPtin
IDArubicin – DOXOrubicin	tiZANidine – tiaGABine
INVanz* – AVINza*	traZODone – traMADol
LaMICtal* – LamISIL*	TRENtal – TEGretol*
lamiVUDine – lamoTRIgine	ZyPREXA* – ZyrTEC*

Table 1. FDA-Approved List of Established Drug Names with Tall Man Letters

acetoHEXAMIDE - acetaZOLAMIDE	hydrALAZINE – hydrOXYzine
buPROPion - busPIRone	medroxyPROGESTERone methylPREDNISolone methylTESTOSTERone
chlorproMAZINE – chlorproPAMIDE	
clomiPHENE – clomiPRAMINE	
cycloSPORINE – cycloSERINE	niCARdipine – NIFEdipine
DAUNOrubicin – DOXOrubicin	predniSONE – prednisoLONE
dimenhyDRINATE – diphenhydrAMINE	sulfADIAZINE – sulfiSOXAZOLE
DOBUTamine – DOPamine	TOLAZamide – TOLBUTamide
glipiZIDE – glyBURIDE	vinBLAStine – vinCRIStine

References: 1) Filik R, Purdy K, Gale A, Gerrett D. Drug name confusion: evaluating the effectiveness of capital ("Tall Man") letters using eye movement data. *Social Science & Medicine* 2004;59(12):2597-2601. **2)** Filik R, Purdy K, Gale A, Gerrett D. Labeling of medicines and patient safety: evaluating methods of reducing drug name confusion. *Human Factors* 2006;48(1):39-47. **3)** Grasha A. Cognitive systems perspective on human performance in the pharmacy: implications for accuracy, effectiveness, and job satisfaction. Alexandria (VA): NACDS; 2000 Report No. 062100.

© ISMP 2008

* Brand names always start with an uppercase letter. Some brand names incorporate tall man letters in initial characters and may not be readily recognized as brand names. An asterisk follows all brand names in Table 2.

Institute for Safe
Medication Practices
www.ismp.org

Select Herbs and Natural Products Used for Medicinal Purposes

Common Name(s)	Scientific Name	Uses	Adverse Reactions	Significant Considerations
Aloe vera	*Aloe vera*	To inhibit infection and promote healing of minor burns and wounds; as a laxative	None significant if used as directed; may cause burning sensation in wound	Rare reports of delayed healing when used in the gel form on a wound. If taken internally as a laxative, do not take longer than 1–3 wk without consulting primary health care provider. Decrease dosage if cramping occurs.
Bilberry	*Vaccinium myrtillus*	For vision enhancement and eye health, microcirculation, spider veins and varicose veins, capillary strengthening before surgery	No adverse effects reported in clinical studies	None.
Black cohosh (black snakeroot, squawroot)	*Cimicifuga racemosa*	For management of some symptoms of menopause and as an alternative to hormone replacement therapy; may be beneficial for hypercholesterolemia or peripheral vascular disease	Overdose causes nausea, dizziness, nervous system and visual disturbances, decreased pulse rate and increased perspiration	Should not be used during pregnancy. Possible interactions with hormone therapy.
Capsicum (hot peppers)	*Capsicum frutescens*	For neuralgic pain relief, bladder pain and hyperreflexia; as an antipruritic for psoriasis	Burning sensation upon application	Creams should be applied with gloves and hands washed thoroughly before touching face or eyes.
Chamomile	*Matricaria chamomilla*	Drunk as an infusion for gastrointestinal (GI) disturbances (e.g., diarrhea, flatulence, stomatitis); as a sedative and as an anti-inflammatory agent	Possible contact dermatitis and, in rare instances, anaphylaxis	Chamomile is a member of the ragweed family and those allergic to ragweed should not take the herb. Avoid use during pregnancy. May enhance anticoagulant effect when administered with anticoagulants. Do not administer to a child without checking with primary health care provider.
Chondroitin	Chondroitin sulfate, chondroitin sulfuric acid, chonsurid	For arthritis—particularly osteoarthritis	None significant if used as directed	Because chondroitin is concentrated in cartilage, theoretically it produces no toxic or teratogenic effects.

(table continues on page 586)

Common Name(s)	Scientific Name	Uses	Adverse Reactions	Significant Considerations
Cranberry	*Vaccinium macrocarpon*	To prevents urinary tract infection (UTI) by acidifying the urine; lower pH also reduces the ammonia odor of urinary incontinence.	Large doses can produce GI symptoms (e.g., diarrhea)	None. Safe for use during pregnancy and while breastfeeding. Inform patient that sugar-free cranberry juice or supplements are available if the patient has diabetes mellitus. Antibiotic is usually needed to treat active UTI.
Eucalyptus oil	*E. globules Labillardiere*	As a decongestant, expectorant for respiratory conditions; topically for antimicrobial effect	Pain, nausea, vomiting; individuals with acute intermittent porphyria should not take	Used in mouthwashes for antimicrobial properties. Adverse reactions of slowing the central nervous system (CNS), drowsiness, seizures and coma when taken orally. Blood sugar levels may decrease with use.
Feverfew	*Tanacetum parthenium*	As an antipyretic; for migraine headaches, asthma, arthritis, relief of menstrual cramps	Most are mild; rash or contact dermatitis may indicate allergy and herb should be withdrawn	Possible interaction with anticoagulants. Patient should be observed for abnormal bleeding. Do not use during pregnancy or lactation.
Flax	*Linum usitatissimum*	As topical emollient, laxative; for diverticulitis, irritable bowel syndrome, possible blood lipid reduction	Few when taken as directed	Advise patient to drink adequate water while taking flax. Advise patient not to take any drug for at least 2 h after taking flax. Advise patient not to take during pregnancy.
Garlic	*Allium sativum*	To lower blood glucose, cholesterol, and lipid levels; as topical antifungal	May cause abnormal blood glucose levels	Increased risk of bleeding in patients taking the warfarin, salicylates, or antiplatelet drugs.
Ginger (ginger root, black ginger)	*Zingiber officinale*	As antiemetic, cardiotonic, antithrombotic, antibacterial, antioxidant, antitussive, anti-inflammatory, prophylaxis for nausea and vomiting; for GI disturbances, colic; to lower cholesterol	Excessive doses may cause CNS depression and interfere with cardiac functioning or anticoagulant activity	Theoretically, ginger could enhance the effects of the antiplatelet drugs, such as coumarin. Observe for excessive bleeding (e.g., nose bleeding, easy bruising) Consult primary health care provider for use during pregnancy.
Ginkgo (maiden hair tree, kew tree)	*Ginkgo biloba*	For cerebral insufficiency dementias, circulatory problems, headaches, macular degeneration, diabetic retinopathy, premenstrual syndrome	Rare if used as directed; possible effects include headache, dizziness, heart palpitations, GI effects, rash, allergic dermatitis	Do not take with antidepressant drugs, such as the monoamine oxidase inhibitors (MAOIs), or antiplatelet drugs, such as coumarin, unless advised to do so by the primary health care provider. Discontinue use at least 2 wk before surgery.

(table continues on page 597)

Common Name(s)	Scientific Name	Uses	Adverse Reactions	Significant Considerations
Ginseng	*Panax quinquefolius Panax ginseng*	For fatigue, lack of concentration, atherosclerosis; to improve cardiovascular or CNS function	Most common: nervousness, excitation, hypoglycemia; Rare: diffuse mammary nodularity, vaginal bleeding	Taking ginseng in combination with stimulants such as caffeine is not advised. Do not use for longer than 3 mo. (Some herbalists recommend use for 1 mo followed by nonuse for 2 mo.)
Goldenseal	*Hydrastis canadensis*	As antiseptic for skin (topical), astringent for mucous membranes (mouthwash), wash for inflamed eyes	Large doses may cause dry or irritated mucous membranes and injury to the GI system	Should not be taken for more than 3–7 d. Contraindicated in pregnancy and hypertension.
Glucosamine (chitosamine)	*2-Amino-2-deoxy-glucose*	As antiarthritic in osteoarthritis	Usually well tolerated; mild adverse reactions such as heartburn, diarrhea, nausea, and itching have been reported	No direct toxic effects have been reported. Cautious use is recommended in diabetes because there is a potential for altering blood glucose levels.
Green tea	*Camellia sinensis*	To reduce cancer risk, lower lipid levels, help prevent dental caries; for antimicrobial and antioxidative effects	Well tolerated; contains caffeine (may cause mild stimulant effects such as anxiety, nervousness, heart irregularities, restlessness, insomnia, and digestive irritation)	No direct toxic effects have been reported. Contains caffeine and should be avoided during pregnancy and by individuals with hypertension, anxiety, eating disorders, insomnia, diabetes, and ulcers. Inform patient to avoid taking green tea with iron supplements because green tea interferes with iron absorption.
Hawthorne	*Crataegus oxyacantha*	For regulation of blood pressure and heart rhythm; to treat atherosclerosis and angina pectoris; as a sedative	Hypotension and sedation (in high doses)	May interfere with serum digoxin effects. Notify primary health care provider and pharmacist if taking the herb.
Kava (kawa, kava-kava, awa yangona)	*Piper methysticum*	For mild to moderate anxiety; as a sedative	Scaly skin rash; disturbances in visual accommodation, habituation	Limit use to no more than 3 mo.
Lemon balm (balm, melissa, sweet balm)	*Melissa officinalis*	For Graves' disease, cold sores (topical); as a sedative, antispasmodic	None significant	None.
melatonin	*melatonin*	For insomnia; topically to protect against ultraviolet light	Headache, depression, possible additive effects when taken with alcohol	Avoid hazardous activities until the CNS effects of this supplement are known. Do not take for prolonged periods, because effects of prolonged use are not known. May interfere with conception.
Passion flower (passion fruit, granadilla, water lemon, apricot vine)	*Passiflora incarnata*	To promote sleep; as a treatment for pain and nervous exhaustion	None if used as directed; excessively large doses may cause CNS depression	May interact with anticoagulants and MAOIs.

(table continues on page 598)

Common Name(s)	Scientific Name	Uses	Adverse Reactions	Significant Considerations
Saw palmetto (cabbage palm, fan palm, scrub palm)	*Serenoa repens*	For symptoms of benign prostatic hypertrophy	Generally well tolerated; occasional GI effects	May interact with hormones such as oral contraceptive drugs and hormone replacement therapy.
St. John's wort (Klamath weed, goatweed, rosin rose)	*Hypericum perforatum*	As an antidepressant or antiviral	Usually mild; may cause dry mouth, dizziness, constipation, other GI symptoms, photosensitivity	May decrease efficacy of theophylline, warfarin, and digoxin; use with other prescriptions is not recommended.
Tea tree oil	*Melaleuca alternifolia*	As topical antimicrobial, antifungal	Contact dermatitis	For topical use only; do not take orally.
Valerian	*Valeriana officinalis*	For restlessness, sleep disorders	Rare if used as directed	May interact with the barbiturates (e.g., phenobarbital), the benzodiazepines (e.g., diazepam), and the opioids, (e.g., morphine).
Willow bark (weidenrinde, white willow, purple osier willow, crack willow)	*Salix alba, S. purpurea, S. fragilis*	As an analgesic	Adverse reactions are those associated with the salicylates	Do not use with aspirin or other nonsteroidal anti-inflammatory drugs. Do not use in patients with peptic ulcers and other medical conditions in which the salicylates are contraindicated.

APPENDIX

D

Less Frequently Used Calculations and Measurements

Body Surface Area Nomograms

Nomogram for Estimating Body Surface Area of Infants and Young Children

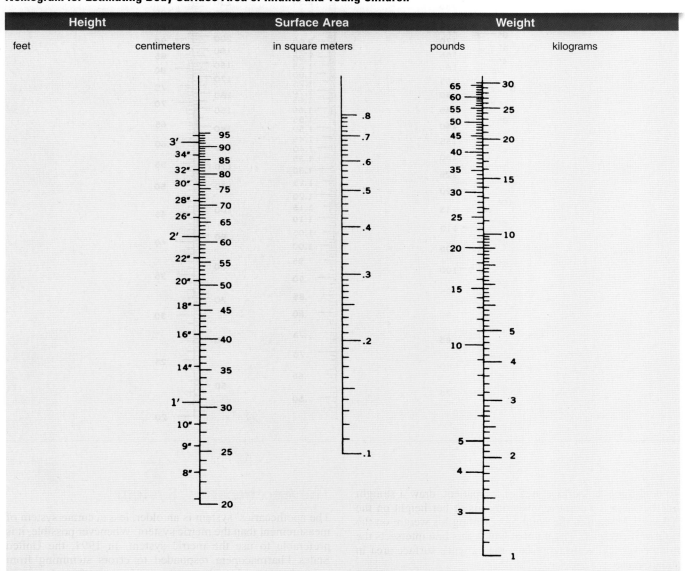

Nomogram for Estimating Body Surface Area of Older Children and Adults

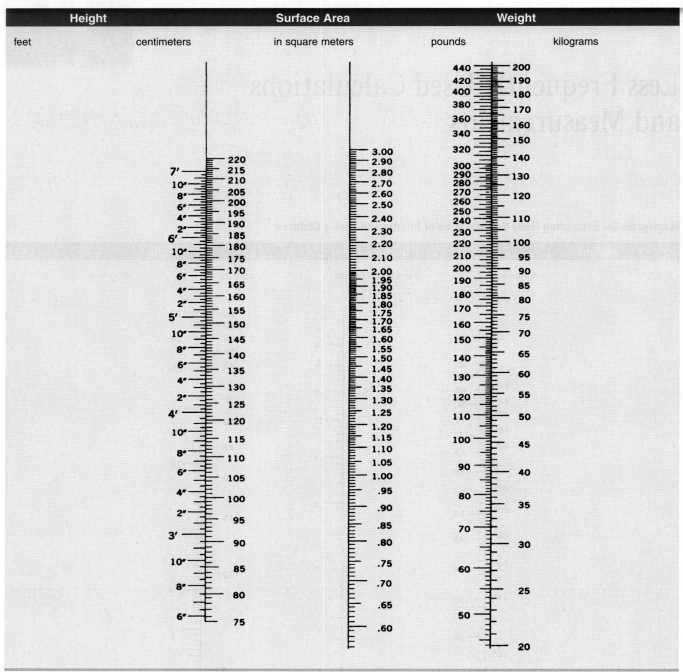

Height		Surface Area	Weight	
feet	centimeters	in square meters	pounds	kilograms

To determine the surface area of the patient, draw a straight line between the point representing his or her height on the left vertical scale to the point representing his weight on the right vertical scale. The point at which this line intersects the middle vertical scale represents the patient's surface area in square meters.

The Apothecaries' System

The apothecaries' system is an older, less accurate system of measurement than the metric system. Whenever possible, it is preferable to use the metric system. In 1994, the United States Pharmacopeia responded to errors stemming from confusion caused by the apothecary system of measurement by eliminating an apothecary system conversion table from its national formulary.

In 2002, the Joint Commission adopted recommendations from the Institute for Safe Medication Practices' list of error-prone medication abbreviations, symbols, and dose designa-

tions for use in its National Patient Safety Goals. It has proven very difficult to convince practitioners of all types to relinquish use of the apothecary system. In keeping with current health care standards, this information is provided for situations in which conversion is necessary.

Approximate Equivalents of Systems of Measurement

Metric	Apothecaries'	Household
Weight		
0.1 mg	gr 1/600	
0.15 mg	gr 1/400	
0.2 mg	gr 1/300	
0.3 mg	gr 1/200	
0.4 mg	gr 1/150	
0.6 mg	gr 1/100	
1 mg	gr 1/60	
2 mg	gr 1/30	
4 mg	gr 1/15	
6 mg	gr 1/10	
8 mg	gr 1/8	
10 mg	gr 1/6	
15 mg	gr 1/4	
20 mg	gr 1/3	
30 mg	gr ss (1/2)	
60 mg	gr 1	
100 mg	gr i ss (1 1/2)	
120 mg	gr ii	
1 g (1000 mg)	gr xv	
Volume		
0.06 mL	min i	
1 mL	min xv or xvi	
4 mL	fluid dram i	1 teaspoon
15 mL	fluid drams iv	1/2 ounce
30 mL	fluid ounce i	1 ounce
500 mL	1 pint	1 pint
1000 mL (1 liter)	1 quart	1 quart

Answers to Review Questions and Medication Dosage Problems

Unit I Foundations of Clinical Pharmacology

Chapter 1 General Principles of Pharmacology

Hints for Thinking Critically - Practice in Pharmacology: Check the table on body system changes and what happens to the pharmacokinetics due to aging.

Review Questions: Test Your Knowledge

1. A
2. B
3. D
4. A

Review Question: NCLEX Prep

1. D

Chapter 2 Administration of Drugs

Hints for Thinking Critically - Practice in Pharmacology: Think about the consequences to the patient's well-being from getting too much of any drug. Relate how question number two would be impacted by what you do in #1.

Review Questions: Test Your Knowledge

1. C
2. C
3. B
4. D

Review Question: NCLEX Prep

1. B

Chapter 3 Calculation of Drug Dosages and Mathematical Review

Questions:

1. Tagamet is the brand name, cimetidine is the generic name
2. The form of the drug is a Tiltab tablet and 400 milligrams is in each tablet of Tagamet
3. Zyprexa and olanzapine are the names; it comes in tablet form and the dose strength is 5 milligrams
4. Lanoxin and digoxin are the names; it comes in tablet form and the dose strength is 250 micrograms or 0.25 milligrams
5. Augmentin and amoxicillin/alavulanate are the names; it comes in liquid form and the dose strength is 250 milligrams in 5 milliliters

Calculations:

1. One tablet after breakfast
2. Two tablets after every meal
3. Two tablets daily
4. Two tablets daily
5. Five milliliters in each dose
6. Patient's weight in kilograms $142 \div 2.2 = 64.5$ kg; Child's weight in kg $43 \div 2.2 = 19.5$ kg

Hints for Thinking Critically - Practice in Pharmacology: Think about the rationale for the redundancy system; is that removed by the advent of a computer system?

Review Questions: Test Your Knowledge

1. B
2. D
3. D
4. C

Review Question: NCLEX Prep

1. C

Chapter 4 The Nursing Process

Hints for Thinking Critically - Practice in Pharmacology: Check Display 4.1 for some reasons that patients have problems staying on medications. What does the patient have or not have control over when taking medications? What does the nurse need to know about patients' habits to be sure they take the prescribed medications?

Review Questions: Test Your Knowledge

1. A & D
2. D
3. C
4. A

Review Question: NCLEX Prep

1. D

Chapter 5 Patient and Family Teaching

Hints for Thinking Critically - Practice in Pharmacology: Reviewing the patients presented, what objective signs might you look for and what subjective symptoms would you ask about to determine priority of the clinic visit?

Review Questions: Test Your Knowledge

1. D
2. A
3. B
4. B

Review Question: NCLEX Prep

1. C

Unit II Anti-Infectives

Chapter 6 Sulfonamides

Hints for Thinking Critically - Practice in Pharmacology: What is the relationship between urinary tract infections, memory, and cognitive processes? Check in Chapter 2 for hints to help her remember to take the medication.

Review Questions: Test Your Knowledge

1. B
2. D
3. A
4. B

Review Question: NCLEX Prep

1. C

Calculate Medication Dosages

1. 10 mL or 2 teaspoons
2. 2 tablets

Chapter 7 Penicillins

Hints for Thinking Critically - Practice in Pharmacology:
1. Check the unit introduction for tests done before selecting anti-infective drugs. Look at information on this drug. Can it be taken with food? How would you approach an active teen about completing the full course of the drug?
2. When is a severe allergic reaction most likely to occur?

Review Questions: Test Your Knowledge

1. A
2. B
3. B
4. D

Review Question: NCLEX Prep

1. B

Calculate Medication Dosages

1. 1 teaspoon (t) = 250 mg of amoxicillin (1 t = 5 mL). The nurse will administer 2 teaspoons (t) or 10 mL of amoxicillin.
2. a. Ninety milliliters (90 mL) of water needed for reconstitution.
   b. Directions for reconstitution: Tap bottle until all powder flows freely. Add approximately 2/3 of the 90 mL of water; shake vigorously to wet powder. Add remaining water and shake vigorously again.

c. Strength of reconstituted solution is 125 mg/5 mL. (The nurse would administer 20 mL.)

Chapter 8 Cephalosporins

Hints for Thinking Critically - Practice in Pharmacology: Think about the important information your patient needs; are any of these items prepared in his native language at the clinic? If not, what resource can you go to?

Review Questions: Test Your Knowledge

1. D
2. B
3. A
4. C

Review Question: NCLEX Prep

1. D

Calculate Medication Dosages

1. 4 mL

Chapter 9 Tetracyclines, Aminoglycosides, Macrolides, and Lincosamides

Hints for Thinking Critically - Practice in Pharmacology: Think about what fecal incontinence means when someone is taking an anti-infective. How do the heart medications interact with anti-infectives?

Review Questions: Test Your Knowledge

1. C
2. B
3. D

Review Question: NCLEX Prep

1. A

Calculate Medication Dosages

1. 2 tablets, 1 tablet
2. 2 mL
3. 20 mL

Chapter 10 Fluoroquinolones and Miscellaneous Anti-Infectives

Hints for Thinking Critically - Practice in Pharmacology: Think about what simple tasks can prevent the spread of infections.

Review Questions: Test Your Knowledge

1. C
2. B
3. A
4. B

Review Question: NCLEX Prep

1. A

Calculate Medication Dosages

1. 1 tablet
2. 15 mL
3. 20 mL

Chapter 11 Antitubercular Drugs

Hints for Thinking Critically - Practice in Pharmacology: Think about the risk factors for TB and what Betty Peterson's perceptions of her living situation are compared to those factors.

Review Questions: Test Your Knowledge

1. D
2. C
3. B
4. D

Review Question: NCLEX Prep

1. A

Calculate Medication Dosages

1. 6 mL
2. 4 tablets

Chapter 12 Antiviral Drugs

Hints for Thinking Critically - Practice in Pharmacology: Think about drug combinations—look at the case study for chapter 9.

Review Questions: Test Your Knowledge

1. A
2. A
3. A
4. B

Review Question: NCLEX Prep

1. C

Calculate Medication Dosages

1. 2 tablets
2. 10 mg
3. 10 mL

Chapter 13 Antifungal and Antiparasitic Drugs

Hints for Thinking Critically - Practice in Pharmacology: Think about safety to the patients and spread of infection in both case study questions.

Review Questions: Test Your Knowledge

1. B
2. B
3. C
4. B

Review Question: NCLEX Prep

1. A

Calculate Medication Dosages

1. (140 lbs = 63.6 kg) 95.4 mg, or 95 if rounded to the nearest whole number
2. 2 tablets
3. 2 capsules

Unit III Drugs Used to Manage Pain

Chapter 14 Nonopioid Analgesics: Salicylates and Nonsalicylates

Hints for Thinking Critically - Practice in Pharmacology: What problems could the aspirin product be causing? If Betty does switch to an acetaminophen product, what other drugs or foods should Betty avoid that might contain salicylates?

Review Questions: Test Your Knowledge

1. C
2. A
3. C
4. C
5. B

Review Question: NCLEX Prep

1. C

Calculate Medication Dosages

1. 1.5 or 1½ mL
2. 2 tablets

Chapter 15 Nonopioid Analgesics: Nonsteroidal Anti-Inflammatory Drugs (NSAIDs) and Migraine Headache Medications

Hints for Thinking Critically - Practice in Pharmacology: In teaching the skilled nursing facility staff, what should they expect with GI-related adverse reactions when using COX-2 inhibitor?

Review Questions: Test Your Knowledge

1. A
2. A
3. D
4. B

Review Question: NCLEX Prep

1. D

Calculate Medication Dosages

1. 10 mL
2. 2 tablets

Chapter 16 Opioid Analgesics

Hints for Thinking Critically - Practice in Pharmacology: Are people with addiction histories less likely to experience pain? What can nurses do to prevent cravings? How would you measure adequate pain relief with regard to heart-related problems?

Review Questions: Test Your Knowledge
1. D
2. C
3. C
4. A

Review Question: NCLEX Prep
1. B

Calculate Medication Dosages
1. 1.2 mL
2. 1 mL

Chapter 17 Opioid Antagonists

Hints for Thinking Critically - Practice in Pharmacology: Think about all components of a pain assessment; which ones were neglected in the patient interview? Who is the opioid-naïve patient, and what steps should the nurse take to facilitate breathing before administering an opioid antagonist?

Review Questions: Test Your Knowledge
1. B

Review Question: NCLEX Prep
1. C

Calculate Medication Dosages
1. 0.8 mL
2. 4 injections

Chapter 18 Anesthetic Drugs

Hints for Thinking Critically - Practice in Pharmacology: Think about the concept of peak action. When would you want these drugs to be at their peak action?

Review Questions: Test Your Knowledge
1. B
2. C
3. A
4. B

Calculate Medication Dosages
1. 1 mL
2. 0.3 mg

Unit IV Drugs That Affect the Central Nervous System

Chapter 19 Central Nervous System Stimulants

Hints for Thinking Critically - Practice in Pharmacology: Did you learn anything about this patient from Chapter 5 that would caution against the use of these drugs?

Review Questions: Test Your Knowledge
1. C
2. A

3. D
4. D

Review Question: NCLEX Prep
1. A

Calculate Medication Dosages
1. 24 mg, yes
2. 2 tablets

Chapter 20 Antianxiety Drugs

Hints for Thinking Critically - Practice in Pharmacology: What are the differences involved in pharmacodynamics of the elderly? Is patient safety an issue with this medication?

Review Questions: Test Your Knowledge
1. A
2. D
3. B
4. C

Review Question: NCLEX Prep
1. B

Calculate Medication Dosages
1. 1 mL
2. 2 tablets, 3 times

Chapter 21 Sedatives and Hypnotics

Hints for Thinking Critically - Practice in Pharmacology: How long and for what reasons should hypnotics be used? Is this an appropriate use of the drug? What other non-pharmacological interventions would be helpful?

Review Questions: Test Your Knowledge
1. C
2. A
3. D
4. C

Review Question: NCLEX Prep
1. A

Calculate Medication Dosages
1. 1 tablet
2. 2 tablets

Chapter 22 Antidepressant Drugs

Hints for Thinking Critically - Practice in Pharmacology: How long does it take for antidepressant medications to take effect? In Chapter 21, we learned that Mr. Phillip was prescribed a hypnotic for sleep; what are the drug interactions when using these medications together?

Review Questions: Test Your Knowledge
1. D

2. C
3. B
4. B

Review Question: NCLEX Prep
1. C

Calculate Medication Dosages
1. 3 tablets
2. 25 mL

Chapter 23 Antipsychotic Drugs

Hints for Thinking Critically - Practice in Pharmacology: Look at the antipsychotic drugs and their uses besides treating psychosis; which ones are nurses on the medical/surgical units likely to see?

Review Questions: Test Your Knowledge
1. C
2. B
3. C
4. D

Review Question: NCLEX Prep
1. B

Calculate Medication Dosages
1. 2 tablets
2. 2 tablets

Unit V Drugs That Affect the Peripheral Nervous System

Chapter 24 Adrenergic Drugs

Hints for Thinking Critically - Practice in Pharmacology: See information in the text of chapters in this unit. How would you explain opposite actions of the autonomic nervous system?

Review Questions: Test Your Knowledge
1. B
2. A
3. D
4. D

Review Question: NCLEX Prep
1. 0.6 mg

Calculate Medication Dosages
1. 1/2 mL

Chapter 25 Adrenergic Blocking Drugs

Hints for Thinking Critically - Practice in Pharmacology: Think about how the drugs work in a manner opposite to those mechanisms discussed in chapter 24.

Review Questions: Test Your Knowledge
1. D
2. D
3. A
4. B

Review Question: NCLEX Prep
1. D

Calculate Medication Dosages
1. 4 tablets

Chapter 26 Cholinergic Drugs

Hints for Thinking Critically - Practice in Pharmacology: Urinary retention can lead to placement of a urinary catheter, putting the patient at risk for infection. What assessments would the nurse conduct for both retention and potential infection?

Review Questions: Test Your Knowledge
1. A
2. B
3. B

Calculate Medication Dosages
1. 10 tablets
2. ½ mL

Chapter 27 Cholinergic Blocking Drugs

Hints for Thinking Critically - Practice in Pharmacology: Review the side effects that can occur with the different cholinergic blocking drugs. What is the impact specifically on the bowels and mobility?

Review Questions: Test Your Knowledge
1. B
2. B
3. D
4. B

Calculate Medication Dosages
1. $^1/_2$ mL
2. 10 mL

Unit VI Drugs That Affect the Neuromuscular System

Chapter 28 Cholinesterase Inhibitors

Hints for Thinking Critically - Practice in Pharmacology: Think about the different stages of the disease. Is the medication losing effectiveness?

Review Questions: Test Your Knowledge
1. B
2. C
3. A
4. D

Review Question: NCLEX Prep
1. C

Calculate Medication Dosages
1. 3 mL
2. 2 tablets

Chapter 29 Antiparkinsonism Drugs

Hints for Thinking Critically - Practice in Pharmacology: What is the cluster of symptoms described in the case study? What are some of the contraindications of medications she has used in the past (Chapter 16)—how will that impact selecting a drug to decrease her symptoms?

Review Questions: Test Your Knowledge
1. A
2. B
3. D
4. B

Review Question: NCLEX Prep
1. D

Calculate Medication Dosages
1. one 500-mg tablet and one 250-mg tablet
2. 3 tablets

Chapter 30 Anticonvulsants

Hints for Thinking Critically - Practice in Pharmacology: What type of seizures do you think Ms. Chase had following her accident? What questions would you ask before you informed the primary health care provider that she is intermittently taking her medications?

Review Questions: Test Your Knowledge
1. D
2. A
3. C
4. B

Review Question: NCLEX Prep
1. B

Calculate Medication Dosages
1. 2 mL
2. 2 tablets
3. 10 mL

Chapter 31 Skeletal Muscle Relaxants and Drugs Used to Treat Bone and Joint Disorders

Hints for Thinking Critically - Practice in Pharmacology: What are the improvements made in treating RA in the last 15 years?

Review Questions: Test Your Knowledge
1. A
2. C

3. D
4. D

Review Question: NCLEX Prep
1. D

Medication Dosage Problems
1. 3 tablets
2. 3 tablets

Unit VII Drugs That Affect the Respiratory System

Chapter 32 Antitussives, Mucolytics, and Expectorants

Hints for Thinking Critically - Practice in Pharmacology: Mrs. Peterson is being treated for depression (MAOIs are antidepressants); how does this influence antitussive/expectorant choices? What questions will the nurse need to ask Mr. Peterson regarding his wife's other prescriptions?

Review Questions: Test Your Knowledge
1. B
2. A
3. D
4. A

Review Question: NCLEX Prep
1. A

Calculate Medication Dosages
1. 5 mL
2. 5 mL

Chapter 33 Antihistamines and Decongestants

Hints for Thinking Critically - Practice in Pharmacology: Janna Wong competes on her school's gymnastic team. How might her abilities be altered due to the influence of either the antihistamine or nasal decongestant?

Review Questions: Test Your Knowledge
1. A
2. C
3. B
4. C

Review Question: NCLEX Prep
1. A

Calculate Medication Dosages
1. 10 mL
2. 2 tablets

Chapter 34 Bronchodilators and Antiasthma Drugs

Hints for Thinking Critically - Practice in Pharmacology: Be sure to place the routine medications and the quick relief medications in the proper areas of the action plan. You have been given the personal best Peak Flow Meter value; calculate the proper values for the yellow/red zones. Check chapter 32 for the medication that the elderly woman had taken.

Review Questions: Test Your Knowledge
1. D
2. D
3. A
4. A

Review Question: NCLEX Prep
1. C

Calculate Medication Dosages
1. 0.25 mL
2. 2 tablets, 40 mg each day

Unit VIII Drugs That Affect the Cardiovascular System

Chapter 35 Antihyperlipidemic Drugs

Hints for Thinking Critically - Practice in Pharmacology: Check the chapter introduction for her baseline information and compare this with the information in the unit introduction. How much has she reduced her risk of a heart attack during the next 10 years? How can you use this information to motivate continued treatment?

Review Questions: Test Your Knowledge
1. C
2. A
3. A
4. B

Review Question: NCLEX Prep
1. C

Calculate Medication Dosages
1. 2 tablets
2. Yes, 200 mg is an appropriate dosage. However, if the patient requires 200 mg, it is preferable to give a 200-mg capsule rather than three 67-mg capsules. The nurse should notify the primary health care provider that only 67-mg capsules are available.

Chapter 36 Antihypertensive Drugs

Hints for Thinking Critically - Practice in Pharmacology: What are the salt supplement restrictions of the SARA medications. What questions do you need to ask Mrs. Chase about flavor preferences?

Review Questions: Test Your Knowledge
1. C
2. C
3. D
4. B

Review Question: NCLEX Prep
1. B

Calculate Medication Dosages
1. 4 tablets
2. 90-mg tablets and give 2 tablets

Chapter 37 Antianginal Drugs

Hints for Thinking Critically - Practice in Pharmacology: Think about the anticipated side effects; how should she modify her activities? When should she replace patches, and what would happen if she forgot to remove an old one?

Review Questions: Test Your Knowledge
1. B
2. B
3. C
4. B

Review Question: NCLEX Prep
1. D

Calculate Medication Dosages
1. 3 tablets
2. 2 tablets

Chapter 38 Anticoagulant and Thrombolytic Drugs

Hints for Thinking Critically - Practice in Pharmacology: Think about what might cause bleeding or increased clotting in the home. What about activities of daily living such as shaving or potential hazards that would cause falls?

Review Questions: Test Your Knowledge
1. D
2. D
3. B
4. A

Review Question: NCLEX Prep
1. B

Calculate Medication Dosages
1. 0.67 mL or 0.7 mL
2. 2 tablets

Chapter 39 Cardiotonics and Miscellaneous Inotropic Drugs

Hints for Thinking Critically - Practice in Pharmacology: Look at the interactions list for digoxin. Think about the patient scenarios; do you remember any of these drugs?

Review Questions: Test Your Knowledge
1. B
2. D
3. A
4. C

Review Question: NCLEX Prep
1. C

Calculate Medication Dosages
1. one 0.5-mg tablet and one 0.25-mg tablet
2. ½ mL

Chapter 40 Antiarrhythmic Drugs

Hints for Thinking Critically - Practice in Pharmacology: As you looked at Internet sites, what types did you find? What information do you get from government, pharmaceutical industry, or individual blog sites?

Review Questions: Test Your Knowledge
1. A
2. D
3. A
4. C

Review Question: NCLEX Prep
1. D

Calculate Medication Dosages
1. 2 tablets
2. 2 tablets

Unit IX Drugs That Affect the Gastrointestinal System

Chapter 41 Drugs That Affect the Upper Gastrointestinal System

Hints for Thinking Critically - Practice in Pharmacology: Antacids—do they actually coat the stomach lining? What do they actually do? Examining the different elements, what should a person reduce in his or her diet when dealing with hypertensive disease? Which elements promote constipation?

Review Questions: Test Your Knowledge
1. C
2. D
3. B
4. C

Review Question: NCLEX Prep
1. B

Calculate Medication Dosages
1. 2 tablets
2. 1 tablet

Chapter 42 Drugs That Affect the Lower Gastrointestinal System

Hints for Thinking Critically - Practice in Pharmacology: Think about what happens with habitual laxative use.

Review Questions: Test Your Knowledge
1. C
2. C
3. A
4. D

Review Question: NCLEX Prep
1. D

Calculate Medication Dosages
1. 3 hours
2. 3 capsules

Unit X Drugs That Affect the Endocrine System

Chapter 43 Antidiabetic Drugs

Hints for Thinking Critically - Practice in Pharmacology: Think the interactions between the drugs used to fight urinary bacterial infections (sulfa) and the oral antidiabetic drugs (sulfonylureas).

Review Questions: Test Your Knowledge
1. C
2. D
3. C
4. B

Review Question: NCLEX Prep
1. C, B, D, A

Calculate Medication Dosages
1. Draw an arrow to the number 45.
2. 2 tablets at each dose; total daily dose 2000 mg
3. 4 tablets
4. Label B

Chapter 44 Pituitary and Adrenocortical Hormones

Hints for Thinking Critically - Practice in Pharmacology: Explain the rationale for consistent early dosing of the drug.

Review Questions: Test Your Knowledge
1. B
2. A
3. B
4. C

Review Question: NCLEX Prep
1. C

Calculate Medication Dosages
1. 2 mL
2. 20 mL

Chapter 45 Thyroid and Antithyroid Drugs

Hints for Thinking Critically - Practice in Pharmacology:
What are the possible limitations to taking radioactive iodine and what precautions should be taken?

Review Questions: Test Your Knowledge
1. B
2. C
3. A
4. C

Review Question: NCLEX Prep
1. B

Calculate Medication Dosages
1. 4 tablets
2. 2 tablets

Chapter 46 Male and Female Hormones

Hints for Thinking Critically - Practice in Pharmacology:
Think about the differences in using hormones to promote sexual organ growth and decreasing tumor cell growth. What are the risks to individuals with steroid use?

Review Questions: Test Your Knowledge
1. C
2. D
3. C
4. B

Review Question: NCLEX Prep
1. A

Calculate Medication Dosages
1. 1.6 mL
2. 1 mL

Chapter 47 Drugs Acting on the Uterus

Hints for Thinking Critically - Practice in Pharmacology:
Think about the role anxiety plays in the birthing process. What would be best to support Betty and her daughter?

Review Questions: Test Your Knowledge
1. D
2. B
3. A
4. C

Review Question: NCLEX Prep
1. D

Calculate Medication Dosages
1. ½ tablet
2. 1 mL

Unit XI Drugs That Affect the Urinary System

Chapter 48 Diuretics

Hints for Thinking Critically - Practice in Pharmacology:
Think about which of the items in Display 48.1 occur with aging.

Review Questions: Test Your Knowledge
1. B
2. C
3. B
4. D
5. C

Review Question: NCLEX Prep
1. B

Calculate Medication Dosages
1. 2 tablets
2. 2.5 mL

Chapter 49 Urinary Tract Anti-Infectives, Antispasmodics, and Other Urinary Drugs

Hints for Thinking Critically - Practice in Pharmacology:
What elements of being alone may contribute to not taking the medication properly?

Review Questions: Test Your Knowledge
1. A
2. D
3. C

Review Question: NCLEX Prep
1. D

Calculate Medication Dosages
1. 2 tablets
2. 10 mL

Unit XII Drugs That Affect the Immune System

Chapter 50 Immunologic Agents

Hints for Thinking Critically - Practice in Pharmacology:
Think about the consequences to the child should he acquire the illness in the timeframe of the delay in immunization.

Review Questions: Test Your Knowledge
1. B
2. A
3. C
4. A

Review Question: NCLEX Prep
1. B

Calculate Medication Dosages

1. 6 vials of the FluLaval vaccine

Hints for Thinking Critically - Practice in Pharmacology:
What is especially frightening to you about cancer? What if you did not have the same knowledge base—how much more frightening would it be?

Review Questions: Test Your Knowledge

1. D
2. B
3. B
4. C

Review Question: NCLEX Prep

1. A

Calculate Medication Dosages

1. 13.7 mg/day
2. 1.375 or 1.4 units

Hints for Thinking Critically - Practice in Pharmacology:
What is the role of the ESA drugs in dialysis and fatigue?

Review Questions: Test Your Knowledge

1. A
2. A
3. A
4. A

Review Question: NCLEX Prep

1. C

Calculate Medication Dosages

1. 0.5 mL
2. 0.2 mL

Unit XIII Drugs That Affect Other Body Systems

Chapter 53 Topical Drugs Used in the Treatment of Skin Disorders

Hints for Thinking Critically - Practice in Pharmacology:
What are the differences in the treatment of HSV and the Varicella-zoster virus?

Review Questions: Test Your Knowledge

1. B
2. B
3. D
4. B

Review Question: NCLEX Prep

1. D

Calculate Medication Dosages

1. 30 mL

Chapter 54 Otic and Ophthalmic Preparations

Hints for Thinking Critically - Practice in Pharmacology:
Appealing to principles of personal growth and development, what would be the best way to interact with and teach Janna?

Review Questions: Test Your Knowledge

1. B
2. C
3. D

Review Question: NCLEX Prep

1. B

Calculate Medication Dosages

1. 5 (gtt) drops

Chapter 55 Fluids, Electrolytes, and Parenteral Therapy

Hints for Thinking Critically - Practice in Pharmacology:
Describe what electrolyte imbalance is occurring as a result of taking sodium bicarbonate for stomach ailments.

Review Questions: Test Your Knowledge

1. D
2. A
3. D
4. A
5. D

Review Question: NCLEX Prep

1. B

Calculate Medication Dosages

1. 100 mL/hour
2. 30 mL

Key to NCLEX-PN Prep

All "Review Question: NCLEX Prep" questions in the book are coded to specific portions of the 2008 NCLEX-PN Detailed Test Plan. Below, you will find how specific questions from each chapter correspond directly to the items of the Detailed Test Plan, Pharnacological and Parenteral Therapies section. By answering these questions, the student will be exposed to sample questions which correspond directly to the items that the NCLEX-PN are built from when students prepare for the examination.

Subcategory: Adverse Effects

Chapter 33 – monitor for actual/potential adverse effects

Chapters 9, 44 – reinforce client teaching on possible adverse effect

Chapter 45 – identify symptoms of an allergic reaction

Chapter 38 – implement procedures to counteract adverse effects of medications

Chapter 8 – withhold medication dose if client experiences adverse effect

Chapter 17 – monitor/document client response to actions taken to counteract adverse effects of medications

Chapters 40, 46 – notify primary health care provider of actual/potential adverse effects of client medications

Subcategory: Contraindication and Compatibilities

Chapter 12 – identify potential/actual incompatibilities of client medications

Chapter 15 – identify contraindication to the administration of medications to a client

Chapter 23 – monitor anticipated interactions among client prescribed medication/fluids

Subcategory: Dosage Calculations

Chapter 24 – perform calculations required for medication administration

Chapters 3, 19 – use clinical decision making when calculating doses

Subcategory: Expected Effects

Chapter 35 – reinforce client teaching on expected effects of prescribed medications

Chapter 4 – identify client expected response to medication

Chapter 11 – monitor client use of medications over time

Chapters 13, 48 – monitor and document client response to medication

Subcategory: Medication Administration

Chapter 2 – follow the rights of medication administration

Chapter 21 – identify client need for PRN medication

Chapter 42 – maintain current and accurate record on the MAR

Chapter 16 – document client medication administration according to policy

Chapter 7 – review pertinent data prior to medication administration

Chapter 50 – monitor transfusion of blood produce

Chapter 47 – monitor client IV site and flow rate

Chapters 5, 10 – administer a medication by the oral route

Chapter 43 – mix client medication from two vials as necessary

Chapter 22 – reinforce client teaching about actions/therapeutic effects of medications

Chapter 36 – reinforce client teaching on administration of medications

Chapter 25 – administer medication by gastrointestinal tube

Chapter 31 – administer a subcutaneous medication

Chapters 6, 54 – administer a medication by the topical route

Chapter 37 – phone in client prescriptions to pharmacy

Chapter 53 – assist in preparing client for insertion of central line

Chapter 28 – dispose of client unused medication according to proper policy

Chapter 1 – count controlled substances

Chapter 50 – regulate client IV rate

Chapter 51 – administer IVPB medications

Subcategory: Pharmacological Actions

Chapters 34, 52 – reinforce client teaching on actions and therapeutic effects

Chapter 41 – use resources to check on purposes and actions of pharmacologic agents

Subcategory: Pharmacological Agents

Chapter 32 - apply knowledge of pathophysiology

Chapter 30 – recognize and report client responses to pharmacological agents

Subcategory: Side Effects

Chapter 39 – monitor and document client side effects to medications

Chapter 14 – review client teaching on management of possible side effects of medications

Chapter 29 – notify primary health care provider of side effects of medications

Chapter 20 – monitor client response to management of medication side effects

Index

Page numbers followed by f, t, and d, indicate figures, tables, and display material respectively.